# GI/LIVER
# SECRETS PLUS

# GI/LIVER SECRETS PLUS

## FOURTH EDITION

**PETER R. McNALLY, DO, FACP, FACG**
CHIEF, GI/HEPATOLOGY
EVANS ARMY HOSPITAL
COLORADO SPRINGS, COLORADO

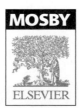

MOSBY

ELSEVIER

1600 John F. Kennedy Blvd.
Ste 1800
Philadelphia, PA 19103-2899

GI/LIVER SECRETS PLUS

ISBN: 978-0-323-06397-5

---

### Notice

Knowledge and best practice in this field are constantly changing. As new research and experience broaden our knowledge, changes in practice, treatment and drug therapy may become necessary or appropriate. Readers are advised to check the most current information provided (i) on procedures featured or (ii) by the manufacturer of each product to be administered, to verify the recommended dose or formula, the method and duration of administration, and contraindications. It is the responsibility of the practitioner, relying on his or her own experience and knowledge of the patient, to make diagnoses, to determine dosages and the best treatment for each individual patient, and to take all appropriate safety precautions. To the fullest extent of the law, neither the Publisher nor the Authors assume any liability for any injury and/or damage to persons or property arising out of or related to any use of the material contained in this book.

The Publisher

---

**Library of Congress Cataloging-in-Publication Data**
GI/liver secrets plus / [edited by] Peter R. McNally. —4th ed.
    p. ; cm. —(Secrets series)
  Rev. ed. of: GI/liver secrets. 3rd ed. c2006.
  Includes bibliographical references and index.
  ISBN 978-0-323-06397-5
  1.  Digestive organs—Diseases—Examinations, questions, etc. I.  McNally, Peter R., 1954-
II.  GI/liver secrets. III.  Series: Secrets series.
  [DNLM: 1.  Digestive System Diseases—Examination Questions. WI 18.2 G4281 2010]
  RC802.G52 2010
  616.30076—dc22

2009053302

Acquisitions Editor: James Merritt
Developmental Editor: Barbara Cicalese
Project Manager: Shereen Jameel
Marketing Manager: Allan McKeown

Printed in Canada

Last digit is the print number:  9  8  7  6  5  4  3  2  1

Working together to grow
libraries in developing countries

www.elsevier.com | www.bookaid.org | www.sabre.org

ELSEVIER   BOOK AID International   Sabre Foundation

*The editor dedicates this book to his wife, Cynthia; to his children, Alex, Meghan, Amanda, Genevieve, and Bridgette; and to his parents, Jeanette and Rusel.*

# CONTRIBUTORS

Sami R. Achem, MD, FACP, FACG, AGAF
Professor of Medicine, Mayo College of Medicine,
Mayo Clinic, Jacksonville, Florida

Amit Agrawal, MD
Fellow of Gastroenterology, Medical University of South
Carolina, Charleston, South Carolina

Scott E. Altschuler, MD
Gastroenterologist, Health Park Medical Center,
Fort Myers, Florida

Francis Amoo, MD
Resident, Internal Medicine, St. Vincent's Medical Center,
Bridgeport, Connecticut

Mainor R. Antillon, MD, MBA, MPH
Professor of Medicine and Surgery, Internal Medicine,
University of Missouri; Internal Medicine, University of
Missouri Hospital and Clinics, Columbia, Missouri

Matthew B.Z. Bachinski, MD, FACP
Attending Physician, Self Regional Hospital, Greenwood,
South Carolina

Bruce R. Bacon, MD
Professor of Internal Medicine and Director of the Division
of Gastroenterology and Hepatology, St. Louis University
School of Medicine and St. Louis University Liver Center;
Professor of Internal Medicine, St. Louis University
Hospital, St. Louis, Missouri

Jamie S. Barkin, MD, MACP, MACG
Professor of Medicine, Miller School of Medicine,
University of Miami, Miami, Florida; Chief, Division
of Gastroenterology, Mt. Sinai Medical Center,
Miami Beach, Florida

David W. Bean Jr., MD
Clinical Associate Professor of Radiology, Sanford School of
Medicine, University of South Dakota, Vermillion, South
Dakota

Major John Boger, MD
Instructor of Medicine, Uniformed Services University of
the Health Sciences, Bethesda, Maryland; Fellow of
Gastroenterology, Department of Medicine, Walter Reed
Army Medical Center, Washington, District of Columbia

Aaron Brzezinski, MD
Gastroenterologist, Center for Inflammatory Bowel Disease,
Cleveland Clinic, Cleveland, Ohio

Christine Janes Bruno, MD
Transplant Hepatologist, Transplant Services, Piedmont
Hospital, Atlanta, Georgia

Donald O. Castell, MD
Professor of Medicine, Medical University of South Carolina,
Charleston, South Carolina

Joseph G. Cheatham, MD
Fellow of Gastroenterology, Walter Reed Army Medical
Center, Washington, District of Columbia; Instructor,
Department of Medicine,  Sciences, Bethesda,
Maryland

James E. Cremins, MD
Robinwood Medical Center, Hagerstown, Maryland

Albert J. Czaja, MD
Professor of Medicine Emeritus, Division of Gastroenterology
and Hepatology, Mayo Clinic and Mayo Clinic College of
Medicine, Rochester, Minnesota

Dirk R. Davis, MD, FACP, FACG
Northern Utah Gastroenterology, Logan, Utah

Amar R. Deshpande, MD
Assistant Professor of Medicine, Division of Gastroenterology,
Miller School of Medicine, University of Miami; Attending
Physician, Division of Gastroenterology, University of Miami
Hospital and Clinics and Jackson Memorial Hospital,
Miami, Florida

John C. Deutsch, MD
Staff Physician, Gastroenterology and Cancer Center,
St. Mary's Duluth Clinic, Duluth, Minnesota

Jack A. DiPalma, MD
Professor and Director, Division of Gastroenterology,
University of South Alabama College of Medicine,
Mobile, Alabama

Gulchin A. Ergun, MD
Clinical Associate Professor of Medicine, Baylor College of
Medicine, Houston, Texas; Clinical Associate Professor
of Medicine, Weill-Cornell Medical College, New York,
New York; Section Chief and Medical Director, Digestive
Disease Department, Reflux Center and GI Physiology
Lab, Department of Medicine, The Methodist Hospital,
Houston, Texas

Henrique J. Fernandez, MD
Senior Fellow of Gastroenterology, University of Miami,
and Jackson Memorial Hospital, Miami, Florida; Senior
Fellow of Gastroenterology, Mt. Sinai Medical Center,
Miami Beach, Florida

James E. Fitzpatrick, MD
Professor and Vice Chair, Department of Dermatology,
University of Colorado Denver, Aurora, Colorado

**Michael G. Fox, MD**
Assistant Professor of Radiology, University of Virginia, Charlottesville, Virginia

**Kevin J. Franklin, MD, FACP**
Assistant Professor, Internal Medicine, Uniformed Services University of the Health Sciences, Bethesda, Maryland; Gastroenterology Fellowship Program Director, San Antonio Uniformed Services Health Education Consortium, Wilford Hall Medical Center, Lackland Air Force Base, San Antonio, Texas

**Stephen R. Freeman, MD**
Associate Professor of Medicine, Division of Gastroenterology and Hepatology, University of Colorado Denver, and University of Colorado Hospital, Aurora, Colorado; Gastroenterology, Denver VA Medical Center and Denver Health Medical Center, Denver, Colorado

**Gregory G. Ginsberg, MD**
Professor of Medicine, University of Pennsylvania School of Medicine; Director of Endoscopic Services, Hospital of the University of Pennsylvania, Philadelphia, Pennsylvania

**John S. Goff, MD**
Clinical Professor of Medicine, University of Colorado Health Sciences Center, Aurora, Colorado; Rocky Mountain Gastroenterology Associates, Lakewood, Colorado

**Seth A. Gross, MD**
Gastroenterologist, Norwalk Hospital, Norwalk, Connecticut

**Carlos Guarner, MD**
Associate Professor of Medicine, Unitat Docent Sant Pau; Director of Gastroenterology and Hepatology, Hospital de la Santa Creu i Sant Pau, Barcelona, Spain

**Stephen A. Harrison, MD**
Associate Professor of Medicine, University of Texas Health Sciences Center, San Antonio; Chief of Hepatology, Department of Medicine, Brooke Army Medical Center, Fort Sam Houston, Texas

**Jorge L. Herrera, MD**
Professor of Medicine, Division of Gastroenterology, University of South Alabama College of Medicine, Mobile, Alabama

**Kent C. Holtzmuller, MD**
Gastroenterology and Hepatology, Carolinas Medical Center, and Staff Physician, Mecklenburg Medical Group, Charlotte, North Carolina; Clinical Assistant Professor of Medicine, University of North Carolina School of Medicine, Chapel Hill, North Carolina

**Lieutenant Colonel J, David Horwhat, MD, FACG**
Assistant Professor of Medicine, Uniformed Services University of the Health Sciences, Bethesda, Maryland; Assistant Chief, Gastroenterology Service, Department of Medicine, Walter Reed Army Medical Center, Washington, District of Columbia

**Jeffrey Hunt, DO**
Visiting Assistant Professor of Medicine, Internal Medicine, Oklahoma State University College of Osteopathic Medicine; Oklahoma State University Medical Center, Tulsa, Oklahoma

**David S. James, DO, FACG**
Chief of the Division of Gastroenterology, Internal Medicine, Oklahoma State University Center for Health Sciences; Director of the Gastrointestinal Center, St. Francis South Medical Center; Director of the Endoscopy Center, Oklahoma State University Medical Center, Tulsa, Oklahoma

**David P. Jones, DO, FACP, FACG**
Associate Professor of Medicine, University of Texas Health Sciences Center, San Antonio; Chief of Gastroenterology and Assistant Chief of Medicine, Brooke Army Medical Center, Fort Sam Houston, Texas

**Ryan W. Kaliney, MD**
Resident, Department of Radiology, University of Virginia Health System, Charlottesville, Virginia

**Sergey V. Kantsevoy, MD, PhD**
Director, Therapeutic Endoscopy Melissa L. Posner Institute for Digestive Health & Liver Disease at Mercy Baltimore, Maryland

**Cynthia W. Ko, MD, MS**
Assistant Professor of Medicine, University of Washington, Seattle, Washington

**Kimi L. Kondo, DO**
Assistant Professor of Radiology, Division of Interventional Radiology, University of Colorado Denver; Attending Physician, Radiology, Division of Interventional Radiology, University of Colorado Hospital, Aurora, Colorado

**Burton I. Korelitz, MD**
Clinical Professor of Medicine, Division of Gastroenterology, New York University School of Medicine; Director of Clinical Research (IBD) and Director Emeritus of Gastroenterology, Department of Medicine, Lenox Hill Hospital, New York, New York

**Michael J. Krier, MD**
Fellow of Gastroenterology and Hepatology, Division of Gastroenterology and Hepatology, Stanford University School of Medicine, Stanford, California

**Miranda Yeh Ku, MD, MPH**
Fellow of Gastroenterology and Hepatology, University of Colorado Health Sciences Center, Denver, Colorado

**Marcelo Kugelmas, MD, FACP**
Gastroenterologist, Center for Diseases of the Liver and Pancreas, Swedish Medical Center; South Denver Gastroenterology PC, Englewood, Colorado

**Stephen P. Laird, MD, MS**
Instructor of Medicine, Gastroenterology, University of Colorado Health Sciences Center, Aurora, Colorado; Denver Health, Denver, Colorado

**Frank L. Lanza, MD, FACG**
Clinical Professor of Medicine, Gastroenterology Section, Baylor College of Medicine; Attending Physician, GI/Endoscopy, Ben Taub General Hospital, Houston, Texas

**Anthony J. LaPorta, MD, FACS**
Clinical Professor of Surgery, University of Colorado Health Sciences Center, Aurora, Colorado

**Nicholas F. LaRusso, MD**
Charles H. Weinman Endowed Professor of Medicine, Biochemistry and Molecular Biology; Director, Center for Innovation, Department of Internal Medicine, Mayo Clinic, Rochester, Minnesota

**Brett A. Lashner, MD**
Professor of Medicine, Gastroenterology, Cleveland Clinic, Cleveland, Ohio

**Randall E. Lee, MD, FACP**
Gastroenterologist, VA Northern California Healthcare System; Associate Clinical Professor of Medicine, University of California at Davis, Sacramento, California

**Sum P. Lee, MD, PhD**
Professor of Medicine, University of Washington; Department of Medicine, VA Puget Sound Health Care System (Seattle Division), Seattle, Washington

**Martin D. McCarter, MD**
Associate Professor of Surgery, Division of GI Tumor and Endocrine Surgery, University of Colorado Denver School of Medicine and Hospital, Aurora, Colorado

**Peter R. McNally, DO, FACP, FACG**
Chief, GI/Hepatology, Evans Army Hospital, Colorado Springs, Colorado; Adjunct Faculty Professor, Center for Human Simulation, School of Medicine, University of Colorado Denver, Aurora, Colorado

**Edgar Mehdikhani, MD**
Fellow of Gastroenterology, Loma Linda University Medical Center, Loma Linda, California

**John H. Meier, MD**
Staff Gastroenterologist, Frye Regional Medical Center and Catawba Valley Medical Center; Partner, Gastroenterology Associates PA, Hickory, North Carolina

**Halim Muslu, MD**
Assistant Professor of Clinical Medicine, Department of Medicine, University of Cincinnati, Cincinnati, Ohio

**James C. Padussis, MD**
Resident, General Surgery, Duke University and Duke University Medical Center, Durham, North Carolina

**Wilson P. Pais, MD, MBA, FACP**
Gastroenterologist and Fellow of Advanced Therapeutic Endoscopy, Division of Gastroenterology, University of Missouri, Columbia, Missouri

**Theodore N. Pappas, MD**
Professor and Vice Chair for Administration, Department of Surgery, Duke University Medical Center, Durham, North Carolina

**Cyrus W. Partington, MD, FACR, FACNM**
Staff Radiologist, Evans Army Hospital, Fort Carson, Colorado

**Pankaj Jay Pasricha, MD**
Chief and Professor of Internal Medicine, Division of Gastroenterology and Hepatology, Stanford University School of Medicine; Chief and Clinician, Medicine– Gastroenterology and Hepatology, Stanford University, Stanford, California

**David A. Peura, MD**
Professor of Medicine, Emeritus, University of Virginia Health System, Charlottesville, Virginia

**Lori D. Prok, MD**
Assistant Professor, Pediatric Dermatology and Dermatopathology, University of Colorado Denver and The Children's Hospital, Aurora, Colorado

**Matthew R. Quallick, MD**
Fellow of Gastroenterology, Division of Gastroenterology, University of Colorado Health Sciences Center, Aurora, Colorado

**Ramona O. Rajapakse, MD, FRCP**
Associate Professor of Clinical Medicine, Division of Gastroenterology, Stony Brook University Medical Center, Stony Brook, New York

**Kevin M. Rak, MD**
Chief of Radiology, Divine Savior Healthcare, Portage, Wisconsin

**Erica N. Roberson, MD**
Fellow of Women's Health, University of Wisconsin School of Medicine and Public Health; University of Wisconsin Hospital, Department of Internal Medicine, Madison, Wisconsin

**Ingram M. Roberts, MD, MBA**
Associate Clinical Professor of Medicine, University of Connecticut School of Medicine, Farmington, Connecticut; Vice Chairman of Medicine and Program Director, Internal Medicine Residency, St. Vincent's Medical Center, Bridgeport, Connecticut

**Arvey I. Rogers, MD, FACP, MACG**
Professor Emeritus, Internal Medicine, Gastroenterology, Miller School of Medicine, University of Miami, Miami, Florida

**Suzanne Rose, MD, MSEd**
Professor of Medical Education and Medicine, Associate Dean for Academic and Student Affairs, and Associate Dean for Continuing Medical Education, Division of Gastroenterology, Mount Sinai School of Medicine, New York, New York

**Kevin B. Rothchild, MD**
Assistant Professor, GI, Tumor, and Endocrine Surgery, University of Colorado Hospital, Aurora, Colorado

**Bruce A. Runyon, MD**
Professor of Medicine, Internal Medicine, Loma Linda University; Chief of Liver Service, Internal Medicine, Loma Linda University Medical Center, Loma Linda, California

**Paul D. Russ, MD, FACR**
Professor, Department of Radiology, University of Colorado Denver, Aurora, Colorado

**Mark W. Russo, MD**
Medical Director of Liver Transplantation, Hepatology Department, Carolinas Medical Center, Charlotte, North Carolina

**Travis J. Rutland, MD**
Instructor in Medicine, Division of Gastroenterology, University of South Alabama College of Medicine, Mobile, Alabama

Richard E. Sampliner, MD
Professor of Medicine, University of Arizona; Chief of Gastroenterology, Southern Arizona VA Health Care System, Tucson, Arizona

Tom J. Sauerwein, MD, FACE
Assistant Professor of Internal Medicine, Uniformed Services University of Health Sciences, Bethesda, Maryland; Endocrinology Fellowship Program Director, Endocrinology, Diabetes, and Metabolism, San Antonio Uniformed Services Health Education Consortium, Wilford Hall Medical Center, Lackland Air Force Base, San Antonio, Texas

Lawrence R. Schiller, MD
Program Director, Gastroenterology Fellowship, Baylor University Medical Center; Attending Physician, Digestive Health Associates of Texas, Dallas, Texas

Jonathan A. Schoen, MD
Assistant Professor of Surgery, GI, Tumor, and Endocrine Surgery, University of Colorado Hospital, Aurora, Colorado

Raj J. Shah, MD
Associate Professor of Medicine and Director of Pancreatic/Biliary/Endoscopic Services, Division of Gastroenterology and Hepatology, School of Medicine, University of Colorado Denver, Aurora, Colorado

Kenneth E. Sherman, MD, PhD
Gould Professor of Medicine and Director of the Division of Digestive Diseases, College of Medicine, University of Cincinnati, Cincinnati, Ohio

Roshan Shrestha, MD
Clinical Professor of Medicine, Mercer University School of Medicine, Savannah, Georgia; Medical Director of Liver Transplantation, Piedmont Hospital, Atlanta, Georgia

Maria H. Sjögren, MD, MPH
Associate Professor, Preventive Medicine, Uniformed Services University of the Health Sciences, Bethesda, Maryland; Director of Hepatology Research, Walter Reed Army Medical Center, and Associate Professor of Medicine, Georgetown University, Washington, District of Columbia

George B. Smallfield, III, MD
Fellow of Gastroenterology, Gastroenterology and Hepatology, University of Alabama and University of Alabama at Birmingham Hospitals, Birmingham, Alabama

Major Won Song, MC
Associate Program Director, Nuclear Medicine, Brooke Army Medical Center, Fort Sam Houston, Texas; Clinical Assistant Professor of Radiology, University of Texas Health Science Center at San Antonio, San Antonio, Texas

Erik Springer, MD
Gastroenterologist, Arapahoe Gastroenterology, PC, Littleton, Colorado

Joel Z. Stengel, MD
Fellow of Gastroenterology, Gastroenterology Service, Brooke Army Medical Center, Fort Sam Houston, Texas

Janet K. Stephens, MD, PhD
Clinical Associate Professor, Department of Pathology, University of Colorado Health Sciences Center, Aurora, Colorado; Staff Pathologist, Department of Pathology, Exempla St. Joseph Hospital, Denver, Colorado

Stephen W. Subber, MD
Associate Professor, Radiology, University of Colorado Health Sciences Center, Aurora, Colorado; Chief of Angiography and Interventional Radiology, Imaging Department, Denver VA Medical Center, Denver, Colorado

Christine M. Surawicz, MD
Professor of Medicine, Division of Gastroenterology, University of Washington, Seattle, Washington

Jayant A. Talwalker, MD, MPH
Associate Professor of Medicine, Gastroenterology and Hepatology; Consultant, Miles and Shirley Fiterman Center for Digestive Diseases, Mayo Clinic, Rochester, Minnesota

Shalini Tayal, MD
Assistant Professor of Pathology, Department of Medicine, Denver Health Medical Center, Denver, Colorado

Christina A. Tennyson, MD
Fellow of Gastroenterology, Mount Sinai School of Medicine, New York, New York

Selvi Thirumurthi, MD, MS
Assistant Professor of Medicine, Division of Gastroenterology and Hepatology, Baylor College of Medicine; Chief of Endoscopy, Division of Gastroenterology and Hepatology, Ben Taub General Hospital, Houston, Texas

John J. Tiedeken, MD
Surgical Resident, Penn State Hershey Medical Center, Hershey, Pennsylvania

Neil W. Toribara, MD, PhD, FACP
Associate Professor of Medicine, University of Colorado Health Sciences Center, Aurora, Colorado; Chief, Division of Gastroenterology and Hepatology, Denver Health Medical Center, Denver, Colorado

Dawn McDowell Torres, MD
Fellow of Gastroenterology, Department of Medicine, Brooke Army Medical Center, Fort Sam Houston, Texas

George Triadafilopoulos, MD
Clinical Professor of Medicine, Division of Gastroenterology and Hepatology, Stanford University School of Medicine, Stanford, California

James F. Trotter, MD
Medical Director, Liver Transplantation, Baylor University Medical Center; Medical Director, Liver Transplantation, Baylor Regional Transplant Institute, Dallas, Texas

Nimish Vakil, MD, FACG
Clinical Professor of Medicine, University of Wisconsin School of Medicine and Public Health, Madison, Wisconsin; Associate Professor, College of Health Sciences, Marquette University, Milwaukee, Wisconsin

*Arnold Wald, MD, AGAF, MACG*
Professor of Medicine, Gastroenterology and Hepatology, University of Wisconsin School of Medicine and Public Health; University of Wisconsin Hospitals, Madison, Wisconsin

*Michael H. Walter, MD*
Associate Professor of Medicine and Gastroenterologist, Internal Medicine, Loma Linda University Medical Center, Loma Linda, California; Gastroenterologist, Internal Medicine, Riverside County Regional Medical Center, Moreno Valley, California

*George H. Warren, MD*
Clinical Associate Professor, Departments of Pathology and Medicine, University of Colorado Health Sciences Center, Aurora, Colorado

*Jill M. Watanabe, MD, MPH*
Associate Professor of Medicine, Division on General Internal Medicine, University of Washington School of Medicine; Harborview Medical Center, Seattle, Washington

*Sterling G. West, MD, MACP, FACR*
Professor of Medicine, Division of Rheumatology, University of Colorado Denver, Aurora, Colorado

*C. Mel Wilcox, MD, MSPH*
Professor of Medicine, Division of Gastroenterology and Hepatology, University of Alabama, Birmingham, Alabama

*Bernard E. Zeligman, MD*
Associate Professor of Radiology, School of Medicine, University of Colorado; Attending Radiologist, University of Colorado Hospital, Aurora, Colorado

*Rowen K. Zetterman, MD*
Dean, School of Medicine, Creighton University, Omaha, Nebraska

*Di Zhao, MD*
Resident, Internal Medicine, St. Vincent's Medical Center, Bridgeport, Connecticut

# PREFACE

To practice the art of medicine, one must learn the secrets of physiology, disease, and therapy. In this text, you will find the answers to many questions about the hepatic and digestive diseases. We hope that medical students, residents, fellows, and, yes, even attending physicians will find the fourth edition of *GI/Liver Secrets Plus* instructive and insightful.

As editor, I am most appreciative of all my contributing authors who have shared their invaluable secrets and made this book an enjoyable, as well as an educational, experience.

**Peter R. McNally, DO, FACP, FACG**

# CONTENTS

# TOP 100 SECRETS

These secrets are 100 of the top board alerts. They summarize the concepts, principles, and most salient details of gastroenterology and hepatology.

1. Lymphocytic gastritis is a rare condition characterized by an increased number of lymphocytes in the gastric epithelium. On average, 3 to 8 lymphocytes occur per 100 epithelial cells in normal gastric mucosa, and a minimum of 30 lymphocytes per 100 epithelial cells is usually required for this diagnosis. Budesonide (9 mg/day) effectively induces clinical remission in patients with lymphocytic colitis and significantly improves histology results after 6 weeks.

2. The anticholinesterase antibody test is about 90% sensitive in diagnosing myasthenia gravis (MG); it is especially helpful in persons without outward clinical features of MG.

3. Swallowing saliva is a key protective mechanism against gastroesophageal reflux injury. Saliva has a neutral pH, which helps to neutralize the gastric refluxate, and the swallowed saliva initiates a peristaltic wave that strips the esophagus of refluxed material (clearance).

4. Screening efforts for adenocarcinoma of the esophagus should be directed toward those at greatest risk of developing cancer: i.e., older white men with more than 5 years of reflux symptoms.

5. Antireflux surgery is an important alternative for patients with medically refractory gastroesophageal reflux disease (GERD). Important preoperative considerations to *tailor* the antireflux surgery include esophageal length, esophageal dysmotility, and prior abdominal surgery. For the short esophagus with normal motility, the surgical options are transthoracic Belsey or Nissen or Collis gastroplasty. For esophagus of normal lenghth, but hypomotility the surgical options are laparoscopic or open Toupet or Hill procedure or transthoracic Belsey procedure.

6. Most cases of achalasia appear to be acquired and it is uncommon before the age of 25, with a clear-cut age-related increase thereafter. Most commonly, the disease occurs in middle adult life (ages 30 to 60) and affects both sexes and all races nearly equally.

7. Sildenafil (Viagra) blocks phosphodiesterase type 5 (the enzyme responsible for degradation of cyclic guanosine monophosphate [cGMP]), which results in increased cGMP levels within smooth muscle and consequent relaxation. The drug is effective in short-term reduction of lower esophageal sphincter (LES) pressures in patients with achalasia.

8. Gastric cancer is one of the tumors found in hereditary nonpolyposis colon cancer syndrome (HNPCC), and about 10% of patients with HNPCC develop gastric cancer. Families with specific mutations in the E-cahedrin gene (*CDH1*) have been reported to have a 100% chance of developing diffuse gastric cancer.

9. Patients identified to have a gastric carcinoid tumor should have the gastrin level checked to evaluate for hypergastrinemia. If the gastrin level is elevated, evaluation for acholorhydria should be conducted, and if gastrin is elevated and the patient is not achlorhydric (atrophic gastritis), an evaluation for Zöllinger-Ellison syndrome (gastrinoma) should be performed.

10. Although identifiable etiologies are apparent in most cases of gastroparesis (see Fig. 13-1), the singular most common cause remains idiopathic at about 35%. This suggests that there may be many yet-to-be-defined inheritable and infectious etiologies.

11. Hepatitis D virus (HDV) infection ONLY occurs in persons previously or co-infected with hepatitis B virus. Do not waste money on HDV tests unless the clinical suspicion is high and HBV is present.

12. Pretreatment characteristics that predict a favorable response to antiviral therapy for hepatitis C include infection with genotype 2 or 3, low viral load (less than 400,000 IU/mL), liver biopsy with little or no fibrosis, age younger than 40 years at time of treatment, and low body weight.

13. Ribavirin is teratogenic, and male and female patients with hepatitis C virus infection should be advised to practice effective contraception during therapy and for 6 months after treatment.

14. When active hepatitis B (HBV) and C (HCV) infections are present, as evidenced by a positive HCV-RNA and high level viremia by HBV-DNA polymerase chain reaction assay, the patient should be treated with the recommended dose of interferon for hepatitis B in conjunction with ribavirin for hepatitis C.

15. In general, if an HBV-infected female is planning pregnancy, it may be best to delay therapy until the third trimester of pregnancy or after delivery if her clinical condition allows. The use of lamivudine can be considered in this situation, with close monitoring for the emergence of HBV resistance.

16. In developed countries, such as the United States, once *Helicobacter pylori* infection has been eliminated, the annual rate of reinfection is very low (less than 1%). Most *reinfection* actually represents recrudescence of original infection resulting from initial treatment failure.

17. Hepatitis A is a preventable infectious disease and the following *at-risk* groups are all considered for vaccination: all children older than 12 months, travelers to countries with high endemicity for hepatitis A virus infection, military personnel, persons with chronic liver diseases of any etiology, homosexually active men, and users of illicit drugs.

18. The presence of cutaneous angiomas and palmar erythrema in a pregnant patient on physical examination is NOT predictive of chronic liver disease. Spider angiomas and palmar erythema are common and appear in about two-thirds of pregnant women without liver disease.

19. The severity of viral hepatitis during pregnancy is dependent on the viral cause. Hepatitis A, B, and C run the similar clinical course among gravid and nongravid females, while hepatitis E and herpes simplex hepatitis tend to be more virulent among gravid females.

20. Acute fatty liver of pregnancy (AFLP) is a genetic disorder. All women with AFLP, as well as their partners and children, should be advised to undergo molecular diagnostic testing. Testing for Glu474Gln only in the mother is not sufficient to rule out long-chain 3 hyroxyacyl CoA dehydrogense (LCHAD) deficiency in the fetus or other family members.

21. The HELLP syndrome (hemolysis, elevated liver enzymes, low platelets) is an uncommon disorder of pregnancy (0.2% to 0.6%), seen more commonly among pregnancies complicated by preeclampsia (4% to 12%). The incidence of HELLP is higher among multiparous, white, and older women, but the mean age of occurrence is around 25 years.

22. The risk for maternal-fetal vertical transmission of viral hepatitis C is approximately 2% for infants of anti-HCV, seropositive women. When a pregnant woman is HCV-RNA positive at delivery, this risk increases to 4% to 7%.

23. Transient arthralgias can occur in 10% of patients during acute hepatitis A viral infection; approximately 25% of patients with hepatitis B antigenemia develop a rheumatic syndrome; up to 50% of patients with hepatitis C develop an autoimmune syndrome. Levels of RNA greater than 1,000,000 copies/ml are reportedly associated with vertical transmission rates as high as 50%. HCV transmission increases up to 20 percent in women co-infected with HCV and HIV.

24. The association between essential mixed cryoglobulemia and viral hepatitis is extremely high. Approximately 80% to 90% of patients with essential mixed cryoglobulinemia (type II and type III) are positive for hepatitis C.

25. Approximately 40% to 75% of patients with hereditary hemochromatosis have a noninflammatory degenerative arthritis, most commonly involving the second and third metacarpophalangeal joints (MCPs), proximal interphalangeal joints (PIPs), wrists, hips, knees, and ankles. Importantly, this arthropathy may be the presenting complaint (30% to 50%) of patients with hemochromatosis and is frequently misdiagnosed in young males as seronegative rheumatoid arthritis.

26. Hepatocellular carcinoma (HCC) should only be considered for liver transplantation when the tumor burden is localized and limited: solitary lesion less than 5 cm or less than 3 nodules, each less than 3 cm and no metastatic or regional lymph node involvement, and no major vascular invasion.

27. Hepatic adenomas are at risk for spontaneous rupture, and intra-abdominal hemorrhage can occur in up to 30% of patients with hepatic adenoma, especially during menstruation or pregnancy.

28. Diphenylhydantoin, para-aminosalicylic acid, sulfonamides, and dapsone are drugs that have been implicated to occasionally cause mononucleosis-like hepatitis.

29. Amoxicillin-clavulanate, chlorpromazine, and erythromycin are drugs that have been associated with acute cholestatic syndromes that mimic acute cholecystitis.

30. Nitrofurantoin and minocyclin are two drugs that can induce hepatitis that mimics clinical autoimmune hepatitis with the presence of autoantibodies, hypergammaglobulinemia, and severe interface hepatitis on liver biopsy.

31. The Maddrey discriminant function (DF) score can be used to assess the risk of death from alcoholic hepatitis and to determine when corticosteroids should be used for those with severe clinical disease. DF = bilirubin (mg/dL) + 4.6 × [prothrombin time in seconds minus the control]. Those patients with DF greater than 32 have associated mortality 50% within 2 months and should be considered for treatment with corticosteroids.

32. The clinical course of non alcoholic steatohepatitis (NASH) is variable but, as a group, natural history studies suggest one-third of NASH patients show disease (fibrosis) progression, one-third have disease regression, and one-third have stable disease over a 5- to 10-year period.

33. Liver transplant recipients are at increased risk to develop cancer. Immunosuppression significantly increases the risk of malignancy and complicates approximately 2% of liver transplants. The most common malignancy following liver transplantation is squamous cell carcinoma of the skin.

34. The serum-ascites albumin gradient (SAAG) is a helpful test to categorize the etiology of ascites. The most common cause of high SAAG (i.e., ≥1.1 g/dL) ascites is cirrhosis, but any cause of portal hypertension leads to a high gradient (e.g., alcoholic hepatitis, cardiac ascites, massive liver metastases, fulminant hepatic failure, Budd-Chiari syndrome, portal vein thrombosis, veno-occlusive disease, myxedema, fatty liver of pregnancy, mixed ascites).

35. The risk for spontaneous bacterial peritonitis (SBP) is increased among cirrhotic patients admitted to the hospital with gastrointestinal hemorrhage.

36. Unlike pyogenic liver abscess, amebic abscess *never* involves the biliary tree. Bile is lethal to amebas; thus, infection of the gallbladder and bile ducts does not occur.

37. There are three gene defects associated with hereditary hemochromatosis (HH). A single missense mutation results in loss of a cysteine at amino acid position 282 with replacement by a tyrosine (C282Y), which leads to disruption of a disulfide bridge and thus to the lack of a critical fold in the alpha1 loop. A second mutation, whereby a histidine at amino acid position 63 is replaced by an aspartate (H63D), is common but less important in cellular iron homeostasis. Recently, a third mutation has been characterized whereby a serine is replaced by a cysteine at amino acid position 65 (S65C).

38. Each unit of blood contains about 200 to 250 mg of iron, depending on the hemoglobin. Therefore, a patient who presents with symptomatic HH and who has up to 20 g of excessive storage iron requires removal of over 80 units of blood, which takes close to 2 years at a rate of 1 unit of blood per week.

39. $\alpha_1$-AT deficiency can lead to cirrhosis and end-stage liver disease. Liver transplant can cure the disease, since the expressed phenotype becomes that of the transplanted liver.

40. Wilson disease is a rare disorder of copper metabolism that can manifest with psychosis, seizures, hemolytic anemia, and hepatitis. Wilson disease is characteristically a disease of adolescents and young adults, and the oldest patient to present with symptoms was in the late 40s.

41. Hepatic granulomas are commonly found in routine liver biopsies (10%). The differential list for hepatic granulomas is long and varied, but tuberculosis and sarcoidosis are the most common causes.

42. Hepatic function usually is not affected by liver cysts in patients with adult polycystic kidney disease (APCK), even when they number in the 1000s. When cysts become symptomatic from infection or hemorrhage, percutaneous cyst drainage may be necessary.

43. Patients with hepatic echinococcosis often unsuspectingly harbor the infection for years before they present with a palpable abdominal mass or other symptoms. The hydatid cyst diameter usually increases by 1 to 5 cm per year, and the symptoms of hepatic cystic echinococcosis are related primarily to the mass effect of the slowly enlarging cyst.

44. About 25% of obese patients undergoing rapid weight loss develop gallstones. Both aspirin and ursodeoxycholic acid may prevent stone formation during rapid weight loss.

45. Black gallstones are associated with chronic hemolysis, long-term total parenteral nutrition, and cirrhosis.

46. Bouveret syndrome refers to the clinical scenario in which gallstones perforate the stomach via a fistulous tract and then obstruct the pylorus.

47. Mirizzi syndrome occurs when a gallstone becomes impacted in the neck of the gallbladder or cystic duct, causing extrinsic compression of the common bile duct. The diagnosis should be considered in patients with cholecystitis who have higher than usual bilirubin levels. Biliary dstP!

48. A porcelain gallbladder is characterized by intramural calcification of the gallbladder wall. The diagnosis can be made by plain abdominal radiographs or abdominal CT. Prophylactic cholecystectomy is recommended to prevent development of carcinoma, which may occur in more than 20% of cases.

49. The infectious etiologies of acute pancreatitis (AP) are more common among children than adults but can occur in any age group. Infectious etiologies of AP include viruses, bacteria, fungi, and parasites.

50. Hypertriglyceridemia is the primary cause of AP in about 3% of all cases. It is a more common cause of AP than hypercalcemia.

51. The most reliable serum marker for diagnosing biliary AP is the serum alanine transaminase (ALT). Elevation of more than 2-fold of normal in patients older than 50 years has a sensitivity of 74% and specificity of 84% in predicting the biliary origin of AP. *gallpaths ↑ALT*

52. Patients with residual gallstones should undergo cholecystectomy after an episode of biliary AP. There is a 20% risk of recurrent biliary complications such as acute pancreatitis, cholecystitis, or cholangitis within 6 to 8 weeks of the initial episode of biliary AP.

53. Courvoisier sign consists of a palpable, distended gallbladder in the right upper quadrant in a patient with jaundice. This usually results from a malignant bile duct obstruction, such as pancreatic cancer with complete obstruction of the distal common bile duct and accumulation of bile in the gallbladder.

54. The most widely used marker to detect pancreatic cancer is the carbohydrate antigen CA 19-9; unfortunately, this marker can be elevated in a number of benign inflammatory disorders of the pancreas, biliary disease, and other intestinal tumors. Using a cutoff of greater than 200 U/mL improves the sensitivity to 97% and specificity to 98% to correctly discriminate pancreatic cancer. *CA19-9*

55. The double-duct sign, noted on endoscopic retrograde cholangiopancreatography (ERCP), demonstrates proximal dilation and distal stenosis of both the common bile and pancreatic ducts within the head of the pancreas. In patients with obstructive jaundice or a pancreatic mass, the double-duct sign has a specificity of 85% in predicting pancreatic cancer.

56. A pancreatic pseudocyst has a low probability of spontaneous resolution if there is concurrent evidence of chronic pancreatitis, such as pancreatic calcifications, or if the pseudocyst is a consequence of traumatic pancreatitis. The strict criteria of drainage required for a pseudocyst whose diameter is greater than 6 cm or that persists for greater than 6 weeks is no longer accepted as absolute.

57. *Hemosuccus pancreaticus* describes the rare phenomenon of major bleeding into the main pancreatic duct from a pseudoaneurysm. Massive gastrointestinal or intra-abdominal bleeding from pseudocyst erosion into a pancreatic or peripancreatic blood vessel occurs in about 5% to 10% of patients with pseudocysts.

58. Microscopic examination of stool using Sudan stain to detect fat is the best screening test for fat malabsorption and has a 100% sensitivity and 96% specificity. The presence of more than 100 globules greater than 6 μm in diameter per high-power field (430×) indicates a definite increase in fecal fat excretion.

59. Whipple disease (tropical sprue) is an infection that can cause diarrhea and mental status changes. It is caused by *Tropheryma whippelii* and can be treated with antibiotics. Tropical sprue is endemic in Puerto Rico, Cuba, the Dominican Republic, and Haiti but not in Jamaica or the other West Indies islands. It is found in Central America, Venezuela, and Colombia. Sprue is common in the Indian subcontinent and Far East, although little information is available from China.

*Tsmet Whipple's*

60. Crohn disease is more common among smokers and tends to have a more virulent clinical course associated with more frequent relapse, more severe complications, and postoperative recurrence.

61. The possibility of Crohn disease should be considered in all patients with chronic diarrhea and recurrent oxylate renal stones. This type of renal stone in more prevalent among Crohn patients, because chronic ileititis and/or ileal resection causes steatorrhea.

62. Extraintestinal manifestations of inflammatory bowel disease (IBD) that run a parallel course with ulcerative colitis include peripheral arthritis, pyoderma gangrenosum, and erythema nodosum. Axial arthritis (ankylosing spondylitis) and primary sclerosing cholangitis tend to run an independent course of bowel activity.

*PSC, AS.*

63. Eosinophilic gastroenteritis (EGE) may cause a variety of gastrointestinal symptoms, and diagnosis requires histologic confirmation of eosinophilic infiltrate. One should be mindful that peripheral eosinophilia is absent in 20% of patients with EGE.

64. The natural protective mechanisms against small intestinal bacterial overgrowth include gastric acid, bile acid, pancreatic enzyme activity, small intestinal motility (migrating motor complex [MMC]), and ileocecal valve.

65. Cancer is the second leading cause of death in the United States (after cardiovascular disease), and colorectal cancer is the second leading cause of death from malignancies (after lung cancer).

66. The prevalence of adenomatous polyps appears to be highly dependent on the population studied. Two colonoscopic studies in asymptomatic populations have reported rates of 23% to 25% prevalence in male and female patients between the ages of 50 and 82 years.

67. Screening recommendation for patients with HNPCC include colonoscopy for all members of the family beginning at age 20 to 25 years, repeated semiannually until age 40, then yearly thereafter.

68. Identification of either high-grade dysplasia or low-grade dysplasia among patients with ulcerative colitis dramatically increases the risk for colon cancer. High-grade dysplasia carries a 40% to 45% risk that a malignancy will be found in a resected specimen and therefore proctocolectomy is recommended. Low-grade dysplasia carries an approximately 20% risk of an existing cancer and an increasing number of clinicians therefore advocate colectomy rather than the traditional program of intensive surveillance (every 3 to 6 months).

69. Any person identified to have sepsis with *Streptococcus bovis* should be evaluated for colon cancer due to a unique clinical association.

70. Dysfunction of the pelvic musculature, also termed anismus, spastic pelvic floor syndrome, or anorectal dyssynergia, can cause functional rectal obstruction. Often there appears to be abnormal coordination of the various muscles involved in defecation.

71. Strictures of the colon are uncommon and the etiologies include cancer, diverticular disease, IBD, and ischemia. The location and length of the stricture can give helpful clues for the etiology. Malignant strictures are usually less than 3 cm in length and associated with abrupt shoulders at either end. Diverticular strictures are longer (3 to 6 cm) with smoother contours. Strictures between 6 and 10 cm are more likely to be due to Crohn disease or ischemia.

72. Both corticosteroids and nonsteroidal anti-inflammatory drugs have been shown to exacerbate diverticulitis. Corticosteroids in high doses have been associated with development of acute diverticulitis. Nonsteroidal anti-inflammatory drugs also have been associated with more severe diverticulitis.

73. The psoas and obturator signs are indication of irritation of the retroperitoneal psoas muscle (pain on right hip extension) or internal obturator muscle (pain on internal rotation of the flexed right hip) by an inflamed retrocecal appendix.

74. Rovsing sign is a clinical sign for appendicitis. The sign is positive when palpation of the left lower quadrant leads commonly to right lower quadrant pain in acute appendicitis.

75. A symptomatic Meckel diverticulum usually follows the *rule of 2*. A congenital omphalomesenteric mucosal remnant that may contain ectopic gastric mucosa, located on the antimesenteric side of the ileum, generally adheres to the rule of 2s: found in 2% of the population, 2 feet from the ileocecal valve, and 2% will develop diverticulitis.

76. When an ovarian tumor is discovered during laparoscopic or open exploration, the normal appendix should be removed after obtaining peritoneal washings and studied for tumor cytology. The ovarian mass itself should not be touched or biopsied.

77. Although most patients with *Clostridium difficile* colitis respond to vancomycin or Flagyl, approximately one-third have recurrent symptoms after stopping therapy. One recurrence makes further recurrences even more likely (up to 40%).

78. Microscopic colitis (MC) involves the colon discontinuously, and the patchy involvement of the normal appearing colon necessitates a minimum of four biopsies to establish the diagnosis of MC.

79. The Forrest classification describes the findings at endoscopy and the risk for ulcer rebleeding: Grade I, active pulsatile bleeding (rebleeding risk of 70% to 90%); Grade Ib, active nonpulsatile bleeding (10% to 20%); Grade IIa, nonbleeding visible vessel (40% to 50%); Grade IIb, adherent clot (10% to 20%); Grade III, no signs of recent bleeding (1% to 2%).

80. UGI hemorrhage due to giant ulcers (greater than 2 cm) is unlikely to be successfully managed with endoscopic methods, as are ulcers with bleeding from major arteries (greater than 2 mm).

81. Clinical history and findings suggestive of a upper gastrointestinal (UGI) source for gastrointestinal hemorrhage include history of ulcer disease, chronic liver disease, use of ASA or nonsteriodal anti-inflammatory drugs (NSAIDs); symptoms of nausea, vomiting or hematemesis; NG aspirate identification of blood or *coffee ground* material; serum blood urea nitrogen (BUN)–to–creatinine ratio greater than 33 is highly suggestive.

82. The most common causes of LGI hemorrhage are diverticulosis and colitis, 30% and 15% respectively; followed by cancer/polyp (13%), angiodysplasia (11%), and small bowel (6%).

83. In 8% of apparent LGI bleeding, the source is found to be from the UGI tract.

84. The natural history of LGI bleeding from colon diverticulosis: about 80% of patients stop bleeding spontaneously; 70% will not rebleed and do not require further treatment; about 60% of those requiring greater than 4 units of blood transfused within 24 hours require surgery; 30% will rebleed and require treatment.

85. It is decidedly uncommon for acute appendicitis to present with nausea, vomiting, or diarrhea *before* abdominal pain. Usually acute appendicitis is heralded by pain and often *followed* by anorexia, nausea, and sometimes single-episode vomiting. Acute appendicitis should be first on the differential diagnosis list in any patient with acute abdominal pain without a prior history of appendectomy.

86. Acute diarrhea cause by seafood is most commonly due to *Vibrio parahaemolyticus* and *Vibrio vulnificus*. Other causes of seafood-induced diarrhea include norovirus, *Plesiomonas shigelloides*, *Campylobacter,* scromboid fish poisoning (fish contains high levels of histamine and heat stable amines), and ciguaters fish poisoning (toxin found in reef fish produced from a dinoflagellate).

87. All persons receiving cytotoxic, anti-TNF-α, or other immunosuppressive therapy for malignancy, organ transplant or rheumatologic/gastrointestinal diseases should be tested for HBV infection (i.e., HBsAg, anti-HBc, and anti-HBs). Prophylactic antiviral therapy can prevent HBV reactivation in HBsAg (+) patients. Those patients with HBsAg (-) & anti-HBc (+) markers should be monitored for HBV replication and started on antiviral therapy when HBV-DNA polymerase is positive.

88. The most common cause of hospital-acquired diarrhea is *C. difficile* infection.

89. The most common causes of esophageal ulceration in acquired immunodeficiency syndrome (AIDS) are cytomegalovirus (CMV) and idiopathic esophageal ulcer (IEU).

90. The key collateral circulatory system between the superior mesenteric artery (SMA) and the inferior mesenteric artery (IMA) is the marginal artery of Drummond, which is a continuous arterial pathway running parallel to the entire colon. The arc of Riolan serves as the collateral communication between the middle colic branch of the SMA and the left colic branch of the IMA.

91. Cowden syndrome is a polyposis syndrome that involves the entire GI tract from the esophagus to rectum. The risk of developing colorectal cancer is generally not increased. Cowden arises from PTEN germline mutation with juvenile polyps the most common type; also seen are hyperplastic polyps, adenomas, lipomas, and rarely ganglioneuromas.

92. Only some foreign bodies in the GI tract need to be removed urgently by endoscopy. Button batteries or magnets, ingested typically by small children, need to be removed urgently if they become lodged. Any sharp object that carries a high risk for perforation should be removed as soon as possible before it passes to a level that is beyond the reach of an endoscope. Objects lodged in the esophagus that compromise the ability to handle oral secretions should be removed urgently to reduce the risk of aspiration.

93. Carnett test is a physical finding that helps to distinguish abdominal wall pain from intraperitoneal pain. The patient should fold the arms across the chest and raise the head off the pillow while the physician palpates the abdomen. If focal tenderness improves or disappears, the etiology is likely visceral in origin. However, if the tenderness is worse with this motion, the origin is the abdominal wall.

94. Tylosis is an uncommon autosomal dominant disorder that is distinguished by thickening of the skin (hyperkeratosis) on the palms and soles, and the syndrome is associated with a 27% incidence of squamous cell carcinoma of the esophagus. The average age at onset of esophageal cancer is 45 years, and death from esophageal cancer can occur in patients as young as 30 years.

95. Terry nails are characterized by uniform white discoloration of the nail, with the distal 1 to 2 mm remaining pink. The white color results from abnormalities in the nail bed vasculature and is most commonly seen in patients with liver cirrhosis, heart disease, and diabetes.

96. Muehrcke nails are characterized by double white transverse lines across the nails that disappear when pressure is applied. These lines are also caused by abnormal vasculature of the nail bed. They are most commonly seen in liver disease associated with hypoalbuminemia.

97. Sister Mary Joseph nodule is umbilical metastases of an internal malignancy. In the largest series reported, the most common primary malignancies were stomach (20%), large bowel (14%), ovary (14%), and pancreas (11%). In 20% of cases the primary could not be established. Umbilical metastases usually indicate advanced disease; the average survival is 10 months.

98. The gastrinoma triangle refers to the three key anatomic landmarks: the cystic duct-common bile duct junction, the second and third portions of the duodenum, and the junction of the neck and body of the pancreas. Approximately 60% to 75% of gastrinomas are found within this triangle.

99. Metabolism of azathioprine/6-MP by the enzyme TPMT (thiopurine methyltransferase) produces the inactive 6-methylmercaptopurine (6-MMP). 6-MMP levels greater than 5700 pmol/8 $\times 10^8$ cells have been associated with hepatotoxicity.

100. Prophylactic antibiotics for laparoscopic cholecystectomy are dispensed for the following reasons: bile spills during laparoscopic cholecystectomy occur in 30% to 50% of cases; normal bile is often colonized with bacteria (30% to 40% of patients); and acute cholecystitis has a 60% rate of bacterbilia after the first 24 hours of inflammation.

# CHAPTER 1

# SWALLOWING DISORDERS AND DYSPHAGIA

*Gulchin A. Ergun, MD*

## 1. What is the most difficult substance to swallow?

Water. Swallowing involves several phases. First, a preparatory phase involves chewing, sizing, shaping, and positioning of the bolus on the tongue. Then, during an oral phase, the bolus is propelled from the oral cavity into the pharynx while the airway is protected. Finally, the bolus is transported into the esophagus. Water is the most difficult substance to size, shape, and contain in the oral cavity. This makes it the hardest to control as it is passed from the oral cavity into the pharynx. Thus, viscous foods are used to feed patients with oropharyngeal dysphagia.

*[handwritten: thick]*

*[handwritten: 1. prep / 2. oral / 3. tspt ES]*

## 2. What sensory cues elicit swallowing?

The sensory cues are not entirely known, but entry of food or fluid into the hypopharynx, specifically the sensory receptive field of the superior laryngeal nerve, is paramount. Swallowing may also be initiated by volitional effort if food is present in the oral cavity. The required signal for initiation of the swallow response is a mixture of both peripheral sensory input from oropharyngeal afferents and superimposed control from higher nervous system centers. Neither is capable of initiating swallowing independent of the other. Thus, swallowing cannot be initiated during sleep when higher centers are turned off or with deep anesthesia to the oral cavity when peripheral afferents are disconnected.

## 3. What is the difference between globus sensation (globus hystericus) and dysphagia?

Globus sensation is the feeling of a lump in the throat. It is present continually and is not related to swallowing. It may even be temporarily alleviated during a swallow. Dysphagia is difficulty in swallowing and is noted by the patient only during swallowing.

*[handwritten: lump throat not d swallow]*

## 4. What are common etiologies of globus sensation?

- Gastroesophageal reflux disease
- Anxiety disorder (must exclude organic disease)
- Early hypopharyngeal cancer
- Goiter

## 5. Do patients accurately localize the site of dysphagia?

Patients with oropharyngeal dysphagia usually recognize that the swallow dysfunction is in the oropharynx. They may perceive food accumulating in the mouth or an inability to initiate a pharyngeal swallow. They can generally recognize aspiration before, during, or after a swallow. Patients with esophageal dysphagia correctly localize the abnormal site only 60% to 70% of time. They report it proximal to the actual site in the remainder. Differentiating between proximal and distal lesions may be difficult based on only the patient's perception. Associated symptoms, such as difficulty with chewing, drooling, coughing, or choking after a swallow, are more suggestive of oropharyngeal than of esophageal dysphagia.

## 6. What are the differences between esophageal and oropharyngeal dysphagia?

See Table 1-1.

## 7. What symptoms can be seen in oropharyngeal dysphagia?

- Inability to initiate a swallow
- Sensation of food getting stuck in the throat
- Coughing or choking (aspiration) during swallowing
- Nasopharyngeal regurgitation
- Changes in speech or voice (nasality)
- Ptosis
- Photophobia or visual changes
- Weakness, especially progressive toward the end of the day

**Table 1-1.** Esophageal Versus Oropharyngeal Dysphagia

| ESOPHAGEAL DYSPHAGIA | OROPHARYNGEAL DYSPHAGIA |
| --- | --- |
| Associated symptoms: chest pain, water brash, regurgitation | Associated symptoms: weakness, ptosis, nasal voice, pneumonia, cough |
| Organ-specific diseases (e.g., esophageal cancer, esophageal motor disorder) | Systemic diseases (e.g., myasthenia gravis, Parkinson disease) |
| Treatable (e.g., dilation) | Rarely treatable |
| Expendable organ (only one function) | Nonexpendable organ (functions include speech, respiration, and swallowing) |

## 8. What are the causes of oropharyngeal dysphagia?

Oropharyngeal dysphagia can be viewed as resulting from propulsive failure or structural abnormalities of either the oropharynx or esophagus. Propulsive abnormalities can result from dysfunction of the central nervous system control mechanisms, intrinsic musculature, or peripheral nerves. Structural abnormalities may result from neoplasm, surgery, trauma, caustic injury, or congenital anomalies. If dysphagia occurs in the absence of radiographic findings, motor abnormalities may be demonstrable by more sensitive methods such as electromyography or nerve stimulation studies. If all studies are normal, impaired swallowing sensation may be the primary abnormality. (See Table 1-2.)

## 9. What causes oropharyngeal dysphagia in the elderly?

Eighty percent of cases of oropharyngeal dysphagia in elderly patients are attributable to neuromuscular disorders. Of these, cerebrovascular accidents account for the vast majority. Parkinson disease, motor neuron disorders, and skeletal muscle disorders are also well known etiologies. Structural disorders are seen in less than 20% of elderly patients with dysphagia.    *80% NM (CVA)*

## 10. Why is a brainstem stroke more likely to cause severe oropharyngeal dysphagia than a hemispheric stroke?

The swallowing center is situated bilaterally, in the reticular substance below the nucleus of the solitary tract, in the brainstem. Efferent fibers from the swallow centers travel to the motor neurons controlling the swallow musculature located in the nucleus ambiguus. Therefore, brainstem strokes are more likely to cause the most severe impairment of swallowing with difficulty in initiating a swallow or absence of the swallow response.

## 11. When is it appropriate to evaluate stroke-related dysphagia?

About 25% to 50% of strokes will result in oropharyngeal dysphagia. Most stroke-related swallowing dysfunction improves spontaneously within the first 2 weeks. Unnecessary diagnostic or therapeutic procedures, such as *PEG* percutaneous gastrostomy, should be avoided immediately after a cerebrovascular accident. If symptoms persist beyond the 2-week period, swallowing function should be evaluated.

## 12. Is a barium swallow examination adequate to evaluate oropharyngeal dysphagia?

A barium swallow focuses on the esophagus, is done in a supine position, and takes only a few still images as the barium passes through the oropharynx. Therefore, aspiration may be missed if a conventional barium swallow is ordered. Oropharyngeal dysphagia is best evaluated with a cineradiographic or videofluoroscopic swallowing study, commonly called the modified barium swallow. Because the oropharyngeal swallow is rapid and transpires in less than 1 second, images must be obtained and recorded at a rate of 15 to 30/sec to adequately capture the motor events. The recorded study can be played back in slow motion for careful evaluation. This study is done with the patient in the upright position and resembles the normal eating position more than does the conventional barium swallow.

## 13. What is the characteristic feature of dysphagia in myasthenia gravis?

*fatiguable*

Myasthenia gravis is an autoimmune disorder characterized by progressive destruction of acetylcholine receptors at the neuromuscular junction. It affects the striated portion of the esophageal musculature. A distinct feature is increasing muscle weakness with repetitive muscle contraction such that dysphagia worsens with repeated swallows or as the meal progresses. Resting to allow reaccumulation of acetylcholine in nerve endings improves pharyngoesophageal functions and symptoms simultaneously. Muscles of facial expression, mastication, and swallowing are frequently involved and dysphagia is a prominent symptom in more than one third of cases. An anticholinesterase antibody test is about 90% sensitive in diagnosing myasthenia gravis. If clinical suspicion is strong, a therapeutic trial with an acetylcholinesterase inhibitor, such as Tensilon, or a cholinomimetic, such as Mestinon, should be considered even in the absence of the anticholinesterase antibody.

**Table 1-2.** Causes of Oropharyngeal Dysphagia

| PROPULSIVE | STRUCTURAL | IATROGENIC |
|---|---|---|
| **Neurologic**<br>Cerebrovascular accident (medulla, large territory cortical)<br>Parkinson disease<br>Amyotrophic lateral sclerosis<br>Multiple sclerosis | **Benign**<br>Cricopharyngeal bars<br>Hypopharyngeal diverticula (Zenker's)<br>Cervical vertebral body osteophytes | **Drug Induced**<br>Steroid myopathy<br>Tardive dyskinesia<br>Mucositis due to chemotherapy |
| **Degenerative Disease**<br>Alzheimer, Huntington, Friedreich ataxia<br>Brain neoplasm (brainstem)<br>Polio and postpolio syndrome<br>Cerebral palsy<br>Cranial nerve palsies<br>Recurrent laryngeal nerve palsy | **Skin Disease**<br>Epidermolysis bullosa, pemphigoid, graft-versus-host disease<br>**Caustic Injury**<br>Lye<br>Pill induced | **Radiation Induced**<br>Xerostomia<br>Myopathy<br>**Prosthetics**<br>Neck stabilization hardware<br>Ill-fitting dental or intraoral prostheses |
| **Muscular**<br>Muscular dystrophy (Duchenne, oculopharyngeal)<br>Myositis and dermatomyositis<br>Myasthenia gravis<br>Eaton-Lambert syndrome | **Infections**<br>Abscess<br>Ulceration<br>Pharyngitis | **Surgery**<br>Oropharyngeal resection |
| **Metabolic**<br>Hypothyroidism with myxedema<br>Hyperthyroidism | **Autoimmune**<br>Oral ulcers in Crohn, Behçet disease | |
| **Inflammatory/Autoimmune**<br>Systemic lupus erythematosus<br>Amyloidosis<br>Sarcoidosis | **Dental**<br>Dental anomalies | |
| **Infectious**<br>AIDS with central nervous system involvement<br>Syphilis (tabes dorsalis)<br>Botulism<br>Rabies<br>Diphtheria<br>Meningitis<br>Viral (coxsackievirus, herpes simplex virus) | **Neoplasms**<br>**Extrinsic Compression**<br>Goiter<br>Lymphadenopathy | |

*mixed = rare* (handwritten)

**14. Why is simultaneous involvement of the oropharynx and esophagus extremely unusual for any disease process other than infection?**

The oropharynx and the esophagus are fundamentally different in respect to musculature, innervation, and neural regulation (Table 1-3). Because most disease processes are specific for a particular type of muscle or nervous system element, it is unlikely that they would involve such diverse systems.

**15. What is Zenker diverticulum?**

Zenker diverticulum is a diverticulum of the hypopharynx. It is located posteriorly in an area of potential weakness at the intersection of the transverse fibers of the cricopharyngeus and the obliquely oriented fibers of the inferior pharyngeal constrictors also called the Killian dehiscence (Fig. 1-1).

**16. Are Zenker diverticula the result of an obstructive or a propulsive defect?**

It was previously believed that the pathogenesis of the diverticulum was due to abnormally high hypopharyngeal pressures caused by defective coordination of upper esophageal sphincter (UES) relaxation during pharyngeal

**Table 1-3.** Comparison of the Oropharynx and the Esophagus

| OROPHARYNX | ESOPHAGUS |
| --- | --- |
| Striated muscle | Striated muscle (proximal), smooth muscle (middle and distal) |
| Direct nicotinic innervation | Myenteric plexus within longitudinal and circular smooth muscles |
| Cholinergic | Cholinergic, nitric oxide, vasoactive intestinal peptide |

bolus propulsion. It is now known that Zenker diverticulum is caused by a constrictive myopathy of the cricopharyngeus (poor sphincter compliance). Increased resistance at the cricopharyngeus and increased intrabolus pressures above this relative obstruction cause muscular stress in the hypopharynx with herniation and diverticulum formation. Thus, Zenker diverticulum is an obstructive rather than a propulsive disease.

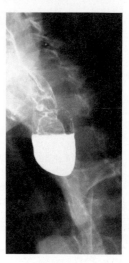

**Figure 1-1.**
Radiograph showing Zenker diverticulum.

**17. What are the treatment options for Zenker diverticula?**

The most common treatments are open surgical diverticulectomy with or without myotomy, rigid endoscopic myotomy, and, recently, cricopharyngeal myotomy using flexible endoscopes. Beware of comorbid conditions causing poor pharyngeal contraction, such as Parkinson disease, because these patients may have poor pharyngeal contraction and may not improve clinically after myotomy.

**18. How does flexible endoscopic therapy differ from standard surgical therapies?**

Surgical therapy usually involves rigid endoscopic therapy in the operating under general anesthesia and requires hyperextension of the neck. The myotomy is done using stapling devices, although laser division has been done.

Endoscopic therapy is usually performed in the endoscopy suite usually with moderate sedation or monitored anesthesia care. During endoscopic therapy, the septum between the diverticulum and esophagus that contains the cricopharyngeus is divided. The septum is reduced to less than 1 cm. Electrocautery is used to divide the muscle, and the usual cutting methods have included needle knife and argon plasma coagulation (APC), although forceps coagulation has been described.

**19. What are the early complications following endoscopy therapy for Zenker diverticulum?**

Complications are those related to aspiration, sedation, perforation, and bleeding. Perforation occurs in up to 23% of patients and usually represents microperforation. Most endoscopists routinely obtain chest radiographs or water-soluble contrast esophagrams after the procedure to look for the presence of mediastinal air or leak from perforation. Bleeding after myotomy occurs in 0% to 10% of patients.

**20. What are the indications and late risks of a cricopharyngeal myotomy?**

See Table 1-4.

**21. When should you consider performing flexible endoscopic therapy for Zenker diverticula?**

Flexible endoscopic treatment may be a better choice for elderly patients who are at high risk for surgery and who may benefit from avoiding general anesthesia and hyperextension of the neck.

**Table 1-4.** Indications and Late Risks of a Cricopharyngeal Myotomy

| INDICATIONS | LATE RISKS |
| --- | --- |
| Zenker diverticulum | Aspiration in patients with gastroesophageal reflux |
| Cricopharyngeal bar with symptoms | Worsening of swallow function |
| Parkinson's disease with impaired upper esophageal sphincter relaxation | |

22. **What is the differential diagnosis of dysphagia in a patient who has had surgery, radiation, and chemotherapy for head and neck cancer?**
   - Radiation myositis and/or fibrosis
   - Xerostomia (hyposalivation)
   - Anatomic defects due to surgery
   - Recurrence of malignancy

23. **Are swallowing disorders related to an increased morbidity and mortality?**
   Yes. Patients with dysphagia have an increased risk of aspiration pneumonia. Relative risk for aspiration is highest in patients with dementia followed by those who are institutionalized. Liquid aspiration is the most common type of aspiration in elderly patients.

24. **What therapies can be used to improve swallowing?**
   The goals of swallow therapy are to help minimize the risk of aspiration and to optimize oral delivery of nutrition.
   - Direct swallow therapies attempt to improve the swallow physiology. Examples include treatment of the primary disease, oral and maxillofacial prosthetics, cricopharyngeal myotomy, and swallow maneuvers such as the supraglottic swallow.
   - Compensatory techniques help eliminate symptoms but do not change the swallowing dysfunction. These techniques include adjustment of the patient's head and neck, changing food viscosity, and optimizing the volume and rate of food delivery.
   - Indirect swallow therapies address the neuromuscular coordination needed for swallowing. Examples include exercise regimens for tongue coordination and chewing.

25. **Which patients are ideal candidates for swallow therapy?**
   Patients who are mentally competent and motivated have the best results with swallow therapy. Therapy is most effective for aspiration (during and after swallow) and unilateral pharyngeal paresis.

26. **What are the etiologies of dysphagia in gastroesophageal reflux disease?**
   - *Inflammation:* 30% of patients with esophagitis experience dysphagia.
   - *Stricture:* Dysphagia occurs when the lumen diameter is less than 11 to 13 mm.
   - *Peristaltic dysfunction:* This is seen with advanced disease.
   - *Hiatus hernia:* Up to 30% of patients with a hiatus hernia may have dysphagia.
   - *Coexisting eosinophilic esophagitis.*

27. **What are the common symptoms and causes of xerostomia?**

| SYMPTOM | CAUSE |
| --- | --- |
| Dysphagia | Sjögren syndrome |
| Dry mouth with viscous saliva | Rheumatoid arthritis |
| Bad taste in mouth | Drugs (e.g., anticholinergics, antidepressants) |
| Oral burning | Radiation therapy |
| Dental decay | Poor oral hygiene, other |
| Bad breath | Multiple |

28. **Why is *cricopharyngeal achalasia* a misnomer? How does it differ from classic achalasia?**
   The UES is a striated muscle that is dependent on tonic excitation to maintain contractility. If innervation to the cricopharyngeus is lost, the UES relaxes and becomes flaccid. This is in contrast to the lower esophageal sphincter (LES). The LES a 3- to 4-cm-long segment of tonically contracted smooth muscle located at the distal end of the esophagus. LES tonic contraction is a property of both the muscle itself and of its extrinsic innervation. Normal resting tone of the LES varies from 10 to 30 mm Hg, being least in the postcibal period and greatest at night. Classic achalasia is caused by loss of the inhibitory myenteric plexus neurons in the distal esophagus, thereby leaving no mechanism to inhibit myogenic contraction (Table 1-5).

29. **When is botulinum toxin (BTx) used for dysphagia?**
   BTx has been best studied in dysphagia caused by achalasia. Achalasia is the result of selective loss of inhibitory neurons at the LES, resulting in unopposed (tonic) excitation of the LES. BTx injection into the distal esophagus can reduce LES pressure by blocking acetylcholine release from the presynaptic cholinergic nerve terminals in the myenteric plexus. Surgical myotomy is the definitive treatment for achalasia, as repeated BTx therapy is required to maintain efficacy. Ideal candidates for BTx are the elderly and those at high operative risk.

**Table 1-5.** Comparison of the Lower and Upper Esophageal Sphincters

|  | LOWER ESOPHAGEAL SPHINCTER | UPPER ESOPHAGEAL SPHINCTER |
|---|---|---|
| Resting tone | Myogenic | None |
| Result of denervation | Contraction | Relaxation |
| Cause of impaired opening | Failure of relaxation | Failure of traction (pulling open) |
| Source of opening force | Bolus | Suprahyoid and infrahyoid musculature |

Endoscopic injection of BTx into the diverticular spur, as an alternative to surgical cricopharyngeal myotomy, has been successful in case reports. The use of BTx in Parkinson disease with dysphagia due to impaired relaxation of the UES has also shown improvement by videofluoroscopic and electromyographic studies. Potential side effects include persistent stenosis and the risk of local BTx diffusion into the larynx or hypopharynx.

## WEBSITES

1. http://www.radiologyassistant.nl/en/440bca82f1b77
2. http://www.nlm.nih.gov/medlineplus/dysphagia.html

### BIBLIOGRAPHY

1. Cook IJ. Diagnostic evaluation of dysphagia. Nat Clin Pract Gastroenterol Hepatol 2008;5:393–403.
2. Cook IJ, Gabb M, Panagopoulos V, et al. Pharyngeal (Zenker's) diverticulum is a disorder of upper esophageal sphincter opening. Gastroenterology 1992;103:1229–35.
3. Cook IJ, Kahrilas PJ. AGA technical review of management of oropharyngeal dysphagia. Gastroenterology 1999;116:455–78.
4. Ferreira A, Simmons DT, Baron TH. Zenker's diverticula: Pathophysiology, clinical presentation, and flexible endoscopic management. Dis Esophagus 2007;21:1–8.
5. Furuta GT, Liacouras C, Collins M, et al. Eosinophilic esophagitis in children and adults: A systemic review and consensus recommendations for diagnosis and treatment. Gastroenterology 2007;133:1342–63.
6. Kolbasnik J, Waterfall WE, Fachnie B. Long term efficacy of botulinum toxin in classical achalasia: A prospective study. Am J Gastroenterol 1999;94:3434–9.
7. Visosky AM, Parke RB, Donovan DT. Endoscopic management of Zenker's diverticulum: Factors predictive of success or failure. Ann Otol Rhinol Laryngol 2008;117:531–7.

# GASTROESOPHAGEAL REFLUX DISEASE

*Peter R. McNally, DO*

CHAPTER **2**

**1. What is gastroesophageal reflux disease (GERD)? How common is it?**

GERD is a pathologic condition of symptoms and injury to the esophagus caused by percolation of gastric or gastroduodenal contents into the esophagus. GERD is extremely common. One survey of hospital employees showed that 7% experienced heartburn daily, 14% experienced symptoms weekly, and 15% experienced symptoms monthly. Other studies have suggested a 3% to 4% prevalence of GERD among the general population, with a prevalence increase to approximately 5% in people older than 55 years. Pregnant women have the highest incidence of daily heartburn at 48% to 79%. The distribution of GERD between the sexes is equal, but men are more likely to have complications of GERD—esophagitis (2–3:1) and Barrett's esophagus (10:1).

**2. What are the typical symptoms of GERD?**

Heartburn is usually characterized as a midline retrosternal burning sensation that radiates to the throat and occasionally to the intrascapular region. Patients often place the open hand over the sternal area and flip the wrist in an up-and-down motion to simulate the nature and location of the heartburn symptoms. Mild symptoms of heartburn are often relieved within 3 to 5 minutes of ingesting milk or antacids. Other symptoms of GERD include the following:

* *Regurgitation* consists of eructation of gastric juice or stomach contents into the pharynx and often is accompanied by a noxious bitter taste. Regurgitation is most common after a large meal and usually occurs with stooping or assuming a recumbent posture.
* *Dysphagia* (difficulty in swallowing) usually is caused by a benign stricture of the esophagus in patients with longstanding GERD. Solid foods, such as meat and bread, are often precipitants of dysphagia. Dysphagia implies significant narrowing of the esophageal lumen, usually to a luminal diameter of less than 13 mm. Prolonged dysphagia, associated with inability to swallow saliva, requires prompt evaluation and often endoscopic removal (see Chapter 61, Fig. 61-1).
* *Water brash* is an uncommon symptom but highly suggestive of GERD. Patients literally foam at the mouth as the salivary glands produce up to 10 mL of saliva per minute as an esophagosalivary reflex response to acid reflux.

**3. Is gastrointestinal (GI) hemorrhage a common symptom of GERD?**

No. Endoscopic evaluation of patients with upper GI hemorrhage has identified erosive GERD as the cause in only 2% to 6% of cases.

**4. What is odynophagia? Is it a common symptom of GERD?**

Odynophagia is a painful substernal sensation associated with swallowing that should not be confused with dysphagia. Odynophagia rarely results from GERD. Instead, odynophagia is caused by infections (monilia, herpes simplex virus, and cytomegalovirus), ingestion of corrosive agents or pills (tetracycline, vitamin C, iron, quinidine, estrogen, aspirin, alendronate [Fosamax], or nonsteroidal anti-inflammatory drugs), or cancer.

**5. What clues about GERD can be gleaned from the physical exam?**

* Severe kyphosis often is associated with hiatal hernia and GERD, especially when a body brace is necessary.
* Tight-fitting corsets or clothing (in men or women) can increase intra-abdominal pressure and may cause stress reflux.
* Abnormal phonation may suggest high GERD and vocal cord injury. When hoarseness is due to high GERD, the voice is often coarse or gravelly and may be worse in the morning, whereas in other causes of hoarseness, excessive voice use or abuse leads to worsening later in the day.
* Wheezing or asthma and pulmonary fibrosis have been associated with GERD. Patients often give a history of postprandial or nocturnal regurgitation with episodes of coughing or choking caused by near or partial aspiration.
* Loss of enamel on the lingual surface of the teeth may be seen in severe GERD, although it is more common in patients with rumination syndrome or bulimia (Fig. 2-1).
* Esophageal dysfunction may be the predominant component of scleroderma or mixed connective tissue disease. Inquiry about symptoms of Raynaud syndrome and examination for sclerodactyly, taut skin, and calcinosis are important.
* Cerebral palsy, Down syndrome, and mental retardation are commonly associated with GERD.
* Children with peculiar head movements during swallowing may have Sandifer syndrome.
* Some patients unknowingly swallow air (aerophagia) that triggers a burp, belch, and heartburn cycle. The observant clinician may detect this behavior during the interview and physical exam.

### 6. Do healthy persons have GERD?

Yes. Healthy persons may regurgitate acid or food contents into the esophagus, especially after a large meal late at night. In normal persons, the natural defense mechanisms of the lower esophageal sphincter (LES) barrier and esophageal clearance are not overwhelmed, and symptoms and injury do not occur. Ambulatory esophageal pH studies have shown that healthy persons have acid reflux into the esophagus during less than 2% of the daytime (upright position) and less than 0.3% of the nighttime (supine position).

### 7. How can swallowing and salivary production be associated with GERD?

Reflux of gastric contents into the esophagus often stimulates salivary production and increased swallowing. Saliva has a neutral pH, which helps to neutralize the gastric refluxate. Furthermore, the swallowed saliva initiates a peristaltic wave that strips the esophagus of refluxed material (clearance). During the awake upright period, persons swallow 70 times an hour; this rate increases to 200 times an hour during meals. Swallowing is least common during sleep (less than 10 times per hour), and arousal from sleep to swallow during GERD may be reduced by sedatives or alcohol ingestion. Patients with Sjögren syndrome and smokers have reduced salivary production and prolonged esophageal acid clearance times.

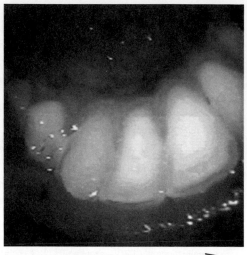

**Figure 2-1.** View of mouth showing the loss of dental enamel on the lingual surface of the teeth in a patient with chronic high gastroesophageal reflux.

### 8. What are the two defective anatomic mechanisms in patients with GERD?

Ineffective clearance and defective GE barrier.

### 9. What clearance defects are associated with GERD?

- *Esophageal.* Normally, reflux of gastric contents into the esophagus stimulates a secondary peristaltic or clearance wave to remove the injurious refluxate from the esophagus. The worst case of ineffective esophageal clearance is seen in patients with scleroderma. The LES barrier is nonexistent, and there is no primary or secondary peristalsis of the esophagus (hence, no clearance).
- *Gastric.* Gastroparesis may lead to excessive quantities of retained gastroduodenal and food contents. Larger volumes of stagnant gastric contents predispose to esophageal reflux.

### 10. How may the GE barrier be compromised?

The normal LES is 3 to 4 cm long and maintains a resting tone of 10 to 30 mm Hg pressure. The LES acts as a barrier against GERD. When the LES pressure is less than 6 mm Hg, GERD is common; however, the presence of *normal* LES pressure does not predict the absence of GERD. In fact, LES pressure of less than 10 mm Hg is found in a minority of people with GERD. Recent studies have shown that transient LES relaxations are important in the pathogenesis of GERD. During transient LES relaxations, the sphincter inappropriately relaxes and free gastric reflux occurs.

### 11. What foods and medications influence resting LES pressure?

See Table 2-1.

| Table 2-1. Increased Versus Decreased Lower Esophageal Sphincter (LES) Pressure | | |
| --- | --- | --- |
| | **INCREASED LES PRESSURE** | **DECREASED LES PRESSURE** |
| Food | Protein | Fat<br>Chocolate<br>Ethanol<br>Peppermint |
| Medication | Antacids<br>Metoclopramide<br>Cisapride<br>Domperidone | Calcium channel antagonists<br>Theophylline<br>Diazepam<br>Meperidine<br>Morphine<br>Dopamine<br>Diazepam<br>Barbiturates |

**12. What other medical conditions may mimic symptoms of GERD?**

The differential diagnosis of GERD includes coronary artery disease, gastritis, gastroparesis, infectious and pill-induced esophagitis, peptic ulcer disease, biliary tract disease, and esophageal motor disorders.

**13. What medical condition clinically presents with dysphagia and is often mistaken for GERD?**

Eosinophilic esophagitis. The condition is usually accompanied by atopy, allergies, or asthma. Symptoms of heartburn are usually mild or nonexistent. Endoscopic findings include *coiled rings*, vertical linear lines, and a narrowed esophageal lumen (Chapter 44, Fig. 44-4). Esophageal biopsy showing greater than 25 eosinophils per high-power field is diagnostic.

*coiled, rings, lines, lumen*     *25 eoph/HPF*

**14. How can GERD be distinguished from coronary artery disease?**

In the evaluation of patients with retrosternal chest pain, the clinician must always be mindful that patients with GERD do not die but patients with new-onset angina or an acute myocardial infarction with symptoms mimicking GERD can. Clues that a patient's chest pain is cardiac in origin include radiation of the pain to the neck, jaw, or left shoulder/upper extremity; associated shortness of breath and/or diaphoresis; precipitation of pain by exertion; and relief of pain with sublingual nitroglycerin. Physical findings of new murmurs or gallops or abnormal rhythms are also suggestive of a cardiac origin. Although positive findings on an electrocardiogram (ECG) are helpful in the evaluation of patients with chest pain, the absence of ischemic ECG changes should not discourage the clinician from excluding a cardiac etiology for the patient's symptoms.

**15. How should patients with symptoms of GERD be evaluated?**

Evaluation of patients with GERD may be guided by the severity of symptoms. Patients without symptoms of high GERD (aspiration or hoarseness) or dysphagia may be given careful instruction about lifestyle modification and a diagnostic trial of $H_2$ blocker therapy and followed clinically. Diagnostic evaluation is warranted when symptoms of GERD are chronic or incompletely responsive to medical therapy. Esophagogastroduodenoscopy (EGD) is the best test for evaluation of GERD. Up to 50% of patients with GERD do not have macroscopic evidence of esophagitis at the time of endoscopy. In this group, more sensitive GERD testing may be necessary or alternative diagnoses considered.

*( Savary Miller )*

**16. Describe a commonly used endoscopic grading system for GERD.** *VS. Los Angeles*

| | |
|---|---|
| Grade 0 | Macroscopically normal esophagus; only histologic evidence of GERD |
| Grade 1 | One or more nonconfluent lesions with erythema or exudate above the GE junction |
| Grade 2 | Confluent, noncircumferential, erosive, and exudative lesions |
| Grade 3 | Circumferential erosive and exudative lesions |
| Grade 4 | Chronic mucosal lesions (ulceration, stricture, or Barrett's esophagus) |

**17. What are the more sophisticated esophageal function tests? How can they be used appropriately in the evaluation of patients with GERD?**

Clinical tests of GERD may be divided into three categories:

- Acid sensitivity
  - Acid perfusion (Bernstein) test
  - 24- to 48-hour ambulatory esophageal pH monitoring
- Esophageal barrier and motility
  - Esophageal manometry
  - GE scintiscanning
  - Standard acid reflux (modified Tuttle) test
  - 24- to 48-hour ambulatory esophageal pH monitoring
- Esophageal acid clearance time
  - Standard acid reflux (clearance) test (SART)
  - 24- to 48-hour ambulatory esophageal pH monitoring

*Acid sens*
*ES barrier/moti*
*ES Hft cl. time*

**18. Do all patients with GERD need esophageal function testing?**

No. Testing should be reserved for patients who fail medical therapy or in whom the correlation of reflux symptoms is in doubt.

**19. What is the use of multichannel intraluminal impedance and pH (MII-pH) technology in the evaluation of GERD?**

The normal pH of the esophagus ranges between 5.0 and 6.8, making it difficult for conventional intraesophageal pH measurements to detect non–acid reflux events. The MMI-pH (impedance) technology is a major advance in esophageal testing that can aid in the detection of both acid and non–acid reflux events.

## 20. When is ambulatory esophageal pH monitoring helpful?

Ambulatory esophageal pH monitoring is helpful in evaluating patients refractory to standard medical therapy. Acid hypersecretion is often seen in patients with GERD, and esophageal pH monitoring may be helpful in titrating the dose of $H_2$ blocker or proton pump inhibitor (PPI). Persistence of acid reflux on *adequate* doses of a PPI should raise the possibility of patient noncompliance or Zöllinger-Ellison syndrome.

The Bravo capsule (Medtronix, Inc.) is a new wireless technology that permits more physiologic intraesophageal monitoring for acid reflux. The Bravo capsule is the size of a gel cap and is placed with or without endoscopic assistance 6 cm above the squamocolumnar junction. The capsule is *stapled* to the esophageal mucosa, permitting more physiologic and prolonged intraesophageal monitoring. Some investigators have begun to staple the capsule in the proximal esophagus to evaluate patients with atypical reflux symptoms, such as hoarseness, throat tightness, asthma, and interstitial lung disease.

*Refr to Rx ES PH mon*

## 21. When are esophageal manometry and scintiscanning helpful?

Esophageal manometry is helpful in evaluating the competency of the LES barrier and the body of the esophagus for motor dysfunction. Severe esophagitis may be the sole manifestation of early scleroderma. When ambulatory pH testing is not available, scintiscanning has been shown to be helpful.

## 22. Define the various types of medical therapy for GERD and give a logical approach to prescription therapy for patients with longstanding GERD.

For patients with mild, uncomplicated symptoms of heartburn, empiric $H_2$ blocker therapy without costly and sophisticated diagnostic testing is reasonable. For patients recalcitrant to conventional therapy or with complications of high GERD (aspiration, asthma, hoarseness), Barrett's esophagus, or stricture, diagnostic and management decisions become more complicated. Medical or surgical therapy depends on patient preference, health care cost, risk of medical or surgical complications, and other related factors (Table 2-2).

**Table 2-2.** Medical Therapy for Gastroesophageal Reflux Disease

| MEDICATION | DOSAGE | SIDE EFFECTS |
|---|---|---|
| **Topicals** | | |
| Antacids | 1–2 tablets after meals and at bedtime, as needed | Diarrhea (magnesium containing) and constipation (aluminum and calcium containing) |
| Sucralfate | 1 g 4 times/day | Incomplete passage of pill, especially in patients with esophageal strictures; constipation; dysgeusia |
| **H2 Blockers** | | |
| Cimetidine | 400–800 mg 2–4 times/day | Gynecomastia, impotence, psychosis, hepatitis, drug interactions with warfarin, theophylline |
| Ranitidine | 150–300 mg 2–4 times/day | Same, less common |
| Famotidine | 20–40 mg 1–2 times/day | Same, less common |
| **PPIs** | | |
| Omeprazole *BAD!* | 20–60 mg/day | Drug interaction due to cytochrome (CYP) P-450 (CYP2C19: warfarin, phenytoin, diazepam, clopedogrel) |
| Lansoprazole | 30 mg/day | CYP-1A2 inducer; decreases theophylline levels |
| Dexlansoprazole | 30–60 mg/day | CYP2C19 inhibition and drug interaction |
| Rabeprazole | 20 mg/day | Probably none |
| Pantoprazole | 40 mg/day | Probably none |
| Esomeprazole | 20–40 mg/day | Probably none |
| **Prokinetic Agents** | | |
| Bethanechol | 10–25 mg 4 times/day or at bedtime | Urinary retention in patients with detrusor-external sphincter dyssynergia or prostatic hypertrophy, worsening asthma |
| Metoclopramide | 10 mg 3 times/day or at bedtime | Extrapyramidal dysfunction, Parkinsonian-like reaction; cases of irreversible tardive dyskinesia have been reported |
| Cisapride | 10–20 mg 3 times/day | FDA recall, because of potential fatal arrhythmia Compassionate use available |

FDA, U.S. Food and Drug Administration; PPI, proton pump inhibitor.

**23. Describe the commonly recommended approach to graded treatment of GERD.**
Stage I—Lifestyle modifications
 Antacids, prokinetics, over-the-counter $H_2$ blockers, or sucralfate
Stage II I—$H_2$ blocker therapy
 Reinforce need for lifestyle modifications
Stage III I—PPIs
 Reinforce need for lifestyle modifications
Stage IV I—Surgical or endoscopic antireflux procedure
    The authors favor initiation of aggressive lifestyle modification (especially weight reduction and dietary changes) and pharmacologic therapy to achieve endoscopic healing of esophagitis (usually a PPI). When esophagitis is healed, the dose of the PPI should be lowered or an effective dose of an intermediate-potency $H_2$ blocker is substituted for the PPI. Then the patient is counseled about the risks, benefits, and alternatives to long-term medical therapy. Surgery is encouraged for the fit patient who requires chronic high doses of pharmacologic therapy to control GERD or dislikes taking medicine. Endoscopic treatments for GERD are very promising, but controlled long-term comparative trials with PPIs and/or surgery are lacking.

**24. Do patients scheduled for surgical antireflux procedures need to undergo sophisticated esophageal function testing before surgery?**
There is no absolute correct answer. However, it is prudent to conduct esophageal motility studies to ensure that esophageal motor disease is not present. Patients with scleroderma may have a paucity of systemic complaints, and the diagnosis may go undetected without esophageal manometry. Generally, surgical antireflux procedures are avoided or modified in such patients. In addition, esophageal motility studies and ambulatory 24-hour pH monitoring may confirm or refute that the patient's symptoms are attributable to GERD before the performance of a surgical procedure.

**25. What are some of the new endoscopic treatments for GERD?**
- Endoluminal gastroplication (ELGP)—Endocinch by CR Bard, Inc., or Endoscopic Suturing Device (ESD), Wilson Cook Inc.
- Single full-thickness plication—NDO Endoplication System by NDO Surgical, Inc.
- Coagulation injury—Stretta by Curon Medical, Inc.
- Polymer injection—Enteryx by Boston Scientific Corp. (recalled from U.S. market, 2005).

**26. How should esophageal strictures be managed?**
- Prevention of peptic stricture with early institution of effective medical or surgical therapy appears to be particularly important for patients with scleroderma.
- For patients with symptoms of dysphagia due to peptic stricture, esophageal dilation is effective. Dilation can be accomplished using mercury-filled polyvinyl Maloney bougies, wire-guided hollow Savary-Gulliard or American dilators, or through-the-scope (TTS) pneumatic balloons. Usually, the esophagus is dilated to a diameter of 14 mm or 42 to 44 French. After successful dilation of a peptic stricture, the patient should be placed on chronic PPI therapy to avoid recurrent stricture formation.
- Surgery is an effective method of managing esophageal strictures. Usually, preoperative and intraoperative dilation is combined with a definitive antireflux procedure.

**27. What is Barrett's esophagus? How is it managed?**
Barrett's esophagus is a metaplastic degeneration of the normal esophageal lining, which is replaced with a premalignant, specialized columnar epithelium. It is seen in roughly 5% to 7% of patients with uncomplicated reflux but in up to 30% to 40% of patients with scleroderma or dysphagia.
    Currently, there is no proven method to eliminate Barrett's esophagus. Preliminary studies of laser or BiCAP ablation of the metaplastic segment followed by alkalization of the GE refluxate are encouraging. The need for cancer surveillance is discussed elsewhere in this book.

**28. List some of the atypical symptoms and signs of GERD.**
Asthma, lingual dental erosions, chest pain, recurrent otitis in children, cough, throat-clearing, hiccups, throat tightness, hoarseness.

**29. Is there an association between obstructive sleep apnea (OSA) and GERD?**
Yes. Nocturnal acid reflux is seen in 54% to 72% of persons with OSA. Administration of nighttime continuous positive airway pressure (CPAP) and/or PPI therapy has been shown to decrease apnea events and acid reflux events.

**30. Does the presence of heartburn symptoms predict a GERD-related cough etiology?**
No. There is poor correlation between symptoms of heartburn and cough. Between 43% and 75% of patients with GERD-related cough do not have heartburn symptoms. Both medical treatment with PPIs and surgical antireflux procedures have been reported to be effective for GERD-related cough. Caveats include the following:

- 35% response rate to omeprazole 40 mg twice a day after 2 weeks
- Results of surgical antireflux procedures are best when preoperative esophageal manometry is normal and response to PPI is positive.

### 31. What is the best method to evaluate for possible GERD-related cough?

The first step is to exclude non–GERD-related etiologies: angiotensin-converting inhibitors, environmental irritants, smoking, parenchymal lung disease, allergic rhinitis and pneumonitis, and asthma and sinusitis, which are often *silent*. Symptom relief after a 2-week trial of high-dose PPI (40 mg twice a day) is a cost-effective approach. Patients who do not respond should be considered for further evaluation, including esophageal manometry/pH testing and/or EGD.

OSA-GERD- Asthma/cough

### 32. What laryngeal conditions are associated with GERD?

The most common laryngeal manifestation of high reflux or esophagopharyngeal reflux (EPR) is hoarseness. Other laryngeal conditions associated with EPR are listed:

- Arytenoid fixation
- Carcinoma of the larynx
- Contact ulcers and granuloma
- Globus pharyngeus
- Hoarseness
- Laryngomalacia
- Pachydermia laryngitis
- Paroxysmal laryngospasm
- Recurrent leukoplakia
- Vocal cord nodules

hireflux

### 33. How often do people with EPR and hoarseness relate symptoms of heartburn?

The prevalence of GERD symptoms among patients with reflux laryngitis is low (6%–43%).

### 34. What is the most efficient, cost-effective method to evaluate hoarse patients for EPR?

The first step in the evaluation of hoarseness should be exclusion of structural ear, nose, and throat (ENT) disorders, including neoplasm. The next step is an empiric trial of double-dose PPI for 2 to 3 months. Most EPR-related hoarseness improves with acid suppression (60%–96%). Patients responding to PPIs may stop the medication and be monitored for recurrence of symptoms. Hoarse patients with a negative ENT evaluation who fail PPI therapy should undergo formal esophageal pH analysis.

r/o ENT    if fail, ESPH
PPI² x 2-3mo

### 35. Can GE reflux worsen asthma?

Yes. Numerous studies have shown that reflux symptoms are common among asthmatics (65%–72%) and that medical and surgical antireflux treatment may improve pulmonary function.

### 36. How does GE reflux worsen asthma?

Several mechanisms are theorized to explain GERD-induced bronchospasm:

- Asthmatic patients with GERD have been shown to have autonomic dysregulation with heightened vagal response, which is presumed to be responsible for the decrease in LES pressure and more frequent transient relaxations of the LES, which promote reflux.    ↑CNS- ↓LES
- Esophageal reflux may incite a vagal-mediated esophagobronchial reflex of airway hyperreactivity.
- Microaspiration of gastric juice has been shown to activate a local axonal reflex involving release of substance P, which leads to airway edema. The finding of lipid-laden alveolar macrophages among asthmatic patients demonstrates aspiration of gastric material into the pulmonary tree.

aspi

### 37. What cytochrome P-450 (CYP-450) systems are involved in the metabolism of PPIs?

All of the PPIs undergo some hepatic metabolism through the CYP-450 system. The CYP-2C19 and CYP-3A4 microsomal enzymes are responsible for the majority of PPI hepatic metabolism. Genetic polymorphism with CYP-2C19 is common; about 5% of Americans and 20% of Asians are deficient in this enzyme. Omeprazole decreases the metabolism of phenytoin and warfarin R-isomer (CYP-2C9), diazepam (CYP-2C19), and cyclosporine (CYP-3A4).

3A4, 2C9 (lefty)

### 38. How do esomeprazole (Nexium) and omeprazole (Prilosec) differ?

Omeprazole is a racemic mixture of both the S- and R-isomers, whereas esomeprazole is a (pure) form of the S-isomer. Less esomeprazole (S-isomer) is metabolized by the CYP-2C19 pathway, leading to greater area under the curve and better intragastric acid suppression for 24 hours. Esomeprazole is the only PPI shown to be statistically superior to omeprazole in healing erosive esophagitis at 8 weeks (90%–94% efficacy rate).

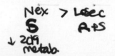

Nex > Losec
S       R+S
↓ 2C19
metabo

**39. Which patients with GERD should be considered for a surgical antireflux procedure?**
Any young, healthy patient with chronic GERD requiring lifelong PPI medical therapy may be considered for an antireflux procedure. Other indications include failed medical therapy, complicated GERD (e.g., bleeding, recurrent strictures), medical success at excessive cost in young, otherwise healthy patients, and problematic symptoms due to regurgitation (asthma, hoarseness, cough).

**40. Which patients are poor candidates for a surgical antireflux procedure?**
- Elderly patients with substantial comorbid disease
- Patients with poor or absent esophageal peristalsis
- Patients with highly functional symptoms

Lack of available surgical expertise is also a contraindication for antireflux procedures.

## WEBSITES

1. http://www.cambridgeconsultants.com
2. http://www.vhjoe.com/Volume2Issue3/2-3-4.htm
3. http://www.vhjoe.com/Volume2Issue3/2-3-3.htm

**BIBLIOGRAPHY**

1. Devault KR. Overview of therapy for the extraesophageal manifestations of gastroesophageal reflux disease. Am J Gastroenterol 2000;95:S39–S44.
2. Devault KR, Castell DO. Updated guidelines for the diagnosis and treatment of gastroesophageal reflux disease. Am J Gastroenterol 2005;100:190–200.
3. Gostout CJ. Endoscopic antireflux. Visible Hum J Endosc (VHJOE) 2003;2:3.
4. Green BT, Broughton WA, O'Connor JB. Marked improvement in nocturnal gastroesophageal reflux in a large cohort of patients with obstructive sleep apnea treated with continuous positive airway breathing. Arch Intern Med 2003;163:41–5.
5. Harding SM, Sontag SJ. Asthma and gastroesophageal reflux. Am J Gastroenterol 2000;95:S23–S32.
6. Irwin RS. Chronic cough due to gastroesophageal reflux disease: ACCP evidence-based clinical practice guidelines. Chest 2006;129(Suppl.):80S–94S.
7. Irwin RS, Richter JE. Gastroesophageal reflux and chronic cough. Am J Gastroenterol 2000;95:S9–S14.
8. Kellog TA, Oelschlanger BK, Pellegrini CA. Laparoscopic antireflux surgery. Visible Hum J Endosc (VHJOE) 2003;2:3.
9. Lazarchick DA, Filler SJ. Dental erosion: Predominant oral lesion in gastrocsophageal reflux disease. Am J Gastroenterol 2000;95:S33–S8.
10. Lichtenstein DR. Standards of Practice Committee: Role of endoscopy in the management of GERD. Gastrointest Endosc 2007;66:219–23.
11. Oelschlager BK, Eubanks T, Oleynikov D, et al. Symptomatic and physiologic outcomes after operative treatment for extraesophageal reflux. Surg Endosc 2002;16:1032–6.
12. Oelschlager BK, Quiroga E, Parra JD, et al. Long term outcomes after laparoscopic antireflux surgery. Am J Gastroenterol 2008;103:280–7.
13. Richter JE. The many manifestations of gastroesophageal reflux disease: Presentation, evaluation, and treatment. Gastroenterol Clin N Am 2007;36:577–99.
14. Senior BA, Khan M, Schwimmer C, et al. Gastroesophageal reflux and obstructive sleep apnea. Laryngoscope 2001;111:2144–6.
15. Spencer CM, Faulds D. Esomeprazole. Drugs 2000;60:321–7.
16. Tutuian R, Castell DO. Use of multichannel intraluminal impedance to document proximal esophageal and pharyngeal nonacidic reflux episodes. Am J Med 2003;115(Suppl. 3A):119S–23S.
17. Ward EM, Devault KR, Bouras EP, et al. Successful oesophageal pH monitoring with a catheter-free system. Aliment Pharmacol Ther 2004;19:449–54.
18. Wong RKH, Hanson DG, Waring PJ, et al. ENT manifestations of gastroesophageal reflux. Am J Gastroenterol 2000;95:S15–S22.

*[handwritten annotations: non CP — GERD dysmotil MSK → BIOPPI + PUD + Bil duct.]*

### 1. When should the clinician consider an esophageal cause of chest pain?

*[handwritten margin note: DES nutcracker HTN LES Achalasia Ineff. motility]*

The concept of the esophagus as the origin of chest pain is not new. More than a century ago, Sir William Osler hypothesized that esophageal spasm represented one cause of chest pain in soldiers during wartime. A recent multicenter study reported that 55% of patients attending the emergency department for chest pain did not have cardiac pain. However, coronary artery disease (CAD) is the most serious and life-threatening cause of chest pain. It should therefore be excluded as a potential diagnosis prior to pursuing esophageal investigations.

### 2. Does history help to discriminate cardiac from esophageal chest pain?

Yes and no. A sharp pain localized by one finger at the fifth intercostal space in the midclavicular line with onset at rest in a 20-year-old woman is unlikely to be caused by coronary artery disease. Certain features in a patient's presenting history help clearly to differentiate between causes. However, many studies have shown sufficient overlap of all features to preclude certain diagnoses on the basis of symptoms alone. The description of pain by some patients with a known esophageal source and no cardiac disease mimics exactly the classic description of angina pectoris, including pain on exertion. One study from Belgium documented normal coronary angiograms in 25% of patients regarded by cardiologists as having myocardial ischemia on the basis of symptoms. In half of these patients, a probable esophageal cause could be identified.

### 3. Does a normal coronary angiogram exclude all cardiac diagnoses?

No. Cardiac abnormalities other than CAD can be found in patients with chest pain, including mitral valve prolapse and microvascular angina. Exclusion of mitral valve prolapse requires echocardiography, whereas microvascular angina can be excluded only by the complicated procedure of measuring coronary artery resistance during stimulation with ergonovine and rapid atrial pacing.

*[handwritten margin note: MVP]*

However, studies suggesting that pain is no more common in patients with mitral valve prolapse or microvascular angina than in the general population question whether these abnormalities produce pain. If they do, the mechanism is unclear. Furthermore, the prognosis is excellent, with the mortality rate being no different from that of the general population. Finally, a positive association between these cardiac abnormalities and esophageal motility disorders suggests a common or associated cause—either a generalized smooth muscle defect or heightened visceral nociception. It is therefore appropriate to search for an esophageal cause, after excluding CAD.

### 4. What are the noncardiac causes of chest pain? How common are they?

Gastroesophageal reflux disease (GERD) is the most frequent esophageal cause of chest pain. In most studies, it accounts for up to 50% of all cases of unexplained chest pain (UCP). Esophageal dysmotility can be diagnosed in another 25% to 30% of cases. Of the remaining 20% to 30%, one third to one half can be explained by a musculoskeletal source, such as costochondritis (Tietze syndrome) and chest-wall pain syndromes. Psychological disorders, acting either independently or as cofactors, are responsible for many of these pain syndromes. Panic disorder, in particular, must be considered.

### 5. Because GERD is the most likely diagnosis, is a trial of acid suppression acceptable?

Yes. A therapeutic trial of acid suppression is relatively inexpensive, noninvasive, and easy to perform and may avoid further investigation. However, adequate doses of appropriate medication must be used. Current studies suggest that a proton pump inhibitor (PPI; omeprazole 20 mg; lansoprazole 30 mg; rabeprazole 20 mg; pantoprazole 40 mg; or esomeprazole 20 mg) be given twice daily before meals for a period of 4 to 8 weeks. This test produces both false-negative and false-positive results. In patients who do not have relief of symptoms, the tendency is to conclude that GERD is not the cause of the pain. This conclusion cannot be made with complete certainty without ambulatory monitoring of intragastric and intraesophageal pH, while the patient continues PPI therapy. False-positive results may occur because of a placebo response that can be particularly high in functional gastrointestinal disorders. One study of patients with presumed esophageal chest pain noted a placebo response of 36%.

## 6. What is the most useful esophageal investigation?

Because GERD is the most common cause of UCP, it should be the first diagnosis considered. Ambulatory pH monitoring of the esophagus is the gold standard for diagnosing GERD and is the test most likely to yield a positive result in patients with UCP. It remains the appropriate initial investigation, even when a trial of acid suppression has appeared ineffective.

If ambulatory pH monitoring is abnormal (see later text), esophagogastroduodenoscopy (EGD) may be indicated to exclude the more serious consequences of GERD, such as esophagitis and Barrett's esophagus. An EGD should be considered when the total esophageal acid exposure for a 24-hour period exceeds 10% or when supine acid exposure is above normal limits. However, diagnostic yield from EGD is low when the only symptom is chest pain. If ambulatory pH monitoring is negative, investigation for esophageal motility abnormalities is indicated.

Unexplained chest pain

↓

Exclude cardiac disease (of epicardial vessels)

↓

Trial of acid suppression

↓

Esophageal pH monitoring*

↓

Baseline manometry and provocation testing

↓

(Bernstein, edrophonium, balloon distention)

↓

Consider other causes

Other more unusual causes of UCP, such as biliary tract disease and gastric or duodenal ulceration, have been reported. Therefore, further gastrointestinal investigation, including abdominal ultrasound, is occasionally warranted, especially if the history points to such diagnoses.

## 7. How is esophageal pH monitoring performed?

Esophageal pH monitoring is performed after an overnight fast. The level of acidity is measured by an intraesophageal electrode of either glass or antimony. The electrode is placed 5 cm above the upper border of the lower esophageal sphincter (LES), as previously determined by manometry.

An antimony electrode is thinner (2-mm diameter) but requires the use of a silver/silver chloride reference electrode either incorporated into the catheter or attached to the patient's chest. The electrode is passed transnasally, and pH is recorded for a minimum of 16 hours. Patients are encouraged to follow their usual routine. Data are recorded on a portable recording device with marker buttons that allow the patient to indicate timing of meals, bed rest, and symptoms. A diary card is also completed to corroborate the timings. All information is transferred to a computer on completion of the study and analyzed both visually and by the use of specialized software.

## 8. What abnormalities may be found with pH monitoring?

Analysis of the tracing includes both duration of esophageal acid exposure (i.e., time when esophageal pH is <4) and its association with symptoms. Objective GERD is diagnosed when the duration of acid exposure for the total time or for either the upright or recumbent periods exceeds the 95th percentile of normal values. In our laboratory, these limits are defined as exposures to a pH <4 for 4.2% of the total time, 6.3% of the upright period, and 1.2% of the recumbent period.

Although an abnormal degree of acid reflux suggests the cause of the patient's symptoms, the case is not proved. Thus, the occurrence of symptoms during the monitoring period is extremely valuable. If symptoms coincide frequently with episodes of acid reflux, the diagnosis can be made even when absolute levels of acid exposure do not exceed the 95th percentile of normal values. Similarly, failure of all symptoms to correlate with acid reflux is strong evidence against reflux-related chest pain.

*EGD is indicated for severe reflux on pH monitoring (see text).

The situation is more difficult when some but not all symptoms are associated with episodes of acid reflux. Various "symptom indices" have been introduced in an attempt to quantify the symptom–reflux association. The simplest index uses the total number of symptoms as its denominator and symptoms that coincide with acid reflux as its numerator:

Symptom index = No. of symptoms occurring during acid reflux / Total No. of symptoms during pH monitoring

A value of 50% or greater (e.g., two of four symptoms occurring during episodes of acid reflux) is regarded as positive (Fig. 3-1). The approach to reflux-induced chest pain is no different from the normal management of GERD (see Chapter 2).

### 9. If reflux has been excluded, which esophageal motility abnormalities may be found in patients with chest pain?

Abnormal esophageal motility may be found in 25% to 30% of patients with UCP. The sooner this can be evaluated relative to an episode of chest pain, the higher is its diagnostic yield. The relative frequency of different diagnoses in these patients with abnormal esophageal manometry is illustrated in Figure 3-2.

1. "Nutcracker esophagus" is the most common manometric abnormality; it has been so named because of the extremely high pressures generated during esophageal peristalsis. The diagnosis requires an average peristaltic amplitude greater than 220 mm Hg during 10 wet swallows over both distal channels (Fig. 3-3).
2. Ineffective esophageal motility is a diagnostic category that includes patients with weak or poorly conducted waves; it is the second most common manometric finding.
3. Diffuse esophageal spasm is diagnosed when at least 2 of 10 water swallows produce simultaneous contractions instead of normal peristalsis. It may also be associated with other abnormalities, such as multipeaked or prolonged duration contractions (Fig. 3-4).
4. An abnormally high basal LES pressure is also associated, on occasion, with UCP—*the hypertensive LES.*
5. Achalasia presents, occasionally, with chest pain and is further discussed in Chapter 4.

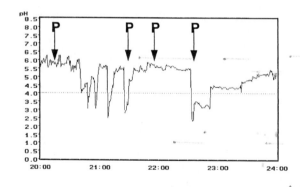

**Figure 3-1.** A 4-hour sample of esophageal pH monitoring. During this period, two of four symptoms (P) were associated with episodes of acid reflux, yielding a symptom index of 2/4 (50%).

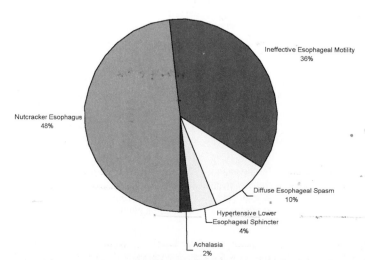

**Figure 3-2.** The relative frequencies of different diagnoses in patients with an esophageal dysmotility cause for chest pain.

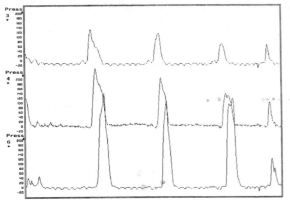

**Figure 3-3.** Nutcracker esophagus. The patient's average peristaltic amplitude was 250 mm Hg. She experienced pain synchronous with most of her swallows.

**Figure 3-4.** Diffuse esophageal spasm. Both simultaneous (S) and peristaltic (P) contractions occur in response to water swallows.

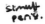

## 10. How can esophageal motility abnormalities cause chest pain?

The mechanism or mechanisms by which motility abnormalities may cause chest pain are poorly understood. Specific mechanoreceptors have been identified in the esophageal mucosal and muscle layers. Abnormal contractions per se may be sufficient to stimulate these receptors and cause pain. Alternatively, the mechanoreceptors may be stimulated by esophageal distention, as a result of failed LES relaxation or retention of the bolus within the esophageal body. Yet another possibility is alteration of the threshold for esophageal sensation, which *tunes in* the patient to changes in esophageal pressure. A further theory Is that high tension in the esophageal wall inhibits esophageal blood flow, causing myoischemia. However, the esophagus has an extensive blood supply, and contractions are unlikely to be sufficiently prolonged to induce ischemia.

It is also possible that dysmotility per se is not the cause of pain. Rather, it may represent an epiphenomenon that, like pain, is induced by another, unrecognized process. This emphasizes that simply diagnosing an esophageal motility disorder does not prove that it is the cause of the patient's pain. Occasionally, during routine manometry, a patient develops pain coincident with abnormal waveforms, demonstrating a closer link between the dysmotility and the pain. More typically, the patient remains asymptomatic.

## 11. Can esophageal pain be provoked during testing?

Yes. In an attempt to provoke symptoms, additional measures analogous to the exercise stress test used by cardiologists may be used to stimulate the esophagus. Options include acid infusion, pharmacologic stimulation, and intraesophageal balloon distention. For many years, it was believed that GERD caused chest pain by inducing dysmotility. Although this theory does not appear to be correct, acid perfusion (Bernstein test) is still used occasionally as a diagnostic test in UCP. Typically, 60 to 80 mL of 0.1N hydrochloric acid is infused into the esophagus at a rate of 6 to 8 mL/min without the patient's knowledge, followed by a similar infusion of saline. The test is positive only if:

1. It reproduces the patient's typical symptoms during acid infusion, and
2. The symptoms disappear or do not recur during saline infusion.

Chemoreceptors are present in the esophageal mucosa. Patients with a positive Bernstein test demonstrate acid sensitivity and should be treated for GERD-induced chest pain. Ambulatory pH monitoring with specific evaluation of symptom associations with pH decreases has largely made the Bernstein test obsolete.

Recent studies have suggested incoordination between the circular and longitudinal muscle layers of the esophageal walls as a mechanism for pain.

Various pharmacologic agents have been used to stimulate the esophageal smooth muscle. The current choice is the cholinesterase inhibitor edrophonium (80 mg/kg intravenously). After injection, even in normal subjects, esophageal smooth muscle responds with increased peristaltic amplitude and duration during swallows. The test is regarded as positive only if it reproduces the patient's typical pain.

Intraesophageal balloon distention (IEBD) involves the graduated inflation of a latex balloon within the esophagus, until pain or a predetermined maximal volume is reached. This test has the advantage of being specific to the esophagus and

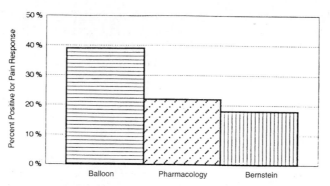

provoke
balloon
edrophonium
acid

**Figure 3-5.** Mean values of seven reported studies of the percentage of positive pain response achieved by provocation with balloon distention, edrophonium, and acid in patients with unexplained chest pain.

may reproduce the pain by a mechanism not dissimilar to that of dysmotility. It is positive only if it induces a patient's typical pain at an inflation volume that does not induce pain in normal subjects. Balloon distention has been shown to be reproducible and has the highest yield of all available provocation tests. Of the three forms of provocation, acid and edrophonium typically induce symptoms in 20% of cases; balloon distention has double this yield (Fig. 3-5).

**12. How does provocation testing compare with combined ambulatory monitoring of both motility and pH?**

All esophageal provocation tests have one major drawback—they are not physiologic. In an attempt to record the motility tracing during spontaneous chest pain, longer periods of manometry have been performed. However, this is used little outside of research institutions.

**13. Are there any emerging technologies for investigation of UCP?**

Yes. Multichannel intraluminal impedance (MII) is a new methodology that can detect intraesophageal events, including the reflux failure of passage of boluses of air or liquid. This has potential benefits for the diagnosis of both nonacid reflux and motility abnormalities.

Monitoring of brain activity in response to esophageal stimulation has advanced our understanding of the central processing of UCP. New technologies in this area include analysis of cerebral-evoked potentials, functional magnetic resonance imaging, and positron emission tomography scanning.

**14. What is visceral hypersensitivity? Define the *irritable esophagus*.**

Many patients with UCP have lower thresholds to pain, in response to IEBD, than normal individuals. This finding is believed to be due to visceral hypersensitivity or altered nociception. For some patients, the problem may not be due to abnormal contractions but rather to abnormal perception of normal events, including peristaltic muscle contractions, physiologic quantities of acid reflux, and luminal distention by air or food. Combined pH and manometric monitoring has identified patients who are sensitive to both acid and motility events. This condition is described as the *irritable esophagus*. Research analyzing cerebral-evoked potential responses to esophageal stimulation suggests that the abnormality is due to central interpretation rather than abnormal firing of the peripheral nociceptors.

**15. Does UCP have a psychological component?**

ψ.

Yes. All disease has a psychological element; illness is interpreted according to personality and previous experiences. This maxim appears to be particularly true for UCP. Psychological abnormalities have been documented in 34% to 59% of patients with UCP and are present in all of the causes described previously. Psychiatric diagnoses are probably most prevalent in patients with esophageal motility abnormalities (84% in one study). Psychological factors, therefore, must be considered in the management of patients with UCP, including the possibility of panic attacks. Patients with high psychological scores are particularly susceptible to an initial placebo response to medication, but, in the long term, treatment is ineffective. If such patients are identified, specific therapies can address the problem. Patients with high psychological scores have a worse prognosis and experience increased disability attributed to the illness.

**16. What are the treatment options for nonreflux esophageal chest pain?**

*Esophageal motility abnormalities.* Calcium antagonists, nitrates, and anticholinergic agents are the primary treatments aimed at motility dysfunction—that is, the spastic component. If the pain is only occasional, short-acting nitrates or calcium antagonists may be taken sublingually as needed. More frequent episodes of chest pain are better managed by regular therapy with a long-acting preparation. Although such medications may have a dramatic effect on esophageal pressures, their symptomatic efficacy is often disappointing. Another therapy that may be considered is peppermint oil. This can also help alleviate chest pain. Benzodiazepines both reduce skeletal muscular contractions and modify sensory pathways. They have had limited success in esophageal motility abnormalities. Management of achalasia is discussed separately in Chapter 4.

*Visceral hypersensitivity.* Drugs used to modify sensory pathways include anxiolytics and antidepressants. The largest body of evidence is for imipramine and other tricyclic antidepressants. They have been shown to be effective in low doses, suggesting that the effect is not due primarily to antidepressant activity.

*Psychological and behavioral therapies.* Various psychological and behavioral therapies have been tried in small-scale studies. Relaxation therapy has met with some success and can be taught easily to patients who are willing to acknowledge the psychological element in their disease. Reassurance is an intervention that is available to all physicians. The ability to demonstrate a definite esophageal abnormality as an explanation for chest pain is of therapeutic benefit. The frequency of both pain and office visits for treatment of pain decreases after such reassurances.

*Additional therapies.* Both empiric dilatation with a bougie and more specific targeting of a hypertensive LES with pneumatic dilatation have had limited success in some patients. Surgical myotomy may be of benefit to some patients with diffuse esophageal spasm or "nutcracker esophagus." However, such interventions have documented complications and should be reserved for the rare, severely disabled patient.

## 17. Are there any emerging treatment options?
Yes. Several studies have demonstrated good symptom response to botulinum toxin injection among patients with chest pain and hypermotility disorders. By contrast, patients with chest pain with ineffective esophageal motility derived little benefit from the 5-hydroxytryptamine (5-HT)$_1$ agonist sumatriptan when it was used to improve muscle contractility. Theophylline significantly increased pain thresholds in patients with functional chest pain, possibly acting by altering adenosine-mediated nociception. Phosphodiesterase inhibitors, such as sildenafil, decrease esophageal contraction pressures through the increased tissue nitric oxide concentrations. They may be effective in patients with regularly recurring chest pain associated with abnormal esophageal contractions. Sildenafil has also been associated with transient esophageal symptoms (mainly dysphagia and odynophagia) in patients without known esophageal disease. Additional novel interventions can be anticipated with the increased understanding of how the brain processes visceral stimuli.

## 18. Can abnormal belching or aerophagia cause chest pain?
Esophageal distention, whether by reflux of gastric contents, impaction of a food bolus, or entrapment of air, can cause chest pain. In several well-documented cases, gaseous esophageal distention was secondary to an abnormal belch reflex. Normally, the upper esophageal sphincter relaxes in response to distention with air. When this response fails, pain may occur.

## 19. What is the prognosis for patients with UCP?
Patients with UCP have a poor functional outcome. Their quality of life is poor compared with healthy control subjects. They continue to consult a physician or visit the emergency department an average of twice per year, with an average of one hospitalization per year. If the patient does not have CAD, making a positive esophageal diagnosis significantly reduces such behavior. Despite ongoing morbidity, the mortality rate of these patients (<1% per annum) is the same as that for the general population.

### BIBLIOGRAPHY

1. Agrawal A, Tutuian R, Hila A, et al. Successful use of phosphodiesterase type 5 inhibitors to control symptomatic esophageal hypercontractility: A case report. Dig Dis Sci 2005;50:2059–62.
2. Bennett J. ABC of the upper gastrointestinal tract. Oesophagus: Atypical chest pain and motility disorders. Br Med J 2001;6:791–4.
3. Cannon RO, Cattau EL, Yakshe PN, et al. Coronary flow reserve, esophageal motility, and chest pain in patients with angiographically normal coronary arteries. Am J Med 1990;88:217–22.
4. Cannon III RO, Quyyumi AA, Mincemoyer R, et al. Imipramine in patients with chest pain despite normal coronary angiograms. N Engl J Med 1994;330:1411–7.
5. Castell DO, Diederich LL, Castell JA. Esophageal Motility and pH Testing. 3rd ed Highlands Ranch, CO: Sandhill Scientific; 2000.
6. Chambers J, Bass C. Chest pain and normal coronary anatomy: A review of natural history and possible etiologic factors. Progr Cardiovasc Dis 1990;33:161–84.
7. Grossi L, Ciccaglione AF, Marzio L. Effect of the 5-HT$_1$ agonist sumatriptan on oesophageal motor pattern in patients with ineffective oesophageal motility. Neurogastroenterol Motil 2003;15:9–14.
8. Johnston BT, Castell DO. Intra-oesophageal balloon distension and oesophageal sensation in humans. Eur J Gastroenterol Hepatol 1995;7:1221–9.

9. Katz PO, Dalton CB, Richter JE, et al. Esophageal testing of patients with noncardiac chest pain or dysphagia: Results of three years' experience with 1161 patients. Ann Intern Med 1987;106:593–7.
10. Lacima G, Grande L, Pera M, et al. Utility of ambulatory 24-hour esophageal ph and motility monitoring in noncardiac chest pain: Report of 90 patients and review of the literature. Dig Dis Sci 2003;48:952–61.
11. Miller LS, Pullela SV, Parkman HP, et al. Treatment of chest pain in patients with noncardiac, nonreflux, nonachalasia spastic esophageal motor disorders using botulinum toxin injection into the gastroesophageal junction. Am J Gastroenterol 2002;97:1640–6.
12. Rao SS, Hayek B, Summers RW. Functional chest pain of esophageal origin: Hyperalgesia or motor dysfunction. Am J Gastroenterol 2001;96:2584–9.
13. Rao SS, Mudipalli RS, Mujica V, et al. An open-label trial of theophylline for functional chest pain. Dig Dis Sci 2002;47:2763–8.
14. Richter JE. Oesophageal motility disorders. Lancet 2001;8:823–8.
15. Sarkar S, Aziz Q, Woolf CJ, et al. Contribution of central sensitisation to the development of non-cardiac chest pain. Lancet 2000;30:1154–9.
16. Shrestha S, Pasricha PJ. Update on noncardiac chest pain. Dig Dis 2000;18:138–46.
17. Smout AJ, DeVore MS, Dalton CB, et al. Cerebral potentials evoked by oesophageal distension in patients with non-cardiac chest pain. Gut 1992;33:298–302.
18. Ward BW, Wu WC, Richter JE, et al. Long-term follow-up of symptomatic status of patients with noncardiac chest pain: Is diagnosis of esophageal etiology helpful? Am J Gastroenterol 1987;82:215–8.

# ACHALASIA

*Michael J. Krier, MD, and*
*Pankaj Jay Pasricha, MD*

*[handwritten: fail relax LES *
aperstalsis body]*

## 1. Define achalasia.

The term *achalasia* (Greek for "lack of relaxation") describes the pathophysiologic hallmark of the disease—failure of the lower esophageal sphincter to relax. This term has replaced the previous designation of *cardiospasm,* which implies an exaggerated state of contraction. The second cardinal feature of achalasia is aperistalsis of the body of the esophagus. However, lower esophageal sphincter (LES) dysfunction is more important because gravity appears to be able to compensate for the lack of pumping ability in the body of the esophagus, in most cases.

## 2. How common is achalasia?

Achalasia is a relatively uncommon disorder, with a prevalence estimated at about 8 cases per 10,000 population and an incidence rate of approximately 0.5 new case per year per 100,000 population. The incidence is increased with age, particularly after the seventh decade, but is equal for men and women.

## 3. What is vigorous achalasia? *[handwritten: simult © No peristaltic © = spasm]*

The term *vigorous* is applied to cases of achalasia in which prominent contractions can be noticed in the body of the esophagus, either on radiography or by manometry. These contractions are simultaneous and therefore fulfill the manometric definition of aperistalsis required for the diagnosis of achalasia. They should be distinguished from isobaric waves, which can be seen in patients with achalasia and represent bolus-induced passive fluctuations in pressure within the common cavity of the dilated esophagus. It is not clear whether vigorous achalasia represents either a variation or an early stage of classic achalasia.

*[handwritten: vigorous ...> classic
DES ...? Operated]*

## 4. What is the relationship between diffuse esophageal spasm (DES) and achalasia?

DES may be regarded as a cousin of achalasia. The primary manometric distinction between DES and vigorous achalasia is the presence of at least some normal peristalsis in the former. LES dysfunction is seen often in DES but to a lesser degree than achalasia. Some evidence suggests that in a small subset (about 5% or less) of patients, DES may evolve into classic achalasia.  *[handwritten: DES Ⓝ perist.]*

## 5. What is the major pathologic lesion in achalasia, and how does it produce the disease?

Although other lesions have been described in these patients, including degeneration of the vagus nerve and changes in its dorsal motor nucleus, it appears that the myenteric plexus is the major site of disease. The characteristic finding here is a loss of ganglion cells, which appears to be selective for inhibitory neurons (those producing nitric oxide and/or vasoactive intestinal peptide [VIP]) with relative sparing of the cholinergic (stimulatory) nerves. Thus, the normal balance of excitatory and inhibitory neural input to smooth muscle is upset. The loss of inhibition, coupled with a relative preservation of the excitatory stimulus, may be responsible for the LES abnormalities.

An inflammatory infiltrate, characteristically mononuclear, is also commonly seen in the myenteric plexus. It is speculated that unchecked inflammation at this site leads to neuronal destruction and, eventually, to the clinical manifestations of achalasia.   *[handwritten: aganglionic + inflam.   tonic Excitate LES (blocked Ach by BTX) loss inh. NO+VIP]*

## 6. What is the suspected cause of achalasia?

Earlier studies raised the possibility of a virus, particularly one belonging to the herpes family (because of the predilection of these viruses for squamous mucosa) and measles virus. A study with DNA hybridization techniques found evidence of the herpes virus in some myotomy specimens from achalasia patients. However, subsequent investigations, using the polymerase chain reaction to detect a variety of different markers, found no evidence for any known viral cause. Attention has also focused on a possible autoimmune basis for this disease, with reports of circulating antimyenteric autoantibodies and immunohistochemical evidence for T-cell inflammatory infiltrates within the myenteric plexus. Autoimmune suspicions have been given further credence by the finding that achalasia may be particularly associated with certain class II human leukocyte antigens (HLAs) such as DQB1, DQA1, and DQw1. Nevertheless, the cause of achalasia remains a mystery.

**7. Is achalasia an acquired or a congenital disease?**

Most cases of achalasia appear to be acquired. Achalasia is uncommon before the age of 25, with a clear-cut age-related increase thereafter. Most commonly, the disease occurs in middle adult life (ages 30–60 years) and affects both sexes and all races nearly equally. Rare cases of familial achalasia have been described. Occasionally, achalasia may be found as part of a congenital syndrome such as the Allgrove or triple-A syndrome (achalasia, alacrima, and resistance to adrenocorticotropic hormone), now noted to be caused by a gene mutation on chromosome 12 (*ALADIN*). Alport syndrome or other rare conditions have also been associated with achalasia.

**8. Describe the dysphagia associated with achalasia.**

In general, the dysphagia due to motor disorders of the esophagus occurs with solids as well as liquids. However, many patients with achalasia complain predominantly, if not exclusively, of solid food dysphagia. The converse, dysphagia for liquids only, is almost never seen. Patients can often localize dysphagia to the region of the LES. Regurgitation of food, either active or induced by the recumbent position or bending, should raise the suspicion of achalasia, particularly if occurring early in the course of symptoms. Patients also often complain of waking up in the mornings with remnants of the previous night's supper in their mouth.

**9. Are there any other symptoms associated with achalasia?**

Weight loss is common but not invariable. Pulmonary symptoms such as recurrent pneumonia and lung abscess from aspiration are much less common today because of earlier diagnosis and treatment. Two surprisingly common symptoms that may lead to the wrong diagnosis are chest pain and heartburn (seen in up to 50% and 25% of patients, respectively). There are at least two different types of chest pain experienced by patients with achalasia. The obstructive type is associated with swallowing a food bolus and resolves with passage of food into the stomach. The second type is unrelated to eating and is more often seen in patients with vigorous achalasia. However, it is not necessarily related to esophageal contractions and may reflect abnormalities in the sensory pathway, similar to what has been described in patients with spastic motility disorders. Heartburn is indistinguishable from that in patients with established gastroesophageal reflux disease (GERD), including a response to antacids. In fact, this symptom has resulted in a mistaken diagnosis of GERD for several years in some patients with achalasia. Whether this is caused by lactic acid production as a result of bacterial breakdown of retained food or a true acid reflux is not clear.

**10. Does achalasia involve any other parts of the gastrointestinal tract?**

Yes. Loss of inhibitory nerves may also involve the stomach and pylorus, but the clinical manifestations may be masked by the esophageal symptoms. Sphincter of Oddi dysfunction has also been reported.

**11. What is the best way to diagnose achalasia?**

Achalasia should always be considered in patients with a history of dysphagia for both solids and liquids. A definite diagnosis requires two steps:

1. Confirmation of the underlying pathophysiology (best done by manometry), and
2. Exclusion of cancer at the gastroesophageal (GE) junction, which can produce a similar picture (pseudo-achalasia); this requires endoscopy with particular emphasis on the retroflexed view.

**12. What are the characteristic radiologic features of achalasia?**

An atonic and dilated body of the esophagus is often seen; however, occasional early cases present with a normal-sized esophagus and prominent (nonperistaltic) contractions. The *sigmoid esophagus* is an elongated, dilated organ seen in patients with longstanding disease. Epiphrenic diverticula may accompany this picture. In most cases of achalasia, the GE junction is smoothly narrowed, giving rise to the classic *bird's beak* and allowing only very small amounts of contrast to pass through to the stomach. Previous dilation or surgery may alter this typical appearance. In early achalasia, these classic features may also be absent in about one third of patients.

**13. What is required for the manometric diagnosis of achalasia?**

Two manometric features:

- Lack of peristalsis in the body (the smooth muscle portion) of the esophagus
- Abnormal or absent LES relaxation in response to swallowing (with normal relaxation being more than 90%).

**14. What is the most important potential pitfall in the manometric diagnosis of achalasia?**

An occasional patient with otherwise typical features of achalasia may demonstrate complete or near-complete relaxation of the LES, but this appearance may be artifactual due to relative movement between the side hole/point sensor in the manometry catheter and the LES. This can be avoided by the use of a Dent sleeve catheter, which incorporates a 6-cm-long sensor device for measurement of LES pressures.

### 15. Describe the typical endoscopic features of achalasia.

Endoscopy may be reported as normal in a surprising number of cases in whom achalasia is not suspected before the procedure. In more obvious cases, esophageal dilation, varying amounts of food material or secretions, and either a lack of contractions or multiple simultaneous contractions are seen. The esophageal mucosa can also demonstrate a variety of changes, from mild erythema to frank erosions or even ulceration. Candidiasis and retained medications may be responsible for some of these lesions; in other cases, stasis of retained material itself may give rise to an edematous and nodular mucosa. A tight but relatively elastic feel as the endoscope passes (or *pops*) through the GE junction is characteristic of achalasia but may be easily overlooked if the diagnosis is not specifically entertained. The inability to pass the scope despite moderate amounts of pressure is highly suggestive of an inflammatory or a neoplastic stricture. Interestingly, resistance can also be encountered at the pyloric outlet in patients with achalasia, giving rise to the *difficult pylorus* sign.

### 16. What is the difference between secondary achalasia and pseudo-achalasia?

Although achalasia is most often idiopathic, it has been described in association with a variety of diseases, such as cancer, Chagas disease, amyloidosis and other infiltrative disorders, mixed connective tissue disorders, endocrine disorders, and intestinal pseudo-obstruction. Such cases are called secondary achalasia; the term is often used interchangeably with *pseudo-achalasia*.

### 17. How can pseudo-achalasia be diagnosed?

A high index of suspicion should be maintained in patients presenting with what looks like achalasia but with *marked weight loss* and *short duration of symptoms*. However, these and other features, such as the age of the patient, are not highly specific and were shown in only one study to have a combined predictive value of 18%. Endoscopy remains the crucial diagnostic test because the clinical history, radiographic appearance of barium study, and even manometric analysis may not distinguish pseudo-achalasia from the idiopathic form. A careful examination of the GE region, including a retroflexed view from the stomach, is absolutely mandatory and biopsy samples should be taken of any suspicious area or lesion. Even so, the sensitivity of this method in excluding underlying cancer is reported to be around 80% or less, and as such, if high clinical suspicion remains, a second endoscopy with repeat biopsy samples may be necessary. Endoscopic ultrasound (EUS) may provide additional value, but this has yet to be convincingly demonstrated.

### 18. Is achalasia a premalignant condition?

Yes. Esophageal cancer may develop in the setting of achalasia, thought to result from longstanding stasis and secondary changes in the epithelium. When cancer develops, it is usually of the squamous variety and arises in the dilated middle part of the esophagus, rendering it relatively silent until a late stage. The overall prevalence of esophageal cancer in achalasia is about 3%, with an incidence of about 197 per 100,000 per year. This incidence significantly increases after 15 years of achalasia. A large population-based study demonstrated only a 16-fold increase of cancer risk during years 2 to 24 after the diagnosis of achalasia. The risk of cancer in most patients with adequate treatment remains very small (see later text).

### 19. Should patients undergo periodic endoscopic surveillance?

Yes and no. A surveillance strategy would require 406 endoscopic procedures to detect one cancer in men and 2220 endoscopic procedures to detect one cancer in women. The American Society of Gastrointestinal Endoscopy recommends the following guidelines for surveillance:

1. There are insufficient data to support routine endoscopic surveillance for patients with achalasia.
2. If surveillance were to be considered, it would reasonable to initiate it 15 years after onset of symptoms, but the subsequent surveillance interval is not defined.

### 20. What are the various treatment options available for achalasia? Describe their rationale.

All of the therapeutic options available for achalasia are palliative. Their goal is to decrease the resistance to bolus transit created by the dysfunctional LES. Traditional pharmacologic therapy such as calcium channel blockers or nitrates does this by inducing smooth muscle relaxation. Botulinum toxin injections block the excitatory neural input to the LES by inhibiting the release of acetylcholine from nerve endings. The theoretical rationale for balloon dilation is to achieve a partial tear of the LES muscle, but this option is somewhat speculative because the few animal studies that were performed to evaluate this method have shown no histologic evidence of damage, despite marked reductions in LES pressure. Surgical myotomy has the most straightforward rationale among all treatment options, but it comes at a price (see later).

*Viagra*

NTG ( isoDN ) > CCB ( Nifedine > dilt )

**21. Discuss the various pharmacologic options available for the palliation of achalasia.**

Nitrates are probably more effective than calcium channel blockers but have significant adverse side effects that lead to discontinuation of the drug in up to one third of cases. Isosorbide dinitrate (5–10 mg sublingually before meals) begins to act within 15 minutes, and its effect may persist for as long as 90 minutes. Symptoms are improved in 75% to 85% of patients. Nifedipine, which may be more effective than diltiazem or verapamil, lowers LES pressure by 30% to 40%. The effects peak within 30 to 45 minutes and last longer than 1 hour. Contrary to popular belief, nifedipine is poorly absorbed sublingually. Oral doses of 10 to 20 mg have been reported to improve symptoms in 50% to 70% of patients. In most cases, however, the use of pharmacotherapy is at best temporizing. Most patients will require additional forms of treatment after 6 months or so because of side effects, progression of disease, or the development of tolerance.

**22. What does Viagra have to do with achalasia?**

Sildenafil (Viagra) blocks phosphodiesterase type 5 (the enzyme responsible for degradation of cyclic guanosine monophosphate [cGMP]), which results in increased cGMP levels within smooth muscle and consequent relaxation. It is effective in short-term reduction of LES pressures in patients with achalasia.

**23. What is the single most permanent treatment of achalasia?**

The answer is clearly surgery with short-term (5 years or less) efficacy around 90%. Long-term results are less positive, with only about two thirds of patients reporting good-to-excellent outcomes. This is probably due, in large part, to the sequelae of the reflux disease that invariably accompanies successful myotomy (see later).

**24. What is the major problem with surgery?**

In the past, surgery was associated with considerable morbidity, whether done via a thoracic or abdominal approach. Recent advances in laparoscopic techniques have enabled a minimally invasive approach to myotomy, with significant reductions in perioperative pain, morbidity and length of hospitalization. However, the major problem with this operation remains unchanged: long-term GE reflux, which can be particularly damaging in an atonic esophagus. Although most surgeons using an abdominal approach will incorporate a *loose* antireflux procedure (anterior or posterior partial fundoplication) along with the myotomy, its effectiveness in preventing GERD remains controversial. Two long-term studies, one with and one without an antireflux procedure, were comparable in that only two thirds of patients in either study were still doing well 10 years and beyond. Although the abdominal approach may be associated with less reflux, long-term results are not yet available after laparoscopic surgery, and patients and physicians should be on the guard for this complication.

GERD
(
PPI

**25. How can postoperative GERD be avoided?**

The best advice to give patients after myotomy is that they need to be followed carefully for GERD. A very low threshold should be used for initiation of antireflux medications. Proton pump inhibitors are effective in preventing postoperative GERD symptoms.

**26. How is balloon dilation of the LES accomplished?**

Using a whalebone as a dilator, Sir Thomas Willis first described dilation of the LES in a patient with achalasia. Forceful dilation of the LES is achieved by stretching it to at least 30 mm or greater (for adults); this obviously requires more than simple bougies and is best accomplished using a specially designed balloon catheter. The most commonly available such device (Rigiflex; Microvasive) is passed over a guidewire and requires fluoroscopic monitoring; a typical starting balloon size for most adults is 30 mm. A less common device is the Witzel dilator, which consists of a polyethylene balloon mounted on a forward viewing endoscope that is inflated under direct visualization (with the endoscope in the retroflexed position in the stomach). It has the advantage of not requiring fluoroscopy. Otherwise, there is little science to dilation. A good stretch requires obliteration of the balloon waist; however, considerations of duration, pressure, number of inflations, and presence of blood on the dilator or induction of chest pain are of little, if any, importance in determining efficacy.

30mm
dil'2

**27. What can be done if symptoms do not respond to the first dilation?**

A larger balloon (available in 5-mm increments from 25 mm to 40 mm) may be used to attempt further stretching of the LES, the so-called progressive method. An alternative method, championed by vanTrappen and colleagues but seldom practiced in the United States, is repeated dilation (regardless of the initial symptomatic response) until certain objective parameters of esophageal emptying (usually determined radiographically) are met. Regardless of the method used, if the patient fails three dilations, most authorities would recommend surgery.

**28. What are the results of pneumatic dilation?**

The overall immediate response to pneumatic dilation is 75% to 80%; long-term results show that up to half of patients will require one or more dilations over a 5-year period. Beyond this time, about 50% to 70% of patients will continue to do well; however, 20% or more may eventually need surgery.

## 29. How does pneumatic dilation compare with surgery?

A classic randomized controlled trial between surgery and dilation clearly favored surgery in terms of long-term results. However, it is not clear whether this is the most cost-effective approach considering the long-term and cumulative costs of surgery (estimated at nearly 2.5 times more than the cost of pneumatic dilation), even in view of the perforation rate and need for retreatment associated with pneumatic dilation.    *LT Sx > P.D.*

## 30. What is the major disadvantage of forceful dilation? How can it be prevented?

The major risk of dilation is perforation (estimated rate, 1% to 10% or even higher). Because of the empiric way in which dilation is performed, this risk appears to be inherent; there are few ways to prevent this complication. It is important to exclude stricture (malignant or benign), to ensure a near-empty esophagus, and to perform all manipulations of the balloon under fluoroscopic control. Relative contraindications cited in the literature include a tortuous sigmoid shape, previous myotomy, epiphrenic diverticula, and large hiatal hernias, but most experts do not view these as absolute. Larger balloons are expected to increase the risk for perforation. GERD is believed to be uncommon after forceful dilation, with an incidence of around 2%.    *perf*

## 31. How is perforation treated in patients with achalasia?

Optimal management following perforation has not been established. Perforations generally occur during the first dilation session and tend to be small and well contained. Thus, many authorities advocate for conservative treatment (i.e., antibiotics and parenteral alimentation) with good results being reported in the literature. However, it is difficult to predict the outcome with this form of treatment in individual cases. Surgery is definitely indicated in patients with large perforations and free flow of contrast into the mediastinum or with evidence of sepsis. When surgery is performed early, the clinical outcome and long-term course appear similar to those for elective myotomy.

## 32. Which patients are particularly likely to respond to dilation?

In general, older patients (older than age 50) do significantly better after dilation than younger patients. Retrospective studies have also shown that young men may require more frequent repeat dilations than young women.

*PD - dd pp + ♀*

## 33. What objective parameters should be followed after dilation?

The most consistent and important parameter determining long-term response after pneumatic dilation is posttreatment LES pressure. The best results are obtained when LES pressure is less than 10 mm Hg. It is theoretically possible that a treatment regimen based on *optimization* of esophageal emptying rather than symptomatic response alone may lead to better long-term results. One study showed that a timed barium esophagram was an important tool to predict long-term results. In this study, about 30% of achalasia patients reported symptoms relived after pneumatic dilation had an abnormally timed barium esophagram study, while 90% of these patients failed within 1 year after treatment.

## 34. How is botulinum toxin type A (BTxA) injection administered?

BTx/A is available through most hospital pharmacies in vials containing 100 U of the lyophilized powder. For use in achalasia, this can be diluted in 5 mL of normal saline to yield a solution containing 20 U/mL. Flexible upper endoscopy is performed using routine sedation, and the toxin injected via a 5-mm sclerotherapy needle into the LES region, piercing the mucosa about 1 cm above the Z-line and slanting the needle approximately 45 degrees. The injections are administered in four aliquots distributed circumferentially in four different quadrants. Initial studies included an empiric dose of 80 U/mL; however, a subsequent prospective study of 78 patients comparing two available formulations of 100 U BTxA (Allergan, Irvine, CA) and 250 U Dysport (Ipsen, Milan, Italy) noted similar efficacy up to 6 months. Precise location of the injection site may not be necessary because diffusion may take care of any minor variations. Others advocate the use of EUS to help guide injections; it is not clear whether EUS results in better outcomes than the "traditional" method just described.

*4 quad scmabae 21, ne*
*2/3 impare > 1 mo exp old rig.*

## 35. What are the results of BTxA treatment?

Only about two thirds of patients sustained improvement (beyond the first month or so). Older patients do better, and patients with vigorous achalasia may have a more favorable response than those with the classic form. Patients who do respond to initial injection remain in remission for several months (range is 4 months to over 1 year). When symptoms return, patients usually respond to repeat injections of BTx. Larger doses of BTxA at the time of initial injection have not been proved to improve the response rate as studies have provided conflicting data.

## 36. What are the major drawbacks of BTx treatment?

Overall, BTxA is a relatively safe and simple treatment with few, if any, major complications. Reported complications are mainly postprocedural and include transient chest pain and heartburn. The major drawback is cost coupled with the need for multiple injections. Some surgical reports suggest that repeat injections of BTxA are somewhat more difficult technically; however, outcomes after surgery appear not to be affected, regardless of whether BTxA has been previously used.

## 37. What is the overall best treatment for achalasia?

Because no treatment is curative, there is no real answer. It is best for the physician to become familiar with the advantages and disadvantages of each option and then present these to the patient. The final choice depends on several factors, including patient preference and risk tolerance, as well as the local availability of technical expertise. However, it is probably fair to say that at the present time, the most permanent treatment is surgical myotomy. Regardless of the treatment, patients need to be followed carefully and therapeutic strategies revisited on a periodic basis.

## ACKNOWLEDGMENT

The authors and editors would like to acknowledge Dr. Xiaotuan Zhao, who provided earlier contributions to this topic review.

## WEBSITES

http://www.nlm.nih.gov/medlineplus/ency/article/000267.htm

http://my.clevelandclinic.org/SearchResults.aspx?k=achalasia&s=Entire+Site&start=0

http://www.emedicine.com/med/TOPIC16.HTM

http://daveproject.org/ViewFilms.cfm?Film_id=488

## BIBLIOGRPAHY

1. Annese V, Bassotti G, Coccia G, et al. Comparison of two different formulations of botulinum toxin A for the treatment of oesophageal achalasia. The Gismad Achalasia Study Group. Aliment Pharmacol Ther 1999;13:1347.
2. Blam ME, Delfyett W, Levine MS, et al. Achalasia: A disease of varied and subtle symptoms that do not correlate with radiographic findings. Am J Gastroenterol 2002;97:1916–23.
3. Bortolotti M, Mari C, Lopilato C, et al. Effects of sildenafil on esophageal motility of patients with idiopathic achalasia. Gastroenterology 2000;118:253–7.
4. Brücher BL, Stein HJ, Bartels H, et al. Achalasia and esophageal cancer: Incidence, prevalence, and prognosis. World J Surg 2001;25:745–9.
5. Cronshaw JM, Matunis MJ. The nuclear pore complex protein ALADIN is mislocalized in triple A syndrome. Proc Natl Acad Sci U S A 2003;100:5823–7.
6. Dunaway PM, Wong RK. Risk and surveillance intervals for squamous cell carcinoma in achalasia. Gastrointest Endosc Clin N Am 2001;11:425–34 ix.
7. Eaker EY, Gordon JM, Vogel SB. Untoward effects of esophageal botulinum toxin injection in the treatment of achalasia. Dig Dis Sci 1997;42:724.
8. Farhoomand K, Connor JT, Richter JE, et al. Predictors of outcome of pneumatic dilation in achalasia. Clin Gastroenterol Hepatol 2004;2:389.
9. Gockel I, Eckardt VF, Schmitt T, et al. Pseudoachalasia: A case series and analysis of the literature. Scand J Gastroenterol 2005;40:378–85.
10. Goodgame RW, Graham DY. Manometry in classic and vigorous achalasia. Gastroenterology 1993;103.
11. Hirota WK, Zuckerman MJ, Adler DG, et al. ASGE guideline: The role of endoscopy in the surveillance of premalignant conditions of the upper GI tract. Gastrointest Endosc 2006;63:570–80.
12. Hoogerwerf WA, Pasricha PJ. Pharmacologic therapy in treating achalasia. Gastrointest Endosc Clin N Am 2001;11:235–48.
13. Mayberry JF. Epidemiology and demographics of achalasia. Gastrointest Endosc Clin N Am 2001;11:235–48.
14. Park W, Vaezi MF. Etiology and pathogenesis of achalasia: The current understanding. Am J Gastroenterol 2005;100:1404–14.
15. Parkman HP, Reynolds JC, Ouyang A, et al. Pneumatic dilation or esophagomyotomy treatment for idiopathic achalasia: Clinical outcomes and cost analysis. Dig Dis Sci 1993;38:75–85.
16. Pasricha PJ, Rai R, Ravich WJ, et al. Botulinum toxin for achalasia: Long-term follow-up and predictors of outcome. Gastroenterology 1996;110:1410–5.
17. Rajput S, Nandwani SK, Phadke AY, et al. Predictors of response to pneumatic dilatation in achalasia cardia. Indian J Gastroenterol 2000;19:126–9.
18. Spiess AE, Kahrilas PJ. Treating acahalasia. From whalebone to laparoscope. JAMA 1998;280:638–42.
19. Triadafilopoulos G, Aaronson M, Sackel S, et al. Medical treatment of esophageal achalasia. Double-blind crossover study with oral nifedipine, verapamil, and placebo. Dig Dis Sci 1991;36:260.
20. Vaezi MF, Baker ME, Achkar E, et al. Timed barium oesophagram: Better predictor of long term success after pneumatic dilation in achalasia than symptom assessment. Gut 2002;50:765–70.
21. Zhao X, Pasricha PJ. Botulinum toxin for spastic GI disorders: A systematic review. Gastrointest Endosc 2003;57:219–35.

# ESOPHAGEAL CANCER

*Nimish Vakil, MD*

**CHAPTER 5**

**1. What is the incidence of esophageal cancer in the United States and is it changing?**

Esophageal cancer is relatively infrequent in the United States. The annual incidence is less than 10 per 100,000 population, whereas in some areas of China the annual incidence is greater than 100 per 100,000. Over the past three decades, the incidence of distal esophageal adenocarcinoma has increased sharply in North America, whereas the incidence of squamous cell carcinoma of the esophagus has fallen. The rise in esophageal adenocarcinoma has been most marked in white men. Recent studies suggest that the incidence of esophageal adenocarcinoma is rising in African American and Hispanic males. For unknown reasons, the disease remains rare in women. Although the absolute numbers of cases of esophageal cancer remains relatively low (approximately 15,500 cases a year), there has been a remarkable rise in the incidence of distal esophageal adenocarcinoma over the past three decades in most developed countries, and it is one of the most rapidly growing cancers in the United States. The decline in distal gastric cancers over the same period has been correlated with a decline in the prevalence of *Helicobacter pylori* infection in the United States.

*↑ Adeno ↓ SCC ↓ gastric.*

**2. What are the risk factors for the development of esophageal cancer?**

Smoking and alcohol use have been associated with the development of squamous cell carcinoma of the esophagus, but they are not major risk factors for the development of esophageal adenocarcinoma. Squamous cell carcinoma is much more frequent in African Americans than in whites, whereas adenocarcinoma is much more frequent in whites. Frequent, longstanding heartburn is an important risk factor for the development of esophageal adenocarcinoma. In some studies, obesity has been shown to be an independent risk factor, and obese patients with reflux disease are at particularly high risk for the development of esophageal cancer. Recent studies have drawn an epidemiologic link between the widespread use of drugs that affect the lower esophageal sphincter and the increasing risk of esophageal cancer. A true cause-and-effect relationship has not been established. Diets low in fresh fruits and vegetables have also been associated with esophageal cancer, and the use of aspirin is associated with a decrease in the incidence of both squamous cell cancers and adenocarcinoma.

*Adeno White? fat w/ GERD > 50y.*

**3. What are the current recommendations for screening and surveillance of esophageal cancer in patients at risk?**

Screening. Currently there is no acceptable screening method for esophageal cancer in the United States. Some economic models have suggested that a one-time screening endoscopy to identify Barrett's esophagus may be cost effective in patients with longstanding reflux esophagitis, but the assumptions for the risk of developing cancer in Barrett's esophagus may be too high. The American College of Gastroenterology guidelines suggest that patients with chronic gastroesophageal reflux disease (GERD) are most likely to have Barrett's esophagus and should undergo endoscopy. The highest yield is in white men older than 50 years of age who have a long history of reflux symptoms.

Surveillance. Surveillance is recommended in patients with Barrett's esophagus and the grade of dysplasia determines the interval for surveillance. In patients with no dysplasia, endoscopy is repeated at 2- to 3-year intervals, but this practice is not based on firm evidence of benefit. A finding of low-grade dysplasia (LGD) requires a follow-up endoscopy within 6 months to ensure that no higher grade of dysplasia is present in the esophagus. If no dysplasia is found, then yearly endoscopy is warranted until dysplasia is demonstrated to be absent on two consecutive annual endoscopies. LGD should be confirmed by an expert pathologist because of the problem of reading variability between pathologists. Approximately 40% of biopsy samples following the recognition of LGD will be negative.

The finding of high-grade dysplasia (HGD) in flat mucosa should be confirmed by an expert gastrointestinal pathologist and a subsequent endoscopy performed within 3 months. Patients with HGD and evidence of endoscopic mucosal abnormalities should be considered for endoscopic mucosal resection or ablation. The risk of developing esophageal adenocarcinoma within 5 years exceeds 30%, if prevalent cases in the first year are not excluded. Due to the high likelihood of prevalent cancer, these patients are often managed as if cancer is present.

*BE q 2-3
LGD 6mo → qy r x 2 ⊙
HGD 3mo → EMR/Abl ə/ Sx*

**4. How is esophageal cancer diagnosed and staged?**

Endoscopy and biopsy are necessary for the diagnosis of esophageal cancer. Staging is of critical importance in the management of patients with esophageal cancer. Staging helps to determine the choice of treatment and is an important determinant of prognosis. Staging should include a clinical examination, blood counts, endoscopy (including bronchoscopy in patients with squamous cell carcinoma), and a computed tomography (CT) scan of the chest and abdomen. In patients who are candidates for surgery, endoscopic ultrasound is essential to assess the depth of invasion (T stage) and lymph node (N stage). Positron emission tomography (PET) may be helpful in identifying otherwise distant metastases.

### 5. Discuss the role of endoscopic ultrasound in the diagnosis and staging of esophageal cancer.

In patients who appear to have limited local disease on CT and no evidence of distant metastases, endoscopic ultrasound may be helpful in regional staging. Esophageal cancer is seen as a hypoechoic interruption of the layers of the esophagus. Endoscopic ultrasound is better than CT at staging the depth of involvement. This factor becomes important in deciding between different methods of curative therapy. For example, patients with cancer localized to the mucosa can be considered for mucosal resection, but deeper levels of invasion make this therapy inappropriate. Endoscopic ultrasound has better results in regional staging than the newest spiral CT scanners. Magnetic resonance imaging (MRI) has not been particularly helpful in imaging the depth of local invasion. Endoscopic ultrasound also may be helpful in the evaluation of mediastinal lymph nodes. Large nodes (less than 10 mm) that are uniformly hypoechoic are suspicious. Fine-needle aspiration under ultrasound guidance may help to establish lymph node involvement.

### 6. How is esophageal cancer staged? Why is staging important?

Esophageal cancer staging is performed according to the tumor–node–metastasis (TNM) classification. Accurate staging is important to establish prognosis and treatment approach. Treatment, as in all malignant disorders, is based on the risk of the therapy balanced against the likelihood of a good outcome. Patient preference and local expertise also may determine the choice of treatment. Rational choices can be based on the stage of esophageal cancer, as discussed below. Survival also correlates with the stage of esophageal cancer (Table 5-1).

**Table 5-1.** Staging of Esophageal Cancer

| STAGE | FINDING |
|---|---|
| **Primary Tumor** | |
| Tx | Primary tumor cannot be assessed |
| T0 | No evidence of primary tumor |
| Tis | Carcinoma in situ |
| T1 | Tumor invades lamina propria or submucosa |
| T2 | Tumor invades muscularis propria |
| T3 | Tumor invades adventitia |
| T4 | Tumor invades adjacent structures |
| **Regional Lymph Nodes** | For the cervical esophagus, cervical and supraclavicular lymph nodes are considered regional; for the thoracic esophagus, mediastinal and perigastric lymph nodes (excluding celiac nodes) are considered regional. |
| Nx | Regional nodes cannot be assessed |
| N0 | No regional lymph node metastases |
| N1 | Regional lymph node metastases |
| **Distant Metastases** | |
| MX | Cannot be assessed |
| M0 | No distant metastases |
| M1 | Distant metastases |
| **Stages** | |
| 0 | Tis N0 M0 |
| 1 | T1 N0 M0 |
| IIA | T2 N0 M0; T3 N0 M0 |
| IIB | T1 N1 M0; T2 N1 M0 |
| III | T3 N1 M0; T4 any N M0 |
| IVA | Any T any N M1a |
| IVB | Any T any N M1b |

Tumors of lower thoracic esophagus: M1a, metastases in celiac lymph nodes; M1b, other distant metastases.
Tumors of the upper thoracic esophagus: M1a, metastases in cervical lymph nodes, M1b: other distant metastases.

### 7. What is the prognosis of esophageal cancer?

Five-year survival rates range from 34% to 60% for patients with stage I or IIA disease and from 15% to 25% for patients with stage IIB or III disease. The prognosis for squamous cell cancer is poorer than that of esophageal adenocarcinoma for a number of reasons, including the location of tumors, their propensity for lymphatic spread, and comorbidities in patients with squamous cell cancer.

### 8. What is the current management of esophageal cancer?

Interdisciplinary planning is essential in the management of patients with esophageal cancer. Surgery is a standard treatment only in patients with localized tumors in patients who are operable. Radiation therapy alone can cure a minority of patients and has been supplanted by combination therapy. Preoperative chemotherapy is of benefit in patients with adenocarcinoma. Preoperative chemoradiation has been shown to confer a survival benefit, and a meta-analysis supports the use of chemoradiation preoperatively. However, postoperative mortality may be increased and the exact population that benefits is not clear. Chemotherapy alone is now increasingly used as an induction therapy before surgery. Stage-directed therapy is changing as new modalities become available.

*Adeno Neoadj CXRX (extensive dz)*

## TREATMENT OF LIMITED DISEASE (STAGE I)  *T1 No Mo*

Patients with early-stage disease generally are treated with curative surgery alone and surgery is the treatment of choice for localized squamous cell carcinoma and adenocarcinoma, particularly if the submucosa or muscularis are involved (T1-2–N0-1). Although controversial, many experts believe that esophagectomy is the preferred treatment for intramucosal superficial cancers as well. Endoscopic mucosal resection or ablation is increasingly used in patients with (Tis-T1a–N0) adenocarcinomas localized to the superficial layers of the esophagus, and the risks and benefits of this less-invasive option need to be discussed with the patient.  *EMR/Abl*

A variety of resection/ablation techniques have been used, such as a suction cap fitted with a snare, to resect mucosa and submucosa. Other ablative therapies also have been used, including electrocautery, argon plasma coagulation, and photodynamic therapy. A recent study of radio frequency ablation showed promising results in patients with HGD and early cancer. Radiofrequency ablation may be another option in the future for these patients.  *RFA.*

Chemotherapy and radiation are not used as adjuvants for early-stage disease. Surgical therapy consists of resection of the tumor with anastomosis of the stomach with the cervical esophagus (gastric pull-up) or interposition of the colon to reestablish gastrointestinal continuity. Results are better in hospitals where this surgery is performed frequently and poorer in small hospitals where this surgery is performed infrequently. Combined modality therapy may be an option for patients who are not surgical candidates and who are unsuitable for endoscopic therapy.

## TREATMENT OF EXTENSIVE DISEASE (STAGE IIA–III)  *IIA T2-3 No Mo → T3 N1; T4*   *triple Rx or CXRX*

Surgery alone is not a standard treatment in these patients because complete tumor resection is not possible in a substantial number of patients, and even when resection is apparently complete, survival rarely exceeds 20%. A recent meta-analysis has shown that a multimodality approach consisting of chemotherapy and radiation followed by surgery (triple therapy) offers the best likelihood of cure. Triple therapy is aggressive and expensive and has a high side effect rate. Patients who are in poor general condition may elect to have palliative therapy after balancing the low probability of cure against the morbidity of treatment. Combined modality therapy using chemoradiation followed by surgery or definitive chemoradiation in patients who cannot or will not undergo surgery are the currently recommended treatments.

## TREATMENT OF DISTANT METASTASES (STAGE IV)  *pall CxRx*

Distant metastases make esophageal cancer incurable; therapy is palliative. Radiation and chemotherapy are frequently used and may offer small increases in survival rates with the tradeoff of systemic side effects. In patients with dysphagia, a number of palliative measures are possible but do not prolong survival.

### 9. What are the endoscopic methods for the palliation of esophageal cancer?

A number of endoscopic methods are available for the palliation of esophageal cancer. Endoscopic dilation causes temporary relief of dysphagia but is not effective as long-term therapy. Expandable metal stents provide rapid palliation of dysphagia, but late complications such as tumor ingrowth can be a problem. Membrane-covered metal stents were developed to prevent the problems associated with tumor ingrowth and have been shown to be superior to uncovered stents. A number of tumor ablative therapies are also available. Injection of absolute alcohol into the tumor has been reported and is inexpensive. There is little control of the degree of necrosis, and tracking of the sclerosant beyond the esophagus can cause perforation and chemical mediastinitis. Argon plasma therapy and Nd:YAG laser can restore luminal patency by tumor ablation. Argon plasma coagulation is considerably less expensive than laser therapy but is as effective. The principal disadvantage of these modalities is that they may require multiple treatments (and therefore multiple visits to the hospital), which is undesirable in patients who have a short time to live. Photodynamic therapy is a recent development in the treatment of esophageal cancer. A light-sensitive drug (Photofrin) is injected intravenously and selectively accumulates in the tumor tissue. Specially developed transendoscopic catheters are used to deliver specific light (usually, 630-nm red laser light) for local activation of Photofrin that is preferentially concentrated in the tumor and causes necrosis of the tumor. The procedure is relatively safe and generally well tolerated. Its principal disadvantages are cost and the development of cutaneous photosensitivity and strictures in the esophagus. The procedure was recently approved by the U.S. Food and Drug Administration and is an important alternative for patients who either do not wish to have surgery or are deemed poor risks for surgery.

*covered SEM*
*APC / EtOH / PDT*

## 10. What does the future hold for patients at risk for the development of esophageal cancer?

The future of esophageal cancer lies in prevention. Symptoms develop late in the disease, and most patients are incurable at presentation. Because of the low absolute numbers of patients who develop the disease, widespread screening programs in the general population are unlikely to be cost-effective. One-time endoscopic screening for Barrett's esophagus has been proposed in patients with chronic reflux disease, as a method for identifying patients at risk, but timing, cost-effectiveness, and efficacy remain unproved. A systematic review of patients taking aspirin or nonsteroidal anti-inflammatory drugs suggested that these agents were protective against adenocarcinoma and squamous cell carcinoma. Chemoprevention of esophageal cancer with aspirin or cyclooxygenase (COX)-2 inhibitors is an exciting new dimension that is undergoing further study. Although definitive evidence is still lacking, many patients with Barrett's esophagus find the risks of aspirin therapy to be acceptable and the potential for decreasing the risk of cancer attractive. Two retrospective, nonrandomized studies have suggested that proton pump inhibitors might reduce the risk of dysplasia in patients with gastroesophageal reflux disease but the data cannot be considered definitive at this time.

## WEBSITES

http://daveproject.org/viewfilms.cfm?film_id=765

http://daveproject.org/ViewFilms.cfm?Film_id=604

https://daveproject.org/ViewFilms.cfm?Film_id=330&View=Radiology

## BIBLIOGRAPHY

1. Inadomi JM, Sampliner R, Lagergren J, et al. Screening and surveillance for Barrett's esophagus in high-risk groups: A cost-utility analysis. Ann Intern Med 2003;138:176–86.
2. Overholt BF, Wang KK, Burdick JS, et al. International Photodynamic Group for High-Grade Dysplasia in Barrett's Esophagus. Five-year efficacy and safety of photodynamic therapy with Photofrin in Barrett's high-grade dysplasia. Gastrointest Endosc 2007;66:460–8.
3. Sadeghi S, Bain CJ, Pandeya N, et al. Australian Cancer Study. Aspirin, nonsteroidal anti-inflammatory drugs, and the risks of cancers of the esophagus. Cancer Epidemiol Biomarkers Prev 2008;17:1169–78.
4. Schembre DB, Huang JL, Lin OS, et al. Treatment of Barrett's esophagus with early neoplasia: A comparison of endoscopic therapy and esophagectomy. Gastrointest Endosc 2008;67:595–601.
5. Siersema PD, Marcon N, Vakil N. Metal stents for tumors of the distal esophagus and gastric cardia. Endoscopy 2003;35:79–85.
6. Stahl M, Olivera J. Esophageal cancer: ESMO clinical recommendations for diagnosis, treatment and follow-up. Ann Oncol 2008;19(Suppl. 2):21–2.
7. Trivers KF, Sabatino SA, Stewart SL. Trends in esophageal cancer incidence by histology, United States, 1998–2003. Int J Cancer 2008.
8. Wang K, Sampliner R. Updated guidelines 2008 for the diagnosis, surveillance and therapy of Barrett's esophagus. Am J Gastroenterol 2008;103:788–97.
9. Wang K, Wongkeesong M, Buttar N. American Gastroenterological Association Medical Position Statement: Role of the gastroenterologist in the management of esophageal carcinoma. Gastroenterology 2005;128:1468–70.

*This pen sucks*

# THE ESOPHAGUS: ANOMALIES, INFECTIONS, AND NONACID INJURIES

*Jeffrey Hunt, DO, John H. Meier, MD, Dirk R. Davis, MD,*
*Matthew B.Z. Bachinski, MD, and David S. James, DO*

# CHAPTER 6

1. **A patient with iron deficiency anemia and dysphagia is found to have a web by barium studies. What disorder must be considered?**
   Esophageal webs can be associated with iron deficiency anemia (Fig. 6-1). This is referred to as Plummer-Vinson syndrome. Brown-Paterson-Kelly syndrome is associated with anemia, esophageal web, and additional features of angular cheilitis and glossitis. Esophageal webs have also been associated with gastric inlet patches (Fig. 6-2) and graft-versus-host disease.

2. **What is the best therapy for the dysphagia?**
   Esophageal bougienage is the preferred therapy, although many webs probably are ruptured unwittingly at endoscopy. Webs are thin, typically less than 2 mm in diameter (Fig. 6-3).

3. **What is the best way to confirm a suspected web?**
   Videofluoroscopy with lateral views. Standard barium swallow allows only brief visualization, and the lesion can be missed.

4. **For which cancer are patients with esophageal webs reportedly at increased risk?**
   Esophageal webs are associated with squamous cell carcinoma of the hypopharynx and upper esophagus, although the degree of risk is not well defined.

5. **Describe the two types of esophageal rings.**
   The two types of esophageal rings are cleverly named A and B. The A ring occurs about 2 cm proximal to the gastroesophageal (GE) junction, is muscular in origin, and is usually asymptomatic. The B ring, also known as a Schatzki ring, is mucosal and occurs at the squamocolumnar junction (Fig. 6-4). In contrast to an esophageal ring, peptic reflux strictures are usually inflammatory and associated with a hiatal hernia (Fig. 6-5).

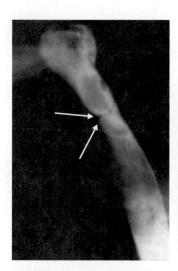

**Figure 6-1.** Barium swallow showing proximal esophageal web (*arrows*). (Courtesy of Peter R. McNally, DO.)

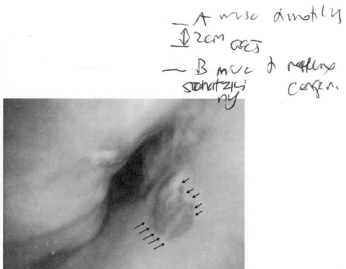

**Figure 6-2.** Endoscopic image of inlet Barrett's esophagus (*arrows*). (Courtesy of Peter R. McNally, DO.)

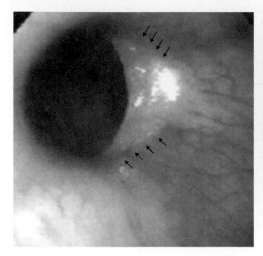

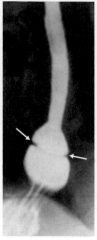

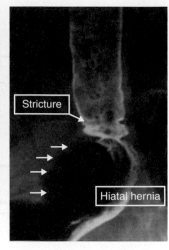

**Figure 6-3.** Endoscopic image showing the thin proximal esophageal web (*arrows*). (Courtesy of Peter R. McNally, DO.)

**Figure 6-4.** Barium swallow radiograph showing a distal esophageal ring consistent with a B or muscular ring (*arrows*). (Courtesy of Peter R. McNally, DO.)

**Figure 6-5.** Barium swallow radiograph showing bulbous hiatal hernia pouch and an irregular inflammatory peptic stricture (*arrows*). (Courtesy of Peter R. McNally, DO.)

### 6. What causes esophageal A and B rings?

The precise cause of these is not known. A rings may be associated with esophageal dysmotility. B rings may be reflux related, but the literature is contradictory. Recent radiology literature suggests that B rings may be more common in children than previously thought, which raises the possibility that they are congenital. Not many children are symptomatic, however, a finding that is unexplained.

### 7. Are all Schatzki rings symptomatic? What is the typical history of the symptomatic patient?

Schatzki rings are usually symptomatic only when the luminal diameter is less than 13 mm. Symptomatic patients usually describe only intermittent solid-food dysphagia induced by hurrying a meal or anxiety. Patients may present initially with foreign-body impaction.

### 8. How are Schatzki rings treated?

Usually with large-diameter bougie. Repeat treatment may be needed over time.

### 9. Describe the three types of esophageal diverticula.

- Upper esophageal, also called Zenker diverticulum (which is arguably a hypopharyngeal lesion—this could be a trick question)
- Mid esophageal, also called a traction or pulsion diverticulum
- Distal esophageal, also called an epiphrenic diverticulum

See Figures 6-6, 6-7, and 6-8.

### 10. What is the typical history of Zenker diverticulum?

Patients may complain of regurgitation of undigested food, bad breath, a visible lump on the side of the neck, and pressure in the lower neck area.

### 11. What causes Zenker diverticulum?

This has been long debated, with initially contradictory studies. The lesion is more common in elderly patients. Impaired cricopharyngeal compliance, usually due to fibrotic changes, causes increased intrabolus pressure with swallowing. Relaxation of the upper esophageal sphincter (UES) is usually normal. The result is increased hypopharyngeal pressure, with herniation at a weak point just above the cricopharyngeus.

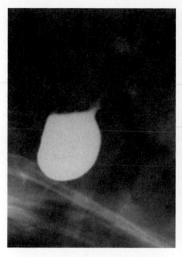

**Figure 6-6.** Barium swallow showing Zenker diverticulum. (Courtesy of Peter R. McNally, DO.)

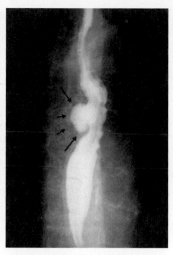

**Figure 6-7.** Barium esophagram showing a midesophageal diverticulum, also called a traction diverticulum (*arrows*). (Courtesy of Peter R. McNally, DO.)

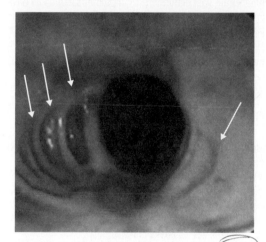

**Figure 6-8.** Endoscopic image showing multiple epiphrenic diverticula (*arrows*). (Courtesy of Peter R. McNally, DO.)

## 12. What is Killian dehiscence?

The weak point just above the cricopharyngeus is called Killian dehiscence. This is in the triangular area where the oblique fibers of the inferior pharyngeal constrictors and the transverse fibers of the cricopharyngeus overlap (Fig. 6-9).

## 13. How is Zenker diverticulum treated?

Symptomatic Zenker diverticula require surgery. Most surgeons perform diverticulectomy because of the small risk of squamous cell carcinoma arising in the pouch remnant. Unilateral cricopharyngeal myotomy should also be done; otherwise, there is a significant recurrence rate.

## 14. Why are midesophageal diverticula called traction diverticula?

It was previously thought that midesophageal diverticula were formed by adhesion of the esophagus to tuberculous mediastinal lymph nodes. Most are now thought to result from esophageal motility disorders called *pulsion diverticulum* or to represent a forme fruste of tracheoesophageal fistula. Few cause symptoms or need treatment.

## 15. Should all epiphrenic diverticula be surgically treated?

No. Unusually large diverticula or those producing symptoms such as regurgitation or aspiration should be resected. Because of the high association with motility disorders, manometry should be performed. Results of manometry will often change the surgical approach to include long myotomy of the lower esophageal sphincter (LES). Recurrence is common with diverticulectomy alone.

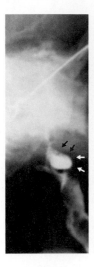
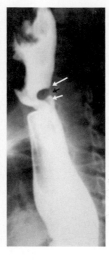

**Figure 6-9.** (Far left) Barium esophagram on lateral projection showing a small Zenker diverticulum protruding through the Killian triangle (*arrows*). (Courtesy of Peter R. McNally, DO.)

**Figure 6-10.** (Near left) Barium swallow, lateral projection, showing the prominence of the cricopharngeus muscle (*arrows*). (Courtesy of Peter R. McNally, DO.)

**16. Is surgery required for the cricopharyngeal *bar* or cricopharyngeal *achalasia* that radiologists sometimes describe?**
No! This finding may or may not be the cause of symptoms (Fig. 6-10). Because the bar can result from poor hypopharyngeal bolus propulsion, hypertrophy, or decreased opening capacity, caution must be exercised before recommending myotomy. Surgery occasionally causes severe reflux. Bougienage can be effective in relieving symptoms in some cases.

**17. Define *dysphagia lusoria*. What is the most common type?**
*Lusoria* means "a trick of nature," and dysphagia lusoria refers to impingement of aberrant vasculature on the proximal esophagus. Most patients with aberrant vasculature are asymptomatic, but some have dysphagia. The most common type involves an aberrant right subclavian artery, which arises from the left side of the aortic arch and compresses the esophagus. Double aortic arch, right aortic arch, and several other anomalies have been reported.

**18. What sort of preoperative evaluation should be done in patients with dysphagia lusoria?**
Magnetic resonance imaging (MRI) is believed to be the most accurate modality for defining the lesion. Patients also should undergo manometry and barium swallow with marshmallow or barium pill to be certain the symptoms are caused by the vascular anomaly.

**19. What causes esophageal atresia with tracheoesophageal fistula?**
Atresia occurs when embryonic foregut fails to recanalize to form an esophagus. The tracheoesophageal (TE) fistula is due to lack of separation of lung bud from the foregut. The exact insult causing these anomalies is not known.

**20. What is the most common type of esophageal atresia with TE fistula? Describe its presentations.**
The most common type of TE fistula with atresia is the lower-pouch fistula. Because the esophagus has not fully formed (atresia), the upper and lower pouches are not in continuity. This anomaly may cause intrauterine polyhydramnios. After birth, regurgitation after feeding and weight loss are seen. The fistula between the distal part of the esophagus and the trachea can cause pneumonia due to reflux of stomach contents.

**21. What is the least common type of esophageal atresia with TE fistula? Describe its presentation.**
The least common form is congenital esophageal stenosis, a forme fruste of atresia, which can present as late as adulthood. The differential diagnosis includes bullous skin disorders, radiation injury to the esophagus, caustic ingestion, and prolonged nasogastric suction. Congenital stenosis typically presents with lifelong dysphagia to solid foods and prolonged meals and low body weight. Barium radiographs may show a fixed segment of narrowing, usually midesophageal (Fig. 6-11). Recent studies suggest that the disorder may in fact be reflux induced rather than congenital.

**22. How is esophageal atresia with TE fistula treated?**
For patients presenting in childhood, surgical repair is usually possible. With modern techniques, mortality is due to associated cardiac anomalies rather than the surgery itself. Congenital esophageal stenosis is generally treatable with cautious bougienage.

**23. What is allergic esophagitis?**
With increasing frequency, persons with solid food dysphagia associated with environmental and food allergies are discovered to have multiple esophageal rings (see Chapter 44, Fig 44-1). Esophageal biopsy samples show greater

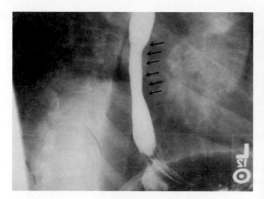

**Figure 6-11.** Barium esophagram showing long smooth distal esophageal stricture, consistent with congenital esophageal stenosis (*arrows*). (Courtesy of Peter R. McNally, DO.)

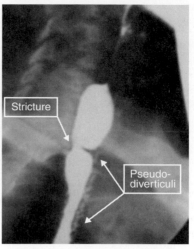

**Figure 6-12.** Barium swallow showing proximal esophageal stricture and multiple small pseudo-diverticula (*arrows*). (Courtesy of Peter R. McNally, DO.)

than 20 to 25 eosinophils per high-power field. The condition is treated with cautious esophageal dilation, as large esophageal tears have been documented with bougienage. Refractory strictures/rings may have been managed with topical budesonide or intralesional triamcinolone (Kenalog) injections. A careful food history should be taken to identify any ingestible allergens.

**24. What is intramural pseudo-diverticulosis?**

Formed by dilation of submucosal esophageal glands, small pseudo-diverticula are commonly associated with *Candida* esophagitis (50%) (Fig. 6-12). Many patients have esophageal motor disorders, and many have esophageal strictures. The inciting event is unknown, but the lesion has been seen after corrosive ingestion. Treatment with stricture dilation and medications can be effective. Some have identified an increased risk of esophageal cancer and recommend periodic surveillance, although the cost-effectiveness of this approach is not established.

## ESOPHAGEAL INFECTIONS

Also see Chapter 8.

**25. What organisms are most commonly identified in esophageal infections?**

The most common etiologies are *Candida albicans*, herpes simplex virus (HSV), and cytomegalovirus (CMV). *Candida* and HSV can be seen in individuals with normal immunity, whereas CMV esophagitis is typically found in an immunocompromised host.

**26. What are the typical presenting symptoms in patients with infectious esophagitis?**

Odynophagia and, to a lesser degree, dysphagia are the most common complaints. Heartburn, chest pain, nausea, dysgeusia, and bleeding can also be symptoms/signs.

**27. What is the most common cause of infectious esophagitis in the general population?**

*C. albicans*. This yeast is virtually ubiquitous and is considered normal oral flora. Esophageal infection occurs by a two-step process. The first step is colonization, which involves adherence to the mucosal surface and proliferation. It is estimated that 20% of asymptomatic individuals have esophageal colonization with *Candida*, and this becomes more common with advanced age. The second step is often associated with impaired host defenses and is identified by mucosal invasion by budding yeast and the presence of mycelial forms on microscopic examination. Adherent creamy white plaque or exudates are the common appearance on endoscopic examination (Fig. 6-13). Barium swallow is a much less sensitive examination for *Candida* esophagitis, but the findings include multiple nodules and diffuse mucosal ulceration.

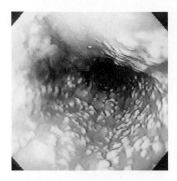

**Figure 6-13.** Endoscopic photograph showing creamy white exudates seen in candidal esophagitis. (Courtesy of Peter R. McNally, DO.)

### 28. List medical conditions known to predispose a person to *Candida* esophagitis.

Conditions compromising normal immune function, primarily human immunodeficiency virus (HIV) infection and hematologic malignancies, increase the incidence of fungal esophagitis. Nonhematologic malignancies, diabetes mellitus, adrenal dysfunction, alcoholism, and advanced age are risk factors as well. Radiation therapy for thoracic malignancies and immunosuppression required in organ transplant recipients is also associated with increased risk. Achalasia and scleroderma esophagus are associated with esophageal stasis and very prone to develop monilial esophagitis.

### 29. What commonly used drugs are associated with fungal esophagitis?

Antibiotics that affect normal oral flora change the competitive milieu, increasing colonization and likelihood of fungal infection. Both systemic and inhaled topical corticosteroids increase risk of infection due to effects on mucosal immunity.

### 30. How is *Candida* esophagitis treated?

- Fluconazole 100 mg/day for 10 to 14 days
- Itraconazole 200 mg/day for 10 to 14 days

Refractory cases (rule out immunodeficiency states)

- Amphoterocin 0.3 to 0.5 mg/kg/day

### 31. Should empiric therapy for *Candida* esophagitis be considered in an at-risk patient presenting with typical symptoms of esophageal infection?

Yes, a therapeutic trial of fluconazole for patients with presumed esophageal candidiasis is a cost-effective alternative to endoscopy. Patients not demonstrating symptomatic improvement within 3 to 5 days should undergo endoscopic evaluation.

### 32. What is the most common viral pathogen-causing esophagitis?

CMV is the most common cause of viral esophagitis in an immunocompromised patient. Because viral esophagitis is rare in individuals with normal immune function, CMV is the most common etiology. Other viral pathogens, including HSV, varicella-zoster virus (VSV), and Epstein-Barr virus (EBV), can also cause esophageal infections in patients with immune dysfunction.

### 33. What is the most common cause of viral esophagitis in patients with normal immunity?

HSV esophagitis, although rare, is the etiology of viral esophagitis in an immunocompetent patient. The infection can be primary or due to reactivation of a latent infection. The finding of orolabial HSV may suggest the diagnosis in patients with acute esophageal symptoms but is present in only about 20% of cases. HSV esophagitis tends to be seen more commonly in males (male-to-female ratio, >3:1).

### 34. How is viral esophagitis diagnosed?

In patients with esophageal ulcers presenting with symptoms of infectious esophagitis, multiple biopsies (10 biopsies are recommended to maximize diagnostic yield) of each ulcer should be obtained. Biopsy samples from the ulcer base and ulcer margins are evaluated for typical cytopathic changes microscopically. Tissue also needs to be sent in medium for viral culture. Tissue culture is more sensitive than microscopic examination. Immunohistochemical stains for HSV and CMV can increase the diagnostic sensitivity as well.

### 35. Differentiate HSV and CMV esophagitis endoscopically.

Early in HSV esophagitis, the typical small vesicles can be seen in the middle-distal esophagus. The vesicles may coalesce, forming well-circumscribed ulcers that have raised yellowish edges—the classic volcano ulcers. HSV esophagitis can cause a diffusely ulcerated mucosa devoid of squamous epithelium in severe infections. CMV ulcers are more often linear, serpiginous lesions in the middle and/or distal esophagus. These ulcers may unite forming giant ulcers and may produce stricturing of the esophageal lumen. Concomitant infections with both organisms have been reported, and in *Candida* esophagitis, a viral coinfection can be present in 20% to 50% of cases. Candidal plaques often obscure viral ulcers.

### 36. How is HSV esophagitis treated?

HSV esophagitis is a self-limited infection in immunocompetent patients and may not require therapy. If the diagnosis is made early in the course of infection, initiating therapy may shorten duration of symptoms. In immunocompromised patients, infection is more serious, may disseminate, and requires treatment. Initial therapy with intravenous acyclovir 250 mg/m$^2$ every 8 hours until the patient is able to swallow normally followed by valacyclovir 100 mg three times daily for a total of 7 to 10 days. Acyclovir-resistant strains of HSV should be treated with foscarnet 40 mg/kg three times daily for 2 weeks.

### 37. Discuss the treatment of CMV esophagitis.

Both ganciclovir and foscarnet are effective drugs in treating CMV. Due to cost, ganciclovir is considered first-line therapy at a dose of 5 mg/kg intravenously for 2 weeks. Granulocytopenia is a potential side effect of ganciclovir.

### 38. Does it make sense to stain for acid-fast organisms in evaluating esophageal ulcers?

A shallow linear ulcer with smooth edges and a necrotic base, usually in the middle third of the esophagus, is suggestive of mycobacterium tuberculosis (TB). TB is seldom a primary infection in the esophagus, but cases have been reported. It more often results from direct extension from adjacent mediastinal lymph nodes in patients with pulmonary tuberculosis. Mycobacterium-avium complex is commonly reported in patients with acquired immunodeficiency syndrome (AIDS) and tends to be widely disseminated at the time of diagnosis. Esophageal involvement is rare but should be considered in the differential diagnosis; appropriate tissue stains and culture should be obtained. As is the case with TB, treatment is difficult requiring multidrug regimens over months.

### 39. Can the diagnosis of Chagas disease be based on classic manometric findings and confirmed by histologic evaluation of deep mucosal biopsies from the distal esophagus?

Chagas disease is caused by infection with *Trypanosoma cruzi*, which is endemic in South America. The organism destroys ganglion cells, and multiple organs are involved. The esophageal abnormalities resemble achalasia but the LES pressure is not elevated and, in fact, may be low. Symptoms typically occur years to decades after the acute infection. Diagnosis requires typical manometric findings, positive serologic tests for the parasite, and evidence of other organ involvement. Mucosal biopsies are of no value in the diagnosis. The esophagus in Chagas disease is more responsive to nitrates and calcium channel antagonists, which improve esophageal emptying. Unlike primary achalasia, Chagas disease is often associated with cardiac, renal, intestinal, and biliary abnormalities.

## PILL AND CORROSIVE ESOPHAGEAL INJURY

### 40. Who is affected by pill-induced esophageal injury?

Anyone of any age who ingests caustic pills is susceptible to pill-induced injury. Reported cases range from 5 to 89 years old. Women outnumber men by a ratio of 1.5:1. It is not uncommon for pills to stick in a normal esophagus during transit. A more sticky gelatin tablet remained in the esophagus for more than 10 minutes in over one-half of normal subjects who ingested the pill in a supine position. Esophageal dysmotility or structural abnormalities, such as rings or strictures, are clearly not required for pill-induced injury.

### 41. What factors contribute to esophageal retention of pills?

- Impaired esophageal clearance
- Supine posture during or immediately after pill ingestion
- Structural defects: rings, stricture, extrinsic compression, etc
- Swallowing pills without sufficient liquid
- Esophageal dysmotility
- Pill characteristics: acidic, basic, sticky, large size

Most common history for pill esophagitis: taking the pill with inadequate fluid and lying down immediately afterward are often the only identifiable risk factors.

### 42. What are the risk factors for pill-induced injury?

Anyone who takes a caustic pill is at risk, but some patients are at particular risk for severe pill-induced esophageal injury, including those with structural abnormalities of the esophagus, both pathologic (stricture, tumor, ring—see Fig. 6-14) and physiologic (hiatal hernia, narrowing of the esophagus secondary to compression from the left

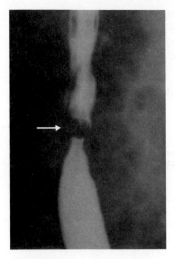

**Figure 6-14.** Barium swallow showing a 12-mm barium pill sticking at an esophageal stricture (*arrow*). (Courtesy of Peter R. McNally, DO.)

atrium, aortic arch, left main stem bronchus). Cardiac disease is a risk factor because of esophageal compression by a <u>dilated left atrium</u> and frequent use of inherently caustic medications (e.g., aspirin, potassium chloride, quinidine).

### 43. Describe the typical presentation of patients with pill-induced injury.
The typical patient has no prior history of esophageal disease and presents with the sudden onset of <u>retrosternal pain</u>, which may have awakened the patient from sleep (particularly if pills were ingested with little liquid just before or while lying down) and may be exacerbated by swallowing. The pain may be mild or so severe that swallowing is impossible. The pain typically increases over the first 3 <u>to 4 days</u> before gradually subsiding. Painless dysphagia is uncommon (20%) and may suggest an alternative diagnosis.

### 44. How is the diagnosis of pill-induced esophageal injury made?
- Clinical suspicion
- Acute onset of odynophagia, dysphagia, and/or <u>chest pain</u>
- Exposure to pills commonly associated with esophageal injury
- Upper endoscopy preferred over barium swallow, as biopsy is often necessary to exclude infectious causes of <u>esophageal ulcer</u>

### 45. What does the typical pill-induced lesion look like at time of endoscopy?
The typical lesion of pill-induced esophageal injury is one or more discrete ulcers with <u>normal surrounding mucosa</u>. Ulcers range in size from pinpoint to circumferential lesions that may be several centimeters long. Most ulcers involve only the mucosa, but deeper penetration can occur and localized perforations have been reported. Ulcers may have local surrounding inflammation. Pill fragments have been seen in ulcer craters.

### 46. How can you remember the many medications that can cause pill-induced esophagitis?
 Know your ABCs: N-O-A-A-B-Cs (Table 6-1).

Doxycycline and tetracycline accounted for 293 of 454 reported cases of pill-induced esophageal injury in one recent review.

### 47. Where are the areas of physiologic narrowing of the esophagus?
- *Esophageal sphincters:* lower and upper sphincters (LES and UES)
- *Strictures*
  - Peptic
  - Webs
  - Rings
- *Extrinsic compression*
  - Aortic arch
  - Left main stem bronchus
  - Left atrium
  - Cervical osteophytes

| Table 6-1. Medications That Can Cause Pill-Induced Esophagitis (NOAABCs) | |
|---|---|
| **CLASS** | **MEDICATION** |
| NSAIDs | Aspirin, naproxen, ibuprofen |
| Others | Quinidine, potassium chloride, ferrous sulfate, ascorbic acid, multivitamins, theophylline |
| Antibiotics | Tetracycline, doxycycline, clindamycin, penicillin |
| Antiviral agents | Zalcitibine, zidovudine, nelfinavir |
| Bisphosphonates | Alendronate, etidronate, pamidronate |
| Chemotherapeutics | Dactinomycin, bleomycin, cytarabine, daunorubicin, 5-fluorouracil, methotrexate, vincristine |

NSAID, nonsteroidal anti-inflammatory drug.

## 48. What are the options for treating pill-induced esophageal injury?

Most pill-induced injuries heal without active intervention in days to several weeks. Avoid the drug responsible for the injury and other caustic drugs. Administration of medications that buffer or decrease production of stomach acid, or create a barrier coat for the esophagus, is frequently prescribed. The use of topical anesthetics in various combinations (Bemylid—Benadryl, Mylanta, and lidocaine in equal parts) may decrease the immediate symptoms of odynophagia, but their use is limited by potential systemic toxicity.

## 49. Discuss the epidemiology of caustic ingestion in the United States.

Chemical ingestion remains an important problem despite improvements in packaging (e.g., child-proof containers), product labeling, and warnings. Approximately 5000 caustic ingestions occur per year. Adolescents and adults who willfully ingest caustic agents as a suicidal gesture in general consume a larger volume and therefore have more serious injury than do children, who ingest the agent accidentally and often expectorate most of it before swallowing. Children often have minimal esophageal damage, but their oral, pharyngeal, and laryngeal injuries may be more severe. Approximately 80% of caustic ingestions occur accidentally in children younger than 5 years, who most often consume household cleaners. Caustic ingestion is the leading cause of esophageal strictures in children.

## 50. What are the common caustic agents? Where are they found?

Caustic agents are present in many common household products. The severity of the damage depends largely on the corrosive properties and concentration of the ingested agents. The caustic agents most often responsible for serious injury are strong alkaline cleaning products, such as drain cleaners and lye soaps. Severe alkaline burns also result from the ingestion of disc batteries that contain concentrated sodium or potassium hydroxide. Concentrated acid compounds also cause severe injury but are not common household items; thus, they are encountered less often. The severity of esophageal and gastric injury secondary to caustic ingestion depends not only on the concentration and corrosive properties of the agent but also on the quantity consumed.

## 51. Describe the pathophysiology of acute alkali esophagitis.

When tissue is exposed to strong alkali, the immediate result is liquefactive necrosis, the complete destruction of entire cells and their membranes. Cell membranes are destroyed as their lipids are saponified and cellular proteins are denatured. Thrombosis of the local blood vessels also contributes to tissue damage. Tissue destruction and organ penetration progress rapidly until the alkali is diluted and neutralized by dilution with tissue fluids.

## 52. The severity of caustic injury to the esophagus can be graded as first, second, or third degree, using the following system.

Endoscopy within the first 24 hours may underestimate the severity of esophageal injury (Table 6-2).

## 53. Describe how an endoscopic grading system guides in management and prognosis of the patient with corrosive injection.

Patients with grade 1 or 2A caustic injury have an excellent prognosis without acute morbidity or chronic stricture formation. For these patients, administration of a liquid diet can be started and advanced to a regular diet after 1 to 2 days. Patients with grade 2B to 3A injury develop strictures in 70% to 100% of cases. Grade 3B carries a 65% early mortality rate and a significant need for esophageal resection. Despite this poor prognosis, there is no evidence that medical therapy with antibiotics or steroids are of any benefit. For difficult strictures, barium swallow may be very helpful in defining anatomy and guiding dilation decisions (Fig. 6-15).

## 54. What is the cancer risk to a patient with stricture after lye ingestion?

The association between esophageal cancer and caustic ingestion is strong. The expected incidence of esophageal carcinoma is higher in patients with caustic ingestion than in the general population. Approximately 1% to 7% of patients with carcinoma of the esophagus have a history of caustic ingestion. The latent period is long, and in one study was an average of 41 years. Vigilance and early endoscopic evaluation of esophageal symptoms are warranted.

**Table 6-2.** Grading Esophageal Injury by Endoscopy

| GRADE | INJURY CHARACTERISTICS |
|---|---|
| 0 | Normal |
| 1 | Mucosal edema |
| 2A | Superficial ulcers, bleeding, exudates |
| 2B | Deep focal or circumferential ulcers |
| 3A | Focal necrosis—deep ulcers with brown, black, or gray discoloration |
| 3B | Extensive necrosis |
| 4 | Perforation |

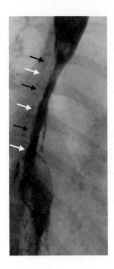

**Figure 6-15.** Barium swallow showing long irregular stricture caused by corrosive ingestion (*arrows*). (Courtesy of Peter R. McNally, DO.)

**55. Describe the emergency department management of a patient with caustic ingestion.**

The initial steps in the management of a suspected caustic injury are similar to those used on an emergency basis to manage any toxic ingestion. First, airway, breathing, and circulation (ABCs) must be controlled. Patients with caustic ingestion may present with respiratory compromise and require endotracheal intubation to protect the airway and to provide adequate oxygenation. Intubation should be performed only under direct visualization and should not be attempted in a blind manner. Next, hypotension must be addressed with adequate fluid support and resuscitation, as needed. If obvious signs of mediastinitis or peritonitis suggest perforation of a viscus, the patient should be prepared for surgery.

**56. What is the role of endoscopic evaluation in patients with caustic ingestion?**

Flexible upper endoscopy has a role in the early, emergent and later, subacute management of caustic ingestion. Patients in whom perforation (diagnosed either radiographically or clinically) requires surgical exploration should undergo complete upper endoscopy to identify the extent of disease. For example, in patients with a normal esophagus but injured stomach, surgery may be limited to the abdomen. The risk of upper endoscopy is acceptable once the decision to operate has been made. If surgery is not indicated, endoscopy still should be performed to identify uninjured patients who do not require prolonged hospital observation and to define the severity of burns in injured patients. Timing of endoscopy is based on clinical suspicion of severe injury. If significant esophageal injury is unlikely, esophagogastroduodenoscopy (EGD) should be performed promptly to provide rapid reassurance and to avoid hospital observation. More than 50% of patients with a history of caustic injury are found on endoscopy to have no injury. If internal injury is likely but signs of perforation are absent, a delay of 48 to 72 hours permits development of the inflammatory reaction (little inflammation may be present in the first 24 hours) and easier assessment of the true extent of injury. Although endoscopic evaluation identifies the location of the mucosal injury, it may not accurately predict the depth of invasion.

## WEBSITES

http://surgery.med.umich.edu/pediatric/clinical/patient_content/a-m/esophageal_atresia_patient.shtml

http://www.learningradiology.com/archives05/COW%20137-Eosphageal%20Atresia/esophatresiacorrect.htm

http://www.mypacs.net/cases/DOXYCYCLINE-INDUCED-ESOPHAGITIS-173438.html

## BIBLIOGRAPHY

1. Achildi O, Grenwal H. Congenital anomalies of the esophagus. Otolaryngol Clin N Am 2007;40:219–44.
2. Assa'ad A. Eosinophilic esophagitis: Association with allergic disorders. Gastrointest Endoscopy Clin N Am 2008;18:119–32.
3. Baehr PH, McDonald GB. Esophageal infections: Risk factors, presentation, diagnosis, and treatment. Gastroenterology 1994;106:509.
4. Colombo-Benkmann M, Unruh V, Krieglstein C, et al. Cricopharyngeal myotomy in the treatment of Zenker's diverticulum. J Am Coll Surg 2003;196:370–78.
5. Dantas RO, Deghaide NH, Donadi EA. Esophageal manometric and radiologic findings in asymptomatic subjects with Chagas' disease. J Clin Gastroenterol 1999;28:245.
6. Donta ST, Engel Jr CC, Collins JF, et al. Benefits and harms of doxycycline treatment for Gulf War Veterans' illness. Ann Intern Med 2004;141:85.
7. Famularo G, De Simone C. Fatal esophageal perforation with alendronate. Am J Gastroenterol 2001;96:3212.
8. Gutschow CA, Hamoir M, Rombaux P, et al. Management of pharyngoesophageal (Zenker's) diverticulum: Which technique? Ann Thorac Surg 2002;74:1677–683.
9. Kikendall JW. Pill-induced esophageal injury. In: Castell DO, Richter JE, eds. The Esophagus. 4th ed. Philadelphia: Lippincott Williams & Wilkins; 2004. p. 572.
10. Lamberti JL, Mainwaring RD. Tracheoesophageal compressive syndromes of vascular origins: Rings and slings. In: Baue A, Geha AS, Hammond GL, et al., eds. Glenn's Thoracic and Cardiovascular Surgery, Vol. 2, 6th ed. Stamford, CT: Appleton & Lange; 1996.
11. Lamireau T, Rebouissoux L, Denis D, et al. Accidental caustic ingestion in children: Is endoscopy always mandatory? J Pediatr Gastroenterol Nutr 2001;33:81–4.
12. Lanas A, Bajador E, Serrano P, et al. Nitrovasodilators, low-dose aspirin, other nonsteroidal anti-inflammatory drugs, and the risk of upper gastrointestinal bleeding. N Engl J Med 2000;343:843.
13. Lanza FL, Hunt RH, Thomson AB, et al. Endoscopic comparison of esophageal and gastroduodenal effects of risedronate and alendronate in postmenopausal women. Gastroenterology 2000;119:886.

14. Lanza FL, Rack MF, Li Z, et al. Placebo-controlled, randomized, evaluator-blinded endoscopy study of risedronate vs. aspirin in healthy postmenopausal women. Aliment Pharmacol Ther 2000;14:1663.

15. Perkins AC, Wilson CG, Frier M, et al. Oesophageal transit, disintegration and gastric emptying of a film-coated risedronate placebo tablet in gastro-oesophageal reflux disease and normal control subjects. Aliment Pharmacol Ther 2001;15:115.

16. Poley JW, Steyerberg EW, Kuipers EJ, et al. Ingestion of acid and alkaline agents: Prognostic value of early upper endoscopy. Gastrointest Endosc 2004;60:372–7.

17. Reed MF, Mathisen DJ. Tracheoesophageal fistula. Chest Surg Clin N Am 2003;13:271–89.

18. Ribeiro A, DeVault KR, Wolfe III JT, et al. Alendronate-associated esophagitis: Endoscopic and pathologic features. Gastrointest Endosc 1998;47:525.

19. Sethumadavan S, Ramanathan J, Rammouni R, et al. Herpes simplex esophagitis in the immunocompetent host: An overview. Am J Gastroenterol 2001;96:2264.

20. Straumann A. The natural history and complications of eosinophilic esophagitis. Gastrointest Endoscopy Clin N Am 2008;18:99–118.

21. Vazquez JA, Sobel JD. Mucosal candidiasis. Infec Dis Clin N Am 2002;16:793–820.

# BARRETT'S ESOPHAGUS

*Richard E. Sampliner, MD*

## 1. What is Barrett's esophagus?

Barrett's esophagus is a metaplastic change in the lining of the normally squamous-lined esophagus that is recognized at endoscopy. As a result of gastroesophageal reflux disease, the esophagus is lined with intestinal metaplasia, a premalignant epithelium.

## 2. How is Barrett's esophagus diagnosed?

The ultimate criterion for histologic diagnosis is the presence of goblet cells. Currently, two techniques are necessary—endoscopy to recognize abnormal appearing esophageal epithelium and biopsy to detect intestinal metaplasia. There have been many technical advances in endoscopic imaging including confocal microendoscopy, spectroscopy, fluorescence imaging, optical coherence tomography, and high-resolution endoscopy. These techniques are expensive and not validated. High-resolution endoscopy is emerging in major centers that treat patients with Barrett's esophagus and may be more widely available, enabling recognition of intestinal metaplasia and high-grade dysplasia (HGD) in the clinical setting by white light endoscopy.

## 3. Why is Barrett's esophagus important?

It is a premalignant lesion for adenocarcinoma of the esophagus and for a proportion of adenocarcinomas of the gastric cardia. Adenocarcinoma of the esophagus in white men is the cancer with the most rapidly rising incidence in the United States and western Europe during the past three decades.

## 4. Does short-segment Barrett's esophagus need to be identified?

Yes. Barrett's esophagus ranges from short tongues of intestinal metaplasia in the distal esophagus to circumferential intestinal metaplasia of nearly the entire length of the esophagus. In the mid 1970s, before the recognition of the importance of intestinal metaplasia, Barrett's esophagus was defined as a *columnar-lined esophagus* of at least 3 cm in length. However, it is now recognized that short-segment Barrett's esophagus can develop dysplasia and adenocarcinoma and is in fact, more common than long segment Barrett.

## 5. What is the risk of cancer associated with Barrett's esophagus?

Recent prospective series have documented a lower risk for the development of cancer than in former series. Rather than a 1% to 2% annual risk, the risk appears to be 0.4% to 0.5% per year. This difference may be due to the larger, prospective series with longer follow-up. This lower incidence has been documented in higher-risk patients, predominantly white men. However, the most important question for the individual patient is his or her specific risk. An evidence-based answer has not yet been developed.

## 6. Who should be screened for Barrett's esophagus?

People at highest risk for the development of adenocarcinoma should be screened. Clues are available from the epidemiology of adenocarcinoma: older white men, patients with long-standing reflux symptoms, smokers, and the obese. Specific criteria to select individual patients have not been defined in prospective studies. In clinical practice, however, the movement has been toward the concept of once-in-a-lifetime endoscopy for patients with chronic gastroesophageal reflux to detect Barrett's esophagus. Focusing on patients at high risk of developing cancer would be more effective (i.e., older white men with more than 5 years of reflux symptoms).

## 7. What is the therapy for Barrett's esophagus?

Standard clinical therapy is pharmacologic (proton pump inhibitor [PPI]) and surgical (laparoscopic fundoplication). Both techniques are highly effective in controlling reflux symptoms and healing erosive esophagitis. For younger patients who are noncompliant or do not wish to take daily medication, surgery is an option. For patients with prominent regurgitation, inadequately controlled with PPIs, surgery should be considered. A higher failure rate for laparoscopic fundoplication has been recognized in patients with Barrett's esophagus compared with those with non-Barrett reflux.

## GOALS OF THERAPY FOR BARRETT'S ESOPHAGUS

- Control reflux symptoms
- Heal erosive esophagitis
- Prevent adenocarcinoma

### 8. Does Barrett's esophagus reverse with medical therapy?

Rarely. In published series, which typically use high doses of PPIs, Barrett's esophagus was eliminated in only 2% of 151 patients. Even if esophageal acid exposure is nearly eliminated, the estimated decrease in the area of Barrett's esophagus over an interval of 2 years is only 8%.

### 9. Does Barrett's esophagus reverse with surgical therapy?

Rarely. Barrett's esophagus was eliminated in less than 4% of 449 patients undergoing surgery in a large series in the 1990s. If the elimination of all refluxate by successful fundoplication does not reverse Barrett's esophagus and eliminate the risk of cancer, it is unlikely that medical therapy other than chemoprevention will do so.

### 10. What is the appropriate surveillance of patients with Barrett's esophagus?

The database for developing guidelines for surveillance of this premalignant mucosa is limited, but gastroenterologists must deal with this issue in everyday practice. Surveillance intervals are based on the detection of dysplasia with the goal of recognition of HGD and early adenocarcinoma to enable intervention to improve survival associated with adenocarcinoma. The surveillance intervals have been increasing and probably will continue to do so with improved understanding of the natural history of dysplasia. Currently, a patient with two endoscopic procedures with systematic biopsies showing no dysplasia can be surveyed every 3 years or longer. If low-grade dysplasia has no greater abnormality on follow-up endoscopy with biopsy and has been confirmed by an expert gastrointestinal pathologist, surveillance can be performed every year for 2 years and then every 2 years until no dysplasia is found.

### 11. Summarize the evolution of Barrett's esophagus to adenocarcinoma.

Intestinal metaplasia → Low-grade dysplasia → High-grade dysplasia → Adenocarcinoma

### 12. Describe the management of HGD.

Management of HGD is one of the most controversial issues in the treatment of Barrett's esophagus. Current alternatives include more frequent surveillance (every 3 months) until cancer is detected, endoscopic reversal therapy, and esophagectomy. The problems with conventional esophagectomy include operative mortality rate, especially in low-volume centers; the high frequency of morbidity; and the permanent impact on eating and nutrition. Endoscopic therapy has now been documented in case-control studies to be as effective as esophagectomy. Many patients are elderly and are not good surgical candidates because of comorbidity. It is also not uncommon for patients to refuse surgery even after consulting with a surgeon.

After the confirmation of HGD by an expert gastrointestinal pathologist, the option of endoscopic therapy should be explained to the patient. Endoscopic therapy includes a combination of endoscopic resection of mucosal irregularities and ablation of the rest of the Barrett with photodynamic therapy (PDT) or a thermal technique. Radiofrequency ablation is emerging as a favorite because of the large surface area that can be readily treated. What is now clear from a large single-center retrospective cohort study of endoscopic therapy versus esophagectomy of Barrett with HGD is that the survival outcome is similar with traditional high-volume surgery or expert endoscopic therapy. With a longer than 5-year mean follow-up, there were no esophageal adenocarcinoma deaths in either group. The reflexive decision for esophagectomy should no longer occur after the documentation of HGD.

### 13. Can the development of adenocarcinoma of the esophagus be prevented in patients with Barrett's esophagus?

Prevention is the major challenge to clinicians. Given the lack of reversal of Barrett's esophagus with standard medical and surgical therapy, it is not clear that the development of adenocarcinoma can be prevented. It has been argued that control of reflux into the esophagus will prevent the progression from metaplasia to dysplasia and subsequent adenocarcinoma. However, this argument is far from proved, and only retrospective data can be brought to bear on the issue. There are exciting developments in endoscopic therapy to eliminate the presence of intestinal metaplasia including endoscopic resection and radiofrequency ablation. Photodynamic endoscopic ablation therapy of patients with HGD can reduce the development of cancer over a follow-up of 5 years, but 13% of patients in the PDT arm still progressed to cancer. The endpoint of endoscopic therapy has to be the elimination of all intestinal metaplasia in the esophagus. The overall reduction of the development of adenocarcinoma in patients with Barrett's esophagus remains a major challenge.

## 14. What advantages can we anticipate in the management of Barrett's esophagus?

Progress in our understanding of the genetic changes involved in the progression of Barrett's esophagus to adenocarcinoma has been dramatic. The technical advances that continue to be made in endoscopy offer the opportunity for major advances in clinical management of Barrett's esophagus. We can look forward to unsedated endoscopy with smaller-caliber endoscopes or nonendoscopic techniques, for less-expensive and easier detection of Barrett's esophagus. Optical methods for identifying dysplasia without biopsy add the possibility of real-time recognition. Newer endoscopic techniques to remove dysplastic and metaplastic epithelium will make current attempts look primitive. Prevention of adenocarcinoma may require validation of biomarkers that define the subgroup of patients at highest risk for the development of cancer. This approach will focus surveillance on patients at higher risk, leading to cost savings and greater clinical effectiveness. Chemoprevention may offer opportunities for cancer prevention that transcend the technical advances.

## WEBSITES

http://www.cancer.gov/

http://www.cancer.gov/cancertopics/types/esophageal/

http://www.nature.com/modpathol/journal/v15/n6/fig_tab/3880574f1.html

## BIBLIOGRAPHY

1. Begg CB, Cramer LD, Hoskins WJ, et al. Impact of hospital volume on operative mortality for major cancer surgery. JAMA 1998;280:1747–51.
2. Corley DA, Kerlikowske K, Verma R, et al. Protective association of aspirin/nsaids and esophageal cancer: A systematic review and meta-analysis. Gastroenterology 2003;124:47–56.
3. Devesa SS, Blot WJ, Fraumeni JF. Changing patterns in the incidence of esophageal and gastric carcinoma in the United States. Cancer 1998;83:2049–53.
4. Drewitz DJ, Sampliner RE, Garewal HS. The incidence of adenocarcinoma in Barrett's esophagus—A prospective study of 170 patients followed 4.8 years. Am J Gastroenterol 1997;92:212–5.
5. Ell C, May A, Pech O, et al. Curative endoscopic resection of early esophageal adenocarcinomas (Barrett's cancer). Gastrintest Endosc 2007;65:3–10.
6. Farrell TM, Smith CD, Metreveli RE, et al. Fundoplication provides effective and durable symptom relief in patients with Barrett's esophagus. Am J Surg 1999;178:18–21.
7. Fass R, Sampliner RE, Malagon IB, et al. Failure of oesophageal acid control in candidates for Barrett's oesophagus reversal on a very high dose of proton pump inhibitor. Aliment Pharmacol 2000;14:597–602.
8. Haag S, Nandurkar S, Talley NJ. Regression of Barrett's esophagus: The role of acid suppression, surgery, and ablative methods. Gastrointest Endosc 1999;50:229–40.
9. Hofstetter WL, Peters JH, DeMeester T, et al. Long-term outcome of antireflux surgery in patients with Barrett's esophagus. Ann Surg 2001;234:532–9.
10. Kara MA, Peters FP, Rosmolen WD, et al. High resolution endoscopy plus chromoendoscopy or narrow band imaging in Barrett's esophagus: A prospective randomized crossover study. Endoscopy 2005;37:929–36.
11. Overholt BF, Wang KK, Burdick JS, et al. Five-year efficacy and safety of photodynamic therapy with photofrin in Barrett's high-grade dysplasia. Gastroenterologist 2007;66:460–8.
12. Peters FTM, Ganesh S, Kuipers EJ, et al. Endoscopic regression of Barrett's oesophagus during omeprazole treatment: A randomised double blind study. Gut 1999;45:489–94.
13. Prasad GA, Wang KK, Buttar NS, et al. Long term survival following endoscopic and surgical treatment of high grade dysplasia in Barrett's esophagus. Gastroenterology 2007;132:1226–33.
14. Sampliner RE Practice Parameters Committee ACG. Updated guidelines for the diagnosis, surveillance, and therapy of Barrett's esophagus. Am J Gastroenterol 2002;97:1888–95.
15. Sharma P, Morales TG, Bhattacharyya A, et al. Dysplasia in short segment Barrett's esophagus—A prospective 3 year follow-up. Am J Gastroenterol 1997;92:2012–6.
16. Sharma P, Morales TG, Sampliner RE. Short segment Barrett's esophagus: The need for standardization of the definition and of endoscopic criteria. Am J Gastroenterol 1998;93:1033–6.
17. Sharma P, Sampliner RE, Camargo E. Normalization of esophageal pH with high dose proton pump inhibitor therapy does not result in regression of Barrett's esophagus. Am J Gastroenterol 1997;92:582–5.
18. Sharma VK, Wang KK, Overholt BF, et al. Balloon-based, circumferential, endoscopic ablation of Barrett's esophagus: 1-Year follow-up of 100 patients. Gastrintest Endosc 2007;65:185–95.
19. Wang K, Sampliner R. Updated guidelines 2008 for the diagnosis, surveillance, and therapy of Barrett's esophagus. Am J Gastroenterol 2008;103:788–97.

# CHAPTER 8

# ESOPHAGEAL AND STOMACH PATHOLOGY

*Shalini Tayal, MD*

## ESOPHAGUS

### 1. Describe a normal esophagus lining.

- Esophagus consists of mucosa, lamina propria, muscularis mucosae, submucosa, muscularis propria, and adventitia (lacks serosa) (Fig. 8-1*A*).
- Sebaceous glands can be seen normally in the submucosa.
- Normal gastroesophageal (GE) junction (Fig. 8-1*B*) shows squamous and columnar epithelium.

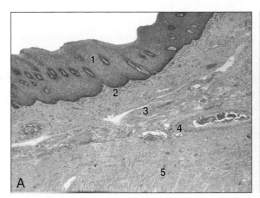
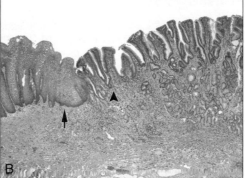

**Figure 8-1.** Photomicrographs of (**A**) Normal esophagus lining. *1*, Mucosa. *2*, Lamina propria. *3*, Muscularis mucosae. *4*, Submucosa. *5*, Muscularis propria (Adventitia is not shown). H&E stain. (**B**) Normal gastroesophageal junction showing squamous mucosa (*arrow*) and columnar mucosa (*arrowhead*). H&E stain.

*' ELMS '*

M
L
MM
SM
MP
A

### 2. What are the histologic features of gastroesophageal reflux disease (GERD) and eosinophilic esophagitis (EE)?

#### GASTROESOPHAGEAL REFLUX DISEASE (Fig. 8-2A)

- Distal esophagus more severe than proximal esophagus
- Basilar hyperplasia
- Elongation of vascular papillae
- Increased intraepithelial neutrophils and eosinophils (~8 per high-power field)
- Balloon cells (enlarged squamous cells with abundant accumulation of plasma proteins) indicate chemical injury.

#### EOSINOPHILIC ESOPHAGITIS (Fig. 8-2B)

- Proximal esophagus more common than distal esophagus. Distribution can be patchy. Need to obtain biopsy samples from upper/mid and distal esophagus.
- Increased intraepithelial eosinophils in upper layers of epithelium (>15 to 20 per high-power field)
- Eosinophilic microabscesses in superficial layers of epithelium
- Extensive degranulation of eosinophils more common
- 30% coexists with GERD; difficult to distinguish histologically

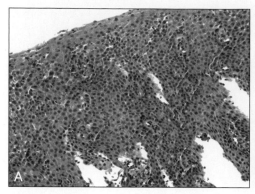
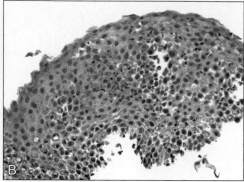

**Figure 8-2.** Photomicrographs of (**A**) Reflux esophagitis (gastroesophageal reflux disease). Basilar hyperplasia and elongated vascular papillae. H&E stain. (**B**) Eosinophilic esophagitis. Note the increased intraepithelial eosinophils in this biopsy sample from the midesophagus. H&E stain. (Courtesy of Dr. K. Capocelli, University of Colorado Denver Health Sciences Center.)

### 3. Discuss the infectious causes of esophagitis.

#### FUNGAL ESOPHAGITIS

- *Candida esophagitis* (Fig. 8-3*A,B*): *Candida albicans* is the most common of the *Candida* spp. Others include *C. glabrata, C. tropicalis, C. parapsilosis,* and *C. krusei.*
  - **Endoscopy:** Whitish raised plaques with erosions or ulcerations
  - **Histology:** Erosion of superficial layers of squamous epithelium or ulceration with yeast and pseudo-hyphal forms (highlighted by special stains such as GMS [Grocott methenamine silver] or PAS [periodic acid–Schiff])
  - **Key:** Presence of pseudo-hyphal forms indicates infection.
  - Presence of only yeast forms suggests oral contamination.
- *Histoplasma:* In the United States, endemic around Mississippi and Ohio River valleys. Also in the central and South America and the Caribbean islands.
  - **Endoscopy:** May appear normal
  - **Histology:** Subepithelial necrotizing granulomas with giant cells that contain organisms of 2- to 4 μm diameter
- *Aspergillus:* Most common species are *Aspergillus fumigatus* and *A. flavus.* Seen as branching (at 45 degrees) septate hyphae 4 μm in diameter.
- *Mucormycosis:* Can be seen in immunocompromised hosts as nonseptate parallel hyphae (10-to 15-μm diameter) that branch at right angles

#### VIRAL ESOPHAGITIS

- *Herpes esophagitis* (Fig. 8-4): Seen in immunocompromised patients
  - **Endoscopy:** May see vesicles or coalesced shallow ulcers
  - **Histology:** Infected epithelial cells show multinucleation with molding and smudged intranuclear inclusions
- *Cytomegalovirus.* Seen in immunocompromised patients. Viral cytopathic effect includes intracytoplasmic and/or intranuclear inclusions seen in endothelial cells, histiocytes, or fibroblasts.

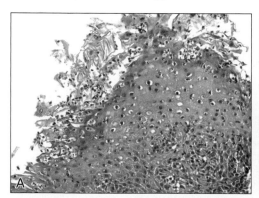
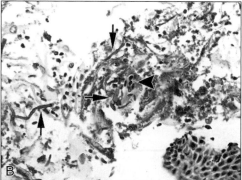

**Figure 8-3.** Photomicrographs of (**A**) *Candida* esophagitis. Note the erosion in the upper layers of squamous mucosa with neutrophilic infiltrate forming microabscesses. H&E stain. (**B**) Yeast (*arrowhead*) and pseudohyphae (*arrows*) highlighted by periodic acid–Schiff stain.

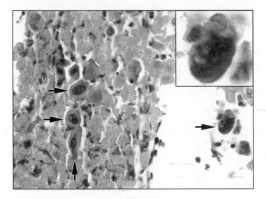

**Figure 8-4.** Photomicrograph of herpes esophagitis. Note the multinucleated cells with molding (*arrows*) and smudged eosinophilic viral inclusions (*inset*). H&E stain.

### 4. What is the most important differential to be considered in biopsy samples to evaluate graft-versus-host disease (GVHD)?

Infectious etiologies must be ruled out with the use of special stains (fungal and viral) and with serology and tissue culture examinations. In general, the upper esophagus is usually affected.

- **Histology:** GVHD is graded as mild, moderate, or severe, based on the degree of damage seen. Apoptotic bodies are seen in the squamous epithelium; there are intraepithelial lymphocytes and basal vacuolization and, in severe cases, ulceration/necrosis.

### 5. What is the histologic prevalence of esophageal Crohn's disease in endoscopically normal studies?

Histologic prevalence varies from 5% to 42% and does not correlate with endoscopic findings. Crohn's esophagitis may be seen with severe cases of ileocolic disease.

- **Histology:** Features vary from mild inflammation with epithelioid non-necrotizing granulomas in the lamina propria to ulcerations and transmural involvement with fistula formation.

### 6. What are other miscellaneous esophageal conditions?

#### GLYCOGEN ACANTHOSIS

- **Endoscopy:** Small, white-gray plaques in the midesophagus. There is an association with Cowden syndrome.
- **Histology:** Squamous cells are distended with increased intracellular glycogen.

#### GASTRIC INLET PATCH

- **Endoscopy:** Patch (2 mm to 3 cm) of gastric-appearing mucosa located just below the cricopharyngeus muscle.
- **Histology:** Consists of oxyntic (parietal)-type mucosa. Intestinal metaplasia may be found.

#### PANCREATIC HETEROTOPIA

- **Endoscopy:** Often not apparent to the eye. This tissue is often seen in biopsy samples at the GE junction or distal esophagus. It may represent metaplasia or ectopic foci of pancreatic tissue.
- **Histology:** Acinar cells with dense, coarse eosinophilic granules are seen.

#### MELANOSIS

- **Endoscopy:** Tiny 1- to 2-mm brown-black spots. Melanocytes may be seen in the basal layer of squamous epithelium. The differential diagnosis is malignant melanoma. The melanocytes in melanosis are benign appearing and mature. Pigment can be seen in upper layers of mucosa and in the adjacent lamina propria.

### 7. List the dermatologic conditions that can affect the esophagus.

Pemphigus vulgaris, bullous pemphigoid, erythema multiforme, Behçet syndrome, lichen planus, dermatitis herpetiformis, scleroderma, and toxic epidermolysis necrosis.

### 8. Discuss the histology of Barrett's esophagus and the grading of dysplasia.

- **Definition:** An endoscopic change in esophageal epithelium of any length, confirmed to have intestinal metaplasia at biopsy (American College of Gastroenterology).
- **Histology:** Normal squamocolumnar junctional mucosa (Fig. 8-1*B*) shows squamous epithelium adjacent to foveolar epithelium. Intestinal metaplasia is recognized by the presence of goblet cells (Fig. 8-5*A*), which stain blue with Alcian blue stain at pH 2.5 (Fig. 8-5*B*).

## Grading Dysplasia in Barrett's Esophagus

*None:* There is no evidence of dysplasia.

*Indefinite for dysplasia:* This grading is assigned when distinction cannot be made between low-grade dysplasia and inflammatory changes. The surface epithelium shows maturation, but the deeper glands show architectural crowding, nuclear hyperchromasia, and occasionally increased mitotic activity.

*Low-grade dysplasia* (Fig. 8-5*C*): Lack of surface maturation and glandular epithelium shows amphophilic cytoplasm with mucin depletion and nuclear hyperchromasia. Architectural crowding is similar to that seen in colonic tubular adenomas.

*High-grade dysplasia:* Lack of surface maturation with cells showing marked cytologic atypia characterized by loss of polarity, high nuclear-to-cytoplasm ratio, irregular nuclear contours, and prominent large nucleoli. The architecture becomes complex with focal areas of cribriforming. Cytologic abnormalities supersede architectural complexity in diagnosing high-grade dysplasia.

*High-grade dysplasia with invasion or intramucosal carcinoma—T1* (Fig. 8-5*D*): Invasion into the lamina propria/muscularis mucosae has prognostic implications in the esophagus unlike in the colon, because of presence of lymphatics in the former. Lymph node metastasis has been reported in 13% of T1 tumors. Duplication of muscularis mucosae can at times be present and should not be mistaken for invasion into the submucosa.

**9. What histologic patterns can be seen in the biopsy samples from the GE junction that do not show typical endoscopic findings of Barrett's esophagus?**
- Gastric-type mucosa without goblet cells—Gastric cardiac mucosa, mostly associated with inflammation (gastric carditis)
- Prominent Z-line showing gastric-cardiac mucosa with goblet cells
- In endoscopically uncertain cases, presence of goblet cells may suggest either Barrett mucosa or gastric cardia with goblet cells.

**10. What is the differential diagnosis of esophageal polypoid lesions?**

## Non-Neoplastic

- Pancreatic heterotopia/metaplasia
  Usually seen at distal esophagus.
  - **Histology:** Pancreatic acinar cells are seen rarely associated with ductal structures.

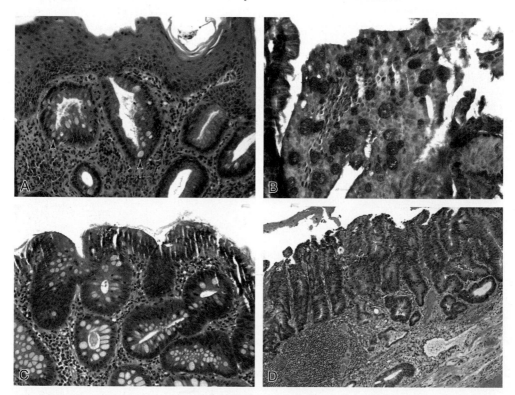

**Figure 8-5.** Photomicrographs of Barrett esophagus (**A**) Intestinal metaplasia is recognized by the presence of goblet cells (*arrows*) in the glandular epithelium. H&E stain. (**B**) Alcian blue stain at pH 2.5 stains the acidic mucin of goblet cells *blue*. (**C**) Barrett's esophagus with low-grade dysplasia. There is lack of surface maturation and the glandular epithelium shows nuclear stratification with hyperchromasia. H&E stain. (**D**) Barrett's esophagus with high-grade dysplasia and invasion into the lamina propria (intramucosal carcinoma) seen next to the lymphoid aggregate. H&E stain.

- Fibrovascular polyp
  Benign, submucosal (fibrovascular and adipose) tissue surrounded by squamous epithelium. Occasionally, atypical stromal cells may be seen.
- Squamous papilloma
  Not uncommon in the esophagus.
  - **Histology:** Lobulated squamous epithelium with fibrovascular cores. Seen in less than 0.1% of endoscopic examinations. Dysplasia is not usually seen. These have been related to human papilloma virus (HPV). Reports also show that most are seen as a result of acid reflux and are not associated with human papillomavirus (HPV). Those that show the presence of HPV are often associated with laryngeal squamous papillomas.

*(handwritten margin notes: PC, FVP, SqP, GCT, LM, GIST, SqCC, Adeno, Melanoma)*

## NEOPLASMS

- *Granular cell tumor:* The esophagus is the most common site in the gastrointestinal (GI) tract, while the most common site in the body is lingual dorsum.
  - **Endoscopy:** Submucosal nodule mostly solitary (multifocal in 10%).
  - **Histology:** Pseudo-epitheliomatous hyperplasia of overlying squamous mucosa is seen with submucosal collection of neoplastic granular cells with granular eosinophilic cytoplasm (Fig. 8-6*A*), which are PAS and S100 reactive (Fig. 8-6*B*). Most are benign; rare cases of malignant metastasis have been reported.
- *Leiomyoma:* Submucosal benign proliferation of spindled smooth muscle cells. Strongly react with muscle markers like smooth muscle actin (SMA) and desmin and are negative for CD117. Its malignant counterpart, leiomyosarcoma, is rare in the esophagus.
- *Gastrointestinal stromal tumor (GIST):* Rare in the esophagus.
  - **Histology:** Shows proliferation of spindle cells that react strongly with CD117 and CD34. Malignant potential depends on the extent of mitotic activity, necrosis, and cytologic atypia.
- *Squamous cell carcinoma* (Fig. 8-7): Midesophagus is the common location.
  - **Histology:** Neoplastic squamous cells with intercellular bridges and keratin overproduction with keratin pearl formation are seen. Involvement of mediastinal structures is common because of a lack of serosal barrier. Subtypes include basaloid squamous cell carcinoma, verrucous carcinoma, and adenosquamous carcinoma.
- *Adenocarcinoma* (Fig. 8-8): Distal esophagus is the common location, if found in midesophagus, usually as a result of Barrett's esophagus. Variants include mucinous and signet ring cell type. The depth of tumor (superficial versus deep) invasion correlates with tumor stage and prognosis. Lymph node metastasis has been reported in 13% of T1 tumors. The presence of lymphovascular invasion predicts worse overall survival and more tumor recurrence and is an independent prognostic factor.
- *Malignant melanoma:* Esophageal melanomas are rare and often larger polypoid lesions involving distal esophagus. Marked cytologic atypia with prominent nucleoli and increased mitotic figures are seen. Malignant cells may show reactivity with one or more of the following antibodies; S100, Melan A, KBA-62, and HMB-45.
- *Other malignant tumors:* Metastatic small cell and sarcomatoid carcinomas are rare.

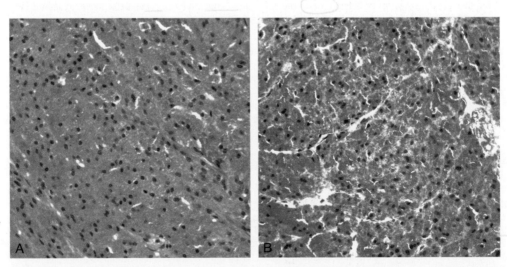

**Figure 8-6.** Photomicrographs of granular cell tumor. (**A**) Note the abundant granular cytoplasm and small round nuclei H&E stain and (**B**) S100 staining in the cytoplasm.

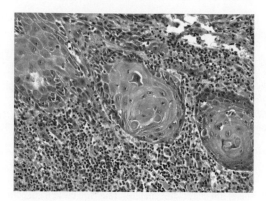

**Figure 8-7.** Photomicrograph of squamous cell carcinoma. Note the infiltrating markedly atypical squamous cell nests, stromal response, and focal keratin pearl formation. H&E stain.

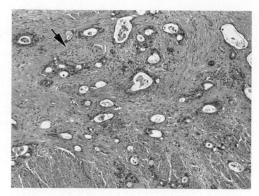

**Figure 8-8.** Photomicrograph of esophageal adenocarcinoma showing infiltrating neoplastic glands with perineural invasion (*arrow*). H&E stain.

## STOMACH

**11. What are the histologic features of the mucosal lining in different parts of the stomach?**
The five layers of the stomach are the:

- **Mucosa**
- **Muscularis mucosae**
- **Submucosa**
- **Muscularis propria** (innermost oblique, inner circular, and outermost longitudinal layer)
- **Serosa**

The mucosa has three zones that vary by function in different locations of the stomach.

**Superficial layer of neutral mucin** secreting foveolar epithelium lines the entire luminal surface of the stomach followed by the isthmus/neck and deep glandular layer.

**Fundus** and **body mucosa** have similar features and contain pyramid-shaped parietal or oxyntic (acid-secreting and intrinsic factor–producing) cells and the chief cells (enzyme producing) in the isthmus/neck and base with scattered endocrine cells. The lining foveolar layer is short. The isthmus/neck also contains mucus-secreting cells.

**Cardia** and **antrum** have similar features and have a broad, superficial zone of foveolar epithelial cells. The gastric antrum also contains gastrin-secreting G cells. The other enteroendocrine cells have been shown to secrete serotonin, somatostatin (D cells), and vasointestinal polypeptide–like (VIP) substance.

**12. What are the histologic patterns of gastritis?**
Two major histologic patterns of gastritis
- **Acute gastritis**—Acute onset. Neutrophilic inflammation, edema, and hemorrhage—any or all of these may be seen. Associated with hemorrhage or erosions/ulceration.
- **Chronic gastritis with or without activity**—Mixed inflammation with predominant mononuclear cell infiltration and foveolar hyperplasia, with or without intestinal metaplasia and atrophy. Activity can be graded based on the extent of acute inflammation present (e.g., mild, moderate, or severe).

**13. What are the various histologic manifestations of *Helicobacter pylori*–associated gastritis?**
Changes may vary from acute to chronic injury patterns: chronic gastritis, chronic active gastritis, multifocal atrophic gastritis, follicular gastritis, ulcers, adenocarcinoma, and mucosa-associated lymphoid tissue (MALT) lymphoma. *H. pylori* organisms are gram-negative, urease-producing, seagull-shaped, curved organisms (Fig. 8-9) that are seen adherent to the superficial foveolar epithelium, entangled in the mucus. These are also seen in the lumens lined by parietal cells. Warthin-Starry (silver stain), Giemsa, Thiazine B, and Diff-Quick are special stains that highlight *H. pylori*. The immunohistochemistry may be helpful in detecting coccoid forms seen in treated gastritis and differentiating it from other causes of gastritis.

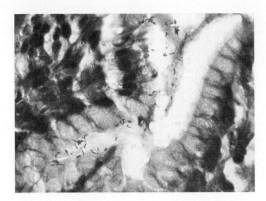

**Figure 8-9.** Photomicrograph of *Helicobacter pylori*. Note the curved, seagull-shaped forms on the epithelial surface (Giemsa stain).

↓ Parietal
↑ ECL
↑ G cell

**14. What is *Helicobacter heilmannii*–associated gastritis?**

*H. heilmannii* (*Gastrospirillum hominis*) is a rare, long, tightly coiled gram-negative, urease-producing bacteria that causes gastritis of mild severity.

**15. What are the types of chronic atrophic gastritis, and how do these differ histologically?**

### AUTOIMMUNE GASTRITIS: TYPE A GASTRITIS

- **Endoscopy:** Typically affects body/fundus
- **Histology:** Advanced disease shows gastric body/fundus mucosa with full-thickness intense chronic inflammation, loss of oxyntic glands with intestinal metaplasia (Fig. 8-10*A*), and hyperplasia (linear or nodular) of enterochromaffin cell-like (ECL) cell (chromogranin stain; Fig. 8-10*B*. Pyloric antrum shows G-cell hyperplasia. Early disease is difficult to diagnose histologically and is indicated by inflammation in the deep glandular layer with antral metaplasia and ECL-cell hyperplasia.

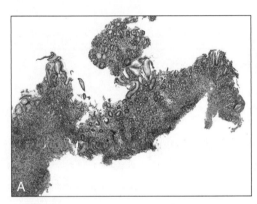

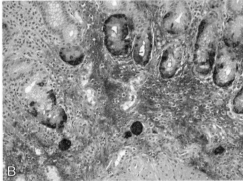

**Figure 8-10.** Photomicrographs of (**A**) Chronic atrophic gastritis. Dense chronic inflammatory infiltrate in the lamina propria and with surface erosions. This biopsy from fundus shows *antral-type* epithelium. There is a loss of parietal cells. H&E stain. (**B**) Chronic atrophic gastritis, *chromogranin stain*, highlights the enterochromaffin cell–like (ECL) cell hyperplasia, both linear and nodular.

### ENVIRONMENTAL GASTRITIS: TYPE B GASTRITIS

- **Endoscopy:** Typically involvement of antrum; body of stomach if severe.
- **Histology:** In the initial stage, chronic inflammatory infiltrate is seen in the superficial zone; the later stages are marked with atrophy and metaplasia.
- **Etiologies:** Associated with *H. pylori*, lack of vitamin C, nitrosamines, and increased salt intake.

**16. What are the salient histologic features of chemical/reactive gastropathy?**

- **Histology:** Foveolar hyperplasia with glandular tortuosity, edema in lamina propria, dilated superficial vessels, vertical muscle fibers in lamina propria, and minimal inflammation (Fig. 8-11).
- **Etiologies:** Nonsteroidal anti-inflammatory drugs (NSAIDs), alcohol, and alkaline reflux (bile).

**17. What is lymphocytic gastritis, and with which disease processes is it associated?**

- **Location:** Fundus and body of stomach, but antrum affected in celiac disease.
- **Histology:** Chronic gastritis pattern with increased intraepithelial lymphocytes. IEL
- **Etiologies:** Celiac disease and *H. pylori* infection are most common. Less common etiologies include varioliform gastritis, lymphocytic gastroenterocolitis, human immunodeficiency virus (HIV) infection, and lymphoma.

## 18. What is the differential diagnosis of granulomatous gastritis?

- **Histology:** Granulomas may be necrotizing or non-necrotizing.
- **Etiologies:** Infectious (tuberculous, fungal), Crohn's disease, sarcoid, drug reaction, vasculitis, or idiopathic (isolated granulomatous gastritis).

## 19. What are the histologic features suggestive of gastric Crohn's disease?

The biopsies show patchy involvement of gastric mucosa by acute and chronic inflammation and pit abscesses (focally active gastritis) with intervening areas of normal mucosa (Fig. 8-12). Occasionally, granulomas can be seen. Although difficult to diagnose in the absence of granulomas, these histologic features may suggest Crohn's disease.

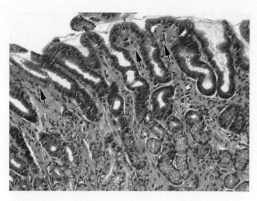

**Figure 8-11.** Photomicrograph of chemical/reactive gastropathy. Note the foveolar hyperplasia, glandular tortuosity, ectatic vessels in the lamina propria (*arrow*), and minimal inflammation. H&E stain.

## 20. Histologically, how do you differentiate gastric antral vascular ectasia (GAVE), portal hypertensive gastropathy, Dieulafoy lesion, and radiation injury?

### GASTRIC ANTRAL VASCULAR ECTASIA

- **Endoscopy:** Red longitudinal stripes usually located in the antrum of the stomach, often referred to as "watermelon stomach."
- **Histology:** Dilated congested vessels, fibrin thrombi and reactive changes like foveolar hyperplasia, strands of muscle fibers in lamina propria.

### PORTAL HYPERTENSIVE GASTROPATHY

- **Endoscopy:** *Tiger skin* pattern of dilated mucosal vessels seen in body and fundus of stomach.
- **Histology:** Biopsy not recommended. Features include dilated ectatic vessels, foveolar hyperplasia, and fibrosis in the lamina propria with minimal inflammation. The lack of fibrin thrombi can distinguish this from GAVE.

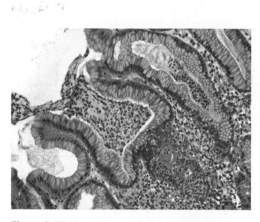

**Figure 8-12.** Photomicrograph of gastric Crohn's disease. Note the neutrophilic infiltrate within the crypt lumens (focally active gastritis). H&E stain.

### DIEULAFOY LESION

- **Endoscopy:** Usually, a *pigmented protuberant vessel* in proximal stomach without mucosal ulceration.
- **Histology:** Abnormal large artery in superficial submucosa, which may erode and cause massive hemorrhage. The histologic features include erosion with fibrin and hemorrhage, and a large vessel in the submucosa.

### RADIATION INJURY

- **Endoscopy:** Numerous mucosal red vascular ectasias located in the radiation port.
- **Histology:** Dilated vessels with hyalinized walls. The epithelial and stromal cells show marked atypia, raising the suspicion of dysplasia. Clinical history is important to rule out other causes of angiectasias like GAVE and portal hypertensive gastropathy.

## 21. What are the histologic features of giant mucosal folds seen in Ménétrier disease and Zöllinger-Ellison syndrome?

- **Endoscopy:** Enlarged gastric folds greater than 8 mm.
- **Histology:** The giant folds are due to hyperplasia of foveolar epithelium or oxyntic epithelium. Ménétrier disease resembles hyperplastic polyp and shows elongated hyperplastic foveolar epithelium with loss of oxyntic glands in the gastric mucosa. Expansion of oxyntic glandular zone resulting in hypertrophic gastropathy is seen in Zöllinger-Ellison syndrome. Large folds can also be seen in *H. pylori*–associated gastritis.

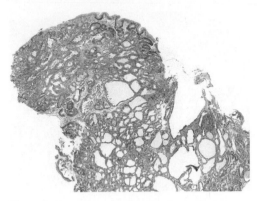

**Figure 8-13.** Photomicrograph of fundic gland polyp showing dilated oxyntic glands. H&E stain.

## 22. What are the histologic features of gastric polyps/polypoid lesions?

### FUNDIC GLAND POLYP

- **Endoscopy:** Located in the fundus and body of stomach. Can be sporadic or seen with familial adenomatous polyposis (FAP).
- **Histology:** Dilated oxyntic glands are seen (Fig. 8-13). The overlying foveolar epithelium is normal or occasionally shows hyperplastic change. Dysplasia is extremely rare in sporadic ones.

### HYPERPLASTIC POLYP

- **Endoscopy:** Usually, a sessile polyp is located in the antrum
- **Histology:** Hyperplastic, dilated foveolar glands within inflamed and edematous lamina propria, often with surface erosions and/or ulceration. The adjacent mucosa generally shows chronic gastritis. Rarely, dysplasia may be seen in these polyps, and rarely these may be present next to an adenocarcinoma. Hyperplastic morphology is seen in the polyps of Cronkhite-Canada syndrome, Ménétrier disease, juvenile polyps, and gastritis cystica profunda (in the postgastrectomy stomach). Isolated gastric hyperplastic polyps are not associated with polyps in the small intestine or colon.

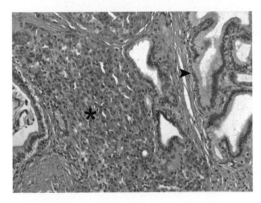

**Figure 8-14.** Photomicrograph of pancreatic heterotopia. Note the acinar cells with dense eosinophilic zymogen granules (*asterisk*) and small ducts lined by cuboidal cells (*arrowhead*). H&E stain.

### PEUTZ-JEGHER POLYP

- **Endoscopy:** Throughout the upper GI tract; more common in the small intestine.
- **Histology:** In the stomach, foveolar hyperplasia is seen prominently with minimal or no inflammation in the lamina propria. Arborizing smooth muscle pattern in the lamina propria is less common at this site.

### PANCREATIC HETEROTOPIA/METAPLASIA

- **Endoscopy:** Most commonly located in the antrum; appearance is that of a submucosal nodule with a central depression ("volcano" lesion).
- **Histology:** It shows ectopic pancreatic acini, ducts, and occasionally islet cells (30%) in varying proportions (Fig. 8-14).

### GASTRIC XANTHOMA

- **Endoscopy:** Flat yellow lesion discovered as an incidental finding.
- **Histology:** Benign collection of lipid containing macrophages in the lamina propria. These have been associated with bile reflux, postgastrectomy stomach, and patients with cholestasis.

### GASTRIC ADENOMA

This is discussed next.

## 23. Compare gastric dysplasia and adenoma.

*Gastric dysplasia* is referred to a flat lesion showing dysplasia (*flat adenoma*). A similar lesion with a polypoid appearance is referred to as an *adenoma*, which consists of tubular, or tubulovillous, architecture. Figure 8-15 depicts a gastric adenoma showing strong immunoreactivity with p53 antibody. The flat lesion is more likely to be multifocal and associated with high-grade dysplasia. Mapping biopsies are required to rule out invasive carcinoma in both. The adenomas can be of intestinal-type (goblet/Paneth cells) or gastric-type morphology. Adenocarcinoma is more commonly associated with intestinal-type morphology. Table 8-1 depicts Vienna classification of gastrointestinal epithelial neoplasia.

### 24. What are the histologic types of gastric adenocarcinoma?

The World Health Organization (WHO) classification describes four histologic patterns:

1. **Tubular**
2. **Papillary**
3. **Mucinous**
4. **Signet ring cell carcinoma**

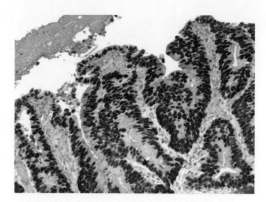

**Figure 8-15.** Photomicrograph of gastric adenoma showing strong nuclear immunoreactivity with p53 antibody. Immunohistochemical stain.

**Table 8-1.** Vienna Classification of Gastrointestinal Epithelial Neoplasia

| | |
|---|---|
| Category 1 | Negative for neoplasia/dysplasia |
| Category 2 | Indefinite for neoplasia/dysplasia |
| Category 3 | Noninvasive low-grade neoplasia (low-grade adenoma/dysplasia) |
| Category 4 | Noninvasive high-grade neoplasia<br>4.1 High-grade adenoma/dysplasia<br>4.2 Noninvasive carcinoma (carcinoma in situ)<br>4.3 Suspicion of invasive carcinoma |
| Category 5 | Invasive neoplasia<br>5.1 Intramucosal carcinoma*<br>5.2 Submucosal carcinoma or beyond |

*Intramucosal carcinoma implies invasion into the lamina propria or muscularis mucosae.
From Schlemper RJ, Riddell RH, Kato Y, et al: The Vienna classification of gastrointestinal epithelial neoplasia. Gut 47:251–255, 2000.

The Laurén system classifies gastric carcinomas into two subtypes:

1. **Intestinal** type (arising in the background of intestinal metaplasia)
2. **Diffuse** type (includes signet ring cell type) (Fig. 8-16)

Rare variants include adenosquamous carcinoma, squamous cell carcinoma, and undifferentiated carcinoma.

### 25. What is the histologic classification of neuroendocrine neoplasms of the stomach?

- **Carcinoid** (well-differentiated neuroendocrine neoplasm)
- **Small-cell carcinoma** (poorly differentiated neuroendocrine neoplasms)
- **Large-cell neuroendocrine neoplasms**

The carcinoids can further be subclassified as:

1. *Enterochromaffin cell-like (ECL) cell carcinoid* associated with autoimmune chronic atrophic gastritis; hypergastrinemia is due to increased gastrin production in the antrum.
2. *Carcinoid tumors* associated with MEN I or Zöllinger-Ellison syndrome.
3. *Sporadic* not associated with hypergastrinemia or autoimmune chronic atrophic gastritis; usually aggressive than the other two.

Aggressive behavior in carcinoids is associated with size greater than 1 cm, invasion of muscularis propria, increased mitotic activity, and angioinvasion.

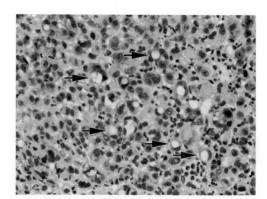

**Figure 8-16.** Photomicrograph of gastric adenocarcinoma with signet ring cell morphology (*arrows*). H&E stain.

## 26. What is the differential diagnosis of gastric stromal tumors?

These are seen as submucosal masses and the differential diagnosis includes schwannoma, leiomyoma, GIST, and inflammatory fibroid polyps. The morphology is similar to that seen in other sites.

*[handwritten notes: Carc, Schw, GIST, LM, IFP]*

## GASTROINTESTINAL STROMAL TUMORS

The most common site in the GI tract is the stomach (50%), followed by the small bowel (25%), the colon and rectum (10%), and the esophagus (5%). Histologically, these can be spindled or epitheloid and show strong reactivity with CD117 (95%) and positive staining with CD34 (60% to 70%). Around one third can also show reactivity with smooth muscle markers (smooth muscle actin). These arise from interstitial cells of Cajal, and *kit* mutations are seen in 85% to 90% of GISTs. Approximately 5% show mutation within the *PDGFRA* gene, and these are seen in gastric GISTs and have epitheloid morphology and a less aggressive clinical course. All the GISTs are potentially aggressive. The clinical behavior can be predicted on the basis of size, mitotic figures, and site. Gastric GISTs have a better prognosis than the small bowel GISTs. The GISTs with exon 11 mutation have a low risk for progressive disease (as opposed to exon 9 mutation) and respond better to imatinib mesylate in the metastatic disease setting.

*[handwritten notes: gleevec   2nd line sunitinib (sutent);   >10cm   >10 MF   5+5]*

## INFLAMMATORY FIBROID POLYPS

Bland spindle cells accentuated around vessels and accompanied by a mixed inflammatory infiltrate in the stroma. These are negative for CD117 and may show immunoreactivity with CD34.

## 27. What are the different types of gastric lymphoma?

MALT lymphomas (also known as extramarginal zone B-cell lymphoma) are low grade and show lymphoepithelial lesions (lymphoma cells infiltrating the gland epithelium). They extend deep into the muscularis mucosae, unlike reactive lymphoid hyperplasia, which is generally more superficial and a major differential diagnosis in these cases. These cells are CD20 (B-cell marker) positive, may coexpress CD43, and are CD5 negative, CD10 negative and positive for bcl-2 protein. *Helicobacter* organisms may be seen. Distinction between reactive infiltrate versus neoplastic can be difficult in small biopsy specimens. Flow cytometry and cytogenetics are other useful studies. Gene rearrangement studies generally help determine the clonality in atypical lymphoid aggregates.

The other lymphomas that can involve the GI tract include mantle cell lymphoma, large B-cell lymphoma, enteropathy-like T-cell lymphoma, and Burkitt lymphoma.

## ACKNOWLEDGMENTS

Special thanks are given to Lisa Litzenberger for her superb photographic technical assistance.

## WEBSITES 🌐

http://www.pathologyoutlines.com/esophaguspf.html

http://library.med.utah.edu/WebPath/webpath.html#MENU

http://www.path.uiowa.edu/virtualslidebox/nlm_histology/content_index_db.html

## BIBLIOGRAPHY

1. Abraham SC, Krasinskas AM, Correa AM, et al. Duplication of muscularis mucosae in Barrett's esophagus: An underrecognized feature and its implications for staging of adenocarcinoma. Am J Surg Pathol 2007;31:1719–25.
2. Carr NJ, Monihan JM, Sobin LH. Squamous cell papilloma of the esophagus: A clinicopathologic and follow-up study of 25 cases. Am J Gastroenterol 1994;98:245.
3. Choudhry U, Boyce HW Jr, Coppola D. Proton pump inhibitor-associated gastric polyps: A retrospective analysis of their frequency, and endoscopic, histologic, and ultrastructural characteristics. Am J Clin Pathol 1998;110:615.
4. Demetri GD, Benjamin RS, Blanke CD, et al. NCCN Task Force report: Management of patients with gastrointestinal stromal tumor (GIST)—Update of the NCCN clinical practice guidelines. JNCCN 2007;5(Suppl. 2):S1–29.

5. Fenoglio-Presiser C, Carneiro F, Correa P, et al. WHO Classification of Tumors: Pathology and Genetics of the Digestive System. Lyon: IARC Press; 2000. p. 43–9.

6. Issacson PG, Muller-Hermelink HK, Piris MA, et al. WHO Classification of Tumors: Tumors of Hematopoietic and Lymphoid Tissues. Lyon: IARC Press; 2001. p. 157–60.

7. Liu L, Hofsetter WL, Rashid A, et al. Significance of depth of tumor invasion and lymph node metastases in superficially invasive esophageal adenocarcinoma. Am J Surg Pathol 2005;29:1079–85.

8. Miettinen M, Lasota J. Gastrointestinal stromal tumors: Pathology and prognosis at different sites. Semin Diagn Pathol 2006;23:111–9.

9. Montgomery EA. Biopsy Interpretation of the Gastrointestinal Tract Mucosa. Philadelphia: Lippincott Williams & Wilkins; 2006.

10. Mosca S, Manes G, Monaco R, et al. Squamous papilloma of the esophagus: Long-term follow up. J Gastroenterol Hepatol 2001;16:857.

11. Noffsinger A, Fenoglio-Presiser C, Maru D, et al. Gastrointestinal Diseases—Atlas of Nontumor Pathology, first series. Washington DC: American Registry of Pathology in collaboration with Armed Forces Institute of Pathology; 2007. p. 104–11,138–51.

12. Oberhuber G, Puspok A, Oesterreicher C, et al. Focally enhanced gastritis: A frequent type of gastritis in patients with Crohn's disease. Gastroenterology 1997;112:698–706.

13. Prasad GA, Buttar NS, Wongkeesong LM, et al. Significance of neoplastic involvement of margins obtained by endoscopic mucosal resection in Barrett's esophagus. Am J Gastroenterol 2007;102:2380–6.

14. Schlemper RJ, Riddell RH, Kato Y, et al. The Vienna classification of gastrointestinal epithelial neoplasia. Gut 2000;47:251–5.

# GASTRITIS

*Selvi Thirumurthi, MD, MS, and*
*Frank L. Lanza, MD, FACG*

## 1. What is gastritis?

Gastritis is inflammation of the gastric mucosa best appreciated on histologic examination. The diagnosis can also be made based on the endoscopic appearance of the stomach. Certain types of gastritis may require the use of endoscopic ultrasound (Ménétrier disease) or serologic studies (chronic autoimmune gastritis) to confirm the diagnosis.

## 2. What are the symptoms of gastritis?

Patients are often diagnosed with gastritis based on their clinical features; however, this correlates poorly with actual endoscopic or histologic findings. Patients can be asymptomatic or may complain of epigastric discomfort or burning pain, postprandial fullness, or nausea. These symptoms can also be seen in other upper gastrointestinal (GI) disorders, such as biliary tract disease, gastric neoplasm, gastroesophageal reflux disease (GERD), or gastroparesis. These diagnoses need to be excluded before symptoms can be attributed to gastritis.

## 3. How is gastritis classified?

The histologic appearance of gastric mucosa determines if gastritis is classified as chronic or reactive. Chronic gastritis (commonly caused by *Helicobacter pylori* infection) is reported more often than reactive (or *acute*) gastritis (caused by aspirin or nonsteroidal anti-inflammatory drug [NSAID] use). Table 9-1 lists other causes of chronic and reactive gastritis.

## 4. What is the endoscopic and histologic appearance of reactive and chronic gastritis?

The endoscopic changes of reactive gastritis are quite characteristic. Areas of hemorrhage may be seen throughout the stomach, and erosions are commonly found in the antrum. Erosions are superficial white-based flat lesions surrounded by a margin of intense erythema. The intervening mucosa is usually normal or simply erythematous. Continued use of the offending agent leads to an increase in the number of erosive lesions and may result in ulcer formation. The mucosa can also become more erythematous, friable, and granular in appearance, and resemble chronic gastritis.

Reactive epithelial changes called foveolar hyperplasia can be seen on histologic examination along with an increased number of smooth muscle fibers in the lamina propria. Erosions appear as focal necrosis to the level of the muscularis mucosa. An acute inflammatory cell infiltrate is not seen; thus, the term *reactive gastritis* rather than *acute gastritis* is used.

The endoscopic appearance of chronic gastritis due to *H. pylori* may be normal or consist of red streaks in the antrum. Biopsy will reveal a chronic inflammatory infiltrate including neutrophils as well as reactive epithelial changes and lymphoid follicles. The bacteria are seen lying in the superficial mucus layer and can be seen on routine hematoxylin and eosin (H&E) stain. Chronic *H. pylori* infection may lead to atrophic changes in the stomach with endoscopy showing a mucosa with a visible vascular pattern, primarily in the fundus, and flattening of the usual rugal folds. These changes may also be seen in autoimmune gastritis due to antiparietal cell and anti–intrinsic factor antibodies resulting in destruction of fundic glands.

**Table 9-1.** Classification of Gastritis

| ACUTE GASTRITIS | CHRONIC GASTRITIS |
|---|---|
| Toxic agents: | *Helicobacter pylori* |
| • Nonsteroidal anti-inflammatory drugs including cyclooxygenase-2 inhibitors and aspirin | Autoimmune |
| • Bisphosphonates | Nonspecific |
| • Potassium | Lymphocytic |
| • Macrolides | Bile reflux |
| • Alcohol | Ménétrier disease |
| Stress | Eosinophilic |
| Viruses | Granulomatous |
| Bacteria | |

**Table 9-2.** Risk Factors for Complications of Acute Nonsteroidal Anti-inflammatory Drug (NSAID)-Related Gastritis

- Prior history of ulcer or upper gastrointestinal bleeding
- Age >65 years
- High-dose NSAID therapy, especially in low–body weight patients
- Concurrent use of other gastrotoxic agents, including a second NSAID or low-dose aspirin

- Anticoagulants
- Corticosteroids
- *Helicobacter pylori*
- Debilitation

**5. How do we treat reactive gastritis, and what can be done to prevent it?**

The most common cause of reactive gastritis is NSAID use. In most cases, cessation of the offending agent leads to rapid normalization of the gastric mucosa. However, in many patients, especially high-risk individuals (Table 9-2), NSAID gastritis can progress to gastric ulcers with a risk of perforation and hemorrhage. If NSAID therapy must be continued in these high-risk patients, concomitant treatment with misoprostol (100 to 200 μg 4 times a day) or daily proton pump inhibitors (PPIs) should be initiated.

Cyclooxygenase (COX) is an enzyme involved in prostaglandin synthesis. COX-1 is important in gastric cytoprotection, and COX-2 is an inducible isoform involved in inflammation. Traditional NSAIDs can affect both COX-1 and COX-2 and have varying potential to harm gastric mucosa. In the late 1990s, several selective COX-2 inhibitors were approved by the U.S. Food and Drug Administration for the treatment of arthritis, with the intent of decreasing gastric toxicity. There is evidence that low-dose aspirin, when taken concurrently with a COX-2 inhibitor, increases the level of gastric toxicity to that of nonselective NSAIDs, thereby losing any protective effect. Given the adverse cardiovascular complications with long-term use, all but one COX-2 inhibitor has been withdrawn from the market. Cotherapy with misoprostol or PPI should be given to high-risk patients on COX-2 inhibitors.

The reactive gastritis seen with use of bisphosphonates, potassium supplements, and macrolide antibiotics is usually mild and limited to the duration of the use of these agents, rarely leading to complications. Alcoholic gastritis can be accompanied by upper GI hemorrhage, but bleeding is more often related to portal hypertensive gastropathy seen when these patients develop cirrhosis.

**6. What are the characteristics of stress gastritis, and how should it be treated?**

Stress gastritis usually occurs in the intensive care unit (ICU) in patients requiring mechanical ventilation and those with coagulopathy, renal failure, central nervous system injury, severe burns, or sepsis. Stress gastritis may develop into frank ulcers leading to hemorrhage or perforation. Prophylactic agents that include $H_2$ blockers, sucralfate, and intravenous PPI may reduce the risk of stress gastritis. PPIs however are able to raise the gastric pH to effective levels to prevent stress gastritis (pH > 4 for 24 hours). This degree of acid inhibition inactivates the proteolytic enzyme pepsin and prevents mucosal injury.

**7. What is the most common etiology of chronic gastritis?**

By far, the most common cause of chronic gastritis is *H. pylori* infection. The prevalence of *H. pylori* infection varies around the world. In developing countries, infection is acquired early in life with 80% of individuals infected by early adulthood. Studies have demonstrated higher prevalence rates among individuals with a lower socioeconomic status during childhood. In developed countries, a pattern of increasing prevalence with age has been described. Although *H. pylori* infection has been linked with a variety of GI and non-GI conditions, the majority of infected individuals remain asymptomatic.

**8. How is chronic gastritis secondary to *H. pylori* infection diagnosed?**

The diagnosis of *H. pylori* gastritis can be made by gastric biopsy or by serology. Biopsy samples obtained at endoscopy can be sent to pathology for routine (H&E) or special staining (Giemsa or Warthin-Starry stains) to visualize the organisms. *H. pylori* can be grown and isolated in culture media. Although considered the gold standard, this is unnecessary unless antibiotic resistance is suspected. Gastric specimens can also be tested with a rapid bedside kit (CLO test, Kimberly-Clark Healthcare). *H. pylori* produce urease, which converts urea to ammonia, raising the pH of the milieu. The CLO test contains a gel that changes color in an alkaline environment, indicating the presence of a urease-producing organism.

Patients will have IgG antibodies against *H. pylori* when chronically infected. IgA antibodies are found in some patients who are IgG negative, and IgM antibodies are found early in the course of infection. Antibody titers will remain elevated for months after eradication treatment and cure of the infection. Therefore, this is a reliable indicator in patients who have not previously been treated for *H. pylori* infection. *H. pylori* has been designated a group I carcinogen by the World Health Organization. Once a physician has detected *H. pylori* infection, he or she must prescribe eradication therapy and follow up with a test of cure. This may include a stool *H. pylori* antigen test or the urea breath test.

For the urea breath test, the patient is given radiolabeled urea to ingest. If the patient is infected with *H. pylori*, urease will convert this urea to labeled carbon dioxide, which will be exhaled by the patient. The urea breath test can be used as a diagnostic tool or as a test of cure with a high degree of specificity and sensitivity. Patients must wait 4 weeks after completion of antibiotic therapy and refrain from PPI use for 2 weeks before testing.

**9. How is chronic gastritis secondary to *H. pylori* infection treated?**

*H. pylori* infection is treated with antibiotics combined with acid suppression for 14 days. Quadruple therapy with bismuth subsalicylate, tetracycline, metronidazole, and PPI therapy is 90% effective in eradication. Triple therapy with amoxicillin (substituted with metronidazole for penicillin-allergic patients), clarithromycin, and PPI is 80% to 90% effective. The most common reason for failure to eradicate infection is patient noncompliance with this complicated drug regimen. There has been recent interest in the literature on sequential drug therapy as well as the use of fluoroquinolones to improve eradication rates.

*OAC*
*OAM (PCN AII)*

**10. What are the long-term implications of *H. pylori* infection?**

Patients chronically infected with *H. pylori* can develop peptic ulcer disease. Although less common, lymphoma and adenocarcinoma of the stomach are also associated with chronic gastritis due to *H. pylori*. Gastritis involving the entire stomach (antrum and corpus) can result in intestinal metaplasia (replacement of gastric mucosa for intestinal goblet cell–laden columnar epithelium) and achlorhydria. Both conditions are associated with gastric ulcer and cancer. MALT (mucosa-associated lymphoid tissue) lymphoma may be related to *H. pylori* infection. The gastric mucosa is normally devoid of lymphoid tissue but chronic *H. pylori* infection may lead to accumulation of lymphoid tissue with subsequent malignant transformation. Superficial, low-grade, nonmetastatic gastric MALT lymphoma may respond to *H. pylori* eradication therapy.

**11. What are the other types of chronic gastritis?**

Autoimmune gastritis, lymphocytic gastritis, and nonspecific gastritis are similar in their endoscopic appearance to the chronic gastritis seen with *H. pylori*. These entities, along with the others listed in Table 9-1, are diagnosed by histology and/or other special studies.

*↓pcell— ↓HCl ↑gastrin ↓B12*
*↓IF*

**12. What is autoimmune gastritis?**

Autoimmune gastritis (AIG) is an uncommon cause of chronic gastritis. This diagnosis can be considered in the evaluation of patients with megaloblastic anemia. Patients with AIG produce antibodies against parietal cells, which affects the secretion of gastric acid and intrinsic factor. Gastric acid, in a negative feedback loop, normally reduces serum gastrin levels. Destruction of parietal cells results in achlorhydria and decreased concentration of intrinsic factor, and leads to high serum gastrin levels and vitamin B$_{12}$ malabsorption. Vitamin B$_{12}$ deficiency also occurs in patients with pernicious anemia who produce antibodies against intrinsic factor and in patients with chronic gastritis, which can lead to decreased production of intrinsic factor. Patients with AIG are often asymptomatic. The endoscopic appearance of AIG is that of severe atrophy with marked flattening of gastric rugae and visible submucosal vasculature. Typical histologic changes are found in the corpus and fundus with marked gastric atrophy and loss of glands. Inflammatory changes are present early in the disease course but resolve over time, being replaced by intestinal metaplasia. Patients with gastric atrophy and parietal cell or intrinsic factor antibodies should be followed carefully for the development of pernicious anemia and with endoscopy for gastric polyps or carcinoma. Upper endoscopy should be performed at 3- to 5-year intervals.

**13. What is lymphocytic gastritis?**

*30ɸ α celiac/ H.P. + HHIV/lymphoma .*

Lymphocytic gastritis is a rare condition characterized by an increased number of lymphocytes in the gastric epithelium. On average, 3 to 8 lymphocytes occur per 100 epithelial cells in normal gastric mucosa. A minimum of 30 lymphocytes per 100 epithelial cells is usually required for this diagnosis. While these patients are usually asymptomatic, some may present with epigastric pain or anorexia. Many cases occur in association with *H. pylori* infection and celiac disease; however, only 2% to 4% of patients with *H. pylori* infection will develop lymphocytic gastritis. There is no specific therapy, but patients with lymphocytic gastritis who are *H. pylori* positive may respond to antimicrobial eradication therapy.

**14. What is chronic nonspecific gastritis?**

Despite the discovery of *H. pylori* and advances in other forms of chronic gastritis, there remains a small group of undiagnosed patients with the endoscopic and histologic features of chronic gastritis. These are usually elderly patients with atrophic gastritis in which autoantibodies or *H. pylori* cannot be found. These patients may represent advanced *H. pylori*–associated gastritis, but no proof of this has been forthcoming.

**15. What is Ménétrier disease, and how does it differ from the other special forms of chronic gastritis?**

Ménétrier disease differs from other forms of chronic gastritis in that it is not associated with significant mucosal inflammation. The disease is usually seen in middle-aged adults who often present with weight loss, diarrhea, edema, and a low protein state. Low acid secretion, loss of parietal cells, and protein-losing gastropathy are typical of this disease. On endoscopy, large gastric folds are seen that do not flatten with maximal insufflation and the diagnosis is made by biopsy. Full-thickness mucosal biopsy samples show the characteristic massive foveolar hyperplasia. Endoscopic ultrasound plays an important diagnostic role in patients with large gastric folds. This technique defines five alternating hyperechoic and hypoechoic layers of the gastric wall, corresponding to mucosa, muscularis mucosa, submucosa, muscularis propria, and adventitia. Ménétrier disease typically produces a thickened mucosal layer. Lymphoma and simple rugal hyperplasia typically involve the mucosal and submucosal layers. The treatment of Ménétrier disease with H$_2$ blockers, prostaglandins, and proton pump inhibitors has generally been unsatisfactory. High doses of anticholinergic agents have reduced albumin loss. Subtotal or total gastrectomy has been performed in patients with severe and intractable symptoms.

## 16. Describe bile reflux gastritis.

Bile reflux gastritis is most commonly seen after gastrectomy, pyloroplasty, or cholecystectomy. Endoscopically, the gastric mucosa is granular and intensely erythematosus with an intense red color or greenish-yellow discoloration. Large amounts of bile are often found in the stomach. Histologic examination of the gastric mucosa reveals elongation and serration of the foveolae, which resembles the histologic changes seen with chronic NSAID or alcohol use. A diverting operation may be a treatment option in patients who fail to respond to medical therapy with sucralfate or ursodeoxycholic acid.

## 17. In what circumstances do granulomatous and eosinophilic gastritis occur?

Granulomatous and eosinophilic gastritis usually occur in conjunction with systemic disease. Granulomatous gastritis can be seen as part of the spectrum of Crohn's disease. The most common clinical presentation is gastric outlet obstruction. Endoscopically, aphthous ulcers are often seen in the antrum, but not the deep rake-like ulcers seen elsewhere in the GI tract. Histologic confirmation is difficult to obtain; however, biopsy samples taken with jumbo forceps can be diagnostic. Granulomatous gastritis can also be seen in sarcoidosis, Wegener granulomatosis, and systemic granulomatosis.

Eosinophilic gastritis is part of the syndrome of eosinophilic gastroenteritis. The stomach and small bowel are usually involved and patients may present with symptoms suggestive of peptic ulcer disease or irritable bowel syndrome. GI symptoms are determined by the depth of eosinophilic involvement in the organ wall. Peripheral eosinophilia is often present and gastric biopsies are diagnostic with more than 20 eosinophils seen per high-power field. No definite therapy is recommended, but there are reports of symptom improvement with corticosteroid therapy.

## BIBLIOGRAPHY

1. Cello JP. Eosinophilic gastroenteritis—A complex entity. Am J Med 1979;67:1097–104.
2. Cook D, Heyland D, Griffith L, et al. Risk factors for clinically important upper gastrointestinal bleeding in patients requiring mechanical ventilation. Crit Care Med 1999;27:2812–7.
3. Dixon MF, O'Connor HJ, Axon AT, et al. Reflux gastritis: Distinct histopathological entity? J Clin Pathol 1986;39:524–30.
4. Dubois RW, Melmed GY, Henning JM, et al. Guidelines for the appropriate use of nonsteroidal anti-inflammatory drugs, cyclo-oxygenase-2-specific inhibitors and proton pump inhibitors in patients requiring chronic anti-inflammatory therapy. Aliment Pharmacol Ther 2004;19:197–208.
5. Graham DY. *H. Pylori* infection in the pathogenesis of duodenal ulcer and gastric cancer: a model. Gastroenterology 1997;113:1983–91.
6. Graham DY, Adam E, Reddy GT, et al. Seroepidemiology of *Helicobacter pylori* infection in India. Comparison of developing and developed countries. Dig Dis Sci 1991;36:1084–8.
7. Graham DY, Lu H, Yamaoka Y. A report card to grade *Helicobacter pylori* therapy. Helicobacter 2007;12:275–8.
8. Hansson LE, Nyren O, Hsing AW, et al. The risk of stomach cancer in patients with gastric or duodenal ulcer disease. N Engl J Med 1996;335:242–9.
9. Hayat M, Arora DS, Dixon MF, et al. Effects of *Helicobacter pylori* eradication on the natural history of lymphocytic gastritis. Gut 1999;45:495–8.
10. Hsing AW, Hansson LE, McLaughlin JK, et al. Pernicious anemia and subsequent cancer: A population-based cohort study. Cancer 1993;71:745–50.
11. International Agency for Research on Cancer. Infection with Helicobacter pylori. Schistosomes, Liver Flukes and Helicobacter pylori. Lyon: International Agency for Research on Cancer, World Health Organization; 1994.
12. Lanza FL, Aspinall RL, Swabb EA, et al. Double-blind, placebo-controlled endoscopic comparison of the mucosal protective effects of misoprostol versus cimetidine on tolmetin-induced mucosal injury to the stomach and duodenum. Gastroenterology 1988;95:289–94.
13. Lanza FL, Schwartz H, Sahba B, et al. An endoscopic comparison of the effects of alendronate and risedronate on upper gastrointestinal mucosae. Am J Gastroenterol 2000;95:3112–7.
14. Larkai EN, Smith JL, Lidsky MD, et al. Gastroduodenal mucosa and dyspeptic symptoms in arthritic patients during chronic nonsteroidal anti-inflammatory drug use. Am J Gastroenterol 1987;82:1153–8.
15. Loffeld BC, van Spreeuwel JP. The gastrointestinal tract in pernicious anemia. Dig Dis 1991;9:70–7.
16. Madura JA. Primary bile reflux gastritis: Which treatment is better, Roux-en-Y or biliary diversion. Am Surgeon 2000;66:417–23.
17. Malaty HM. Epidemiology of *Helicobacter pylori* infection. Best Pract Res Clin Gastroenterol 2007;21:205–14.
18. Meuwissen SG, Ridwan BU, Hasper HJ, et al. Hypertrophic protein-losing gastropathy. A retrospective analysis of 40 cases in The Netherlands. The Dutch Menetrier Study Group. Scand J Gastroenterol Suppl 1992;194:1–7.

19. Oberhuber G, Bodingbauer M, Mosberger I, et al. High proportion of granzyme B-positive (activated) intraepithelial and lamina propria lymphocytes in lymphocytic gastritis. Am J Surg Pathol 1998;22:450–8.
20. Parsonnet J, Issacson PG. Bacterial infection and MALT lymphoma. N Engl J Med 2004;350:213–5.
21. Scolapio JS, DeVault K, Wolfe JT. Eosinophilic gastroenteritis presenting as a giant gastric ulcer. Am J Gastroenterol 1996;91:804–5.
22. Shapiro JL, Goldblum JR, Petras RE. A clinicopathologic study of 42 patients with granulomatous gastritis. Is there really an idiopathic granulomatous gastritis. Am J Surg Pathol 1996;20:462–70.
23. Silverstein FE, Faich G, Goldstein JL, et al. Gastrointestinal toxicity with celecoxib vs nonsteroidal anti-inflammatory drugs for osteoarthritis and rheumatoid arthritis: The CLASS study: A randomized controlled trial. Celecoxib Long-term Arthritis Safety Study. JAMA 2000;284:1247–55.
24. Stemmermann GN, Hayashi T. Intestinal metaplasia of the gastric mucosa: A gross and microscopic study of its distribution in various disease states. J Natl Cancer Inst 1968;41:627–34.
25. Terdiman JP, Ostroff JW. Gastrointestinal bleeding in the hospitalized patient: A case-control study to assess risk factors, causes and outcomes. Am J Med 1998;104:349–54.
26. Wolfsen HC, Carpenter HA, Talley NJ. Menetrier's disease: A form of hypertrophic gastropathy or gastritis? Gastroenterology 1993;104:1310–9.

# GASTRIC CANCER

*John C. Deutsch, MD*

### 1. What are the histologic types of gastric cancer?

Over 80% of gastric cancers are adenocarcinomas. Less common are gastric lymphomas, gastric stromal tumors, leiomyosarcomas, carcinoid tumors, and metastatic tumors (e.g., melanoma, breast cancer) (Fig. 10-1).

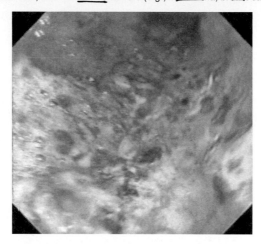

*adeno*
*LM*
*Carc*
*GIST*
*NHL*
*meta mel/Br*

**Figure 10-1.** Endoscopic image of massive diffuse ulcerated gastric cancer.

### 2. What is a signet ring cell carcinoma?

Signet ring carcinomas are adenocarcinomas in which more than 50% of the malignant cells in a tumor have intracytoplasmic mucin. Signet ring cell carcinoma tends to infiltrate and produces a desmoplastic (fibrous stromal) reaction. In general, signet ring carcinoma is a very aggressive subtype.

### 3. What is the ethnic and geographic distribution of distal gastric adenocarcinoma?

Distal gastric adenocarcinoma is one of the most common malignancies worldwide. Approximately 600,000 deaths per year are caused by gastric cancer worldwide. There is a high incidence in Asia and South America. Scandinavian countries have a higher incidence than the United States.

### 4. What is the role of diet in the development of gastric cancer?

Dietary factors appear to be important in the development of gastric cancer. In general, the incidence of gastric cancer is higher when a higher proportion of the diet is obtained from salted or smoked meats or fish. Fruits and vegetables appear to be protective. Tobacco smoking appears to increase the risk of gastric cancer. Dietary factors are thought to explain a large part of the variation in incidence of gastric cancers from country to country. Immigration from high-incidence countries to lower-incidence countries decreases the risk of gastric cancer risk.

### 5. What inherited genetic alterations are associated with gastric adenocarcinoma?

*FAP*
*HNPCC 10x*
*CDH1*

About 10% of gastric cancer appears to be familial, independent of *Helicobacter pylori* status. Familial adenomatous polyposis patients have a 10-fold increase in gastric cancer over the population at large. Gastric cancer is one of the tumors found in hereditary nonpolyposis colon cancer syndrome, and about 10% of patients with hereditary nonpolyposis colorectal cancer (HNPCC) develop gastric cancer. Families with specific mutations in the E-cahedrin gene (*CDH1*) have been reported to have a 100% chance of developing diffuse gastric cancer.

### 6. What is the role of *H. pylori* in gastric adenocarcinoma?

The medical literature generally supports the notion that *H. pylori* infection appears to increase the lifetime risk of gastric cancer. Infected persons have about a 2-fold increase in the risk of acquiring gastric adenocarcinoma. However, the chance of an *H. pylori*–infected person contracting cancer is very low.

**7. What mechanism is proposed for *H. pylori* causing an increased risk of gastric cancer?**

*H. pylori* infection results in a rather marked inflammatory state in the stomach, which can eventually lead to atrophic gastritis and achlorhydria. Some reports suggest that host factors, including a *proinflammatory host genotype,* favor achlorhydria and gastric cancer development.

**8. What is the role of achlorhydria in gastric cancer?**

Achlorhydria is generally caused by immune destruction of the parietal cells. Antiparietal cell antibodies and elevated gastrin levels can be found in the serum, and patients have associated $B_{12}$ deficiency. Other causes include destruction after long bouts of infection with *H. pylori*. People with achlorhydria have a 4- to 6-fold increase in the incidence of gastric cancers, possibly related to the associated elevation in gastrin levels, as well as the inflammation that leads to the parietal cell destruction.

**9. Should *H. pylori* infection be eradicated to prevent gastric cancer from occurring?**

Despite the epidemiologic link between *H. pylori* infection and gastric cancer, the data do not appear to support *H. pylori* eradication as a cancer preventive strategy at this point in time. The reasons for this include the relatively low incidence of cancer development in *H. pylori*–infected individuals and the variety of other factors related to cancer development, including the host's genetic propensity and the genetic makeup of different *H. pylori* strains. Furthermore, there seems to be important environmental factors such as tobacco use and diet that modulate the potential carcinogenic effects of *H. pylori*.

**10. Who should be screened for gastric cancer?**

Screening is performed in Japan in middle-aged people and is recommended on an annual basis over the age of 50 years. There are no screening recommendations for distal gastric adenocarcinoma in the United States, and no recommendations are widely accepted for the screening of immigrants from high-risk areas. Screening for proximal gastric cancer is probably warranted in people with a longstanding history of reflux symptoms.

**11. What is gastric stump cancer?**

After partial gastric resection, the incidence of gastric cancers at the site of the intestinal-gastric anastomosis appears to be increased by about 2-fold. However, this increase is not apparent until at least 15 years after surgery. In the initial 5 years after partial gastrectomy, there may be an actual decrease in cancer risk. These data suggest a certain background rate of gastric cancer formation. If part of the stomach is removed, less mucosa is at risk for malignant transformation. However, the surgery then imparts a procancer effect, and over time more and more cancers start to form in the remaining mucosa.

**12. What is early gastric cancer?**

Early gastric cancer is when a gastric adenocarcinoma has been found that is confined to the mucosa or submucosa, independent of nodal status (Fig. 10-2).

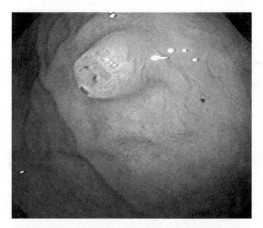

**Figure 10-2.** Endoscopic image of early gastric cancer.

**13. How is the incidence of gastric adenocarcinoma changing?**

Gastric adenocarcinoma has two major sites of presentation—either proximally in the stomach near the esophagogastric junction or distally in the stomach in the antrum. Worldwide, adenocarcinoma of the distal stomach is one of the most common malignancies; in the United States, however, this presentation has markedly decreased over the past several decades. Conversely, proximal gastric adenocarcinoma has been increasing rapidly increasing in the United State, probably in relation to reflux of gastric contents.

### 14. What is the staging scheme for gastric adenocarcinoma?

Tumor-node-metastasis (TNM) staging is generally used. T stage is primarily determined by the relation of the tumor to the muscularis propria (above, into, or through). N stage is determined by the number and location of affected nodes (local versus distant). M stage is determined by whether distant metastases are present.

### 15. How does staging help in treating gastric cancer?

Survival after gastrectomy for gastric cancer is directly correlated with stage. For instance, Stage-stratified 5-year/10-year relative survival rates in a study of over 50,000 cases of gastric cancer in the United States were as follows:

- Stage IA—78%/65%
- Stage IB—58%/42%
- Stage II—34%/26%
- Stage IIIA—20%/14%
- Stage IIIB—8%/3%
- Stage IV—7%/5%

Therapy, prognosis, and follow-up can be tailored based on the initial staging.

### 16. What is the role of endoscopic ultrasonography in staging gastric cancer?

Endoscopic ultrasonography (EUS) is a technique in which an ultrasound probe is attached to an endoscope. As a rule, it is the most accurate method of T and N staging gastrointestinal tumors and has the advantage of biopsy capability. EUS can detect small amounts of ascites in staging gastric cancer, which suggests unresectability (Fig. 10-3).

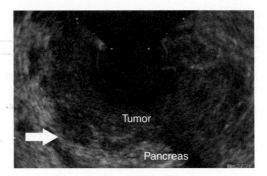

Tumor

Pancreas

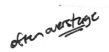
*often overstage*

**Figure 10-3.** Endoscopic ultrasonography showing massive gastric cancer infiltrating the pancreas.

However, the accuracy of EUS in staging gastric cancer is still relatively low for certain tumor stages, including T2 lesions, which tent to be overstaged. Lymph node staging is about 80% accurate in most studies and may be lower with the general application of EUS in the medical community. EUS imaging can provide a roadmap but, in general, biopsy-proof or surgical staging should be performed.

### 17. What is the role of endoscopy in the treatment of early gastric cancer?

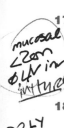
*mucosal
<2cm
0LN in
future*

Early gastric cancer, less than 2 cm across, is amenable to endoscopic removal. If the tumor shows no evidence of lymphovascular invasion, is confined to the mucosa, and has intestinal histology, the chance of cure can be greater than 95%. EUS is a valuable adjunct to endoscopic resection, because abnormal adenopathy precludes definitive endoscopic management of the tumor.

### 18. What is the role of surgery in treating localized gastric adenocarcinoma?

*D0 LY
D1 LY+OY
D2 ELY+OY*

Surgery is a potential curative therapy for localized gastric adenocarcinoma. The prognosis is based on TNM staging. The extent of resection is somewhat controversial. Japanese literature suggests that an extended lymphadenectomy plus omentectomy (D2 operation) is superior to a limited lymphadenectomy with omentectomy (D1 procedure) or limited lymphadenectomy (D0 procedure). In a randomized European study, patients undergoing D2 resection had twice the operative mortality as those undergoing D1 resection. There was no survival benefit.

*+ ADJ.
CxRT*

### 19. What is the role of neoadjuvant therapy in gastric adenocarcinoma?

Neoadjuvant therapy is treatment given before an attempt at curative surgical resection, to make the primary tumor smaller and possibly to treat small foci of disease outside the operative field. Although the concept is attractive, definitive studies demonstrating the utility of neoadjuvant therapy for gastric cancer have not been performed.

**20. What is the role of adjuvant therapy in gastric adenocarcinoma?**

Adjuvant therapy is additional treatment given to patients after attempted curative surgery. Adjuvant treatment is given if there is no evidence of remaining disease. A 2001 report has shown the effectiveness of neoadjuvant therapy in treating gastric cancer in U.S. patients. In this large randomized study, fluorouracil, leucovorin, and radiation therapy provided a significant survival advantage over observation following surgery. There was a 33% increase in median survival. More recently, a 2007 trial of adjuvant therapy with the oral fluoropyrimidine S1 in surgically resected stage II and III patients in Japan has been shown to significantly improve survival at 3 years.

**21. What is the usual therapy for metastatic gastric adenocarcinoma?**

Chemotherapy can be used with modest benefits. Several regimens have activity in gastric adenocarcinoma, using drugs such as 5-fluorouracil, etoposide, platinum-containing drugs, and taxanes.  *5FU/cisplatin.*

**22. What is a MALT lymphoma?**

MALT lymphomas are mucosal-associated lymphoid tumors. They can occur in any mucosal location, both within and outside the gastrointestinal tract. MALT lymphomas are often low-grade B-cell lymphomas but they also may be high-grade aggressive tumors.

**23. What is special about gastric MALT lymphomas?**

Gastric MALT lymphomas, unlike MALT lymphomas in other locations, often are associated with infection by *H. pylori*. Lymphoid tissue is not a normal part of gastric epithelium, and infection with *H. pylori* seems to drive lymphoid proliferation and tumor development.  *lymphoid*

**24. What is the role of antibiotic therapy in gastric MALT lymphomas?**

Treatment of *H. pylori* infection usually leads to regression of low-grade B-cell gastric MALT lymphomas. It is believed that the low-grade tumors retain responsiveness to *H. pylori* antigen stimulation. Complete responses can take up to 18 months after antibiotic therapy. In general, high-grade gastric MALT lymphomas and those with more acquired chromosomal abnormalities do not respond well to antibacterial therapy.

**25. Describe the staging scheme for gastric lymphoma.**

Several staging systems are used for gastric lymphoma, including TNM staging (as for gastric adenocarcinoma). A clinical staging system used for non-Hodgkin's lymphoma (the Ann Arbor Classification) is also available. The Ann Arbor system identifies the primary site of lymphoma as nodal or extranodal and assesses extent of disease based on number of sites involved, relation of the tumor to the diaphragm, and whether disease has metastasized to nonlymphoid organs. In the Ann Arbor system, a lymphoma involving both the stomach and a lymph node may be stage 2E (two sites with extranodal primary) or stage 4 (nodal primary with metastasis to the stomach). A new staging system that combines TNM staging with Ann Arbor criteria was recommended in 1994 for gastrointesintal lymphomas.

**26. What is the best therapy for aggressive (non-MALT) gastric lymphoma?**

Therapy is determined somewhat by stage. For most cases of Ann Arbor stages I and II, surgery can be curative. However, data in a 1999 report suggest that chemotherapy with or without radiation therapy can be equally effective. T stage is also important because of the possibility of perforation when chemotherapy is used for T3 or T4 tumors. The trend is away from surgery for all stages.  *>1cm = more px*  *>2cm mets*

**27. What are gastric carcinoid tumors?**  *S. chromogranin*

Gastric carcinoid tumors are growths of neuroendocrine cells that may be benign or malignant. They stain for chromogranin. As a rule, even the malignant tumors are slow growing. Tumors greater than 1 cm in diameter are generally more dangerous, whereas smaller tumors are not and may represent endochromagraffin cell hyperplasia. Tumors larger than 2 cm often have metastasized. As a rule, large tumors often require gastrectomy, whereas smaller tumors can be managed endoscopically.  *<2cm*

**28. What causes gastric carcinoid tumors?**

Two processes appear to lead to gastric carcinoid—de novo malignant transformation and loss of normal growth regulation in response to chronic elevation of serum gastrin levels. Tumors arising from de novo malignant transformation are usually single, larger, and more aggressive, whereas those arising from elevated gastrin levels are often multiple and smaller. It is important to distinguish between the two types.

**29. What should be done when a gastric carcinoid has been identified?**

Patients should have a gastrin level checked to see if the carcinoid tumor is associated with hypergastrinemia. If the gastrin level is elevated, evaluation for atrophic gastritis should be carried out, with assessment for vitamin $B_{12}$ levels, and consideration of gastric biopsy to look for the presence of parietal cells, and evaluation for serum antiparietal cell antibodies. If gastrin is elevated, and the patient does not appear to have atrophic gastritis, an evaluation for Zöllinger-Ellison syndrome (gastrinoma) should be performed.

*? ZE + AG.*

## 30. What is a gastric GIST?

GIST, or gastrointestinal stromal tumor, is a tumor that develops in the gastric wall from the interstitial cells of Cajal. The tumor can be benign or malignant. Generally, malignancy correlates with size (greater than 3 to 5 cm in cross section) and histologic features, such as the number of mitoses per 10 high-power fields. These tumors resemble leiomyomas, and the distinction between gastric leiomyomas and GIST can be difficult without special histocytochemistry. GIST marks with an antibody against surface KIT, which is a tyrosine kinase. KIT is otherwise known as CD117. It has been shown that GIST responds to a specific tyrosine kinase inhibitor, imatinib mesylate or STI 571, although resistance seems to eventually develop. Sunitinib is being used in imatinib-resistant patients.

> 3-5cm

CD117 = KIT ⊕ (GIST)

# WEBSITES

http://www.cancer.gov/cancerinfo/types/stomach/

http://www.carcinoid.org

http://www.nlm.nih.gov/medlineplus/stomachcancer.html

http://www.stomachcancer.org

http://www.vhjoe.org

## BIBLIOGRAPHY

1. American Joint Committee on Cancer. Handbook for Staging of Cancer. In: Greene FL, Page DL, Fleming ID, et al., editors. The Manual for Staging of Cancer. 6th ed. New York: Springer Publishers; 2002. p. 111–6.
2. Badalamenti G, Rodolico V, Fulfaro F, et al. Gastrointestinal stromal tumors (gists): Focus on histopathological diagnosis and biomolecular features. Ann Oncol 2007;18(Suppl. 6):vi136–40.
3. Bretagne JF. Could *Helicobacter pylori* treatment reduce stomach cancer risk?. Gastroenterol Clin Biol 2003;27(3 Pt 2):440–52.
4. Chen CH, Yang CC, Yeh YH. Preoperative staging of gastric cancer by endoscopic ultrasound: The prognostic usefulness of ascites detected by endoscopic ultrasound. J Clin Gastroenterol 2002;321–7.
5. Crump M, Gospodarowicz M, Shepherd FA. Lymphoma of the gastrointestinal tract. Semin Oncol 1999;26:324–337.
6. De Silva CM, Reid R. Gastrointestinal stromal tumors (GIST): C-kit mutations, CD117 expression, differential diagnosis and targeted cancer therapy with imatinib. Pathol Oncol Res 2003;13–9.
7. Devesa SS, Blot WJ, Fraumeni Jr JF. Changing patterns in the incidence of esophageal and gastric carcinoma in the United States. Cancer 1998;83:2049–53.
8. El-Omar EM, Rabkin CS, Gammon MD, et al. Increased risk of noncardia gastric cancer associated with proinflammatory cytokine gene polymorphisms. Gastroenterology 2003;1193–201.
9. El-Serag HB, Sonnenberg A. Ethnic variations in the occurrence of gastroesophageal cancers. J Clin Gastroenterol 1999;28:135–9.
10. Gylling A, Abdel-Rahmen WM, Juhola M, et al. Is gastric cancer part of the tumour spectrum of hereditary non-polyposis colorectal cancer? A molecular genetic study. Gut 2007;56:926–33.
11. Humar B, Toro T, Graziano F, et al. Novel germline CDH1 mutations in hereditary diffuse gastric cancer families. Hum Mutat 2002;19:518–25.
12. Hundahl SA, Phillips JL, Menck HR. The National Cancer Data Base Report on poor survival of U.S. gastric carcinoma patients treated with gastrectomy: Fifth edition. American Joint Committee on Cancer staging, proximal disease, and the different disease hypothesis. Cancer. 2000; 921–32.
13. Lauffer JM, Zhang T, Modlin IM. Review article: Current status of gastrointestinal carcinoids. Aliment Pharmacol Ther 1999;13:271–87.
14. Lynch HT, Grady W, Suriano G, et al. Gastric cancer: New genetic developments. J Surg Oncol 2005;90:114–33.
15. Macdonald JS, Smalley SR, Benedetti J, et al. Chemoradiotherapy after surgery compared with surgery alone for adenocarcinoma of the stomach or gastroesophageal junction. N Engl J Med 2001;345:725–730.
16. Moradi T, Delfino RJ, Bergstrom SR, et al. Cancer risk among Scandinavian immigrants in the US and Scandinavian residents compared with US whites, 1973-89. Eur J Cancer Prev 1998;7:117–25.
17. Morgner A, Schmelz R, Thiede C, et al. Therapy of gastric mucosa associated lymphoid tissue lymphoma. World J Gastroenterol 2007;13:3554–66.
18. Moss SF, Malfertheiner P. Helicobacter and gastric malignancies. Helicobacter 2007;12(Suppl. 1):23–30.
19. Oda I, Saito D, Tada M, et al. A multicenter retrospective study of endoscopic resection for early gastric cancer. Gastric Cancer 2006;9:262–70.
20. Roderick R, Davies R, Raftery J, et al. Cost-effectiveness of population screening for *Helicobacter pylori* in preventing gastric cancer and peptic ulcer disease, using simulation. J Med Screen 2003;10:148–56.
21. Rohatiner A, d'Amore F, Coiffier B, et al. Report on a workshop convened to discuss the pathological and staging of GI tract lymphomas. Ann Oncol 1994;5:397–400.
22. Sakuramoto S, Sasako M, Yamaguchi T, et al. Adjuvant chemotherapy for gastric cancer with S-1, an oral fluoropyrimidine. N Engl J Med 2007;357:1810–20.
23. Sankhala KK, Papadopoulos KP. Future options for imatinib mesilate-resistant tumors. Expert Opin Investig Drugs 2007;16:1549–60.

# CHAPTER 11

# HELICOBACTER PYLORI AND PEPTIC ULCER DISEASE

Scott Altschuler, MD, and
David A. Peura, MD

### 1. Why is *Helicobacter pylori* a unique bacterium?

*H. pylori* is a spiral-shaped, gram-negative bacterium that is 0.5 μm in width and 2 to 6.5 μm in length. It is distinguished by its multiple-sheathed, unipolar flagella and potent urease activity; urease accounts for more than 1% of the organism's protein weight. Its shape and flagella allow penetration of and movement through the gastric mucus layer, while its urease activity appears essential for colonization and survival. *H. pylori* is unique in its ability to survive within the hostile acid environment of the stomach. Although gastric bacteria were described as early as at the turn of the century, their importance in peptic ulcer disease and chronic gastritis was not appreciated until the 1980s. *H. pylori* was first successfully cultured in 1982 by Drs. Barry Marshall and Robin Warren, an accomplishment for which they shared the 2005 Nobel Prize in Medicine and Physiology.

### 2. What is the prevalence of *H. pylori*?

*H. pylori* infects more than 50% of the world's adult population, possibly making it the most common chronic human bacterial infection. Its geographic distribution closely correlates with socioeconomic development (Fig. 11-1). In developing countries, the prevalence of infection may reach levels of 80% to 90% by 20 years of age, and this prevalence remains constant for the rest of adult life. In contrast, in developed countries, the prevalence of *H. pylori* infection is less than 20% in people younger than age 25 years and increases about 1% per year to about 50% to 60% by age 70. Most infection is acquired during childhood, usually by the age of 5 years, in both developing and developed countries. Antibodies against *H. pylori* can be detected in neonates, but they probably represent placental transfer of maternal antibodies rather than primary infection. Familial clustering of infection is common, and siblings and parents of infected children are more likely to be infected. Members of the same family can be infected with the same strain of the organism. Prevalence data from developing countries appear to be subject to generational bias; primary infection is acquired during childhood, but each successive birth cohort is less likely to develop infection. Within a given geographic area, infection rate appears to be affected by racial, ethnic, and economic factors. For example, in the United States, blacks and Hispanics acquire infection earlier in life and more frequently than do whites, and living in poverty increases the likelihood of infection.

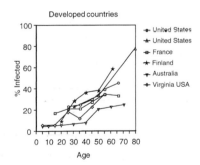 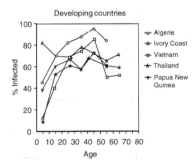

**Figure 11-1.** Seroprevalence of *Helicobacter pylori* infection in developed and developing countries. (From Marshall BJ, McCallum RW, Guerrant RL: *H. pylori* in Peptic Ulceration and Gastritis. Boston, Blackwell, 1991, pp 46–58. Reprinted with permission of the American Digestive Health Foundation.)

### 3. How is infection transmitted?

The exact method of transmission is not known, but most data support fecal-oral or oral-oral routes and best explain the high rate of infection in young children. The bacterium has been cultured from the stool of individuals with acute diarrheal disease. The higher-than-anticipated prevalence in institutionalized individuals, familial clustering of infection, association with crowded living conditions, and documented transmission from contaminated devices such as endoscopes also support person-to-person spread. Humans appear to be the major reservoir of *H. pylori*, although the organism has been isolated from domestic pets and primates. The organism remains viable in water for several days, and thus contaminated water may serve as a source of infection. While *H. pylori* can be isolated from houseflies, insect transmission remains unproved and unlikely. There is no evidence to support sexual transmission of infection.

## 4. Where in the gastrointestinal (GI) tract does *H. pylori* live?

The organism lives within or beneath the gastric mucus layer, somewhat protected from stomach acid. *H. pylori* has potent urease activity, which hydrolyzes urea to ammonia and bicarbonate and increases its resistance to the stomach's low pH environment. Organisms recognize and bind to specific receptors expressed by gastric epithelial cells and, therefore, are able to adhere tightly to the epithelial cell surface. This attachment process may morphologically or functionally alter the epithelial cell. The organism has been found adherent to ectopic gastric epithelium throughout the GI tract—that is, esophagus (Barrett's esophagus), duodenum (gastric metaplasia), small intestine (Meckel diverticulum), and rectum (ectopic patches of gastric mucosa).

## 5. How does *H. pylori* produce mucosal damage?

The organism generally does not directly invade the epithelial cells but indirectly makes the gastric mucosa more vulnerable to acid peptic damage by disrupting the mucous layer, liberating a variety of enzymes and toxins, and adhering to and altering the gastric epithelium. In addition, the host immune response to *H. pylori* incites an inflammatory reaction, which further perpetuates tissue injury. This chronic inflammation upsets gastric acid secretory physiology to varying degrees and leads to chronic gastritis, which, in most individuals, is asymptomatic but in some will lead to ulcers and even gastric cancer.

## 6. What endoscopy-based (invasive) tests can be used to diagnose *H. pylori* infection?

*Histopathologic examination* is widely available, and specimens are easy to store. Organisms can be detected with standard hematoxylin and eosin stains or special stains, such as Giemsa or Warthin-Starry, which make the organisms easier to identify. Immune stains specific for the organism are now widely used to improve detection in biopsy specimens. The sensitivity and specificity of histopathology for *H. pylori* are greater than 95% but may be influenced by sampling error, number of organisms present, use of proton pump inhibitors (PPIs), and experience of the pathologist.

*Rapid urease testing* relies on the potent urease activity of *H. pylori*. A gastric biopsy specimen is placed in medium containing urea and a colored pH indicator, and if organisms are present in the specimen, their urease hydrolyzes urea to bicarbonate and ammonia, increasing the pH and changing the color of the pH indicator. The number of organisms present, use of certain medications such as PPIs, and sampling error may influence urease testing. The sensitivity of the rapid urease test is about 90%; its specificity is 100%.

*Culture of gastric biopsy* specimens for *H. pylori* is occasionally performed but is difficult, requiring incubation for 3 to 5 days in special medium in a controlled microaerophilic environment. With easier diagnostic methods available, culture is not clinically useful for diagnosis and is reserved for determining antibiotic sensitivities in treatment-resistant infections.

## 7. How is *H. pylori* diagnosed noninvasively?

**Serology**. IgG antibodies directed at various bacterial antigens can be detected by enzyme-linked immunosorbent assay (ELISA) in the serum of infected individuals. In addition, several office-based serology methods are commercially available. Serologic methods detect primary *H. pylori* infection in infected people with sensitivity and specificity of greater than 90%. Although antibody levels may fall after successful bacterial eradication, they remain elevated for many years. This serologic scar limits the usefulness of serology in assessing treatment and determining reinfection, as well as reducing the positive predictive value of the test, especially in areas of the world, such as the United States, where prevalence of infection is low. For this reason, a positive serology result should be confirmed with a test of active infection such as a stool or urea breath test before treatment is initiated.

**Urea breath tests** are ideally suited to make a primary diagnosis of infection, to monitor treatment response, and to assess reinfection, because they are positive only in a setting of active infection. The patient ingests a small amount of carbon-labeled ($^{13}C$ or $^{14}C$) urea. The urease of *H. pylori* hydrolyzes the urea and liberates labeled carbon dioxide. Labeled carbon dioxide can be collected and quantified in breath samples. Sensitivity and specificity of urea breath testing are greater than 95%. Certain medications, such as antibiotics, bismuth-containing compounds, and PPIs, can influence test results and should be discontinued for 1 to 2 weeks before testing.

**Stool antigen testing** is becoming increasingly popular. It is accurate (sensitivity and specificity of 90% and 98%, respectively) and inexpensive. The test is based on ELISA of specific *H. pylori* antigens that are excreted in stool samples. An office-based stool antigen test is also available but it uses monoclonal antibodies and is less sensitive than the lab-based technology. Stool antigen testing is useful in primary diagnosis and confirmation of eradication of the organism after antibiotic treatment. As with urea breath testing, antibiotics, bismuth-containing compounds, and PPIs can influence test results (Table 11-1).

**Table 11-1.** Diagnostic Tests for *Helicobacter pylori*

| TEST | SENSITIVITY (%) | SPECIFICITY (%) | RELATIVE COST |
|---|---|---|---|
| Noninvasive (nonendoscopic) | | | |
| Serology | 88–99 | 86–95 | $ |
| Urea breath test | 90–97 | 90–100 | $$ |
| Stool antigen test | 90 | 98 | $ |
| Invasive (endoscopic) | | | |
| Rapid urease assay | 89–98 | 93–98 | $$$$* |
| Histology | 93–99 | 95–99 | $$$$$* |
| Culture | 77–92 | 100 | $$$$$* |

*Includes cost of endoscopy.
Data from the Foundation for Digestive Health and Nutrition.

8. **What is the association of *H. pylori* with histologic gastritis?**

   Infection with *H. pylori* produces an active chronic gastritis with intraepithelial and interstitial neutrophils in addition to lymphocytes and plasma cells. In many people, gastritis remains primarily confined to the antrum. In others, however, it may progress to involve the entire stomach. Patients with antral gastritis alone produce more acid and are more likely to develop subsequent duodenal ulcers, whereas patients with pangastritis, especially in association with atrophy and intestinal metaplasia, produce less acid and are at risk for gastric ulcers and adenocarcinoma. Genetic differences in the host's inflammatory cytokine profile appear to determine which pattern of gastritis and which potential clinical outcome result from infection.

   While all infected people develop histologic evidence of active chronic gastritis, only a minority develop clinically obvious symptoms. At present, it is unknown whether host factors, such as immune response or genetic susceptibility, or infection with more virulent bacterial strains is the major determinant of clinical illness. Data suggest that specific polymorphisms of genes related to the innate and acquired immune responses, including nucleotide-binding oligomerization domain containing 2 (NOD2), cyclooxygenase-2 (*COX-2*), and toll-like receptor 4 (TLR-4), and inflammatory cytokines such as Interleukin 1 β (IL1B) can confer a genetic risk for those infected with *H. pylori*, resulting in low acid output and subsequent development of gastric cancer.

9. **What is the association of *H. pylori* with peptic ulcer disease?**

   Many gastric ulcers occur in the setting of *H. pylori* gastritis. *H. pylori* makes the gastric mucosal layer more susceptible to acid injury through various mechanisms, including cell disruption due to adherence of the organism to the epithelium, ammonia production catalyzed by the organism's urease enzyme, and direct damage of epithelial cell membranes mediated by bacterial cytotoxins. The local and systemic inflammatory response to infection further disrupts the protective mucus barrier, rendering the underlying mucosal surface more susceptible to acid injury.

   The association between *H. pylori* and duodenal ulcer disease is also quite strong. Infection increases gastrin secretion, which results in increased gastric acid production by parietal cells. Excessive acid production over time can lead to damage of duodenal mucosa with subsequent development of duodenal gastric metaplasia. *H. pylori* may infect these duodenal *patches* of gastric mucosa, leading to duodenitis and eventual duodenal ulceration. Elimination of either gastric acid or infection can prevent duodenal ulcers due to *H. pylori*.

   ↑gastrin

10. **What may cause ulcers besides *H. pylori*?**

    Most *H. pylori*–negative gastric ulcers are associated with nonsteroidal anti-inflammatory drugs (NSAIDs); however, both gastric adenocarcinoma and lymphoma can cause ulceration and should be ruled out. As the prevalence of *H. pylori* decreases, *H. pylori*–negative duodenal ulcers are more commonly encountered and now account for the majority of duodenal ulcers in persons in the United States. Hypersecretory conditions such as Zöllinger-Ellison syndrome or unusual manifestations of conditions such as Crohn's disease are other causes. True idiopathic duodenal ulcers may be genetically determined and are characterized by hypersecretion of acid, rapid gastric emptying, poor response to traditional treatment, frequent recurrence, and clinical complications.

11. **Does *H. pylori* cause symptoms in patients with functional dyspepsia?**

    Functional (or nonulcer) dyspepsia is a poorly defined clinical entity, probably with multiple causes. Evidence that *H. pylori* gastritis causes dyspepsia in the absence of an ulcer has been difficult to obtain, because no specific symptoms separate *H. pylori*–related dyspepsia from other forms of functional dyspepsia. In addition, the effect of treatment for *H. pylori* infection on dyspeptic symptoms has been inconsistent. Nevertheless, a subset of patients with functional dyspepsia certainly has symptoms related to infection and responds to antibiotic treatment.

## 12. Does *H. pylori* play a role in gastric cancer?

Gastric cancer is the second most common cancer in the world. Unfortunately, it still carries a poor prognosis, and treatment options are limited. Patients with *H. pylori* infection have been repeatedly reported to have a 3- to 6-fold higher incidence of gastric cancer. The World Health Organization has classified *H. pylori* as a group I carcinogen. The chronic gastritis produced by *H. pylori* results in increased DNA turnover and free radical generation. Infection with *H. pylori* also results in decreased secretion of vitamin C, a known antioxidant, in gastric juice. Over time, these factors can lead to mutation of gastric epithelial cells and development of adenocarcinoma. Recent studies suggest that eliminating *H. pylori* in high-risk people can obviate the development of subsequent gastric cancer, especially if treatment is initiated before more advanced histologic changes (i.e., atrophy, metaplasia) have developed.

There is also a strong association with *H. pylori* and MALT (mucosa-associated lymphoid tissue) lymphoma. It is believed that the chronic inflammation produced by the organism (T-cell response to bacterial antigens) can lead to a monoclonal (B-cell) neoplasm of inflammatory cells. MALT tumor cells express surface membrane immunoglobulins and B-cell–associated antigens such as CD20. Identification of cytogenetic abnormalities such as t(11;18) by conventional chromosomal analysis or by fluorescence in situ hybridization (FISH) can also be used to identify low-grade MALT lymphomas. When a MALT tumor is superficial and of low histologic grade, eradication of *H. pylori* infection results in regression or cure in 90% of patients.

## 13. In what situation is it appropriate to eradicate *H. pylori* infection?

Anyone with active or past ulcer disease should be tested for *H. pylori* and treated if positive. Those who experience any ulcer-related complication also should be tested and treated if positive. Patients with low-grade MALT lymphoma should be tested and treated because eradication of *H. pylori* may result in a cure of the lymphoma. More controversial yet reasonable treatment situations include young patients with dyspepsia prior to proceeding with invasive diagnostic studies, patients at increased risk of gastric cancer (i.e., positive family history or gastric metaplasia on prior biopsies), or older patients beginning NSAID therapy. Treatment decisions in these situations should be made on a case-by-case basis. Current data are insufficient to recommend screening and treating asymptomatic people to prevent subsequent ulcer disease or gastric neoplasia.

## 14. What treatment regimens have been used to eradicate *H. pylori*?

The current preferred initial treatment for *H. pylori* infection is a 10- to 14-day course of proton pump inhibitor (PPI) triple therapy (PPI, amoxicillin 1000 mg, and clarithromycin 500 mg, all given twice daily) and this can successfully cure infection in more than 75% of individuals. Metronidazole 500 mg an be substituted for amoxicillin, but this should be done only in penicillin-allergic individuals because of the high prevalence of metronidazole-resistant organisms. Another effective eradication strategy involves 10-day sequential treatment with PPI and amoxicillin (1 g), each administered twice daily for the first 5 days, followed by PPI, clarithromycin (500 mg), and tinidazole (500 mg), each administered twice daily for an additional 5 days. This treatment has been shown to be more effective than standard PPI triple therapy, especially in those harboring clarithromycin-resistant bacteria. Recently, a combination capsule containing bismuth subsalicylate (525 mg), metronidazole (125 mg), and tetracycline (125 mg) was approved for use in the United States and Canada. Three such combination capsules administered four times daily along with a PPI twice daily for 10 days is another treatment option proven to be as effective as PPI triple therapy. Once therapy for *H. pylori* eradication is complete, cure of the infection should be confirmed noninvasively. Urea breath testing and stool antigen testing are appropriate for this purpose but should be performed sooner than 4 to 8 weeks after completion of treatment.

Those who fail initial therapy (positive stool, breath, or endoscopic test after treatment) should not be retreated with clarithromycin because of presumed acquired macrolide resistance. An appropriate second-treatment regimen is a 2-week course of quadruple therapy (PPI BID plus bismuth subsalicylate [Pepto-Bismol] 2 tablets, tetracycline 500 mg, and metronidazole 500 mg QID) or combination capsule treatment as described earlier. While third and even fourth courses of such therapies are sometimes successful in curing persistent infection, quinolone-, rifabutin-, or furazolidone-based therapies may be more suitable for particularly refractory cases (Table 11-2).

## Table 11-2.  Therapy for *Helicobacter pylori* Infection

**FIRST-LINE TRIPLE THERAPY: 10–14 DAYS**

| DRUG 1 (PROTON PUMP INHIBITOR) | DRUG 2 | DRUG 3 |
| --- | --- | --- |
| Omeprazole 20 mg BID *or* lansoprazole 30 mg BID *or* pantoprazole 40 mg BID *or* rabaprazole 20 mg BID *or* esomeprazole 40 mg BID | Clarithromycin 500 mg BID | Amoxicillin 1000 mg BID (can be substituted by metronidazole 500 mg BID in patient sensitive to penicillin) |

**SEQUENTIAL THERAPY: 10 DAYS**

| DRUG 1 | DRUG 2 | DRUG 3 |
| --- | --- | --- |
| 5 Days of: Proton pump inhibitor | Amoxicillin 1 g BID | |
| Followed by 5 days of: Proton pump inhibitor | Clarithromycin 500 mg BID | Tinidazole 500 mg BID |

**QUADRUPLE THERAPY: 14 DAYS**

| DRUG 1 | DRUG 2 | DRUG 3 | DRUG 4 |
| --- | --- | --- | --- |
| Proton pump inhibitor (BID) | Tetracycline 500 mg QID | Metronidazole 500 mg QID | Bismuth subsalicylate 2 tablets QID |

*[handwritten annotations]* Seq OA x5 + OTC x5    Quad  O TMB

### 15. Is reinfection a common problem?

Rates of reinfection after eradication vary geographically, but even in developing countries the annual recurrence rate is typically less than 5%. In developed countries, such as the United States, once infection has been eliminated, the annual rate of reinfection is very low (less than 1%). Most *reinfection* actually represents recrudescence of original infection resulting from initial treatment failure.

### 16. What is the role of vaccination in the prevention of *H. pylori*?

Vaccines against *H. pylori* have proven effective in preventing infection in animals, but no safe vaccine is currently available for large-scale human use. Development of a preventive or therapeutic vaccine remains an important area of research.

### 17. What role does *H. pylori* play in gastroesophageal reflux disease (GERD)?

There is no evidence that *H. pylori* causes GERD; in fact, it may be protective or reduce its severity. Some patients who have no reflux symptoms of disease may actually develop GERD once treated with an eradication regimen for *H. pylori*. The bacteria also appear to augment the effect of antisecretory drugs, $H_2$ blockers, and proton pump inhibitors, used to treat reflux.

### 18. Is *H. pylori* associated with any diseases outside the GI tract in humans?

There appears to be a small but consistent excessive risk of ischemic heart disease in patients infected with *H. pylori*. It is theorized that higher serum cytokine levels induced by *H. pylori* infection lead to increased systemic inflammatory responses and atherosclerosis. Idiopathic chronic urticaria, as well as acne rosacea and alopecia areata, has been linked to *H. pylori* infection. In some patients, urticaria has improved with the eradication of *H. pylori*, but the results with alopecia and rosacea are less striking. Raynaud phenomenon and migraine headaches have been observed to improve with treatment of *H. pylori*, although no controlled studies have been performed in these or any other extraintestinal conditions. Idiopathic thrombocytopenic purpura (ITP) and "refractory" iron deficiency anemia have also been liked to infection with resolution of these conditions in some individuals following treatment of *H. pylori*. *H. pylori* has also recently been shown to be associated with conjunctival MALToma.

## WEBSITES

http://www.cdc.gov/ulcer/keytocure.htm

http://www.consensus.nih.gov

### BIBLIOGRAPHY

1. Amieva MR, El-Omar EM. Host-bacterial interaction in *Helicobacter pylori* infection. Gastroenterology 2008;134:306–23.
2. Chang MC, Wu MS, Wang HP, et al. *Helicobacter pylori* stool antigen (HpSA) test: A simple, accurate, and non-invasive test for detection of *Helicobacter pylori* infection. Hepatogastroenterology 1999;46:299–302.
3. Chey WD, Wong BC. American College of Gastroenterology guideline on the management of *Helicobacter pylori* infection. Am J Gastroenterol 2007;102:1808–25.
4. Ciocola AA, McSorley DJ, Turner K, et al. *Helicobacter pylori* infection rates in duodenal ulcer patients in the U.S. may be lower than previously estimated. Am J Gastroenterol 1999;94:1834–40.
5. Cremonini F, Di Caro S, Delagado-Aros S, et al. Meta-analysis: the relationship between *Helicobacter pylori*. infection and oesophageal reflux disease. Aliment Pharmacol Ther 2003;18:279–89.
6. El-Omar EM, Carrington M, Chow WH, et al. Interleukin-1 polymorphisms associated with increased risk of gastric cancer. Nature 2000;404:398–40.
7. Ernst PB, Peura DA, Crowe SE. The translation of *Helicobacter pylori* basic research to patient care. Gastroenterology 2006;130:188–206.
8. Fallone CA, Barkun AN, Friedman G, et al. Is *Helicobacter pylori* eradication associated with gastroesophageal reflux disease?. Am J Gastroenterol 2000;95:914–20.
9. Go M. Review article: Natural history and epidemiology of *Helicobacter pylori* infection. Aliment Pharmacol Ther 2002;16(Suppl.):3–15.
10. Huang JQ, Sridhar S, Hunt RH. Role of *Helicobacter pylori* infection and non-steroidal anti-inflammatory drugs in peptic-ulcer disease: A meta-analysis. Lancet 2002;359:14–22.
11. Lee SB, Yang JW, Kim CS. The association between conjunctival MALT lymphoma and *Helicobacter pylori*. Br J Ophthalmol 2008;92:534–6.
12. Makola D, Peura DA, Crowe SE. *Helicobacter pylori* infection and related gastrointestinal diseases. J Clin Gastroenterol 2007;41:548–58.
13. Marshall BJ, Warren JR. Unidentified curved bacilli in the stomach of patients with gastritis and peptic ulceration. Lancet 1984;1:1311–5.
14. McColl L, El-Omar E, Gillen D. *Helicobacter pylori* gastritis and gastric physiology. Gastrointenterol Clin North Am 2000;29:687–703.
15. McMahon BJ, Hennessy TW, Bensler JM, et al. The relationship among previous antimicrobial use, antimicrobial resistance, and treatment outcomes for *Helicobacter pylori* infections. Ann Intern Med 2003;139:463–9.
16. Moayyedi P, Soo S, Deeks J, et al. Systematic review and economic evaluation of *Helicobacter pylori* eradication treatment for non-ulcer dyspepsia. BMJ 2000;321:659–64.
17. Moss SF, Malfertheiner P. *Helicobacter* and gastric malignancies. Helicobacter 2007;12(Suppl. 1):23–30.
18. Sanders MA, Peura DA. *Helicobacter pylori* associated diseases. Curr Gastroenterol Rep 2002;4:448–54.
19. Spiegel B, Vakil N, Ofman J. Dyspepsia management strategies in primary care: A decision analysis of competing strategies. Gastroenterology 2002;122:1270–85.
20. Sutton P, Lee A. Review article: *Helicobacter pylori* vaccines—The current status. Aliment Pharmacol Ther 2000;14:1107–18.
21. Uemora N, Okamoto S, Yamamoto S, et al. *Helicobacter pylori* infection and the development of gastric cancer. N Engl J Med 2001;345:784–9.
22. Vaira D, Gatta L, Ricci C, et al. Review article: Diagnosis of *Helicobacter pylori* infection. Aliment Pharmacol Ther 2002;16(Suppl. 1):16–23.
23. Van Leerdam ME, Tytgat GN. Review article: *Helicobacter pylori* infection in peptic ulcer hemorrhage. Aliment Pharmacol Ther 2002;16(Suppl. 1):66–78.

# CHAPTER 12

# GASTRIC POLYPS AND THICKENED GASTRIC FOLDS

*Gregory G. Ginsberg, MD*

**1. What are gastric polyps, and what are the most commonly observed types of gastric polyps?**

Gastric polyps are any abnormal growth of epithelial tissue arising from the otherwise smooth surface of the stomach. Gastric polyps may be sessile or pedunculated. *Fundic gland* polyps (Fig. 12-1) are now the most commonly observed gastric polyp in Western populations, superseding *hyperplastic* gastric polyps in prevalence (Fig. 12-2). Together, they account for greater than 90% of gastric polyps; *adenomatous* and *hamartomatous* polyps make up the remainder. Early *gastric cancers* may present as polypoid lesions. Gastric polyps may be singular or multiple. Although endoscopic features may predict histology, accurate discrimination of polyp type can be achieved only with tissue sampling and, in some cases, only after complete resection of the polyp.

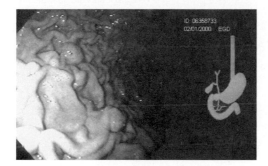

**Figure 12-1.** Two fundic gland polyps are seen among normal-appearing gastric rugae in the fundus.

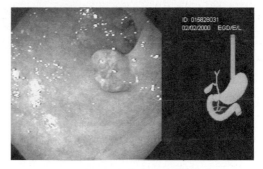

**Figure 12-2.** Sessile hyperplastic polyp, with superficial inflammatory changes, is seen in the antrum.

**2. Describe the endoscopic features typical of each type of gastric polyp.**

*Fundic gland* polyps are typically numerous (greater than 5, often too numerous to count), small (3 to 5 mm), pale, and hemispherical arising in the gastric fundus. Larger fundic gland polyps may develop a pedicle. *Hyperplastic* polyps are more typically pedunculated and erythematous, vary more in number (1 to many) and size (5 to 20 mm), and may occur anywhere throughout the stomach. *Adenomatous* gastric polyps are more apt to be singular and 5 to 20 mm in size. They may be sessile or pedunculated and otherwise indistinguishable from hyperplastic polyps. Endoscopically, *hamartomas*, too, are indistinguishable from hyperplastic and adenomatous polyps.

**3. Describe the histologic features of each type of gastric polyp.**

*Fundic gland* polyps are composed of hypertrophied fundic gland mucosae.

*Hyperplastic* polyps consist of hyperplastic, elongated gastric glands with abundant edematous stroma. There is often cystic dilation of glandular portions but no alteration of the original cellular configuration.

*Adenomatous* polyps are true neoplastic growths composed of dysplastic epithelium not normally present in the stomach. They are composed of cells with hyperchromatic, elongated nuclei arranged in picket-fence patterns with increased mitotic figures.

*Hamartomatous* polyps have branching bands of smooth muscle surrounded by glandular epithelium; the lamina propria is normal.

**4. What is the risk of malignancy associated with gastric polyps?**

*Adenomas* are true neoplasms. The risk of malignant transformation is as high as 75% and size dependent; size greater than 2.0 cm is critically significant, although carcinoma arising in adenomatous polyps less than 2.0 cm is well reported. The risk of malignant transformation in *hyperplastic* polyps is low (0.6% to 4.5%). Because hyperplastic and adenomatous gastric polyps occur against a background of chronic gastritis, the risk of cancer in the gastric mucosa apart from the polyp is increased. Therefore, in addition to removing all polyps, a careful exam should be performed to evaluate the remaining mucosa for early gastric cancer. *Fundic gland* polyps and gastric *hamartomas* are thought to have no malignant potential.

### 5. How should gastric polyps be managed?

Because polyp histology cannot be reliably distinguished by endoscopic appearance, gastric epithelial polyps should be excised endoscopically when feasible. Forceps biopsy alone may result in sampling error. Small gastric epithelial polyps (diameter 3 to 5 mm) may be removed entirely by forceps biopsy resection. Sessile and pedunculated polyps greater than 5.0 mm in diameter should be excised by *snare resection* and tissue retrieved for histologic inspection. Large polyps that cannot be safely removed endoscopically should undergo surgical excision. When gastric polyps are too numerous to count (as is commonly the case with fundic gland polyps and in some polyposis syndromes), resection or biopsy should be performed on the largest lesions, and a sufficient number sampled to confirm benignity and uniformity of histology.

*>/ 5mm snare*

### 6. Is surveillance indicated for patients with gastric polyps?

Although data are insufficient to demonstrate a long-term benefit from endoscopic surveillance, in selected patients it is appropriate. The detection of intestinal metaplasia in the surrounding gastric mucosa—and even more so, atypia or dysplasia—should be taken into consideration. Endoscopic surveillance, if undertaken, should be performed no more frequently than every 2 to 3 years in the absence of dysplasia.

### 7. Describe the relationships between gastric polyps and other conditions.

Fundic gland polyps are promoted by the long-term use of proton pump inhibitors; however, the causal mechanism is unclear. Gastric adenomas and hyperplastic polyps commonly appear against a background of chronic gastritis and are late manifestations of *Helicobacter pylori* infection or type A chronic gastritis (pernicious anemia). Mucosal biopsy samples should be obtained to determine the presence and severity of underlying gastritis and the presence and type of intestinal metaplasia. *H. pylori* eradication should be undertaken for patients with *H. pylori* gastritis and gastric polyps. *H. pylori* eradication may reduce polyp recurrence. Gastric hyperplastic, adenomatous, and fundic gland polyps have an increased prevalence in patients with familial adenomatous polyposis (FAP) and attenuated FAP syndromes.

### 8. What is meant by thickened gastric folds?

Thickened gastric folds appear larger than normal and do not flatten with insufflation of air at endoscopy. Radiographically, large gastric folds are greater than 10 mm in width after distention of the stomach with contrast material during upper gastrointestinal (GI) series.

*fold >1cm*

### 9. List the differential diagnosis for intrinsic causes of thickened gastric folds.

See Table 12-1.

| **Table 12-1.** Intrinsic Causes of Thickened Gastric Folds | |
| --- | --- |
| Lymphoma | Lymphocytic gastritis |
| Mucosa-associated lymphoid tissue (MALT) | Eosinophilic gastritis |
| Linitis plastica | Granulomatous gastritis |
| Gastric adenocarcinoma | Gastritis cystica profunda |
| Ménétrier disease | Gastric anisakiasis |
| Gastric antral vascular ectasia (GAVE) syndrome | Kaposi sarcoma |
| *H. pylori* gastritis (acute) | Gastric varices |
| Zöllinger-Ellison syndrome | Sentinel fold |

### 10. What systemic diseases may be associated with thickened gastric folds or granulomatous gastritis?

Gastric Crohn's disease and sarcoidosis are the most commonly encountered granulomatous gastropathies. Other potential causes of granulomatous gastritis include histoplasmosis, candidal infection, actinomycoses, and blastomycoses. Secondary syphilis may present with *Treponema pallidum* infiltration, producing a perivascular plasmacytic response in the gastric mucosa. Disseminated mycobacteria in tuberculosis may result in gastric infiltration. Systemic mastocytosis, in addition to facial flushing, may be associated with hyperemic thickened gastric folds. Rarely, amyloidosis may cause gastric wall infiltration with thickened gastric folds.

**11. Endoscopic ultrasound (EUS) displays the gastric wall in five alternating hyperechoic and hypoechoic bands. Histologically, to what wall layers do they correlate?**

See Table 12-2.

| **Table 12-2.** Correlation of Endoscopic Ultrasound (EUS) Bands and Wall Layers | | |
|---|---|---|
| WALL LAYER | EUS BANDS | HISTOLOGIC CORRELATION |
| 1st | Hyperechoic | Superficial mucosa |
| 2nd | Hypoechoic | Deep mucosa, including the muscularis mucosa |
| 3rd | Hyperechoic | Submucosa |
| 4th | Hypoechoic | Muscularis propria |
| 5th | Hyperechoic | Serosa |

**12. Describe the role of EUS in the evaluation of thickened gastric folds.**

EUS is the most accurate diagnostic imaging study for the evaluation of thickened gastric folds. EUS allows selection of patients in whom further investigation is warranted with large-particle endoscopic biopsy, snare biopsy, EUS-guided fine-needle aspiration, or full-thickness biopsy at laparotomy. Gastric varices are readily recognized by EUS as serpiginous anechoic structures within and beyond the gastric wall. When EUS demonstrates mural thickening limited to the superficial layers, multiple large-capacity forceps biopsies are apt to provide a histologic diagnosis. Conversely, when EUS documents thickening and wall layer disruption of the deeper layers (i.e., the submucosa or muscularis propria), endoscopic biopsies are not apt to be diagnostic. This appearance on EUS is highly suggestive for malignancy and full-thickness biopsy is recommended when endoscopic tissue sampling is negative (Fig. 12-3).

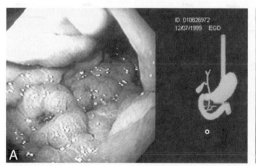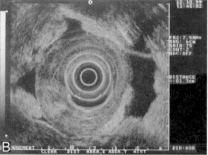

**Figure 12-3.** Thickened gastric folds in a patient with linitis plastica. (**A**) The gastric lumen fails to distend on insufflation, and the folds do not flatten out. (**B**) Endoscopic ultrasound may show wall thickening (13 mm), elimination of the normal wall-layer pattern, and ascites, as seen here.

**13. What are the clinical features of high-grade non-Hodgkin's gastric lymphoma?**

High-grade non-Hodgkin's gastric lymphomas account for 3% of all gastric malignancies but make up the largest group second to adenocarcinoma. The stomach is the most common site of extranodal lymphoma, accounting for 10%. B-cell lymphomas make up the largest pathologic group of gastric lymphomas, followed by T-cell phenotype and other varieties. Endoscopically they may present as a discrete polypoid lesion, an ulcerated mass, or a diffuse submucosal infiltration with enlarged rugal folds. The most common presenting symptoms are abdominal pain, weight loss, nausea, anorexia, and bleeding. When gastric lymphoma is suspected large-particle biopsies should be attempted. EUS is useful in identifying abnormalities of the submucosal wall layers and in establishing nodal involvement (Fig. 12-4). When endoscopic biopsy techniques are unrevealing, full-thickness biopsy should be obtained.

**14. Define MALToma.**

Low-grade gastric mucosa-associated lymphoid tissue (MALT) lymphoma (MALToma) is classified as an extranodal marginal zone lymphoma. MALT is characterized histologically by numerous enlarged lymphoid follicles, a dense B-cell lymphocytic infiltrate, infiltrates of plasma cells, and the presence of lymphoepithelial lesions. Gastric MALTomas may present with bleeding due to ulceration or simply as thickened folds seen on endoscopy or computed tomography (CT) scan (Fig. 12-5). Mucosal biopsy samples, preferably from large-particle forceps, are usually satisfactory for diagnosis. The majority (greater than 80%) of gastric MALT lymphomas are associated with *H. pylori* infection. The median age of detection is in the fifth decade, but it can occur at any age. The majority of MALTomas are low grade and run an indolent course; however, they may bleed and/or progress to invasive lymphoma.

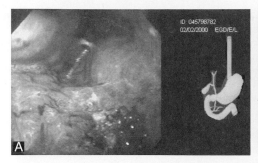
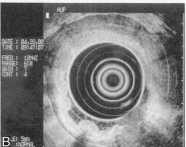

**Figure 12-4.** (**A**) In a patient with gastric lymphoma, endoscopy demonstrates expansive focal thickening of folds, erosions, and hyperemia. (**B**) Endoscopic ultrasound demonstrates focal mural thickening (12 mm) and disruption of the normal wall-layer pattern superiorly. The normal wall-layer pattern and thickness (5.4 mm) are preserved inferiorly.

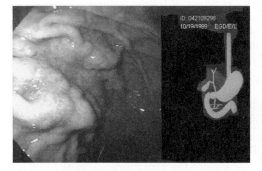

**Figure 12-5.** MALToma detected on endoscopy in a patient with dyspeptic symptoms. There is focal thickening of the folds in contrast to normal surrounding gastric mucosa.

### 15. How are MALTomas managed?
Gastric mapping should be done to assess for *H. pylori* and distribution of the MALT. EUS should be performed to assess the depth of wall-layer involvement and presence of wall-layer disruption. Low-grade MALTomas demonstrate only focal thickening of the mucosal and submucosal layers without wall-layer disruption or surrounding adenopathy. Transmural thickening and wall-layer disruption indicates high-grade MALToma. Treatment options include surgery, radiation, chemotherapy, and *H. pylori* eradication. Numerous studies indicate that if *H. pylori* infection is eradicated in low-grade disease limited to the submucosa, regression of tumor occurs in 60% to 75% of patients. EUS is useful to measure regression of disease objectively.

### 16. Define Ménétrier disease.
Ménétrier disease is a rare condition characterized by giant gastric rugal folds that often spare the antrum. The histologic features are marked foveolar hyperplasia with cystic dilations that may penetrate into the submucosa. Symptoms include abdominal pain, weight loss, gastrointestinal blood loss, and hypoalbuminemia. The cause is unclear. The diagnosis can be confirmed by EUS findings of thickening of the deep mucosal layer and large-particle biopsy specimens demonstrating the characteristic histology. Treatment with monoclonal antibody therapy has been effective in some patients (Fig. 12-6).

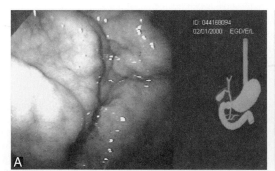
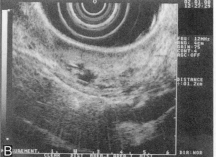

**Figure 12-6.** In Ménétrier disease, giant gastric folds are commonly seen. (**A**) They are soft and pliable on palpation with a probe. (**B**) Endoscopic ultrasound demonstrates marked thickening of the submucosa (12 mm) with cystic dilations.

**17. How is Ménétrier disease different in children and adults?**

Unlike Ménétrier disease in adults, which is characterized by chronicity of symptoms, Ménétrier disease in children is generally self-limited. Recurrence and sequelae are rare. Clinically, pediatric patients present with abrupt onset of vomiting associated with abdominal pain, anorexia, and hypoproteinemia. Gradual onset of edema and ascites results from this protein-losing enteropathy. Hypoalbuminemia, peripheral eosinophilia, and mild normochromic, normocytic anemia are often seen. Radiographic findings include thickened gastric folds in the fundus and body of the stomach, often with antral sparing. Such findings are confirmed by an upper GI barium meal, ultrasonography, and endoscopy. Histologically, the gastric mucosa is hypertrophic with elongation of gastric pits and glandular atrophy. In children, however, intranuclear inclusion bodies consistent with cytomegalovirus (CMV) infection are common; culture of gastric tissue is often positive for CMV. Pediatric patients generally respond to supportive, symptomatic treatment with complete resolution.  *Kids —CMV*

**18. What is the differential diagnosis for a subepithelial mass seen on endoscopy?**

See Table 12-3.

Extrinsic compression by normal or abnormal liver, spleen, gallbladder, lymph nodes, or surrounding vasculature occurs in 30% of cases.

*Submucosal.*

**Table 12-3.** Differential Diagnosis for a Subepithelial Mass Seen on Endoscopy

| COMMON | LESS COMMON | RARE |
|---|---|---|
| Gastrointestinal stromal tumor (GIST) | Leiomyoma | Leiomyoblastoma |
| Lipoma | Granular cell tumor | Liposarcoma |
| Pancreatic rest | Leiomyosarcoma | Schwannoma |
| Carcinoid | Duplication cyst | Fibroma |
| Submucosal cyst | Neurofibroma | Glomus tumor |

**19. What role does EUS play in evaluating submucosal lesions?**

EUS is accurate in differentiating intramural lesions from extraluminal compression. Although EUS does not provide a histopathologic diagnosis, it can suggest the nature of certain submucosal lesions based on their wall layer location and echotexture (Fig. 12-7). Cysts and varices are anechoic; fatty tumors are hyperechoic; and stromal tumors are hypoechoic. Gastrointestinal stromal tumors (GISTs) are seen as hypoechoic structures arising, most commonly, from the fourth (hypoechoic) sonographic layer, which corresponds to the muscularis propria. Although no unique sonographic differences in size, shape, or appearance distinguish benign from malignant GISTs, the risk of malignancy is considered low if the lesion is less than 3 cm in diameter. Gastric lipomas appear as hyperechoic lesions within the submucosal layer. Gastric wall cysts are seen as echo-free structures within the submucosa. Varices are serpiginous. Less common submucosal lesions, such as pancreatic rests, carcinoids, fibromas, and granular cell tumors, can also be recognized.

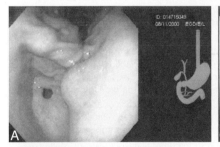
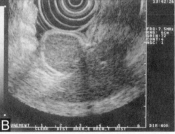

*>3cm GIST in MP*

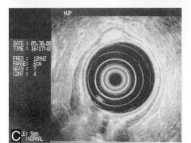

**Figure 12-7.** (**A**) Multiple large and small submucosal lesions are seen on endoscopy. Endoscopic ultrasound demonstrates typical characteristics of leiomyoma (**B**) and lipoma (**C**).

**20. What is a GIST?**

*grow, >3cm ➝OR or invade*

GISTs are the most commonly identified intramural subepithelial mass in the upper GI tract, and the stomach is the most common location. GISTs were once thought to be smooth muscle tumors (leiomyoma and leiomyosarcoma); however, they are now believed to be arise from the interstitial cells of Cajal and express c-kit protein (CD117) on immunohistochemical staining. GISTs most commonly arise in the muscularis propria layer and are usually asymptomatic. All GISTs have malignant potential. Large (greater than 3 cm) and symptomatic lesions should be resected, as should lesions that increase in size or invade surrounding tissue. When the lesion is well circumscribed, small (less than 3 cm), and without evidence of surrounding tissue invasion or adenopathy, it may be followed for interval stability.

**21. A 65-year-old woman presents with self-limited, coffee-grounds emesis. Endoscopy reveals a single, pedunculated, 1-cm polyp in the gastric body. What is the best option for management?**

While most gastric epithelial polyps are asymptomatic, gastric polyps may cause abdominal pain or bleeding. Complete removal of the lesion by snare polypectomy for histologic evaluation is both diagnostic and curative. Snare polypectomy is generally safe and well tolerated, although bleeding occurs more commonly than with colonoscopic polypectomy. Glucagon may be used to inhibit peristalsis aiding in specimen retrieval. An overtube or a retrieval net should be used to avoid accidental dislodgement of the resected specimen into the airway during retrieval. A 6- to 8-week course of a proton pump inhibitor is generally recommended to promote healing.

**22. A patient with FAP has multiple gastric polyps on surveillance endoscopy. What is the most likely histology of such polyps? What is their malignant potential? What other significant upper GI lesions may be detected at the time of upper endoscopy?**

Nearly all patients with FAP have polyps in the upper GI tract. Most polyps are found in the proximal stomach or fundus; they are small, multiple, and hyperplastic. Although they carry no risk for carcinomatous conversion, they may cause bleeding. From 40% to 90% of patients, however, have adenomatous polyps in the distal stomach, antrum, or duodenum, particularly in the periampullary region. Risk of adenocarcinoma of the gastric antrum is not increased in U.S. families with adenomatous polyposis but appears to be increased in Japanese families. The relative risk of duodenal, particularly periampullary, cancer is markedly increased in patients with FAP and duodenal or ampullary adenomas.

**23. Describe the manifestations of gastric polyps in the other hereditary GI polyposis syndromes.**

*Gardner - HP*
*PJS/JPS*
*hamart.*

Patients with Gardner syndrome have a preponderance of hyperplastic polyps in the proximal stomach. Patients with Peutz-Jeghers syndrome and juvenile polyposis syndromes may have hamartomatous polyps in the stomach. Although hamartomas may cause bleeding, an increased cancer risk is not apparent.

**24. A 40-year-old man has a history of chronic pancreatitis complicated by pseudocysts requiring drainage. He presents with a self-limited upper GI bleed. Endoscopy demonstrates a normal esophagus and duodenum. What is the most likely diagnosis? What therapeutic options should be considered?**

The patient has isolated gastric varices secondary to splenic vein thrombosis. Splenic vein thrombosis is a potential complication of acute and chronic pancreatitis, pancreatic carcinoma, lymphoma, trauma, and hypercoagulable states. The left gastric veins empty via the splenic vein. Esophageal venous flow is unaffected. Gastric varices are submucosal or deep to the submucosa, whereas the esophageal varices lie superficial in the lamina propria. Among patients with cirrhotic portal hypertension, gastric variceal bleeding accounts for 10% to 20% of acute variceal hemorrhage, and the incidence of gastric variceal bleeding is 10% to 20% among patients with bleeding from esophagogastric varices. Bleeding from isolated gastric varices attributable to splenic vein thrombosis alone is less common. Acute gastric variceal bleeding may be treated endoscopically with injection sclerotherapy. However, rebleeding is the rule, and the mortality rate is as high as 55%. When endoscopic therapy is not effective, splenectomy is required.

*SV ➝ LGV*

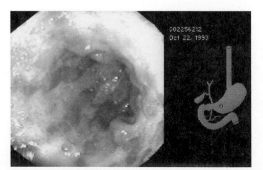

002256212
Oct 22, 1993

**Figure 12-8.** What do these endoscopic findings suggest?

**25. A 65-year-old woman is referred for evaluation of chronic iron deficiency anemia and hemoccult-positive stool. Colonoscopy and upper GI series are negative. Findings of an upper endoscopy are noted in Figure 12-8. Identify the immediately apparent diagnosis and appropriate treatment.**

The raised red folds that radiate spokelike from a pylorus displaying friable vascular malformations are characteristic of gastric antral vascular ectasia (GAVE), also known as *watermelon stomach*. GAVE is a source of chronic occult

GI bleeding. It occurs more frequently in women and often is associated with autoimmune or connective tissue disorders. Underlying atrophic gastritis with hypergastrinemia and pernicious anemia may be present. The pathogenesis is unclear. Histologic features include dilated mucosal capillaries with focal thrombosis; dilated, tortuous submucosal venous channels; and fibrous fibromuscular hyperplasia. Chronic GI blood loss responds to endoscopic contact or noncontact coagulation therapy. Lesions may recur but usually respond to repeat endoscopic therapy.

*APC*

*\* focal thrombi (not in PHG)*

## WEBSITE 🌐

http://www.vhjoe.org

## BIBLIOGRAPHY

1. Al-Haddad M, Ward EM, Bouras EP, et al. Hyperplastic polyps of the gastric antrum in patients with gastrointestinal blood loss. Dig Dis Sci 2007;52:105.
2. Archimandritis A, Spiliadis C, Tzivras M, et al. Gastric epithelial polyps. Ital J Gastroenterol 1996;28:387.
3. Aull MJ, Buell JF, Peddi VR, et al. MALToma: A *Helicobacter pylori*-associated malignancy in transplant patients: A report from the Israel Penn International Transplant Tumor Registry with a review of published literature. Transplantation 2003;75:225.
4. Caletti GC, Brocchie E, Baraldini M, et al. Assessment of portal hypertension by endosonography. Gastrointest Endosc 1988;34:154–5.
5. Fischbach W, Goebeler-Kolve ME, Greiner A. Diagnostic accuracy of EUS in the local staging of primary gastric lymphoma: Results of a prospective, multicenter study comparing EUS with histopathologic stage. Gastrointest Endosc 2002;56:696.
6. Frucht H, Howard JM, Slaff JL, et al. Secretin and calcium provocative tests in Zollinger-Ellison syndrome. Ann Intern Med 1989;111:697–9.
7. Geller A, Gostout CJ, Balm RK, et al. Development of hyperplastic polyps following laser therapy for watermelon stomach. Gastrointest Endosc 1996;43:54.
8. Ginsberg GG, Al-Kawas FH, Fleischer DE, et al. Gastric polyps: Relationship of size and histology to cancer risk. Am J Gastroenterol 1996;91:714–7.
9. Hirota WK, Zuckerman MJ, Adler DG, et al. ASGE guideline: The role of endoscopy in the surveillance of premalignant conditions of the upper GI tract. Gastrointest Endosc 2006;63:570.
10. Hwang JH, Kimmey MB. The incidental upper gastrointestinal subepithelial mass. Gastroenterology 2004;126:301–7.
11. Jalving M, Koornstra JJ, Wesseling J, et al. Increased risk of fundic gland polyps during long-term proton pump inhibitor therapy. Aliment Pharmacol Ther 2006;24:1341.
12. Koch P, del Valle F, Berdel WE, et al. Primary gastrointestinal non-Hodgkin's lymphoma: I. Anatomic and histologic distribution, clinical features, and survival data of 371 patients registered in the German Multicenter Study GIT NHL 01/92. J Clin Oncol 2001;19:3861.
13. Mendis RE, Gerdes H, Lightdale CJ, et al. Large gastric folds: A diagnostic approach using endoscopic ultrasonography. Gastrointest Endosc 1994;40:437–41.
14. Muehldorfer SM, Stolte M, Martus P, et al. Diagnostic accuracy of forceps biopsy versus polypectomy for gastric polyps: A prospective multicentre study. Gut 2002;50:465.
15. Nobre-Leitao C, Lage P, Cravo S, et al. Treatment of gastric MALT lymphoma by *Helicobacter pylori* eradication: A study controlled by endoscopic ultrasonography. Am J Gastroenterol 1998;93:732–6.
16. Ohkusa T, Takashimizu I, Fujiki K, et al. Disappearance of hyperplastic polyps in the stomach after eradication of *Helicobacter pylori*. A randomized clinical trial. Ann Intern Med 1998;129:712–5.
17. Okada M, Iizuka Y, Oh K, et al. Gastritis cystica profunda presenting as giant gastric mucosal folds: The role of endoscopic ultrasonography and mucosectomy in the diagnostic work-up. Gastrointest Endosc 1994;40:640–4.
18. Settle SH, Washington K, Lind C, et al. Chronic treatment of Menetrier's disease with Erbitux: Clinical efficacy and insight into pathophysiology. Clin Gastroenterol Hepatol 2005;3:654.
19. Steinbach G, Ford R, Glober G, et al. Antibiotic treatment of gastric lymphoma-associated lymphoid tissue: An uncontrolled trial. Ann Intern Med 1999;131:88–95.
20. Stolte M, Sticht T, Eidt S, et al. Frequency, location, age and sex distribution of various types of gastric polyps. Endoscopy 1994;26:659.

# GASTROPARESIS

*Edgar Mehdikhani, MD, and Michael Walter, MD*

## 1. Define *gastroparesis*.

It is a symptomatic chronic disorder of gastric motility characterized by delayed gastric emptying without evidence of mechanical obstruction. The disorder is estimated to have 5% prevalence in the United States. Symptoms of gastroparesis are due to failure of the stomach to properly empty its contents into the duodenum.

| SYMPTOM | PREVALENCE IN GASTROPARESIS |
|---|---|
| Nausea | 92% |
| Vomiting | 84% |
| Bloating | 75% |
| Early satiety | 60% |
| Upper abdominal discomfort | 46% |

## 2. What are the factors that determine gastric motility and emptying?

The interplay of physiologic, neural, and hormonal factors influences gastric emptying (Tables 13-1 and 13-2). Once in the stomach, liquids tend to empty without a lag phase. Solids, however, must undergo trituration (grinding) until approximately 1 mm in size.

**Table 13-1.** Physiologic Factors That Influence Gastric Emptying

| DELAY | PROMOTE |
|---|---|
| Solid meal | Liquid meal |
| Fat content | Carbohydrates |
| Cold | Tepid |
| Large volume | Small volume |
| Hyperosmolality | Iso-osmolar |
| Hyperglycemia | Hypoglycemia |
| Smoking | Exercise |

*small CHO meals + exercise*

**Table 13-2.** Neural and Hormonal Factors That Influence Gastric Emptying

| DELAY | PROMOTE |
|---|---|
| Cholecystokinin (CCK) | Motilin |
| Vasoactive intestinal peptide | Serotonin |
| Somatostatin | Acetylcholine |
| Opioids | Substance P |
| Progesterone (pregnancy) | Thyroid |

## 3. Describe the electric pacesetter in the stomach.

The rate of contraction of the stomach is controlled by a *pacesetter* located at a site along the greater curvature in the proximal and middle corpus. The *pacesetter* is composed of a concentration of specialized, fibroblastic-like cells called interstitial cells of Cajal (ICCs) that lie between the axonal plexuses of the gut and the smooth muscle to mediate impulse conduction. ICCs have three major functions:

*ICC*

1. Acting as pacemaker cells in the generation of autorhythmicity of gut muscle
2. Conducting the active propagation of electrical events
3. Mediating enteric neurotransmission

Throughout the gastrointestinal tract, a repetitive, highly regular electrical pattern, known as *slow waves,* occurs at different frequencies. In the stomach, slow waves occur at a frequency of 3 cycles per minute. These slow waves migrate in both circumferential and longitudinal directions. Action potentials occur only at the summit of slow waves, resulting in muscular contraction.

### 4. What is the migrating motor complex?    *MMC 3phases .*
In the fasting state, motor activity is organized into distinct cyclical sequence of events known as the *migrating motor complex.* Cyclical contractions occur in the stomach and small bowel with cycle lengths of 90 to 120 minutes. This cycle consists of three phases. Phase I is the quiescence phase where there is little activity. During the dominant phase II, irregular muscle contractions begin to appear and culminate to a point of maximal contractility (phase III), which lasts about 5 minutes. Phase III is a forceful burst of contractions that sweep the antrum and continue along the entire gastrointestinal (GI) tract to the ileocecal valve. Each repetition of phases I, II, and III is known as the *migrating motor complex* (MMC). The MMC functions to eliminate the small intestine of food, bacteria, and debris between meals.

### 5. Describe gastric motility and emptying.
The stomach serves as a reservoir for food and allows it to pass into the duodenum at a controlled rate. The stomach can be divided into three distinct regions: proximal stomach (cardia, fundus, and proximal stomach), distal stomach (distal corpus and antrum), and pylorus. In the proximal portion, receptive relaxation occurs with distention of the esophagus and/or stomach to accommodate food. In the distal two thirds, forceful contractions by circumferential bands of muscles culminate in terminal antral contractions that grind food into 1-mm pieces (trituration). Liquids rapidly disperse throughout the stomach and begin to empty without a lag period, thus following first-order kinetics. Solids empty in two phases: an initial lag phase when there is no emptying followed by a prolonged linear phase. Overall, gastric emptying is controlled by the activity in the proximal and distal halves of the stomach as well as the pyloric outlet, all of which act in sequence with one another.

### 6. What is idiopathic gastroparesis?    *Y9 ♀.*
The term *idiopathic gastroparesis* has been used to describe patients who present with sudden or insidious onset of postprandial pain, bloating, nausea, vomiting, and early satiety. Despite normal endoscopic exams and lack of prior surgery or other identifiable primary cause, these patients have delayed gastric emptying. Women younger than age 50 comprise 80% to 90% of cases. Nausea, fever, myalgias, and diarrhea may be present in some cases, suggesting viral etiologies. Those patients whose illness begins with a viral prodrome are more likely to do well in the long term and to respond to prokinetic agents in the short term (Fig. 13-1).

### 7. What is diabetic gastroparesis?
Diabetic gastroparesis is one of the most recognizable disorders of delayed gastric emptying with a prevalence of 27% to 58% in long-standing type 1 diabetes mellitus (DM). It encompasses a spectrum of gastric motor abnormalities that include both accelerated and delayed emptying, as well as abnormalities in proximal gastric function and gastric sensation, thus making the term *diabetic gastroenteropathy* more appropriate than gastroparesis. Prominent symptoms

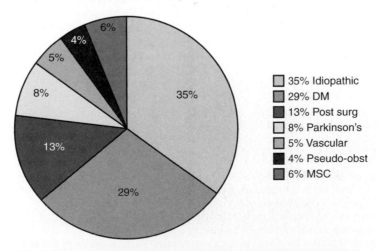

**Figure 13-1.** Etiologies of gastroparesis. DM, diabetes mellitus; MSC, miscellaneous.

among patients with diabetic gastroparesis include early satiety, nausea, and vomiting. It was previously thought that gastroparesis was a complication of diabetes (usually type 1) of more than 10 years' duration with concomitant peripheral and autonomic neuropathy. However, it is seen in as many as 30% of patients with type 2 DM, even with the absence of neuropathy.

## 8. What is the pathogenesis of diabetic gastroparesis?

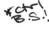

Under normal circumstances, intramural nerves under the influence of the vagus nerve predominantly control gastric motility. A diseased vagus nerve is thought to be the cause of impaired gastric motility in diabetics. For example, diabetics produce only one third of the normal gastric acid output in response to sham feeding, a vagally mediated reflex. However, periods of hyperglycemia in the absence of neuropathy have been correlated with delays in emptying, suggesting that the motor defect is not fixed. A strong correlation exists with delayed gastric emptying of liquids and when the *blood glucose exceeds 270 mg/dL*. Likewise, delays in solid emptying are observed during periods of hyperglycemia in type 1 diabetics, which improve during euglycemia.

## 9. What surgical procedures are associated with postoperative gastroparesis?
Gastroparesis can be seen after the following surgical conditions:

- **Gastric atony after vagotomy:** Approximately 5% of patients who undergo vagotomy and drainage for peptic ulcer disease or malignancy experience nausea, vomiting, and early satiety caused by postoperative gastric stasis in the absence of an anatomic obstruction. Some patients who undergo highly selective vagotomy, including those performed by a laparoscopic approach, may develop gastroparesis. Studies suggest that vagotomy-related gastroparesis tends to resolve over time; however, persistent postsurgical gastric motor dysfunction presents a formidable management challenge and may require complete gastrectomy in resistant cases.
- **Roux stasis syndrome:** Some patients may experience intractable nausea, vomiting, and abdominal pain after construction of a Roux-en-Y gastrojejunostomy. Symptoms of retention may result from either gastric, spastic, or retroperistaltic Roux limb motor abnormalities.
- **Delayed gastric emptying in association with fundoplication:** Although the usual effect of fundoplication is to accelerate, rather than delay, gastric emptying, instances of gastroparesis have been described in 4% to 40% of patients following laparoscopic or open antireflux surgery.
- **Gastric stasis after gastric bypass surgery:** Gastroplasty and gastric bypass are performed in some morbidly obese patients who fail dietary methods of weight control. *Gastroplasty* (gastric partitioning) creates a 50-mL fundic pouch, which is continuous with the distal stomach through a 10-mm stoma. *Gastric bypass* divides the stomach in two with the proximal compartment draining through a 12-mm gastroenterostomy. These procedures produce delayed gastric emptying of solids and fundic distention leading to early satiety, loss of appetite, and weight reduction.
- **Gastroparesis after other surgeries:** Esophagectomy with colonic interposition or gastric pull-through into the thoracic cavity may be curative for esophageal malignancy, but delays in gastric emptying are reported. Pylorus preserving Whipple procedures performed for pancreatic cancer and chronic pancreatitis are complicated by delayed gastric emptying in up to 50% of cases. Gastroparesis is a common sequela of lung and heart-lung transplantation and may predispose to microaspiration into the transplanted lung.

## 10. What conditions cause selective gastric motor dysfunction leading to gastroparesis?
- **Gastroparesis in association with gastroesophageal reflux disease (GERD):** Delays in solid or liquid phase gastric emptying can be seen in some patients with GERD. Delays in gastric emptying in patients with GERD correlate poorly with symptoms, lower esophageal sphincters pressure, and 24-hour pH monitoring results.
- **Radiation-induced gastric stasis:** Severe nausea, vomiting, and intolerance of both liquid and solid meals are common after abdominal irradiation.
- **Delayed gastric emptying with atrophic gastritis:** Delayed gastric emptying of solids but not liquid meals may be seen in patients with atrophic gastritis with or without pernicious anemia. This may be caused, in part, by poor intragastric processing of food due to decreased secretion of digestive enzymes, which in turn prolong the time needed to fragment solid foods.

## 11. Which disorders with diffuse abnormalities of gastrointestinal motor activity cause gastroparesis?
- **Rheumatologic disorders:** Scleroderma (40% to 70%), polymyositis, dermatomyositis, and systemic lupus erythematosus (SLE)
- **Chronic intestinal pseudo-obstruction** (CIPO): CIPO is often familial and presents with symptoms caused by gastric and small bowel hypomotility. The diagnosis is suggested by delayed transit and luminal dilation and confirmed by full-thickness biopsy of the small bowel.
- **Infectious disorders:** *Trypanosoma cruzi* (Chagas disease), varicella zoster, Epstein-Barr virus, *Clostridium botulinum,* and human immunodeficiency virus (HIV)
- **Miscellaneous conditions with diffuse motor abnormalities:** Myotonic dystrophy and progressive muscular dystrophy, and primary or secondary amyloidosis

## 12. Which drugs affect gastric emptying?

Many prescription and over-the-counter medications can modify gastric emptying rates (Table 13-3).

### Table 13-3. Effects of Medications on Gastric Emptying

| DELAYS GASTRIC EMPTYING | ACCELERATES GASTRIC EMPTYING |
| --- | --- |
| Alcohol (high concentration) | β-Blockers |
| Aluminum hydroxide antacids | Diazepam |
| Atropine | Domperidone |
| β-Agonist | Erythromycin |
| Calcitonin | Histamine $H_2$ |
| Calcium channel blockers | Metoclopramide |
| Dexfenfluramine | Naloxone |
| Diphenhydramine | Prostaglandin $E_2$ |
| Dopamine | |
| Glucagon | |
| Interleukin 1 | |
| Levodopa | |
| Lithium | |
| Omeprazole | |
| Ondansetron | |
| Opiates | |
| Phenothiazine | |
| Potassium | |
| Progesterone | |
| Sucralfate | |
| Theophylline | |
| Tobacco | |
| Tricyclic antidepressants | |

## 13. List the conditions that have an established association with delayed gastric emptying.

- **Diabetes mellitus**
- **Anorexia nervosa**
- **Gastric surgery:** Gastric atony may occur after gastric surgery. Surgery should not be done acutely on a dilated, obstructed stomach as atony is more likely to occur.
- **Parkinson disease:** Responsible for 7% of cases of gastroparesis. **IMPORTANT:** Avoid metoclopramide as a treatment in the patient group, as this may provoke a parkinsonian crisis even in those with mild preclinical disease!
- **Connective tissue disease:** Especially scleroderma (up to 40% to 70%)

## 14. What associations are likely to be important in gastroparesis?

- **Gastric dysrhythmias:** Usually of an idiopathic nature, dysrhythmias may delay gastric emptying. Various dysrhythmias have been described and may be measured with electrogastrography.
- **Tachygastria** is associated with delayed gastric emptying. No contractions occur during periods of tachygastria. Secondary gastric dysrhythmias are associated with anorexia nervosa and motion sickness. They have also been reported in gastric ulcers and gastric cancers (Fig. 13-2).
- **Obesity** appears to slow gastric emptying, because there is an inverse relationship between body size and gastric emptying. This may relate to insulin resistance.
- **Stress** from pain and anxiety can alter gastric emptying through the central nervous system (CNS).
- **Neurologic disorders,** including strokes, brain tumors, headaches, and high intracranial pressures, can alter gastric emptying.
- **Diseases that involve the gastric wall** may slow gastric emptying, including scleroderma, amyloidosis, SLE, and dermatomyositis.
- **Abdominal cancer** may delay gastric emptying via direct involvement of the stomach wall or by invading the surrounding nerves. Gastroparesis also may be a paraneoplastic effect.

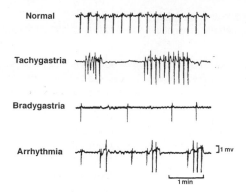

**Figure 13-2.**  Gastric arrhythmias that may delay gastric emptying are measured with electrogastrography.

## 15. Which part of the history and physical exam is important in establishing a diagnosis of gastroparesis?

Nausea may be insidious and without vomiting. When present, the timing of vomiting is important as patients with gastroparesis may vomit undigested food several hours after eating. Patients with regurgitation do not have true nausea; therefore, other diagnoses should be considered. Associated symptoms, such as pain, fever, and diarrhea, may be indicative of other causes. A review of the surgical history is crucial. Medication lists need to be reviewed as some may slow gastric emptying, including pain medications and any drug with anticholinergic properties. A psychological history is also important because patients with bulimia and anorexia nervosa may be difficult to identify. Ruling out gastric outlet obstruction and its causes is necessary before making a diagnosis of gastroparesis.

## 16. What modalities are available for diagnosing gastroparesis?

- *Gastric emptying* of a solid-phase meal by scintigraphy is considered the gold standard for the diagnosis of gastroparesis. Because gastric emptying of solids is a better indicator of disease, solid-meal study is the method of choice. Most centers use a standardized test meal: toast, jam, EggBeaters labeled with $^{99m}$Tc-sulfur colloid. With this technique, scintigraphic gastric retention greater than 60% at 2 hours and greater than 10% at 4 hours are considered consistent with gastroparesis. However, it is important to continue scanning for at least 4 hours, as this improves accuracy and specificity in identifying gastroparesis.
- *Isotope breath test* is an indirect means of measuring gastric emptying. Most commonly $^{13}$C-labeled octanoate, a medium-chain triglyceride, is incorporated into a solid meal. After ingestion, the isotope is rapidly absorbed in the small bowel and metabolized into $^{13}CO_2$, which is expelled from the lungs during respiration. The rate-limiting step for the signal appearing in the breath is the rate of solid gastric emptying. The test assumes normal small bowel, pancreas, liver, and pulmonary functions. With this protocol, the test is reproducible, although comparisons with scintigraphy have revealed variable results, and its use in the clinical setting remains limited.
- *Ultrasonography* has been used to measure gastric emptying and has been shown to be equivalent to scintigraphy. However, its widespread application has been limited by the high level of expertise required to perform and interpret the study.
- *Electrogastrography* (EGG) records gastric myoelectrical activity. An abnormal EGG is defined when the percent time in dysrhythmia exceeds 30% of the recording time and/or when meal ingestion fails to elicit an increase in signal amplitude. Gastric dysrhythmias, including tachygastria (greater than 4 cycles per minute), bradygastria (less than 2 cycles per minute), and decreased amplitude responses to meal ingestion, have been characterized in patients with gastroparesis. The clinical role of EGG remains to be established, although currently it is considered to be an adjunct to gastric emptying in patients suspected of having gastroparesis.
- *Antroduodenal manometry* measures phasic pressure changes due to contractions and provides information about coordination of gastric, pyloric, and duodenal motor function in the fasting and postprandial periods. In gastroparesis, antroduodenal manometry can exhibit a decreased frequency and amplitude of antral contractions. However, this test is often difficult to perform and is usually reserved for the refractory patient evaluated at tertiary referral centers.

## 17. Outline an approach to the diagnosis of gastroparesis.

See Figure 13-3.

---

- Lab tests: HCG, CBC, chemistry, TSH
- Structural exam:
  - –EGD & / or
  - –UGI and small bowel
- Functional exam:
  - –2 and 4 hr solid phase emptying  (scintigraphy)
- Tobacco smokers & paraneoplastic syndrome
  - –Chest X-ray (80% normal CXR)
  - –80% IgG Ab to myenteric neurons
  - –(+) IgG anti-ANNA or (+) IgG anti-Hu

---

**Figure 13-3.** Tests to evaluate for gastroparesis.

## 18. Once gastroparesis is diagnosed, how should it be treated?

Correction of any reversible causes of gastroparesis is the first step in management. Electrolyte abnormalities should be corrected, and drugs that potentially slow gastric emptying should be stopped. In diabetics, tight glycemic control is imperative and needs to be emphasized. A diet consisting of small, frequent, low-fat meals should be started. Several prokinetic drugs that facilitate gastric motility are available:

- *Bethanechol:* A cholinergic drug that stimulates muscarinic receptors. A slight increase in amplitude and a slight decrease in frequency of antral contractions were seen. Its usefulness in gastroparesis is limited.
- *Metoclopramide:* A dopamine antagonist with potent cholinergic effects. It acts mainly on the proximal GI tract. In the stomach, it increases antral contractions and relaxes the pylorus. It also has antiemetic properties. The usual dosage is 10 mg 4 times a day and it may be given orally or intravenously. Side effects, such as drowsiness, dystonic reactions, and nervousness, are common and can limit its use. Moreover, it is effective in the short term and long-term utility has not been proved.
- *Cisapride:* A benzamide derivative that facilitates acetylcholine release at the myenteric plexus. It affects the entire GI tract and does not have the CNS side effects of metoclopramide. Cisapride was recently taken off the market due to life-threatening arrhythmias, and QT-interval prolongation in some patients, but it may be obtained directly from Janssen Pharmaceutica, if certain criteria are met.
- *Domperidone:* A benzimidazole derivative with clinical effects similar to metoclopramide. It acts primarily on the proximal GI tract and has fewer side effects than metoclopramide. It is available in the United States through an FDA-approved process.
- *Erythromycin:* Given in doses of 50 mg intravenously, erythromycin induces phase III contractions in the antrum and upper small bowel. It is most effective in an acute setting. It stimulates motilin and cholinergic receptors and induces dumping of food from the stomach. Efficacy with long-term oral administration has not been established and may be complicated by the risks associated with long-term antibiotic use.
- *Tegaserod:* A serotonin (5-HT$_4$) receptor partial agonist was found to improve gastric emptying compared to placebo in healthy men. It also improved gastric emptying in patients with gastroparesis complaining of dyspeptic symptoms. In 2007, the Food and Drug Administration (FDA) requested that tegaserod be withdrawn from the market due to increased risk of heart attack and stroke.

## 19. What are the complications of gastroparesis?

Gastroparesis can have a significant impact on a patient's quality of life. Severe nausea and vomiting may lead to significant weight loss, malnutrition, gastrointestinal hemorrhage from Mallory-Weiss tears, and aspiration pneumonia. Nutritional deficiencies are commonly seen in patients with postvagotomy gastric stasis. A common complication is development of phytobezoar in the stomach, which can lead to ulcerations, small intestinal obstruction, and gastric perforation.

## 20. What is the surgical management for medically refractory gastroparesis?

Surgery is performed only as a last resort in carefully evaluated patients with profound gastroparesis. Surgical jejunostomy with enteric feeding can improve overall health, gastrointestinal symptoms, and nutritional status and reduce hospitalization rates. Additional gastrostomy placement can drain gastric secretions during severe symptom flares. Vomiting, need for parenteral nutrition, and retained food in the stomach predict poor outcome following surgery. Diabetic patients with gastroparesis and renal failure have shown greater improvement in gastric function after combined pancreas-kidney transplantation than after kidney transplantation alone, suggesting that the enhancement of glycemic control provided by the pancreatic graft provides significant beneficial effects.

## 21. What is the role of botulinum toxin injection in refractory gastroparesis?

Botulinum toxin is a potent inhibitor of neuromuscular transmission. Intrapyloric injection of Botox has been reported to be efficacious in gastric emptying, although symptoms typically persist and effects are short lived. Thus far, the data available do not support the widespread application of this treatment modality in gastroparesis.

## 22. What is gastric electrical stimulation?

Gastric electrical stimulation (GES) was first introduced more than 40 years ago, although little progress was made until recent years. The basic components required for GES include electrodes mounted on a single lead or a pair of leads and an implantable pulse generator. Although the pulse generator is commonly placed in the subcutaneous pouch in the abdomen, different methods for placement of the stimulation electrodes are used, including open surgical placement under general anesthesia; minimally invasive laparoscopic placement, which does not require hospitalization; or endoscopic placement. The electrical stimuli delivered can be classified into long pulses (low frequency, high energy), which are on the order of milliseconds, and short pulses (high frequency, low energy), which are on the order of microseconds, and trains of short pulses. Long pulses are needed to alter the functions of gastric smooth muscle to normalize dysrhythmias. At the present, no commercially available implantable pulse generator is capable of producing pulses with a width of greater than 1 ms.

## 23. What is the role of gastric electrical stimulation in refractory gastroparesis?

GES received FDA Humanitarian Use Device approval in 2000. The device includes a neurostimulator (Enterra Therapy system) and two intramuscular leads. The beneficial effects of GES have been documented, most notably in a multicenter Worldwide Antivomiting Electrical Stimulation Study (WAVESS), which established the positive short-term effects of low energy, high frequency GES on symptom reduction. Most studies to date have documented improvement of nausea and vomiting with minimal effects on the rate of gastric emptying using GES.

More recently, however, the focus has switched to using multichannel (two or four) stimulation, also known as *gastric pacing*, to attempt to entrain or modulate the rate of the intrinsic gastric pacemaker. Animal studies have shown promising results in improving emetic responses, acceleration of gastric emptying, and normalization of gastric dysrhythmias using multichannel pacers. Multichannel gastric electric pacing delivers electrical pulses to multiple locations along the greater curvature of the stomach. The use of synchronized multichannel gastric electrical pacing was recently studied in patients with diabetic gastroparesis. Improvement in both gastric emptying (accelerated gastric emptying) and symptoms were observed. Therefore, gastric electrical pacing may represent a promising approach to managing patients with refractory symptoms. However, gastric pacing remains experimental and is not approved by the FDA.

## WEBSITES

http://www.medtronic.com/neuro/gastro/enterra/enterra.html

http://www.medscape.com/viewarticle/460632

## BIBLIOGRAPHY

1. Abell T, McCallum R, Hocking M, et al. Gastric electrical stimulation for medically refractory gastroparesis. Gastroenterology 2003;125: 421.
2. Anand C, Al-Juburi A, Familoni B, et al. Gastric electrical stimulation is safe and effective: A long-term study in patients with drug-refractory gastroparesis in three regional centers. Digestion 2007;75:83–9.
3. Bitytskiy LP, Soykan I, McCallum RW. Viral gastroparesis: A subgroup of idiopathic gastroparesis clinical characteristics and long-term outcomes. Am J Gastroenterol 1997;92:1501.
4. Cucchiara S, Salvia G, Borrelli O, et al. Gastric electrical dysrhythmias and delayed gastric emptying in gastroesophageal reflux disease. Am J Gastroenterol 1997;92:1103.
5. Cutts TF, Luo J, Starkebaum W. Is gastric electrical stimulation superior to standard pharmacologic therapy in improving GI symptoms, healthcare resources, and long-term health care benefits? Neurogastroenterol Motil 2005;17:35–43.
6. Degen L, Matzinger D, Merz M, et al. Tegaserod, a 5-HT4 receptor partial agonist, accelerates gastric emptying and gastrointestinal transit in healthy male subjects. Aliment Pharmacol Ther 2001;15:1745.
7. Fujuwara Y, Nakagawa K, Tanaka T, et al. Relationship between gastroesophageal reflux and gastric emptying after distal gastrectomy. Am J Gastroenterol 1996;91:75.
8. Guo JP, Maurer AH, Fisher RS, et al. Extending gastric emptying scintigraphy from two to four hours detects more patients with gastroparesis. Dig Dis Sci 2001;46:24.
9. Guorcerol G, Leblanc I, Leroi AM, et al. Gastric electrical stimulation in medically refractory nausea and vomiting. Eur J Gastroenterol Hepatol 2007;19:29–35.
10. Hasler WL. Gastroparesis: Symptoms, evaluation and treatment. Gastroenterol Clin N Am 2007;36:619–47.
11. Jones MP, Maganti K. A systematic review of surgical therapy for gastroparesis. Am J Gastroenterol 2003;98:2122.

12. Kashyap P, Farrugia G. Enteric autoantibodies and gut motility disorders. Gastroenterol Clin N Am 2008;37:397–410.
13. Konturek JW, Fischer H, van der Voort IR, et al. Disturbed gastric motor activity in patients with human immunodeficiency virus infection. Scand J Gastroenterol 1997;32:221.
14. Maranki J, Lytes V, Meilahn JE, et al. Predictive factors for clinical improvement with Enterra gastric electric stimulation treatment for refractory gastroparesis. Dig Dis Sci 2008;53:2072–8.
15. Park MI, Camilleri M. Gastroparesis: clinical update. Am J Gastroenterol 2006;101:1129–39.
16. Patrick A. Review: gastroparesis. Aliment Pharmcol Ther 2008;27:724–40.
17. Patterson D, Abell T, Rothstein R, et al. A double-blind multicenter comparison of domperidone and metoclopramide in the treatment of diabetic patients with symptoms of gastroparesis. Am J Gastroenterol 1999;94:1230.
18. Tougas G, Eaker EY, Abell TL, et al. Assessment of gastric emptying using low fat meal and establishment of international control values. Am J Gastroenterol 2000;95:1456–62.
19. Yin J, Chen J. Implantable gastric electrical stimulation: Ready for prime time? Gastroenterology 2008;134:665–7.
20. Zhang J, Chen DZ. Systematic review: Applications and future of gastric electrical stimulation. Aliment Pharmacol Ther 2006;24:991–1002.

# 14 CHAPTER

# EVALUATION OF ABNORMAL LIVER TESTS

*Kenneth E. Sherman, MD, PhD*

### 1. What are *liver tests*?

Usually the term refers to the routine chemistry panel that includes alanine aminotransferase (ALT), aspartate aminotransferase (AST), γ-glutamyl transpeptidase (GGT), alkaline phosphatase (AP), bilirubin, albumin, and protein. Other terms for the same tests are *liver function tests* (LFTs) and *liver-associated enzymes* (LAEs), but neither is totally accurate. Only the first four are properly called enzymes, and only the last two provide a measure of liver function. These tests help to characterize injury patterns and provide a crude measure of the synthetic function of the liver. Various combinations can be helpful in diagnosing specific disease processes, but generally these tests are not diagnostic. Other LFTs are described later. Finally, certain tests help to define specific causes of liver disease. They may be serologic (e.g., hepatitis C antibody) or biochemical (e.g., $\alpha_1$-antitrypsin level) but generally are not used as screening assays or as part of general health profiles.

### 2. What are the true *liver function tests*?

True LFTs evaluate the liver's synthetic capacity or measure the ability of the liver either to uptake and clear substances from the circulation or to metabolize and alter test reagents. *Albumin* is the most commonly used indicator of synthetic function, although it is not highly sensitive and may be affected by poor nutrition, renal disease, and other factors. In general, low albumin levels indicate poor synthetic function. The *prothrombin time* (PT) is another simple measure of the liver's capacity to synthesize clotting factors. The PT may be related to decreased synthetic ability or vitamin K deficiency. A high PT that does not correct with oral administration of vitamin K (5 to 10 mg for 3 days) may indicate liver disease, unless ductal obstruction or intrahepatic cholestasis prevents bile excretion into the duodenum and thus limits absorption of vitamin K. Administration of a subcutaneous or intravenous injection of vitamin K (10 mg) may correct the defect and suggests that vitamin K absorption rather than synthetic dysfunction is responsible for the PT abnormality.

Various uptake and excretion tests profess to define liver function, including bromosulfothalein (BSP), indocyanine green, aminopyrine, caffeine, monoethylglycinexylidide (MEGX), and the cholate shunt. Research laboratories frequently use such tests to determine severity of liver disease and to predict survival outcomes, but currently they are not part of routine clinical practice.

### 3. What is the difference between cholestatic and hepatocellular injury?

The two main mechanisms of liver injury are damage or destruction of liver cells, which is classified as *hepatocellular,* and impaired transport of bile, which is classified as *cholestatic*. Hepatocellular injury is most often due to viral hepatitis, autoimmune hepatitis, and various toxins and drugs. Transport of bile may be impaired by extrahepatic duct obstruction (e.g., gallstone, postsurgical stricture), intrahepatic duct narrowing (e.g., primary sclerosing cholangitis), bile duct damage (e.g., primary biliary cirrhosis), or failed transport at the canalicular level (e.g., chlorpromazine effect). In some cases, elements of both types of damage are involved; this scenario is often called a *mixed injury* pattern.

### 4. What is the most specific test for hepatocellular damage?

The most specific test for hepatocellular damage is the ALT level. The AST level also may be elevated but is not as specific.

### 5. How is cholestatic injury best diagnosed?

Cholestatic injury is best diagnosed by an elevated AP level. Bile acids stimulate AP production, but duct obstruction or damage prevents bile acid excretion into the duodenum. Therefore, the AP level in serum rises dramatically. Serum AP levels may be slightly increased in early hepatocellular disease, but this increase is due to release of cellular enzyme without excessive stimulation of new enzyme. Because AP can be derived from other body tissue (e.g., bone, intestine), a concurrent elevation of GGT or 5′-nucleotidase helps to support a cholestatic mechanism. Alternatively, some clinical laboratories can fractionate alkaline phosphatase into component fractions (e.g. liver, bone, intestine).

### 6. What are serum transaminases?

The two serum transaminases commonly assayed in clinical practice are ALT and AST. Many laboratories still use older terminology that refers to ALT as serum glutamic pyruvate transaminase (SGPT) and to AST as SGOT (serum glutamic oxaloacetic transaminase). The newer terms reflect more accurately their enzymatic action, which involves the transfer of amino groups from one structure to another. As noted earlier, elevation of ALT and/or AST reflects the presence of hepatocellular injury. It is important to understand how the assays are performed and what confounding factors may alter interpretation of test results.

## 7. How is ALT assessed?

The most commonly used test reaction for ALT is as follows:

$$\text{Alanine} + \text{alpha-ketoglutarate} \rightarrow \text{pyruvate} + \text{L-glutamate}$$

This reaction requires ALT and pyridoxal phosphate (vitamin $B_6$). A crucial point is that enzyme assays do not measure how much enzyme is present; instead, they indirectly measure the catalytic activity of the enzyme in performing a particular function. Therefore, the assay does not indicate how much ALT is present but how quickly it causes the above reaction to take place. The assumption is that the faster the reaction, the greater is the amount of ALT. To complicate matters further, the assay does not measure the amount of reaction product that is created. Instead, a linked enzyme reaction is used:

$$\text{Pyruvate} \rightarrow \text{L-lactic acid}$$

This reaction occurs in the presence of another enzyme, lactate dehydrogenase. The reaction requires the oxidation of reduced nicotinamide adenine dinucleotide (NADH) and creates the unreduced form ($NAD^+$) as an additional reaction product. $NAD^+$ absorbs light at a 340-nm wavelength. This absorption, as measured by a spectrophotometer, is used to determine ALT activity. Therefore, the end-point measurement is several steps removed from the quantitative measurement of interest. The speed of a reaction, however, may be affected by several components of the process, including temperature, substrate concentration, amount of enzymes or cofactors, interfering substances in the reaction mix, and sensitivity of the spectrophotometer. For example, if a patient is deficient in pyridoxal phosphate and this cofactor is not added in excess of the amount needed for the test reaction, the reaction rate is slowed, and the final result is a falsely low ALT activity. This confounding effect is probably common in malnourished alcoholics, in whom deficiency of vitamin $B_6$ rather than ALT level is the limiting step in the reaction.

## 8. How are normal and abnormal levels of ALT determined?

This determination is generally made by the local laboratory in an arbitrary manner. A small set of so-called healthy patients is selected, often from a blood bank. The ALT is determined in all members, and a mean and standard deviation are calculated. Arbitrary cutoffs are assigned, usually at values representing the top and bottom 2.5% of the sample population. This technique is unfortunate, because many demographic factors play a role in ALT level. Men have higher ALT levels than do women, obese women have higher ALT levels than do people close to ideal body weight, and certain racial groups have higher ALT activity than do others. In addition, patients who donate blood may not in fact be free of liver disease. Therefore, if the random test population consists mainly of thin white women who donate blood at an office drive, the cutoff values may be very low. Thus, many overweight men may have ALT levels in the *high* range, even in the absence of disease. This problem applies to all of the enzyme tests described in this chapter. Therefore, the farther a test result is from normal, the more likely it is that disease in fact exists. Conversely, patients with significant silent liver disease may have normal ALT levels. Recent population studies suggest that the relationship between ALT and liver injury and that local laboratory normal values almost always understate the presence of liver disease. These studies suggest that clinicians should define abnormal as ALT greater than 30 IU/L for men and greater than 19 IU/L for women regardless of the local laboratory normal values.

The ALT level, therefore, is an imperfect marker of the liver process. In diseases that involve massive liver damage, such as acute viral hepatitis, acetaminophen or solvent toxicity, or amanita mushroom poisoning, ALT may be increased to very high levels. For example, an ALT value of 2000 IU/L (50 times the upper limit of normal) is frequently seen in significant acetaminophen overdoses. This value reflects significant loss of ALT from damaged hepatocytes. In patients with chronic viral hepatitis, levels tend to be lower and frequently are 2 to 10 times normal values.

## 9. What makes the AP level rise?

AP is a group of enzymes that catalyze the transfer of phosphate groups. Different isoenzymes can be identified from multiple sites in the body, including liver, bone, and intestine. Most hospital labs do not have the facilities to identify the source. This inability may pose a problem for clinicians. In one large study of hospitalized patients, only about 65% of elevated AP was from the liver. When the source is the liver, the mechanism appears to be related to stimulation of enzyme synthesis associated with local increases in bile acids. This finding results from drug-associated cholestasis and intrahepatic and extrahepatic obstruction. The problems associated with determining enzyme activity and establishing a normal range are analogous to those described for serum transaminases. The association of elevated AP with either GGT or 5′-nucleotidase helps to establish a liver source and suggests the presence of a cholestatic process.

## 10. What does an elevated bilirubin mean?

Bilirubin, a breakdown product of red blood cells, exists in two forms: conjugated and unconjugated. Unconjugated bilirubin appears in the serum when blood is broken down at a rate that overwhelms the processing ability of the liver. This finding is most common in patients with hemolysis. Several genetically acquired enzyme deficiencies result in improper or incomplete bilirubin conjugation in the liver. The most common is Gilbert's syndrome, which is characterized by a relative deficiency of uridine diphosphate–glucuronyl transferase. Recently, the specific gene polymorphism that accounts for a significant proportion of the observed phenotypic abnormality was described. Patients often have high-normal to borderline-elevated bilirubin levels. When they fast or decrease caloric intake (e.g., patients with viral gastroenteritis), the bilirubin rises, primarily because of increases in the unconjugated form. If a bilirubin fractionation is not done, a patient with abdominal pain, nausea and vomiting, and an elevated bilirubin level may be misdiagnosed as having cholecystitis. The resulting cholecystectomy could easily have been avoided by obtaining the fractionation.

## 11. How is bilirubin level determined?

The most common test for bilirubin involves running a biochemical reaction over time. Many clinical labs report only total bilirubin. By stopping the reaction at a particular time and subtracting the result from the total bilirubin, the lab arrives at the indirect bilirubin, which is an approximation of unconjugated bilirubin. Exact measurement requires the use of chromatography, which is not routinely performed in clinical labs. Conjugated bilirubin is elevated in many diseases, including viral, chemical, and drug- and alcohol-induced hepatitis; cirrhosis; metabolic disorders; and intrahepatic and extrahepatic biliary obstruction.

## 12. What tests are used to evaluate hemochromatosis?

Hemochromatosis is a disease of iron overload in the liver and other organs. The defect is probably in a regulatory mechanism for iron absorption in the small intestine. Over many years, patients build up stored iron in the liver, heart, pancreas, and other organs. The most common screening test for hemochromatosis is *serum ferritin*; an elevated level suggests the possibility of iron overload. Unfortunately, ferritin is also an acute-phase reactant and may be falsely elevated in various inflammatory processes (including alcohol abuse). If ferritin is elevated (usually greater than 400 μg/L), serum iron and total iron-binding capacity (TIBC) should be assessed. If the serum iron value divided by the TIBC value is greater than 50% to 55%, hemochromatosis should be strongly suspected instead of secondary iron overload (hemosiderosis).

Until recently, the definitive test was a quantitative assessment of iron. A *liver biopsy* specimen is used to determine the amount of iron in liver tissue. From a calculation based on the patient's age and iron content in liver, an index, called the *iron-age index,* was used to determine the presence or absence of hemochromatosis. This test may not be as reliable as previously thought, based on the recent availability of genetic testing. Three major *gene defects* have been described. They involve single amino acid mutations, which result in altered iron absorption. The most important gene is designated *C282Y; H63D* also may have a role in some populations. These genes are biallelic; that is, each parent contributes one half of the patient's complement. Therefore, patients may be homozygote wild-type, heterozygote, or homozygote with mutation. Only patients with both mutated alleles are thought to have genetic hemochromatosis. However, only about 85% of patients with hemochromatosis will have one of the commonly identified mutations.

Studies suggest that *magnetic resonance imaging* of the liver also may be helpful in evaluating hepatic iron content and in the future may reduce the need for liver biopsy. However, most radiologists are not trained to interpret the results.

## 13. Describe the role of $\alpha_1$-antitrypsin.

$\alpha_1$-Antitrypsin is an enzyme, made by the liver, that helps to break down trypsin and other tissue proteases. Multiple variants are described in the literature. The variant is expressed as an allele from both parents. Therefore, a person may have one or two forms of $\alpha_1$-antitrypsin in the blood. One particular variant, called Z because of its unique electrophoretic mobility on gel, is the product of a single amino acid gene mutation from the wild-type protein (M). The Z protein is difficult to excrete from the liver cell and causes local damage that may result in hepatitis and cirrhosis.

## 14. What three tests are used to diagnose $\alpha_1$-antitrypsin deficiency?

1. *Serum protein electrophoresis (SPEP).* When blood proteins are separated on the basis on electrical migration in gel, several bands are formed. One of these, the $\alpha_1$ band, consists mostly of $\alpha_1$-antitrypsin. Therefore, an $\alpha_1$-antitrypsin deficiency results in a flattening of the $\alpha_1$ band on SPEP.
2. *Direct assay* that uses a monoclonal antibody against $\alpha_1$-antitrypsin. The degree of binding can be measured in a spectrophotometer by rate nephelometry.
3. $\alpha_1$-*Antitrypsin phenotype.* Only a few labs in the United States run this test, which designates the allelic protein types in the serum (e.g., MM, ZZ, MZ, FZ). Patients with protein of the ZZ type are said to be homozygotic for Z-type $\alpha_1$-antitrypsin deficiency. This is the form most frequently associated with significant liver disease. If Z protein is trapped in hepatocytes, it can be seen in liver tissue as small globules that stain with the periodic acid–Schiff (PAS) reaction and resist subsequent digestion with an enzyme called diastase. An immunostain is also available in some institutions.

## 15. What is Wilson's disease?

Wilson disease, a disorder of copper storage, is associated with deficiency of an enzyme derived from liver cells. Like iron, copper may accumulate in many tissues in the body. Its storage sites are somewhat different, however. Deposition may be seen in the eye (Kayser-Fleischer rings) and parts of the brain. Many cholestatic diseases of the liver (e.g., primary biliary cirrhosis) also result in aberrant copper storage but not to the degree seen in true Wilson disease.

## 16. How is Wilson's disease diagnosed?

The main screening test is the serum ceruloplasmin level, which is low in over 95% of patients with Wilson disease. Ceruloplasmin is also an acute-phase reactant and may be falsely elevated into a low-normal range in patients with an inflammatory process. Follow-up tests include assessments of urine and serum copper levels. A quantitative assessment of copper in liver tissue from liver biopsy provides definitive diagnosis. Copper is stained in the tissue with special stain processes (e.g., rhodanine stain).

## 17. Summarize the tests for common metabolic disorders of the liver.

There are numerous other hereditary diseases of the liver, including Gaucher disease, Niemann-Pick disease, and hereditary tyrosinemia. These rare diseases are usually diagnosed in children. Specific tests are beyond the scope of this chapter. See Table 14-1.

**Table 14-1.** Tests for Common Metabolic Disorders of the Liver

| DISEASE | PRIMARY TEST | SUPPORTIVE TEST | DEFINITIVE TEST |
|---|---|---|---|
| Hemochromatosis | Serum ferritin >400 µg/L | Iron saturation >55% Iron age index >2 | C282Y, H63D homozygosity |
| $\alpha_1$-Antitrypsin | SPEP or $\alpha_1$-antitrypsin level | Phenotype (Pi type) | Liver biopsy with PAS–positive diastase-resistant granules |
| Wilson's disease | Ceruloplasmin <10 mg/dL | Urine copper >80 µg/24 hr | Liver biopsy with quantitative copper >50 µg/g wet weight |

PAS, periodic acid–Schiff test; SPEP, serum protein electrophoresis.

## 18. What are autoimmune markers?

Autoimmune markers are tests used to determine the presence of antibodies to specific cellular components that have been epidemiologically associated with the development of specific liver diseases. Autoimmune markers include antinuclear antibody (ANA), anti–smooth muscle antibody (ASMA; also called *anti-actin antibody*), liver-kidney microsomal antibody type 1 (LKM-1), anti–mitochondrial antibody (AMA), soluble liver antigen (SLA), and anti–asialoglycoprotein receptor antibody. ANA, ASMA, and AMA are the most readily available tests and help to define the probability of the more common classes of autoimmune liver disease. Currently, SLA is not easily obtained in the United States.

## 19. How are the common antibody tests performed and interpreted?

The common antibody tests are performed by exposure of the patient's serum to cultured cells and labeling with a fluorescein-tagged antibody against human antibodies. The cells are examined by fluorescent microscopy and graded according to intensity of the signal and which part of the cell binds the antibody. Therefore, reading of antibody levels and determination of positive or negative results are highly subjective, and most hepatologists require positive results in dilution titers greater than 1:80 or 1:160 before considering the tests as part of a diagnostic algorithm. Newer assays permit determination of an antibody level directly. ANA and ASMA are particularly common in older people, women, and patients with a wide spectrum of liver diseases. Therefore, the diagnosis of autoimmune liver disease depends on a broad clinical picture that takes into account age, sex, presence of other autoimmune processes, γ-globulin levels, and liver biopsy findings. In addition, the overlap in antibodies in different autoimmune liver diseases is considerable. Table 14-2 provides a crude representation of one classification scheme. A newer scoring system that tries to take into account the variables noted above also has been proposed.

**Table 14-2.** Classification of Autoimmune Liver Disease

| DISEASE | ANTIBODY |
|---|---|
| Type I classic lupoid hepatitis | Antinuclear antibody and/or anti–smooth muscle antibody |
| Type II autoimmune hepatitis | Liver-kidney microsomal antibody type I |
| Type III autoimmune hepatitis | Soluble liver antigen |
| Primary biliary cirrhosis | Antimitochondrial antibody |

## 20. When should screening or diagnostic tests be ordered for patients with suspected liver disease?

The transaminases, bilirubin, and AP serve as screening tests when liver disease is suspected. The history, physical exam, and estimation of risk factors help to determine which specific diagnostic tests should be ordered.

Some patients have occult liver disease with normal or near-normal enzymes, and occasionally patients with isolated enzyme elevations have no identifiable disease. In general, patients should have at least two sets of liver enzyme tests to eliminate lab error before a full workup for liver disease is begun. Many diseases (hepatitis B and hepatitis C) generally require proof of chronicity (abnormality greater than 6 months) before therapy is initiated or confirmatory and staging liver biopsy samples are obtained. The severity of enzyme abnormality and the likelihood of finding a treatable process may modify the typical waiting period. For example, a female patient with transaminase levels 10 times normal, a history of autoimmune thyroid disease, and an elevated globulin fraction probably has a flare of previously unrecognized chronic autoimmune hepatitis. An autoimmune profile and early liver biopsy may help to support this hypothesis and lead to prompt treatment with steroids and other immunosuppressants.

## 21. What are noninvasive markers of fibrosis, and what is their utility?

Noninvasive markers of fibrosis fall into three major categories. These include serum biomarkers, imaging techniques to evaluate degree of fibrosis, and transient elastography, which uses sound waves to evaluate liver stiffness. It has been known for some time that there is a positive correlation between markers of early portal hypertension and the presence or absence of advanced liver fibrosis. Platelet counts below normal in a patient with liver disease often indicate the presence of fibrosis, which has caused portal hypertension, splenomegaly, and platelet sequestration. Recently, more or less complex indices that include platelet count and other serum tests have been described. These include AST to platelet ratio index (APRI), FIB-4, Fibrotest, and Fibrosure. All are highly correlated with degree of fibrosis observed on liver biopsy but are relatively poor at close comparison (e.g., F2 versus F3). They are moderately reliable in identifying cirrhosis and absence of fibrosis, although error rates of 20% to 30% have been reported. Imaging modalities include ultrasound, computed tomography, magnetic resonance imaging (MRI), and single-photon emission computed tomography. Of these, only MRI, using special equipment and unique algorithms, has reproducibly predicted fibrosis stage at a level that is clinically useful. The most recent development is transient elastography, which determines liver stiffness and not just fibrosis. Results are significantly affected by the presence or absence of inflammation and, to a lesser degree, steatosis and hepatic iron concentration. Widely accepted as a substitute for histology in Europe, the device was not approved or available in the United States in August 2009.

## 22. What is the role of liver biopsy?

Liver biopsy is used to confirm suspected diagnoses and to evaluate prognostic finding in a patient with a known disease process (e.g., degree of fibrosis and inflammation in a patient with chronic hepatitis C virus infection). Rarely, biopsy may be used to evaluate etiologies when there is uncertainty regarding etiology. The value of the biopsy is highly dependent on two factors—provision of an adequate specimen, defined as an intact liver slice containing more than 11 portal areas, and review by a qualified pathologist or hepatologist. Unfortunately, small fragmented specimens are often provided by clinicians or radiologists and few pathologists have significant experience in the interpretation of liver biopsy findings. Liver biopsy provides important prognostic information in many patients with chronic hepatitis B virus and hepatitis C virus infection and in those with autoimmune hepatitis, nonalcoholic steatohepatitis (NASH), and various metabolic diseases of the liver.

## WEBSITES

http://www.aasld.org/

http://www.eurowilson.org

http://www.liverfoundation.org

**BIBLIOGRAPHY**

1. Bacon BR, Olynyk JK, Brunt EM, et al. HFE genotype in patients with hemochromatosis and other liver disease. Ann Intern Med 1999;130:953–62.
2. Bassett ML, Halliday JW, Powell LW. Value of hepatic iron measurements in early hemochromatosis and determination of the critical iron level associated with fibrosis. Hepatology 1986;6:24–9.
3. Bejarano PA, Koehler A, Sherman KE. Am J Gastroenterol 2001;96:3158–64.
4. Brensilver HL, Kaplan MM. Significance of elevated liver alkaline phosphatase in serum. Gastroenterology 1975;68:1556–62.
5. Buffone GS, Beck JR. Cost-effectiveness analysis for evaluation of screening programs: hereditary hemochromatosis. Clin Chem 1994;40:1631–6.
6. Eriksson S, Carlson J, Velez R. Risk of cirrhosis and primary liver cancer in alpha-1 antitrypsin deficiency. N Engl J Med 1983;314:736–9.

7. Gressner OA, Weiskirchen R, Gressner AM. Clin Chim Acta 2007;381:107–13.
8. Kaplan MM. Laboratory Tests in Diseases of the Liver. 6th ed. Philadelphia: JB Lippincott; 1987.
9. Prati D, Taloli E, Zanella A, et al. Updated definitions of healthy ranges for serum alanine aminotransferase levels. Ann Intern Med 2002;139:1–9.
10. Scharschmidt BF, Goldberg HI, Schmid R. Approach to the patient with cholestatic jaundice. N Engl J Med 1983;308:1515–9.
11. Sherman KE. Alanine aminotransferase in clinical practice: A review. Arch Intern Med 1991;151:260–5.
12. Wroblewski F. The clinical significance of transaminase activities of serum. Am J Med 1959;27:911–23.

# CHAPTER 15

# VIRAL HEPATITIS

*Halim Muslu, MD*

### 1. What are the types of hepatitis viruses?

There are currently five identifiable forms of viral hepatitis: A, B, C, D, and E (Table 15-1). All of these viruses are hepatotrophic; that is, the liver is the primary site of infection. Other viruses also infect the liver, but this is not their primary site of replication, and cellular damage. Examples include cytomegalovirus (CMV), herpes simplex virus (HSV), Epstein-Barr virus (EBV), and many of the arthropod-borne flaviviruses. Then there are some other viruses such as hepatitis G/GB-C, which also belong to the flavivirus family. However, the replication primarily takes place in the bone marrow and the spleen. This virus is not primarily hepatotrophic. Hence, the name itself may be considered a misnomer. Interestingly, hepatitis GB virus may even be considered potentially beneficial for individuals infected with human immunodeficiency virus (HIV). Transfusion-transmitted virus (TTV), a DNA virus classified as an anellovirus, also appears to be associated with some liver disease among some patient groups (e.g., HIV infected), but its exact role in acute and chronic liver disease remains controversial.

**Table 15-1.** Key Characteristics of the Hepatitis Viruses

| TYPE | NUCLEIC ACID | GENE SHAPE | ENVELOPE | SIZE (NM) |
|------|--------------|------------|----------|-----------|
| A | RNA | Linear | No | 28 |
| B | DNA | Circular | Yes | 42 |
| C | RNA | Linear | Yes | (?) 40–50 |
| D | RNA | Circular | Yes | 43 |
| E | RNA | Linear | No | 32 |

### 2. What is the difference between acute and chronic hepatitis?

All hepatitis viruses can cause *acute infection*, which is defined as the presence of clinical, biochemical, and serologic abnormalities for up to 6 months. Hepatitis A and E are cleared from the body within 6 months and do not cause persistent infection. In contrast, hepatitis B, C, and D can lead to chronic infection, which is more likely to be associated with development of cirrhosis. An increased risk of primary hepatocellular carcinoma occurs in patients chronically infected with hepatitis B, C, and D.

### 3. How common is chronicity in hepatitis B?

The risk of chronicity for hepatitis B is highly dependent on the person's age at infection and immunologic status. Neonates infected with hepatitis B have a chronicity rate approaching 100%. The rate decreases to about 70% for young children. Healthy young adults probably have chronicity rates less than 1%, but persons taking steroids or with chronic illness (e.g., HIV, renal disease) are less likely to clear the viral infection.

### 4. When does chronic hepatitis D develop?

Hepatitis D chronicity occurs only in the presence of simultaneous hepatitis B infection. In patients with chronic hepatitis B who become superinfected with hepatitis D, the risk of chronicity approaches 100%.

### 5. How common is chronic hepatitis C?

From 150 to 200 million people are infected with hepatitis C worldwide. Hepatitis C may become chronic in 40% to 85% of those who present with acute hepatitis C. The outcome of chronic hepatitis C is a result of a complex interaction between host immune and viral factors. A small number of patients may have a chronic, nonfibrotic carrier state.

### 6. How are hepatitis viruses transmitted?

Hepatitis A and E are transmitted via a fecal-oral route. Both agents are prevalent in areas where sanitation standards are low. Large epidemics of both diseases frequently occur after floods and other natural disasters that disrupt already marginal sanitation systems. Hepatitis A is endemic in the United States and much of the world. Large outbreaks of hepatitis E have been seen in Central and South America, Bangladesh, and India. The fecal-oral transmission route includes not only direct contamination of drinking water and food but also viral concentration and enteric acquisition by eating raw shellfish from sewage-contaminated waters. There is growing evidence that pigs in the United States may serve as a reservoir for hepatitis E infection, but the potential of this strain for human pathogenesis remains unclear.

## 7. Describe the symptoms of hepatitis.

The classic symptoms of acute viral hepatitis include anorexia, nausea, vomiting, severe fatigue, abdominal pain, mild fever, jaundice, dark urine, and light stools. Some patients may have a serum sickness–like presentation that includes arthralgia, arthritis, and skin lesions; this presentation is more common in hepatitis B than in other forms of acute viral hepatitis and may be seen in up to 20% of infected patients. It is associated with the formation of immune complexes between the antigen and antibody. Many patients with acute viral hepatitis do not have disease-specific symptoms. All forms of viral hepatitis may present as a mild-to-moderate flulike illness. In a recent national survey of the U.S. population, approximately 30% of participants had serologic evidence of past *hepatitis A* infection, but few were diagnosed with hepatitis A or reported an illness with classic hepatitis features. On the other hand, the clinician should be able to recognize the clinical signs of fulminant hepatitis. Examples of such clinical signs are mental status changes attributable to hepatic encephalopathy, prothrombin time greater than 3 seconds over control, or development of ascites. In such situations, timely referral to a transplant center can be lifesaving.

Acute viral hepatitis in special populations such as persons with acquired or congenital immunodeficiency states may be caused by atypical viruses. CMV, HSV, and EBV may play a role here, so patients may have to be screened for these as well.

Patients with chronic hepatitis B or C report fatigue as the leading symptom. Other common manifestations include arthralgias, anorexia, and vague, persistent right upper quadrant pain. Jaundice, easy bruisability, or prolonged bleeding after shaving or other small skin breaks usually marks the development of end-stage liver disease and often signifies the presence of scarring and irreversible liver dysfunction.

## 8. What biochemical abnormalities are associated with viral hepatitis?

Elevation of serum transaminases (alanine aminotransferase [ALT], aspartate aminotransferase [AST]) is the hallmark of acute liver damage and identifies the presence of various processes caused by viral hepatitis. ALT is more specific than AST, as AST may be elevated in association with muscle injury. In patients with acute hepatitis A, B, D, or E, elevations of transaminases to several thousand are not uncommon; they usually are accompanied by more modest increases in alkaline phosphatase and γ-glutamyl-transpeptidase (GGT). As the disease progresses, the transaminases decrease. As the levels decrease slowly over a period of weeks, bilirubin often rises and may peak weeks after the transaminases peak. Bilirubin levels usually subside by 6 months after infection. Hepatitis C is not as frequently associated with a notable acute hepatitis, and transaminases rarely exceed 1000 IU/L. Viral hepatitis seldom is associated with elevations of transaminases in excess of 7000 to 8000 IU/L. Other etiologies, including concomitant toxic exposure or hepatic ischemia, must be considered when this is observed. An important subset of hepatitis C virus (HCV)-infected patients have persistently normal serum ALT levels. This is more common among women than among men. Many of these patients have active liver disease on liver biopsy.

## 9. What biochemical findings indicate chronic infection?

Abnormalities that persist for longer than 6 months define the process as chronic. In this stage of disease, transaminases range from mildly elevated to 10 to 15 times the upper limit of normal. Bilirubin is often normal or mildly elevated, as are alkaline phosphatase and GGT. Sudden elevations of transaminases in the chronic period often signify a viral flare rather than development of a new process superimposed on the preexisting chronic viral state. However, superinfection with hepatitis D in a patient with chronic hepatitis B may be observed in some parts of the world.

## 10. How is hepatitis A diagnosed?

The diagnosis of hepatitis A depends on identifying a specific immunoglobulin M (IgM) antibody directed against the viral capsid protein. This is often identified as hepatitis A viral antibody-IgM (HAVAB-M) class test on lab order sheets. The IgM antibody appears early in infection and persists for 3 to 6 months and rarely can be detected up to a year. This condition, however, does not imply chronicity. The other available lab test detects the immunoglobulin G (IgG) form of the antibody, which provides diagnosis of past infection or vaccination. Some laboratories offer a combined (total) IgM + IgG, which represents current or past exposure, and therefore complicates interpretation of positive results.

## 11. How is hepatitis B diagnosed?

The incorrect interpretation of hepatitis B serologic markers is common and leads to many inappropriate lab tests and specialty consultations. It is important to understand the sequence of marker appearance and disappearance and the information that each marker provides. Tests of hepatitis B include both serologic and molecular markers: hepatitis B surface antigen (HBsAg) and hepatitis B surface antibody (HBsAb), hepatitis B anticore antibody (HBcAb), hepatitis B e antigen (HBeAg) and hepatitis B e antibody (HBeAb), branched-chain DNA (bDNA) assays, and polymerase chain reaction (PCR).

## 12. Describe the HBsAg and HBsAb tests.

HBsAg, a protein that forms the outer coat of the hepatitis B virus, is produced in great excess during viral replication and aggregates to form noninfectious spherical and filamentous particles in the serum. It is detected by a radioimmunoassay (RIA) or enzyme-linked immunosorbent assay (ELISA) and indicates the presence of either acute or chronic infection. Its disappearance from the serum indicates viral clearance.

The HBsAb test detects an antibody directed against the surface antigen. This neutralizing antibody binds with and helps to clear the virus from the circulation. Its presence, therefore, indicates past infection with hepatitis B, which has been successfully cleared. The surface antibody also may appear in patients who are successfully vaccinated with the currently available recombinant hepatitis B vaccines. Its presence at a titer greater than 10 mIU/mL of serum confers protection against active infection.

## 13. How is the HBcAb test interpreted?

This test detects antibody formation against the core protein of the hepatitis B virus. The core protein surrounds the viral DNA and is surrounded by HBsAg in the complete virion, which is called the Dane particle. No commercial assay for HB core antigen is available. An ELISA is used to detect the antibody (HBcAb). The specific test comes in three forms, which must be differentiated to understand the meaning of the results: an IgG form, an IgM form, and a total form that measures both IgG and IgM. Most laboratories include the total test in hepatitis screening profiles, but it is important to find out which test is routinely run. A positive total HBcAb indicates either current or past hepatitis B infection. A positive HB anti-HBc IgM usually indicates an acute hepatitis B infection, although it also may indicate viral reactivation associated with immunosuppression or chronic illness. In contrast, a positive HB anticore IgG is consistent with either resolved past infection or, if present in conjunction with HBsAg, a chronic carrier state. Rarely, the presence of anti-HBc without anti-HBs suggests an occult infectious process. This finding requires further evaluation with an HBV DNA assay.

## 14. What do the HBeAg and HBeAb tests indicate?

The e antigen is a soluble protein encoded by the precore portion of the coding domain. Its presence indicates the presence of wild-type hepatitis B suggesting active replication. HBeAg is seen in both acute and actively replicating hepatitis B. In patients with acute infection, ordering of the test is not necessary. Only when HBsAg is present and chronic liver disease is suspected, this test helps in decision making related to treatment and treatment outcomes. In a patient with resolved acute hepatitis B or relatively inactive chronic hepatitis B either as natural progression or as the result of medical therapy HBeAg disappears and HBeAb appears. Some patients, who may have been infected with a virus that has a point mutation in the precore region of the virus genome, do not produce either HBeAg or HBeAb in their serum. However, this does not affect the viral replication, and precore mutant virus still has the potential to cause significant liver disease and progress to hepatocellular cancer. In clinical practice, a patient who has developed HBeAb and loses HBeAg may still show high titers of HBV viral DNA. In this circumstance, a precore mutant virus should be suspected. In such an event, the treatment end point is not clear due to the lack of an observable HBeAb response. In these patients, the goal of therapy is viral suppression rather than HBe antigen to HBe antibody conversion.

## 15. Describe the bDNA assay.

In this hybridization assay the viral nucleic acid hybridizes with complementary bDNA attached to a microtiter well. The hybridized viral DNA is then further hybridized to specific complementary DNAs in a reaction mixture, which are arrayed in a manner analogous to a multibranched tree. On the tree are pods of a marker molecule that emit light in a chemiluminescent reaction that can be detected by a luminometer. Because the light emission is proportionate to the amount of bound DNA, the test provides a highly reliable quantitative assay that is more sensitive than older hybridization assays.

## 16. What are HBV PCR assays?

The bDNA assay amplifies the signal generated by hybridization, but PCR amplifies a portion of the DNA itself and makes it more detectable. PCR is the most sensitive technique available for the detection of hepatitis DNA. The commercial version of this assay is a highly sensitive quantitative marker of infection. While all hepatitis B chronic carriers are positive on this assay, the titer for those with nonreplicative disease is low. New generations of real-time PCR with a large dynamic range and high sensitivity are now commercially available. Sensitivity may be as low as 20 IU/mL.

## 17. How is hepatitis C diagnosed?

The screening assay for hepatitis C is an ELISA (also called EIA) that detects the presence of antibody to two regions of the hepatitis C genome. The currently available assay is in its third generation, and future modifications are likely. The test is highly sensitive but not specific; therefore, it gives many false-positive reactions. In populations with a low pretest probability of carrying hepatitis C, more than 40% of repeatedly reactive specimens are false positives. The antibody that is detected is nonneutralizing; that is, its presence does not confer immunity. If antibody is detected and the reaction is not a false positive, the patient almost always has active viral infection. Clearly, it is important to separate false positives from true positives. The cause of most false-positive reactions is binding of nonspecific immunoglobulin on the ELISA well surface. To avoid the use of serum, which requires obtaining drawn blood, oral fluid collection has been demonstrated to be an alternative screening modality to screen populations for hepatitis C virus.

## 18. How is a positive result on the ELISA confirmed?

To support a true-positive reaction, the most commonly used test is a recombinant immunoblot assay (RIBA), which involves exposing the patient's serum to a nitrocellulose strip impregnated with bands of antigen. The currently available version (HCV RIBA 3.0; Chiron Corp.) has multiple antigens on the test strip as well as controls for nonspecific immunoglobulin binding and superoxide dismutase antibodies, which may confound the test results. The RIBA is not as sensitive as the ELISA, however, and therefore should not be used as a screening test for hepatitis C infection.

## 19. What nucleic acid assays are available for hepatitis C?

Other assays in specialized laboratories include a bDNA quantitative assay for hepatitis C RNA and a PCR assay (see earlier hepatitis B tests). In the past, both bDNA assays and PCR-based assays were reported in terms of copies of HCV RNA/mL. Now, a World Health Organization (WHO) standard defined as an international unit (IU) is used for reporting purposes. The presence of hepatitis C RNA in serum or liver tissue is the gold standard for the diagnosis of hepatitis C infection. Quantitative evaluation of hepatitis C RNA levels in serum has prognostic value in determining who is likely to respond to therapeutic intervention and in following the course of a treatment cycle. The most sensitive nucleic acid assay is performed by a method called transcription-mediated amplification (TMA). This technique is sensitive to approximately 5 IU/mL. Real-time PCR approaches this sensitivity and permits a broad quantitative dynamic range.

## 20. How is hepatitis D diagnosed?

Hepatitis D is diagnosed by an ELISA that detects the presence of antibody to hepatitis D in serum or plasma. The presence of the antibody in serum correlates with ongoing hepatitis D replication in the liver. Detection of hepatitis D antigen in liver tissue generally adds little to the diagnostic process. Early in the course of infection, acute hepatitis D may be detectable only by performing a test for the IgM form of the antibody. A PCR-based assay also may be performed to detect the presence of RNA from hepatitis D in serum or tissue. This assay is not commercially available, and its use seems to add little to the antibody testing. Because hepatitis D occurs only with concurrent acute hepatitis B infection or as a superinfection of chronic hepatitis B, there is little utility in testing for its presence at the initial workup for viral causes of liver enzyme abnormalities.

## 21. How is hepatitis E diagnosed?

There should be a high index of suspicion in patients who have an acute hepatitis A–like illness, have test negative for hepatitis A antibody IgM, and have traveled to an endemic area. Hepatitis E can be diagnosed using a commercial serologic assay and evaluating for the present of IgM antibody.

## 22. Are there other hepatitis viruses not yet discovered?

Probably. Several lines of evidence suggest that there are more hepatotrophic viruses than are currently recognized. Epidemiologic studies suggest that a small percentage of posttransfusion cases and a higher percentage of community-acquired cases of hepatitis have no identifiable viral infection, even when molecular detection techniques are used. Forms of liver disease (e.g., giant cell hepatitis) have been associated with paramyxovirus infection, although its role remains speculative at best. The cause of fulminant hepatic failure, hepatitis-associated aplastic anemia, and cryptogenic cirrhosis cannot be defined in a significant proportion of cases. Such findings point to the presence of one or more as yet unidentified agents. In recent years, two new agents have been extensively studied: the TTV and SEN-V. All may be associated with serum transaminase abnormalities in certain circumstances, but their exact role in acute and chronic disease has not been delineated.

## 23. What is the treatment of acute hepatitis B and hepatitis D?

The primary treatment of acute hepatitis of any type is mainly supportive. Patients generally do not require hospitalization unless the disease is complicated by significant hepatic failure, as evidenced by encephalopathy, coagulopathy with bleeding, renal failure, or inability to maintain adequate nutrition and fluid intake. Efforts must be made to identify the form of hepatitis and, if necessary, to ensure that the patient is removed from situations in which he or she is a high risk to others. For example, a food-handler should be removed from the workplace when hepatitis A is diagnosed, and health authorities must be notified. There are some case reports and a pilot study in which lamivudine was used to treat severe acute hepatitis B with beneficial results. Unfortunately, a recently published larger randomized controlled trial was unable to confirm better clinical outcome despite improved biochemical and virologic parameters. In respect to acute hepatitis D, interferon, which plays a role in treatment of its chronic infection, has been found to be unsuccessful. When this disease runs a fulminant course, liver transplantation may be the only viable option.

## 24. What is the treatment of acute hepatitis C?

Following high-risk exposure, patients should be monitored every 4 weeks for seroconversion or development of HCV RNA viremia. From the time of identification of acute infection, the patients should be followed for 12 weeks. A percentage (15% to 30%) will spontaneously clear HCV in this time and will not require treatment. Those who do not clear should immediately be started on pegylated interferon with or without ribavirin for 24 weeks. This will prevent the development of chronic infection in most patients.

### 25. Is chronic viral hepatitis treatable?

Yes. Hepatitis B, C, and D have been studied with regard to a number of treatment modalities. One thing remains common for all these viruses—interferon alpha has antiviral activity against all of them with varying success rates. The combination of interferon alpha and ribavirin has been studied and approved for the treatment of chronic hepatitis C. In addition to these antiviral therapies, small molecules including protease, polymerase, and helicase inhibitors are currently being investigated in respect to their use in combination with the existing drug therapy against hepatitis C virus. Against hepatitis B, fortunately there are some newer agents besides lamivudine, such as the nucleotide and nucleoside analogs of entecavir, telbivudine, emtricitabine, adefovir, and tenofovir. Lamivudine is the least expensive agent against hepatitis B. Unfortunately, the long-term use of this agent is not recommended due to the high incidence of resistant strains emerging following relatively short courses of therapy.

### 26. Does lamivudine have any clinical relevance in this day and age?

Lamivudine still has clinical utility in the treatment of expectant mothers with active hepatitis B. Due to its widespread use in the prevention of perinatal transmission of HIV and its proven safety and its cost, lamivudine is the cheapest and perhaps the safest alternative in rapid reduction of HBV viral loads, thereby decreasing the transmission of hepatitis B to the newborn. However, the drug needs to be initiated in the latter part of the second trimester to achieve efficacy at the time of delivery.

### 27. Which patients with chronic hepatitis B are candidates for therapy?

Patients with chronic hepatitis B, well-compensated liver disease, and evidence of viral replication (HBV DNA or HBeAg) are candidates for therapy. The goal of therapy is to reduce the level of replication and to change the infection to a relatively inactive disease. The clearance of HBsAg is not the immediate goal of therapy, although some evidence suggests that this may occur more frequently in successfully treated patients than in those that do not respond over subsequent years. Patients with decompensated liver disease due to hepatitis B may also benefit for nucleoside/nucleotide analog treatment, but this should be provided under the direction of an experienced hepatologist in a transplant center setting.

### 28. Describe the standard treatment and its side effects.

There are several factors that are taken into consideration when deciding how to treat patients with hepatitis B. Pegylated interferon alpha is superior to lamivudine alone in achieving seroconversion. HBeAg-negative patients may also benefit from interferon alpha. Genotypes A and B appear to be especially susceptible to interferon therapy. Interferons are associated with neuropsychiatric side effects, bone marrow depression, activation of autoimmune syndromes, hyperthyroidism or hypothyroidism, and a flulike illness following the administration of the drug, among many others. Therefore, for long-term therapy or patients who may not be candidates for interferon, nucleoside/nucleotide monotherapy is an option. These drugs are usually far better tolerated than interferon. Due to viral resistance, there is growing concern about the validity of monotherapy. When monotherapy has resulted in the appearance of drug-resistant hepatitis B virus, the addition of an appropriate second agent may be considered. For instance, after lamivudine resistance occurs, adefovir may be added for salvage therapy.

### 29. What is the response rate to treatment of chronic hepatitis B?

Interferon-based therapy has a success rate of seroconversion about 25% to 32%. HBV DNA virus clearance rates following 52 weeks of therapy with lamivudine, entecavir, telbivudine, and adefovir are roughly 70%, 90%, 88%, and 51%, respectively, among patients with HBeAg-negative hepatitis. Liver inflammation correlates with HBV DNA levels. Therefore, maintaining a low or undetectable DNA level is crucial to see histologic improvement. HBsAg clearance is rare but does occur, particularly following interferon-based therapy.

### 30. Describe the treatment of chronic hepatitis C. How effective is it?

Treatment of chronic hepatitis C is interferon based. Current treatment standards include the use of weekly pegylated interferon alpha and weight-based ribavirin 1000 to 1200 mg, which is split into a twice-daily dosing regimen. Treatment response rates depend on both host and viral factors. The viral factors include virus genotype and viral load. Genotype alone is the most important predictor of treatment success. Genotype 1 is the most common type among patients with hepatitis C in the United States and is also the one that is associated with the least successful outcome of therapy after 48 weeks of duration (40% to 50%). Genotypes 2 and 3 are associated with far better outcome (70% to 80%) following 24 weeks of therapy. Host factors that influence the treatment response in hepatitis C include the subject's age, gender, body mass index, presence or absence of an acquired or a congenital immunodeficiency state, HIV, or organ transplantation. Race is also a key factor. Genotype 1 African Americans are less likely to clear virus than are Caucasians.

### 31. Describe the side effects of ribavirin.

Certain patients may be at risk of complications with ribavirin use. Ribavirin causes a dose-dependent hemolysis in approximately 80% of treated patients. This anemia may be ameliorated with use of epopoietin or other growth factors. Patients with underlying cardiac disease who cannot tolerate anemia may not be suitable candidates. Furthermore, ribavirin is teratogenic. Adequate birth control should be used during and for 6 months after treatment.

## 32. What is PEG-interferon?

Addition of a polyethylene glycol (PEG) moiety to interferon results in a PEG-interferon product that has a prolonged half-life with higher potency against the hepatitis C virus.

## 33. What happens if the patient fails to clear the hepatitis C virus?

In some cases, the best alternative therapy may be a strategy of cautious waiting. This may be especially true for patients who have relative contraindications to treatment with interferon. Relative other risk factors need to be identified and be minimized. This may include alcohol abstinence, weight reduction, and optimization of therapy against HIV. The exact stage of the liver disease may have to be delineated by a repeat liver biopsy. If the decision has been made to re-treat the patient, then another form of interferon such as consensus interferon in combination with ribavirin may be used. As long as the viral clearance is not achieved, long-term continuation of interferon (maintenance therapy) does not seem to improve the outcome and is contraindicated.

## 34. What alternative therapies for hepatitis C are under investigation?

Newer-generation therapies, including protease/helicase inhibitors, RNA-dependent RNA polymerase inhibitors, ribozymes, and antisense therapy, are under development. Immune modulation with agents including thymosin alpha-1 and study of antifibrotic therapy ($\gamma$ interferon) are under active evaluation.

## 35. How is hepatitis D treated?

Hepatitis D also may be treated with interferon. Both standard and pegylated forms of interferon have been tried with varying success rates. The addition of another agent such as lamivudine, ribavirin, or a similar agent does not change the overall outcome. Therefore, an interferon-based monotherapy of 12 months' duration is the usual method of treating this disease. Virologic relapse is common following such therapy, but the clinical outcome is significantly better when patients are treated with interferon alpha. Treatment of hepatitis B virus with nucleoside/nucleotide analog may also mitigate hepatic inflammation.

## 36. Can hepatitis C be prevented?

No vaccine is available for hepatitis C. Because of rapid mutation in the envelope region of the genome, a multivalent vaccine probably will be required and may take several years to develop and test before it is available for routine use. There is some interest in development of virus-free pooled globulin products, which may mitigate the infectious process, particularly in patients infected with hepatitis C virus after liver transplant.

## CONTROVERSY

## 37. Should all patients with hepatitis C undergo liver biopsy?

*For:* Liver biopsy is the gold standard for evaluation of activity and fibrosis in the liver. Surrogate markers, including imaging with liver-spleen scan, single-photon emission computed tomography, computed tomography, magnetic resonance imaging, and ultrasonography, as well indices derived from laboratory tests, have not been reliable, with error rates of greater than 20%. Standard liver tests are also frequently not helpful. A liver biopsy helps to:

1. Determine whether treatment should be started
2. Decide aggressiveness of therapy
3. Provide factual evidence of an otherwise often asymptomatic condition, which encourages patients to continue treatment

The risk of biopsy in experienced hands is low, and until treatments are highly effective in all treated patients, it should be a mandatory part of the workup.

*Against:* Almost all patients with hepatitis C virus infection deserve at least one course of therapy, regardless of the level of activity or fibrosis. Biopsies are a barrier to treatment, relegating patient care to a limited pool of practitioners who perform liver biopsies. Therefore, liver biopsy is not indicated in routine management. Furthermore, noninvasive assays such as Fibroscan, based on ultrasound technology to measure liver stiffness, are highly concordant with liver biopsy findings.

## WEBSITE

http://www.aasld.org/

## BIBLIOGRAPHY

1. Abraham P. GB virus C/hepatitis G virus—Its role in human disease redefined? Indian J Med Res 2007;125:717–9.
2. Alter MJ, Margolis HS, Krawczynski K, et al. The natural history of community-acquired hepatitis C in the United States. N Engl J Med 1992;327:1899–905.
3. Berg T, von Wagner M, Nasser S. Extended treatment duration for hepatitis C virus type 1: Comparing 48 versus 72 weeks of peginterferon-alfa-2a plus ribavirin. Gastroenterology 2006;130:1086–97.
4. Blackard JT, Shata MT, Shire NJ. Acute hepatitis C virus infection: a chronic problem. Hepatology 2008;47:321–31.
5. Centers for Disease Control. Hepatitis B virus: A comprehensive strategy for eliminating transmission in the United States through universal childhood vaccination: Recommendations of the Immunization Practices Advisory Committee (ACIP). Mortal Morb Wkly Rep MMWR 1991;40(RR-13).
6. Chen CH, Lee CM, Hung CH. Clinical significance and evolution of core promoter and precore mutations in HBeAg-positive patients with HBV genotype B and C: A longitudinal study. Liver Int 2007;27:806–15.
7. Choo QL, Richman KH, Han JH, et al. Genetic organization and diversity of the hepatitis C virus. Proc Natl Acad Sci USA 1991;88:2451–5.
8. Conjeevaram HS, Fried MW, Jeffers LJ. Peginterferon and ribavirin treatment in African American and Caucasian American patients with hepatitis C genotype 1. Gastroenterology 2006;131:470–7.
9. Cooper CL. An overview of HIV and chronic viral hepatitis co-infection. Dig Dis Sci 2008;53:899–904.
10. Dawson GJ, Chau KH, Cabal CM, et al. Solid phase enzyme linked immunosorbent assay for hepatitis E virus IgG and IgM antibodies utilizing recombinant antigens and synthetic peptides. J Virol Meth 1992;38:175–86.
11. Deterding K, Pothakamuri SV, Schlaphoff V. Clearance of chronic HCV infection during acute delta hepatitis. Infection 2009;37:159–62.
12. Dienstag JL, Schiff ER, Wright TL, et al. Lamivudine as initial treatment for chronic hepatitis B in the United States. N Engl J Med 1999;341:1256–63.
13. Everson GT, Balart L, Lee SS. Histological benefits of virological response to peginterferon alfa-2a monotherapy in patients with hepatitis C and advanced fibrosis or compensated cirrhosis. Aliment Pharmacol Ther 2008;27:542–51.
14. Everson GT, Hoefs JC, Seeff LB. Impact of disease severity on outcome of antiviral therapy for chronic hepatitis C: lessons from the HALT-C trial. Hepatology 2006;44:1675–84.
15. Farci P. Treatment of chronic hepatitis D: New advances, old challenges. Hepatology 2006;44:536–9.
16. Fried MW, et al. Peginterferon alfa-2a plus ribavirin for chronic hepatitis C virus infection. N Engl J Med 2002;347:975–82.
17. Jaeckel E, Cornberg M, Wedemeyer H, et al. Treatment of acute hepatitis C with interferon alfa-2b. N Engl J Med 2001;345:1452–7.
18. Jeon MJ, Shin JH, Suh SP. TT virus and hepatitis G virus infections in Korean blood donors and patients with chronic liver disease. World J Gastroenterol 2003;9:741–4.
19. Kamal SM, Moustafa KN, Chen J. Duration of peginterferon therapy in acute hepatitis C: A randomized trial. Hepatology 2006;43:923–31.
20. Keeffe EB. Hepatitis B: Explosion of new knowledge. Gastroenterology 2007;133:1718–28.
21. Kemmer N, Neff GW. Managing chronic hepatitis C in the difficult-to-treat patient. Liver Int 2007;27:1297–310.
22. Koretz RL, Abbey H, Coleman E, et al. Non-A, non-B post-transfusion hepatitis: Looking back in the second decade. Ann Intern Med 1993;119:110–5.
23. Kubitschke A, Bader C, Tillmann HL. Injuries from needles contaminated with hepatitis C virus: How high is the risk of seroconversion for medical personnel really? Internist (Berl) 2007;48:1165–72.
24. Kumar M, Satapathy S, Monga R. 1: A randomized controlled trial of lamivudine to treat acute hepatitis B. Hepatology 2007;45:97–101.
25. Lau GK, Piratvisuth T, Luo KX. Peginterferon alfa-2a, lamivudine, and the combination for HBeAg-positive chronic hepatitis B. N Engl J Med 2005;352:2682–95.
26. Leevy CB. Consensus interferon and ribavirin in patients with chronic hepatitis C who were nonresponders to pegylated interferon alfa-2b and ribavirin. Dig Dis Sci 2008;53:1961–6.
27. Lok AS, McMahon BJ. AASLD practice guidelines. Hepatology 2007;45(2):507–39.
28. Mangia A, Minerva N, Bacca D. Individualized treatment duration for hepatitis C genotype 1 patients: a randomized controlled trial. Hepatology 2008;47:43–50.
29. Manns MP, McHutchison JG, Gordon SC, et al. Peginterferon alfa-2b plus ribavirin compared with interferon alfa-2b plus ribavirin for initial treatment of chronic hepatitis C: A randomised trial. Lancet 2001;358:958–65.
30. Mushahwar IK. Hepatitis E virus: Molecular virology, clinical features, diagnosis, transmission, epidemiology, and prevention. J Med Virol 2008;80:646–58.
31. Papatheodoridis GV, Manolakopoulos S, Dusheiko G, et al. Therapeutic strategies in the management of patients with chronic hepatitis B virus infection. Lancet Infect Dis 2008;8:167–78.
32. Reijnders JG, Janssen HL. Potency of tenofovir in chronic hepatitis B: mono or combination therapy? J Hepatol 2008;48:383–6.
33. Sánchez-Tapias JM, Diago M, Escartín P. Peginterferon-alfa2a plus ribavirin for 48 versus 72 weeks in patients with detectable hepatitis C virus RNA at week 4 of treatment. Gastroenterology 2006;131:451–60.
34. Sherman KE, Creager RL, O'Brien J, et al. The use of oral fluid for hepatitis C antibody screening. Am J Gastroenterol 1994;89:2025–7.
35. Sherman KE, Fleischer R, Laessig K. Development of novel agents for the treatment of chronic hepatitis C infection: Summary of the FDA Antiviral Products Advisory Committee recommendations. Hepatology 2007;46:2014–20.
36. Shiffman ML, Ghany MG, Morgan TR. Impact of reducing peginterferon alfa-2a and ribavirin dose during retreatment in patients with chronic hepatitis C. Gastroenterology 2007;132:103–12.
37. Shiffman ML, Suter F, Bacon BR. Peginterferon alfa-2a and ribavirin for 16 or 24 weeks in HCV genotype 2 or 3. N Engl J Med 2007;357:124–34.
38. Starkel P. Genetic factors predicting response to interferon treatment for viral hepatitis C. Gut 2008;57:440–2.
39. Thomas HC. Best practice in the treatment of chronic hepatitis B: A summary of the European Viral Hepatitis Educational Initiative (EVHEI). J Hepatol 2007;47:588–97.
40. Yurdaydin C, Bozkaya H, Onder FO. Treatment of chronic delta hepatitis with lamivudine vs lamivudine + interferon vs interferon. J Viral Hepat 2008;15:314–21.

# ANTIVIRAL THERAPY FOR HEPATITIS C INFECTION

# CHAPTER 16

*Jorge L. Herrera, MD*

**1. What are the indications for antiviral therapy in patients with chronic hepatitis C?**

Hepatitis C progresses in all chronically infected patients but at different rates. The average time for development of cirrhosis is 30 years, but there is a wide range of variability. Only about 20% of patients progress to cirrhosis. Because it is difficult to predict who will progress, everyone who is chronically infected should be evaluated for possible treatment. Many factors can speed progression of fibrosis, including alcohol consumption, coinfection with hepatitis B or human immunodeficiency virus (HIV), iron overload, and concomitant liver disease such as $\alpha_1$-antitrypsin deficiency, Wilson disease, or autoimmune hepatitis. Patients with fatty liver, in particular with nonalcoholic steatohepatitis and the metabolic syndrome, progress at a faster rate and have decreased response rates to treatment. In general, antiviral therapy should be offered to all infected patients who have no contraindication to therapy.

Patients with extrahepatic manifestations of hepatitis C infection should be considered for antiviral treatment regardless of the severity of the liver disease. Mixed cryoglobulinemia, leading to leukocytoclastic vasculitis, may be a systemic manifestation of hepatitis C infection and may respond to antiviral therapy. Renal disease, joint inflammation, or central nervous system complications may result from microvascular injury.

**2. What is the recommended evaluation of patients with chronic hepatitis C before therapy is begun?**

The initial history and physical exam should include identification of possible risk factors in an effort to assess the duration of infection. Laboratory evaluation is geared toward confirming viremia, establishing the hepatitis C virus (HCV) genotype, excluding other possible causes of liver disease, and detecting coinfection. Recommended laboratory tests are listed in Table 16-1.

Testing for immunity against hepatitis B (hepatitis B surface antibody [HBsAb]) and hepatitis A (anti-HAV) is recommended. Patients who are not immune should be vaccinated to prevent hepatitis A and B. In the absence of obvious advanced disease, a liver biopsy is advised to assess severity of disease, estimate prognosis, and determine urgency of antiviral therapy (Table 16-1).

**Table 16-1.** Recommended Pretreatment Evaluation of Patients With Chronic Hepatitis C Infection

| TEST | PURPOSE |
|---|---|
| HCV-RNA by PCR | Confirm viremia. |
| Serum albumin, bilirubin, PT | Assess liver function. |
| Iron, transferrin, ferritin | Assess for iron overload. |
| Antinuclear antibody | Detect autoimmune hepatitis. |
| $\alpha_1$-Antitrypsin phenotype | Detect $\alpha_1$-antitrypsin deficiency. |
| Ceruloplasmin (age <45 years) | Detect Wilson disease. |
| HBsAg, HIV antibody test | Detect viral coinfection. |
| Hepatitis C genotype | Assess likelihood of response to therapy. |
| Liver biopsy | Determine severity of disease and urgency for therapy. |
| Hepatitis B surface antibody | Determine need for hepatitis B vaccination. |
| Hepatitis A antibody (total) | Determine need for hepatitis A vaccination. |

HBsAg, hepatitis B surface antigen; HCV, hepatitis C virus; HIV, human immunodeficiency virus; PCR, polymerase chain reaction; PT, prothrombin time.

### 3. Should hepatitis C genotype testing be performed before initiation of therapy?

Based on genomic sequencing of the HCV, several genotypes (or strains) have been identified. They are classified as genotypes 1 through 6, with several subtypes denoted as 1a, 1b, 2a, and so forth. The various genotypes exhibit geographic variability. In the United States, genotype 1 accounts for approximately 70% of infections. Genotypes 2 and 3 account for the remaining 30%. In Europe, the proportion of genotype 2 and 3 infections is greater than in the United States. In the Middle East, genotype 4 predominates, and genotype 6 is seen most commonly in Asia.

Determining the genotype before therapy is important because it helps to predict likelihood of response and length of antiviral therapy. For example, patients infected with genotype 2 without cirrhosis have a greater than 80% chance of achieving a sustained response and need to be treated for only 6 months. In contrast, the probability of response to therapy is less likely in genotype 1 infections, which require treatment for at least 1 year to maximize the chance of sustained remission. The genotype, however, has no value in predicting severity of disease or likelihood of progression to cirrhosis and should not be determined in patients that are not candidates for antiviral therapy.

### 4. Is a liver biopsy mandatory before initiation of antiviral therapy?

A liver biopsy is not required to diagnose or treat chronic hepatitis C but it is used to evaluate the level of hepatic inflammation and fibrosis. No other test makes this determination with the same accuracy. Liver function tests, such as prothrombin time and albumin or bilirubin level, become abnormal only when extensive damage has occurred. Likewise, liver enzymes, viral load, and genotype do not correlate with severity of liver disease. An adequate biopsy sample is the best way to assess the severity of liver disease and helps the patient and clinician in deciding whether to proceed with therapy. Findings on liver biopsy that would favor antiviral therapy include the presence of significant portal or lobular inflammation or fibrosis extending beyond the portal triads. The presence of steatosis or steatohepatitis would indicate an increased risk of progression without therapy and a decreased likelihood of response to antiviral therapy.

### 5. What are the treatment options for hepatitis C infection?

The immune modulator interferon (IFN) was the first medication approved by the U.S. Food and Drug Administration (FDA) for the treatment of hepatitis C. Three different types—IFNα-2a, IFNα-2b, and consensus IFN differing in amino acid configuration—are available. They require subcutaneous administration 3 or more times per week, and the antiviral efficacy is lower than newer forms of IFN therapy.

To increase the half-life of the IFN molecule, increase its antiviral efficacy, and reduce the number of injections per month, a polyethylene glycol (PEG) molecule was covalently attached to IFN. The size and shape of the PEG molecule affect the biological properties of the IFN. Currently, two types of pegylated IFN are approved by the FDA for the treatment of chronic hepatitis C infection. Pegylated IFNα-2b is covalently attached to a linear 12-kDa PEG molecule. Pegylated IFNα-2a is attached to a larger, branched 40-kDa PEG molecule. Both of these compounds are self-administered by patients as a once-a-week subcutaneous injection.

Ribavirin, an oral nucleoside analog, is approved for the treatment of hepatitis C. Used alone, it is not effective as an antiviral agent against hepatitis C, but in combination with IFNα, the antiviral activity of IFN is greatly enhanced.

At present, combination therapy with peginterferon and ribavirin is the treatment of choice for patients who have not been previously treated. Selected patients who failed to respond to IFN monotherapy or to combination IFN ribavirin therapy may also benefit from a trial of peginterferon and ribavirin combination therapy.

### 6. How are the antiviral agents dosed?

Pegylated IFNα-2b is dosed by weight and administered as a single subcutaneous injection once a week. Pegylated IFNα-2a is administered as 180 μg subcutaneously once a week regardless of the patient's weight. Ribavirin should be dosed by weight, particularly when treating patients infected with genotype 1 infection. Currently, patients who weigh less than 75 kg should receive 1000 mg of ribavirin daily, and those who weigh more than 75 kg receive 1200 mg daily. Clinical research has demonstrated the importance of maximizing ribavirin dosing. Recently, the FDA has approved a weight-based dosing scale of ribavirin in combination with pegylated IFNα-2b for patients infected with genotype 1 virus. This new dosing scale includes a dose of 800 mg for patients weighing less than 65 kg, 1000 mg daily for those weighing between 65 and 85 kg, 1200 mg for those weighing 86 to 105 kg, and a higher dose of 1400 mg per day for those weighing over 105 kg. The total daily ribavirin dose should be administered in two divided doses. Patients infected with genotype 2 or 3 may be treated with a fixed ribavirin dose of 800 mg daily regardless of the patient's weight; however, weight-based ribavirin may enhance results. The duration of therapy is determined by the patient's genotype and early virologic response.

### 7. How is response to antiviral therapy assessed?

A decrease or normalization of liver enzymes usually indicates a positive response and is classified as a biochemical response to treatment. Such changes correlate with decreased hepatic inflammation as assessed by repeat liver biopsy. A biochemical response to treatment is not always associated with a virologic response. Liver enzymes should be monitored monthly, and viral load should be assessed at 3 and 6 months of treatment. Early virologic response is measured at 12 weeks of therapy and is defined as loss of detectable virus or a decrease in viral load of greater than 2 logs from baseline. At 6 months, a favorable response to therapy is defined as no detectable virus in blood using a qualitative or highly sensitive quantitative HCV-RNA assay. Patients who do not achieve these milestones have a less than 2% chance of achieving a sustained response to antiviral therapy; discontinuation of therapy should be considered. In contrast, those who achieve the expected response have a greater than 65% chance of sustained viral response. Recent research has shown that response at week 4 of treatment may help guide therapy. Patients who fail to achieve at least 1-log decrease in viral load during the first 4 weeks of therapy are unlikely to clear virus. Those who clear virus in the first 4 weeks have a greatly increased chance of sustained response with completion of therapy. Patients who have no detectable virus at the end of treatment are considered virologic responders. If detectable virus appears after treatment is stopped, the patient is considered a relapser. In contrast, if virus remains undetectable 6 months after discontinuation of therapy, the patient is considered a sustained responder and has a very high likelihood of remaining virus free for the foreseeable future.

## 8. How often should viral load be measured during treatment?

Baseline quantitation of HCV-RNA using a PCR-based assay should be performed before initiation of therapy, and it is recommended that the same laboratory and assay be used to monitor response to therapy over time. At 4 and 12 weeks of therapy, a repeat quantitative HCV-RNA assay should be obtained to assess for early viral response. If the expected response is achieved, antiviral therapy should be continued. At 24 weeks of therapy, a high-sensitivity HCV-RNA PCR assay (with a lower limit of detection of less than 50 IU/mL) should be obtained. If no detectable virus is found, a repeat assay should be obtained at the end of therapy to document an end-of-treatment response. Six months after discontinuation of therapy, a repeat highly sensitive HCV-RNA assay should be obtained to determine if a sustained virologic response was achieved.

## 9. What pretreatment characteristics predict a favorable response to antiviral therapy?

1. Infection with genotype 2 or 3
2. Low viral load (less than 400,000 IU/mL)
3. Liver biopsy with little or no fibrosis
4. Age younger than 40 years at time of treatment
5. Low body weight
6. Ethnicity—African Americans are less likely to respond than are whites.

Genotype is the most important predictive factor of response to therapy. Patients infected with genotype 2 or 3 without fibrosis on liver biopsy need to receive combination therapy for only 6 months.

## 10. What is the efficacy of combination peginterferon and ribavirin?

Efficacy of therapy is highly dependent on genotype. Patients infected with genotype 2 or 3 have an 80% to 85% chance of a sustained response after completing 24 weeks of therapy. Failure to clear virus by the fourth week of therapy identifies patients with a lower response rate; only 35% to 40% of these patients will achieve a sustained response with 24 weeks of therapy. Genotype 1 patients are more difficult to eradicate—40% to 50% will achieve a sustained response after 48 weeks of therapy. In genotype 1 patients, failure to clear virus by week 12 of therapy predicts a low likelihood of sustained response; only about 30% of these patients will clear virus after 48 weeks of therapy. Recent research has shown that for slow responders (those who have a greater than 2-log drop in viral load by week 12 of therapy but have not cleared virus), extending total treatment duration to 72 weeks increases the likelihood of a sustained response.

## 11. How can response to antiviral therapy be maximized?

To maximize sustained response rates, ribavirin should be dosed by weight and adherence to medications should be promoted. Patients who are unable to take 80% of their medications for 80% of the time are much less likely to achieve a sustained response. To minimize dose reduction and dose interruptions, it is crucial that side effects be monitored and aggressively treated. Whenever possible, dose reduction should be avoided.

## 12. What are the side effects of IFN therapy? How should the patient be monitored?

IFN suppresses the bone marrow, potentially resulting in leukopenia or thrombocytopenia. Complete blood counts are monitored periodically, and the dose is adjusted as needed. To avoid dose reductions, use of growth factors such as filgrastim for neutropenia should be considered. Other side effects that can diminish quality of life include flulike symptoms, headaches, fever, depression, anxiety, sexual dysfunction, hair loss, insomnia, and fatigue. Evening administration and preinjection acetaminophen or ibuprofen can reduce the flulike symptoms.

Depression requires close monitoring. Patients with a history of severe depression or suicidal ideation or attempts should not be treated with IFN. Patients who have required pharmacologic therapy for mild depression in the past may benefit from initiation of antidepressants before treatment with IFN. Selective serotonin reuptake inhibitors usually are successful in reversing IFN-associated depression. Close monitoring for suicidal ideation is mandatory.

Hypothyroidism is an irreversible side effect of IFN. Levels of thyroid-stimulating hormone (TSH) should be determined before initiation of therapy and at regular intervals during treatment. IFN is contraindicated during pregnancy.

### 13. What are the side effects of ribavirin therapy? How should the patient be monitored?

Ribavirin can cause hemolysis and may rapidly lead to symptomatic anemia. A reduction in hemoglobin to 10 g/dL or less, if associated with symptoms, should trigger corrective action. Use of epoetin alfa to treat anemia is preferred to ribavirin dose reduction to maximize treatment efficacy. If the hemoglobin decreases to 8.5 g/dL or less, temporary discontinuation of therapy is advised. For patients with known ischemic cardiac disease, closer monitoring is recommended, with reduction or discontinuation of therapy if the hemoglobin decreases by more than 2 g/dL compared with baseline.

Other side effects from ribavirin include rash, shortness of breath, nausea, sore throat, cough, and glossitis. The rash may be severe and require discontinuation of the medication. The other side effects are generally not life-threatening and can be treated symptomatically.

Because ribavirin is teratogenic, both male and female patients should be advised to practice effective contraception during therapy and for 6 months after completion.

### 14. What are the contraindications to IFN therapy?

1. IFN should not be used in patients who already have leukopenia or thrombocytopenia because of the potential for bone marrow suppression. It is not recommended for patients with decompensated cirrhosis because it is rarely effective and may cause further decompensation of liver disease.
2. Patients with severe depression, history of suicide attempt or ideation, psychosis, or personality disorders should not be treated or should receive treatment only under the close monitoring of a psychiatrist. Patients with manic depression do poorly with IFN therapy and should not be treated unless their psychiatric condition is well controlled and they are under the care of a psychiatrist.
3. Patients who continue to drink alcohol on a daily basis respond less to antiviral therapy. Complete abstinence from alcohol during therapy is recommended. For patients who drink excessive amounts of alcohol, abstinence for a minimum of 6 months before initiation of therapy is required to maximize benefits of therapy.
4. Autoimmune diseases such as rheumatoid arthritis, sarcoidosis, and systemic lupus erythematosus pose a relative contraindication to therapy. Psoriasis can worsen during therapy.
5. IFN therapy should not be administered during pregnancy. If hepatitis C infection is diagnosed during pregnancy, treatment should be initiated only after delivery and breastfeeding have been completed.
6. Patients with advanced comorbid conditions should not be offered antiviral therapy for hepatitis C. Hepatitis C infection progresses slowly over time. If the patient has a life expectancy of less than 5 to 10 years, treating the hepatitis C infection is not likely to be of benefit.
7. Patients who have received an organ transplant other than liver should not receive IFN as the risk of rejection is increased.

### 15. What are the contraindications to ribavirin therapy?

Because ribavirin must be used with IFN, all contraindications to IFN apply to treatment with ribavirin. In addition, there are specific contraindications to ribavirin:

1. Pregnancy is an absolute contraindication because of the teratogenic potential.
2. Anemia and hemoglobinopathies should be considered relative contraindications. Extreme care should be exercised in treating such patients. As a rule, females with a hemoglobin less than 12 g/dL or males with less than 13 g/dL before therapy are at high risk of developing severe anemia during therapy.
3. Patients with known ischemic heart disease should be treated with caution and monitored closely.
4. Patients with renal insufficiency should not be treated with ribavirin because the development of severe, long-lasting, and life-threatening hemolysis is common.

### 16. Should patients with cirrhosis secondary to hepatitis C infection be treated with antiviral therapy?

Patients with compensated cirrhosis (normal albumin and bilirubin levels, normal prothrombin time, and no ascites, encephalopathy, or history of variceal bleeding) are excellent candidates for antiviral therapy. They are most likely to benefit from viral eradication. Once liver insufficiency develops or complications of portal hypertension become clinically evident, antiviral therapy is relatively contraindicated. Evaluation for liver transplantation is a better option for such patients.

For patients with compensated disease, the main concern about antiviral therapy is worsening of preexisting thrombocytopenia or leukopenia due to hypersplenism. Although sustained viral response in patients with cirrhosis is less common than in noncirrhotic patients, normalization of liver enzymes and reduction in viral load during treatment may result in overall improvement of liver disease and possibly delayed need for liver transplantation or development of hepatocellular carcinoma.

### 17. Should patients with hepatitis C and normal liver enzyme levels be treated with antiviral therapy?

As a group, patients who test positive for HCV-RNA in blood and have persistently normal levels of alanine aminotransferase over time tend to have mild disease on liver biopsy. Such is not the case in all patients, however, and up to 20% may have evidence of significant necroinflammatory disease on biopsy or even fibrosis. For this reason, the approach should be individualized. In general, the natural history of the disease should be discussed with the patient. A liver biopsy should be offered to stage severity of disease. If the liver biopsy shows mild or minimal disease, continued observation without therapy is a reasonable option. For patients who wish to be treated or those with more advanced disease on liver biopsy, antiviral therapy has been shown to be as effective as in patients with elevated liver enzymes. Most patients who present with normal liver enzymes on initial evaluation will demonstrate elevated enzymes on subsequent testing.

### 18. Should patients with HCV/HIV coinfection receive antiviral therapy for hepatitis C infection?

Coinfection with HIV and HCV results in marked acceleration of progression of liver disease. With the advent of newer, more effective antiretroviral agents, patients infected with HIV are living longer, and more are developing end-stage liver disease from HCV infection. For this reason, patients coinfected with HIV and HCV should be considered candidates for antiviral therapy against HCV.

Anti-HCV therapy is most likely to be effective if the patient is first placed on antiretroviral therapy, the HIV viral load is controlled, and the CD4 count is reconstituted. In general, patients with a CD4 count of less than 250/mm$^3$ are less likely to respond to antiviral therapy for HCV.

Anti-HCV therapy in patients receiving anti-HIV medications is complicated by the additive bone marrow suppression as well as other gastrointestinal side effects. Interactions between ribavirin and several antiretroviral agents may increase the risk of lactic acidosis; cotherapy with didanosine or stavudine plus ribavirin is strongly discouraged due to increased risk of lactic acidosis. Zidovudine, although not contraindicated when used with IFN and ribavirin, will enhance bone marrow suppression and increase the need for growth factor therapy to correct anemia and leukopenia. Close monitoring of blood counts and chemistries is needed. Lower dose of ribavirin (800 mg daily) is recommended when treating patients coinfected with HIV to decrease the incidence of severe anemia.

### 19. How should patients with HCV/HBV coinfection be treated?

Because most patients with HCV/HBV coinfection have quiescent hepatitis B infection, the antiviral therapy need be directed only at the HCV. If active hepatitis B and C infection are present, as evidenced by a positive HCV-RNA and high level viremia by HBV-DNA PCR assay, the patient should be treated with the recommended dose of IFN for hepatitis B in conjunction with ribavirin for hepatitis C. A flare of hepatitis is not unusual when treating patients with hepatitis B infection. Alternatively, treatment with pegylated IFN, ribavirin, and a nucleoside or nucleotide analog active against hepatitis B infection could be considered (see Chapter 17).    *Both IFN + RBV use HepC similarly*

### 20. What are the options for patients who did not respond to combination therapy with nonpegylated IFN and ribavirin?

Chances of response to retreatment with pegylated IFN and ribavirin differ depending on the type of nonresponse noted with prior therapy. Research has shown that patients who respond to nonpegylated IFN and ribavirin therapy and then relapse have a 45% to 55% chance of a sustained response if retreated with peginterferon and ribavirin therapy for 48 weeks; these patients should be offered retreatment. In contrast, those patients who do not achieve a virologic response with IFN and ribavirin have only a 10% to 15% chance of sustained response after retreatment with peginterferon and ribavirin. The decision to retreat prior nonresponders should be individualized taking into consideration the histologic severity of disease, the side effects experienced by the patient during the initial therapy and the patient's enthusiasm for retreatment. Antiviral products aimed directly at the HCV genome, such as protease and polymerase inhibitors, are currently under development and may increase the percentage of patients who achieve a sustained response to therapy when retreated.

### 21. What is the role of antiviral therapy in acute hepatitis C?

The role for antiviral therapy in acute hepatitis C is unclear. Acute infections are usually asymptomatic and found incidentally, such as needlestick injuries in health care workers. It is not clear what percentage of these cases become chronic. Some studies have shown that early treatment with IFN or combination therapy decreases the chronicity rate in patients with acute hepatitis C. More recent data suggest that as many as 50% of acute hepatitis C cases acquired via a needlestick injury may clear virus within 6 months. Although the current antiviral regimens for hepatitis C are not FDA approved for the treatment of acute hepatitis C, strong consideration should be given to early initiation of antiviral therapy when acute hepatitis C is diagnosed, particularly if the virus has not cleared within 6 months. Patients who present with symptomatic acute hepatitis C infection are more likely to clear virus spontaneously compared with those without symptoms.

## 22. Are there new treatments on the horizon for hepatitis C?

Extensive research is ongoing to develop new therapies for hepatitis C infection. Currently, the most promising compounds are protease and polymerase inhibitors, some of which have advanced to phase 3 clinical research. Development of resistance is common when protease or polymerase inhibitors are used as monotherapy. Combination with IFN and ribavirin increases efficacy of therapy and decreases the risk of resistant mutants. The protease inhibitors currently under development will be used in combination with pegylated IFN and ribavirin. Triple therapy promises enhanced response rates with a shorter treatment period; however, toxicity will likely be the same or worse with the new triple-drug regimen under development. In the distant future, cocktails of protease and polymerase inhibitors may allow an IFN- and/or ribavirin-free treatment regimen with lower toxicity.

## WEBSITES

http://www.aasld.org

http://www.cdc.gov/ncidod/diseases/hepatitis

### BIBLIOGRAPHY

1. Blackard JT, Shata MT, Shire NJ, et al. Acute hepatitis C virus infection: A chronic problem. Hepatology 2008;47:321–31.
2. Ferreira-Gonzalez A, Shiffman ML. Use of diagnostic testing for managing hepatitis C infection. Semin Liver Dis 2004;24:9–18.
3. Jacobson IM, Brown RS, Freilich B, et al. Peginterferon alfa-2b and weight-based or flat dose ribavirin in chronic hepatitis C patients: A randomized trial. Hepatology 2007;46:971–81.
4. Mallat A, Hezode C, Lotersztajn S. Environmental factors as disease accelerators during chronic hepatitis C. J Hepatol 2008;48:657–65.
5. McHutchison JG, Bartenschlager R, Patel K, et al. The face of future hepatitis C antiviral drug development: Recent biological and virologic advances and their translation to drug development and clinical practice. J Hepatol 2006;44:411–21.
6. McLean OR, Herrera JL. Acute hepatitis C: Diagnosis and management. Pract Gastroenterol 2007;31:66–77.
7. Pearlman BL, Ehleben C, Saifee S. Treatment extension to 72 weeks of peginterferon and ribavirin in hepatitis C genotype 1 infected slow responders. Hepatology 2007;46:1688–94.
8. Russo MW, Fried MW. Side effects of therapy for chronic hepatitis C. Gastroenterology 2003;124:1711–9.
9. Soriano V. Treatment of chronic hepatitis C in HIV-positive individuals: Selection of candidates. J Hepatol 2006;S44–8.
10. Strader DB, Wright T, Thomas DL, et al. Diagnosis, management and treatment of hepatitis C. Hepatology 2004;39:1147–71.
11. Vallet-Pichard A, Pol S. Natural history and predictors of severity of chronic hepatitis C virus (HCV) and human immunodeficiency virus (HIV) co-infection. J Hepatol 2006;44:S28–34.
12. Wong W, Terrault N. Update on chronic hepatitis C. Clin Gastroenterol Hepatol 2005;3:507–20.

# ANTIVIRAL THERAPY FOR HEPATITIS B

*Jorge L. Herrera, MD*

CHAPTER 17

## 1. Is antiviral therapy recommended for acute hepatitis B?

No. Acute hepatitis B, defined as a positive test for hepatitis B surface antigen (HBsAg) and the presence of hepatitis B core antibody–immunoglobulin M (HBcAb-IgM), is a self-limited disease in 90% to 95% of adults and resolves without specific antiviral therapy within 3 to 6 months after the onset of clinical symptoms. For this reason, only supportive care is offered to patients with acute hepatitis B infection. Antiviral therapy is considered only for patients with chronic hepatitis B (positive HBsAg test for longer than 6 months). For patients with severe acute hepatitis B with evidence of liver dysfunction such as coagulopathy or encephalopathy, antiviral therapy may be considered; in this situation, expert consultation is advised.

## 2. Do all patients with chronic hepatitis B benefit from therapy?

No. Only patients with detectable viremia and evidence of ongoing hepatic necrosis, such as elevated liver enzyme levels and/or liver biopsy demonstrating active inflammation or fibrosis, are most likely to benefit from therapy. Typical candidates for antiviral therapy test positive for hepatitis B e antigen (HBeAg) and negative for HBe antibodies (HBeAb); they also have high levels of hepatitis B virus DNA by polymerase chain reaction (HBV-DNA by PCR) assays. In contrast, chronic hepatitis B carriers (HBsAg-positive), who are characterized by normal levels of liver enzymes, negative HBeAg, positive HBeAb, and nondetectable or low levels of HBV-DNA by PCR, do not require antiviral therapy, but should be monitored for evidence of disease reactivation (Table 17-1).

**Table 17-1.** Antiviral Therapy for Patients With Chronic Hepatitis B Infection

| SEROLOGIC PATTERN | INTERPRETATION | COURSE OF ACTION |
|---|---|---|
| HBsAg positive, HBcAb-IgM positive | Acute hepatitis B | Observe; resolution likely in 90-95% of adults |
| HBsAg positive >6 mo, HBeAg positive, HBeAb negative, HBV-DNA positive, elevated ALT level | Chronic infection with wild virus | Initiate antiviral therapy |
| HBsAg positive >6 mo, HBeAg negative, HBeAb positive, ALT normal, HBV DNA negative, or low-level viremia (<2000 IU/mL) | Chronic carrier | Observe |
| HBsAg positive >6 mo, HBeAg negative, HBeAb positive, HBV-DNA positive, elevated ALT level | Chronic infection with HBeAg mutant | Initiate antiviral therapy |

HBsAg, hepatitis B surface antigen; HBcAb-IgM, hepatitis B core antibody-immunoglobulin M; HBeAg, hepatitis B e antigen; HBeAb, hepatitis B e antibody; HBV-DNA, hepatitis B virus DNA by PCR; ALT, alanine aminotransferase; IU, international units.

## 3. How should the HBV-DNA PCR assay results be used to make therapy decisions?

Hepatitis B infection is almost never totally eradicated. Instead, it can be controlled with medications. Low levels of HBV-DNA are not associated with progressive liver disease and do not require therapy. The upper limit of HBV-DNA levels that are consistently associated with inactive disease has not been clearly established, but it is generally agreed that nondetectable HBV DNA or levels consistently below 2000 IU/mL, associated with normal alanine aminotransferase (ALT) levels or a liver biopsy showing no inflammation do not require treatment. It is important to note that in some cases, particularly in HBeAg-negative disease, viral levels can fluctuate over time and multiple measurements may be necessary to confirm that levels remain below 2000 IU/mL. In patients with advanced liver disease, particularly decompensated cirrhosis, treatment should be considered if any detectable virus is noted, regardless of how low the reading may be.

## 4. Is liver biopsy required before therapy is started?

A liver biopsy is not needed to establish the diagnosis of hepatitis B infection; however, it is the only tool available to determine severity of disease. Treatment decisions are different for patients with advanced fibrosis and cirrhosis compared with those with mild histologic disease. The risk of liver cancer and the intensity of surveillance for liver cancer would be greater for those patients with cirrhosis. The detection of cirrhosis on liver biopsy selects a group of patients who require closer observation as well as screening for esophageal varices. A liver biopsy is also important for patients that have high viral load (>2000 IU) but normal liver enzymes. The presence of inflammation or fibrosis on biopsy would be a strong indicator that therapy should be considered.

## 5. What are the options for treating chronic hepatitis B infection?

Currently, six medications have been approved for the treatment of chronic hepatitis B infection: interferon α2b, pegylated interferon α2a, lamivudine, adefovir dipivoxil, entecavir, and telbivudine (Table 17-2). In addition, two other medications with activity against hepatitis B are available by prescription but are not approved by the U.S. Food and Drug Administration (FDA) for treatment of hepatitis B: tenofovir and emtricitabine. Interferon is an injectable immunomodulatory medication that enhances clearance of the hepatitis B virus by improving the immune response. The pegylated form of interferon α2a is most often used and is dosed as 180 μg subcutaneously once a week for 52 weeks. Lamivudine, telbivudine, and entecavir are oral nucleoside analogs that directly inhibit viral replication without stimulating an immune response. Lamivudine is dosed at 100 mg/day, telbivudine at 600 mg once daily, and entecavir at 0.5 mg/day in treatment-naïve patients. Adefovir dipivoxil is an oral nucleotide analog of adenosine monophosphate. It inhibits both the reverse transcriptase and DNA polymerase activity and is incorporated into viral DNA, causing chain termination. Adefovir is given as a single 10-mg daily dose. Oral nucleoside/nucleotide analogs differ in potency and resistance profile. Lamivudine is of intermediate potency but has an inferior resistance profile, with 20% of patients becoming resistant by the first year of therapy and up to 70% by the fourth year. For this reason, lamivudine is no longer recommended as monotherapy for the treatment of hepatitis B infection. Entecavir and telbivudine have higher potency. Entecavir has the best resistance profile, with no resistance in the first year and 1% by the fourth year. Adefovir has a good resistance profile but lower potency. HBV-DNA declines slower and primary non-response is more common with adefovir therapy.

**Table 17- 2.** Comparison of Approved Antiviral Treatments for Chronic Hepatitis B

|  | PEGYLATED INTERFERON | LAMIVUDINE | ADEFOVIR | ENTECAVIR | TELBIVUDINE |
|---|---|---|---|---|---|
| Potency | ++ | +++ | ++ | ++++ | ++++ |
| e-Antigen seroconversion (1 yr) | ≈30% | ≈12–20% | ≈15–20% | ≈15–25% | ≈15–25% |
| Duration of treatment |  |  |  |  |  |
|   HBeAg (+) chronic hepatitis | 52 wk | ≥1 yr | ≥1 yr | ≥1 yr | ≥1 yr |
|   HBeAg (-) chronic hepatitis | 52 wk | Indefinite | Indefinite | Indefinite | indefinite |
| Route | Subcutaneous | Oral | Oral | Oral | Oral |
| Dose | 180 μg weekly | 100 mg daily* | 10 mg daily | 0.5 mg daily† | 600 mg daily |
| Side effects | Common and expected | Uncommon | Uncommon, rare renal toxicity | Uncommon | Uncommon, rare myopathy |
| Drug resistance | None reported | ≈20% by 1 yr ≈70% by 4 yr | 3% by 2 y, 29% by 5 y In LAM resistance 20% after 2 yr | 1% by 4 yr In LAM resistance 40% after 4 yr | 9–22% by 2 yr |

*For persons coinfected with HIV, 150 mg twice daily along with other antiretroviral medications.
†1.0 mg daily for lamivudine-resistant infection or prior nonresponse to the 0.5-mg dose.
HBeAg, hepatitis B e antigen; LAM, lamivudine.

## 6. What are the endpoints of antiviral therapy?

The goals of antiviral therapy are to drastically reduce viremia, ideally to undetectable levels. For patients who are e-antigen positive at the initiation of therapy, induction of e-antigen seroconversion (defined as achieving HBeAg-negative, HBeAb-positive status) signals response to therapy. After e-antigen seroconversion is achieved, antiviral therapy is continued for an additional 24 to 48 weeks and then may be discontinued. Remission is usually long-lasting, but as long as the patient continues to test positive for hepatitis B surface antibody enclose in parens: HBsAb, he or she is at risk of reactivation and should be monitored closely.

Patients who are viremic but e-antigen negative at initiation of therapy will likely require life-long therapy. Even after 5 or more years of nondetectable HBV-DNA levels on therapy, discontinuation of therapy results in reactivation of disease in the majority of patients; thus, when a decision is made to treat e-antigen–negative disease, treatment is usually lifelong or until the patient loses HBsAg and acquires hepatitis B surface antibody (HBsAb), which is a rare event.

HBsAg rarely clears during antiviral therapy. With continued follow-up after successful antiviral therapy, however, a percentage of patients lose HBsAg and develop HBsAb. HBsAg clearance occurs in less than 5% of patients within the first year after treatment and is most often seen in patients treated with interferon.

## 7. What is the expected response to interferon therapy?

Because interferon stimulates the immune response, increased clearance of the hepatitis B virus is expected during therapy. Clearance of the virus is achieved by necrosis of infected hepatocytes. Thus, a flare of hepatitis is common during treatment with interferon. Usually it occurs soon after initiation of interferon therapy and is manifested by elevated levels of ALT and aspartate aminotransferase (AST). The flare may be accompanied by jaundice and signs and symptoms typical of acute viral hepatitis but usually is associated with reduction or disappearance of HBV-DNA in blood. As the liver enzyme levels return to normal, the HBeAg assay becomes negative, followed by seroconversion to positive HBeAb. The virologic response is usually long-lasting if e-antigen seroconversion is achieved. Positive predictors of response to interferon therapy include HBeAg-positive patients, low viral levels, elevated ALT levels (>150 IU), infection with hepatitis B virus genotype A, and absence of cirrhosis. Seroconversion to HBeAg-negative and HBeAb-positive status occurs in about 30% of patients treated with interferon; the majority of responders have a durable response.

## 8. What is the expected response to oral nucleoside/nucleotide therapy?

In contrast to interferon, nucleosides and nucleotides inhibit viral replication but do not stimulate immune clearance of the virus. For this reason, immune-mediated hepatocyte necrosis is unusual, and biochemical flare of hepatitis is rarely seen with these agents. In most patients, the HBV-DNA serum levels decrease dramatically or become undetectable soon after initiating therapy, depending on the initial viral load and the potency of the drug being used. This decrease is associated with normalization of liver enzyme levels. Seroconversion from HBeAg-positive to HBeAg-negative status and from HBeAb-negative to HBeAb-positive status is less common than with interferon therapy and often requires prolonged therapy for several years.

Prolonged therapy with nucleosides/nucleotides has been associated with the emergence of resistant escape mutants; development of resistance is defined as an increase in viral load of >1 log over the nadir, confirmed at least on two different occasions. Risk of resistance is highest with lamivudine and lowest with entecavir. Prompt viral suppression after initiation of therapy is associated with a lower risk of resistance.

## 9. What are the advantages of interferon therapy for chronic hepatitis B infection?

Therapy with interferon is of finite duration (52 weeks in most cases) and is successful in 25% to 40% of selected patients. Successful response is durable, and relapses are rare once interferon is discontinued. Once the HBV infects the liver cell, the HBV genome localizes to the nucleus of the hepatocyte and is converted to covalently closed circular DNA (cccDNA). Clearance of this HBV-DNA is needed to achieve HBsAg seroconversion and can be achieved only by immune-mediated lysis of infected hepatocytes. Cases of HBsAg seroconversion (HBsAg status becomes negative and HBsAb status becomes positive) have been documented years after inducing e-antigen seroconversion by interferon. Finally, *interferon escape mutants* have not been described.

## 10. What are the disadvantages of interferon therapy?

Interferon therapy is associated with significant side effects, including flulike syndrome, fever, depression, insomnia, irritability, and bone marrow suppression (see Chapter 16). The interferon-induced flare of hepatitis may be severe and is particularly dangerous in patients with advanced liver disease and cirrhosis, who may not be able to tolerate a flare of hepatitis. For this reason, interferon therapy is relatively contraindicated in patients with cirrhosis caused by chronic hepatitis B infection.

Another disadvantage is that patients with persistently normal liver enzyme levels, those who acquired the disease at birth, and those infected with HBV genotype C or D are unlikely to respond to interferon therapy. Finally, patients infected with the hepatitis B e-antigen mutant are less likely to achieve a lasting response to interferon.

## 11. Which parameters predict a good response to interferon therapy?

Patients likely to respond to interferon therapy are characterized by elevated liver enzymes (ALT >150 U/dL), low viral load (HBV-DNA <$10^9$ IU), hepatitis B virus genotype A, positive HBeAg status, female sex, and acquisition of infection during adulthood. Such patients have a 30% to 40% chance of achieving e-antigen seroconversion after a 52-week course of interferon. In contrast, patients with normal or minimal elevations of liver enzymes have a less than 5% chance of achieving sustained remission.

**12. What are the advantages of oral nucleoside/nucleotide therapy?**

Oral agents are taken once daily and are associated with minimal to no side effects. They have potent antiviral activity and in most cases induce a profound decrease in viremia with normalization of the liver enzymes. Oral agents can be safely used in patients with decompensated liver disease at times with dramatic responses.

**13. What are the disadvantages of oral nucleoside/nucleotide therapy?**

The treatment course is long; most patients require treatment for multiple years; and in the case of e-antigen–negative disease, treatment is lifelong. The cost of these medications is significant. The development of resistant mutants increases with longer duration of therapy, and once resistance develops to one drug, the chances of developing resistance to other drugs increases. Finally, oral agents have a lower rate of HBsAg seroconversion compared to interferon; however, with prolonged therapy, surface antigen seroconversion rates approach those of interferon therapy.

**14. Should patients with advanced, decompensated cirrhosis secondary to hepatitis B receive antiviral therapy or be referred for liver transplantation without a trial of therapy?**

Although patients with decompensated disease cannot be treated with interferon, treatment with nucleoside or nucleotide analogs is beneficial and often lifesaving. In many such patients, evidence of severe decompensation reverses, and patients no longer need to be listed for liver transplantation after a response to antiviral therapy. In addition, oral therapy, when continued after transplantation in conjunction with hepatitis B immune globulin, is associated with a decreased chance of recurrence of infection in the graft. In general, patients with severe liver disease due to hepatitis B infection, even if listed for transplantation, should be treated with oral nucleosides or nucleotides. Once a response is achieved, lifelong therapy is recommended as flares induced by discontinuation of antiviral therapy could be fatal in these patients.

**15. How should response to therapy be monitored?**

After initiation of therapy, repeat viral load should be performed at 3 months. Failure of the viral load to decrease greater than 1 log indicates either primary nonresponse or lack of compliance. Patients who have an initial response should be tested again at 6 months of therapy. Those who are receiving drugs that have a low genetic barrier (i.e., higher risk of escape mutants, such as lamivudine or telbivudine) should have nondetectable virus by week 24 of therapy; otherwise, the chance of developing resistant mutants is greatly increased. In contrast, those receiving therapy with drugs that have a high genetic barrier (adefovir or entecavir) can continue therapy as long as the viral load at week 24 of therapy is less than 2000 IU/mL. Those patients continuing therapy should be retested at 9 and 12 months. By 12 months of therapy, patients should have nondetectable HBV-DNA. Failure to achieve these milestones may require addition of a second antiviral agent or change to a more potent drug; expert advice should be obtained.

**16. How is resistance diagnosed and how should it be managed?**

Development of resistance to nucleoside/nucleotide therapy is always a concern. Resistance is more likely to develop when using drugs that have a low genetic barrier (e.g., lamivudine and telbivudine) or if patients do not become virus negative after 24 to 48 weeks of therapy. Antiviral drug resistance has been reported in up to 70% of patients after 4 years of lamivudine therapy and in 9% to 22% of patients after 2 years of telbivudine therapy. Of the agents currently approved by the FDA, adefovir and entecavir have the highest genetic barrier and the lowest rates of resistance—1% resistance occurs after 4 years of entecavir, and up to 29% after 4 years of adefovir. Resistance rates to adefovir and entecavir are substantially higher in patients who have already developed resistance to lamivudine.

Regardless of the agent used, patients need to be monitored to detect the emergence of resistant mutants. Levels of HBV-DNA should be monitored every 3 months as long as detectable virus is present, and then every 6 months after viral negativity is achieved. Viral breakthrough is defined as a rise of greater than 1 log from nadir in serum HBV-DNA during treatment. Viral breakthrough should be confirmed on two separate occasions and patients should be questioned closely regarding compliance with therapy; trials have shown that 30% to 35% of breakthroughs are associated with poor compliance and not emergence of resistant mutants. Tests to detect resistant HBV mutants are commercially available and may be helpful in differentiating noncompliance from the emergence of mutant strains. Current resistance panels, however, have limitations and the absence of detectable resistant mutants does not always indicate lack of compliance.

Once resistance is detected, a second drug without cross resistance should be added. The initial drug should be continued. Sequential therapy (i.e., stopping the first drug and switching to a different drug) is not recommended as it is likely to result in the selection of multidrug-resistant hepatitis B virus. In general, adefovir should be added to the antiviral regiment of patients who develop resistance to lamivudine or telbivudine, and telbivudine, lamivudine, or entecavir should be added to adefovir in those patients who develop adefovir resistance. Entecavir at a higher dosage of 1.0 mg/day may be used to treat patients with lamivudine resistance; however, the potency of entecavir is significantly reduced in this situation and the likelihood of entecavir-resistant mutations is increased. Thus, entecavir should not be the treatment of choice for lamivudine-resistant patients.

### 17. Should patients with chronic hepatitis B be treated if they are to undergo immune suppression?

The immune system plays a pivotal role in the control of hepatitis B infection. Patients who are HBsAg positive but have no detectable viremia or low level of virus can promptly reactivate if immunosuppressed. If immunosuppression is planned (i.e., cancer chemotherapy, anti–tumor necrosis factor therapy, high-dose corticosteroid therapy), patients should be screened for HBsAg. If positive, initiation of antiviral therapy with a nucleoside/nucleotide analog should be strongly considered even if HBV-DNA is nondetectable. Antiviral therapy should be started 2 to 4 weeks before or at the time of the introduction of the immunosuppressant and continued for at least 6 to 12 months after completion of immunosuppression. Patients who would have met criteria for hepatitis B therapy before immunosuppression (i.e., high viral load, elevated ALT) should continue on long-term antiviral therapy until traditional endpoints of treatment are achieved.

### 18. How should HBV infection be treated in patients coinfected with the human immunodeficiency virus (HIV)?

Most of the antiviral agents currently available for the treatment of hepatitis B have activity against HIV. Initiation of monotherapy for HBV in patients with known or undiagnosed HIV can lead to emergence of HIV-resistant mutants. All patients infected with HBV should be tested for HIV. If coinfected with HIV, they should be evaluated for highly active antiretroviral therapy (HAART). Current HIV treatment guidelines consider the presence of hepatitis B infection an indication to initiate HAART. Selection of a HAART regimen that includes at least two drugs active against HBV (i.e., tenofovir and emtricitabine or lamivudine) is recommended. Patients coinfected with HBV/HIV should not receive lamivudine as the only HBV-active drug in the HAART cocktail.

For patients in whom HAART is contraindicated or not desired, therapeutic options for treating HBV are very limited. Lamivudine, entecavir, emtricitabine, and tenofovir all have activity against HIV and are not recommended as monotherapy for HBV in this situation. Telbivudine does not appear to be active against HIV but has not been thoroughly tested. Only pegylated interferon is active against HBV and does not affect the resistance profile of HIV. Adefovir, at the HBV dose of 10 mg/day, is not active against HIV but has a low potency and is less likely to be effective in HIV/HBV-coinfected individuals.

### 19. Should hepatitis B be treated during pregnancy?

Hepatitis B infection is vertically transmitted. The introduction of the hepatitis B vaccine and hepatitis B immune globulin injection for babies born to HBsAg-positive mothers has markedly decreased vertical transmission of HBV but has not eliminated the risk. A high maternal viral load ($>10^7$ IU/mL) has been associated with an increased risk of vertical transmission even to babies who receive the appropriate passive and active immunization at birth. Limited clinical research suggests that lowering the viral load during the last trimester of pregnancy further decreases the risk of vertical transmission.

The choice of antiviral agent to use during pregnancy is difficult. Pegylated interferon is contraindicated. Lamivudine, entecavir, and adefovir are classified as Class C pregnancy drugs by the FDA. Telbivudine and tenofovir are Class B pregnancy drugs. Extensive experience exists with lamivudine therapy during pregnancy in HIV-infected patients. This experience indicates that lamivudine appears safe and not associated with birth defects. Although tenofovir and telbivudine are classified as Class B pregnancy drugs, clinical experience is very limited during human pregnancy. Given these uncertainties, most authorities recommend treatment with lamivudine starting in the third trimester for pregnant patients with high HBV-DNA viral load. After delivery, if continued maternal therapy is required, switching to a drug with a more favorable resistance profile should be considered. All nucleoside/nucleotide analogs are excreted in breast milk and breastfeeding should be avoided if the mother is taking these drugs.

The safety of antiviral agents during the first trimester of pregnancy is not known, with the exception of the clinical experience of lamivudine in HIV-infected patients. In general, if an HBV-infected female is planning pregnancy, it may be best to delay therapy until the third trimester of pregnancy or after delivery if her clinical condition allows. The use of lamivudine can be considered in this situation, with close monitoring for the emergence of resistance. Patients who become pregnant while on interferon, adefovir, or entecavir therapy should discontinue antiviral therapy as soon as the pregnancy is diagnosed and either be monitored off therapy or switched to lamivudine depending on the clinical situation.

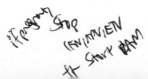

## WEBSITES

http://www.aasld.org/

http://www.hbvadvocate.org

## BIBLIOGRAPHY

1. Andreani T, Serfaty L, Mohand D, et al. Chronic hepatitis B virus carriers in the immunotolerant phase of infection: Histologic findings and outcome. Clin Gastroenterol Hepatol 2007;5:636–41.
2. Benhamou Y. Treatment algorithm for chronic hepatitis B in HIV-infected patients. J Hepatol 2006;44:S90–4.
3. Dusheiko G, Antonakopoulous N. Current treatment of hepatitis B. Gut 2008;57:105–24.
4. Gambarin-Gelwan M. Hepatitis B in pregnancy. Clin Liver Dis 2007;11:945–63.
5. Keeffe EB, Dieterich DT, Han SH, et al. A treatment algorithm for the management of chronic hepatitis B virus infection in the United States: An update. Clin Gastroenterol Hepatol 2006;4:936–62.
6. Keeffe EB, Zeuzem S, Koff RS, et al. Report of an international workshop: Roadmap for management of patients receiving oral therapy for chronic hepatitis B. Clin Gastroenterol Hepatol 2007;5:890–7.
7. Landreneau SW, Herrera JL. Chronic hepatitis B: Who and how to treat. Pract Gastroenterol 2007;31:25–40.
8. Lok AS, McMahon BJ. Chronic hepatitis B. Hepatology 2007;45:507–39.
9. McMahon MA, Benjamin BS, Jilk L, et al. The HBV drug entecavir—Effects on HIV-1 replication and resistance. N Engl J Med 2007;356:2614–21.
10. Mindikoglu AL, Regev A, Schiff ER. Hepatitis B virus reactivation after cytotoxic chemotherapy: The disease and its prevention. Clin Gastroenterol Hepatol 2006;4:1076–81.
11. Pawlotsky JM, Dusheiko G, Hatzakis A, et al. Virologic monitoring of hepatitis B virus therapy in clinical trials and practice: Recommendations for a standardized approach. Gastroenterology 2008;134:405–15.
12. Peters MG, Andersen J, Lynch P, et al. Randomized controlled study of tenofovir and adefovir in chronic hepatitis B virus and HIV infection: ACTG A5127. Hepatology 2006;44:1110–6.
13. Tsang PS, Trinh H, Garcia RT, et al. Significant prevalence of histologic disease in patients with chronic hepatitis B and mildly elevated serum alanine aminotransferase levels. Clin Gastroenterol Hepatol 2008;6:569–74.
14. Zoulim F, Perillo R, Hepatitis B. Reflections on the current approach to antiviral therapy. J Hepatol 2008;48:S2–S19.

# CHAPTER 18

# AUTOIMMUNE HEPATITIS: DIAGNOSIS AND PATHOGENESIS

Albert J. Czaja, MD

## 1. What is autoimmune hepatitis?

Autoimmune hepatitis is an unresolving inflammation of the liver of unknown cause that is characterized by interface hepatitis on histologic examination, autoantibodies, and hypergammaglobulinemia. Cirrhosis, portal hypertension, liver failure, and death are possible consequences. There are no specific diagnostic features, and the designation requires the exclusion of other conditions that can resemble it, especially chronic viral hepatitis, Wilson disease, drug-induced hepatitis (most commonly, minocycline or diclofenac toxicity), alcoholic and nonalcoholic fatty liver disease, and other immune-mediated liver diseases, such as primary biliary cirrhosis and primary sclerosing cholangitis (Table 18-1).

## 2. What are its predominant features?

Autoimmune hepatitis affects mainly women (71%). It may occur at any age (9 months to 77 years) but typically it is diagnosed before the fourth decade. Concurrent immunologic diseases are present in 38%, and they include autoimmune thyroiditis, ulcerative colitis, Graves disease, and synovitis (Table 18-2). Smooth muscle antibodies (SMAs) and antinuclear antibodies (ANAs) are the most common serologic markers. In 64% of patients, SMAs and ANAs occur together. Autoantibody titers fluctuate, and they may disappear. Serologic features may also change during the disease, and one autoantibody may disappear as another appears. There is no minimum titer of significance, but autoantibody titers greater than 1:80 increase diagnostic confidence. Hypergammaglobulinemia, especially abnormal elevation of the

## Table 18-1. Differential Diagnosis and Discriminative Tests

| POSSIBLE DIAGNOSES | SCREENING TESTS | DIAGNOSTIC FINDINGS |
|---|---|---|
| Wilson disease | Copper studies | Low ceruloplasmin<br>Low serum copper level<br>High urinary copper level<br>Increased hepatic copper |
| | Slit lamp eye exam | Kayser-Fleischer rings |
| Primary sclerosing cholangitis | Cholangiography<br>Liver biopsy | Focal biliary strictures<br>Fibrous obliterative cholangitis |
| Primary biliary cirrhosis | Antimitochondial antibodies<br><br>Liver biopsy | AMA titer ≥1:40<br>Anti-pyruvate dehydrogenase-E2<br>Florid duct lesion<br>Increased hepatic copper |
| Chronic hepatitis C | Viral markers<br><br>Liver biopsy | Anti-HCV positive<br>HCV RNA present<br>Portal lymphoid aggregates<br>Steatosis |
| Drug-induced hepatitis | Clinical history | Exposure to minocycline, diclofenac, isoniazid, nitrofurantoin, propylthiouracil, α-methyldopa |
| Hemochromatosis | Genetic testing<br>Transferrin saturation<br>Liver biopsy | *C282Y, H63D* mutations<br>Increased<br>Iron overload<br>Hepatic iron index >1.9 |
| α₁-Antitrypsin deficiency | Phenotype<br>Liver biopsy | ZZ or MZ<br>Hepatic inclusions |
| Nonalcoholic steatohepatitis | Clinical findings<br><br>Ultrasonography<br>Liver biopsy | Obesity, diabetes, drugs, hyperlipidemia<br>Hepatic hyperechogenicity<br>Macrosteatosis |

AMA, antimitochondial antibodies; HCV, hepatitis C virus; RNA, ribonucleic acid; C282Y, substitution of tyrosine for cysteine at amino acid position 282 in $\alpha_3$ loop; H63D, substitution of histidine for aspartate at amino acid position 63 in $\alpha_1$ loop; ZZ or MZ, major protease inhibitor ($P_i$) deficiency phenotypes.

**Table 18-2.** Immunological Diseases Associated With Autoimmune Hepatitis

| | |
|---|---|
| Autoimmune sclerosing cholangitis | Lichen planus |
| Autoimmune thyroiditis* | Myasthenia gravis |
| Celiac disease | Neutropenia |
| Coombs-positive hemolytic anemia | Pericarditis |
| Cryoglobulinemia | Peripheral neuropathy |
| Dermatitis herpetiformis | Pernicious anemia |
| Erythema nodosum | Pleuritis |
| Fibrosing alveolitis | Pyoderma gangrenosum |
| Focal myositis | Rheumatoid arthritis* |
| Gingivitis | Sjögren syndrome |
| Glomerulonephritis | Synovitis* |
| Graves disease* | Systemic lupus erythematosus |
| Idiopathic thrombocytopenic purpura | Ulcerative colitis* |
| Insulin-dependent diabetes | Urticaria |
| Intestinal villous atrophy | Vitiligo |
| Iritis | |

*Most common association.

serum immunoglobulin G (IgG) level, is a hallmark of the disease, and the diagnosis is suspect without it. Marked cholestatic features are incompatible with the diagnosis, and serum alkaline phosphatase levels more than 3-fold the upper limit of normal, pruritus, hyperpigmentation, and bile duct lesions on histologic examination suggest other diseases, such as primary biliary cirrhosis or primary sclerosing cholangitis.

### 3. What are the symptoms of autoimmune hepatitis?

The major symptoms of autoimmune hepatitis are fatigue and arthralgia. Autoimmune hepatitis is asymptomatic in 25% to 34% of patients. Asymptomatic patients are typically men, and they have lower serum aspartate aminotransferase (AST) levels at presentation than do symptomatic patients. Histologic features are similar between symptomatic and asymptomatic patients, including the occurrence of cirrhosis. As many as 70% of asymptomatic patients become symptomatic during the course of the disease, and all asymptomatic patients must be monitored closely for changes in disease severity.

### 4. What are the characteristic histologic findings in autoimmune hepatitis?

Interface hepatitis is the *sine qua non* for the diagnosis of autoimmune hepatitis. The limiting plate of the portal tract is completely disrupted by a mononuclear inflammatory infiltrate, which spills into the acinus (Fig. 18-1). Interface hepatitis may be seen in acute and chronic hepatitis associated with viruses, drugs, alcohol, and toxins, and its presence does not compel the diagnosis of autoimmune hepatitis. Panacinar (*lobular*) hepatitis is characterized by prominent cellular infiltrates that line sinusoidal spaces in association with degenerative or regenerative changes, and it is another common but nondiagnostic histologic manifestation (Fig. 18-2). Plasma cells are present in 66% of liver tissue specimens, and they support the diagnosis of autoimmune hepatitis but they are neither specific nor required for it (Fig. 18-3). A centrilobular or

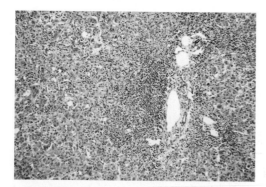

**Figure 18-1.** Interface hepatitis. The limiting plate of the portal tract is disrupted by inflammatory infiltrate (hematoxylin and eosin, original magnification ×100).

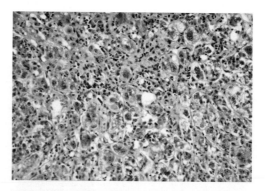

**Figure 18-2.** Panacinar hepatitis. Inflammatory cells line the sinusoidal spaces in association with liver cell regenerative or degenerative changes (hematoxylin and eosin, original magnification ×200).

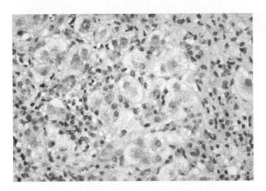

**Figure 18-3.** Plasma cell infiltration. Plasma cells, identified by the cytoplasmic haloes about their nucleus, infiltrate the periportal region (hematoxylin and eosin, original magnification ×400).

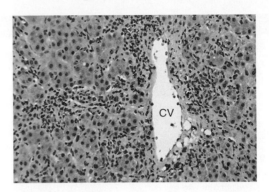

**Figure 18-4.** Centrilobular (zone 3) necrosis. Inflammatory and degenerative changes concentrate around the central vein (CV) and involve the centrilobular or Rappaport zone 3 region of the liver tissue (hematoxylin and eosin, original magnification, ×200).

Rappaport zone 3 necrosis may represent an early acute form of autoimmune hepatitis as sequential liver tissue examinations have demonstrated its transition to interface hepatitis during the course of the disease (Fig. 18-4). Prominent portal lymphoid aggregates and steatosis suggest the diagnosis of chronic hepatitis C (Fig. 18-5); ground-glass hepatocytes are characteristic of chronic hepatitis B; and marked bile duct damage or loss connotes a cholestatic disease.

## 5. Can autoimmune hepatitis have a fulminant presentation?

Yes. Autoimmune hepatitis can have an acute severe or fulminant presentation that can be mistaken for an acute viral or toxic hepatitis, and misdiagnosis can delay or defer the institution of potentially life-saving treatment. Corticosteroid therapy can be effective in suppressing the inflammatory activity in 36% to 100% of these patients, whereas delay in treatment can have a strong negative impact on outcome. Furthermore, unrecognized chronic disease can have a spontaneous exacerbation and appear acute. These latter patients invariably die if there has been no response to corticosteroid therapy after 2 weeks. Liver transplantation is an important management option for these individuals.

## 6. Are there patients who may be underdiagnosed?

Yes. Infants, elderly individuals, patients with acute severe or fulminant presentations, and nonwhite patients may be underdiagnosed because the disease is unsuspected, confused with other diseases, or atypical in its manifestations. Twenty-three percent of adults with autoimmune hepatitis are older than 60 years, and these patients commonly have thyroid or rheumatic diseases (42%) that may mask their underlying liver disease. Furthermore, elderly patients may have an acute onset, which may be mistakenly ascribed to their medication. African American patients have a higher frequency of cirrhosis at presentation than white North Americans. Alaskan natives have a higher occurrence of acute icteric disease than nonnative counterparts; Arab patients frequently have cholestatic features; Asians have late onset, mild disease; and South American patients are commonly young children with severe disease. The diverse presentations of the same disease in different ethnic groups are important to recognize to ensure a prompt and accurate diagnosis. The different clinical phenotypes in nonwhite patients probably reflect ethnic differences in the genetic predisposition for the disease or regional differences in the etiologic basis for the condition.

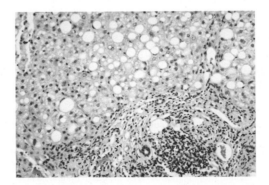

**Figure 18-5.** Chronic hepatitis C. Small lymphocytes aggregate in the portal tract and vacuoles of lipid are present within the cytoplasm of hepatocytes (hematoxylin and eosin, original magnification ×200).

**Table 18-3.** Types of Autoimmune Hepatitis

| FEATURES | TYPE 1 | TYPE 2 |
|---|---|---|
| Autoantibodies | Smooth muscle<br>Nucleus<br>Actin<br>Soluble liver antigen<br>Atypical pANCA | Liver/kidney microsome type 1<br>Liver cytosol type 1<br>Liver/kidney microsome type 3 |
| Organ-specific antibodies | Common (antibodies to thyroid) | Common (antibodies to thyroid, parietal cells, islets of Langerhans) |
| Autoantigen | Unknown | CYP2D6 (P450 IID6) |
| HLA phenotype | B8, DR3, DR4 | DR7, B14, DR3 |
| Susceptibility alleles | *DRB1\*0301, DRB1\*0401* (North American and northern Europe)<br>*DRB1\*04* alleles (Japan, China, Mexico)<br>*DRB1\*1301* (South America) | *DQB1\*0201* (principal determinant)<br>*DRB1\*0701* (anti-LKM1 expression)<br>*DRB1\*03*<br>*C4A-Q0* |
| Predominant age | Adult | Childhood (2–14 years) |
| Fulminant onset | Possible | Possible |
| Concurrent immune disease | 38% | 34%<br>Autoimmune sclerosing cholangitis |
| Low IgA level | No | Possible |
| Progression to cirrhosis | 36% | 82% |
| Corticosteroid responsive | Yes | Yes |

HLA, human leukocyte antigen; pANCA, perinuclear anti-neutrophil cytoplasmic antibodies; LKM1, liver/kidney microsome type 1; IgA, immunoglobulin A

## 7. What are the different types of autoimmune hepatitis?

Three types of autoimmune hepatitis have been proposed based on distinctive serologic markers, but only two continue to be described (Table 18-3). These classifications do not define clinically valid subgroups of different etiology or prognosis, and the designations have not been endorsed by the International Autoimmune Hepatitis Group. Nevertheless, they continue to be used as clinical descriptors and in research settings. In the former instance, they convey a clinical and serological phenotype, and in the latter instance, they help maintain homogeneity of study populations. The designations do not identify independent pathologic entities, and they should not be used as formal diagnoses.

- *Type 1 autoimmune hepatitis* is characterized by SMA or ANA, and it is the most common form worldwide. Antibodies to actin (antiactin), a subgroup of SMA, also support the diagnosis.
- *Type 2 autoimmune hepatitis* is characterized by antibodies to liver/kidney microsome type 1 (anti-LKM1). Patients with type 2 autoimmune hepatitis are typically young (ages, 2 to 14 years) and European. They frequently have concurrent immunological diseases, such as autoimmune thyroiditis, vitiligo, and insulin-dependent diabetes, and they may have low serum concentrations of immunoglobulin A (IgA). Type 2 autoimmune hepatitis is found in only 4% of white adults with autoimmune hepatitis in North America.
- *Type 3 autoimmune hepatitis* was characterized by the presence of antibodies to soluble liver antigen (anti-SLA). Since 16% of patients with type 1 autoimmune hepatitis have anti-SLA and patients with anti-SLA cannot be distinguished from patients without anti-SLA, the designation of type 3 autoimmune hepatitis has been largely abandoned.

## 8. What are the clinical criteria for diagnosis?

The diagnostic criteria for autoimmune hepatitis have been codified by an international panel. The *definite diagnosis* requires histologic evidence of interface hepatitis with or without panacinar (lobular) hepatitis or bridging necrosis and absence of biliary lesions, granulomas, copper deposits, or other changes suggestive of a different etiology. The serum aspartate (AST) or alanine aminotransferase (ALT) level must be abnormally increased, and it must dominate the biochemical profile. Total serum globulin, gamma globulin, or IgG levels must be greater than 1.5-fold the upper limit of normal, and serum titers of SMA, ANA, or anti-LKM1 must be greater than 1:80. There must be no history of parenteral exposure to blood or blood products, recent use of hepatotoxic drugs, or excessive alcohol consumption (<35 g/day in men and <25 g/day in women). Active viral infection must be excluded, and serum levels of $\alpha_1$-antitrypsin, copper, and ceruloplasmin must be normal. The *probable diagnosis* is made when there are similar findings that are less pronounced. A cholestatic form of autoimmune hepatitis is not recognized.

## 9. What are the diagnostic scoring systems and how are they used?

A scoring system for the diagnosis of autoimmune hepatitis was first developed in 1992 as a research tool, and it was revised in 1999 to ensure the comparability of study populations in clinical trials. The revised original scoring system has subsequently been applied in clinical practice to enable the systematic assessment of the key clinical features of the disease. It evaluates 12 clinical components and renders 27 possible scores, thereby providing an objective measure of the net strength of the diagnosis and preventing any single manifestation from swaying the judgment (Table 18-4). Response to corticosteroid therapy is scored, and the treatment outcome can upgrade the diagnosis.

A simplified scoring system has been proposed recently to ease clinical application. It evaluates only four clinical components and renders seven possible grades (Table 18-5). The simplified scoring system has been validated in diverse ethnic groups and liver diseases, and it is based on the presence and level of autoantibody expression, serum IgG concentration, typical or compatible histologic features, and the absence of viral markers. The revised original scoring system has greater sensitivity for the diagnosis of autoimmune hepatitis than the simplified scoring system (100% versus 95%), but the simplified scoring system has superior specificity (90% versus 73%) and predictability (92% versus 82%). The original scoring system is useful in evaluating patients with absent or atypical features where every component of the disease must be assessed. In this context, it may reclassify patients with cryptogenic chronic hepatitis as having autoimmune hepatitis. The simplified scoring system is useful in excluding autoimmune hepatitis in patients with other conditions who have confusing concurrent immune features, such as patients with virus-induced or drug-related hepatitis or a cholestatic syndrome. Each system has its own virtues that can be exploited in different clinical situations, and one system does not replace the other.

### Table 18-4. Scoring System for the Diagnosis of Autoimmune Hepatitis*

| CLINICAL FEATURES | SCORE | CLINICAL FEATURES | SCORE |
|---|---|---|---|
| Female | +2 | Average alcohol intake | |
| | | <25 g/day | +2 |
| Alkaline phosphatase:aspartate aminotransferase ratio | | >60 g/day | −2 |
| <1.5 | +2 | Histologic findings | |
| 1.5–3.0 | 0 | Interface hepatitis | +3 |
| >3.0 | −2 | Lymphoplasmacytic infiltrate | +1 |
| | | Rosette formation | +1 |
| | | None of above | −5 |
| Serum γ-globulin or immunoglobulin G level above normal limit | | Biliary changes | −3 |
| | | Other changes | −3 |
| >2.0 | +3 | Concurrent immune disease | +2 |
| 1.5–2.0 | +2 | | |
| 1.0–1.5 | +1 | Novel autoantibodies | +2 |
| <1.0 | 0 | HLA DR3 or DR4 | +1 |
| ANA, SMA, or anti-LKM1 | | | |
| >1:80 | +3 | Response to corticosteroids | |
| 1:80 | +2 | Complete | +2 |
| 1:40 | +1 | Relapse after drug withdrawal | +3 |
| <1:40 | 0 | | |
| AMA positive | −4 | Aggregate score pretreatment | |
| | | Definite autoimmune hepatitis | >15 |
| | | Probable autoimmune hepatitis | 10–15 |
| Hepatitis markers | | Aggregate score posttreatment | |
| Positive | −3 | Definite autoimmune hepatitis | >17 |
| Negative | +3 | Probable autoimmune hepatitis | 12–17 |
| Drug history | | | |
| Positive | −4 | | |
| Negative | +1 | | |

*Adapted from the revised original scoring system of the International Autoimmune Hepatitis Group. J Hepatol 31:929–938, 1999.
AMA, antimitochondrial antibodies; ANA, antinuclear antibodies; HLA, human leukocyte antigen; LKM1, liver/kidney microsome type 1; SMA, smooth muscle antibodies.

**Table 18-5.** Simplified Scoring System of the International Autoimmune Hepatitis Group*

| VARIABLE | RESULT | POINTS |
|---|---|---|
| **Autoantibodies** | | |
| Antinuclear antibodies or smooth muscle antibodies | ≥1:40 | +1 |
| | ≥1:80 | +2 |
| Antibodies to liver/kidney microsome type 1 | ≥1:40 | +2 |
| Antibodies to soluble liver antigen | Positive | +2 |
| **Immunoglobulin Level** | | |
| Immunoglobulin G | >Upper limit of normal | +1 |
| | >1.1 times upper limit of normal | +2 |
| **Histologic Findings** | | |
| Morphologic features | Compatible with autoimmune hepatitis | +1 |
| | Typical of autoimmune hepatitis | +2 |
| **Viral Disease** | | |
| Absence of viral hepatitis | No viral markers | +2 |

*Adapted from the simplified scoring system of the International Autoimmune Hepatitis Group: Hepatology 48:169–176, 2008.

## 10. What is the standard serologic battery for diagnosis?

ANAs, SMAs, and anti-LKM1 are the standard serologic markers of autoimmune hepatitis (Table 18-6). They are useful in diagnosis, but they lack pathogenicity and specificity. Furthermore, their behavior does not correlate with disease activity or treatment response. The classification of ANA reactivity into homogeneous, speckled or other patterns by indirect immunofluorescence (IIF) has no diagnostic or prognostic value, and this practice has been largely abandoned.

**Table 18-6.** Autoantibodies Associated With Autoimmune Hepatitis

| AUTOANTIBODY SPECIES | IMPLICATION(S) |
|---|---|
| Nuclear | Type 1 autoimmune hepatitis<br>Reactive to multiple nuclear antigens |
| Smooth muscle | Type 1 autoimmune hepatitis<br>Reactive to actin and nonactin components<br>Frequently concurrent with antinuclear antibodies |
| Actin | Type 1 autoimmune hepatitis<br>Diagnostic specificity<br>Commonly young patients<br>Possibly more aggressive disease<br>Unsettled assay |
| Liver/kidney microsome 1 | Type 2 autoimmune hepatitis<br>Inhibits CYP2D6 in vitro<br>May occur in chronic hepatitis C |
| Asialoglycoprotein receptor | Generic marker of autoimmune hepatitis<br>Correlates with inflammatory activity<br>Possible barometer of treatment response<br>Associated with propensity to relapse |
| Liver cytosol type 1 | Type 2 autoimmune hepatitis<br>Young patients<br>Possibly worse prognosis<br>Directed against formiminotransferase cyclodeaminase |
| Soluble liver antigen | Antigenic target is tRNP[(ser)sec]<br>Useful in evaluating seronegative autoimmune hepatitis<br>Associated with *DRB1*0301* and relapse after treatment<br>High specificity but low sensitivity for autoimmune hepatitis |
| Chromatin | Coexists with antinuclear antibodies<br>Associated with relapse after treatment |
| Atypical perinuclear anti-neutrophil cytoplasm | Common in type 1 autoimmune hepatitis<br>Absent in type 2 autoimmune hepatitis<br>Useful in evaluating seronegative autoimmune hepatitis |

tRNP[(ser)sec], transfer ribonucleoprotein (serine) selenocysteine.

## 11. What serologic assays are best for detecting the standard autoantibodies?

The International Autoimmune Hepatitis Group endorses assays based on indirect immunofluorescence (IIF) as the gold standards of serologic diagnosis in liver disease. Clinical laboratories, however, are replacing the time- and labor-intensive immunofluorescence assays with commercial enzyme immunoassays (EIA) based on recombinant antigens, and the serologic tests by IIF are becoming obsolete despite their endorsement by hepatic serologists. Intraobserver interpretative error can be eliminated; antigen-specific reactivity can be measured; and test results can be obtained quickly by using the available EIA kits for ANA and anti-LKM1. The antigens recognized by the semiautomated EIA kits, however, may not be the same antigens detected by IIF, and the strength of the reactivities and their clinical implications may not correlate with those obtained by IIF. There are no conversion formulae that render the result of one method into the result of another method. International serum exchange workshops with calibrated reference sera have been proposed to standardize methods of serologic testing and minimize discrepancies between laboratories and clinical experiences. Currently, serologic methods and results can vary between institutions, and the presence or absence of the autoantibody is more reliable and meaningful than the strength of its reaction.

## 12. What other autoantibodies may have diagnostic and prognostic importance?

Multiple autoantibodies have been described in autoimmune hepatitis, but none has been incorporated into the conventional diagnostic algorithm. New antibodies continue to be characterized in the hope that they will improve diagnostic specificity and have prognostic value. Their characterization may also help identify the autoantigens responsible for the disease. Commercial EIA kits are available for the detection of anti-SLA, antiactin, antichromatin, anti–asialoglycoprotein receptor, and atypical perinuclear antineutrophil cytoplasmic antibodies (pANCAs) (see Table 18-6). The autoantibodies that have most promise as prognostic markers are antibodies to soluble liver antigen (anti-SLA).

- *Antibodies to soluble liver antigen (anti-SLA)* are directed against a 50-kDa cytosolic protein, which has been identified as a transfer ribonucleoprotein complex [tRNP$^{(ser)sec}$] involved in selenocysteine metabolism. Anti-SLAs have high specificity (99%) for autoimmune hepatitis, but they occur in only 16% of individuals with the disease. Patients with anti-SLA have more severe disease than do patients without anti-SLA, and they more commonly relapse after corticosteroid withdrawal. Antibodies to SLA have a strong association with *DRB1*0301*, which is the principal susceptibility allele for autoimmune hepatitis, and they may be surrogate markers of a genetic propensity for relapse after drug withdrawal. Antibodies to SLA have been found in cryptogenic chronic hepatitis, and the assay for anti-SLA may be useful in reclassifying these patients as having autoimmune hepatitis.
- *Antibodies to actin (antiactin)* are a subset of SMA that react predominantly against polymerized F-actin, and they have greater specificity for the diagnosis of autoimmune hepatitis than SMA. The lack of consensus regarding the best assay for their detection has delayed their incorporation into conventional diagnostic strategies. Patients with antiactin have an earlier age of disease onset, poorer response to corticosteroid therapy, and higher frequency of death from liver failure or requirement for liver transplantation than do patients with ANA but not antiactin. These prognostic implications have not been found with all assays for antiactin, and not all patients with autoimmune hepatitis and SMA have antiactin. Assays that detect antibodies to the $\alpha$-actinin domain on the actin molecule identify patients with severe clinical and histologic disease when they are present with antibodies to filamentous actin. The assessment of reactivity against select small molecular sequences rather than the large epitopes may have prognostic value, and the development of these assays promises to extend the clinical value of testing for antiactin.
- *Antibodies to chromatin (ant-chromatin)* are found in 39% of patients with autoimmune hepatitis, and they occur more commonly in men than women (33% versus 15%, respectively; $p = .0008$). Antibodies to chromatin occur only in patients with ANA, and they may define a subgroup prone to relapse after drug withdrawal. They commonly disappear during corticosteroid therapy, and they are more frequent during active than inactive disease (32% versus 19%, $p = .01$).
- *Antibodies to liver cytosol type 1 (anti-LC1)* have specificity for autoimmune hepatitis, and they occur mainly in young patients, typically less than 20 years old. Antibodies to LC1 are detected in 32% of patients with anti-LKM1, and their presence has been associated with severe disease. They may be the sole serologic findings in 14% of patients with autoimmune hepatitis, and they may be useful in evaluating young patients who lack conventional autoantibodies. Formiminotransferase cyclodeaminase has been proposed as the target autoantigen.
- *Antibodies to asialoglycoprotein receptor (anti-ASGPR)* are specific for autoimmune hepatitis. They are present in 82% of patients with SMA or ANA, 67% of patients with anti-LKM1, and 67% of patients with anti-SLA. The autoantibodies are directed against a transmembrane hepatocytic glycoprotein that can capture, display, and internalize potential antigens, induce T-cell proliferation, and activate cytotoxic T -cells. Antibodies to ASGPR are present when inflammation is detected in the liver tissue, and they disappear when this activity subsides. Patients with anti-ASGPR relapse after drug withdrawal, whereas those in whom the autoantibodies disappear sustain their remission without treatment. Antibodies to ASGPR may define a treatment end point and avoid the need for liver tissue confirmation of an inactive inflammatory process.
- *Atypical perinuclear antineutrophil cytoplasmic antibodies (pANCAs)* are directed against antigens within the nucleus of neutrophils, and they colocalize with the proteins of the nuclear membrane (lamins A, B1, and C and the lamin B receptor). These antibodies are present in 92% of patients with ulcerative colitis, primary sclerosing cholangitis, and autoimmune hepatitis. Their most valuable clinical application may be in the assessment of patients with presumed autoimmune hepatitis who lack the conventional autoantibodies. Their colocalization with the nuclear membrane has justified the proposal that they be designated as *antineutrophil nuclear antibodies* (ANNAs) rather than *antineutrophil cytoplasmic antibodies*.

### 13. What investigational antibodies have promise as clinical tools?

Investigational efforts continue to characterize novel immune reactions in autoimmune hepatitis in the hope of discovering pertinent target antigens, improving diagnostic algorithms, and providing prognostic information. Autoantibodies in the early phases of characterization are investigational, and they may never be incorporated into conventional diagnostic strategies for autoimmune hepatitis. Antibodies to lactoferrin, cyclic citrullinated peptide, *Saccharomyces cerevisiae,* and liver/kidney microsome type 3 are in this category.

- *Antibodies to lactoferrin* are directed against an iron binding protein with putative anti-inflammatory and immune modulatory actions. Lactoferrin is present in the granules of granulocytes, and it prevents complement activation by inhibiting the C3 pathway. Antibodies to lactoferrin occur in ulcerative colitis, primary sclerosing cholangitis, rheumatoid arthritis, primary biliary cirrhosis, and autoimmune hepatitis. The role of antibodies to lactoferrin in the pathogenesis, diagnosis, and management of autoimmune hepatitis remains uncertain.
- *Antibodies to cyclic citrullinated peptide (anti-CCP)* are highly specific for rheumatoid arthritis, and their strong association with erosive joint destruction suggests that they have pathogenic properties. Antibodies to CCP occur in 11% of patients with autoimmune hepatitis, and 60% of these patients do not have rheumatoid arthritis. Patients with anti-CCP have a significantly greater occurrence of histologic cirrhosis at presentation (47% versus 20%, $p = .01$) and death from hepatic failure than patients without anti-CCP (25% versus 9%, $p = .04$). Furthermore, patients with anti-CCP and concurrent rheumatoid arthritis invariably have cirrhosis. Antibodies to CCP may define a subgroup of patients with a severe aggressive liver disease.
- *Antibodies to Saccharomyces cerevisiae (ASCA)* are directed against a species of baker's or brewer's yeast, and they occur in 22% to 28% of patients with autoimmune hepatitis. Their association with inflammatory bowel disease and celiac disease suggests that they may reflect disruption of the gastrointestinal mucosal barrier and sensitization against an environmental agent. In autoimmune hepatitis, ASCA are associated with high serum IgA levels, and they may indicate heightened mucosal immunity within the gastrointestinal tract. ASCA may contribute to the diagnosis of concurrent mucosal diseases in autoimmune hepatitis.
- *Antibodies to liver/kidney microsome type 3 (anti-LKM3)* are directed against uridine diphosphate glucuronosyl transferase, and they are markers of type 2 autoimmune hepatitis and chronic hepatitis D (which is associated with the hepatitis delta virus). They are of investigational interest mainly to explore the relationship between the virus and the autoimmune disease.

### 14. What is the significance of antimitochondrial antibodies in autoimmune hepatitis?

Antimitochondrial antibodies (AMAs) can be demonstrated by IIF in 20% of patients with autoimmune hepatitis, but serum titers are typically low (<1:160 in 88% of instances). The histologic findings in such patients are indistinguishable from those of patients without AMA, and copper stains of the liver tissue are negative or only mildly positive. Patients with low titer AMA and histologic features of typical autoimmune hepatitis respond to corticosteroid treatment, and the presence of AMA does not change the diagnosis of autoimmune hepatitis or its treatment.

Patients with high titer AMA by IIF (>1:160) may have primary biliary cirrhosis, a variant syndrome with mixed features of autoimmune hepatitis and primary biliary cirrhosis, or anti-LKM1 that has been mistaken for AMA. Recognition of AMA by IIF requires reactivity to the distal tubules of the murine kidney and parietal cells of the murine stomach. Recognition of anti-LKM1 requires reactivity to the proximal tubules of the murine kidney and murine hepatocytes. An exuberant reaction against the renal tubule may obscure the distinction between proximal and distal tubule, and anti-LKM1 reactivity may be reported as AMA positivity. Enzyme immunoassays based on recombinant mitochondrial and LKM1 antigens have reduced the interpretative errors associated with assays dependent on patterns of IIF.

The antibodies that are specific against the mitochondrial antigens of primary biliary cirrhosis are the E2 subunits of pyruvate dehydrogenase and branched-chain ketoacid dehydrogenase. These occur in only 8% of patients with autoimmune hepatitis by enzyme immunoassay, and they may indicate an incorrect original diagnosis, a variant disorder with mixed features, or a rare instance of false positivity.

### 15. Can autoimmune hepatitis exist in the absence of conventional autoantibodies?

Yes. Thirteen percent of adults with chronic hepatitis lack a confident diagnosis, and they are frequently classified as having *cryptogenic chronic hepatitis.* Some may have autoimmune hepatitis that has escaped detection by conventional serological testing, and a more appropriate designation may be *autoantibody-negative autoimmune hepatitis.* Patients with cryptogenic chronic hepatitis are frequently similar by age, gender, human leukocyte antigen (HLA) phenotype, laboratory findings, and histologic features to patients with autoimmune hepatitis. They may also respond as well to corticosteroid therapy, entering remission as commonly (83% versus 78%) and failing treatment as infrequently (9% versus 11%) as patients with conventional markers. Some patients may express SMA or ANA later in their course or have less conventional autoantibodies, such as anti-SLA, anti-LC1, or pANCA. Others may have chronic hepatitis associated with celiac disease, and they may be recognized after testing for IgA antibodies to endomysium (EMA) or tissue transglutaminase (anti-tTG). The revised original diagnostic scoring system (see Table 18-4) is the best method of securing the diagnosis of autoimmune hepatitis. Patients with the features of autoimmune hepatitis except for the autoantibodies should be treated with corticosteroids.

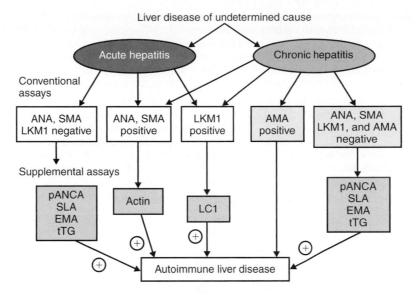

**Figure 18-6.** Serologic testing sequence for diagnosing autoimmune liver disease in patients with acute or chronic hepatitis of undetermined cause. The conventional serological battery includes antinuclear antibodies (ANA), smooth muscle antibodies (SMA), antibodies to liver/kidney microsome type 1 (LKM1), and antimitochondrial antibodies (AMA). Supplemental serological tests to confirm or further direct the diagnosis include atypical perinuclear antineutrophil cytoplasmic antibodies (pANCA), antibodies to soluble liver antigen (SLA), antibodies to liver cytosol type 1 (LC1), and antibodies for celiac disease, including immunoglobulin A antibodies to endometrium (EMA) and tissue transglutaminase (tTG).

**16. What is the appropriate testing sequence for the autoantibody determinations?**

All patients with acute and chronic hepatitis of undetermined cause should be assessed for ANAs, SMAs, and anti-LKM1. Adults with chronic hepatitis of undetermined cause should also be assessed for AMA. These assessments constitute the initial diagnostic battery (Fig. 18-6). Patients who lack these serologic markers should undergo a second battery of tests that include determinations of pANCAs, antibodies to soluble liver antigen (anti-SLA) and immunoglobulin A antibodies to endomysium (IgA EMA) or tissue transglutaminase (IgA tTG). Patients strongly suspected of having bile duct disease who are AMA negative by IIF should be assessed for antibodies to the E2 subunits of the pyruvate dehydrogenase complex by enzyme immunoassay. These assessments constitute the supplemental diagnostic battery (Fig. 18-6). Patients who still lack serologic markers of autoimmune hepatitis should be graded by the revised original diagnostic scoring system (see Table 18-4), and patients with scores of at least 10 points should treated as *autoantibody-negative autoimmune hepatitis*. The conventional battery of ANAs, SMAs, and anti-LKM1 should be repeated in the patients who lack all markers at presentation since these autoantibodies may be expressed later in the course of the disease.

**17. In what other clinical situation should autoimmune hepatitis be considered?**

Graft dysfunction after liver transplantation. Autoimmune hepatitis recurs in at least 17% of patients who are transplanted for autoimmune hepatitis, and it develops de novo in 3% to 5% of children and adults who undergo liver transplantation for nonautoimmune diseases. In the former instance, the recurrence is typically mild in individuals who are inadequately immunosuppressed, and the disease is easily managed by adjustments in the immunosuppressive regimen. In unusual instances, progression to cirrhosis and graft loss may occur. In the latter instance, the disease may be unsuspected and aggressive in nature leading to graft failure. Timely therapy with immunosuppressive medication, especially corticosteroids, is important to manage this condition. Autoimmune hepatitis must be considered in all patients with graft dysfunction after liver transplantation.

**18. What are the variant (*overlap*) syndromes of autoimmune hepatitis?**

Patients with autoimmune hepatitis may have features of primary sclerosing cholangitis (PSC), primary biliary cirrhosis (PBC), or a cholestatic syndrome in the absence of PSC or PBC. Variant syndromes are important because they are common (18%), and they can respond poorly to corticosteroid therapy. Their presence should be considered in all patients with autoimmune hepatitis who have cholestatic features or a poor response to corticosteroid treatment. Multicenter, collaborative clinical studies are needed to validate these entities as distinct diagnoses, codify diagnostic criteria, and establish confident treatment algorithms.

The variant syndromes are commonly dubbed *overlap syndromes*, thereby implying that two distinct entities coexist in the same patient. The outer boundary when a classic diagnosis can no longer be considered is undefined, and a discriminative diagnostic index that can draw the limits between different diseases does not exist. Variant syndromes are unlikely to reflect different ends of a continuous pathologic spectrum or distinctive pathogenic mechanisms. They are more likely to represent atypical cases of the classic disease.

### 19. Is autoimmune hepatitis in children different from that of adults?

Yes. Children with autoimmune hepatitis are commonly asymptomatic, and their serologic markers may be weakly expressed. The presence of ANAs, SMAs, or anti-LKM1 in any titer should be considered pathologic in children, and those with autoimmune hepatitis are more likely to express anti-LKM1 than are adults. Children may have concurrent *autoimmune sclerosing cholangitis* even in the absence of inflammatory bowel disease or a cholestatic clinical syndrome. Retrograde endoscopic cholangiography is preferred to magnetic resonance cholangiography to make this diagnosis since the biliary changes may be subtle. Since corticosteroid therapy can be effective in these children and their biliary changes are unassociated with a distinctive clinical syndrome, the concurrent biliary disease has been distinguished from PSC. Children also seem to be more treatment-dependent than adults.

### 20. What are the pathogenic mechanisms?

Two hypotheses have been proposed for the pathogenesis of autoimmune hepatitis, and they are probably interrelated (Fig. 18-7). One theory proposes an *antibody-dependent cell-mediated form of cytotoxicity*. A defect is postulated in the modulation of B-cell production of immunoglobulin G. The immunoglobulin adheres to normal hepatocytic membrane proteins and creates an antigen-antibody complex on the hepatocyte surface. This complex is then targeted by natural killer cells (NKTs) that have Fc receptors for the immunoglobulin. The NKTs do not require previous exposure to the target antigen for activation, and they accomplish liver cell injury by cytolysis.

The other theory proposes a *cellular form of cytotoxicity*. A disease-specific autoantigen is displayed on the surface of antigen presenting cells in association with HLA class II antigens. Immunocytes that are HLA restricted are sensitized to the self-antigen, and clonal expansion of the antigen-primed lymphocytes follows. Activated cytotoxic T-lymphocytes infiltrate the liver tissue and destroy the hepatocytes displaying the target autoantigen. Lymphokines facilitate cell-to-cell communication, promote neo-expression of HLA class II antigens, enhance autoantigen presentation, activate the immunocytes, and intensify tissue damage by direct action.

Common to both theories are a host predisposition for heightened immune reactivity that is genetically determined, uncertainty about the nature of the triggering antigen, and disruption of normal homeostatic immune response

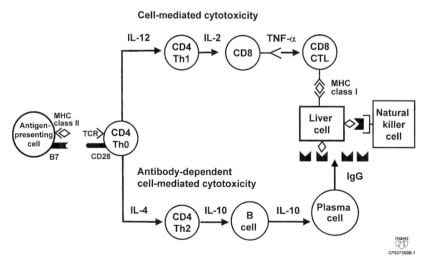

**Figure 18-7.** Putative pathogenic mechanisms. Activation of CD4 T helper cells requires ligation of its T-cell antigen receptor (TCR) with the antigenic peptide displayed by the class II molecule of the major histocompatibility complex (MHC) (first signal) and coupling of B7 and CD28 (second signal). The activated CD4 T helper cell (Th0) then differentiates in accordance with the predominant cytokine milieu. Cell-mediated cytotoxicity is favored by a type 1 (Th1) cytokine response mediated by interleukin (IL)-12, IL-2, and tumor necrosis factor-$\alpha$ (TNF-$\alpha$). Cytotoxic T lymphocytes (CD8 CTL) undergo activation by interaction with processed antigenic peptides presented by class I MHC molecules. Sensitized cytotoxic T lymphocytes accomplish liver cell injury by the release of lymphokines. Antibody-dependent cell-mediated cytotoxicity is favored by a type 2 (Th2) cytokine response mediated by IL-4 and IL-10. Plasma cells are activated to produce immunoglobulin G (IgG), which forms complexes with normal membrane constituents of the hepatocyte. The Fc receptors of natural killer cells bind to the antigen-antibody complexes and cause cytolysis.

networks. Defects in the counter-regulatory cytokine milieu may reflect the failure of T-regulatory (T-reg) cells (CD4+CD25+ cells) to modulate CD8 T-cell proliferation and cytokine production or NKTs to modulate the apoptosis of altered hepatocytes. Viral infections, drug exposures, and environmental factors have been evoked as triggering mechanisms that can activate a final common pathway of pathogenesis. Molecular mimicry between foreign and self-antigens is the most popular hypothesis for loss of self-tolerance, and antibodies (but not immunocytes) that cross-react against foreign and host antigens have been demonstrated.

## 21. What are the autoantigens?
Cytochrome monooxygenase, CYP2D6 (P450 IID6), is the target autoantigen of type 2 autoimmune hepatitis. The target autoantigen of type 1 autoimmune hepatitis is unknown. CYP2D6 (P450 IID6) is a 50-kDa microsomal enzyme that metabolizes at least 25 different drugs, including antihypertensive agents, β-blockers, antiarrhythmic drugs, and antidepressants. It is capable of transforming a variety of peptides into immunoreactive molecules.

## 22. Can viruses cause autoimmune hepatitis?
Yes. Multiple viruses can trigger a clinical syndrome that resembles autoimmune hepatitis. Since autoimmune hepatitis is defined as a disease of unknown cause, conditions with a known etiologic agent are designated by that agent and not classified as autoimmune hepatitis. Hepatitis A virus, hepatitis B virus, and hepatitis C virus can each produce a syndrome that resembles autoimmune hepatitis, and this syndrome can be self-perpetuating even in the absence of the virus. Furthermore, antiviral therapy in rare instances can clear the inciting virus and change the clinical phenotype of the disease to that of autoimmune hepatitis, which is then responsive to corticosteroid therapy. The lack of a confident animal model for the disease, the long lag time between exposure to the etiological agent and discovery of the disease, and the likely persistence of autoimmune hepatitis after disappearance of its trigger have hampered efforts to fully define etiologic factors. Homologies have been demonstrated between amino acid sequences in the CYP2D6 molecule and the genomes of the hepatitis C virus, cytomegalovirus, and herpes simplex virus type 1, and these molecular mimicries have resulted in cross-reacting antibodies between the autoimmune and viral diseases. These findings support the hypothesis that repeated viral infections with agents that have similar epitopes may eventually overwhelm self-tolerance and cause the disease. The multiplicity of viruses that have been implicated as triggers suggests that there is a final common pathway of pathogenesis that can be initiated by a variety of agents. The triggering epitope is likely to be small and commonly shared.

## 23. Can drugs cause autoimmune hepatitis?
Yes. Drugs can produce a clinical syndrome that resembles autoimmune hepatitis, and they must be excluded at the time of presentation. Like virus-induced disease, drug-induced syndromes resembling autoimmune hepatitis are designated by the drug that causes the disorder. Drug-related and virus-induced autoimmune syndromes are not true autoimmune hepatitis, which by definition lacks a cause. The drug-related syndromes are typically self-limited and nonrecurrent after discontinuation of the medication. Minocycline is the most common drug that can produce a clinical syndrome identical to that of classic autoimmune hepatitis, and diclofenac and herbal remedies must also be considered. Other medications that can produce a liver disease that mimics autoimmune hepatitis are less commonly used, and they include nitrofurantoin, isoniazid, propylthiouracil, and α-methyldopa.

## 24. Are there genetic predispositions for autoimmune hepatitis? *HLA DR3+4*
Susceptibility In white northern Europeans and North Americans relates to HLA DR3 and DR4. HLA DR3 is the principal risk factor, and HLA DR4 is a secondary but independent risk factor. Eighty-five percent of North American patients with type 1 autoimmune hepatitis have HLA DR3, DR4, or both DR3 and DR4. HLA DR7 characterizes patients with type 2 autoimmune hepatitis, and HLA DR13 is associated with the disease in South America. The HLA phenotype identifies patients with a predisposition for autoimmune hepatitis, but it does not predict emergence of the disease. Autoimmune hepatitis does not have a strong penetrance in families, and familial occurrence is rare.

## 25. Does autoimmune hepatitis have a Mendelian pattern of inheritance?
No, with one exception. Most cases of autoimmune hepatitis are nonsyndromic, complex, polygenic disorders. The one exception is the autoimmune hepatitis found in 15% of the patients with autoimmune polyendocrinopathy-candidiasis-ectodermal dystrophy (APECED). The gene responsible for this syndrome is located on chromosome 21q22.3, and its gene encodes an autoimmune regulator that modulates the negative selection of autoreactive T cells by the thymus. Deficiencies in this regulator can result in the escape of autoreactive T cells that can cause the syndrome by targeting CYP1A2 and CYP2A6. APECED is an autosomal recessive disease that does not have a gender predilection, and it is most common among individuals of Finnish or Sardinian ancestry.

## 26. What are the susceptibility alleles?
The principal susceptibility alleles for nonsyndromic autoimmune hepatitis reside on the *DRB1* gene. High resolution DNA-based techniques have indicated that *DRB1*0301* is the principal risk factor and *DRB1*0401* is the secondary risk factor in white northern Europeans and North Americans. In contrast, *DRB1*1501* protects against the disease in these

populations. Susceptibility alleles for type 1 autoimmune hepatitis in various ethnic groups are different, and they include *DRB1*0405* in Japan and mainland China, *DRB1*0405* in Argentine adults, *DRB1*1301* in Argentine children and Brazilian patients, and *DRB1*0404* in Mestizo Mexicans.

### 27. How do different susceptibility alleles produce the same disease?

Each susceptibility allele for autoimmune hepatitis encodes an amino acid sequence in the antigen binding groove of the HLA DR molecule, and this sequence influences recognition of the autoantigen by the T-cell antigen receptor (TCR) of CD4 T helper cells. The sequence is six amino acids long and in a critical position on the lip of the antigen binding groove where it is in contact with the autoantigen and the TCR. The sequence encoded by *DRB1*0301* and *DRB1*0401* in white northern Europeans and North Americans is denoted as LLEQKR at positions 67 to 72 of the DRβ polypeptide chain. Lysine (K) at position DRβ71 is the critical residue. Different susceptibility alleles that encode the same or similar short amino acid sequence in this critical location carry the same risk for autoimmune hepatitis.

*DRB1*0404* in the Mestizo Mexicans and *DRB1*0405* in the Japanese and mainland Chinese encode an arginine for a lysine at position DRβ71. Arginine is positively charged like lysine, and its substitution would have little effect on the presentation of antigenic peptide. In contrast, *DRB1*1501* encodes an alanine for a lysine at DRβ71, and the substitution of this nonpolar amino acid for either lysine or arginine at DRβ71 would alter antigen binding and TCR recognition. As a result, a single amino acid substitution in a critical location may protect against the disease.

### 28. How do regional factors affect disease occurrence?

Certain regions may have indigenous agents that can trigger the disease, and individuals within that environment may have certain genetic predispositions that favor an immune response to that agent. *DRB1*1301* has been associated with protracted hepatitis A virus infection, and the hepatitis A virus has been implicated as a cause of autoimmune hepatitis. Hepatitis A virus infection is endemic in South America, and the high association between autoimmune hepatitis and children with *DRB1*1301* in this region may reflect the protracted exposure of these patients to viral and hepatic antigens. Other geographic regions may have other indigenous etiologic agents that select patients with different genetic phenotypes.

### 29. Why do patients with the same HLA have different clinical phenotypes?

Other factors than HLA contribute to disease expression and severity. These factors may be genetically acquired and not disease specific. Multiple polymorphisms have been described that can influence the clinical phenotype and behavior of type 1 autoimmune hepatitis. The implicated polymorphisms in white North American and northern European patients include *TFNA*2*, which may result in high inducible and constitutive levels of tumor necrosis factor-α and favor expansion of cytotoxic T cells; *cytotoxic T lymphocyte antigen-4 (CTLA-4)*, which may unleash the cellular immune response; and *TNFRSF6*, which is a *Fas* gene polymorphism that may impair the apoptosis of immunocytes and extend the immune attack. Other implicated modifiers of the immune response include polymorphisms of *interleukin (IL)-2, IL-4*, and *IL-6, interferon* γ (IFNγ), *transforming growth factor-*β (TGF-β), and the *vitamin D receptor (VDR)* gene. A point mutation of the *tyrosine phosphatase CD45* gene has also been described. These autoimmune modifiers may act singly, in various combinations, or in synergy (epistasis) with the principal drivers of the disease.

### 30. Do the HLA phenotypes influence disease expression and outcome?

Yes. Both HLA DR3 and HLA DR4 and the associated alleles, *DRB1*0301* and *DRB1*0401*, have been associated with different clinical manifestations and outcomes in white North American and northern European patients (Table 18-7). Individuals with HLA DR3 (*DRB1*0301*) develop their disease at an early age, and they have more active disease, as assessed by serum aminotransferase levels and histologic features, than patients with other HLA. They also relapse more frequently after corticosteroid withdrawal, enter remission less commonly, deteriorate more often, and require liver transplantation more frequently. In contrast, patients with HLA DR4 (*DRB1*0401*) are older and more commonly women than patients with HLA DR3 (*DRB1*0301*). They have higher serum levels of gamma globulin, a greater frequency of concurrent immunologic diseases, and a greater likelihood of entering remission during therapy.

### 31. Should HLA typing be part of the standard diagnostic algorithm?

No. HLA DR3 and DR4 are common in the general population of white North American and northern European patients, and they would be expected to occur coincidentally in 19% and 16%, respectively, of patients with other liver diseases. Furthermore, their presence would not change immediate management; the diagnostic scoring systems can make the diagnosis without HLA determinations; and HLA typing is expensive.

**Table 18-7.** Effects of Class II MHC Alleles on Disease Expression and Behavior in White North American and Northern European Patients With Type 1 Autoimmune Hepatitis

| DISEASE EXPRESSION AND BEHAVIOR | ASSOCIATED CLASS II MHC ALLELES | |
|---|---|---|
| | *DRB1*0301* | *DRB1*0401* |
| Young age of onset | + | − |
| Severe liver tissue inflammation and/or cirrhosis | + | − |
| Lower frequency of remission during therapy | + | − |
| Higher frequency of treatment failure | + | − |
| Higher frequency of relapse after drug withdrawal | + | − |
| More frequent liver transplantation | + | − |
| Associated with polymorphism of *tumor necrosis factor-α* gene (*TNFA*2*) involving adenine→guanine substitution at position −308 | + | − |
| Associated with polymorphism of *cytotoxic T lymphocyte antigen-4* gene involving guanine for adenine substitution at position 49 in the first exon | + | − |
| Older age onset | − | + |
| More commonly women | − | + |
| Frequently associated with concurrent immune disorders | − | + |
| Higher frequency of remission during therapy | − | + |

MHC, major histocompatibility complex.

## WEBSITE

http://www.aasld.org/

## BIBLIOGRAPHY

1. Carpenter HA, Czaja AJ. The role of histologic evaluation in the diagnosis and management of autoimmune hepatitis and its variants. Clin Liver Dis 2002;6:685–705.
2. Czaja AJ. Autoantibodies in autoimmune liver disease. Adv Clin Chem 2005;40:127–64.
3. Czaja AJ. Autoimmune hepatitis—Part A: Pathogenesis. Exp Rev Gastroenterol Hepatol 2007;1:113–28.
4. Czaja AJ. Autoimmune hepatitis—Part B: Diagnosis. Exp Rev Gastroenterol Hepatol 2007;1:129–43.
5. Czaja AJ. Frequency and nature of the variant syndromes of autoimmune liver disease. Hepatology 1998;28:360–5.
6. Czaja AJ. Genetic factors associated with the occurrence, clinical phenotype and outcome of autoimmune hepatitis. Clin Gastroenterol Hepatol 2008;6:379–88.
7. Czaja AJ. Performance parameters of the diagnostic scoring systems for autoimmune hepatitis. Hepatology 2008;48:1540-48.
8. Czaja AJ, Carpenter HA. Optimizing diagnosis from the medical liver biopsy. Clin Gastroenterol Hepatol 2007;5:898–907.
9. Czaja AJ, Freese DK. Diagnosis and treatment of autoimmune hepatitis. Hepatology 2002;36:479–97.
10. Hennes EM, Zeniya M, Czaja AJ, et al. Simplified diagnostic criteria for autoimmune hepatitis. Hepatology 2008;48:169–76.

# AUTOIMMUNE HEPATITIS: TREATMENT

*Albert J. Czaja, MD*

## 1. What therapies are effective for patients with autoimmune hepatitis?

Prednisone in combination with azathioprine or a higher dose of prednisone alone are the established therapies. Both regimens are equally effective in inducing clinical, laboratory, and histologic remission and prolonging immediate life expectancy. The combination regimen is associated with a lower frequency of drug-related side effects than the regimen using higher doses of prednisone alone (10% versus 44%), and it is preferred. Azathioprine has a corticosteroid-sparing action in the treatment of autoimmune hepatitis, and its combination with prednisone achieves the same results as twice the dose of prednisone alone (Table 19-1).

**Table 19-1.** Recommended Treatment Regimens

| INTERVAL DOSE ADJUSTMENTS | SINGLE-DRUG THERAPY | COMBINATION THERAPY | |
|---|---|---|---|
| | PREDNISONE (MG DAILY) | PREDNISONE (MG DAILY) | AZATHIOPRINE (50 MG DAILY) |
| Week 1 | 60 | 30 | 50 |
| Week 2 | 40 | 20 | 50 |
| Week 3 | 30 | 15 | 50 |
| Week 4 | 30 | 15 | 50 |
| Daily maintenance dose until endpoint | 20 | 10 | 50 |

Postmenopausal women and patients with labile hypertension, brittle diabetes, emotional instability, exogenous obesity, acne, or osteoporosis are candidates for the combination regimen (Table 19-2). Women who are pregnant or contemplating pregnancy and patients with active neoplasia or severe cytopenia are candidates for the single-drug regimen. The single-drug regimen also may be used in patients in whom a short treatment trial (≤6 months) is anticipated and in patients with thiopurine methyltransferase deficiency. Azathioprine has a delayed onset of action (≥3 months), and its advantages as a corticosteroid-sparing agent are evident only after protracted treatment.

**Table 19-2.** Indications for Corticosteroid Therapy and Criteria for Treatment Selection

| INDICATIONS FOR TREATMENT | CRITERIA FOR TREATMENT SELECTION |
|---|---|
| **Absolute** | **Single Drug (Prednisone) regimen** |
| AST ≥10-fold normal | Severe cytopenia |
| AST ≥5-fold normal and γ-globulin ≥2-fold normal | Thiopurine methyltransferase deficiency |
| Histologic findings of bridging necrosis or confluent necrosis | Pregnancy or contemplation of pregnancy |
| Incapacitating symptoms | Active neoplasia |
| | Short-term (≤6 months) trial |
| **Relative** | **Combination Regimen** |
| Persistent symptoms | Preferred therapy |
| Disease progression | Postmenopausal women |
| Mild-moderate laboratory changes | Obesity |
| | Osteopenia |
| **None** | Brittle diabetes |
| Inactive or minimally active cirrhosis | Labile hypertension |
| Liver failure with minimal inflammatory activity | Acne |
| | Long-term (>6 months) treatment |

## 2. How do the medications work?

Corticosteroids limit T-cell activation by inhibiting cytokine production and the expression of adhesion molecules. They are lipophilic and can diffuse into the cytosol of cells to bind the glucocorticoid receptor. The complex of drug and receptor then translocates to the nucleus, where it inhibits cytokine gene expression, including the production of key mediators such as interleukin (IL)-2, IL-4, IL-5, IL-6, IL-8, IL-12, interferon-$\gamma$, and tumor necrosis factor-$\alpha$. The activity of nuclear factor-$\kappa$B, which is an important transcription factor that promotes RNA polymerase activity and cytokine production, is also reduced. Type 1 and type 2 cytokine pathways are affected, and corticosteroids can thereby impair both cellular and humoral immune responses. Continuous administration of corticosteroids is required to achieve these results since the drug has a short biological half-life.

Azathioprine is a purine antagonist that blocks the proliferation of lymphocytes. It is converted to 6-mercaptopurine in blood via a nonenzymatic, glutathione-based pathway, and this metabolite is in turn converted to 6-thioguanines by hypoxanthine guanine phosphoribosyl transferase. The 6-thioguanines are the active metabolites that interfere with purine nucleotide synthesis within the cell cycle, and they thereby impair proliferation of rapidly dividing T and B lymphocytes. Competing enzymatic pathways can convert 6-mercaptopurine to either 6-thiouric acid by xanthine oxidase or 6-methyl mercaptopurine by thiopurine methyltransferase. Each end product is inactive, and the integrity of the enzymatic routes responsible for their production influences the erythrocyte concentrations of the active 6-thioguanine nucleotides. Drugs that inhibit xanthine oxidase activity, such as allopurinol, or deficiencies in thiopurine methyltransferase activity can increase the therapeutic efficacy or the toxicity of the 6-thioguanine metabolites. The immunosuppressive action of azathioprine is slow to achieve because of the drug transformations and nuclear incorporations that are required to limit immunocyte proliferation. Azathioprine is also a selective inhibitor of inflammatory gene expression in activated T lymphocytes and a powerful inducer of T cell apoptosis.

## 3. What are the side effects of the medication?

Prednisone induces cosmetic changes, such as facial rounding, dorsal hump formation, striae, weight gain, acne, alopecia. and facial hirsutism, in 80% of patients after 2 years of treatment (Table 19-3). Severe side effects include osteopenia with vertebral compression, diabetes, cataracts, emotional instability, pancreatitis, opportunistic infection, and hypertension. Severe complications are uncommon, but if they do develop, it is usually after protracted therapy

**Table 19-3.** Side Effects Associated With Prednisone and Azathioprine Therapy

| PREDNISONE-RELATED SIDE EFFECTS | | AZATHIOPRINE-RELATED SIDE EFFECTS | |
|---|---|---|---|
| *TYPE* | *FREQUENCY* | *TYPE* | *FREQUENCY* |
| Cosmetic (usually mild)<br>Facial rounding<br>Weight gain<br>Dorsal hump<br>Striae<br>Hirsutism<br>Alopecia | 80%<br>(after 2 years) | Hematologic (mild)<br>Cytopenia | 46% (especially with cirrhosis) |
| Somatic (severe)<br>Osteopenia<br>Vertebral compression<br>Cataracts<br>Diabetes<br>Emotional instability<br>Hypertension | 13%<br>(treatment ending) | Hematologic (severe)<br>Leukopenia<br>Thrombocytopenia | 6% (treatment ending) |
| Inflammatory/neoplastic<br>Pancreatitis<br>Opportunistic infection<br>Malignancy | Rare | Somatic (usually mild)<br>Nausea<br>Emesis<br>Rash<br>Fever<br>Arthralgias | 5% |
| | | Neoplastic<br>Nonhepatic cell types | 3% (after 10 years) |
| | | Hematologic/enteric<br>Bone marrow failure<br>Villous atrophy and malabsorption | Rare (treatment ending) |
| | | Vascular<br>Sinusoidal obstruction syndrome<br>Nodular regenerative hyperplasia | Not yet reported |

(>18 months) and on the single-drug (prednisone) schedule. Corticosteroid-related side effects are the most common causes for premature drug withdrawal in autoimmune hepatitis. Of the 13% of patients who are prematurely withdrawn from therapy because of side effects, 47% have intolerable cosmetic changes or obesity, 27% have osteoporosis with vertebral compression, and 20% have brittle diabetes.

Azathioprine can induce cholestatic liver injury, nausea, emesis, rash, pancreatitis, opportunistic infection, arthralgias, and cytopenia (see Table 19-3). Five percent of patients treated with azathioprine develop early adverse reactions (nausea, vomiting, arthralgias, fever, skin rash, or pancreatitis), which warrants its discontinuation. The overall frequency of azathioprine-related side effects in patients treated with 50 mg daily is 10%, and the side effects typically improve after the dose is reduced or the therapy is discontinued. Cytopenia is the most common consequence of treatment, and bone marrow failure is rare but possible. Cytopenia occurs in 46% of patients, and the occurrence of severe hematological abnormalities is 6% (see Table 19-3). These toxicities are not predictable by either genotyping or phenotyping for thiopurine methyltransferase activity, and the most common association with cytopenia in these patients is cirrhosis and presumed hypersplenism associated with portal hypertension. The incidence of extrahepatic neoplasm is 1 per 194 patient-years; the probability of tumor occurrence is 3% after 10 years; and the risk of malignancy is 1.4-fold greater than normal.

Adjuvant therapies instituted prior to treatment can pre-empt the occurrence of complications related to the medications and the disease. A bone maintenance regimen, consisting of calcium (1-1.5 grams daily), vitamin D3 (400 units daily), an active exercise schedule and bisphosphonates, should be instituted in all corticosteroid-treated patients, especially the elderly. Vaccination against the hepatitis B and hepatitis C viruses prior to treatment is also important if there has been no previous vaccination or susceptibility to these viruses has been shown.

## 4. Can azathioprine be used during pregnancy?
Probably, but there are theoretical risks that do not justify its use. Azathioprine has been administered successfully in pregnant women with autoimmune hepatitis, pregnant mothers with inflammatory bowel disease, and women who have conceived while taking azathioprine after liver transplantation. Nevertheless, azathioprine has been associated with congenital malformations in pregnant mice, and these defects have included cleft palate, skeletal anomalies, hydrops fetalis, reduced thymic size, anemia, and hematopoietic depression. Furthermore, the placenta is only a partial barrier to the metabolites of azathioprine, and low levels of the 6-thioguanine nucleotides are detectable in the newborns of mothers treated for Crohn's disease. The odds ratio of having a child with congenital malformations while taking azathioprine for inflammatory bowel disease is 3.4. Since azathioprine is not an essential medication in the treatment of autoimmune hepatitis, it can be discontinued during pregnancy and the disease managed by adjustments in the dose of prednisone. The U.S. Food and Drug Administration (FDA) has rated azathioprine as a category D drug in pregnancy

## 5. What are the indications for treatment?
Severe liver inflammation or incapacitating symptoms. The benefits of corticosteroid therapy have been demonstrated by controlled clinical trial only in patients with severe, immediately life-threatening disease. Therapy in patients with less active disease has an uncertain benefit:risk ratio. The absolute indications for treatment are sustained severe laboratory abnormalities that reflect aggressive hepatic inflammation, incapacitating symptoms, and/or bridging necrosis or multilobular necrosis on histologic examination (see Table 19-2). Other findings do not compel immediate therapy. Autoimmune hepatitis is by nature an aggressive disease of fluctuating severity, and it is uncertain if mild disease remains mild long term. Treated patients have a greater 10-year survival than untreated asymptomatic patients with mild disease, and treatment is now favored in all patients with disease activity. Treatment is not indicated in patients with inactive or minimally active cirrhosis and in patients with decompensated liver disease and mild or no inflammatory activity.

## 6. What are the indices that reflect disease severity?
The degree of serum aspartate (AST) or alanine (ALT) aminotransferase abnormality, the serum gamma globulin or immunoglobulin G (IgG) concentration, and the histologic findings of confluent hepatic necrosis (see Table 19-2). Sustained serum AST activity of at least 10-fold the upper normal limit (UNL) or more than 5-fold UNL in conjunction with a hypergammaglobulinemia of at least twice UNL is associated with a 3-year survival of 50% and 10-year survival of 10% if not treated. Lesser degrees of laboratory activity are associated with better prognoses. In such patients, the 15-year survival exceeds 80%, and the probability of progression to cirrhosis is less than 50%. Asymptomatic patients with minimal or no inflammatory activity have 10-year survival expectations without therapy that approximate 80% even if cirrhosis is present.

Extension of the inflammatory process between portal tracts or between portal tracts and central veins (bridging necrosis) is associated with a 5-year mortality of 45% and an 82% frequency of cirrhosis if untreated. Similar consequences occur in untreated patients who have destruction of entire lobules of liver tissue at presentation (multilobular necrosis). The 5-year mortality of untreated cirrhosis with active inflammation is 58%, and 20% die of variceal hemorrhage within 2 years. In contrast, patients with interface hepatitis on histological examination and few other findings have a normal 5-year life expectancy and a low frequency of cirrhosis (17%) without treatment. Spontaneous resolution of inflammatory activity may occur unpredictably in 13% to 20% of patients, and autoimmune hepatitis may have a natural burnout, albeit frequently with the consequence of inactive cirrhosis.

### 7. Are there any predictors of response to treatment?

Yes, but they have limited predictability. There are no findings at presentation that predict the response to treatment or preclude improvement during therapy, including cirrhosis, ascites, and mild hepatic encephalopathy. The Model of End-stage Liver Disease (MELD) is useful in identifying patients who are likely to fail corticosteroid therapy, die of liver failure, or require liver transplantation. A MELD score of at least 12 points at presentation has 97% sensitivity and 68% specificity for treatment failure. Patients with human leukocyte antigen (HLA) DR3 (*DRB1*0301*) have a higher frequency of treatment failure than patients with other HLAs, and individuals with antibodies to soluble liver antigen (anti-SLA) are likely to have severe disease and requirement for continuous therapy. HLA phenotype, serologic markers, and histologic findings, including cirrhosis, are not highly predictive of treatment failure, and they do not alter the initial management strategy or expectations.

### 8. Does the rapidity of the response to treatment have prognostic value?

Yes. The principal laboratory manifestations of response are improvements in the serum levels of AST, bilirubin, and gamma globulin. At least 90% of patients demonstrate improvement in at least one parameter within 2 weeks of therapy. This response rate predicts survival with 98% accuracy. Failure to improve a pretreatment hyperbilirubinemia within 2 weeks of therapy in a patient with multilobular necrosis at presentation predicts death within 6 months, and these patients should be considered for liver transplantation. Patients who fail to enter remission within 2 years of treatment have a 43% frequency of subsequent hepatic decompensation, and the frequency of decompensation increases to 69% after 4 years of continuous therapy without remission. The first feature of decompensation is the formation of ascites, and this occurrence during therapy is an indication to consider liver transplantation. Elderly patients (aged >60 years) respond more quickly to corticosteroid therapy than young adults (aged ≤30 years). A rapid treatment response (within 24 months) has been associated with lower frequencies of progression to cirrhosis and requirement for liver transplantation.

### 9. What are the results of therapy?

Sixty-five percent of patients achieve clinical, laboratory, and histologic remission within 2 years after start of treatment (Fig. 19-1). The average duration of therapy until remission is 22 months. The probability of entering remission increases at a constant annual rate during the first 3 years of therapy, and the majority of individuals who enter remission (87%) do so within this period. Patients with and without histologic cirrhosis at presentation have 10-year life expectancies that exceed 80%. Their survival is similar to that of age- and sex-matched normal individuals from the same geographic region.

Thirteen percent of patients develop drug-related side effects that prematurely limit treatment (drug toxicity) (Table 19-3). The most common complication is intolerable obesity or cosmetic change (47%). Osteoporosis with vertebral compression (27%), and brittle diabetes (20%) restrict therapy less frequently. Patients with cirrhosis develop serious side effects more commonly than others, possibly because they have higher serum levels of unbound prednisolone as a consequence of prolonged hyperbilirubinemia and/or hypoalbuminemia. No findings at presentation predict a serious side effect, and all previously treated patients, including postmenopausal women, should be managed similarly. All patients should be started on a pre-emptive bone maintenance regimen, and susceptible patients should be vaccinated against hepatitis B and hepatitis C viruses prior to therapy.

Deterioration despite compliance with therapy (treatment failure) develops in 9% of patients, and an incomplete response occurs in 13% (see Fig. 19-1). Cirrhosis develops in 36% of patients within 6 years. Relapse after drug withdrawal occurs in as many as 79% of individuals who enter remission, and only 21% of patients have sustained inactivity after cessation of therapy.

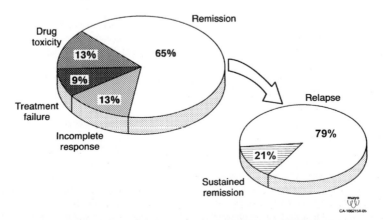

**Figure 19-1.** Responses to initial course of corticosteroid therapy.

## 10. What are the endpoints of treatment?

Initial treatment should be continued until remission, drug toxicity, disease progression (treatment failure), or stalled improvement (incomplete response). Remission connotes absence of symptoms, resolution of all laboratory indices of active inflammation, and histologic improvement to normal liver tissue or inactive cirrhosis. Liver tissue evaluation before drug withdrawal is essential to establish remission since histologic activity may be present in 55% of patients who satisfy other requirements. Typically, histologic improvement lags behind clinical and laboratory resolution by 3 to 8 months, and treatment should be extended for at least this period. Patients with normal serum AST and gamma globulin levels and normal liver biopsy findings immediately prior to drug withdrawal have a significantly lower frequency of relapse after drug withdrawal than patients with near-normal tests and tissue (60% versus 90%, $p < .001$). Only 40% of treated patients, however, are able to improve to this degree. Treatment failure connotes progressive worsening of laboratory tests, persistent or recurrent symptoms, ascites formation, or features of hepatic encephalopathy despite compliance with therapy. The emergence of serious drug-related side effects and the failure to induce remission after protracted treatment (incomplete response) also compel modifications in the initial treatment regimen. The risk of serious drug toxicity exceeds the likelihood of inducing remission after 3 years of continuous therapy, and a decreasing benefit:risk ratio justifies termination of conventional treatment in these patients.

## 11. When should a liver biopsy be performed?

At presentation before therapy to establish the diagnosis and stage the disease, after satisfaction of clinical and laboratory criteria for remission during initial therapy, and at any time when the disease worsens and the basis for its behavior is uncertain. Liver tissue examination is not necessary to diagnose relapse if it occurs within 6 months of drug withdrawal, and the serum AST level has increased from normal to at least 3-fold UNL. Alternatively, liver biopsy evaluation is essential to evaluate treatment failure, especially to exclude corticosteroid-related fatty liver disease or a previously unrecognized or emerging cholestatic syndrome such as primary biliary cirrhosis or primary sclerosing cholangitis.

## 12. Does corticosteroid treatment prevent or reverse fibrosis?

Yes. Corticosteroid therapy reduces hepatic fibrosis in 53% of patients or prevents its progression in 26% during a mean observation interval of 5 years. By suppressing inflammatory activity, corticosteroids eliminate metalloproteinase inhibitors, stimulate degradation of the fibrotic liver matrix, and enhance apoptosis of hepatic stellate cells. Corticosteroids have been reported to reverse cirrhosis in autoimmune hepatitis, but cirrhosis is a complex anatomic transformation, and its disappearance during treatment remains controversial. Thirty-six percent of patients still develop cirrhosis within 6 years, usually during the early, most active, stages of the disease. The mean annual incidence of cirrhosis is 11% during the first 3 years of illness and 1% thereafter despite relapse and retreatment. The presence of histological cirrhosis during or after treatment does not diminish survival or increase morbidity.

## 13. What precautions can be undertaken to reduce the frequency side effects?

Select patients who can benefit from treatment, pursue realistic treatment goals, anticipate side effects in vulnerable patients, institute comprehensive counseling before therapy, and introduce preemptive management schedules (Table 19-4).

## 14. What is the most common treatment problem?

Relapse after drug withdrawal. Fifty percent of patients who enter remission relapse within 6 months after termination of treatment, and 70% relapse within 3 years. The frequency of relapse can be as high as 86%, and it increases after each subsequent retreatment and drug withdrawal. The risk of relapse diminishes with duration of sustained remission, but it never disappears. A sustained remission of at least 6 months is associated with only an 8% frequency of subsequent relapse.

## 15. What are the consequences of relapse and retreatment?

Progression to cirrhosis, death from liver failure, requirement for liver transplantation, and drug-induced side effects. Repeated relapse and retreatment have a cumulative morbidity and mortality. Cirrhosis develops more commonly (38% versus 4%, $p = .004$); death from hepatic failure or need for liver transplantation occurs more often (20% versus 0%, $p = .008$); and drug-induced side effects are more frequent (70% versus 30%, $p = .01$) in individuals who relapse than in those who sustain remission after drug withdrawal. The frequencies of each complication increases with each subsequent relapse and retreatment. The optimal time to interrupt this sequence is after the first treatment and relapse. At this time, a different treatment strategy must be implemented.

## 16. Does determination of serum thiopurine methyltransferase activity predict azathioprine toxicity?

No. Genotypic and phenotypic screening for serum thiopurine methyltransferase activity has not reduced the frequency of azathioprine-induced side effects in autoimmune hepatitis compared to unscreened patients, nor has the occurrence of these side effects been associated with below normal levels of thiopurine methyltransferase activity. The most important association with cytopenia in azathioprine-treated patients is advanced fibrosis and cirrhosis. Near-zero enzyme activity occurs rarely in normal individuals (0.3% to 0.5%), and the value of screening to detect this unusually low enzyme deficiency remains uncertain, especially if not everyone with low levels exhibits azathioprine toxicity. Bone marrow failure has occurred during azathioprine treatment, and this consequence is catastrophic but not reliably predicted. Testing for serum thiopurine methyltransferase activity seems most appropriate in patients with preexistent or progressive cytopenia and in individuals subjected to doses of azathioprine higher than the conventional schedule of 50 mg daily. Avoidance of azathioprine in patients with preexistent or progressive cytopenia (leukocyte counts $<2.5 \times 10^9/L$ or platelet counts $<50 \times 10^9/L$) and close monitoring (3-month intervals) of the blood leukocyte and platelet counts in all patients taking the drug may be the best preventive strategy (Table 19-4).

**Table 19-4.** Management Strategies to Reduce Treatment-Related Side Effects

| CLINICAL SITUATION | MANAGEMENT STRATEGY |
| --- | --- |
| Uncertain benefit:risk ratio | • Apply strict indications for therapy.<br>• Limit treatment trials if weak indications for therapy.<br>• Use combination regimen if treatment prolonged. |
| Unrealistic treatment goals | • Maintain realistic objectives recognizing that some patients may never have full response.<br>• Avoid protracted and repeated therapy.<br>• Individualize dosing schedules early if drug intolerant or slow response. |
| Preexistent cytopenia | • Assess thiopurine methyltransferase activity and avoid azathioprine if near zero enzyme activity.<br>• Avoid azathioprine treatment if leukocyte counts below $2.5 \times 10^9/L$ or platelet counts below $50 \times 10^9/L$ regardless of thiopurine methyltransferase activity.<br>• Monitor leukocyte and platelet counts at 3-month intervals even if counts are normal pretreatment.<br>• Discontinue azathioprine if leukocyte counts decrease below $2.5 \times 10^9/L$ or platelet counts below $50 \times 10^9/L$. |
| Pregnancy | • Provide early counseling about potential hazards to mother and fetus.<br>• Use prednisone instead of azathioprine.<br>• Reduce prednisone dose to lowest level possible.<br>• Anticipate flare in disease activity after delivery and adjust treatment before delivery to prevent it. |
| Osteopenia or its possibility | • Institute bone maintenance regimen in all patients on long-term corticosteroid treatment (≥12 months).<br>• Encourage calcium supplements 1 to 1.5 g daily, vitamin $D_3$ 400 IU daily, alendronate 70 mg each week, and an active exercise program.<br>• Assess bone density every 12 months on corticosteroid treatment. |

### 17. How should relapse be managed?

By instituting a long-term maintenance regimen with azathioprine, 2 mg/kg daily. Therapy with prednisone and azathioprine is restarted after the initial relapse until clinical and laboratory resolution is again achieved. The dose of azathioprine is then increased to 2 mg/kg daily as the dose of prednisone is withdrawn. Azathioprine is then continued indefinitely as a chronic maintenance therapy. Eighty percent of patients are able to sustain remission in this fashion over a 10 year period of observation. Azathioprine-induced cytopenia compels dose reduction in 9% of patients; corticosteroid-related side effects improve; and arthralgias associated with corticosteroid withdrawal eventually resolve (but may be protracted). Malignancy reflecting diverse cell types develops in 7% of patients, but its association with the drug is disputed.

### 18. Do patients receiving azathioprine maintenance therapy ever get off treatment?

Yes. Twelve percent of patients treated with long-term azathioprine maintenance regimens achieve this result. Drug withdrawal should be attempted in all patients with inactive disease on long-term treatment schedules since relapse in these situations can be closely monitored and easily treated. Relapse is generally well tolerated, and it is typically manifested by laboratory rather than clinical instability with an increase in the serum AST level to at least 3-fold UNL. Withdrawal attempts can be repeated each year of inactive disease on treatment. Indefinite azathioprine therapy is a possibility, but the continued need for the drug must be demonstrated on a repeated basis to justify its risks.

### 19. How should treatment failure be managed?

High-dose prednisone (60 mg daily) or prednisone (30 mg daily) in conjunction with azathioprine (150 mg daily) induces clinical and laboratory remission in 75% of patients within 2 years (Fig. 19-2). The doses of medication are reduced each month of clinical and laboratory improvement until conventional doses are achieved (see Table 19-1). Histologic remission occurs in less than 20% of patients, and the majority who fail treatment become corticosteroid dependent and at risk for disease progression and drug-related complications. Limited studies have suggested the advantage of 6-mercaptopurine (6-MP) over azathioprine in treatment failure. The drug may have different absorption characteristics or metabolic pathways that favor its use. The initial dose of 6-MP is 12.5 to 25 mg daily, and it is then increased as tolerated to 1.5 mg/kg daily. Pharmacokinetic studies in patients with cirrhosis have not demonstrated a sufficient

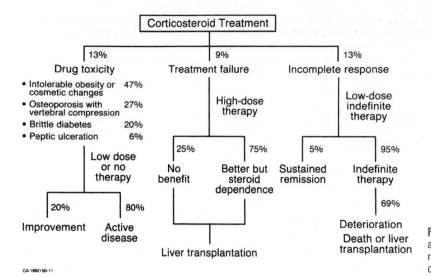

**Figure 19-2.** Frequency, treatment, and consequences of suboptimal responses to conventional corticosteroid regimens.

disturbance in the conversion of prednisone to prednisolone to justify a preference for prednisolone. Decompensations unresponsive to high-dose corticosteroid therapy compel a liver transplantation evaluation. Emerging drugs for treatment failure include cyclosporine, tacrolimus, and mycophenolate mofetil (Table 19-5). These agents have been used empirically for problematic patients, and preliminary results have been encouraging. None has been studied rigorously or incorporated into a standard management algorithm. Additional clinical trials are necessary to establish their target populations, dosing schedules, safety profiles, monitoring mechanisms, and long-term results.

## Table 19-5. Promising New Drugs for Autoimmune Hepatitis

| AGENT | PUTATIVE ACTIONS | EXPERIENCE |
|---|---|---|
| Cyclosporine | Calcineurin inhibitor that impairs lymphokine release and prevents cytotoxic T-cell expansion | Anecdotal use in corticosteroid-intolerant or refractory disease<br>Uncertain target population, dosing schedule, monitoring mechanisms, safety profile, and long-term results |
| Tacrolimus | Calcineurin inhibitor that prevents cytotoxic T-cell expansion, inhibits interleukin-2 receptor, and impairs antibody production | Small anecdotal experience<br>Stimulates experimental fibrogenesis<br>Uncertain target population, dosing schedule, monitoring mechanisms, safety profile, and long-term results |
| Mycophenolate mofetil | Purine antagonist that impairs creation of new RNA and DNA<br>Prevents lymphocyte proliferation and activation<br>Independent of thiopurine methyltransferase metabolic pathway | Anecdotal success in small experiences<br>May allow corticosteroid withdrawal<br>Uncertain target population, dosing schedule, monitoring mechanisms, safety profile, and long-term results |
| 6-Mercaptopurine | Purine antagonist that is active metabolite of azathioprine<br>Possibly better intestinal absorption or different metabolic pathways than parent drug | Anecdotal success in treatment failure and corticosteroid intolerance |
| Budesonide | Second-generation steroid<br>High hepatic first-pass clearance<br>Metabolites devoid of glucocorticoid activity | Controlled clinical trial shows clinical and laboratory improvement in treatment-naïve mild disease<br>Preserves bone integrity<br>No advantage as salvage therapy<br>Glucocorticoid side effects possible |

## 20. How effective is liver transplantation for decompensated disease?

It is excellent. The 5-year life expectancy of patient and graft after transplantation ranges from 83% to 92%, and the actuarial 10-year survival after transplantation is 75%. The autoantibodies and hypergammaglobulinemia disappear within 2 years. Disease recurs in at least 17% of patients, usually as a result of inadequate immune suppression, and it is controlled by adjustments in this regimen. Progression to cirrhosis and graft failure have been reported, and patients with autoimmune hepatitis may be at increased risk to develop acute rejection, steroid-resistant rejection, and chronic rejection. Corticosteroid withdrawal may be difficult, and its continued use for at least 1 year after surgery may be necessary.

### 21. What strategy is best for patients with drug toxicity or incomplete response?

Management is empiric, and outcomes must be closely monitored (see Fig. 19-2). For drug toxicity, the dose of the offending medication is reduced to the lowest possible level or withdrawn fully. Disease activity is controlled by the medication (prednisone or azathioprine) that has been tolerated, and its dose is adjusted to suppress disease activity. For an incomplete response, the medication is reduced to the lowest level possible to prevent symptoms and maintain the serum AST level below 3-fold UNL. Inadequately controlled patients eventually may require liver transplantation.

### 22. Does hepatocellular carcinoma occur?

Yes, but it is unusual. The 10-year probability of hepatocellular carcinoma is 2.9%, and its incidence is 4 cases per 1000 patient-years. Hepatocellular carcinoma develops only in patients with longstanding cirrhosis, and risk factors for its occurrence include male gender, portal hypertension, history of blood transfusions, immunosuppressive therapy for at least 3 years, treatment failure, and cirrhosis of at least 10 years' duration. The mean age of diagnosis is 65 years, and the risk becomes apparent mainly after the age of 40 years. These risk factors can identify a subset of patients that might benefit from close surveillance with at least hepatic ultrasonography at 6-month intervals. The median survival at 1 year after diagnosis is 63% regardless of treatment.

### 23. How are variant syndromes managed?

By treating the predominant manifestations of the disorder with the appropriate medication (Fig. 19-3). The degree of cholestasis reflected mainly in the serum alkaline phosphatase level determines the need for adjuvant therapy with ursodeoxycholic acid (13 to 15 mg/kg daily). Autoimmune hepatitis with concurrent features of primary sclerosing cholangitis warrants a treatment trial with high-dose ursodeoxycholic acid (25 mg/kg daily) in addition to prednisone, and autoimmune hepatitis with concurrent features of primary biliary cirrhosis and a serum alkaline phosphatase level above 2-fold UNL or florid duct lesions of histologic examination warrants therapy with ursodeoxycholic acid in conjunction with prednisone or budesonide (Fig. 19-3). Management strategies are empiric, and multicenter collaborative studies are necessary to codify diagnostic criteria and treatment algorithms for these variants.

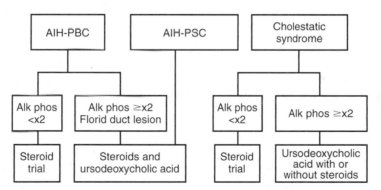

**Figure 19-3.** Treatment algorithm for variant syndromes. Variant syndromes combine features typically associated with separate diseases. They include patients with autoimmune hepatitis and primary biliary cirrhosis (AIH-PBC), autoimmune hepatitis and primary sclerosing cholangitis (AIH-PSC), and autoimmune hepatitis with cholestatic findings in the absence of PBC and PSC (cholestatic syndrome). The degree of cholestasis as reflected in whether the magnitude of the serum alkaline phosphatase level is less than 2-fold the upper limit of normal (alkaline phosphatase [Alk phos] <×2) or 2-fold the upper limit of normal or higher (Alk phos >×2) determines if corticosteroid therapy is sufficient or should be combined with ursodeoxycholic acid.

### 24. How are patients with mixed autoimmune and viral features managed?

By treating the predominant manifestations of the disorder with the appropriate medication (Fig. 19-4). Most patients with mixed autoimmune and viral features have true viral infection and low titer autoantibodies that have no diagnostic, clinical, or therapeutic relevance. These patients have chronic viral hepatitis with autoimmune features, and antiviral therapy should be instituted as indicated (Fig. 19-4). Rarely, patients with autoimmune hepatitis have either false positive markers for viral infection or true coincidental viral infection. Patients with false-positive viral markers respond well to corticosteroids. Patients with true viral infection, high titers of smooth muscle antibodies (SMA) and/or antinuclear antibodies (ANA) (titers >1:320), and histologic changes of moderate-to-severe interface hepatitis with plasmacytic infiltration have autoimmune hepatitis with coincidental viral infection. Treatment must be directed against the predominant disorder, and corticosteroid therapy is justified. Antiviral therapy may be instituted later if viral-predominant manifestations emerge. Antiviral and immunosuppressive therapies should not be combined, and the nondominant drug should be discontinued.

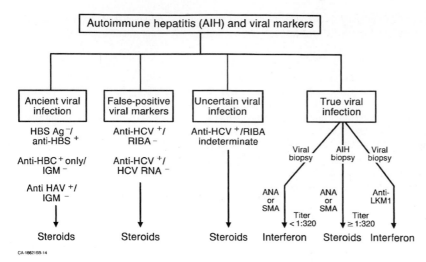

**Figure 19-4.** Treatment strategies for patients with autoimmune hepatitis (AIH) and viral markers. Patients with true viral infection require liver biopsy assessment to establish the presence of histologic patterns consistent with viral infection (viral biopsy) or AIH biopsy. Clinical, laboratory, and histologic changes of AIH, including high titer autoantibodies, support the diagnosis of AIH with coincidental viral infection. Empiric treatment with corticosteroids can be instituted and monitored closely.

## 25. What new drug therapies are promising?

The drugs that are emerging mainly as salvage therapies for patients who are intolerant or refractory to treatment with prednisone and azathioprine include calcineurin inhibitors and purine antagonists (Table 19-5). Budesonide is a glucocorticoid with a high first-pass clearance by the liver and metabolites devoid of glucocorticoid activity. It has been used successfully as frontline therapy for treatment-naïve patients with mild autoimmune hepatitis, and its major advantage may be the preservation of bone density.

## 26. What new site-specific molecular interventions are promising?

The promising new molecular treatments have site-specific actions that interrupt key pathways for autoantigen presentation and immunocyte activation, differentiation and expansion (Table 19-6). As the pathogenic mechanisms of autoimmune hepatitis are further defined, the number of these interventions will increase. Some treatments are already being tested in the rheumatic diseases, but none has been applied or endorsed in autoimmune hepatitis (Table 19-6).

**Table 19-6.** Promising New Therapies Based on Site-Specific Molecular Interventions

| AGENT | PUTATIVE ACTIONS | EXPERIENCE |
|---|---|---|
| Blocking peptides | Displaces autoantigenic peptide from antigen binding groove of class II HLA DR molecule | Tested in rheumatic diseases Untried in autoimmune hepatitis |
| Soluble CTLA-4 | Blocks ligation of B7 to CD28 and prevents CD4 T helper cell activation | Successful in preventing rejection after mismatched bone marrow transplantation |
| Adoptive transfer of T-regulatory cells | Suppression of key cytokine pathways | Untried in autoimmune hepatitis |
| Oral tolerance | Induces nonresponsiveness to fed antigen Causes suppression or clonal anergy depending on antigen dose | Limited success in experimental and human autoimmune encephalitis, diabetes, rheumatoid arthritis Untried in autoimmune hepatitis |
| Recombinant interleukin-10 or rituximab | May downregulate cytotoxic type 1 cytokine response. Alters cytokine type 2 response | Tested in human chronic hepatitis C Anti-B cell monoclonal antibody successful in one patient with autoimmune hepatitis |
| Antibodies to TNF-α | Suppresses proinflammatory cytokine May impair cytotoxic type 1 cytokine response | Used in inflammatory bowel disease Untried in autoimmune hepatitis |
| Autologous or mesenchymal stem cell transplantation | Engrafts in damaged liver Differentiates into functioning hepatocytes Restores hepatic function | Successful rescue therapy in immune-deficient mice with hepatic failure Untried in autoimmune hepatitis |

CTLA, cytotoxic T lymphocyte antigen; HLA, human leukocyte antigen; TNF, tumor necrosis factor.

# WEBSITE

http://www.aasld.org

## BIBLIOGRAPHY

1. Czaja AJ. Clinical features, differential diagnosis and treatment of autoimmune hepatitis in the elderly. Drugs Aging 2008;25:219–39.
2. Czaja AJ. Emerging treatments for autoimmune hepatitis. Curr Drug Targets Inflamm Allergy 2002;1:317–26.
3. Czaja AJ. Safety issues in the management of autoimmune hepatitis. Exp Opin Drug Saf 2008;7:319–33.
5. Czaja AJ. Treatment of autoimmune hepatitis. Semin Liver Dis 2002;22:365–77.
6. Czaja AJ. Treatment strategies in autoimmune hepatitis. Clin Liver Dis 2002;6:799–824.
7. Czaja AJ, Carpenter HA. Thiopurine methyltransferase deficiency and azathioprine intolerance in autoimmune hepatitis. Dig Dis Sci 2006;51:968–75.
8. Montano-Loza A, Carpenter HA, Czaja AJ. Consequences of treatment withdrawal in type 1 autoimmune hepatitis. Liver Int 2007;27:507–15.
9. Montano-Loza AJ, Carpenter HA, Czaja AJ. Features associated with treatment failure in type 1 autoimmune hepatitis and predictive value of the model of end stage liver disease. Hepatology 2007;46:1138–45.
10. Montano-Loza A, Carpenter HA, Czaja AJ. Improving the end point of corticosteroid therapy in type 1 autoimmune hepatitis to reduce the frequency of relapse. Am J Gastroenterol 2007;102:1005–12.
11. Montano-Loza AJ, Carpenter HA, Czaja AJ. Predictive factors for hepatocellular carcinoma in type 1 autoimmune hepatitis. Am J Gastroenterol 2008;103:1944-51.
12. Montano Loza A, Czaja AJ. Current therapy for autoimmune hepatitis. Nature Clin Pract Gastroenterol Hepatol 2007;4:202–14.
13. Czaja AJ. Current and future treatments of autoimmune hepatitis. Expert Rev Gastroenterol Hepatol 2009;3:269–91.

# 20 CHAPTER

# PRIMARY BILIARY CIRRHOSIS AND PRIMARY SCLEROSING CHOLANGITIS

*Jayant A. Talwalkar, MD, MPH, and Nicholas F. LaRusso, MD*

### 1. Define *primary biliary cirrhosis* (PBC) and *primary sclerosing cholangitis* (PSC).

PBC and PSC are chronic cholestatic liver diseases of unknown etiology in adults. PBC mainly affects women in the sixth decade of life and is characterized by destruction of interlobular and septal bile ducts. PSC mainly affects men in the fifth decade of life and is characterized by diffuse inflammation and fibrosis of the intrahepatic and extrahepatic bile ducts. Both PBC and PSC may eventually progress to end-stage liver disease requiring consideration for liver transplantation.

### 2. Is PBC an autoimmune disorder?

The underlying cause of PBC is unknown. Evidence for an autoimmune etiology includes the following:

- Frequent association with other autoimmune diseases such as Sjögren syndrome, rheumatoid arthritis, scleroderma/ CREST (the syndrome consisting of **c**alcinosis, **R**aynaud phenomenon, **e**sophageal disease, **s**clerodactyly, and **t**elangiectasia), thyroiditis, lichen planus, discoid lupus, and pemphigoid
- Presence of circulating serum autoantibodies, such as antimitochondrial antibodies (AMA), antinuclear antibody (ANA), anti–smooth muscle antibody (ASMA), extractable nuclear antigen (ENA), rheumatoid factor, thyroid-specific antibodies, and elevated serum immunoglobulin M (IgM) levels
- Histologic features, including lymphoplasmacytic cholangitis with portal tract expansion indicative of immunologic bile duct destruction
- Familial clustering among patients with PBC, including evidence for genetic transmission from mothers to daughters
- Increased prevalence of circulating serum autoantibodies in relatives of patients with PBC
- Increased frequency of class II major histocompatibility complex (MHC) antigens in PBC

### 3. Is PSC an autoimmune disorder?

The evidence supporting an immunogenic origin for PSC includes the following:

- The 70% to 80% prevalence of inflammatory bowel disease among patients with PSC in Europe and North America
- Increased incidence of PSC and chronic ulcerative colitis in families of patients with PSC
- Evidence for immune system dysregulation, including increased serum levels of IgM, serum autoantibodies such as ANA, ASMA, and peripheral antineutrophil cytoplasmic antigen (pANCA), circulating immune complexes, and abnormalities in peripheral blood lymphocyte subsets
- Increased frequency of human leukocyte antigens (HLA) B8, DR3a, and DR4
- Aberrant expression of HLA class II antigen on bile duct epithelial cells

### 4. Do viral infections have a role in the development of PSC?

Viral agents such as respiratory enteric orphan (REO) virus type III and cytomegalovirus, which are capable of infecting the biliary tree, have been implicated in the development of PSC. A hypothesis of virus-mediated immune system activation with subsequent immunologically mediated bile duct destruction has been proposed. However, no direct evidence has linked these or other viruses to the development of PSC.

### 5. What are the clinical features of PBC and PSC?

The clinical presentations of both PBC and PSC may be similar, although some demographic and clinical characteristics differ. From 85% to 90% of patients with PBC are women presenting in the fourth to sixth decade of life, whereas 70% of patients with PSC are men with an approximate age of 40 years at diagnosis. Despite an increasing frequency of asymptomatic or subclinical disease greater than 40%, affected patients with either condition generally present with the gradual onset of fatigue and pruritus. Right upper quadrant pain and anorexia also may be observed at diagnosis. Although uncommon, steatorrhea in PBC and PSC is usually due to bile salt malabsorption, pancreatic exocrine insufficiency, or coexisting celiac disease. Jaundice as a primary manifestation of PBC is uncommon but strongly associated with the presence of advanced histologic disease. In PSC, the development of bacterial cholangitis characterized by recurrent fever, right upper quadrant pain, and jaundice may occur. A history of previous reconstructive biliary surgery, the presence of dominant extrahepatic biliary strictures, or the development of a superimposed cholangiocarcinoma may also be responsible. The symptoms of end-stage liver disease, such as gastrointestinal bleeding, ascites, and encephalopathy, occur late in the course of both diseases.

### 6. What are the common findings on physical examination?
Physical examination may reveal jaundice and excoriations from pruritus in both disorders. Xanthelasmas (raised lesions over the eyelids from cholesterol deposition) and xanthomas (lesions over the extensor surfaces) are occasionally seen in the late stages of both diseases, particularly PBC. Hyperpigmentation, especially in sun-exposed areas, and vitiligo may be present. The liver usually is enlarged and firm to palpation. The spleen may also be palpable if portal hypertension from advanced disease has developed. Characteristics of end-stage liver disease, including muscle wasting and spider angiomata, appear in the advanced stages of both diseases.

### 7. What diseases are associated with PBC?
Up to 80% of patients with PBC also have coexistent extrahepatic autoimmune diseases. The most common extrahepatic autoimmune disease is sicca (Sjögren) syndrome. Other conditions described in association with PBC include autoimmune thyroiditis, scleroderma/CREST, rheumatoid arthritis, dermatomyositis, mixed connective tissue disease, systemic lupus erythematosus, renal tubular acidosis, and idiopathic pulmonary fibrosis.

### 8. What diseases are associated with PSC?
Chronic ulcerative colitis (CUC) and, less frequently, Crohn's colitis are present in at least 70% to 80% of patients with PSC. The disease activity of CUC in PSC is usually quiescent; in 80% of patients, CUC is either asymptomatic or mildly symptomatic when PSC is diagnosed. CUC may also be diagnosed after the recognition of PSC. Although reports of CUC have been described in association with PBC, this is still considered quite uncommon.

### 9. What important biochemical abnormalities are associated with PBC and PSC?
In both disorders, serum alkaline phosphatase is elevated at least 3 to 4 times the upper limit of normal with mild-to-moderate elevations in alanine aminotransferase (ALT) and aspartate aminotransferase (AST). In PBC, serum total bilirubin values are usually within normal limits at diagnosis. In PSC, serum bilirubin values are modestly increased in up to 50% of patients at the time of diagnosis. Tests reflective of synthetic liver function, including serum albumin and prothrombin time, remain normal unless advanced liver disease is present. Serum immunoglobulin M (IgM) levels are elevated in 90% of patients with PBC. Tests related to copper metabolism are virtually always abnormal in both diseases, reflecting the influence of chronic cholestasis. Based on the widespread use of automated blood chemistries, an increasing number of asymptomatic patients with PBC and PSC are being diagnosed.

### 10. What is the lipid profile in patients with PBC? Are they at increased risk for developing coronary artery disease?
Serum cholesterol levels are usually elevated in PBC. In the early stages of disease, increases in high-density lipoprotein (HDL) cholesterol exceed those of low-density lipoprotein (LDL) and very-low-density lipoprotein (VLDL). With liver disease progression, the concentration of HDL decreases while LDL concentrations become markedly elevated. An increased risk for atherosclerotic disease has not been demonstrated among patients with persistent hyperlipidemia in association with PBC.

### 11. What serum autoantibodies are associated with PBC?
Serum AMA is found in up to 95% of patients with PBC. Although considered non–organ specific as well as non–species specific, serum AMA usually is detected by an enzyme-linked immunosorbent assay (ELISA). However, antibodies directed against a specific group of antigens on the inner mitochondrial membrane (M2 antigens) are present in 98% of patients with PBC. This subtyping of serum AMA increases the sensitivity and specificity for disease detection.

Other AMA subtypes related to PBC react with antigens on the outer mitochondrial membrane. Anti-M4 occurs in association with anti-M2 in patients with overlap syndromes of autoimmune hepatitis and PBC. Anti-M8, when present with anti-M2, may be associated with a more rapid course of disease progression in selected patients. Anti-M9 has been observed with and without anti-M2 and may be helpful in the diagnosis of early-stage PBC.

### 12. What serum autoantibodies are associated with PSC?
In PSC, serum AMA is rare and, if present, is usually seen in very low titers. However, detectable titers of serum ANA, ASMA, and antithyroperoxidase antibodies have been found in up to 70% of patients with PSC. pANCA has been observed in up to 65% of patients with PSC. However, the finding of pANCA among patients with ulcerative colitis and no evidence of PSC limits its diagnostic utility. Anticardiolipin antibodies are also increased in patients with PSC.

## 13. What are the cholangiographic features of the biliary tree in PSC?

Evaluation of the biliary tree in PSC by endoscopic or percutaneous transhepatic cholangiography may reveal diffuse stricturing of both intrahepatic and extrahepatic ducts with saccular dilatation of intervening areas. These abnormalities result in the characteristic *beads-on-a-string* appearance seen with PSC. Exclusive intrahepatic and hilar involvement occurs in only 20% of patients. Hepaticolithiasis is observed in 10% to 20% of cases. The presence of a dominant stricture should raise the question of cholangiocarcinoma as a complication of PSC. Increasing experience with magnetic resonance cholangiography (MRC) suggests that this non-invasive diagnostic approach is accurate in more than 90% of cases diagnosed as PSC compared with invasive cholangiography (Fig. 20-1).

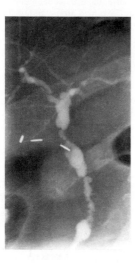

**Figure 20-1.** Retrograde cholangiogram exhibiting classic features of PSC, including diffuse stricturing and beading of intrahepatic and extrahepatic bile ducts. (From LaRusso NF, Wiesner RH, Ludwig J, et al: Current concepts. Primary sclerosing cholangitis. N Engl J Med 310:899–903, 1984, with permission.)

## 14. Is it important to evaluate the biliary tree in PBC?

In PBC, an ultrasound examination of the biliary tree is usually adequate to exclude the presence of extrahepatic biliary obstruction. However, in patients with atypical features such as male sex, AMA seronegativity, or associated inflammatory bowel disease, a cholangiogram should be considered to distinguish PBC from PSC and other disorders causing biliary obstruction.

## 15. What are the hepatic histologic features of PBC and PSC?

Histologic abnormalities on liver biopsy are highly characteristic of both PBC and PSC in the early stages of disease. In PBC, the diagnostic finding is described as a *florid duct lesion*, which reveals bile duct destruction and granuloma formation. A severe lymphoplasmacytic inflammatory cell infiltrate in the portal tracts is accompanied by the segmental degeneration of interlobular bile ducts (also termed chronic nonsuppurative destructive cholangitis) (Fig. 20-2).

Early histologic changes in PSC include enlargement of portal tracts by edema, increased portal and periportal fibrosis, and proliferation of interlobular bile ducts. The diagnostic morphologic abnormality in PSC is termed *fibrous obliterative*

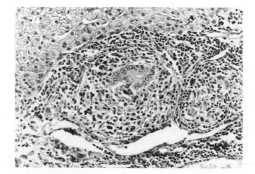

**Figure 20-2.** Florid duct lesion (granulomatous bile duct destruction) in PBC. A poorly formed granuloma surrounds and destroys the bile duct in an eccentric fashion.

*cholangitis*, which leads to the complete loss of interlobular and adjacent septal bile ducts from fibrous chord and connective tissue deposition. This histologic feature, however, occurs in only 10% of known cases. The histologic findings of end-stage liver disease for PBC and PSC are characterized by a paucity of bile ducts and biliary cirrhosis (Fig. 20-3).

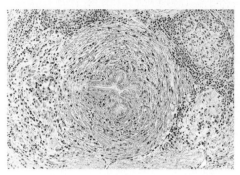

**Figure 20-3.** Fibrous obliterative cholangitis in PSC. The interlobular bile duct shows a typical fibrous collar, and epithelium seems undamaged.

### 16. Do asymptomatic patients with PBC have a normal life expectancy?
Most patients with PBC experience a progressive clinical course resulting in eventual cirrhosis. Asymptomatic patients have a longer median survival than symptomatic patients. However, a reduced median survival in asymptomatic PBC patients compared with age- and sex-matched healthy populations is observed. Estimates of overall median survival without liver transplantation range between 10 and 12 years from the time of diagnosis; advanced histologic disease imparts a median survival approaching 8 years. Elevations of total bilirubin above 8 to 10 mg/dL have been associated with a median life expectancy of 2 years without liver transplantation.

### 17. Do asymptomatic patients with PSC have a normal life expectancy?
Although some patients with PSC show no evidence for disease progression for many years, most published investigations support the contention that PSC is a progressive disease which can ultimately lead to liver failure and death without liver transplantation. A median survival of 9 to 12 years from the time of diagnosis in all patients with PSC appears to be independent of geographic and environmental influences.

### 18. What is the role of mathematical models in estimating survival for PBC and PSC?
The development of mathematical models for both PBC and PSC has improved the ability to predict rates of disease progression and survival without liver transplantation on an individual basis. They are useful for stratifying patients by survival risk, developing endpoints of treatment failure, and designing therapeutic trials. The use of these models in defining the optimal selection of patients and timing for liver transplantation has been the subject of several investigations.

A prognostic model for PBC developed at the Mayo Clinic relies on clinical and biochemical parameters including serum total bilirubin, albumin, prothrombin time, presence or absence of peripheral edema, and patient age. In PSC, the important variables that predict survival include patient age, serum total bilirubin, presence of splenomegaly, and histologic stage by liver biopsy. A revision of the Mayo Clinic PSC model (substituting a history of variceal bleeding for histologic stage) continues to provide similar prognostic information without the need for invasive procedures such as a liver biopsy. Similar results about prognosis have also been observed using the Model for End-stage Liver Disease (MELD).

### 19. What vitamin deficiencies are associated with PBC and PSC?
Patients with PBC and PSC are susceptible to fat-soluble vitamin deficiencies, especially in advanced stages of disease. The occurrence of diminished visual acuity at night can be attributed to vitamin A deficiency. Vitamin D deficiency occurs commonly in association with marked steatorrhea, which is related to a decrease in duodenal bile acid concentration. The development of metabolic bone disease in PBC and PSC is associated in part with vitamin D deficiency. Prolongation of serum prothrombin time is associated with vitamin K deficiency. Finally, vitamin E deficiency occurs uncommonly but when present results in neurologic abnormalities affecting the posterior spinal columns, leading to areflexia, loss of proprioception and ataxia.

### 20. What bone disease is associated with PBC and PSC?
Metabolic bone disease (i.e., hepatic osteodystrophy), which may lead to disabling pathologic fractures, is a serious complication of both PBC and PSC. Clinical manifestations include osteopenia, osteoporosis, and fracture. Both vitamin D

deficiency and smoking have been implicated as risk factors for metabolic bone disease. Risk factors for osteoporosis include advancing age, low body mass index, previous history of fractures, and advanced histologic disease. Severe bone pain in an acute or chronic setting related to avascular necrosis (AVN) may occur in PBC and PSC.

### 21. What liver-related complications are specific to PSC?

Complications specific to PSC include recurrent bacterial cholangitis, dominant stricturing of the extrahepatic bile ducts, and cholangiocarcinoma. Bacterial cholangitis is frequent in patients with a history of previous biliary surgery or dominant stricture formation. Dominant strictures occur in approximately 15% to 20% of patients with PSC during the natural course of disease. They often involve the hilum but can equally affect both hepatic ducts as well as the common bile duct. Dominant strictures are frequently associated with asymptomatic elevations in serum liver biochemistries or the acute onset of symptoms including jaundice, pruritus, and bacterial cholangitis.

From 10% to 15% of patients with PSC will develop cholangiocarcinoma during the course of disease. The risk for cholangiocarcinoma is estimated between 1% and 1.5% per year. Between 30% and 50% of patients are diagnosed with cholangiocarcinoma within 2 years of identifying PSC. Early detection of cholangiocarcinoma remains difficult based on the insensitivity of mucosal biopsy and brush cytology. The detection of elevated serum CA-19-9 levels greater than 100 IU/L may herald the existence of clinically detectable cholangiocarcinoma in patients with PSC. Advanced molecular cytologic techniques have facilitated the early detection of cholangiocarcinoma in patients with PSC.

### 22. What is the differential diagnosis of PBC and PSC?

The differential diagnosis of PBC and PSC includes other causes of chronic cholestasis, including extrahepatic biliary obstruction due to choledocholithiasis, iatrogenic strictures, and tumors. Although ultrasound or computed tomography may suggest the presence of biliary dilation, the performance of cholangiography is required to render a definitive diagnosis of PSC. Drug-induced cholestasis secondary to phenothiazines, estrogens, azoles, and a number of other drugs also should be considered as alternative diagnoses.

### 23. Define *autoimmune cholangitis*. How is it related to PBC?

Recent observations have documented a group of patients with PBC and no detectable serum AMA. The presence of significant titers (greater than 1:40) of serum ANA and/or ASMA has been observed in this setting as well. The terms *autoimmune cholangitis* and *AMA-negative PBC* have been applied to such patients. The clinical course and response to therapy with ursodeoxycholic acid (UDCA), however, are the same as in patients with AMA-positive PBC.

### 24. What is meant by an overlap or a variant syndrome in PBC and PSC?

The presence of features consistent with both autoimmune hepatitis (AIH) and PBC is defined as an overlap or a variant syndrome. Both serum ANA and AMA are present with increased titers by serologic testing. Lymphocytic piecemeal necrosis and coexistent portal inflammation with bile duct destruction are commonly seen. This group appears to benefit from either UDCA monotherapy, immunosuppressive treatment, or a combination of both treatments, in addition to UDCA. Using strict criteria, less than 20% of patients with PBC actually have objective evidence for an overlap syndrome with AIH. Recent data confirm that patients with typical PBC can develop autoimmune hepatitis years later despite successful therapy with UDCA.

Similar overlap occurs in PSC and AIH in both adult and pediatric populations. The multifocal biliary stricturing and dilation typical of PSC are often accompanied by histologic lesions seen in AIH. In patients with features of AIH and inflammatory bowel disease, cholangiography is recommended to exclude PSC, especially in the presence of abnormal serum liver biochemistries reflective of cholestasis. Patients with AIH-PSC overlap syndrome may benefit from immunosuppressive therapy. Using strict criteria, less than 5% of patients with PSC will have objective evidence for an overlap syndrome with AIH.

### 25. What is meant by *small duct PSC*?

*Small duct PSC* is defined by the presence of chronic cholestatic liver test abnormalities, liver histology compatible with PSC, and a normal biliary tree by cholangiography. Most patients also have a concurrent diagnosis of inflammatory bowel disease, but this may not be absolutely required in some cases. Approximately 30% to 40% of patients will progress to typical PSC over time. Histologic disease progression may occur without biliary tract involvement and can lead to hepatic failure necessitating liver transplantation. The median survival of patients with small duct PSC is favorable compared with individuals with typical PSC but reduced compared with the general population.

## 26. Describe the treatment of pruritus in patients with PBC and PSC.

Pruritus is a frequent complication of both diseases and creates difficult management options for patients with moderate to severe involvement. Cholestyramine relieves the itching associated with PBC and PSC by reducing serum bile acid levels in patients with cholestasis. In addition, it increases the intestinal excretion of bile acids by preventing their absorption. It is administered in 4-g doses (mixed with liquids) with meals or after breakfast for a total daily dose of 12 to 16 g. Cholestyramine should be given 1½ hours before or after other medications to avoid nonspecific binding and diminished intestinal absorption. Once the itching remits, the dosage should be reduced to the minimal amount that maintains relief.

Rifampin at a dosage of 300 to 600 mg/day also has been effective in relieving pruritus due to either p450 enzyme induction or inhibition of bile acid uptake. For refractory cases, phenobarbital may be added in a dose of 120 to 160 mg/day. Novel approaches for the treatment of severe or refractory pruritus include sertraline, ondansetron, naltrexone, and molecular adsorbent recirculation system (MARS) therapy for the removal of bile acids. Intractable pruritus is an indication for liver transplantation, which results in symptomatic relief.

## 27. How is osteopenia treated in patients with PBC and PSC?

There is no identified effective therapy for metabolic bone disease associated with PBC and PSC. As mentioned earlier, this is most often due to osteoporosis and infrequently to osteomalacia. However, low serum vitamin D levels can be corrected by administering 50,000 units up to 3 times/week or 1000 units daily.

Estrogen replacement therapy (ERT), especially when instituted soon after menopause, has been associated with the slowing of bone loss in women. In cholestatic patients, ERT was previously thought to be contraindicated because of the risk for drug-induced cholestasis. However, this problem does not appear to be associated with standard ERT, which was shown to improve osteoporosis in a recent retrospective study. It is prudent, however, to institute clinical and biochemical monitoring of treated patients within 2 to 3 months after starting estrogen therapy. Recent concerns about the safety of ERT, though, have resulted in diminished enthusiasm for its use. Positive early studies demonstrate significant increases in bone mineral density with alendronate. However, none of these studies has used fracture rate as a primary endpoint.

## 28. Describe the treatment of fat-soluble vitamin deficiency in PBC and PSC.

Problems with night vision due to vitamin A deficiency may be alleviated by oral replacement therapy. Decreased serum levels can be corrected with the oral administration of vitamin A (25,000 to 50,000 units) 2 or 3 times per week. Because excessive vitamin A intake has been associated with hepatotoxicity, serum levels should be frequently monitored. In patients with low vitamin E levels, oral replacement therapy with 400 units/day can be instituted, although replacement is not always effective. If prothrombin time (PT) levels improve after a trial of water-soluble vitamin K (5 to 10 mg/day for 1 week), patients should be maintained on this regimen indefinitely. Prolongation of PT may be associated with hepatic failure in treatment unresponsive cases.

## 29. Do lipid-lowering agents have a role in treatment of PBC and PSC?

Because patients with PBC and PSC do not appear to have an increased risk of atherosclerotic disease despite high serum cholesterol levels, lipid-lowering agents usually are not recommended. However, the decision to use lipid-lowering agents needs to be individualized as patients with PBC may still be at risk for coronary artery disease based on family history. Furthermore, there is no increased risk for hepatotoxicity with lipid-lowering agents in patients with PBC compared with the general population. In some patients with xanthelasma, cholestyramine may stabilize or even decrease the size of subcutaneous lipid deposits.

## 30. Describe the treatment of bacterial cholangitis in PSC.

Bacterial cholangitis in PSC should be treated with broad-spectrum parenteral antibiotics. The administration of ciprofloxacin results in high biliary concentrations and has broad gram-negative and gram-positive coverage. Similar results can be observed with other fluoroquinolones, such as norfloxacin and levofloxacin. Prophylactic therapy with oral fluoroquinolone therapy may reduce the frequency of recurrent cholangitis, although no controlled trial has been performed to support this conclusion.

## 31. What are the therapeutic options for biliary strictures in PSC?

Balloon dilation of dominant strictures by either transhepatic or endoscopic approaches can relieve biliary obstruction in PSC. Balloon dilation is most effective in patients with acute elevations of serum total bilirubin level or recent onset of bacterial cholangitis. It appears less effective in patients with longstanding jaundice or a history of recurrent bacterial cholangitis. The role for long-term endoscopic stent placement and exchange for recurrent PSC-related strictures, however, has not been assessed in a prospective controlled trial setting. Concerns regarding an increased rate of stent-related infection suggest their cautious use at this time. For malignant strictures related to cholangiocarcinoma, the use of expandable metal stents and/or photodynamic therapy have been recently employed for palliative treatment.

**32. Describe the role of transjugular intrahepatic portosystemic shunt (TIPS) in PBC and PSC.**

TIPS rapidly decompresses the portal system with subsequent reduction in local venous pressure within both esophageal and gastric varices. TIPS placement is indicated for refractory variceal bleeding or recalcitrant ascites from end-stage liver disease. In patients with PSC who have undergone proctocolectomy because of CUC, the development of peristomal varices with subsequent transfusion-dependent bleeding has been shown to resolve after TIPS placement. Serial Doppler ultrasound examinations every 3 to 6 months are required to exclude the possibility of TIPS shunt stenosis or occlusion.

**33. What medical agents have been tried for the treatment of PBC?**

A number of potential treatments for PBC have been evaluated to date with the primary goal of stabilizing or halting disease progression. Pharmacologic agents such as colchicine, corticosteroids, cyclosporine, azathioprine, methotrexate, and mycophenolate mofetil have demonstrated marginal clinical benefit and significant adverse effects. The efficacy of ursodeoxycholic acid (UDCA) as medical therapy for PBC has recently been questioned in a meta-analysis of randomized controlled trials. In five of the largest randomized, placebo-controlled clinical trials, UDCA in dosages of 13 to 15 mg/kg/day is associated with an estimated 30% risk reduction in the time to treatment failure or liver transplantation compared with placebo or inactive therapy. In contrast, there have been several cohort studies documenting increased short- and medium-term survival for patients with early-stage PBC responding to UDCA compared with the general population. However, an estimated 30% to 40% of patients still do not achieve a complete biochemical response after 6 to 12 months of UDCA, which places them at increased risk for histologic disease progression. UDCA has also been shown to reduce the risk of developing esophageal varices.

**34. What medical agents have been tried for the treatment of PSC?**

Because of the variable nature of disease progression in PSC, the development of randomized clinical trials for the assessment of medical therapies in PSC has been difficult. As a potential consequence, no identified effective treatment is available. As with PBC, the use of pharmacologic agents such as d-penicillamine, colchicine, corticosteroids, and immunosuppressive agents such as mycophenolate mofetil has not conferred significant clinical benefit. UDCA in standard doses (13 to 15 mg/kg/day) appears to improve biochemical parameters, but no significant effect on histology or survival has been observed. While higher doses of UDCA (20 to 30 mg/kg/day) were observed to improve biochemical, cholangiographic, and Mayo risk scores in two pilot investigations, a large prospective randomized, double-blind controlled trial in Europe failed to confirm these initial results. Results from a North American trial using even higher doses of UDCA also failed to demonstrate a survival benefit and raised concerns about safety in this population.

**35. Describe the mechanism of action for UDCA in PBC.**

UDCA is a hydrophilic, nonhepatotoxic compound that acts by attenuating the effect of endogenous hydrophobic bile acids, some of which are believed to be hepatotoxic. Alterations in the bile acid pool may occur by competition for ileal uptake sites or by direct action at the hepatocyte level. In addition, UDCA may reduce Class I and Class II HLA antigen expression on hepatocytes and biliary epithelial cells.

**36. What is the role of reconstructive biliary tract surgery in PSC?**

Choledochoduodenostomy and choledochojejunostomy are palliative measures to alleviate symptoms related to biliary obstruction. Reconstructive surgery does not have a beneficial effect on the natural history of PSC, particularly in patients with advanced liver disease. The development of postoperative bacterial cholangitis occurs in greater than 60% of patients. In addition, an increased risk for technical difficulty, increased blood product use, and mortality during liver transplantation has been associated with previous biliary reconstructive surgery At most centers, however, reconstructive biliary tract surgery is rarely performed for PSC because of improvements in endoscopic approaches to therapy.

**37. Does proctocolectomy in patients with PSC and CUC favorably affect hepatobiliary disease?**

Proctocolectomy has not been shown to have a beneficial effect on clinical outcome or survival in PSC. Currently, there is no indication to remove the colon in a patient with PSC in anticipation of a beneficial effect on liver disease. If carcinoma or precancerous lesions in the colon develop, a proctocolectomy is indicated. The development of peristomal varices after ileostomy creation is associated with considerable morbidity after proctocolectomy. Creation of an ileal pouch–anal anastomosis is recommended to avoid this significant complication.

**38. Do patients with PBC and PSC have an increased risk for hepatocellular carcinoma (HCC)?**

Recent information is controversial regarding the rate of HCC development in patients with end-stage liver disease from PBC. Screening and surveillance procedures, including abdominal ultrasound with serum alpha fetoprotein (AFP) levels every 6 months, may be useful for the early detection of HCC. An increased risk for HCC in patients with PSC also occurs in the setting of end-stage liver disease.

## 39. What is the role of liver transplantation in PBC and PSC?

The treatment of choice for patients with end-stage PBC and PSC is liver transplantation. Five- and 10-year survival rates of 85% and 70%, respectively, are among the highest for all individuals after liver transplantation. Factors that influence the consideration for liver transplantation are deteriorating hepatic synthetic function (defined as a Child-Turcotte-Pugh score $\geq 7$), intractable symptoms, and diminished quality of life. Refractory ascites, progressive hepatic encephalopathy, uncontrolled or recurrent variceal bleeding, spontaneous bacterial peritonitis, and hepatorenal syndrome are also indications for consideration of liver transplantation. Patients with PSC may also be considered for liver transplantation based on the development of recurrent bacterial cholangitis despite maximum medical therapy. In addition to increased survival, improvements in health-related quality of life after liver transplantation for patients with PBC and PSC have been documented in a number of published reports. A specialized protocol involving external beam and internal brachytherapy radiation, combined with chemotherapy and subsequent liver transplantation, has produced excellent short- and medium-term results for selected patients with early-stage cholangiocarcinoma from PSC.

## 40. Do PBC and PSC recur after liver transplantation?

Serum AMA levels decline then increase to baseline levels in most patients with PBC after liver transplantation. The cumulative incidence of recurrent PBC is between 15% and 30% over 10 years based on strict clinical and histological criteria. No significant impact on survival, however, has been associated with recurrent histologic disease. Tacrolimus-based immunosuppression is associated with a shorter time-to-recurrence than cyclosporine-based therapy. While initial data suggest a potentially useful role for UDCA in slowing disease progression among liver transplant recipients with early-stage, recurrent PBC, further studies are required to verify this initial observation.

Recurrent allograft disease with PSC has been reported, yet its true prevalence depends on establishing well-defined diagnostic criteria and the rigor of excluding patients with chronic ischemic biliary tract strictures from those with other causes. These include the presence of chronic ductopenic rejection, ABO incompatibility, prolonged cold ischemia time, cytomegalovirus infection, and hepatic artery thrombosis. Nevertheless, recent data suggest that approximately 20% to 30% of patients transplanted for PSC will develop recurrent disease over a 10-year period with some individuals requiring consideration for hepatic retransplantation.

## 41. What are the complications in PSC patients after liver transplantation?

Patients with PSC appear to have an increased incidence of chronic ductopenic rejection and ischemic biliary duct stricturing. Individuals with concurrent inflammatory bowel disease are at increased risk for increased colonic disease activity (30% to 40%), colonic dysplasia, and carcinoma.

## WEBSITES ⊕

http://www.aasld.org/

http://www.guideline.gov

## BIBLIOGRAPHY

1. Boberg KM, Bergquist A, Mitchell S, et al. Cholangiocarcinoma in primary sclerosing cholangitis: Risk factors and clinical presentation. Scand J Gastroenterol 2002;37:1205–11.
2. Charatcharoenwitthaya P, Pimentel S, Talwalkar JA, et al. Long-term survival and impact of ursodeoxycholic acid treatment for recurrent primary biliary cirrhosis after liver transplantation. Liver Transpl 2007;13:1236–45.
3. Dickson ER, Grambsch PM, Fleming TR, et al. Prognosis in primary biliary cirrhosis: Model for decision making. Hepatology 1989;10:1–7.
4. Fulcher AS, Turner MA, Franklin KJ, et al. Primary sclerosing cholangitis: Evaluation with MR cholangiography: A case-control study. Radiology 2000;215:71–80.
5. Graziadei IW, Wiesner RH, Batts KP, et al. Recurrence of primary sclerosing cholangitis following liver transplantation. Hepatology 1999;29:1050–6.
6. Graziadei IW, Wiesner RH, Marotta PJ, et al. Long-term results of patients undergoing liver transplantation for primary sclerosing cholangitis. Hepatology 1999;30:1121–7.
7. Heimbach JK, Haddock MG, Alberts SR, et al. Transplantation for hilar cholangiocarcinoma. Liver Transpl 2004;10:S65–8.
8. Kim WR, Therneau TM, Wiesner RH, et al. A revised natural history model for primary sclerosing cholangitis. Mayo Clin Proc 2000;75:688–94.
9. Lazaridis KN, Juran BD, Boe GM, et al. Increased prevalence of antimitochondrial antibodies in first-degree relatives of patients with primary biliary cirrhosis. Hepatology 2007;46:785–92.
10. Lindor KD, Dickson ER, Baldus WP, et al. Ursodeoxycholic acid in the treatment of primary biliary cirrhosis. Gastroenterology 1994;106:1284–90.
11. Menon KV, Angulo P, Weston S, et al. Bone disease in primary biliary cirrhosis: Independent indicators and rate of progression. J Hepatol 2000;35:316–23.

12. Moreno Luna LE, Kipp B, et al. Advanced cytologic techniques for the detection of malignant pancreatobiliary strictures. Gastroenterology 2006;131:1064–72.
13. Nichols JC, Gores GJ, LaRusso NF, et al. Diagnostic role of CA 19-9 for cholangiocarcinoma in patients with primary sclerosing cholangitis. Mayo Clin Proc 1993;68:874–9.
14. Olsson R, Boberg KM, de Muckadell OS, et al. High-dose ursodeoxycholic acid in primary sclerosing cholangitis: A 5-year multicenter, randomized, controlled study. Gastroenterology 2005;129:1464–72.
15. Parés A, Caballería L, Rodés J. Excellent long-term survival in patients with primary biliary cirrhosis and biochemical response to ursodeoxycholic acid. Gastroenterology 2006;130:715–20.
16. Talwalkar JA, Keach JC, Angulo P, et al. Overlap of autoimmune hepatitis and primary biliary cirrhosis: An evaluation of a modified scoring system. Am J Gastroenterol 2002;97:1191–7.
17. Talwalkar JA, Lindor KD. Primary biliary cirrhosis. Lancet 2003;362:53–61.

# HEPATITIS VACCINES AND IMMUNOPROPHYLAXIS

*Maria H. Sjögren, MD, COL (R), MC, and*
*Joseph G. Cheatham, MD, CPT, MC*

# CHAPTER 21

## 1. Discuss the concept of immunization (vaccination).

During the past century, major progress in the control of infectious diseases has become possible because of the remarkable developments in microbiology. The success of immunization in humans rests on one major concept: humans have specific immunologic mechanisms that can be programmed to provide a defense against infectious agents. The body's immune mechanism is stimulated by direct introduction of infectious agents or smaller components in the form of vaccines.

## 2. Outline briefly the history of vaccination.

In 1798, Edward Jenner described his work with cowpox vaccination. He demonstrated that a person inoculated and infected with cowpox was protected against smallpox. The procedure, which he termed *vaccination*, represented the first use of a vaccine for prevention of disease. The word *vaccine* is derived from the Latin word for "cow"; cows were host to the first true vaccine virus, cowpox. The evolution into the golden era of vaccine development began in 1949 with the discovery of virus propagation in cell culture. The first product developed by using the new cell culture technique was the Salk trivalent formalin-inactivated polio vaccine. After its success, vaccines to prevent human hepatitis A and B were developed rapidly, considering that the viral agents were discovered in 1973 and 1965, respectively.

## 3. Distinguish between active and passive immunization.

- *Active immunization* involves the introduction of a specific antigen to provoke an antibody response that will prevent disease.
- *Passive immunization* or *immunoprophylaxis* is the introduction of antibodies produced in an animal or human host by immunization or prior natural infection to prevent or modify the natural infection in a susceptible person.

## 4. What are the major categories of vaccines?

Two categories of vaccines are widely available:

- *Inactivated or killed vaccines*, in which the infectious agent is incapable of multiplying in the host but retains antigenic properties and evokes an antibody response
- *Live, attenuated vaccines,* which are prepared with live bacteria or viruses that have been altered making them incapable of inducing clinical disease. The end result is development of antibodies and prevention of infection. The live vaccines generally contain relatively low concentrations of the infectious agent. Ideally, only one administration is required with live vaccines, and the immunity is long-lasting. With killed vaccines, the immunologic response correlates with the concentration of the antigenic component. Inactivated vaccines commonly require a series of doses to stimulate a long-lasting immunologic response.

## 5. Describe the basic characteristics of immunoprophylaxis.

Immunoprophylaxis affords a relatively brief period of protection (weeks to a few months). Before the development of hepatitis A and B vaccines, immunoprophylaxis was the mainstay of preventing infection. Passive immunization occurs naturally in humans when maternal antibodies of the immunoglobulin G (IgG) class are passed to neonates. Such antibodies provide protection against many communicable bacterial and viral diseases for a period of months, during the period when the immune system has not yet fully developed. They disappear within the first year of life.

At the beginning of passive immunization therapy, the antibody-containing serum (e.g., horse serum) was administered directly. Currently, the antibody of interest is fractionated from serum and concentrated.

## 6. Which Igs are available for human use?

See Table 21-1.

**Table 21-1.** Immunoglobulins for Hepatitis Prophylaxis

| PRODUCT | SOURCE | USE |
|---|---|---|
| Immune serum globulin | Pooled human plasma | Prevents measles Prevents hepatitis A |
| Measles immunoglobulin | Pooled human plasma | Prevents measles |
| Hepatitis B immunoglobulin | Pooled plasma donors with high antibody titer | Used in accidental needlestick or sexual exposure |
| Rabies immunoglobulin | Pooled plasma from hyperimmunized donors | Immunotherapy for rabies |
| Botulism | Specific equine antibody | Treatment and prophylaxis for botulinum toxin |

## 7. Which viral agents are mainly responsible for acute and chronic viral hepatitis?

See Table 21-2.

**Table 21-2.** Viral Agents Responsible for Acute and Chronic Hepatitis

| ACUTE HEPATITIS | CHRONIC HEPATITIS | MAIN ROUTE OF TRANSMISSION | VACCINE STATUS |
|---|---|---|---|
| Hepatitis A virus (HAV) | No | Fecal-oral | Commercially available |
| Hepatitis B virus (HBV) | Yes | Bloodborne | Commercially available |
| Hepatitis C virus (HCV) | Yes | Bloodborne | Not available |
| Hepatitis D virus (HDV) | Yes | Bloodborne | Not available |
| Hepatitis E virus (HEV) | No | Fecal-oral | IND status |

IND, investigational new drug.

## 8. When should Ig be used?

Ig should be used to provide short-term protection in persons who require immediate immunity and are not ideal candidates for the vaccine (younger than 1 or older than 40 years of age, immunocompromised, or allergic) and in those requiring immediate immunity who have chronic liver disease. A single dose of hepatitis A monovalent vaccine or an accelerated dosing schedule of the bivalent TWINRIX vaccine (combination hepatitis A and hepatitis B vaccine) has been shown to be equally effective for preexposure immediate immunity compared with Ig. The monovalent vaccines are also now recommended as first line therapy for postexposure prophylaxis by the Centers for Disease Control and Prevention's Advisory Committee on Immunization Practices (ACIP), after a recent study comparing the vaccine to Ig (Ig) for postexposure prophylaxis met their noninferiority criteria (currently not approved by the U.S. Food and Drug Administration). The long-term protection gained if the booster doses of the vaccines are given according to schedule and the cost savings are clear advantages of the vaccine compared to Ig. Although considered safe, Ig may cause fever, myalgias, and considerable pain at injection sites. Ig reduces the individual's response to live attenuated virus (i.e., measles-mumps-rubella [MMR] and varicella) and adjustments to standard schedules must be made.

The recommended dose of IgG for adults is 0.02 mL/kg for preexposure when the period of exposure will not exceed 3 months. If the period of exposure is prolonged, 0.06 mL/kg every 5 months is recommended. Within 2 weeks after exposure to hepatitis A virus (HAV), 0.02 mL/kg of Ig is approximately 80% to 90% effective in preventing hepatitis A.

## 9. What vaccines are available for hepatitis A?

Two monovalent vaccines are commercially available in the United States:

- VAQTA, manufactured by Merck & Co., Inc.
- HAVRIX, manufactured by GlaxoSmithKline

A single dose of VAQTA has 100% protective efficacy. The initial trial included 1037 children, aged 2 to 16 years, and took place in an upstate New York community with a 3% annual incidence of acute hepatitis A. Children were randomized to receive one intramuscular injection of a highly purified, formalin-inactivated HAV vaccine or placebo. From day 50 until day 103 after injection, 25 cases of clinically apparent hepatitis developed in the placebo group and 0 developed in the vaccine group ($p < 0.001$). The vaccine gave a calculated 100% efficacy rate.

HAVRIX, when tested against placebo in more than 40,000 Thai children, gave a calculated 97% rate of protective efficacy after three doses. Two doses of either vaccine provide long-term immunity. Both are approved in the United States for subjects older than 12 months.

One combination vaccine containing both hepatitis A and hepatitis B antigens, TWINRIX, manufactured by GlaxoSmithKline, is currently licensed in the United States Three doses of TWINRIX administered on a 0-, 1-, and 6- month schedule produces equivalent antibody responses seen after the single monovalent vaccines are given separately on standard schedules. Due to lower seroconversion rates seen in children compared with the monovalent vaccines, it is restricted for use in individuals older than 18 years.

## 10. Compare the major characteristics of VAQTA, HAVRIX, and TWINRIX.
See Table 21-3.

**Table 21-3.** Comparison of VAQTA, HAVRIX, and TWINRIX Vaccines

|  | VAQTA | HAVRIX | TWINRIX |
|---|---|---|---|
| Type | Inactivated vaccine | Inactivated vaccine | Inactivated both A and B |
| HAV strain | Attenuated CR326F | Attenuated HMI75 | Attenuated HMI75 |
| Cell culture | Cultured in MRC-5 cells | Cultured in MRC-5 cells | Cultured in MRC-5 cells |
| Adjuvant | Aluminum hydroxide | Aluminum hydroxide | Aluminum hydroxide |
| Standards met | FDA, WHO | FDA, WHO | FDA, WHO |
| Immunity | Serum anti-HAV | Serum anti-HAV | Serum Anti-HAV and Anti-HBV |
| Route of administration | Intramuscular | Intramuscular | Intramuscular |
| Standard Adult doses | 1 ml (50 U) at 0 and 6 months | 1 ml (1440 U) at 0 and 6–12 months | 1 ml (720 U) at 0, 1 and 6 months |
| Pediatric doses (2–17 yr) | 0.5 ml (25 U) at 0 and 6–18 months | 0.5 ml (720 U) at 0 and 6–12 months | Not approved |
| Accelerated schedule | 1 dose ≥2 weeks prior to travel* | 1 dose ≥2 weeks prior to travel^ | 1 dose at 0, 7, and 21–30 days* |
| Postexposure prophlaxis | 1 dose <2 weeks after exposure*† | 1 dose <2 weeks after exposure*† | Not recommended |

*Boosters must be given for long-term protection: VAQTA at 6 mo, HAVRIX at 6–12 mo, and TWINRIX at 12 mo.
†ACIP but not FDA approved.
FDA, U.S. Food and Drug Administration; WHO, World Health Organization.

## 11. Who should be immunized against hepatitis A?
- All children older than 12 months
- Travelers to countries with high endemicity for hepatitis A virus infection
- Military personnel
- Persons with chronic liver diseases of any etiology
- Homosexually active men
- Users of illicit drugs
- Residents of communities experiencing a hepatitis A outbreak
- Persons with clotting factor disorders
- Certain institutional workers
- Employees of child day-care centers

## 12. What side effects have been observed with the hepatitis A vaccine?
- *1%–10%:* local reactions at injection site, such as induration, redness, and swelling; systemic reactions, such as fatigue, fever, or malaise; anorexia; nausea
- *Less than 1%:* hematoma at injection site, pruritus, skin rash, pharyngitis, upper respiratory tract infections, abdominal pain, diarrhea, vomiting, arthralgia, myalgia, lymphadenopathy, insomnia, photophobia, vertigo
- Hepatitis A vaccine should not be administered to persons with a history of hypersensitivity reactions to alum or, for HAVRIX, to the preservative 2-phenoxyethanol. The safety of hepatitis A vaccination during pregnancy has not been determined.

### 13. Do nonresponders to hepatitis A vaccine exist?

HAV vaccines are highly immunogenic in most healthy people. Some nonhealthy populations have a shown a lower anti-HAV titer after immunization, such as HIV-infected people and people with chronic liver disease.

### 14. What is the lowest protective anti-HAV serum level after immunization?

The lowest anti-HAV protective titer has not been established, but the ACIP defines the minimum as 20 mIU/mL.

### 15. Does the concurrent administration of hepatitis A vaccine influence the immune response to other traveler's vaccines?

Recent studies of 396 travelers who received vaccines against hepatitis A, poliomyelitis, hepatitis B, diphtheria, tetanus, yellow fever, Japanese encephalitis, typhoid fever, or rabies (according to individual needs) showed that concurrent administration of hepatitis A vaccine did not compromise the immune response to the hepatitis A or other vaccines.

### 16. What kind of immunoprophylaxis is available for hepatitis B?

- *Active immunization:* hepatitis B vaccine, first licensed in the United States in 1981, is recommended for both preexposure and postexposure prophylaxis.
- *Passive immunization:* hyperimmune globulin (HBIG) provides temporary passive protection and is indicated in certain postexposure situations.

### 17. What is the recommended dose of HBIG for adults and children?

HBIG contains high concentrations of anti-HBs, whereas regular Ig is prepared from plasma with varying concentrations of anti-HBs. In the United States, HBIG has an anti-HBs titer greater than 1:100,000 by radioimmunoassay.
See Table 21-4.

**Table 21-4.** Recommended Treatment after Exposure to Hepatitis B Virus

| | HBIG | | | VACCINE | |
| EXPOSURE | DOSE | TIMING | DOSE | TIMING |
| --- | --- | --- | --- | --- |
| Perinatal | 0.5 mL IM | Within 12 hours of birth | 0.5 mL at birth | Within 12 hr of birth; repeat at 1 and 6 mo |
| Sexual | 0.6 mL/kg IM | Single dose within 14 days of sexual contact | Same time as HBIG | Start immunization at once |

IM, intramuscularly; HBIG, hyperimmune globulin.

### 18. How many hepatitis B vaccines are available in the United States? Are they comparable?

Three vaccines have been licensed in the United States. For practical purposes, they are comparable in immunogenicity and efficacy rates, although the preparations are different:

- *Heptavax-B* (Merck & Co., Inc.) became available in 1986 and is no longer manufactured in the United States. It consists of hepatitis B surface antigen (HBsAg) purified from the plasma of chronically infected humans and evokes antibodies to the group a determinant of HBsAg, effectively neutralizing the various subtypes of HBV. Abundant evidence supports its efficacy, but it is expensive to prepare, and a number of physical and chemical inactivation steps are needed for purification and safety. Because of these problems, alternate approaches based on recombinant DNA technology were developed. Each milliliter of plasma-derived vaccine contains 20 mg of HBsAg.
- *Recombivax-HB*, also manufactured by Merck & Co., Inc., became available in 1989. It is a noninfectious, nonglycosylated HBsAg vaccine, subtype adw, made by recombinant DNA technology. Yeast cells (*Saccharomyces cerevisiae*) expressing the HBsAg gene are cultured, collected by centrifugation, and broken by homogenization with glass beads. HBsAg particles are purified and absorbed in aluminum hydroxide. Each milliliter contains 10 mg of HBsAg.
- *Engerix-B*, manufactured by GlaxoSmithKline Biologicals, is a noninfectious recombinant DNA vaccine. It contains purified HBsAg obtained by culturing genetically engineered *Saccharomyces cerevisiae* cells, which carry the surface antigen gene of HBV. This surface antigen is purified from the cells and adsorbed on aluminum hydroxide. Each milliliter has 20 mg of HBsAg.

### 19. What is the immunization schedule for HBV vaccine in adults and children?

See Table 21-5.

**Table 21-5.** Immunization Schedule for Hepatitis B Virus Vaccine in Adults and Children

| GROUP | FORMULATION | INITIAL | 1 MONTH | 6 MONTHS |
|---|---|---|---|---|
| **Recombivax-HB Vaccine** | | | | |
| Birth to 10 yr | Pediatric dose: 0.5 mL | 0.5 mL | 0.5 mL | 0.5 mL |
| Adults and older children | Adult dose: 10 mg/1.0 mL | 1.0 mL | 1.0 mL | 1.0 mL |
| Dialysis patients | Special dose: 40 mg/1.0 mL | 1.0 mL | 1.0 mL | 1.0 mL |
| **Engerix-B Vaccine** | | | | |
| Birth to 10 yr | Pediatric dose: 10 mg/0.5 mL | 0.5 mL | 0.5 mL | 0.5 mL |
| Adults and older children | Adult dose: 20 mg/1.0 mL | 1.0 mL | 1.0 mL | 1.0 mL |
| After needlestick injury | 20 mg/1.0 mL | 1.0 mL at 0, 1, and 2 mo | | |
| Hemodialysis patients | 40 mg/2.0 mL | 2.0 mL at 0, 1, 2, and 6 mo | | |

### 20. What is the recommended regimen for infants born to HBsAg-positive mothers?

Infants born to HBsAg-positive mothers should receive HBIG (0.5 mL) and the first dose of hepatitis B vaccine within 12 hours of birth. Females admitted for delivery without HBsAg test results should have blood drawn for testing. While test results are pending, the infant should receive hepatitis B vaccine without HBIG within 12 hours of birth (standard practice). See Table 21-6.

**Table 21-6.** Recommended Regimen for Infants Born to Hepatitis B Surface Antigen–Positive Mothers

| TREATMENT | BIRTH | WITHIN 7 DAYS | 1 MONTH | 6 MONTHS |
|---|---|---|---|---|
| Recombivax-HB (pediatric dose) | 0.5 mL | 0.5 mL | 0.5 mL | 0.5 mL |
| HBIG | 0.5 mL | None | None | None |

HBIG, hyperimmune globulin.

### 21. Is a booster needed after immunization? If so, how often?

Booster shots are not recommended for healthy adults or children. For immunocompromised patients (e.g., hemodialysis patients), a booster dose should be administered when anti-HBs levels drop to 10 mIU/mL or less.

### 22. Summarize the evidence for long-term immunization after vaccination.

The persistence of antibody directly correlates with the peak level achieved after the third dose. Follow-up of adults who were immunized with plasma-derived hepatitis B vaccine demonstrated that the antibody levels had fallen to undetectable or very low levels in 30% to 50% of recipients. Long-term studies of adults and children indicate that protection lasts at least 9 years, despite loss of anti-HBs in serum. After 9 years of follow-up, anti-HBs loss ranged from 13% to 60% in a group of homosexual men and Alaskan Eskimos, two groups at high risk of infection. However, vaccine recipients were virtually 100% protected from clinical illness, despite the absence of booster immunization. Among people without detectable anti-HBs, breakthrough infections have been noted in later years, based on the detection of hepatitis B core antibody. However, clinical illness did not occur, and HBsAg was not detected. The infection is assumed to be without consequence and to confer permanent immunity.

### 23. Is it possible that the vaccine will not protect against HBV infection?

Hepatitis B vaccines effectively evoke neutralizing antibodies to the group a determinant of HBsAg, which is believed to be formed by the highly conformational structure between amino acids 124 and 127. Some diversity has been demonstrated but probably does not affect neutralization of HBsAg. Hepatitis B mutants have been reported. Probably they arose randomly and were not corrected because of an intrinsic failure of the polymerase enzyme. Significant variants have been described in HBV vaccines, initially in Italy but also in Japan and Gambia. Italian investigators reported that 40 of 1600 immunized children showed evidence of HBV infection despite adequate antibody response to the HBV vaccine. The mutant virus had substitutions in amino acids 145 (Italy), 126 (Japan), and 141 (Gambia). Whether HBV mutants have substantial clinical significance is not known. Large-scale epidemiologic studies of the incidence, prevalence, and clinical correlation have not been performed.

### 24. Is it harmful to give hepatitis B vaccine to known hepatitis B carriers?

No deleterious effects were observed in 16 chronic carriers of HBsAg who received at least six monthly injections of hepatitis B vaccine. The vaccine was administered in an attempt to eliminate the chronic carrier status. However, no such result was observed. None of the volunteers lost HBsAg or developed anti-HBs. This finding simplified the design of hepatitis B vaccination programs.

### 25. Is it appropriate to use the therapeutic vaccines to Hepatitis B?

A recent study with inactive HBsAg carriers (patients had never received prior antiviral therapies) showed that the recombinant HBV vaccine had no great effect in enhancing the rate of HBsAg seroconversion in inactive HBsAg carriers.

### 26. Is it possible to immunize people simultaneously against hepatitis A and B?

To date, more than 1000 subjects have received a combined product of both vaccines. TWINRIX, which is commercially available in the United States and Europe, elicits antibodies to HAV and HBV in more than 80% of recipients by the second month. Limited long-term follow-up reports a 100% anti-HAV and a 95% anti-HBV response by 2 years after immunization. The combined vaccine appears to be safe, well tolerated, and highly immunogenic. The side effect profile is reportedly similar to that of the individual vaccines.

### 27. Is immunoprophylaxis advisable for hepatitis C?

No firm recommendation can be made for postexposure prophylaxis for hepatitis C. Study results are equivocal. Some experts recommend administration of Ig (0.06 mg/kg) after a bona fide percutaneous exposure. The Ig should be administered as soon as possible. However, work in chimpanzees has shown a lack of protectiveness when animals that received prophylaxis with Ig were challenged with HCV. Moreover, recent data show that in humans the neutralizing antibody evoked after infection with HCV is short-lived and does not protect against reinfection. Immunoprophylaxis for hepatitis C seems to be quite difficult. To date, there is no effective vaccine against HCV infection. Efforts to develop an HCV vaccine are complicated by the extensive genetic and possible antigenic diversity among HCV strains, the absence of a robust immunity after natural infection, and the lack of tissue culture systems and small animal models.

### 28. Is a vaccine available for hepatitis E?

At present, no commercially available vaccines exist for the prevention of hepatitis E. However, several studies for the development of an effective vaccine against hepatitis E are in progress.

A 56-kDa recombinant HEV-derived ORF2 protein has been used to vaccinate rhesus monkeys against different strains of hepatitis E virus (HEV). Recent studies demonstrated that recombinant hepatitis E vaccine suitable for clinical evaluation was highly immunogenic and efficacious in preventing hepatitis E and even infection in rhesus monkeys following intravenous challenge with three different genotypes of HEV. Two doses of vaccine were essential for optimal protection. The titers of anti-HEV that were protective in this study were quantified against a World Health Organization (WHO) standard. The results of this preclinical trial of a candidate hepatitis E vaccine strongly suggest that it will be highly efficacious for preventing hepatitis E in the field trial of this vaccine that is currently in progress in Nepal (an endemic setting).

### 29. Should patients with chronic liver disease be immunized against hepatitis A and hepatitis B?

- Acute hepatitis A has resulted in higher morbidity and mortality rates in healthy people older than 40 years of age and in people with chronic hepatitis C. HAV vaccine is safe and effective in people with chronic liver disease and may prevent additional injury to an already compromised liver.
- Acute hepatitis B has not been shown to induce high mortality rates in people with chronic liver disease; however, preventing further hepatic injury seems logical and wise. A recent review showed that the cost-effective analyses have yielded encouraging results regarding the immunization to prevent HAV infection in all patients with chronic liver disease.

## WEBSITE

http://www.cdc.gov/ncidod/diseases/hepatitis/b/

**BIBLIOGRAPHY**

1. Bock HL, Kruppenbacher JP, Bienzle U, et al. Does the concurrent administration of an inactivated hepatitis A vaccine influence the immune response to other travelers' vaccines? J Travel Med 2000;7:74–8.
2. Carman WF, Zanetti AR, Karayaiannis P, et al. Vaccine-induced escape mutants of hepatitis B virus. Lancet 1990;336:325–9.

3. Centers for Disease Control and Prevention. Hepatitis B virus: A comprehensive strategy for eliminating transmission in the United States through universal childhood vaccination. MMWR 1991;40/RR-13:10.
4. Centers for Disease Control and Prevention. Prevention of hepatitis A through active or passive immunization. Recommendations of the Advisory Committee on Immunization Practices. MMWR 2006;55/RR-07:1–23.
5. Centers of Disease Control and Prevention. Update: Prevention of hepatitis A after exposure to hepatitis A virus and in international travelers. Updated recommendations of the Advisory Committee on Immunization Practices (ACIP). MMWR 2007;56:1080–4.
6. Centers for Disease Control and Prevention. Update: Recommendations to prevent hepatitis B virus transmission—United States. MMWR 1999;48:33–4.
7. Chen HL, Chang MH, Ni YH, et al. Seroepidemiology of hepatitis B virus infection in children: Ten years of mass vaccination in Taiwan. JAMA 1996;276:906–8.
8. Connor BA, Blatter MM, Trofa AF, et al. Rapid and sustained immune response against hepatitis A and B achieved with combined vaccine using an accelerated administration schedule. J Travel Med 2007;14:9–15.
9. Diaz-Mitoma F, Law B, Hoet B. Long-term antibody persistence induced by a combined hepatitis A and B vaccine in children and adolescents. Vaccine 2008;26:1759–63.
10. Emerson SU, Purcell RH. Running like water—The omnipresence of hepatitis E. N Engl J Med 2004;351:2367–8.
11. Fan PC, Chang MH, Lee PI, et al. Follow-up immunogenicity of an inactivated hepatitis A vaccine in healthy children: Results after 5 years. Vaccine 1998;16:232–5.
12. Hadler SC, Francis DP, Maynard J, et al. Long-term immunogenicity and efficacy of hepatitis B vaccine in homosexual men. N Engl J Med 1986;315:209–14.
13. Keefe EB, Iwarson S, McMahon BJ, et al. Safety and immunogenicity of hepatitis A vaccine in patients with chronic liver disease. Hepatology 1998;27:881–6.
14. Lee PI, Chang LY, Lee CY, et al. Detection of hepatitis B surface gene mutation in carrier children with or without immunoprophylaxis at birth. J Infect Dis 1997;176:427–30.
15. Nothdurft HD, Dietrich M, Vollmar J, et al. A new accelerated vaccination schedule for rapid protection against hepatitis A and B. Vaccine 2002;20:1157–62.
16. Parkman PD, Hopps HE, Meyer HM. Immunoprevention of infectious diseases. In: Nohmias AJ, O'Reilly RJ, editors. Immunology. New York: Plenum; 1982. p. 561–83.
17. Plotkin S, Plotkin S. A short history of vaccine. In: Plotkin S, Mortimer E, editors. Vaccines. 2nd ed Philadelphia: WB Saunders; 1988. p. 1–7.
18. Prevention and control of infections with hepatitis viruses in correctional settings. MMWR 2003;52/RR-18:34.
19. Purcell RH, et al. Pre-clinical immunogenicity and efficacy trial of a recombinant hepatitis E vaccine. Vaccine 2003;2:2607–15.
20. Qiao M, Murata K, Davis AR, et al. Hepatitis C virus-like particles combined with novel adjuvant systems enhance virus-specific immune responses. Hepatology 2003;37:52.
21. Ryan ET, Kain K. Health advice and immunization for travelers. N Engl J Med 2000;342:1716–25.
22. Siberry G, Coller R, Hutten A, et al. Antibody response to hepatitis A immunization among human immunodeficiency virus-infected children and adolescents. Pediatr Infect Dis J 2008;27:465–8.
23. Sjogren M. Immunization and the decline of viral hepatitis as a cause of acute liver failure. Hepatology 2003;38:554–6.
24. Surveillance for acute viral hepatitis, United States—2006. MMWR Morb Mortal Wkly Rep 2008;57:1–24.
25. Taliani G, et al. Hepatitis A: Post-exposure prophylaxis. Vaccine 2003;21:2234–7.
26. Thoelen S, Van Damme P, Leentvaar-Kuypers A, et al. The first combined vaccine against hepatitis A and B: An overview. Vaccine 1999;17:1657–62.
27. Victor JC, Monto AS Margolis HS. Hepatitis A vaccine versus immune globulin for postexposure prophylaxis. N Engl J Med 2007;357:1685–94.
28. Wainwright RD, McMahon B, Bulkow L, et al. Duration of immunogenicity and efficacy of hepatitis B vaccine in a Yupik Eskimo population. JAMA 1989;261:2362–6.
29. Whittle HC, Inskip H, Hall AJ, et al. Vaccination against hepatitis B and protection against viral carriage in the Gambia. Lancet 1991;337:747–50.
30. Yalcin K, Acar M, Degertekin H, et al. Specific hepatitis B vaccine therapy in inactive HbsAg carriers: A randomized controlled trial. Infection 2003;31:221–5.

# PREGNANCY AND LIVER DISEASE

*Christine J. Bruno, MD, and*
*Roshan Shrestha, MD*

## NORMAL ANATOMICAL AND PHYSIOLOGIC CHANGES DURING PREGNANCY

**1. What are the structural and functional hepatic adaptations during pregnancy?**

Liver size and histology do not change. Maternal blood volume and cardiac output increase significantly, without a corresponding increase in hepatic blood flow, with a net decrease in fractional blood flow to the liver. An enlarging uterus makes venous return via the inferior vena cava progressively more difficult toward term. Blood is shunted via the azygous system with possible development of esophageal varices.

**2. Does liver function change during pregnancy?**

Hepatic function remains normal during pregnancy, but the normal range of laboratory values changes because of hormonal changes and an increase in blood volume with subsequent hemodilution. Aspartate aminotransferase (AST), alanine aminotransferase (ALT), γ-glutamyl transpeptidase (GGTP), bilirubin, and prothrombin remain within normal limits. Total alkaline phosphatase (AP) is elevated. The placenta is the major source of AP; levels return to normal within 20 days after delivery. Estrogen increases the synthesis of fibrinogen, as well as other coagulation proteins (factors VII, VIII, IX, and X). Attributed also to estrogen's effects are significant increases in serum concentrations of major lipid classes (triglycerides, cholesterol, and low- and very-low-density lipoproteins). These levels may be twice the normal limit of nonpregnant women of the same age. Serum albumin decreases slightly, contributing to the approximately 20% decline in serum protein concentration. Plasma concentrations of other serum proteins (ceruloplasmin, corticosteroids, testosterone, serum binding protein for thyroxine), as well as vitamin D and folate, also increase during pregnancy.

## DISEASES DURING PREGNANCY

- Coincident occurrence of liver disease (viral hepatitis, alcoholic hepatitis, gallstone disease, autoimmune hepatitis)
- Intrahepatic cholestasis of pregnancy (IHCP)
- Acute fatty liver of pregnancy (AFLP)
- Hemolysis, elevated liver enzymes, and low platelet count (HELLP syndrome)

**3. Can gestational age differentiate between different liver diseases in pregnancy?**

Most definitely. Hyperemesis gravidarum presents in the first trimester of pregnancy. Patients have severe nausea and vomiting, and about one-half have associated elevations of bilirubin, AST, or ALT. Cholestasis of pregnancy, viral hepatitis, and abnormal liver chemistries due to cholelithiasis may present at any point in gestation, from the first to the third trimester. AFLP and preeclamptic liver disease (HELLP, hepatic infarct, and hepatic rupture) are specifically encountered in the third trimester of pregnancy. Both herpes simplex virus and hepatitis E virus are exacerbated in pregnancy and usually present in the third trimester. The presentation may be a mild elevation in transaminases or severe hepatic failure. Budd-Chiari syndrome presents from the second half of pregnancy to 3 months postpartum.

## COINCIDENT OCCURRENCE

**4. Can we assume the presence of chronic liver disease in a pregnant patient with angiomas and palmar erythema on physical examination and small esophageal varices detected endoscopically?**

No. Spider angiomas and palmar erythema are common and appear in about two-thirds of pregnant women without liver disease. Small esophageal varices are present in approximately 50% of healthy pregnant women without liver disease because of the increased flow in the azygous system.

**5. What is the most common cause of jaundice in pregnancy?**

Viral hepatitis.

**6. How severe is the course of viral hepatitis acquired during pregnancy?**
- *Hepatitis A, B, and C* run a similar course in pregnant and nonpregnant patients.
- *Hepatitis E* runs a different course in pregnancy. It is fulminant in up to 20% of patients, compared with less than 1% of nonpregnant women. The fatality rate is 1.5% during the first trimester, 8.5% during the second trimester, and up to 21% during the third trimester compared with 0.5% to 4% in nonpregnant women. Fetal complications and neonatal deaths are increased if infection is acquired in the third trimester of pregnancy.
- *Herpes simplex hepatitis* can be fulminant in pregnancy and associated with high mortality rates. Patients present in the third trimester with fever, systemic symptoms, and possibly vesicular cutaneous rash. Associated pneumonitis or encephalitis may be present. Liver biopsy is characteristic, showing necrosis and inclusion bodies in viable hepatocytes, along with few or no inflammatory infiltrates. Response to acyclovir therapy is prompt; there is no need for immediate delivery of the baby.

**7. What signs and symptoms suggest the diagnosis of Budd-Chiari syndrome?**
The clinical triad of sudden onset of abdominal pain, hepatomegaly, and ascites, near term or shortly after delivery. Ascitic fluid shows a high protein content in about one-half of cases. Biopsy typically shows centrilobular hemorrhage and necrosis, along with sinusoidal dilation and erythrocyte extravasation into the space of Disse. Hepatic scintigraphy and computed tomography (CT) typically show compensatory hypertrophy of the caudate lobe due to its separate drainage into the inferior vena cava. Doppler analysis of portal and hepatic vessels and magnetic resonance imaging (MRI) establish hepatic vein occlusion.

**8. Is the serum ceruloplasmin level a good diagnostic marker in pregnant women at term who are suspected of having Wilson disease?**
No. Ceruloplasmin levels increase gradually during pregnancy, reaching the maximum at term. Because of this, a patient with Wilson disease who usually has a low level of ceruloplasmin may have it increase misleadingly into the normal range (greater than 20 mg/dL) during pregnancy.

**9. Can we maintain a woman with Wilson disease on therapy during pregnancy?**
Absolutely. Therapy must continue during pregnancy; otherwise, the mother is at risk for hemolytic episodes associated with fulminant hepatic failure. Agents approved by the U.S. Food and Drug Administration are D-penicillamine, trientine, and zinc. Evidence indicates that penicillamine and trientine (tissue copper-chelating agents) are teratogenic in animal studies, and there are reports of penicillamine effects in humans, including cutis laxis syndrome or micrognathia, low-set ears, and other abnormalities. According to the current consensus, penicillamine and trientine are safe in doses of 0.75 to 1 g/day during the first two trimesters; the dosage should be reduced to 0.5 g/day during the last trimester and in nursing mothers. Zinc therapy is an attractive alternative with a different mechanism of action; it induces synthesis of metallothionein, which sequesters copper in enterocytes, blocking its absorption. No teratogenic effects have been reported in animals or humans. The recommended doses are 50 mg 3 times/day for patients with 24-hour urinary copper values greater than 0.1 mg and 25 mg 3 times/day for patients with lower urinary copper values. Close monitoring of urinary copper and zinc levels is suggested; the zinc dose should be adjusted accordingly.

## INTRAHEPATIC CHOLESTSIS OF PREGNANCY

**10. What is the most common liver disorder unique to pregnancy?**
Intrahepatic cholestasis of pregnancy (IHCP).

**11. What is the major clinical manifestation of IHCP?**
Severe pruritus with onset in the second or, more commonly, third trimester (more than 70% of cases).

**12. What biochemical changes are noted in IHCP?**
Serum bile acids, often measured as cholylglycine, increase by 10- to 100-fold. Serum levels of AP rise by 7- to 10-fold, along with a modest rise in serum levels of 5′-nucleotidase (confirming the hepatic source of AP). AST, ALT, and direct bilirubin also rise. No evidence of hemolysis is found. GGTP is usually normal, as is prothrombin time (PT), unless cholestyramine treatment leads to malabsorption.

**13. What is the expected clinical and biochemical course after delivery for patients with IHCP?**
Pruritus should improve promptly after delivery (within 24 hours). Jaundice is rare and, if present, may persist for days. Biochemical abnormalities may persist for months.

14. **What is a possible cause for abnormal bleeding in a postpartum woman previously diagnosed with IHCP? What is the treatment?**

    Malabsorption of liposoluble vitamins, including vitamin K, especially in patients treated with cholestyramine for pruritus. The international normalized ratio (INR) corrects with parenteral administration of vitamin K.

15. **What is the effect of IHCP on the fetus?**

    Fetal distress requiring cesarean section develops in about 30% to 60% of cases. Prematurity occurs in about 50% of cases and fetal death in up to 9% of affected pregnancies. All of these effects are more likely if the disorder begins early in pregnancy.

16. **What is the therapy for IHCP?**

    Alleviating pruritus is the main goal. Therapeutic agents include:

    - Ursodeoxycholic acid, ≈15 mg/kg/day; up to 24 mg/kg/day studied with good results
    - Cholestyramine, 4 g 4 or 5 times/day (bile acid–binding resin)
    - Hydroxyzine hydrochloride (Atarax) or pamoate (Vistaril) (antihistamines); Atarax 25-50 mg every 6 hours as needed, Vistaril 15-30 mg every 6 hours as needed
    - Phenobarbital, 100 mg/day (choleretic and centrally acting sedative)
    - Phototherapy with ultraviolet B light as directed by a dermatologist

    Vitamin K before delivery is highly recommended to minimize the risk of postpartum hemorrhage. Mother and fetus should be observed closely. Elective induction is recommended at 36 weeks (severe cases) or 38 weeks (average cases) if the fetal lungs have matured.

17. **Can IHCP recur?**

    Yes. About 40% to 70% of subsequent pregnancies show evidence of mild intrahepatic cholestasis. The same pattern can be seen with use of estrogen-containing contraceptives.

18. **What atypical signs and symptoms make the diagnosis of IHCP doubtful?**

    Fever, hepatosplenomegaly, pain, jaundice preceding or without pruritus, and pruritus after delivery or before 21 weeks of pregnancy, especially with a singleton pregnancy, should prompt the search for an alternate diagnosis.

19. **What biochemical changes suggest an alternate diagnosis?**
    - Normal AST and ALT levels
    - Elevated AP and GGTP (i.e., biliary disease)
    - Predominantly unconjugated hyperbilirubinemia (i.e., hemolysis)

## ACUTE FATTY LIVER OF PREGNANCY

20. **What are the clinical and laboratory features of AFLP?**

    AFLP is a rare disorder with an incidence of 1 in 13,000 to 1 in 16,000 pregnancies. Onset occurs in the second half of pregnancy, usually during the third trimester, although occasionally postpartum onset is reported. Clinical manifestations include nausea and vomiting, jaundice, malaise, thirst, and altered mental status. Severe cases progress rapidly to hypoglycemia, disseminated intravascular coagulation (DIC), renal insufficiency, coma, and death. Signs of coexistent preeclampsia may be present, such as moderately increased arterial blood pressure, proteinuria, and hyperuricemia. Laboratory abnormalities consist of moderate AST/ALT elevations (usually less than 1000), conjugated hyperbilirubinemia, elevated PT, fibrin split products, and D-dimers, along with low platelet count, elevated levels of ammonia and serum uric acid, and leukocytosis. Hypoglycemia is a sign of extreme severity; blood glucose levels must be monitored closely.

21. **How do we diagnose and treat AFLP?**

    High clinical suspicion is crucial for early recognition and appropriate management. AFLP is suggested by hepatic failure at or near term or shortly after delivery in the absence of risk factors or serology suggesting viral hepatitis. Thirst, a symptom of underlying vasopressin-resistant diabetes insipidus, is characteristic to AFLP or HELLP syndrome. Liver biopsy, if feasible, is diagnostic in the appropriate clinical context. Treatment consists of admission to hospital, close monitoring by a multidisciplinary team (hepatologist, maternal-fetal medicine specialist, intensive care specialist) and immediate delivery. Recovery is usually complete, although it may be delayed in patients with significant clinical complications before delivery (e.g., DIC, renal failure, infections).

22. **Is biopsy pathognomonic for AFLP?**

    Biopsy is confirmatory but not pathognomonic or indispensable in making the diagnosis. Histology is characterized by microvesicular fatty infiltration, mostly in centrilobular zones. In general, lobular and trabecular architecture is preserved, and inflammatory infiltrates and cell necrosis are mild, if present at all. AFLP is a systemic disorder. Similar fatty changes have been noted in pancreatic acinar cells and tubular epithelial cells of the kidneys. The same prominent microvesicular steatosis is seen in other conditions such as Reye syndrome, sodium valproate toxicity, Jamaican vomiting sickness, and congenital defects of urea cycle enzymes or beta-oxidation of fatty acids.

### 23. Describe the pathogenesis of AFLP.

Pathogenesis remains somewhat unclear. AFLP seems to be a fetal-maternal interaction. In some cases the fetus has an isolated deficiency of long chain 3-hydroxyacyl-CoA dehydrogenase (LCHAD), which leads to a disorder of mitochondrial fatty acid oxidation. The inheritance pattern is recessive and involves a mutation from glutamic acid to glutamine at amino acid residue 474 (Glu474Gln) on at least one allele. It is hypothesized that in the presence of this mutation in homozygous or compound heterozygote fetuses, long-chain fatty acid metabolites produced by the fetus or placenta accumulate in the mother and are highly toxic to the maternal liver. The mother is phenotypically normal; her genotype does not correlate with development of AFLP.

### 24. What is the outcome of a child whose mother has AFLP?

Previously reported fetal mortality rates of 75% to 90% have been significantly reduced by better awareness, earlier diagnosis, availability of neonatal intensive care units, and institution of close monitoring and dietary treatment through childhood. In pregnancies associated with LCHAD defects, children present at a mean age of 7.6 months (range, 0 to 60 months) with acute hepatic dysfunction (incidence of 79%). They may experience hypoketotic hypoglycemia, hypotonia, hepatomegaly, hepatic encephalopathy, high transaminase levels, and fatty liver. The condition may progress rapidly to coma and death. Frequent feedings of a low-fat diet in which the fats are medium-chain triglycerides prevent hypoketotic hypoglycemic liver dysfunction. According to recent studies, 67% of children treated with dietary modification are alive, and most attend school.

### 25. Does AFLP recur in subsequent pregnancies?

In the cases associated with LCHAD defects, the disorder is recessive, affecting one in four fetuses. The rate of recurrence of maternal liver disease is 15% to 25%.

### 26. Is genetic testing indicated in women diagnosed with AFLP?

All women with AFLP, as well as their partners and children, should be advised to undergo molecular diagnostic testing. Testing for Glu474Gln only in the mother is not sufficient to rule out LCHAD deficiency in the fetus or other family members.

## HEMOLYSIS, ELEVATED LIVER ENZYMES, AND LOW PLATELETS (HELLP)

### 27. What is the spectrum of liver involvement in preeclampsia?

Liver involvement in preeclampsia ranges from subclinical, with biopsy evidence of fibrinogen deposition along hepatic sinusoids, to several possibly severe disorders. In patients with HELLP syndrome, the chief complaint is abdominal pain, which usually presents in the second half of gestation but may occur up to 7 days after delivery (almost 30% of affected women). Hepatic infarction is another rare manifestation of liver involvement in preeclampsia. Patients present in the third trimester or early after delivery with unexplained fever, leukocytosis, abdominal or chest pain, and extremely elevated aminotransferases (greater than 3000). The diagnosis depends on visualization of hepatic infarcts on CT contrast images or MRI. Subcapsular hematomas and hepatic rupture are life-threatening complications with high morbidity and mortality rates. A high index of suspicion and early CT imaging allow diagnosis and prompt intervention.

### 28. How common is HELLP syndrome?

The incidence of HELLP syndrome is 0.2% to 0.6% in all pregnancies and 4% to 12% in preeclamptic patients. The incidence is higher in multiparous, white, and older women, but the mean age of occurrence is around 25 years.

### 29. Describe the incidence and prognosis of spontaneous intrahepatic hemorrhage.

Spontaneous intrahepatic and subcapsular hemorrhage occurs in about 1% to 2% of patients with preeclampsia, with an estimated incidence of 1 in 45,000 live births. Prognosis improves with awareness, early diagnosis by imaging studies, and aggressive surgical management. Recent reported maternal mortality rates range from 33% to 49%. Fetal mortality remains high (≈60%).

### 30. What findings typically lead to the diagnosis of HELLP syndrome?

Diagnosis relies on typical laboratory evidence of liver involvement with associated thrombocytopenia. Not all patients have clinical hypertension or proteinuria at presentation. Liver test abnormalities are hepatocellular. Liver function is normal. Thrombocytopenia is present, usually less than 100,000/mm$^3$. Hemolysis is mild, with microangiopathic findings on peripheral smear. Biopsy is characteristic but may be extremely risky and is not needed for diagnosis. It shows periportal hemorrhage, fibrin deposition, and necrosis, possibly with steatosis and/or deposition of fibrinogen along sinusoids with focal parenchymal necrosis. A normal biopsy does not exclude the diagnosis, because involvement may be patchy.

## 31. What is the treatment for severe preeclamptic liver disease?

The initial priority is to stabilize the mother, by administering intravenous fluids, correcting any concurrent coagulopathy, administering magnesium for seizure prophylaxis, and treating severe hypertension. Early hepatic imaging is indicated to rule out infarcts or hematomas. Fetal functional status should be determined. Fetal outcome is related mostly to gestational age. Beyond 34 weeks of gestation with evidence of fetal lung maturity, delivery is the recommended therapy. If fetal lungs are immature, the fetus can be delivered 48 hours after administration of two doses of steroids. Termination of pregnancy should be attempted immediately with evidence of fetal or maternal distress. In cases of ruptured subcapsular hematoma, massive transfusions and immediate surgical intervention are required. In cases where surgical intervention is not possible and there are of signs and symptoms of acute liver failure liver, transplantation should be considered for survival.

## 32. Does HELLP recur in subsequent pregnancies?

Possibly. Studies report recurrence risks as low as 3.4% and as high as 25%.

## 33. What information helps to differentiate AFLP from HELLP?

At presentation, AFLP and HELLP may be difficult to differentiate. Hypertension is usually but not invariably associated with HELLP syndrome. Patients with HELLP have mild, predominantly unconjugated hyperbilirubinemia due to hemolysis, along with severe thrombocytopenia, but no laboratory values suggestive of hepatic failure. Laboratory abnormalities are significantly more severe in AFLP; evidence of hepatic synthetic failure manifests as prolonged PT and significant hypoglycemia in advanced stages. Fibrinogen is low, and ammonia is elevated. Biopsy shows microvesicular steatosis, predominantly in the central zone, in patients with AFLP, whereas patients with HELLP show predominantly periportal fibrin deposition, necrosis, and hemorrhage.

## 34. Is prospective screening necessary in pregnancies complicated by AFLP or HELLP?

From 15% to 20% of pregnancies complicated by AFLP and less than 2% of pregnancies complicated by HELLP syndrome are associated with fetal LCHAD deficiency. Newborns should be screened prospectively at birth in all pregnancies complicated by AFLP. Homozygosity and heterozygosity for the Glu474Gln would indicate the need for avoidance of prolonged fasting and replacement of dietary long-chain fatty acids with medium-chain fatty acids. Parents and physicians should be educated in the risk of metabolic crises and sudden death and instructed in the need for early intervention with intravenous glucose during episodes of vomiting, lethargy, and even minor illnesses.

Recent results do not justify routine screening of newborns in pregnancies complicated by HELLP syndrome. Molecular diagnostic testing should, however, be considered in women with recurrent HELLP syndrome in multiple pregnancies.

## CARE OF PATIENTS WITH PREEXISTING LIVER DISEASE

### BEFORE AND DURING PREGNANCY

- Contraception
- Management of underlying liver disease
- Management of portal hypertension
- Management in the setting of transplantation
- Prevention of vertical transmission

### CONTRACEPTION

## 35. What methods of contraception are available for patients with liver disease?

Patients with advanced or untreated liver disease commonly experience amenorrhea and infertility. If clinical improvement leads to restoration of fertility, multiple methods of contraception are available, including barrier methods and intrauterine devices. Tubal ligation may be used in women who have completed their families. Estrogen-based contraceptive agents are generally contraindicated, especially for patients with acute liver disease, but progestin contraceptives are safe alternatives. Combination contraceptives are absolutely contraindicated in patients with cholestatic jaundice of pregnancy or jaundice with prior use, and World Health Organization is listing them as category 4 type of drugs for patients with decompensated cirrhosis of any etiology. Numerous formulations and delivery systems are available.

# MANAGEMENT OF UNDERLYING LIVER DISEASE

## 36. How should patients with preexisting liver disease be managed if pregnancy occurs?

Patients are best managed by a multidisciplinary team that includes a maternal-fetal medicine specialist, perinatologist, and hepatologist. They have an increased risk for maternal complications along with a higher incidence of fetal wastage and prematurity. In general, patients should be maintained on the previous therapy that was successful in controlling liver disease and restoring fertility. Women with autoimmune hepatitis should be continued on corticosteroids alone or in combination with azathioprine, which is not teratogenic at the usual dose. Patients with Wilson disease should be continued on the anticopper agent. Patients with portal hypertension should have a baseline endoscopy. If they have never bled and medium or large varices are present, they are at increased risk for variceal hemorrhage during pregnancy. Primary prophylaxis with a nonselective beta blocker or isosorbide mononitrate should be instituted. The fetus should be monitored for bradycardia or growth retardation if the mother is maintained on beta blockers. Variceal bleeding is safely managed with variceal band ligation or sclerotherapy. Octreotide in customary doses is safe in pregnancy. Performing surgical portacaval shunts for patients with well-preserved liver function is possible. Placement of a transjugular intrahepatic portosystemic shunt and splenectomy (in patients with massive splenomegaly, varices, and thrombocytopenia) also have been reported.

# MANAGEMENT OF PORTAL HYPERTENSION

## 37. What are the effects of pregnancy on the mother with portal hypertension?

The morbidity rate is 30% to 50% because of possible onset of hepatic encephalopathy, spontaneous bacterial peritonitis, and progressive liver failure. The incidence of variceal hemorrhage is 19% to 45%, especially in the second trimester and during labor. Postpartum hemorrhage is seen in 7% to 10% of women, most frequently in those with cirrhotic portal hypertension; thrombocytopenia plays a major role. The mortality rate of these complications is 4% to 7% in noncirrhotic and 10% to 18% in cirrhotic patients with portal hypertension. Data regarding this topic originate mostly from case series and prospectively acquired data are few.

## 38. What is the effect of maternal portal hypertension on pregnancy?

Spontaneous abortion rates for patients with cirrhosis range from 15% to 20%. Most cases occur in the first trimester. Of interest, patients with extrahepatic portal hypertension and patients with well-compensated cirrhosis who underwent surgical shunting before conception have abortion rates similar to the general population. The incidence of premature termination of pregnancy in the second and third trimesters is similar in all of the above groups. Fetal mortality rates are around 50% if the mother requires emergent surgical intervention for variceal hemorrhage. Perinatal mortality rates in cirrhotic mothers are as high as 11% to 18% because of premature delivery, stillbirth, and neonatal death, but they are similar to those for the general population in noncirrhotic patients with portal hypertension and patients who underwent previous portal surgical decompressive procedures.

# MANAGEMENT IN THE SETTING OF ORTHOTOPIC LIVER TRANSPLANTATION

## 39. When can a liver transplant recipient actively seek conception?

At least a 1-year waiting period is advisable. Case reports suggest that conception close to the transplant date may result in increased maternal and fetal morbidity and mortality. Contraception should be instituted before resuming sexual relations, preferably with barrier methods.

## 40. Is pregnancy possible after liver transplantation?

Pregnancy will become possible once normal menstrual cycles resume. In women with chronic liver disease, most pretransplant amenorrhea resolves in approximately 3 to 10 months following liver transplantation.

## 41. What are the possible complications of pregnancies occurring after liver transplantation?

Hypertensive complications, preterm delivery, infection and fetal growth restriction. Immunosuppressive agents used such as cyclosporine and tacrolimus cause hypertension and renal insufficiency, as well as impairment of placental amino acid transport systems, leading to fetal growth restriction. Cytomegalovirus (CMV) infection can cause congenital anomalies and liver disease if the mother was infected early in the pregnancy. Risk for CMV infection is greatest immediately after transplant or in case of increased immunosuppression due to rejection episodes. Rejection is a rare complication; only about 10% of the reported pregnancies have been complicated by biopsy-proved rejection.

**42. What is recommended in the management of a pregnancy occurring post liver transplantation?**

Management as high-risk pregnancy by a specialist in maternal-fetal medicine is preferred. Immunosuppression should be continued with close monitoring of blood levels. Abnormal liver function tests should be evaluated aggressively. Percutaneous liver biopsy is not contraindicated but should be performed under ultrasound guidance. Monitoring for maternal and fetal CMV infection is indicated. Quantitative CMV immunoglobulins or detection of CMV viremia and viruria in the mother are adequate tests, and even amniotic fluid analysis could be used if there is suspicion of fetal infection. Deliveries should be via cesarean section if there are active herpes simplex lesions present. Prophylactic antibiotics should be used for deliveries in general.

**43. What are pregnancy safety data regarding maintenance immunosuppressive agents used in orthotopic liver transplantation (OLT)?**

- **Category B** (no evidence of risk in humans): prednisone
- **Category C** (risks cannot be ruled out): cyclosporine, tacrolimus (FK506), rapamycin (Sirolimus), OKT3, antithymocyte globulin, antilymphocyte globulin
- **Category D** (evidence of risk): azathioprine
- **Category D with black box warning** (high risk: mutagenic/teratogenic): mycophenolate mofetil (CellCept, Myfortic). It is advised that anyone pregnant or wishing to become pregnant be changed to azathioprine.

**44. Is breastfeeding permitted after delivery in a liver transplant recipient?**

At this time, it is believed that breastfeeding should be discouraged. A woman administered immunosuppressive drugs should not breast feed. Calcineurin inhibitors could cause immunosuppression and nephrotoxicity, and no recommendation can be made at this time regarding azathioprine-based regimens because there is extremely limited experience. Manufacturer recommends against breastfeeding in mothers administered interferon therapy, ribavirin, ganciclovir, or lamivudine. No specific recommendation can be made regarding foscarnet. No data are available regarding ursodeoxycholic acid excretion in breast milk.

**45. Are immunosuppressive agents safe during pregnancy?**

Corticosteroids, azathioprine, cyclosporine, tacrolimus, and OKT3 have no apparent teratogenic potential. All may contribute to low birth weights and fetal prematurity. Tacrolimus crosses the placenta and may contribute to transient perinatal hyperkalemia and mild, reversible renal impairment. There are no reports of allograft loss as a result of pregnancy in the tacrolimus-treated group of 35 patients at the University of Pittsburgh. The Philadelphia-based cyclosporine registry reports an allograft rejection rate of 17% and a graft loss rate of 5.7% in 35 patients taking cyclosporine during gestation and post partem period.

## PREVENTION OF VERTICAL TRANSMISSION

**46. How may vertical transmission of viral hepatitis A be prevented?**

Maternal infection with the hepatitis A virus (HAV) is not associated with fetal wastage or teratogenic effects. Vertical transmission of HAV is rare. There are no restrictions concerning breastfeeding. Passive immunization with immunoglobulin for urgent postexposure prophylaxis, and HAV vaccine is safe and recommended in pregnant women at risk for acquiring the disease, such as women traveling to endemic areas.

**47. How may vertical transmission of viral hepatitis B be prevented?**

The hepatitis B virus (HBV) may be transmitted vertically. If the mother acquires HBV in the first trimester of pregnancy, there is a 10% risk that the infant will test positive for hepatitis B surface antigen (HBsAg) at birth. The percentage dramatically increases to 80% to 90% if the acute maternal infection develops during the third trimester. In mothers who have chronic hepatitis B and test positive for the hepatitis Be antigen (HBeAg), 90% of neonates develop chronic hepatitis B without prophylaxis. If the mother has HBeAg- and HBeAb-negative chronic hepatitis B, 40% of neonates develop chronic hepatitis B infection without prophylaxis. The rate decreases to less than 5% if the mother is HBeAg negative and HBeAb positive. Antepartum serum HBsAg testing is mandatory. Neonates of HBsAg-positive mothers or HBsAg status–unknown mothers are treated with HBV human hyperimmune globulin (HBIG), 0.5 mL intramuscularly, at delivery. At the same time, they are given the first dose of HBV vaccine. The second dose is administered at 1 month of age, and the third dose at 6 months of age. If the mother is HBsAg negative, the child should be vaccinated only with the three-dose regimen, with the first inoculation at birth. The regimen is about 85% effective in preventing chronic hepatitis B in neonates and is ineffective in cases of hematogenous transplacental transmission, which are seen in about 15% of pregnancies as a result of small placental tears. Active and passive immunization at birth reduces also possibility of viral transmission by breastfeeding. Hepatitis B vaccination is safe in pregnant women. Lamivudine administered in the last month of pregnancy was recently shown to be safe and efficacious in decreasing risk of vertical transmission. Telbivudine has similar safety profile during pregnancy in animal studies.

## 48. What about vertical transmission of viral hepatitis C?

The risk of perinatal transmission is approximately 2% for infants of anti-HCV seropositive women. When a pregnant woman is HCV RNA positive at delivery, this risk increases to 4% to 7%. Higher HCV RNA levels appear to be associated with a greater risk. Levels of RNA of 1 million copies/mL are reportedly associated with vertical transmission rates as high as 50%. HCV transmission increases up to 20% in women coinfected with HCV and HIV. There are currently no data to determine whether antiviral therapy reduces perinatal transmission. Immunoglobulin therapy is ineffective. Rate of infection is similar among first- and second-born children.

## 49. Is it possible to prevent vertical transmission of viral hepatitis D and G?

Perinatal transmission of the hepatitis D virus (HDV) is rare. There are no documented cases of vertical transmission of HDV in the United States. No clinical data about hepatitis G infection during pregnancy are available, and no studies of vertical transmission have been done. Due to the lack of data on HDV, recommendations regarding breastfeeding are unknown.

## 50. Are HCV-infected women allowed to breastfeed?

HCV-infected women should be told that hepatitis C transmission via breastfeeding has not been documented. Current available studies show that the average rate of infection is 4%, similarly for breastfed and bottle-fed infants. According to the Centers for Disease Control and Prevention (CDC) and to a 1997 consensus statement from the National Institutes of Health (NIH), "Breastfeeding is not contraindicated for HCV-positive mothers," and "the maternal to baby transmission of HCV infection through breast milk has not been documented." Risk of transmission by breastfeeding was not found to be significant unless coinfection with HIV was present.

## 51. Does the mode of delivery influence hepatitis C transmission?

Current data are limited but indicate that infection rates are similar in infants delivered vaginally and cesarean-delivered infants. There are no prospective studies evaluating the use of elective cesarean section for the prevention of mother-to-infant transmission of HCV. However, avoiding fetal scalp monitoring and prolonged labor after rupture of membranes may reduce the risk of transmission to the infant.

## 52. How can perinatal HCV infection be diagnosed?

Infants passively acquire maternal antibodies that can persist for months. Anti-HCV antibodies after 15 months of age or positive HCV-RNA, which can be detected as early as 1 or 2 months, are diagnostic of perinatal transmission of HCV. A recent NIH consensus conference recommends that infants born to HCV-positive mothers be tested for HCV infection by HCV-RNA tests on two occasions between the ages of 2 and 6 months and/or have tests for anti-HCV after 15 months of age. Positive anti-HCV in infants prior to 15 months of age may be due to transplacental transfer of maternal anti-HCV antibody.

## WEBSITES

http://www.aasld.org

http://www.liverfoundation.org

### BIBLIOGRAPHY

1. Armenti VT, Herrine SK, Radomski JS, et al. Pregnancy after liver transplantation. Liver Transpl 2000;6:671–85.
2. Barton JR, Sibai BM. HELLP and the liver diseases of preeclampsia. Clin Liver Dis 1999;3:31–49.
3. Brewer GJ, Johnson VD, Dick RD, et al. Treatment of Wilson's disease with zinc. XVII: Treatment during pregnancy. Hepatology 2000;31:364–70.
4. Carr DB, Larson AM, Schmucker BC, et al. Maternal hemodynamics and pregnancy outcome in women with prior orthotopic liver transplantation. Liver Transpl 2000;6:213–21.
5. Connoly TJ, Zuckerman AL. Contraception in the patient with liver disease. Semin Perinatol 1998;22:178–82.
6. European Pediatric Hepatitis C Virus Network. Effects of mode of delivery and infant feeding on the risk of mother-to-child transmission of hepatitis C virus. Br J Obstet Gynaecol 2001;108:371–7.
7. Everson GT. Liver problems in pregnancy: Distinguishing normal from abnormal hepatic changes. Medscape Women's Health 1998;3:3.
8. Ibdah JA, Yang Z, Bennett MJ. Liver disease in pregnancy and fetal fatty acid oxidation defects. Mol Genet Metab 2000;71:182–9.
9. Jain A, Venkataramanan R, Fung JJ, et al. Pregnancy after liver transplantation under tacrolimus. Transplantation 1997;64:559–65.
10. Misra S, Sanyal AJ. Pregnancy in a patient with portal hypertension. Clin Liver Dis 1999;3:147–63.
11. National Institutes of Health. Consensus Development Conference Statement: Management of Hepatitis C. 2002.
12. Oral contraceptives. An update on health benefits and risks. J Am Pharm Assoc 2001;41:875–86.
13. Polywka S, Schröter M, Feucht H-H, et al. Low risk of vertical transmission of hepatitis C virus by breast milk. Clin Infect Dis 1999;29:1327–9.

14. Reinus JF, Leikin EL. Viral hepatitis in pregnancy. Clin Liver Dis 1999;3:115–31.
15. Riely CA. Contraception and pregnancy after liver transplantation. Liver Transpl 2001;7(Suppl. 1):S74–6.
16. Riely CA, Fallon HJ. Liver diseases. In: Burrow GN, Duffy TP, editors. Medical Complications During Pregnancy. 5th ed Philadelphia: WB Saunders; 1999. p. 269–94.
17. Rinaldo P, Raymond K, Al-Odaib A, et al. Clinical and biochemical features of fatty acid oxidation disorders. Curr Opin Pediatr 1998;10:615–21.
18. Sandhu BS, Sanyal AJ. Pregnancy and liver disease. Gastroenterol Clin North Am 2003;32:407–36.
19. Sheikh RA, Yasmeen S, Pauly MP, et al. Spontaneous intrahepatic hemorrhage and hepatic rupture in the HELLP syndrome. J Clin Gastroenterol 1999;28:323–8.
20. Van Nunen AB, De Man RA, Heijtink RA, et al. Lamivudine in the last 4 weeks of pregnancy to prevent perinatal transmission in highly viremic chronic hepatitis B patients. J Hepatol 2000;32:1040–1.
21. World Health Organization. Hepatitis B and breastfeeding. J Int Assoc Physicians AIDS Care 1998;4:20–1.
22. Yang Z, Yamada J, Zhao Y, et al. Prospective screening for pediatric mitochondrial trifunctional protein defects in pregnancies complicated by liver disease. JAMA 2002;288:2163–6.
23. Zanetti AR, Ferroni P, Magliano EM, et al. Perinatal transmission of the hepatitis B virus and of the HBV-associated delta agent from mothers to offspring in Northern Italy. J Med Virol 1982;9:139–48.

# CHAPTER 23

# RHEUMATOLOGIC MANIFESTATIONS OF HEPATOBILIARY DISEASES

*Sterling G. West, MD*

## VIRAL HEPATITIS

**1. How often is viral hepatitis associated with rheumatic manifestations?**

Approximately 25% of patients with hepatitis B antigenemia develop a rheumatic syndrome. Up to 50% of patients with hepatitis C develop an autoimmune syndrome. Transient arthralgias can occur in 10% of patients during acute hepatitis A viral infection.

**2. What are the most common extrahepatic rheumatologic manifestations of hepatitis B infection?**

- Acute polyarthritis-dermatitis syndrome
- Polyarteritis nodosa
- Membranous or membranoproliferative glomerulonephritis
- Cryoglobulinemia—usually associated with hepatitis C. Only 5% of all essential mixed cryoglobulinemia is due to hepatitis B alone.

**3. Describe the clinical characteristics of the polyarthritis-dermatitis syndrome associated with hepatitis B infection.**

In the preicteric prodromal period of acute hepatitis B infection, up to 25% of patients develop a polyarthritis that is acute, severe, and symmetric, involving both small (fingers) and large (knees, ankles) joints. A classically urticarial rash frequently (40%) accompanies the arthritis. Both the arthritis and rash can precede the onset of jaundice and/or elevated liver-associated enzymes by several days. The arthritis improves with nonsteroidal anti-inflammatory drugs (NSAIDs) and usually subsides soon after the onset of jaundice. Patients who develop chronic hepatitis B viremia may subsequently have recurrent arthralgias/arthritis. The etiology of this syndrome is due to deposition of circulating HBsAg-HBsAb immune complexes in the joints and skin.

**4. What is the typical presentation of hepatitis B–associated polyarteritis nodosa (PAN)?**

Up to 25% of all patients with PAN have positive hepatitis B serologies and evidence of viral replication (HBeAg, hepatitis B virus [HBV] DNA). They may present with a combination of fever, arthritis, mononeuritis multiplex, abdominal pain, renal disease, and/or cardiac disease. Although liver-associated enzymes may be abnormal, symptomatic hepatitis is not a prominent feature.

**5. How is PAN associated with hepatitis B antigenemia diagnosed?**

The diagnosis is made on the basis of a consistent clinical presentation coupled with an abdominal or renal angiogram showing vascular aneurysms and corkscrewing of blood vessels (Fig. 23-1). The gold standard is a tissue biopsy showing medium-vessel vasculitis.

**6. What is the treatment of hepatitis B–associated PAN?**

Patients are typically very ill and will die without aggressive therapy. Antiviral agents and plasmapheresis are used early to control the acute symptoms and antigenemia. Corticosteroids are also used early to control inflammation acutely. Once the acute process is controlled, corticosteroids are tapered (usually over 2 to 3 weeks) since they alone or in combination with cytotoxic drugs can enhance viral replication. Patients older than 50 years of age and those with renal insufficiency, cardiac, gastrointestinal, or central nervous system involvement have the worst prognosis. The overall 5-year survival rate is 50% to 70%.

**7. What are the most common hepatitis C virus (HCV)-related autoimmune disorders?**

- Mixed cryoglobulinemia (40% to 60% of HCV patients have cryoglobulins but only 5% develop vasculitis)
- Systemic polyarteritis nodosa–like vasculitis (<1% of HCV patients)
- Membranoproliferative glomerulonephritis

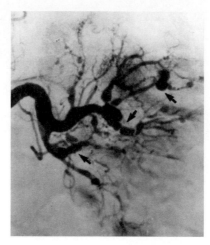

**Figure 23-1.** Renal angiogram showing vascular aneurysms in a patient with hepatitis B–associated polyarteritis nodosa (*arrows*).

- Nonerosive polyarthritis (2% to 20%)—Patients with acute hepatitis C infection can have an acute (usually transient) polyarthritis resembling rheumatoid arthritis with involvement of hands, wrists, shoulders, knees, and hips symmetrically. Although these patients are frequently rheumatoid factor (RF) positive, they do not have anti–cyclic citrullinated peptide (anti-CCP) antibodies. Other patients have an intermittent, monoarthritis or oligoarthritis affecting large and medium-sized joints.
- Autoantibody production (40% to 65%)—rheumatoid factor, antinuclear antibodies (ANA), anticardiolipin antibodies, anti-smooth muscle antibodies (SMA), anti-LKM1, and antithyroid antibodies
- Sjögren's-like syndrome with dry eyes and dry mouth (5% to 19%)—due to a lymphocytic sialadenitis. Anti–SS-A(Ro) and anti–SS-B(La) antibodies are negative.
- Autoimmune thrombocytopenia, myasthenia gravis, and sarcoidosis have been rarely associated with HCV infection or its therapy.

8. **What is the relationship between viral hepatitis and cryoglobulinemia?**
   Approximately 80% to 90% of patients with essential mixed cryoglobulinemia (type II and type III) are positive for hepatitis C. Hepatitis C virus is concentrated up to 1000-fold in the cryoprecipitate. Hepatitis C–infected patients are prone to develop autoimmune and lymphoproliferative diseases (35× higher risk). This is due to HCV's predilection to bind to B lymphocytes via CD81. This binding lowers the activation threshold for these cells, facilitating autoantibody production and cryoglobulinemia. Also, HCV infects B cells, causing proto-oncogene, *bcl-2*, recombination, which inhibits apoptosis, leading to extended lymphocyte survival. This results in cryoglobulinemia and neoplastic transformation (non–Hodgkin B-cell lymphomas).

9. **Describe the typical clinical features of cryoglobulinemia associated with hepatitis C infection.**
   Cryoglobulins are one or more immunoglobulins that precipitate at temperatures below 37° C and redissolve with rewarming. They precipitate in blood vessels in patients, causing a variety of symptoms. Patients present with a combination of fever, arthritis (which can be confused with rheumatoid arthritis), renal disease, paresthesias from peripheral neuropathy, and a predominantly lower extremity petechial rash, positive rheumatoid factor, and low complement levels (especially C4). Hepatitis is not a prominent feature. Patients have been successfully treated with combined corticosteroids, Peg-interferon α-2b/ribavirin combination, and plasmapheresis. Recently, rituximab (anti-CD20) has been used successfully to deplete the B-cell population making the cryoglobulins.

## AUTOIMMUNE AND OTHER LIVER DISEASES

10. **What is lupoid hepatitis?**
    Lupoid hepatitis is now called type I (classic) autoimmune hepatitis (AIH). Type I AIH can occur in all age groups, but most patients are young and predominantly female (70%). Many patients have clinical (arthralgias [50%]) and laboratory manifestations that may resemble systemic lupus erythematosus (SLE). Patients commonly have positive ANAs, antibodies against smooth muscle antigen (80%) frequently with specificity against F1 actin, and occasionally lupus erythematosus (LE) cells. They do not have antibodies against dsDNA. Type I AIH has been described in patients with

Sjögren's syndrome, SLE, mixed connective tissue disease, and limited systemic sclerosis. Patients with type I AIH can have other autoantibodies including anti–soluble liver/liver pancreas antigen (anti-SLA/LP), atypical perinuclear antineutrophil cytoplasmic antibodies (pANCAs), and anti-CCP antibodies.

**11. To what degree is type I AIH similar to SLE?**
See Table 23-1.

| Table 23-1. Comparison of Type I AIH and SLE | | |
|---|---|---|
| | SLE | TYPE I AIH |
| Young women | + | + |
| Polyarthritis | + | + |
| Fever | + | + |
| Rash | + | + |
| Nephritis | + | − |
| Central nervous system disease | + | − |
| Photosensitivity | + | − |
| Oral ulcers | + | − |
| ANA | 99% | 70–90% |
| LE cells | 70% | 40–50% |
| Polyclonal gammopathy | + | + |
| Anti-Smith antibodies | 25% | 0 |
| + Anti-dsDNA | 70% | Rare |
| + Anti–F1 actin | Rare | 60–95% |

AIH, autoimmune hepatitis; ANA, antinuclear antibody; LE, lupus erythematosus; SLE, systemic lupus erythematosus.

**12. What is the difference between anti-Sm and anti-SM antibodies?**
Anti-Sm antibodies are antibodies against the Smith antigen, which is an epitope on small nuclear ribonuclear proteins. It is highly diagnostic of SLE. The anti-SM antibody is an antibody against the smooth muscle antigen (which is frequently F1 actin). It is highly diagnostic of type I autoimmune hepatitis (Table 23-2).

| Table 23-2. Anti-Sm Versus Anti-SM Antibodies | | |
|---|---|---|
| | SLE | TYPE I AIH |
| Anti–Smith (Sm) antibodies | Yes | No |
| Anti–smooth muscle (SM) antibodies | No | Yes |

AIH, autoimmune hepatitis.

**13. List the common autoimmune diseases associated with primary biliary cirrhosis (PBC).**
Up to 80% of patients with PBC have one or more of the following disorders:

- Keratoconjunctivitis sicca (Sjögren syndrome)—66%
- Autoimmune thyroiditis (Hashimoto disease)—20%
- Scleroderma/Raynaud disease—20%
- Rheumatoid arthritis—10%
- Limited scleroderma (calcinosis, Raynaud phenomenon, esophageal, telangiectasia [CREST]) occurs in 4% of PBC patients and antedates PBC by 14 years.

**14. Compare and contrast the arthritis that may occur with PBC and rheumatoid arthritis.**
See Table 23-3.

**Table 23-3.** Primary Biliary Cirrhosis (PBC) Arthritis Versus Rheumatoid Arthritis (RA)

|  | PBC ARTHRITIS | RA |
|---|---|---|
| Frequency in patients | 10% develop RA | 1–10% develop PBC |
| No. of joints* | Polyarticular | Polyarticular |
| Symmetry | Symmetric | Symmetric |
| Inflammatory | Yes | Yes |
| Rheumatoid factor | Sometimes | Yes (85%) |
| Erosions on radiograph | Rare | Common |

*PBC can involve distal interphalangeal joints of fingers, whereas RA does not involve these joints.

### 15. What other musculoskeletal manifestations may occur in patients with PBC?
- Osteomalacia due to fat-soluble vitamin D malabsorption (low 25-OH vitamin D level)
- Osteoporosis due to renal tubular acidosis
- Hypertrophic osteoarthropathy

### 16. What autoantibodies commonly occur in patients with PBC?
- Antimitochondrial antibodies—80%
- Anticentromere antibodies—20%*
- *Most patients also have manifestations of the CREST variant of scleroderma.

### 17. How commonly does arthritis occur in patients with hereditary hemochromatosis?
Approximately 40% to 75% of patients have a noninflammatory degenerative arthritis, most commonly involving the second and third metacarpophalangeal joints (MCPs), proximal interphalangeal joints (PIPs), wrists, hips, knees, and ankles. Of importance, this arthropathy may be the presenting complaint (30% to 50%) of patients with hemochromatosis and is frequently misdiagnosed in young males as seronegative rheumatoid arthritis.

### 18. Describe the radiographic features suggestive of hemochromatotic arthropathy.
Suggestive radiographic features include subchondral sclerosis, cyst formation, irregular joint space narrowing, and osteophyte formation consistent with degenerative arthritis of involved joints. The key is finding degenerative changes in the MCP joints (typically second and third) with hooklike osteophytes (Fig. 23-2). This finding is important, because the MCPs and wrists rarely develop degenerative joint disease without an underlying cause such as hemochromatosis.

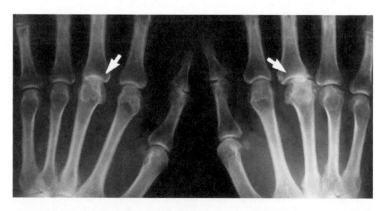

**Figure 23-2.** Radiographs of hands showing degenerative arthritis with hooklike osteophytes of the second and third metacarpophalangeal joints in a patient with hemochromatosis (*arrows*).

### 19. What is the relationship between calcium pyrophosphate disease and hemochromatosis?
Chondrocalcinosis of the triangular fibrocartilage at the ulnar side of the wrist and the hyaline cartilage of the knees is seen in 20% to 50% of patients with hemochromatosis. Crystals of calcium pyrophosphate may shed into the joints, causing superimposed flares of inflammatory arthritis (i.e., pseudogout).

### 20. Discuss the genetics of hereditary hemochromatosis.
Hereditary hemochromatosis is among the most common genetic disorders in whites of northern European descent. Between 80% and 90% of patients are homozygous for the same mutation (C282Y) in the hemochromatosis (*HFE*) gene. The homozygote frequency in this white population is 0.3% to 0.5% and carrier frequency is 7% to 10% (i.e., heterozygotes). The *HFE* gene is located on chromosome 6 near the major histocompatibility (MHC) locus. It encodes for an MHC Class I–like protein that complexes with $\beta_2$-microglobulin and the transferrin receptor. This protein

complex on the surface of duodenal crypt cells can bind to transferrin-bound iron in the circulation, enabling these cells to sense body iron stores. A proposed but controversial mechanism for hereditary hemochromatosis is that the C282Y mutation inactivates the HFE protein through its inability to bind $\beta_2$-microglobulin, leading to impaired cellular trafficking, reduced incorporation into the cell membrane, and reduced association with the transferrin receptor. This reduced association with the transferrin receptor results in a protein complex that does not bind well to transferrin. Consequently, the duodenal crypt cells sense that the body is low in iron and in turn upregulate their divalent metal transporter 1 protein, which facilitates iron absorption from the intestinal lumen. However, not all patients homozygous for this HFE mutation develop clinical manifestations of iron overload (28% of male homozygotes over 12 years). This suggests that a mutation in a concomitant second gene such as *HAMP* (hepcidin), *HJV* (hemojuvelin), ferroportin, or transferrin receptor 2 gene is necessary for the full expression of hereditary hemochromatosis.

**21. Compare and contrast the features of hemochromatotic arthropathy (HA) and rheumatoid arthritis (RA).**
See Table 23-4.

**Table 23-4.** Comparison of Hemochromatotic Arthropathy and Rheumatoid Arthritis

|  | HEMOCHROMATOTIC ARTHROPATHY | RHEUMATOID ARTHRITIS |
| --- | --- | --- |
| Sex | M>F (10:1) | F>M (3:1) |
| Age of onset | >35 years | All ages |
| Joints | Polyarticular | Polyarticular |
| Symmetry | Symmetric | Symmetric |
| Inflammatory signs and symptoms | Only if pseudogout attack | Yes |
| Rheumatoid factor | Negatlve | Positive (85%) |
| Gene | HFE (90%) | HLA DR4 (70%) |
| Synovial fluid | Noninflammatory | Inflammatory |
| Radiographs | Degenerative changes | Inflammatory, erosive disease |

F, female; HFE, hemochromatosis; HLA, human leukocyte antigen; M, male.

**22. How effective is phlebotomy in halting the progression of hemochromatotic arthropathy?**
Phlebotomy does not halt the progression of the arthropathy.

**23. What is the correlation between the severity of arthropathy and severity of liver disease in hemochromatosis?**
There is no correlation.

**24. Why does hemochromatosis cause a degenerative arthritis?**
The arthropathy is characterized by hemosiderin deposition in synovium and chondrocytes. The presence of iron in these cells may lead to increased production of destructive enzymes (e.g., matrix metalloproteinases), free radical generation, or crystal deposition that causes cartilage damage. Other mechanisms also may be possible; the precise pathway by which chronic iron overload leads to tissue injury has not been fully established.

**25. What other musculoskeletal problems may occur in patients with hemochromatosis?**
- Osteoporosis due to gonadal dysfunction from pituitary insufficiency caused by the iron overload state (low follicle-stimulating hormone [FSH], luteinizing hormone [LH], and testosterone).
- Osteomalacia due to vitamin D deficiency due to liver disease (low 25-OH vitamin D level).
- Hypertrophic osteoarthropathy—cirrhosis of any cause including hemochromatosis can be associated with periosteal reaction involving shafts of long bones.

**BIBLIOGRAPHY**

1. Allen KJ, Gurrin LC, Constantine CC, et al. Iron-overload-related disease in HFE hereditary hemochromatosis. N Engl J Med 2008;358:221–30.
2. Cacoub P, Delluc A, Saadoun D, et al. Anti-CD20 monoclonal antibody (rituximab) treatment for cryoglobulinemic vasculitis: Where do we stand? Ann Rheum Dis 2008;67:283–7.
3. Cacoub P, Poynard T, Ghillani P, et al. Extrahepatic manifestations of chronic hepatitis C. Arthritis Rheum 1999;42:2204–12.

4. Camaschella C. Understanding iron hemostasis through genetic analysis of hemochromatosis and related disorders. Blood 2005;106:3710–7.
5. Culp KS, Fleming CR, Duffy J, et al. Autoimmune associations and primary biliary cirrhosis. Mayo Clin Proc 1982;57:365–70.
6. Czaja AJ. Autoantibodies in autoimmune liver disease. Adv Clin Chem 2005;40:127–64.
7. Farrell GC, Teoh NC. Management of chronic hepatitis B virus infection: A new era of disease control. Intern Med J 2006;36:100–13.
8. Guillevin L, Mahr A, Callard P, et al. Hepatitis B virus-associated polyarteritis nodosa: Clinical characteristics, outcome, and impact of treatment in 115 patients. Medicine (Baltimore) 2005;84:313–22.
9. Hall S, Czaja AJ, Kaufman DK, et al. How lupoid is lupoid hepatitis? J Rheumatol 1986;13:95–8.
10. Krawitt EL. Autoimmune hepatitis. N Engl J Med 2006;354:54–66.
11. Marx WJ, O'Connell DJ. Arthritis of primary biliary cirrhosis. Arch Intern Med 1979;139:213–6.
12. Pietrangelo A. Hereditary hemochromatosis: A new look at an old disease. N Engl J Med 2004;350:2383–97.
13. Saadoun D, Resche-Rigon M, Thibault V, et al. Antiviral therapy for hepatitis C virus-associated mixed cryoglobulinemic vasculitis: A long-term follow-up study. Arthritis Rheum 2006;54:3696–706.
14. Trepo C, Guillevin L. Polyarteritis nodosa and extrahepatic manifestations for HBV infection. J Autoimmunity 2001;16:269–74.

# EVALUATION OF FOCAL LIVER MASSES

Mark W. Russo, MD, and
Roshan Shrestha, MD

**CHAPTER 24**

## 1. Describe the initial workup for a patient with a liver mass.

The first step is an accurate history and physical examination. Age, sex, and birthplace are important clues to etiology. Risk factors for viral hepatitis or a history of cirrhosis increases the possibility of a primary malignant process. A previously diagnosed neoplasm heightens suspicion for metastatic disease. Use of oral contraceptives or anabolic steroids, alcohol intake, and potential occupational exposure to carcinogens should be noted. Hepatomegaly and/or splenomegaly, abdominal pain, or stigmata of chronic liver disease, such as palmar erythema, spider angiomata, or gynecomastia, may be present.

Liver-associated enzymes, with the exception of gamma-glutamyl transpeptidase (GGT), are usually normal with benign liver tumors. Serum alkaline phosphatase levels are often elevated with hepatic metastases, but not in all cases. An increase in serum transaminases may signify chronic hepatitis or cirrhosis. Positive hepatitis B or C serologies or iron studies may identify an underlying cause of liver dysfunction or cirrhosis (Table 24-1).

**Table 24-1.** Differential Diagnosis of Focal Liver Masses in Adults

| BENIGN | MALIGNANT |
|---|---|
| **Epithelial Tumors** | |
| Hepatic adenoma | Hepatocellular carcinoma |
| Bile duct adenoma | Cholangiocarcinoma |
| Biliary cystadenoma | Biliary cystadenocarcinoma |
| **Mesenchymal Tumors** | |
| Cavernous hemangioma | Angiosarcoma |
| | Primary hepatic lymphoma |
| **Other Lesions** | |
| Focal nodular hyperplasia | Metastatic tumors |
| Liver abscess | |
| Macroregenerative nodules in cirrhosis | |
| Focal fatty infiltration | |
| Simple hepatic cyst | |

Modified from Kew MC: Tumors of the liver. In Zakim D, Boyer TD (eds): Hepatology: A Textbook of Liver Disease, 2nd ed. Philadelphia, W.B. Saunders, 1990, pp. 1206-1239.

## 2. What tumor markers are useful in the evaluation of focal liver lesions?

Serum alpha-fetoprotein (AFP) and tumor-associated antigen CA 19-9 are markers of primary hepatic malignancy and are used when radiographic studies indicate a focal neoplasm originating in the liver.

*AFP* is the best diagnostic marker for hepatocellular carcinoma (HCC) and also plays a role in screening programs of at-risk populations. AFP levels above 200 ng/mL are highly suggestive of HCC, whereas lesser elevations may be due to benign chronic hepatitis. A universally accepted cutoff value for AFP in the diagnosis of HCC has not been established, and some authorities use a level greater than 500 ng/mL. Not all hepatomas secrete AFP, and approximately one-third of patients have a normal AFP value, especially when the tumor is smaller than 2 cm. AFP levels should decrease or normalize with successful treatment. Other tumor markers that appear to be promising for the detection of hepatocellular carcinoma include AFP-L3% and des-gamma-carboxyprothombin (DCP). The sensitivity and specificity of AFP-L3% and DCP for HCC have been reported to be 56% and 90% and 87% and 85%, respectively.

*CA 19-9* is used in the diagnosis of cholangiocarcinoma, a malignancy originating in the bile ducts. CA 19-9 levels greater than 100 U/mL are found in over 50% of patients and values greater than 1000 suggest unresectability. This marker is more sensitive in patients with primary sclerosing cholangitis, a risk factor for cholangiocarcinoma. Significant false-positive elevations in CA 19-9 can occur with bacterial cholangitis. CA 19-9 also serves as a tumor marker for pancreatic carcinoma.

### 3. What imaging modalities are used in the detection and characterization of focal liver masses?

Recent advances in computed tomography (CT) and magnetic resonance imaging (MRI) allow detailed assessment of focal liver lesions. These imaging studies have largely supplanted previously used nuclear medicine–based protocols for the characterization of liver masses.

*Triphasic CT,* which is now widely available, offers substantial improvement in hepatic imaging because of its rapid scan time within a single breath-hold. This feature eliminates respiratory motion and allows contrast injection to be viewed in unenhanced, arterial (early) and portal venous phases of perfusion. Lesions that derive their vascular supply from the hepatic artery, such as HCC and hypervascular metastases, are prominent during the arterial phase. The venous or portal phase of helical CT provides maximal enhancement of normal liver parenchyma and optimizes detection of hypovascular lesions, such as colon, gastric, and pancreatic metastases.

*MRI* has undergone similar refinements, with breath-hold T1-weighted images and fast (turbo) spin-echo T2-weighted sequences that eliminate motion artifacts and make use of contrast agents in a manner analogous to triphasic CT. Gadolinium-enhanced MRI should be considered in patients with contraindications to iodine-based CT, such as contrast allergies or renal insufficiency.

*Contrast-enhanced ultrasonography* has been studied outside of the United States as a modality to distinguish benign from malignant lesions. This modality may decrease costs and exposure to radiation but is not widely used in the United States.

Many focal liver masses are found incidentally on *ultrasound* examination of the abdomen. Although liver ultrasound often cannot fully characterize the lesion, it has a role in verifying simple hepatic cysts, which may have nonspecific radiographic patterns on CT or MRI. Intraoperative ultrasound remains the best modality for defining hepatic metastases.

### 4. What is the most common benign cause of a focal liver lesion?

Cavernous hemangiomas are the most common benign hepatic tumor, occurring in up to 20% of the population. They occur in all age groups, more commonly in women, as solitary (60%) or multiple asymptomatic masses. Most are less than 3 cm and usually occur in the posterior segment of the right hepatic lobe. The term *giant hemangioma* is sometimes used when the size exceeds 5 cm. Microscopically, hemangiomas consist of blood-filled vascular sinusoids separated by connective-tissue septae. Occasionally, hemangiomas are large enough to cause abdominal pain, but the risk of tumor growth or bleeding is minimal and does not justify surgical removal unless the patient is significantly symptomatic.

### 5. Why is oral contraceptive use important in the differential diagnosis of focal liver masses?

Most cases of hepatic adenomas directly relate to the use of oral contraceptive pills (OCPs). This benign tumor was rarely seen before oral contraceptive agents came into common usage in the 1960s. Risk correlates with duration of use and age older than 30 years. Hepatic adenomas most commonly occur in young and middle-aged women, with an incidence of 3 to 4 per 100,000. Men infrequently develop adenomas, although cases have been reported with anabolic steroid use.

Hepatic adenomas are well-demarcated, fleshy tumors with prominent surface vasculature. Microscopically, they consist of monotonous sheets of normal or small hepatocytes with no bile ducts, portal tracts, or central veins.

### 6. Why is surgical resection of hepatic adenomas recommended?

Spontaneous rupture and intra-abdominal hemorrhage can occur in up to 30% of patients with hepatic adenoma, especially during menstruation or pregnancy. HCC also can develop within adenomas. Approximately 50% of patients with these tumors have abdominal pain, sometimes as a result of bleeding within the adenoma. Adenomas have been known to regress with discontinuation of birth control pills, which should be recommended, but surgical resection remains the management of choice.

### 7. What is focal nodular hyperplasia (FNH)?

FNH is a round, nonencapsulated mass, usually exhibiting a vascular central scar. Fibrous septae radiate from the scar in a spokelike fashion. Hepatocytes are arranged in nodules or cords between the septae, and the mass includes bile ductules, Kupffer cells, and chronic inflammatory cells. FNH are considered the result of a hyperplastic response to increased blood flow secondary to vascular malformations.

FNH is the second most common benign liver tumor. More than 90% of cases occur in women and usually are diagnosed between 20 and 60 years of age. OCPs are not considered a causative agent of FNH but occasionally may enhance their growth; therefore, some authorities recommend discontinuing OCPs in women if FNH is diagnosed.

**8. List the differences between hepatic adenomas and FNH.**
See Table 24-2.

**Table 24-2.** Hepatic Adenomas Versus Focal Nodular Hyperplasia

| | HEPATIC ADENOMA | FOCAL NODULAR HYPERPLASIA |
| --- | --- | --- |
| Size (mean) | 10 cm | < 5 cm |
| Kupffer cells | No | Yes |
| Central scar | Rare | Common |
| Symptoms | Common | Rare (only with large lesions) |
| Complications | Bleeding, malignancy | Rare lesions may grow in size |
| Treatment | Surgical resection | Resection not necessary |
| Sulfur-colloid liver scan | Cold defect | Positive uptake in 60% to 70% |

**9. What is the most frequent malignancy in the liver?**
Metastatic disease to the liver is much more common than primary hepatic tumors in the United States and Europe. Cancers arising in the colon, stomach, pancreas, breast, and lung are the most likely to metastasize to the liver. Esophageal, renal, and genitourinary neoplasms also should be considered when searching for the primary site. Multiple defects in the liver suggest a metastatic process: only 2% present as solitary lesions. Involvement of both lobes is most common; 20% are confined to the right lobe alone and 3% to the left lobe.

**10. What is the most common primary liver cancer?**
HCC is by far the most common malignancy originating in the liver, accounting for approximately 80% of primary liver cancers. The incidence in the United States ranges from 2 to 3 cases per 100,000 and has doubled over the past two decades. The recent increase in HCC in the United States over the past decade is directly attributable to the rising incidence of hepatitis C infection. Geographic location influences both the age of peak occurrence (older than 55 years in the United States) and male-to-female incidence ratios. High-incidence areas in Asia and Africa, related to hepatitis B, have a much younger average age of onset and a higher male predominance. Worldwide, men are more likely than women to develop HCC by a factor of 4:1. HCC usually occurs within a cirrhotic liver; approximately 80% of patients diagnosed with HCC have cirrhosis.

**11. Describe the various presenting forms of HCC.**
- *Nodular:* most common; multiple nodules of varying size scattered throughout the liver.
- *Solitary* (or *massive*): occurs in younger patients; large, solitary mass, often in the right lobe.
- *Diffuse:* rare; difficult to detect on imaging; widespread infiltration of minute tumor foci.

**12. What types of cirrhosis are most commonly associated with HCC?**
Autopsy studies indicate that 20% to 40% of patients dying with cirrhosis harbor HCC. The etiologies of cirrhosis most commonly related to HCC, in order of decreasing risk, are as follows:

1. Chronic hepatitis C (greater than 5 years; 7% of patients with HCV cirrhosis develop HCC)
2. Chronic hepatitis B
3. Hemochromatosis
4. $\alpha_1$-Antitrypsin deficiency
5. Alcoholic cirrhosis (alcohol potentiates the carcinogenic risk in viral cirrhosis)
6. Nonalcoholic fatty liver disease (1% to 3% over 10 to 15 years)

**13. What clinical and laboratory findings should raise suspicion for HCC?**
1. New abdominal pain or weight loss
2. Hepatomegaly
3. Hepatic bruit
4. Acute hemoperitoneum
5. Blood-tinged ascitic fluid
6. Persistent fever
7. Sudden increase in serum alkaline phosphatase
8. Increasing ratio of aspartate aminotransferase to alanine aminotransferase
9. Polycythemia or persistent leukocytosis
10. Hypoglycemia

11. Hypercalcemia
12. Hypercholesterolemia

Findings 9–12 are paraneoplastic syndromes associated with HCC.

### 14. What primary liver tumor occurs in young adults without underlying cirrhosis?

The fibrolamellar variant of HCC is a distinctive, slow-growing subtype of hepatic neoplasm, occurring at a mean age of 26 years. Patients seldom have a history of prior liver disease. Unlike typical HCC, men and women are equally affected. Fibrolamellar tumors usually present with abdominal pain, due to a large, solitary mass, most often in the left lobe (75%). The AFP level is normal.

The term *fibrolamellar* characterizes the microscopic appearance of this lesion; thin layers of fibrosis separate the neoplastic hepatocytes. A *fibrous central scar* may be seen on imaging studies. Recognition of this variant is important because nearly one-half are resectable at the time of diagnosis.

### 15. What factors predispose to the development of cholangiocarcinoma?

Cholangiocarcinomas, which account for about 10% of primary liver cancers, arise as adenocarcinomas from bile duct epithelium. Jaundice is the most frequent clinical presentation of this tumor. Risk factors for cholangiocarcinoma include:

- Primary sclerosing cholangitis
- Liver fluke infestation
- Chronic ulcerative colitis
- Congenital cystic liver diseases
- Choledochal cysts

### 16. What is a Klatskin tumor?

Cholangiocarcinomas at the hilar bifurcation of the hepatic ducts are referred to as Klatskin tumors. Peripheral (or intrahepatic) and extrahepatic bile duct cholangiocarcinomas are other subtypes. The characteristic desmoplastic reaction accompanying these tumors often makes them poorly visible on imaging studies and difficult to diagnose on biopsy. Delayed tumor enhancement on CT after intravenous (IV) contrast is noted in approximately 75% of intrahepatic cholangiocarcinomas. In recent years, definitive diagnosis can be made with direct visualization and biopsy of the intraductal mass using cholangioscopy via a SpyGlass Probe/Scope (Boston Scientific Corporation). Only about 25% of cholangiocarcinomas occur in the setting of cirrhosis. Most are unresectable when diagnosed and thus require palliative drainage of obstructive jaundice by endoscopic, percutaneous, or surgical methods.

### 17. When should liver transplantation be considered in patients with HCC?

Solitary lesion less than 5 cm
*Or*
Fewer than 3 nodules, each less than 3 cm
*And*
No metastatic or regional lymph node involvement and no major vascular invasion

### 18. When should resection be considered in patients with HCC?

HCC is resectable in only ≈10% of patients in the United States. Five-year survival rates with surgical treatment range between 17% and 40%. Most patients succumb to intrahepatic recurrence of tumor. The multifocal nature of HCC carcinogenesis explains this poor prognosis. Selection criteria for resectability of HCC include:

- Child-Pugh class A cirrhosis
- Solitary lesion less than 5 cm
- Hepatic wedge pressure gradient less than 10 mm Hg
- Lack of vascular invasion or extrahepatic spread

### 19. What palliative therapies are available for the management of HCC?

Radiofrequency ablation is a direct application of thermal energy by percutaneous or surgical means, which destroys unresectable areas of HCC. Radiofrequency ablation appears to offer some benefit over percutaneous ethanol injection by decreasing local recurrence rates and enhancing directed tissue necrosis, although both modalities are now commonly used.

Transarterial chemoembolization involves the selective administration of chemotherapy, followed by embolization, into the hepatic artery branch feeding the tumor. Recent reports suggest this technique may improve survival, as well as local tumor control. It is frequently used to delay tumor progression in patients awaiting liver transplantation.

**20. Who should be screened for HCC? Describe a typical screening strategy.**
Patients with cirrhosis, especially those at high risk of HCC, should be screened. Screening is done routinely in people with virus-induced cirrhosis (hepatitis B and C) and cirrhosis related to metabolic liver disease.

Serial AFP measurements and hepatic ultrasound studies are the most commonly used screening tools. Optimal screening intervals are not established, but AFP levels and ultrasound every 6 months are common practice. Although surveillance may not have a definite impact on mortality rate, it allows more tumors to be amenable to curative resection.

**21. What benign tissue abnormality may simulate a focal liver mass?**
Focal fatty infiltration may appear similar to the focal hepatic lesions described above. Focal fatty liver is often seen in alcoholism, obesity, diabetes mellitus, malnutrition, corticosteroid excess or therapy, and acquired immunodeficiency syndrome (AIDS). MRI may be necessary to fully characterize this entity. An interesting aspect of focal fat is its rapid disappearance once the inciting disease process is corrected.

**22. What new imaging techniques are under development to evaluate focal liver masses?**
- MRI angiography, which permits the rapid acquisition of arterial and venous sequences, has shown promise in the detection of small HCCs missed by triphasic CT scanning.
- Positron emission tomography (PET scanning) is currently being studied to improve the difficult detection of cholangiocarcinoma. PET scans are also playing an increasing role in the detection of hepatic metastases from colorectal cancer when liver resection is contemplated.
- Endoscopic ultrasound with fine needle aspiration (FNA) has also been reported to aid in the diagnosis of suspected cholangiocarcinoma when other tissue sampling methods such as intraductal cytology have failed to provide a diagnosis.
- Cholangioscopy with direct visualization of biliary tree and forceps biopsy of intraductal lesions using SpyGlass technology provide much higher sensitivity and specificity in diagnosing cholangiocarcinoma and other various biliary lesions (biliary papillomatosis, stones).

**23. Why is fine-needle biopsy of hepatic masses controversial?**
Establishing a diagnosis for a focal liver mass by FNA cytology is more problematic than one would think, owing to subtle histopathologic differences between normal hepatocytes and benign lesions or even well-differentiated hepatomas. The literature reveals a wide range of sensitivity for FNA-based diagnosis of primary hepatic lesions. The most optimistic studies report sensitivities and specificities greater than 90%. Hemangiomas, FNH, and HCC appear to be more difficult to diagnose accurately by FNA; sensitivity ranges between 60% and 70% in many series. Rigorous protocols making use of two or more imaging studies to characterize a benign lesion can have an accuracy and sensitivity as high as 80% to 90%. When HCC is suspected, the use of MRI, CT, and angiography (in selected cases) can confirm the diagnosis in greater than 95% of patients without the use of FNA.

Another controversy regarding the use of FNA in HCC is the risk of needle-track seeding and tumor spread into the circulation, a risk that may be as high as 5%. With the increasing use of liver transplantation in the treatment of HCC, this complication can have grave consequences.

FNA plays a dominant role in the setting of suspected metastatic disease to the liver and inoperable primary cancers. When surgical resection of a lesion, based on clinical and imaging findings, is deemed necessary, preoperative biopsy is generally not advocated.

**24. What should be done when small incidental liver lesions are found?**
Lesions less than 1 cm are common incidental findings on liver imaging. In the vast majority of cases, they represent benign entities such as small cysts or hemangiomas. Their small size makes further characterization by other radiographic studies or percutaneous biopsy problematic, and usually impossible.

Simple, thin-walled hepatic cysts, regardless of size, need no further follow-up when definitively documented by ultrasound. Otherwise, clinical follow-up by repeating the imaging study in 6 months is recommended. This provides verification that the lesion has not grown in size. Interval growth of such lesions should prompt further workup.

**25. Outline a logical approach to the evaluation of a focal hepatic mass.**

The workup of a focal liver mass must occur in the context of a carefully considered differential diagnosis. Associated symptoms, presence of underlying liver disease or extrahepatic malignancy, drug and occupational exposures, and laboratory abnormalities must be assessed before proceeding with further radiographic studies. Symptomatic lesions and lesions noted incidentally are likely to have different etiologies. The patient's age and sex are important clues. Cirrhosis requires a modified approach because of the increased likelihood of HCC.

## INCIDENTAL LESIONS

Small lesions less than 1 cm → repeat study in 6 months

Simple cysts → verify with ultrasound

Hemangiomas → triphasic CT with contrast → $^{99m}$Tc-labeled red blood cell scan (for lesions greater than 2 cm) or gadolinium-enhanced MRI

FNH → triphasic CT with contrast → gadolinium-enhanced MRI → ? biopsy

Hepatic adenoma → history of OCPs → rule out hemangioma and FNH → resection (outlined above)

## SYMPTOMATIC LESIONS

Hepatic adenoma → history of OCPs → rule out hemangioma/FNH → resection

Liver abscess → sepsis → ultrasound → triphasic CT (rim enhancement)

## CIRRHOSIS OR RISK FACTORS FOR CHOLANGIOCARCINOMA

HCC → AFP → triphasic CT → MRI with contrast or MRI angiography

Cholangiocarcinoma → CA 19-9 → triphasic with delayed-phase CT → ? MRCP or PET scan

## HISTORY OF MALIGNANCY

Metastases → triphasic CT with contrast → if resection is considered → PET scan (to rule out multiple metastases)

## WEBSITE

http://www.bostonscientific.com

### BIBLIOGRAPHY

1. de Groen PC, Gores GJ, LaRusso NF, et al. Biliary tract cancers. N Engl J Med 1999;341:1368–78.
2. Durazo FA, Blatt LM, Corey WG, et al. Des-gamma-carboxyprothrombin, alpha-fetoprotein and AFP-L3 in patients with chronic hepatitis, cirrhosis and hepatocellular carcinoma. J Gastroenterol Hepatol 2008; 23:1541-8.
3. Ekstedt M, Franzen LE, Mathiesen UL, et al. Long term follow up of patients with NAFLD and elevated liver enzymes. Hepatology 2006;44:802–5.
4. El-Serag HB. Epidemiology of hepatocellular carcinoma in the USA. Hepatol Res 2007;37(Suppl. 2):S88–94.
5. Giannitrapani L, Soresi M, LaSpada E, et al. Sex hormones and risk of liver tumor. Ann N Y Acad Sci 2006;1089:228–36.
6. Hanna RF, Aguirre DA, Kased N, et al. Cirrhosis-associated hepatocellular nodules: Correlation of histologic and pathologic MR imaging features. Radiographics 2008;28:747–69.
7. Heinken JP. Distinguishing benign from malignant liver tumors. Cancer Imaging 2007;7(Suppl .A):S1–14.
8. Ibrahim S, Chen CL, Wang SH, et al. Liver resection for benign liver tumors: Indications and outcome. Am J Surg 2007;193:5–7.
9. Ishak KG, Goodman Z, Stocker JT. Tumors of the liver and bile ducts. In: Atlas of Tumor Pathology. 3rd ed. Washington, DC: Armed Forces Institute of Pathology; 2001.
10. Kim TK, Jang HJ, Wilson SR. Hepatic neoplasms: Features on grayscale and contrast enhanced ultrasound. Ultrasound Clin 2007;2:333–54.
11. Lanka B, Jang HJ, Kim TK, et al. Impact of contrast-enhanced ultrasonography in a tertiary clinical practice. J Ultrasound Med 2007;26:1703–14.
12. Lizardi-Cervera J, Cuellar-Gamboa L, Motola-Kuba D. Focal nodular hyperplasia and hepatic adenoma: A review. Ann Hepatol 2006;5:206–11.
13. Mor E, Kaspa RT, Sheiner P, et al. Treatment of hepatocellular carcinoma associated with cirrhosis in the era of liver transplantation. Ann Intern Med 1998;129:643–53.
14. Patel AH, Harnois DM, Klee GG, et al. The utility of CA 19-9 in the diagnosis of cholangiocarcinoma in patients without primary sclerosing cholangitis. Am J Gastroenterol 2000;95:204–7.
15. Peng YC, Chan CS, Chen GH. The effectiveness of serum a-fetoprotein level in anti-HCV positive patients for screening hepatocellular carcinoma. Hepato-Gastroenterol 1999;46:3208–11.

16. Rebouissou S, Bioulac-Sage P, Zucman-Rossi J. Molecular pathogenesis of focal nodular hyperplasia and hepatocellular adenoma. J Hepatol 2008;48:163–70.
17. Siegel MJ, Chung EM, Conran RM. Pediatric liver focal masses. Magn Reson Imaging Clin N Am 2008;16:437–52.
18. Souto E, Gores GJ. When should a liver mass suspected of being a hepatocellular carcinoma be biopsied? Liver Transpl 2000;6:73–5.
19. Takamori R, Wong LL, Dang C, et al. Needle-tract implantation from hepatocellular cancer: Is needle biopsy of the liver always necessary?. Liver Transpl 2000;6:67–72.
20. Terkivatan T, Hussain SM, de Man RA, et al. Diagnosis and treatment of benign focal liver lesions. Scand J Gastroenterol 2006;243:102–15.
21. van den Bos IC, Hussain SM, de Man RA, et al. Magnetic resonance imaging of liver lesions: Exceptions and atypical lesions. Curr Probl Diagn Radiol 2008;37:95–103.
22. Verslype C, Libbrecht L. The multidisciplinary management of gastrointestinal cancer. The diagnostic and therapeutic approach for primary solid liver tumors in adults. Best Pract Res Clin Gastroenterol 2007;21:983–96.

# DRUG-INDUCED LIVER DISEASE

*Peter R. McNally, DO, FACP, FACG*

### 1. How common is drug-induced liver disease?

More than 600 medicines have been reported to cause liver injury. Drug-induced hepatic injury is the most frequent reason cited for the withdrawal from the market of an approved drug, and it also accounts for 2% to 5% of hospital admissions for jaundice and more than 50% of the cases of acute liver failure in the United States today.

### 2. How are the three patterns of drug-induced liver injury distinguished?

Hepatocellular, cholestatic, and mixed injury patterns typically are distinguished by alanine aminotransferase (ALT) and alkaline phosphatase (AP) values and ratios (Table 25-1).

**Table 25-1.** Patterns of Drug-Induced Liver Disease

| ALT | ALP | ALT:ALP | PHOSPHORUS RATIO |
|---|---|---|---|
| Hepatocellular injury | ≥2-fold increase | Normal | High (≥5) |
| Cholestatic injury | Normal | ≥2-fold increase | Low (≤2) |
| Mixed injury | ≥2-fold increase | ≥2-fold increase | 2–5 |

ALT, alanine aminotransferase; ALP, alkaline phosphatase.

### 3. Describe the typical chronologic association between drug exposure and onset of hepatitis or cholestasis.

Cholestatic or hepatocellular liver injury typically occurs 5 to 90 days after initial exposure. On withdrawal of the drug, biochemical improvement in hepatocellular injury usually is seen within 2 weeks, whereas cholestatic or mixed injury may not improve for 4 weeks. Persistence of abnormal liver biochemistries beyond these intervals suggests a coexistent or independent cause of liver disease (e.g., viral or autoimmune liver disease, primary biliary cirrhosis, primary sclerosing cholangitis).

### 4. What is the differential diagnosis of drug-induced liver disease?

Diagnosis of a drug-induced cause of liver injury requires exclusion of viral, toxic, cardiovascular, inheritable, and malignant causes. Careful history, review of past laboratory testing, and physical examination are often helpful. When drug-induced liver injury is suspected, withdrawal of the offending agent and close observation often provide adequate circumstantial evidence for the diagnosis. Liver biopsy should be reserved for situations in which discontinuation of the medication is not followed by prompt improvement, the cause of liver disease remains in question, or the severity necessitates intervention (organ transplantation, corticosteroids).

### 5. Explain the two most common mechanisms of drug-induced liver injury.

1. *Intrinsic* (hepatotoxin with direct or indirect toxicity to hepatocytes). Examples include phosphorus, carbon tetrachloride, acetaminophen, and chloroform. Intrinsic hepatotoxins cause direct damage to the liver by covalently binding to cellular macromolecules, such as hydrogen peroxide, hydroxyl radicals, or lipid peroxides. These, in turn, interrupt cell membranes or inactivate critical cellular enzyme systems.
2. *Idiosyncratic hyperimmune reaction.* Examples include phenytoin, isoniazid, ticrynafen, halothane, and valproic acid. Idiosyncratic hepatotoxins are dose independent, and hepatic injury cannot be reproduced in animal models. Clinical features of hypersensitivity (rash, fever, and eosinophilia) are common.

### 6. What variables appear to influence susceptibility to drug-induced hepatic injury?

* *Age.* Young people are more susceptible to aspirin and valproic acid. Old people are more susceptible to isoniazid, halothane, and acetaminophen.
* *Sex.* Women are more susceptible to all drug-induced liver disease, probably because of lower body mass and susceptibility to autoimmune hepatitis (e.g., alcohol, methyldopa, nitrofurantoin).

- *Inducers of hepatic enzymes.* Phenobarbital, phenytoin, ethanol, cigarette smoke, and grapefruit juice have all been shown to induce the hepatic cytochrome P-450 system causing either rapid or competitive metabolism of drugs.
- *Route of administration.* Tetracycline toxicity occurs primarily with the parenteral route.
- *Drug-drug interactions.* Valproic acid increases chlorpromazine-induced cholestasis. Rifampin potentiates isoniazid hepatotoxicity. Chronic alcohol ingestion potentiates acetaminophen and isoniazid hepatotoxicity.
- *Malnutrition.* Low glutathione level potentiates acetaminophen hepatotoxicity.

**7. Name the two most common causes of drug-induced liver disease.**
Alcohol and acetaminophen.

**8. How is acetaminophen toxic to the liver?**
Acetaminophen is toxic to the liver only in excessive doses or when the protective-detoxifying pathway (cytochrome P450 2E1) in the liver is overwhelmed. Accumulation of the toxic metabolite *N*-acetyl-*p*-benzoquinone-imine (NAPQI) is responsible for the death of hepatocytes. Acetaminophen is the second most common cause of death from poisoning in the United States.

**9. At what dose is acetaminophen toxic?**
Acetaminophen is hepatotoxic in nonalcoholic patients at doses greater than 7.5 g. A potentially lethal effect is seen with ingestion greater than 140 mg/kg (10 g in a 70-kg man). Chronic alcoholics are at greater risk of acetaminophen injury because of alcohol induction of the cytochrome P450 2E1 system and attendant malnutrition with low levels of glutathione, an intracellular protectant naturally found in hepatocytes.

**10. How is acetaminophen toxicity treated?**
The Rumack-Matthew nomogram helps to predict the likelihood of liver injury from acetaminophen and to direct therapy. The antidote for acetaminophen overdose is *N*-acetylcysteine (NAC). The oral dose of NAC is 140 mg/kg, followed by 17 maintenance doses of 70 mg/kg every 4 hours. NAC can be administered intravenously for 48 hours with equal or better efficacy than the oral route. Ipecac is given if the time of ingestion can be verified to be less than 4 hours. Use of activated charcoal is controversial, because it can interfere with the adsorption of oral NAC.

**11. Describe the clinical features of allergic hepatitis.**
Phenytoin causes allergic hepatitis, cholestasis, granulomatous liver disease, and even frank fulminant hepatic failure. Symptoms of hepatotoxicity usually occur within the first 8 weeks of administration. The incriminated metabolite is arene oxide. Systemic symptoms include pharyngitis, lymphadenopathy, and atypical lymphocytosis (so-called pseudolymphoma syndrome). There are some favorable reports of treating acute phenytoin hepatitis with corticosteroids.

**12. What drugs have been reported to cause chronic hepatitis and cirrhosis?**
Isoniazid, methotrexate, methyldopa, nitrofurantoin, oxyphenisatin, perhexiline maleate, and trazodone.

**13. Name the two types of cholestatic drug-induced hepatic injury.**
Inflammatory and bland cholestasis.

**14. List the common causes of drug-induced cholestasis.**

| Inflammatory Cholestasis | Bland Cholestasis |
| --- | --- |
| Allopurinol | Anabolic steroids |
| Amitriptyline | Androgens |
| Azathioprine | Estrogens |
| Captopril | Oral contraceptives |
| Carbamazepine | Phenytoin |

**15. List the drugs associated with the mixed cholestatic-hepatitis type of liver injury.**

| | | |
| --- | --- | --- |
| Amitriptyline | Flutamide | Ranitidine |
| Amoxicillin | Ibuprofen | Sulfonamides |
| Ampicillin | Imipramine | Sulindac |
| Captopril | Nitrofurantoin | Toxic oil syndrome |
| Carbamazepine | Phenylbutazone | Trimethoprim-sulfamethoxazole |
| Cimetidine | Quinidine | Naproxen |

**16. Which drugs cause the three types of drug-induced steatosis (*fatty liver*)?**
See Table 25-2.

**Table 25-2.** Three Types of Drug-Induced Steatosis

| MICROVESICULAR STEATOSIS | MACROVESICULAR STEATOSIS | PHOSPHOLIPIDOSIS |
|---|---|---|
| Aspirin (Reye syndrome) | Acetaminophen | 4,4'-Diethylaminoethylhexestrol |
| Ketoprofen | Cisplatin | Perhexiline maleate |
| Tetracycline | Corticosteroids | Amiodarone |
| Valproic acid | Methotrexate | Trimethroprim-sulfamethoxazide |
| Zidovudine (AZT) | Tamoxifen | Parenteral nutrition |

## 17. Which three vascular injuries to the liver can be caused by drugs?

- *Hepatic veno-occlusive disease (VOD):* pyrrolizidine alkaloids, antineoplastic drugs
- *Peliosis hepatis:* anabolic steroids, oral contraceptives
- *Hepatic vein thrombosis:* oral contraceptives

## 18. What are the three most common drug-induced hepatic neoplasms?

- *Hepatocellular carcinoma:* anabolic steroids, oral contraceptives, thorium oxide (Thorotrast), vinyl chloride
- *Angiosarcoma:* thorium oxide (Thorotrast), vinyl chloride, arsenic, anabolic steroids
- *Hepatic adenoma:* oral contraceptives,* anabolic steroids

## 19. More than 50 drugs have been cited as causing hepatic granulomas. Name the most common.

| | | |
|---|---|---|
| Allopurinol | Nitrofurantoin | Diazepam |
| Quinidine | Gold Aspirin | Sulfonamides |
| Penicillin | Oral contraceptives | Phenytoin |
| Mineral oil | Tolbutamide | Quinine |
| Diltiazem | Isoniazid | Oxacillin |
| Phenylbutazone | Chlorpromazine | |

## 20. What antiarthritic drugs have been reported to cause liver injury?

- *Aspirin.* Dose-dependent hepatocellular injury. Risk factors include high salicylate levels, female, youth, underlying rheumatoid arthritis, SLE, and possibly coexistent liver disease.
- *Sulindac (Clinoril).* Over 400 cases of sulindac-induced hepatitis have been reported. A cholestatic hepatitis is seen in most patients. Common clinical manifestations include fever, rash, and Stevens-Johnson syndrome. A "trapped" common bile duct causing cholestasis has been reported after sulindac-induced pancreatitis.
- *Bromfenac (Duract).* Acute hepatitis and liver failure. More common in women, those older than 50 years; treatment longer than 90 days. The U.S. Food and Drug Administration removed this drug from the U.S. market in June 1998.
- *Diclofenac (Voltaren).* The pattern of injury, uniquely more common in women than men, is primarily hepatitis. Fulminant hepatitis and death have been reported. Steroids may be helpful in severe cases.
- *Phenylbutazone (Butazolidin).* An immunologic type of injury is usually seen, with fever, rash, and eosinophilia. Illness usually starts within 6 weeks of initiating the drug. The hepatic injury seen is variable; acute hepatitis, cholestasis, and granulomatous hepatitis have been reported.
- *Ibuprofen (Motrin, Advil).* Hepatic injury due to ibuprofen is relatively uncommon. Over-the-counter doses of ibuprofen have not been reported to cause clinically apparent liver injury.
- *Piroxicam (Feldene).* Lethal hepatitis and cholestasis have been reported, but overall liver injury appears to be uncommon.
- *Celecoxib (Celebrex).* Acute pancreatitis and hepatitis have been reported. Women are more susceptible and an increased risk for those with preexisting sulfa allergy is controversial.

## 21. How should patients receiving chronic methotrexate (MTX) be monitored for chronic hepatitis and cirrhosis?

MTX has been used in patients with refractory psoriasis and rheumatoid arthritis. In patients with psoriasis, many advocate an index liver biopsy after 2 to 4 months of MTX therapy, followed by serial repeat biopsies after every 1.0 to 1.5 g of cumulative dose. In patients with rheumatoid arthritis, MTX appears to be somewhat less hepatotoxic. The American College of Rheumatology does not recommend a pretreatment liver biopsy in the absence of preexisting liver disease, but liver-associated enzymes should be monitored. Reevaluation of MTX safety is advised when aspartate aminotransferase (AST) or ALT levels exceed 3 times the baseline values. Liver biopsies are advised every 2 or 3 years (or every 1.5 g of cumulative dose).

*Before the availability of oral contraceptives, hepatic adenomas were rare. After 5 years of oral contraceptive use, the relative risk of developing a hepatic adenoma has been estimated to increase 116-fold. Hepatic adenomas often regress when exogenous estrogen is removed and can recur during pregnancy. Anabolic steroids also have been reported to cause hepatic adenomas. Hepatic adenomas are usually asymptomatic but can be associated with abdominal fullness, pain, hepatomegaly, and hemorrhage.

**22. What are the histologic grades of MTX liver injury?**
See Table 25-3.

**Table 25-3.** Histologic Grades of Methotrexate Liver Injury

| GRADE | FIBROSIS | FATTY INFILTRATION | NUCLEAR VARIABILITY | PORTAL INFLAMMATION |
|-------|----------|--------------------|--------------------|--------------------|
| I | None | Mild | Mild | Mild |
| II | None | Moderate to severe | Moderate to severe | Portal expansion, lobular necrosis |
| IIIB | Moderate to severe | Moderate to severe | Moderate to severe | Portal expansion, lobular necrosis |
| IV | Cirrhosis | | | |

**23. Outline the recommendations for change in MTX therapy based on liver biopsy findings.**
**I** Continue therapy; repeat biopsy after 1 to 1.5 g of cumulative dose.
**II** Continue therapy; repeat biopsy after 1 to 1.5 g of cumulative dose.
**IIIA** Continue therapy, but repeat biopsy in 6 months.
**IIIB** No further MTX; exceptional cases need close histologic follow-up.
**IV** No further MTX; exceptional cases need close histologic follow-up.

**24. What are the clinical findings of chlorzoxazone hepatotoxicity?**
Chlorzoxazone (Parafon Forte) is a centrally acting muscle relaxant. Hepatotoxic effects are rare, but severe hepatitis, including fulminant hepatic failure, has been reported. Onset of injury may occur within 1 week of initiation or up to several years later. The transaminase elevation may exceed 1000 IU/L. Most patients also exhibit hyperbilirubinemia. Discontinuation of the medication is usually the only intervention necessary.

**25. Which drugs commonly used to treat endocrine disease have been reported to cause liver injury?**
- *Thiazolidinediones* (TZDs) are a class of compounds specifically designed to reduce insulin resistance by increasing peripheral glucose disposal and decreasing glucose production. The TZDs include troglitazone, rosiglitazone, and pioglitazone. Ninety-four cases of acute liver failure were reported to be caused by troglitazone, causing the drug to be removed from the U.S. market in March 2000. Case reports of hepatotoxicity caused by rosiglitazone (4) and pioglitazone (3) have been published, but the rate of hepatotoxicity is far less common than with troglitazone. FDA recommendations for baseline and then monthly monitoring of liver tests during the first year of treatment with -glitazone agents is of unproved value and infrequently performed by health care providers.
- *Sulfonylureas* include chlorpropamide, glipizide, tolazamide, tolbutamide acetohexamide, and glyburide. The pattern of injury is cholestatic for chlorpropamide, glipizide, tolazamide, and tolbutamide and hepatocellular or mixed with the remainder. A hypersensitivity reaction is thought to be responsible. Hypersensitivity to chlorpropamide does not predict the same response to tolbutamide.
- *Thiourea derivatives* (propylthiouracil, methimazole) may cause hepatocellular or cholestatic injury.
- *Steroid derivatives* (anabolic steroids, oral contraceptives, tamoxifen, danazol, glucocorticoids) are reported to cause cholestasis or canalicular type of liver injury.
- *Lipid-lowering agents* include niacin and HMG-CoA reductase inhibitors. Niacin (nicotinic acid) may cause mixed cholestatic-hepatic injury. Injury is more common with the sustained-release form or at doses greater than 3 g/day for the regular-release form. Serial monitoring of liver enzymes is recommended, and the drug should be discontinued if elevations are detected. Lovastatin is the most commonly prescribed of the HMG-CoA reductase inhibitors used to treat hypercholesterolemia. Mild elevations in aminotransferases are common, but levels usually return to normal on drug withdrawal.

**26. What commonly used cardiovascular drugs have been reported to cause liver injury?**
- *Quinidine.* Liver injury has been reported after a single dose. The predominant injury is hepatocellular with focal necrosis, but diffuse granulomas also have been seen.
- *Procainamide.* Injury to the liver is rare, but hepatocellular, cholestatic, and granulomatous injuries have been reported.
- *Verapamil* and *nifedipine.* Hepatitis has been reported to develop within 2 to 3 weeks of drug administration. Cholestatic, hepatocellular, and mixed injuries have been reported. A pseudo-alcohol pattern of steatosis and Mallory hyaline has been reported with use of nifedipine.
- *Hydralazine.* Hepatocellular and granulomatous injury have been reported.
- *Captopril.* Hypersensitivity symptoms usually herald jaundice. Cholestasis usually ameliorates rapidly after drug removal.
- *Enalapril.* Scattered cases of hepatitis and cholestasis have been reported.

- *Ticrynafen.* This uricosuric diuretic was removed from the U.S. market shortly after its introduction because of the significant incidence of liver injury. The hepatitis can be fatal.
- *Amiodarone.* This iodine-containing benzofuran used as an antianginal and antiarrhythmic agent, accumulates within the hepatic lysosome, where it complexes with phospholipids and inhibits lysosomal phospholipases.

## 27. What are the clinical features of methyldopa (Aldomet) hepatocellular injury?

Liver injury usually occurs within 6 to 12 weeks of initiation of methyldopa therapy. Aminotransferase values should be obtained periodically during the first 4 months of drug administration. Women appear to be more susceptible to methyldopa hepatotoxicity, and the clinical presentation may mimic autoimmune lupoid hepatitis.

## 28. What commonly used antimicrobial agents have been shown to cause liver injury?

- *Tetracycline.* Liver injury is seen almost exclusively with parenteral administration and is more common in women, especially during pregnancy. Microvesicular steatosis is the characteristic histologic finding.
- *Erythromycin estolate.* Initially liver injury was thought to occur only with the estolate form, but the ethylsuccinate form has recently been implicated as a cause of cholestatic hepatitis. A hypersensitivity picture is usually seen within days to 2 weeks after exposure.
- *Chloramphenicol.* Rare cases of cholestasis and jaundice have been reported.
- *Penicillin.* Both cholestatic and hepatitis-like patterns have been reported. Hypersensitivity is the mechanism of injury.
- *Amoxicillin, clavulanic acid.* Cholestatic hepatitis has been seen during or within weeks of administration.
- *Sulfonamides* cause mixed hepatocellular injury that usually is heralded by rash, fever, and eosinophilia.
- *Pyrimethamine-sulfadoxine.* Hepatocellular injury is most common, but fulminant hepatitis and death have been reported.
- *Sulfasalazine,* which is used to treat inflammatory bowel disease, may cause the same injury as sulfonamides.
- *Nitrofurantoin.* Hallmarks of hypersensitivity are common, with both cholestatic and hepatocellular injury reported. Chronic active hepatitis has been reported, usually in women older than 40 years with HLA-B8 histocompatibility.
- *Rifampin* potentiates the hepatotoxicity of isoniazid, presumably by induction of cytochrome P450. Women older than 50 years are especially susceptible.
- *Griseofulvin.* Hepatitis is rare, but the drug can precipitate attacks of acute intermittent porphyria.
- *Ketoconazole.* Toxic hepatitis more common in women older than 40 years. Fulminant hepatitis has been reported. Periodic monitoring of liver enzymes is recommended to detect early injury.
- *Flucytosine.* Transaminase elevations are common; significant hepatitis is rare.

## 29. Who is at risk for liver toxicity from isoniazid (INH) therapy?

INH hepatitis may present insidiously from 4 to 6 months after initiation of therapy. Some patients experience influenza-like symptoms. Abnormal AST and ALT elevations develop in up to 20% of patients taking INH, but aminotransferase activity usually subsides to normal spontaneously. The risk for frank hepatitis is 0.3% at ages 20 to 34 years, 1.2% at ages 35 to 49 years, and 2.3% at ages over 50 years. Coadministration of rifampin increases the likelihood of INH toxicity. Acetaminophen toxicity is increased by INH because it induces the cytochrome P450 enzyme system.

## 30. How is INH toxicity prevented?

Current recommendations include screening patients for ethanol abuse and preexisting liver or renal disease. The presence of chronic liver disease is not an absolute contraindication to the use of INH, but the indications should be scrutinized and therapy monitored more closely. The American Thoracic Society recommends dispensing only 1 month's supply of INH to ensure close monitoring. Patients should be advised to report prodromal symptoms immediately. All patients older than 35 years should have serial monitoring of ALT, and the use of INH should be reconsidered when ALT elevations persist or remain greater than 100 IU/L.

## 31. What commonly used recreational drugs are associated with hepatotoxicity?

- *Cocaine.* An estimated 30 million Americans have experimented with cocaine, and 5 million abuse it habitually. Patients with cocaine hepatotoxicity may present with jaundice or fatigue and generalized malaise. The aminotransferase elevations can be in the 5000-IU/L range. Cocaine toxicity also may cause coagulopathy, rhabdomyolysis, and disseminated intravascular coagulation (DIC). The mechanism of hepatotoxicity is unknown. Liver biopsy typically shows zone III injury, suggesting related ischemia. In this setting, liver injury may be multifactorial and include coexistent viral liver disease (hepatitis B, C, and delta) and acetaminophen or alcohol use.
- *Ecstasy.* This synthetic amphetamine (3,4-methylene dioxymethamphetamine) is commonly used as a weekend drug. It makes users euphoric and more sociable and eliminates fatigue. Initially thought to have little toxicity, Ecstasy has been reported to cause various systemic effects, including cardiac arrhythmias, DIC, acute renal failure, hyperthermia, and fulminant hepatitis. Physicians should suspect Ecstasy use in a young adult with acute hepatitis but no identifiable cause.

**32. What anesthetic agents are associated with hepatocellular injury?**

Halothane, enflurane, methoxyflurane, and isoflurane. Whenever hepatitis occurs postoperatively, nonanesthetic causes must be considered (e.g., viral hepatitis, drug-induced hepatitis, bile duct injury, cholestasis of total parenteral nutrition or sepsis, transfusion hepatitis, ischemic hepatopathy).

The risk for halothane hepatitis is 1 in 10,000 patients but increases to 7 in 10,000 after two or more exposures. More than 75% of patients with halothane liver injury present within 2 weeks of exposure with fever, nausea, rash, arthralgias, and diffuse abdominal discomfort. Laboratory abnormalities include eosinophilia, AST and ALT elevations in the range of 500 to 1000 IU/L, and AP elevation (usually less than 2 times normal). The mechanism appears to be related to development of sensitization to both the oxidative metabolite of halothane, trifluoroacetyl halide, and autoantigens (including CYP2D6). Prognostic factors for poor outcome include a short latent period from exposure to jaundice, obesity, age older than 40 years, hepatic encephalopathy, and prolongation of the prothrombin time. Corticosteroids and exchange transfusions are not helpful, and the mortality rate of fulminant halothane hepatitis is nearly 80% without liver transplantation.

**33 Can herbal therapies injure the liver?**

Yes and no. Because the composition of herbal remedies is variable and unregulated, persons with preexisting liver disease should be cautious and consult their doctor.

- *Safe herbs:* Milk thistle (Silybum marianum) is a safe substance that has been used for centuries to remedy liver disease. Many patients with liver disease self-medicate with milk thistle. Although aminotransferase levels commonly improve, no good evidence suggests that it improves the liver disorder. Silymarin plus thioctic acid and penicillin has been successfully used in the treatment of Amanita mushroom poisoning.
- *Potentially hepatotoxic herbs*
  - Autoimmune hepatitis: *Syo-saiko-to, Ma-huang,* germander
  - Cirrhosis: *Syo saiko-to,* chaparral, greater celandine, *Jin Bu Huan*
  - Cholestasis hepatitis: *Cascara sagrada,* chaparral, greater celandine, kava, *Syo-saiko-to*
  - Fulminant hepatic failure: *Atractylis gummifera,* chaparral, cocaine, germander, kava
  - Veno-occlusive disease: pyrolizidine alkaloids (teas), Skullcap

# WEBSITES

http://www.fda.gov/cder/livertox/

http://www.livertransplant.org

# BIBLIOGRAPHY

1. Andrade RJ, Lucena MI, Fernández MC, et al. Drug-induced liver injury: An analysis of 461 incidences submitted to the Spanish registry over a 10-year period. Gastroenterology 2005;129:512–21.
2. Bhardwaj SS, Chalasani N. Lipid lowering agents that cause drug-induced hepatotoxicity. Clin Liver Dis 2007;11:597–613.
3. Bromer MQ, Black M. Acetaminophen hepatotoxicity. Clin Liver Dis 2003;7:351–67.
4. Chang CY, Schiano TD. Review article: Drug hepatotoxicity. Aliment Pharmacol Ther 2007;25:1135–51.
5. Cunha BA. Antibiotic therapy: Antibiotic side effects. Med Clin North Am 2001;85:149–85.
6. Gunawan BK, Kaplowitz N. Mechanisms of drug-induced liver disease. Clin Liver Dis 2007;11:459–75.
7. Hussaini SH, Farrington EA. Idiosyncratic drug-induced liver injury: An overview. Exp Opin Drug Saf 2007;6:673–84.
8. Junaidi O, Di Bisceglie A. Aging liver and hepatitis. Clin Geriatr Med 2007;23:889–903.
9. Lee WM. Drug induced hepatotoxicity. N Engl J Med 2003;349:474–85.
10. Lewis JH. 'Hy's law,' 'the Rezulin Rule,' and other predictors of severe drug-induced hepatotoxicity. Pharmacoepidemiol Drug Saf 2006;15:221–9.
11. Maddrey WC. Drug-induced hepatotoxicity. J Clin Gastroenterol 2005;39(Suppl. 2):S83–9.
12. Nathwani RA, Kaplowitz N. Drug hepatotoxicity. Clin Liver Dis 2006;10:207–17.
13. Seeff LB. Herbal hepatotoxicity. Clin Liver Dis 2007;11:577–96.
14. Teoh NC, Farrell GC. Hepatotoxicity associated with non-steroidal anti-inflammatory drugs. Clin Liver Dis 2003;7:401–13.
15. Tolman KG, Chandramouli J. Hepatotoxicity of the thiazolidinediones. Clin Liver Dis 2003;7:369–79.
16. Tostmann A, Boeree MJ, Aarnoutse RE, et al. Antituberculosis drug-induced hepatotoxicity: Concise up-to-date review. J Gastroenterol Hepatol 2008;23:192–202.
17. West SG. Methotrexate hepatotoxicity. Rheum Dis Clin North Am 1997;23:883–915.
18. Yew WW, Leung CC. Antituberculosis drugs and hepatotoxicity. Respirology 2006;11:699–707.
19. Zapater P, Moreu R, Horga JF. The diagnosis of drug-induced liver disease. Curr Clin Pharmacol 2006;1:207–17.

# ALCOHOLIC LIVER DISEASE

*Rowen K. Zetterman, MD, MACP, MACG*

### 1. How does the liver metabolize ethanol?

The liver is the principal site of ethanol metabolism. Following ingestion, ethanol is absorbed from the stomach and the proximal small intestine. Although a small amount of alcohol dehydrogenase (ADH) is present in the stomach mucosa, ethanol is largely oxidized to acetaldehyde within the liver by ADH. Some ethanol is also metabolized by the microsomal ethanol oxidizing system (MEOS) through microsomal P450 enzymes (CYP2EI) and by catalase. The role of CYP2EI in ethanol metabolism is greater when large quantities of ethanol are consumed. The metabolism of ethanol by P450 enzymes results in formation of reactive oxygen species and causes lipid peroxidation that can result in hepatocyte injury.

$$\underset{\text{(Ethanol)}}{C_2H_5OH} + 2[O] \xrightarrow[\text{MEOS}]{\text{ADH}} \underset{\text{(Acetaldehyde)}}{CH_3COOH} + H_2O$$

Consequences of chronic ethanol detoxification include:

- Ketosis
- Hypoglycemia
- Hypertriglyceridemia
- Hyperuricemia
- Insulin resistance
- Mitochondrial inhibition of oxidative phosphorylation

Some Japanese patients with cirrhosis are more likely to have a variant of ADH enzyme leading to greater formation of acetaldehyde. Aldehyde dehydrogenase (ALDH) within the mitochondria metabolizes the majority of acetaldehyde to acetate. A variant of ALDH, ALDH2*2 reduces the conversion of acetaldehyde to acetate. Homozygous ALDH2*2 patients accumulate acetaldehyde because of reduced conversion to acetate with occurrence of offensive symptoms such as flushing. Up to 50% of patients from the Far East are homozygous for AIDH2*2 and develop symptoms from ethanol consumption.

### 2. How common is alcohol abuse in the United States?

Approximately 6% to 7% of the American population meets the criteria for diagnosis of alcohol abuse or alcohol dependence, representing approximately 2 million Americans. More than 70% of the annual U.S. consumption of alcohol is used by only 10% of the population and, of these, approximately three quarters are male.

### 3. How can I screen a patient for alcoholism during an office visit?

The diagnosis of alcohol dependence can be based on *DSM-IV-TR* criteria with positive findings in at least three of seven categories, including tolerance, withdrawal, consuming more ethanol over time, having a desire to cut down on ethanol consumption, time spent in obtaining alcohol, giving up of important activities to drink ethanol, and continuing to drink despite knowledge of personal impairment.

The CAGE questionnaire mnemonic is a quick and simple test that can help identify alcohol dependence. It includes four questions:

| | |
|---|---|
| **C** | Have you ever tried to cut down on drinking? |
| **A** | Are you annoyed when people criticize you for drinking? |
| **G** | Do you feel guilty about your drinking? |
| **E** | Do you need an eye opener in the morning? |

A positive response to two or more of these questions suggests a high likelihood of alcohol dependence with the diagnostic accuracy of approximately 80%.

The Michigan Alcoholism Screening Test (MAST) can also be used and includes 25 "yes or no" questions that are scored with the diagnostic accuracy of approximately 90% for alcoholism.

## 4. What are the signs and symptoms of alcohol withdrawal syndrome?

Signs and symptoms of ethyl alcohol withdrawal can be divided into four time intervals (Table 26-1).

**Table 26-1.** Signs and Symptoms of Ethyl Alcohol Withdrawal

| SYMPTOMS OF ALCOHOL WITHDRAWAL | ΔTIME FROM CESSATION TO ONSET OF SYMPTOM | PEARLS |
|---|---|---|
| Insomnia, tremulousness, mild anxiety, GI upset, headache, diaphoresis, palpation, anorexia | 6 to 12 hr | |
| Alcohol hallucinations: visual, auditory, or tactile | 12 to 24 hr | These symptoms usually resolve in 48 hr. |
| Withdrawal seizures: generalized tonic-clonic type. They can be very difficult to treat; avoid medications that lower seizure threshold. | 24 to 48 hr | Do not be fooled; seizures can occur as early as 2 hr after cessation of alcohol. |
| Delirium tremens: hallucinations (predominately visual), disorientation, tachycardia, hypertension, low-grade fever, agitation, diaphoresis | 48 to 72 hr | These symptoms peak at 5 days. |

GI, gastrointestinal.

## 5. How should I manage alcohol withdrawal in the alcoholic patient?

Chronic ethanol ingestion enhances the effect of γ-aminobutyric acid (GABA) on brain neuroreceptors resulting in decreased brain excitability. With abrupt withdrawal of ethanol, brain hyperexcitability develops producing the symptoms of withdrawal. Early symptoms of withdrawal include tremulousness, insomnia, anxiety, palpitations, sweating, anxiety, agitation, tremor, and nausea and vomiting. Approximately 24 hours after ethanol withdrawal, generalized seizures may develop. Alcohol withdrawal seizures are more common in those with multiple prior alcohol withdrawal episodes. At 48 to 72 hours following withdrawal, hallucinations, tachycardia, hypertension, fever, and agitation typically become manifest.

The evaluation of an alcoholic patient with suspected withdrawal should include a careful history and physical to identify complicating conditions. Other clinical conditions that may mimic alcohol withdrawal include thyrotoxicosis, anticholinergic drug poisoning, amphetamine or cocaine excess, and other drug withdrawal.

## 6. How is alcohol detoxification best managed?

Detoxification management will reduce complications and improve rehabilitation of the alcoholic. Detoxification includes initiating abstinence from ethanol, treating withdrawal symptoms, and maintaining abstinence treatment to prevent recidivism. Of those going through alcohol withdrawal, approximately 10% to 20% will require inpatient treatment. You should consider hospitalization for any patient with a previous history of severe alcohol withdrawal, prior seizures during withdrawal, concomitant medical or psychiatric illness, and lack of reliable home support.

## 7. What are the usual steps taken for in-hospital treatment of withdrawal?

### STEP 1. SUPPORTIVE CARE

- Quiet room, soft lighting and supportive care
- Intravenous fluids (dehydration)
- Correction of electrolyte disturbance (↓K, ↓glucose, and ↓Mg)
- *Parenteral* thiamine, 100 mg then daily

Pearl: Give thiamine before glucose to prevent Wernicke-Korsakoff syndrome, and remember oral thiamine is poorly absorbed.

- Folic acid (malnutrition)
- Antiemetics for nausea
- Acid blockers for gastrointestinal (GI) upset

### STEP 2. WITHDRAWAL SYMPTOMS (Tremulousness, hallucinations, agitation, autonomic hyperactivity)

- Benzodiazepine drugs will reduce the severity of withdrawal symptoms.
- Longer half-life ($T_{1/2}$): chlordiazepoxide and alazepam (caution among elderly)
- Shorter $T_{1/2}$: lorazepam and oxazepam (renal clearance safer in liver failure)

### Step 3. Other Treatments

- Seizures: diazepam, phenytoin, or carbamazine
- Agitation or hallucinations: haloperidol
- Tachycardia: γ-blockers or clonidine

Either a fixed dose schedule of daily benzodiazepines or symptom-triggered regimens can be used. When symptom-triggered regimens are recommended, the use of an algorithm to establish the frequency of benzodiazepine doses for withdrawal symptoms and signs (e.g., CIWA-Ar with a score higher than 10 points) should be considered. The use of symptom-triggered regimens often results in less total drug does than standard or fixed regimens of withdrawal therapy. With time, benzodiazepine doses should be reduced as withdrawal symptoms improve.

### 8. What treatments help in the long term for alcohol dependency?

Long-term abstinence should include referral to a substance use disorder clinic, as both cognitive and behavioral therapy is required to sustain ethanol abstinence. Those with repeated detoxification frequently have increased alcohol craving, which increases the severity of subsequent withdrawal episodes. Recidivism is common and pharmacologic agents to encourage abstinence can be used. Disulfiram is an aldehyde dehydrogenase inhibitor that prevents acetaldehyde metabolism and increases circulating acetaldehyde levels to produce symptoms of flushing, dizziness, and vomiting if ethanol is consumed. This aversion therapy can decrease ethanol intake. Other agents that can be used to encourage abstinence include acamprosate or naltrexone. Naltrexone, an opioid antagonist, can also be administered intramuscularly. If pharmacologic therapy is used, behavioral therapy should be included. Despite adequate detoxification, only one-third of patients will be abstinent or have limited ethanol consumption at 1-year follow-up.

### 9. What are the different types of alcoholic liver disease (ALD)?

End-stage liver disease (ESLD) due to ethanol is the most common cause of cirrhosis of the Western world. Several morphologic manifestations of alcohol consumption may be observed, although some patients with chronic alcoholism will have no histologic evidence of liver injury at liver biopsy.

- *Fatty metamorphosis* of the liver is the most common histologic finding and the earliest manifestation following ethanol ingestion. Fat accumulation in hepatocytes can develop within 2 days of excessive ethanol consumption and clear within 2 weeks of cessation. Fatty metamorphosis is macrovesicular with large droplet fat that displaces the nucleus of centrilobular hepatocytes. The finding of fatty liver in the alcoholic can be an indicator for future risk of developing alcoholic cirrhosis if ethanol intake continues.
- *Microvesicular steatosis* or alcoholic foamy degeneration is an infrequent complication of alcohol consumption. It appears to be a consequence of mitochondrial dysfunction from ethanol, largely developing within centrilobular hepatocytes, and results in hyperbilirubinemia, hepatic encephalopathy, and death.
- *Alcoholic hepatitis* occurs in approximately 10% to 20% of chronic alcoholics and is the pathway for the development of cirrhosis for most patients with chronic alcohol intake. The diagnosis is established by a typical history of long-term daily ethanol consumption, appropriate laboratory findings, and a liver histology that includes centrilobular hepatocellular necrosis, polymorphonuclear leukocyte inflammation, and the presence of Mallory hyaline.
- *Alcoholic cirrhosis* is the ESLD of ALD that follows alcoholic hepatitis or veno-occlusive alcoholic liver injury. Alcoholic cirrhosis develops as micronodular cirrhosis. With cessation of ethanol intake, many patients will transform to macronodular (larger regenerative nodules) cirrhosis. Alcoholic hepatitis may coexist with cirrhosis in those continuing to consume ethanol. Alcoholic cirrhosis is also a predisposing lesion for hepatocellular carcinoma (HCC).

### 10. How does ALD differ from nonalcoholic fatty liver disease?

Nonalcoholic fatty liver disease (NAFLD) develops in patients who have metabolic syndrome associated with obesity, hyperlipidemia, and type 2 diabetes mellitus. The histologic manifestations of NAFLD are similar to ALD and its diagnosis is dependent on the exclusion of significant ethanol intake. Most use a criterion of less than 20 g of absolute ethanol equivalent daily to establish the diagnosis of nonalcoholic fatty liver disease. This would be equivalent to two bottles of beer or one shot of spirits daily.

### 11. What is the natural history of ALD?

As alcoholic patients are a heterogeneous population, the prevalence of liver injury from alcohol varies from person to person and a direct correlation of advanced liver disease from excessive alcohol consumption is not always observed. In general, there is a direct correlation between the consumption of ethanol and subsequent liver-related mortality. Patients with fatty metamorphosis of the liver from alcohol are more likely to progress to end-stage cirrhosis with continued ethanol consumption than those lacking fatty change of hepatocytes. Fatty liver also correlates with increased all-cause mortality. Of those who consume daily excess alcohol for 12 or more years, more than 20% will develop cirrhosis. Risk factors for development of ALD are listed in Table 26-2.

**Table 26-2.** Risk Factors for Development of Alcoholic Liver Disease

| RISK FACTOR | QUALIFIER | RELATIVE RISK |
| --- | --- | --- |
| Quantity of ethyl alcohol (EtOH) | | |
| ♂ | 80 g/day × 10+ yr | ↑↑↑ |
| ♀ | 40 g/day × 10+ yr | ↑↑↑ |
| Consumption pattern | Continuous > periodic | ↑↑ |
| Malnutrition | | ↑↑ |
| Ethnicity | Hispanic and African American > white American | ↑ |
| Genetics | Japanese AHD gene A1DH2*2 | ↑↑ |
| Obesity | High fat content Empty calories from EtOH | ↑↑ |
| HCV infection | PCR positive, viral replicator | ↑↑↑ |
| Hemochromatosis | Homozygous gene | ↑↑↑ |
| Age >65 yr | Varies with general health and nutrition | ↑ |

PCR, polymerase chain reaction.

## 12. What is the epidemiology of ALD?
In the United States, 11% of men and 4% of women or a total of more than 6% of Americans are alcoholics. Approximately 15% to 30% of alcoholics who continue to drink daily will develop cirrhosis. Alcoholic cirrhosis accounts for 28% to 50% of total deaths from cirrhosis with an age-adjusted rate of 3.8 per 100,000 population.

## 13. What is the pathogenesis of ALD?
The pathogenesis of ALD is not well established. A number of factors have been identified and discussed in this chapter, including the total dose of alcohol consumed over a long period, the genetic polymorphism of alcohol metabolizing enzymes and their potential effect on levels of both ethanol and acetaldehyde, genetic factors in which monozygotic twins have a 3-fold increase of alcoholism in both compared with dizygotic or fraternal twins, the effect of high-fat/low-carbohydrate diets and of obesity, the greater susceptibility of women to effects of alcohol, and the additive effects of hepatitis C virus (HCV) and alcohol in producing ESLD.

Although fatty liver is often considered a benign condition, it may play a direct role in progression as those who develop fatty liver from alcohol or more likely to progress to alcoholic cirrhosis with continued drinking than those who do not. Fatty metamorphosis may change the intrahepatic immune milieu permitting greater effects of tumor necrosis factor-α (TNFα) or of acetaldehyde-adduct formation that results in progressive liver injury.

Possible immune mechanisms leading to advanced ALD are complex. Consumption of ethanol results in generalized immunosuppression, yet ALD may be a consequence of increased cellular immunity. A cellular immune response seems evident by the increase of CD8-positive cells in the peripheral blood and liver tissue of patients with alcoholic hepatitis and increased natural killer (NK) cells are also noted. Alcohol directly increases intestinal permeability to bacterial endotoxins. Circulating endotoxin levels are increased in patients with advanced ALD. Endotoxin binds to the CD14 receptor on Kupffer cells to enhance transcription of proinflammatory cytokines such as TNFα, transforming growth factor-β (TGFβ), and interleukin (IL)-6. Each of these cytokines could play a role in the inflammatory process of alcoholic hepatitis and their levels correlate with both endotoxinemia and with the severity of liver disease. TNFα will enhance transcription of cytokines such as IL-1 and IL-8 that increase inflammation and recruitment of white cells to the site of liver injury in alcoholic hepatitis. TNFα may play a role in that hemodynamic changes occurring in patients with severe alcoholic hepatitis. TGFβ may prepare hepatocytes to undergo apoptosis, a mechanism of cellular death.

Hypergammaglobulinemia is common in patients with advanced ALD. Circulating antibodies to acetaldehyde-protein adducts also develop. Acetaldehyde binds to lysine residues on proteins to form adducts within centrilobular hepatocytes that may initiate cellular immune responses to produce hepatocyte injury and liver fibrosis. Lipid peroxidation also occurs during ethanol metabolism resulting in the formation of malondialdehyde. Malondialdehyde-acetaldehyde protein adducts have been observed in patients with alcoholic cirrhosis and alcoholic hepatitis but not in alcoholics who lack advanced liver injury. While conclusive evidence is not available to confirm their role, these adducts may be a factor in causing liver injury.

The initial injury of the liver in alcoholic hepatitis is centrilobular or perivenular in location. Pericellular fibrosis develops at the site of maximal liver injury, eventually progressing to bridging fibrosis from central-to-central and central-to-portal areas, resulting in cirrhosis. Recruitment of inflammatory cells with secretion of cytokines causes sinusoidal stellate cell activation and production of collagen. Products of lipid peroxidation such as malondialdehyde and reactive oxygen species can activate collagen production by stellate cells. Circulating acetaldehyde can up regulate the transcription of collagen I. Kupffer cells that are activated by endotoxin can release cytokines such as TGFβ to induce collagen synthesis by stellate cells with deposition of extracellular matrix proteins. These events appear to lead to fibrosis at the site of maximum alcoholic injury.

## 14. What are the clinical findings in the patient with ALD?

The diagnosis of ALD is assisted by a careful clinical history and physical examination. Physical findings include enlarged liver (often tender hepatomegaly), jaundice, spider angiomata, hypogonadism, gynecomastia, Dupuytren contracture, and palmar erythrema.

## 15. What are the laboratory findings in patients with ALD?

- Elevated triglycerides
- Elevated uric acid
- Elevated γ-glutamyl transpeptidase (GGT)
- Elevated mean corpuscular volume (MCV)

## 16. Patients with alcoholic fatty liver may lack any laboratory signs, although aminotransferase levels and GGT can be elevated.

Patients with alcoholic hepatitis typically have elevated aspartate aminotransferase (AST) levels that are typically higher than alanine aminotransferase (ALT) levels but usually of less than 250 IU/mL. Alcoholic hepatitis is a cholestatic disease with elevation of alkaline phosphatase, GGT, and serum bilirubin levels. Complete blood counts can include leukocytosis. White cell counts are typically modest, 12,000 to 14,000/μL, although leukemoid levels are observed. Red blood cell levels may be normal or reduced and have macrocytic due to alcohol or be microcytic from iron deficiency due to blood loss. Hemolysis can occur with reticulocytosis, plasma hemoglobin levels, and peripheral blood smears demonstrating helmet cells and acanthocytes. Platelet counts may be reduced by a direct effect of ethanol on the bone marrow or by splenic sequestration from hypersplenism. Coagulopathy occurs from impaired hepatic production of coagulation factors. The international normalized ratio (INR) for prothrombin times is often abnormal. Electrolyte disturbances including hypokalemia and hypomagnesemia can be present.

Alcoholic cirrhosis can also result in elevation of aminotransferase levels including an AST/ALT ratio of greater than 1. In the abstinent patient, aminotransferase levels are only modestly elevated or are normal. In compensated cirrhosis, all liver tests can be normal. Hypoalbuminemia and hypergammaglobulinemia with elevation of IgG and IgA may be present. Some patients with alcoholic cirrhosis and continuing ethanol consumption will have coexisting alcoholic hepatitis.

## 17. How does radiographic imaging help in evaluation of the patient with ALD?

Findings on radiographic imaging of the liver in ALD are nonspecific. Changes of fatty liver are common, but indistinguishable from other causes of fatty liver and non–alcoholic liver disease (NASH). Gallstones are more common in ALD, but no different from that seen in other patients with cholelethiasis. Findings of an enlarged portal vein, splenomegaly, and a nodular liver are consistent with cirrhosis and not specific to ALD. The reader is referred to Chapter 70 for a detailed discussion of noninvasive gastrointestinal imaging.

## 18. What are the characteristic histologic features of ALD?

Liver histology can be obtained percutaneously, laparoscopically, by open biopsy, or by transvenous biopsy across the hepatic veins. Before a percutaneous liver biopsy is carried out, significant coagulopathy should be excluded. Most clinicians recommend that there be at least 80,000 platelets/μL with an INR of less than 1.5. For patients whose coagulation profile cannot be normalized, transvenous liver biopsy may be used.

See Chapter 33 for the gamut of histologic findings seen with ethyl alcohol (EtOH) liver injury:

Alcoholic fatty liver → Alcoholic hepatitis → Cirrhosis

Pearls: The histologic picture of EtOH liver disease can look identical to that of NASH, including cirrhotic liver disease! Identification of Mallory hyaline on liver biopsy is not specific to alcoholic hepatitis and can be seen in NASH, Wilson disease, autoimmune hepatitis, Indian childhood cirrhosis, and primary biliary cirrhosis (PBC).

## 19. What is the treatment for ALD?

### STEP 1. SUPPORTIVE CARE

- EtOH abstinence
- Substance use disorder programs
- Nutrition
- Vitamin supplements: folate and thiamine

### STEP 2. IDENTIFY HIGH-RISK ACUTE ALCOHOLIC HEPATITIS

- Bilirubin and prothrombin INR levels are predictive of outcome.
- The patient with alcoholic hepatitis and a bilirubin level of less than 5 mg/dL usually does well.
- The Maddrey discriminant function (DF) score can be used to assess the risk of death from alcoholic hepatitis and to determine when corticosteroids should be used for those with severe clinical disease.

$$DF = bilirubin (mg/dL) + 4.6 \times (prothrombin\ time\ [in\ seconds]\ - the\ control)$$
DF ≥32, associated mortality 50% within 2 months
DF <32, associated mortality 15% within 2 months

Administration of corticosteroids can improve 30-day survival in those whose DF is greater than 32 or those with spontaneous encephalopathy in the presence of alcoholic hepatitis. Other treatments of acute alcoholic hepatitis are listed in Table 26-3.

**Table 26-3.** Proposed Treatments for Acute Alcoholic Hepatitis.

| TREATMENT | IMPROVEMENT IN SURVIVAL | QUALIFYING FACTORS |
|---|---|---|
| Corticosteroids | Yes<br>No | DF ≥32<br>DF <32 |
| Nutrition | Yes | ↓ Spontaneous bacterial peritonitis<br>May improve histology |
| Anabolic steroids | Yes<br>No | Improve long-term survival<br>Short-term survival p=NS |
| Pentoxifylline | Yes | 40% |
| TNF-α medications | Perhaps | Not FDA approved<br>Concern of ↑ infection risk |
| Propylthiouracil (PTU) | No | |
| Colchicine | No | |
| Liver transplant | Yes | 6 mo abstinence required; account for 25% of all transplants and do well! |

DF, Maddrey discriminant function score; FDA, U.S. Food and Drug administration.

## 20. What is the prognosis of patients with ALD?

The prognosis of the patient with fatty liver who stops ethanol consumption is excellent. However, those with fatty liver who continue to drink are more likely to progress to cirrhosis. Alcoholic hepatitis has a broad range of mortality of 15% to 55% depending on the severity of liver disease. Alcoholic hepatitis may continue to progress for the first weeks or months after abstinence. Those with encephalopathy have a poor outcome as do those with a Maddrey DF greater than 32. A Model for End-Stage Liver Disease (MELD) score greater than 21 is also a predictor of increased mortality. Recently, the Glasgow Alcoholic Hepatitis Score has been used to assess severity and prognosis (Table 26-4).

For those with alcoholic cirrhosis, the 5- and 10-year survival is 23% and 7%, respectively. For those who maintain abstinence and lack evidence of portal hypertension, a life expectancy similar to that of age-matched controls may occur.

**Table 26-4.** Glasgow Alcoholic Hepatitis Score
A total score of more than 9 equates to poor prognosis.

| VARIABLE | SCORE (IN POINTS) |
| --- | --- |
| Age <50 yr | 1 |
| Age >50 yr | 2 |
| WBC <15,000/μL | 1 |
| WBC >15,000/μL | 2 |
| BUN <5 mg/dL | 1 |
| BUN >5 mg/dL | 2 |
| INR <1.5 | 1 |
| INR 1.5 to 2.0 | 2 |
| INR >2.0 | 3 |
| Bilirubin <7.4 mg/dL | 1 |
| Bilirubin 7.4 to 14.8 mg/dL | 2 |
| Bilirubin >14.8 mg/dL | 3 |

WBC, white blood cells; BUN, blood urea nitrogen; INR, international normalized ratio.
From Forrest EH, Evans CDJ, Stewart S, et al. Analysis of factors predictive of mortality in alcoholic hepatitis and derivation and validation of the Glasgow Alcoholic Hepatitis Score. Gut 2005; 54:1174–9.

### 21. Does HCV infection increase the risk of cirrhosis in the alcoholic?

For the patient with alcohol consumption of greater than 60 g of ethanol daily who also is a HCV carrier, there is an increased risk of developing cirrhosis over that of either condition alone. Continuing ethanol use during interferon and ribavirin therapy for HCV will reduce response to treatment.

### 22. Does alcoholic cirrhosis predispose a patient to development of HCC?

Alcoholic cirrhosis is associated with the development of HCC with a median interval of 4 to 5 years following its diagnosis. The combination of obesity, hepatitis B virus (HBV) or HCV infection, and alcoholic cirrhosis may add to the risk of HCC development. HCC can develop in alcoholic patients in the absence of cirrhosis.

### 23. How should I screen patients with alcoholic cirrhosis for HCC?

Patients with alcoholic cirrhosis should be screened for HCC on a regular basis. At a minimum, and alpha-fetoprotein level should be determined every 6 months and an ultrasound of the liver obtained annually.

### 24. Can the patient with end-stage ALD undergo liver transplantation?

Patients with decompensated alcoholic cirrhosis and complications such as variceal hemorrhage, encephalopathy, or ascites are good candidates for liver transplantation. Their outcome is similar to that of patients with other forms of end-stage liver disease.

Continued alcoholism is the most common reason for not being considered a candidate for liver transplantation. A period of 6 months of ethanol abstinence is generally recommended prior to liver transplantation coupled with careful evaluation for factors that may predict recidivism. For those who deny alcoholism, post-transplant resumption of ethanol is more likely. A relapse of alcoholism while awaiting transplantation is a contraindication to liver transplantation.

Following liver transplantation, patients transplanted for alcoholic cirrhosis need continued support to prevent resumption of alcoholism. Abstinence should remain the goal of care, and continued involvement in a substance use disorder clinic should be recommended. Despite best efforts, more than 20% of patients transplanted for alcoholic cirrhosis return to excessive ethanol consumption with a graft loss in 5% of those transplanted. In one study, at 5 years post liver transplantation, 42% of those transplanted for alcoholic cirrhosis had used alcohol at least once, with the first drink occurring during the first year post transplant in 22%. Twenty-six percent resumed binge drinking. A resumption of drinking is associated with significant post transplant mortality.

## BIBLIOGRAPHY

1. Akriviadis E, Botla R, Briggs W, et al. Pentoxifylline improves short-term survival in severe acute alcoholic hepatitis: A double-blind, placebo-controlled trial. Gastroenterology 2000;119:1637–48.
2. Cabre E, Rodriguez-Iglesias P, Caballeria J, et al. Short-and long-term outcome in severe alcohol-induced hepatitis treated with steroids or enteral nutrition: A multicenter randomized trial. Hepatology 2000;32:36–42.
3. Carithers Jr RL, Herlong HF, Diehl AM, et al. Methylprednisolone therapy in patients with severe alcoholic hepatitis: A randomized multicenter trial. Ann Intern Med 1989;110:685–90.
4. Ceccanti M, Attili A, Balducci G, et al. Acute alcoholic hepatitis. J Clin Gastroenterol 2006;40:833–41.
5. Crabb DW, Edenberg HJ, Bosron WF, et al. Genotypes for aldehyde dehydrogenase deficiency and alcohol sensitivity. The inactive ALDH2(2) allele is dominant. J Clin Invest 1989;83:314–6.
6. Day CP. Treatment of alcoholic liver disease. Liver Trans 2007;13:S69–75.
7. Dunn W, Jamil LH, Brown LS, et al. MELD accurately predicts mortality in patients with alcoholic hepatitis. Hepatology 2005;41:353–8.
8. Forrest EH, Evans CDJ, Stewart S, et al. Analysis of factors predictive of mortality in alcoholic hepatitis and derivation and validation of the Glasgow Alcoholic Hepatitis Score. Gut 2005;54:1174–9.
9. Freiberg MS, Vasan RS, Cabral HJ, et al. Alcohol consumption and the prevalence of the metabolic syndrome in the U.S.: A cross-sectional analysis of data from the Third National Health and Nutrition Examination Survey. Diabetes Care 2004;27:2954–9.
10. Kim WR, Brown Jr RS, Terrault NA, et al. Burden of liver disease in the United States: Summary of a workshop. Hepatology 2002;36:227–42.
11. Kosten TR, O'Connor PG. Management of drug and alcohol withdrawal. N Engl J Med 2003;348:1786–95.
12. Li TK, Hewitt BG, Grant BF. Is there a future for quantifying drinking in the diagnosis, treatment and prevention of alcohol use disorders? Alcohol 2007;42:57–63.
13. Maddrey WC, Boitnott JK, Bedine MS, et al. Corticosteroid therapy of alcoholic hepatitis. Gastroenterology 1978;75:193–9.
14. Mathurin P, Mendenhall CL, Carithers Jr RL, et al. Corticosteroids improve short-term survival in patients with severe alcoholic hepatitis (AH): Individual data analysis of the last three randomized placebo controlled double blind trials of corticosteroids in severe alcoholic hepatitis. J Hepatol 2002;36:480–7.
15. Mayo-Smith F. Pharmacological management of alcohol withdrawal. A meta-analysis and evidence-based practice guideline. JAMA 1997;278:144–51.
16. Ntais C, Pakos E, Kyzas P, et al. Benzodiazepines for alcohol withdrawal. Cochrane Database Syst Rev 2005; CD005063.
17. Pfitzmann R, Schwenzer J, Rayes N, et al. Long-term survival and predictors of relapse after orthotopic liver transplantation for alcoholic liver disease. Liver Transpl 2007;13:197–205.
18. Polycarpou A, Papanikolau P, Ioannidis JPA, et al. Anticonvulsants for alcohol withdrawal. Cochrane Database Syst Rev 2005; CD005064.
19. Raynard B, Balian A, Fallik D, et al. Risk factors of fibrosis in alcohol-induced liver disease. Hepatology 2002;35:635–8.
20. Rouault TA. Hepatic iron overload in alcoholic liver disease. Why does it occur and what is its role in pathogenesis. Alcohol 2003;30:103–6.
21. Stewart SH. Racial and ethnic differences in alcohol-associated aspartate aminotransferase and gamma-glutamyltransferase elevation. Arch Int Med 2002;162:2236–9.
22. Sullivan JT, Sykora K, Schneiderman J, et al. Assessment of alcohol withdrawal: The revised Clinical Institute Withdrawal Assessment for Alcohol scale (CIWA-Ar). Br J Addict 1989;84:1353–7.
23. Tilg H, Jalan R, Kaser A, et al. Anti-tumor necrosis factor-alpha monoclonal antibody therapy in severe alcoholic hepatitis. J Hepatol 2003;38:419–25.
24. You M, Crabb DW. Recent advances in alcoholic liver disease. II. Minireview: Molecular mechanisms of alcoholic liver disease. Am J Physiol 2004;287:G1–6.
25. Zakhari S, Li T-K. Determinants of alcohol use and abuse: Impact of quantity and frequency patterns on liver disease. Hepatology 2007;46:2032–9.
26. Zetterman RK. Liver transplantation for alcoholic liver disease. Clin Liver Dis 2005;9:171–81.

# 27 | CHAPTER

# VASCULAR LIVER DISEASE

*Marcelo Kugelmas, MD, FACP*

*(handwritten margin notes):* HDA ↓ CA ↓ HA → L, PV → L, SINUS. RHV→IVC, LHV+MHV→X, SMV, IMV, SpIV

## 1. Describe the principal vascular anatomy of the liver.

The liver constitutes 5% of body weight in adults and receives 20% of cardiac output via the hepatic artery and portal vein. The *hepatic artery* is a branch of the celiac artery via the hepaticoduodenal artery. It delivers approximately 30% of the hepatic afferent flow but more than 50% of the necessary oxygen in the resting state. Oxygen delivery to the biliary tree derives almost exclusively from the hepatic artery.

Conversely, the *portal vein* carries nearly 70% of total liver blood flow and delivers less than 50% of the needed oxygen. The portal vein derives its name from being one of two portal systems in the human body, with the other located in the pituitary gland. Its first set of venules drains blood from intestinal and splenic capillaries, forming the superior and inferior mesenteric veins and the splenic vein. These veins join to form the portal vein that in turn divides into tributaries and a net of fenestrated capillaries (sinusoids) in the liver. Despite its low oxygen content, portal venous blood delivers intestinal nutrients, drugs, and inflammatory mediators directly to the liver.

At the end of the sinusoid, blood enters the central venules, which drain directly into the right, middle, and left *hepatic veins*. The right hepatic vein drains directly into the inferior vena cava (IVC), while the left and middle hepatic veins usually merge before draining into the IVC via a common trunk. Vascular anatomy divides the liver into eight segments, each with its own afferent and efferent blood flow (Fig. 27-1). This anatomy is particularly important in the surgical resection of liver masses. The caudate lobe drains directly into the vena cava through dorsal hepatic veins, which explains its compensatory hypertrophy in hepatic outflow obstructive states such as Budd-Chiari syndrome (BCS).

## 2. Describe the microcirculation of the liver.

The basic element in the liver architecture is the cell plate, which consists of 15 to 20 hepatocytes between the portal area and central (hepatic) vein lined up between sinusoids (Fig. 27-2). Blood flows unidirectionally from the portal venule and hepatic arteriole through the sinusoid and bathes hepatocytes before emptying into the central venule.

Rappaport's concept of the liver lobule divides it into three zones (Fig. 27-3).

- **Zone I** refers to hepatocytes surrounding the portal triad.
- **Zone II** refers to the intermediate hepatocytes between the periportal and perivenular areas.
- **Zone III** refers to perivenular hepatocytes.

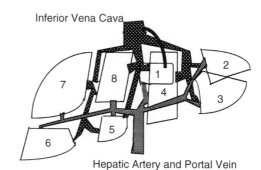

**Figure 27-1.** Vascular and surgical anatomy of the liver. According to Couinaud there are eight functional segments in the liver, which receive blood supply via the portal vein and hepatic artery. Efferent drainage is through the right, middle, and left hepatic veins. The caudate lobe (segment 1) has a separate and direct outflow into the vena cava via the dorsal hepatic veins.

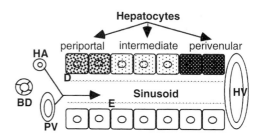

**Figure 27-2.** Hepatic microarchitecture. Blood from the portal vein (PV) and hepatic artery (HA) traverses the sinusoids, eventually leaving the liver from the hepatic veins (HV). The low-pressure circulation in the sinusoids allows plasma to pass through the fenestrated epithelium (E) and reach the Space of Disse (D), where exchange of nutrients and metabolites occurs. The hepatocytes near the portal triad are called periportal and those near the hepatic vein are called perivenular or pericentral.

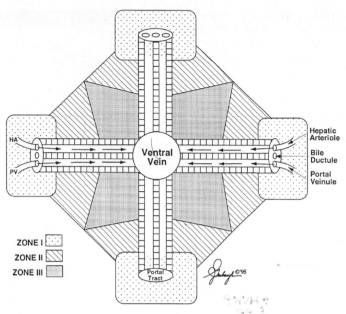

ZONE I
ZONE II
ZONE III

**Figure 27-3.** Rappaport hepatic lobule with portal (zone I), sinusoidal (zone II), and pericentral hepatocytes (zone III).

There are no absolute boundaries between these zones; however, the metabolic function and susceptibility to injury significantly vary according to the zone. For example, in congestive diseases such as right-sided heart failure or BCS, the outflow is impeded and zone III hepatocytes are the first to be damaged, as a result of their relative hypoxia.

### 3. What makes the liver resistant to ischemic and vascular disease?

The liver benefits from an extremely rich blood supply of fully oxygenated blood from the hepatic artery and partially oxygenated blood from the portal vein. Between these sources the liver receives over 20% of the cardiac output, one third of which comes from the hepatic artery. The liver can autoregulate its blood flow in the setting of portal venous or hepatic artery insufficiency via vasoconstriction of the affected vessel, closure of intrasinusoidal sphincters, and vasodilation of the other vessel. Oxygen extraction is also enhanced and autoregulated in the liver, probably because of short diffusion distances and properties of the hepatocyte itself. Finally, the regenerative capacity of hepatocytes allows liver function to continue and recover rapidly after severe ischemia.

### 4. What is Budd-Chiari syndrome?

George Budd described three cases of hepatic venous thrombosis in 1845, and Hans Chiari added the first pathologic description in 1899.

BCS results from obstruction of the hepatic venous outflow tract from any etiology including thrombosis, tumor, abscess, or vascular anomaly. Obstruction of at least two of three hepatic veins is generally required to cause clinical symptoms. Hepatic veno-occlusive disease and congestive heart failure are not included in this category. IVC webs are the leading causes in developing countries, whereas thrombosis is the predominant cause in Europe and the United States (Fig. 27-4). The majority of thrombotic cases are associated with an underlying coagulation disorder such as polycythemia rubra vera, factor V Leiden deficiency, or

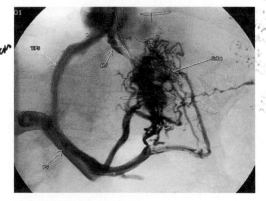

**Figure 27-4.** Hepatic venogram indicating central hepatic vein obstruction (web) with marked collateral development and flow, with 25-mm pressure gradient across weblike stenosis at central hepatic veins.

paroxysmal nocturnal hemoglobinuria. Less common inheritable disorders include protein C/S deficiencies, antithrombin III deficiency, and the antiphospholipid antibody syndrome. Additional risk factors include oral contraceptives, cancer, dehydration, and trauma.

### 5. How is BCS diagnosed?

The onset of ascites, abdominal pain, hepatosplenomegaly, or unexplained liver failure in a patient should raise the suspicion of BCS, particularly if there are risk factors for thrombosis. Doppler ultrasonography usually shows hepatomegaly and decreased or absent flow in the hepatic veins. Contrast-enhanced computed tomography (CT) or magnetic resonance imaging (MRI) may additionally show nonvisualization of the main hepatic veins or a mosaic perfusion pattern of the liver parenchyma. Another key imaging finding is caudate lobe hypertrophy (Fig. 27-5). Transjugular hepatic venography confirms the site and extent of thrombosis, may demonstrate collateral formation in a *spider web* distribution, allows for biopsy, and may direct intravascular therapy. Typically, pressure readings reveal increased wedged hepatic venous pressure, portal pressure, and gradient.

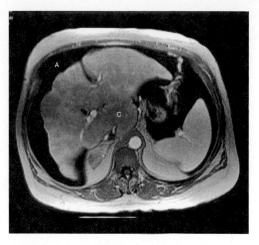

**Figure 27-5.** Magnetic resonance image showing features of Budd-Chiari syndrome including hepatomegaly with caudate lobe hypertrophy, ascites, and splenomegaly. A, ascites; C, caudate lobe.

### 6. Why do some patients with BCS have an enlarged caudate lobe?

Approximately one half of patients with BCS develop hypertrophy in the caudate lobe of the liver (see Fig. 27-5). This finding occurs because dorsal hepatic veins drain the caudate lobe and empty directly into the IVC. Usually, the obstruction does not affect these veins, and the caudate lobe hypertrophies in a compensatory fashion. The hypertrophy may be marked, cause a characteristic indentation in the inferior cava venogram, or result in significant IVC stenosis.

### 7. What are the histopathologic findings in BCS?

A nearly universal finding on liver biopsy is centrilobular congestion with dilation of the perivenular sinusoids. In severe acute and chronic forms, massive hepatocyte necrosis may occur, most prominently in zone III. Ongoing hepatic venous outflow obstruction may lead to centrilobular fibrosis after 4 to 6 weeks, with fibrosis and/or cirrhosis developing later. As fibrosis becomes more extensive it may contribute to occlusion of the outflow tract and liver failure. Examination of the hepatic veins and IVC may reveal concentric thickening in the vessel wall, but intravascular thrombosis is uncommon.

### 8. What is the treatment for BCS?

Except for occasional reports of cases improving with medical therapy alone, BCS is generally progressive without definitive therapy. Diuretics may control ascites, and anticoagulants are useful to limit clot burden. The underlying hematologic disorder should be treated accordingly. Ultimately, most patients require decompression of the hepatic veins to preserve liver function.

In the acute setting, percutaneous transluminal angioplasty, stenting, and thrombolytic therapy have been used successfully. The evidence supporting thrombolytic therapy is limited to case reports and uncontrolled series.

Portosystemic shunt surgery (portocaval, mesocaval, or mesoatrial) is effective in improving symptoms, parameters of liver function, and liver histology. However there is significant surgical morbidity, and shunts may become thrombosed in the long term. Patients with cirrhosis or liver failure may have limited benefit.

Transjugular intrahepatic portosystemic shunting (TIPS; Fig. 27-6) has been used to stabilize liver function and bridge patients to transplantation. Most patients have long-term, symptomatic benefit with compensated liver function, and shunt patency problems have been significantly improved with the use of covered stents. TIPS placement does not interfere with candidacy for, or outcome after, liver transplantation.

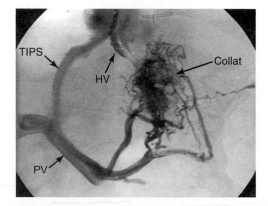

**Figure 27-6.** Hepatic venography with transjugular intrahepatic portosystemic shunt (TIPS) insertion. HV, hepatic vein; PV, portal vein; Collat, venous collateral formation within liver.

Liver transplantation is the treatment of choice for those patients with acute liver failure that does not improve after TIPS and for those with chronic BCS and decompensated liver function due to longstanding cirrhosis. Recently, graft and patient survival rates have dramatically improved compared with older series (80.6% and 84.9% for 3-year graft and patient survival, respectively).

### 9. Which patients with BCS should be considered for liver transplantation?

Patients with BCS and signs of liver failure should be evaluated for liver transplantation. Fulminant liver failure is an indication for urgent transplantation, and patients with this presentation may benefit from TIPS, thrombolytics, or angioplasty until an allograft is available. Patients with persistent symptoms or liver dysfunction despite shunting or intravascular therapy should also be considered for liver transplantation. Patients with a known clotting factor deficiency may be cured by liver transplantation. The presence of decompensated liver cirrhosis warrants a transplant evaluation; however, patients with compensated cirrhosis may have long-term benefit from other therapies.

### 10. What is the pathogenesis of hepatic veno-occlusive disease (VOD)?

A better term for VOD may be *sinusoidal obstruction syndrome* since the initial injury involves the perivenular endothelium and hepatocytes. Although no specific mechanism has been identified, risk factors include chemotherapy (particularly cyclophosphamide and busulfan-containing regimens), stem cell transplantation, hepatic irradiation and radioembolization with yttrium 90–labeled microspheres, and ingestion of pyrrolizidine alkaloids. Initially, the sinusoidal endothelium becomes leaky with extravasation of red blood cells into the space of Disse and edema in zone III hepatocytes. Perivenular necrosis, fibrosis, and fibrin deposition usually follow, causing outflow obstruction and congestion. The central vein may not be involved. Histologically, sinusoidal dilation and pericentral necrosis are typical, which can mimic BCS or congestive hepatopathy.

*CXRX, SCTx, RMTX*

### 11. What are the clinical features of VOD?

The typical presentation of right upper quadrant pain and weight gain 1 to 5 weeks after chemotherapy or bone marrow transplantation may be subtle. Alternatively, patients can develop rapidly progressive jaundice. Physical examination may reveal jaundice, tender hepatomegaly, and/or ascites. The most common lab abnormality is a conjugated hyperbilirubinemia, although thrombocytopenia and elevated prothrombin time may also occur from spleen and liver congestion. Mild-moderate elevations in aspartate aminotransferase (AST) and alanine aminotransferase (ALT) suggest hepatocyte necrosis. A serum AST greater than 750 or rapidly rising bilirubin portends a poor prognosis. Elevated creatinine occurs in less than 50% of patients.

*RUQ AP, ↑wt/ascites, ↑DBili, ↑ALT/AST, ARF*

### 12. How is VOD diagnosed?

Any patient with risk factors and unexplained weight gain, abdominal pain, hepatomegaly, or jaundice should raise the suspicion for VOD. Ultrasonography may show ascites, hepatomegaly, or venous dilation although it is most helpful for excluding other diseases such as BCS or gallstones. MRI and CT add little information if the sonogram is adequate. Liver biopsy remains the gold standard for diagnosis of VOD and should complement the clinical picture. It is usually done by the transjugular route to minimize bleeding risk and to allow measurement of hepatic venous pressures. Histologic findings typically include edema and/or necrosis of zone III hepatocytes and sinusoidal congestion. Centrilobular fibrosis is uncommon.

### 13. Describe the clinical features of ischemic hepatitis

Also known as shock liver, ischemic hepatitis is diagnosed clinically by a sudden, profound elevation in liver enzymes shortly after a drop in cardiac output and/or blood pressure. It mostly affects elderly patients with underlying cardiac disease, often in the setting of surgery, trauma, or sepsis. Tender hepatomegaly and anorexia are common exam findings. The elevation in serum transaminases may be abrupt and marked (greater than 1000) reflecting hepatocyte necrosis. Serum bilirubin and prothrombin time are modestly elevated, and many patients have elevated creatinine, usually from acute tubular necrosis (ATN). The liver function tests and coagulopathy improve over the ensuing days as the patient's hemodynamic status is restored.

*↓BP/CO vascular path ↑AP, ↑INR/Bili, ↑↑ALT/AST, ARF (ATN)*

### 14. What is the pathogenesis of ischemic hepatitis?

A drop in cardiac output may result from various etiologies including sepsis, hypovolemia, cardiac tamponade, pulmonary embolism, and left or right ventricular failure. Hypoperfusion mostly affects the perivenular hepatocytes since they receive oxygen-poor blood. Histologically, the typical finding of centrilobular necrosis reflects mechanism. As many patients have chronic underlying heart disease, hepatic congestion or fibrosis may be present.

### 15. What are the clinical manifestations of congestive hepatopathy?

The underlying cardiac disease dominates the presentation with dyspnea, fatigue, edema, and weight gain. Many patients will report right upper quadrant pain and/or fullness, which is thought to result from distention of Glisson capsule. Jaundice is less common, and encephalopathy and variceal bleeding are rare. Physical exam may reveal ascites, hepatosplenomegaly, or hepatojugular reflux.

*by nutmeg liver fibrosis (cirrhosis uncommon)*

*@ CHF /constricts Ascites Puls path, mild ↑AP - Rx ♥ dz ↑INR if ↑↑ ALT/AST*

**16. What liver chemistry abnormalities are found in congestive hepatopathy?**

Elevated prothrombin time is the most common lab abnormality. Chronic passive congestion alone rarely causes significant elevations of ALT, or AST. Markedly increased transaminases in the setting of heart disease suggest acute ischemia caused by low cardiac output rather than congestion. Unconjugated hyperbilirubinemia and mildly elevated alkaline phosphatase occur in less than half of patients. The biochemical abnormalities tend to improve with treatment of the underlying cardiac disease.

**17. Describe the pathologic changes associated with congestive hepatopathy.**

Grossly, the liver is enlarged and darkened. The classic cross-sectional appearance, termed *nutmeg liver*, represents lighter, less affected periportal areas surrounding the darkened, congested areas around central venules. Microscopically there is centrilobular and sinusoidal dilation. Adjacent hepatocytes usually appear atrophic, compressed, or necrotic. Fibrosis occurs in the majority of patients with chronic disease, but cardiac cirrhosis is uncommon.

**18. What is the most frequent vascular complication following liver transplantation?**

Hepatic artery thrombosis occurs with an incidence of 2% to 10% following orthotopic liver transplantation and carries over 50% mortality. Roughly half of cases present early (within 1 week), although some may present after months to years. Risk factors include old donor age, prolonged cold ischemia time, the use of an aortic conduit, and early use of rapamycin in the immunosuppressive regimen. Although a minority of patients are asymptomatic with abnormal liver tests or imaging, most develop cholestasis and cholangitis secondary to ischemic bile duct injury. Imaging by Doppler ultrasound may suggest the diagnosis, although confirmatory angiography is usually necessary. Surgical thrombectomy and revascularization may salvage selected grafts but does not always reverse the underlying cholangiopathy. Otherwise, retransplantation remains the treatment of choice.

**19. What are the risk factors for portal vein thrombosis (PVT)?**

Cirrhosis (with portal hypertension) with or without hepatocellular carcinoma is the most common risk factor for PVT, presumably by causing sluggish portal blood flow and/or decreased synthesis of clotting inhibitors. Inherited or acquired prothrombotic disorders such as protein C/S deficiencies, the antiphospholipid syndrome, polycythemia vera, and estrogen use or pregnancy are independent risk factors. Cancer, particularly pancreatic and hepatocellular carcinomas, predisposes the portal vein to thrombosis through extrinsic compression, direct invasion, or an underlying thrombophilia. Surgery or trauma involving the portal or splenic veins similarly increases the risk.

**20. What treatments options are available for PVT?**

In the acute setting, thrombolytics, angioplasty and/or TIPS, or surgical thrombectomy may restore portal flow, although controlled studies demonstrating their safety and long-term efficacy are lacking. Otherwise, heparinization and long-term warfarin therapy usually allow repermeation in acute PVT. The first-line treatment of chronic PVT involves endoscopic and medical obliteration of esophageal varices. Shunt surgery and splenectomy carry surgical risk but may be helpful in patients with preserved liver function and refractory complications of portal hypertension. Long-term anticoagulation may benefit noncirrhotic patients with underlying thrombophilia, although the benefit needs to be weighed carefully against the risk of bleeding.

**21. What is the most common vascular tumor of the liver?**

Cavernous hemangioma is the most common benign liver tumor with autopsy series indicating a prevalence of 2% to 20%. It is typically small (less than 5 cm), asymptomatic, and found incidentally in adults during hepatic imaging. However, larger lesions are not uncommon and may cause significant abdominal pain. Hemangiomas larger than 10 cm are at risk for rupture, internal bleeding, or causing disseminated intravascular coagulation (Kasabach-Merritt syndrome). Tumors tend to be more common and larger in females, so estrogen sensitivity may play a role. Ultrasound, CT scan, or red blood cell scans may suggest the diagnosis, but MRI has evolved into the most specific and sensitive test. Fine needle biopsy may confirm the diagnosis but carries a significant risk of bleeding and is not recommended. Treatment options including surgical enucleation, resection, or liver transplantation are reserved for large, painful tumors or complications (Fig. 27-7).

**22. What is hepatic hemangioendothelioma?**

It is a rare vascular neoplasm with variable malignant potential that may occasionally involve the liver. It grows more commonly in soft tissue or bone. Histologic examination with endothelium-specific (FVIII-rAg) staining is diagnostic. It is nearly always multifocal and slow growing; however, it is resistant to chemotherapy and may recur following liver transplantation. The overall prognosis is poor.

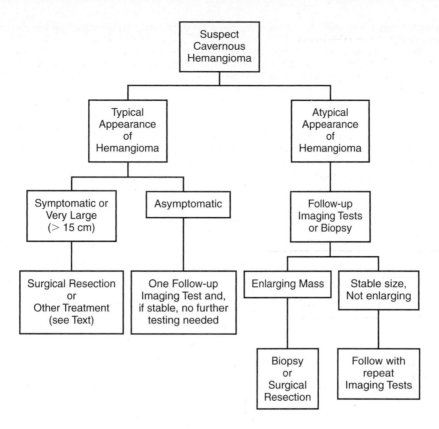

**Figure 27-7.** Approach to management of hemangioma. (From Everson GT, Trotter JT: Benign focal lesions of the liver. Clin Liver Dis 5:17–42, 2001.)

## BIBLIOGRAPHY

1. Attwell A, Ludkowski M, Nash R, et al. Treatment of Budd-Chiari syndrome in a liver transplant unit: The role of transjugular intrahepatic porto-systemic shunt and liver transplantation. Aliment Pharmacol Ther 2004;20:867–73.
2. Bacon BR, Joshi SN, Granger DN. Ischemia, congestive failure, Budd-Chiari syndrome, and veno-occlusive disease. In: Kaplowitz N, editor. Liver and Biliary Diseases. 2nd ed. Baltimore: Williams & Wilkins; 1992. pp. 469–81.
3. Bynum TE, Biotnott JK, Maddrey WC. Ischemic hepatitis. Dig Dis Sci 1979;24:129–35.
4. Chalasani N, Cummings OW. The liver in systemic illness. In: Boyer TD, Zakim D, editors. Hepatology: A Textbook of Liver Disease. 4th ed. Philadelphia: Saunders; 2003. pp. 1561–5.
5. DeLeve LD, Shulman HM, McDonald GB. Toxic injury to hepatic sinusoids: Sinusoidal obstruction syndrome. Semin Liver Dis 2002;22:27–41.
6. Eid A, Lyass S, Venturero M, et al. Vacular complications post orthotopic liver transplantation. Transplant Proc 1999;31:1903–4.
7. Fuchs S, Bogomolski-Yahalom V, Paltiel, et al. Ischemic hepatitis: Clinical and laboratory observations in 34 patients. J Clin Gastroenterol 1998;26:183–6.
8. Kugelmas M. Budd-Chiari syndrome. Treatment options and the value of liver transplantation. Hepatogastroenterology 1998;45:1381–6.
9. Kumar S, DeLeve LD, Kalamath PS, et al. Hepatic veno-occlusive disease after hematopoietic stem cell transplantation. Mayo Clin Proc 2003;78:589–98.
10. Mahmoud AEA, Mendoza A, Meshikhes AN, et al. Clinical spectrum, investigations, and treatment of Budd-Chiari syndrome. Q J Med 1996;89:37–43.
11. McCuskey RS, Reilly FD. Hepatic microvasculature: Dynamic structure and its regulation. Semin Liver Dis 1993;13:1–12.
12. Myers RP, Cerini R, Sayegh R, et al. Cardiac hepatopathy: Clinical, hemodynamic, and histologic characteristics and correlations. Hepatology 2003;37:393–400.
13. Orloff MJ, Daily PO, Orloff SL, et al. A 27-year experience with surgical treatment of Budd-Chiari syndrome. Ann Surg 2000;3:340–52.
14. Ross RM. Hepatic dysfunction secondary to heart failure. Am J Gastroenterol 1981;7:511–7.
15. Sangro B, Gil-Alzugaray B, Rodriguez J, et al. Liver disease induced by radioembolization of liver tumors. Cancer 2008;112:1538–46.
16. Sarin SK, Agarwal SR. Extrahepatic portal vein obstruction. Semin Liver Dis 2003;22:43–55.
17. Seeto RK, Fenn B, Rockey DC. Ischemic hepatitis: Clinical presentation and pathogenesis. Am J Med 2000;109:109–13.
18. Segev DL, Nguyen GC, Locke JE, et al. Twenty years of liver transplantation for Budd-Chiari syndrome: A national registry analysis. Liver Transpl 2007;13:1285–94.
19. Sobhonslidsuk A, Reddy KR. Portal vein thrombosis: A concise review. Am J Gastroenterol 2002;97:535–41.
20. Tesser TS, Sze DY, Jeffrey RB. Imaging and Intervention in the hepatic veins. Am J Radiol 2003;180:1583–91.
21. Tilanus HW. Budd-Chiari syndrome. Br J Surg 1995;82:1023–30.

22. Torras J, Lladó L, Figueras J, et al. Diagnostic and therapeutic management of hepatic artery thrombosis after liver transplantation. Transplant Proc 1999;31:2405.
23. Trotter JF, Everson GT. Benign focal lesions of the liver. Clin Liver Dis 2001;5:17–42.
24. Uchimara K, Nakamuta M, Osoegawa M, et al. Hepatic epithelioid hemangioendothelioma. J Clin Gastroenterol 2001;32:431–4.
25. Valla DC. Hepatic vein thrombosis. Semin Liver Dis 2002;22:5–14.
26. Valla DC, Condat B. Portal vein thrombosis in adults: Pathophysiology, pathogenesis, and management. J Hepatol 2000;32:865–71.
27. Zimmerman MA, Cameron AM, Ghobrial RM. Budd Chiari syndrome. Clin Liver Dis 2006;10:259–73.

# NONALCOHOLIC FATTY LIVER DISEASE AND NONALCOHOLIC STEATOHEPATITIS

# CHAPTER 28

*Dawn M. Torres, MD, and*
*Stephen A. Harrison, MD*

**1. What is the difference between nonalcoholic fatty liver disease (NAFLD) and nonalcoholic steatohepatitis (NASH)?**

Nonalcoholic fatty liver disease (NAFLD) is an umbrella classification for a group of diseases marked by intrahepatic fat (steatosis), usually as the result of insulin resistance without significant alcohol use (typically thought to be two or three drinks per day in a male and one or two drinks per day in a female). Nonalcoholic steatohepatitis (NASH) is a subset of NAFLD that in addition to hepatic steatosis has histologic evidence of hepatocyte injury to include lobular inflammation, ballooning degeneration, with or without Mallory hyaline and perivenular and perisinusoidal fibrosis. While isolated fatty liver (the majority of patients with NAFLD) has a generally favorable prognosis with low risk for progression to cirrhosis, the clinical course of NASH patients is more variable. Natural history studies suggest one third of NASH patients show disease (fibrosis) progression, one third have disease regression, and one third have stable disease over a 5- to 10-year period.

**2. How do patients with NAFLD present?**

Patients with NAFLD are often noted to have elevated serum aminotransferases on routine blood work, which prompts a gastroenterology referral. The vast majority of these patients are asymptomatic, although a small but clinically notable fraction of patients complain of right upper quadrant discomfort. This symptom, which can range in presentation from a dull ache to sharp severe pain, has been attributed to capsular swelling in the setting of hepatomegaly, although it is not always associated with liver enlargement and does not correlate with disease severity. Often these patients will have undergone extensive negative evaluations for alternative causes of abdominal pain with only fatty liver on imaging and moderate (1.5 to 3 times normal) elevations of serum aminotransferases. Alkaline phosphatase is less frequently elevated but has been shown to be the sole abnormality in a select cohort of predominantly female patients.

Serologic workup in patients with NAFLD is typically negative with normal levels of ceruloplasmin and $\alpha_1$-antitrypsin and negative viral hepatitis panels. Antinuclear antibody (ANA) and anti–smooth muscle antibody (ASMA) may be positive in up to one third of cases. As a marker of inflammation, serum ferritin may also be elevated in NAFLD patients, and further study to assess for genetic markers of hereditary hemochromatosis (HH) or hepatic iron overload (via liver biopsy) should be considered.

**3. Describe the typical NAFLD patient.**

Most patients with NAFLD are overweight middle-aged adults, although the disease can present in childhood with a rising incidence secondary to the increasing numbers of obese children. While there was initially thought to be a female predominance, it appears to be evenly distributed between males and females. The majority of patients already have met criteria for the metabolic syndrome with at least three of the following:

- Increased waist circumference (men, greater than 40 inches; women, greater than 35 inches)
- Fasting serum triglycerides of 150 mg/dL
- High-density lipoprotein (HDL) of 40 mg/dL in men or 50 mg/dL in women
- Systolic blood pressure of 130 mm Hg
- Diastolic blood pressure of 85 mm Hg
- Fasting glucose of 100 mg/dL

Patients may already be on medications to improve these metabolic profiles such as HMG-CoA reductase inhibitors and present when serum aminotransferases are found to be elevated during routine blood work.

## 4. What is the prevalence of NAFLD and NASH?

While the exact prevalence of NAFLD is unknown, it is easily the most common chronic liver disease in the developed world. Prevalence studies suggest upward of 30% of the United States population has NAFLD. Somewhat lower prevalence rates of 18% to 25% have been noted in non-American populations. National Health and Nutrition Examination Survey (NHANES) data from 1999–2002 describe a prevalence of elevated serum aminotransferases (aspartate aminotransferase (AST) greater than 40 or alanine aminotransferase (ALT) greater than 43) of 9.8%, which suggests a much higher actual prevalence if using the mean ALT cutoffs of less than 20s for male patients and less than 30s for females.

Higher prevalence is seen in type 2 diabetic patients, where NAFLD prevalence has been documented to be as high as 70% to 75%. Given the lack of histologic data in most prevalence studies, the rates of NASH within the larger NAFLD population are uncertain although autopsy data suggest an overall NASH prevalence of 3% to 6%. Among morbidly obese patients undergoing bariatric surgery, prevalence rates of 91% for NAFLD and 37% for NASH have been demonstrated. Preliminary evidence also suggests increased prevalence in Hispanic populations and a lower prevalence in African American individuals despite similar rates of comorbid conditions.

## 5. How can you distinguish between NAFLD and NASH?

The short answer to this is liver biopsy—it remains the gold standard and is the only test that can provide clear-cut evidence of steatohepatitis. Imaging studies, such as ultrasound (US), computed tomography (CT), and magnetic resonance imaging (MRI), are very good at diagnosing steatosis with upward of 95% sensitivity and 80% specificity, although the accuracy of US is reduced in the morbidly obese. However, these studies are unable to distinguish NASH from isolated fatty liver. Recent advances that may prove useful are US and MRI transient elastography, which show promise in noninvasively identifying advanced fibrosis (stage 3 and 4) (Fig. 28-1).

Serum biomarkers (adipocytokines, hyaluronic acid, C-reactive protein, cytokeratin 18) used alone or in combination with other noninvasive testing are also intriguing and may be used routinely in the future but are not ready for use in clinical practice at this point. Several research centers have developed scoring systems that use a combination of serum biomarkers, basic laboratories, or clinical indices in an effort to predict either the presence of NASH or advanced fibrosis. No one scoring system has proven universally appicable in clinical practice. General indicators suggestive of advanced disease that may sway clinicians toward liver biopsy include AST:ALT ratio greater than 0.8, presence of diabetes, morbid obesity, or age over 50 years.

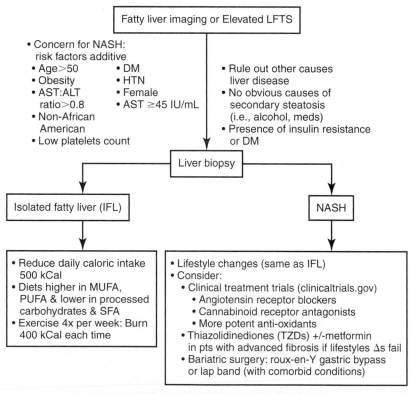

MUFA = mono-unsaturated fatty acid, PUFA = poly-unsaturated fatty acid, SFA = saturated fatty acid

**Figure 28-1.** NAFLD algorithm.

## 6. How is the severity of disease determined in patients with NASH?

While hepatic histology is the ultimate indicator of disease severity, biochemical parameters that are often tracked in research trials include serum aminotransferases, fasting insulin and serum glucose, and adipocytokines such as leptin and adiponectin.

The Brunt classification system is the predominant system used to assess hepatic histology and is based on a grade and stage system where grade is defined by degree of steatosis and inflammation and stage is based on degree of fibrosis.

### NECROINFLAMMATORY ACTIVITY

- **Grade 1**: Up to 66% steatosis with only minimal ballooning hepatocytes predominantly in zone 3, scattered polymorphonuclear neutrophils (PMNs) and possibly intra-acinar lymphocytes with no or mild portal inflammation
- **Grade 2**: Steatosis of greater than 33% to exceeding 66% with more prominent PMNs and obvious ballooning hepatocytes; mild to moderate portal and intra-acinar chronic inflammation are also present
- **Grade 3**: Marked steatosis with marked ballooning, intra-acinar inflammation with PMNs that are associated with ballooned hepatocytes, portal chronic inflammation of mild to moderate severity

### FIBROSIS

- **Stage 1**: Zone 3 perisinusoidal/pericellular fibrosis to a mild-moderate degree
- **Stage 2**: Zone 3 perisinusoidal/pericellular fibrosis with focal or extensive periportal fibrosis
- **Stage 3**: Zone 3 perisinusoidal/pericellular fibrosis and portal fibrosis with focal or extensive bridging fibrosis
- **Stage 4**: Cirrhosis

## 7. Are there other causes of fatty liver beside insulin resistance/obesity/metabolic syndrome?

Alcohol is the leading secondary cause of steatohepatitis. Alcohol-induced steatohepatitis (ASH) is indistinguishable from NASH on liver biopsy, but a lifetime adult drinking history of greater than 20 g/day in men or greater than 10 g/day in women supports alcohol as the primary cause of the patient's liver disease. A combination of lower alcohol intake, even as low as 40 g/week, with coexisting insulin resistance may also lead to steatohepatitis.

Other comparatively rare causes of hepatic steatosis with or without steatohepatitis include certain drugs such as tamoxifen, amiodarone, or methotrexate; copper toxicity (Wilson disease); jejunoileal bypass or other condition causing rapid profound weight loss; parenteral nutrition; abetalipoproteinemia; or bacterial overgrowth. Human immunodeficiency virus (HIV) infection therapy with antiretroviral medication such as didanosine and stavudine also results in hepatic steatosis, and coinfection with hepatitis C virus further contributes to the deposition of triglycerides in hepatocytes.

Chemotherapy-associated steatohepatitis (CASH) is another important entity that has been seen with the addition of new chemotherapeutic agents such as irinotecan and oxaliplatin. Recent study has shown administration of these in combination with 5-fluorouracil (5-FU) prior to surgical resection of isolated liver metastasis from colon cancer improves survival but can result in severe steatohepatitis. While these conditions (Table 28-1) are thought to comprise less than 5% of cases of hepatitis steatosis or steatohepatitis, they are important to recognize given their specific and unique treatments.

## 8. What is the relationship between hepatic steatosis and hepatitis C virus infection?

Hepatitis C virus (HCV) infection is associated with hepatic steatosis, particularly in genotype 3 infections, although even genotype 1 constructs have been shown to promote triglyceride accumulation in hepatocytes. In genotype 3 infection, successful eradication of HCV infection results in a marked reduction in hepatic steatosis suggesting direct viral involvement in this process.

Alternatively, preexisting NAFLD unrelated to primary HCV infection has important implications for the severity of disease and portends the development of advanced hepatic fibrosis. In additional, coexisting NAFLD suggests a decreased responsiveness to antiviral therapy with pegylated interferon and ribavirin. Therefore, NAFLD has a cause-and-effect relationship with HCV infection.

## 9. What is the cause (pathogenesis) of NAFLD, in particular NASH?

Insulin resistance is thought to be the common denominator in an intricate multistep pathway that begins with accumulation of lipids in hepatocytes and ends with the activation of stellate cells that promote collagen deposition and fibrosis development. The intervening steps are the subject of intense research and are thought to involve oxidative stress with increased levels of proinflammatory cytokines such as tumor necrosis factor-$\alpha$ (TNF$\alpha$), decreased levels of cytoprotective cytokines such as adiponectin, mitochondrial dysfunction, endoplasmic reticulum stress, and upregulation of endocannabinoid receptors.

**Table 28-1.** Causes of Hepatic Steatosis or Steatohepatitis

| CAUSE | COMMENT |
|---|---|
| **Drugs** | |
| *Associated With Steatohepatitis* | |
| Tamoxifen (and other estrogen agonists) | Steatosis (more frequently) and rarely steatohepatitis<br>Can occur with normal serum aminotransferases<br>Three months into treatment up until 4 years after stopping |
| Amiodarone | 1% to 3% of patients<br>Usually reverses on discontinuation of drug<br>Rare cases of cirrhosis or acute liver failure |
| Calcium channel blockers | Controversial association |
| Glucocorticoids | Mediated by ↑ serum triglycerides and glucose |
| Methotrexate | Pseudo-alcoholic steatohepatitis |
| Irinotecan | Chemotherapy-associated steatohepatitis (CASH) |
| Oxaliplatin | |
| *Associated With Steatosis* | |
| Valproic acid | |
| Ibuprofen | |
| Aspirin | |
| Tetracycline | |
| Zidovudine/didanosine/stavudine | |
| **Surgery** | |
| Jejunal-ileal bypass | |
| Biliopancreatic diversion | |
| Extensive small bowel resection | |
| **Miscellaneous** | |
| Total parenteral nutrition | |
| Bacterial overgrowth | Jejunal diverticulosis |
| Abetalipoproteinemia | |
| Hepatitis C virus | |

10. **How do you treat patients with isolated fatty liver (i.e., NAFLD patients without histologic evidence of NASH)?**

    As these patients are not at a substantially increased risk of chronic liver disease (i.e., cirrhosis and liver cancer), lifestyle changes are the mainstay of therapy. Moderate reduction in caloric intake of about 500 calories per day along with exercise designed to expend 400 kCal four times per week are thought to be adequate to produce biochemical and histologic improvement, although large well-designed studies are lacking.

11. **What is the optimal treatment of patients with biopsy-proved NASH?**

    No single treatment has been shown to be universally efficacious and applicable to all patients in the treatment of NASH. Treatments are typically grouped into lifestyle interventions, pharmacologic therapies, or surgical interventions.

    Lifestyle interventions resemble those advocated for isolated fatty liver patients including caloric reduction and increased activity level. In addition, there is some evidence to suggest diet composition modification may be helpful including low glycemic index diets as well as high intake of polyunsaturated fatty acids (PUFAs) and a lower intake of saturated fatty acids (SFAs). While these interventions are safe and efficacious, they are difficult to sustain over long periods of time and are difficult to apply to clinical practice.

    Pharmacotherapy is appealing as a treatment for this chronic medical condition as many of these patients are already taking medications for coexisting hypertension or hyperlipidemia. Numerous agents, including antioxidants, cytoprotective agents such as ursodeoxycholic acid, lipid-lowering medications, weight-loss agents, and diabetic medications, have all been evaluated, although most in small, uncontrolled pilot studies.

    While the theory behind the use of antioxidants, cytoprotective agents, and lipid-lowering agents appears sound, preliminary studies have been disappointing in showing a benefit over placebo. Weight loss agents such as Xenical have been equally disappointing, although likely this is because of limited efficacy in producing sustained significant weight loss. Future study into more potent weight loss agents such as the cannabinoid receptor antagonists is ongoing.

Diabetic medications have shown the most promise in producing biochemical and histologic improvement. The thiazolidinediones (TZDs) in particular have been shown to improve markers of insulin resistance as well as hepatic steatosis, inflammation, and even fibrosis with 9 to 12 months of therapy. As this benefit does not appear to be sustained with cessation of medication, the long-term side effects of the TZDs, which include weight gain, peripheral edema, and potentially increased rates of myocardial infarction, have limited their universal use.

Other diabetic medications such as metformin and glyburide do not appear beneficial as monotherapy in NASH, although metformin may have a benefit in combination with a TZD, possibly through amelioration of the weight gain seen with TZD monotherapy. Other newer diabetic agents such as incretin analogs are under study.

Preliminary evidence in pilot animal and human trials suggests a benefit to treatment with angiotensin receptor blockers (ARBs) in NASH where both insulin resistance and hepatic fibrinogenesis may be affected. However, these results need to be confirmed in larger, randomized controlled trials.

While pharmacotherapeutic agents as monotherapy or in combination are still being investigated, studies in patients undergoing bariatric surgery for morbid obesity have suggested surgical weight loss may improve NASH histology. Early studies in patients undergoing biliopancreatic diversion showed some concern over worsening of hepatic fibrosis, but the vast majority of studies using either Roux-en-Y gastric bypass or laparoscopic band placement have shown significant improvement in hepatic histology, with even total resolution of steatohepatitis reported. These studies offer compelling evidence that bariatric surgery in morbidly obese patients improves steatohepatitis. It would seem these invasive procedures offer a viable alternative for those with comorbid conditions that are amenable to an invasive surgical approach.

In patients with cirrhosis who become decompensated or develop hepatocellular carcinoma, liver transplantation is the primary treatment modality.

## 12. How many patients diagnosed with NASH go on to require liver transplants?

The often-quoted rate of progressive liver disease in NAFLD populations is on the order of 15% to 20%. A much smaller portion goes on to require liver transplant secondary to NASH cirrhosis. United Network for Organ Sharing (UNOS) data from 2007 specify that 5.2% of patients underwent liver transplantation as cryptogenic cirrhosis and 5.0% as fatty liver–specific cirrhosis.

## 13. What is the role of hepatic steatosis in liver transplant donors?

Up to 30% of all livers evaluated for transplant show some steatosis, and livers with less than 30% hepatic steatosis are generally considered acceptable for transplantation, while moderate (30% to 60%) steatosis is regarded with caution and livers with greater than 60% steatosis are considered unsuitable by many centers. Two recent studies revealed that moderate and even severe steatosis shows comparable short- and long-term mortality to patients with absent or mild steatosis although with longer initial intensive care unit stays.

## 14. Does NAFLD/NASH recur after liver transplant?

Most of the data pertaining to NASH post transplantation are limited to case reports or series of recurrence of preexisting NASH or de novo steatohepatitis. The development of NAFLD/NASH post OLT is likely multifactorial with some contribution from host metabolic factors and some from post transplant immune suppressive medications such as prednisone and tacrolimus, which promote the development of diabetes. Retrospective data on 68 OLT patients followed for a mean of 28 ± 18 months showed 18% of patients developed de novo NAFLD and 9% of patients developed de novo NASH.

## WEBSITES

www.aasld.org

www.clinicaltrials.gov

www.liverfoundation.org

www.unos.org

## BIBLIOGRAPHY

1. Adams LA, Sanderson S, Lindor KD. The histological course of nonalcoholic fatty liver disease: A longitudinal study of 103 patients with sequential liver biopsies. J Hepatol 2005;42:132–8.
2. Belfort R, Harrison SA, Brown K, et al. A placebo controlled trial of pioglitazone in subjects with nonalcoholic steatohepatitis. N Engl J Med 2006;355:2297–307.
3. Brunt EM. Pathology of fatty liver disease. Mod Pathol 2007;20:S40–8.
4. de Alwis NMW, Day CP. Nonalcoholic fatty liver disease: The mist gradually clears. J Hepatol 2008;48:S104–1112.
5. Ekstedt M, Franzen LE, Mathiesen UL, et al. Long-term follow-up of patients with NAFLD and elevated liver enzymes. Hepatology 2006;44:865–73.
6. Fan JG, Zhu J, Li XJ, et al. Prevalence of and risk factors for fatty liver in a general population of Shanghai. China J Hepatol 2005;43:508–14.
7. Fernandez FG, Ritter J, Goodwin JW, et al. Effect of steatohepatitis associated with irinotecan or oxaliplatin pretreatment on resectability of hepatic colorectal metastasis. J Am Coll Surg 2005;200:845–53.
8. Harrison SA, Day CP. Benefits of lifestyle modification in NAFLD. Gut 2007;56:1760–9.
9. Harrison SA, Torgerson S, Hayashi PH. The natural history of nonalcoholic fatty liver: A clinical histopathological study. Am J Gastroenterol 2003;98:2042–7.
10. Ioannou GN, Boyko EJ, Lee SP. The prevalence and predictors of elevated serum aminotransferase activity in the United States in 1999-2002. Am J Gastroenterol 2006;101:76–82.
11. Kurita S, Takamura T, Ota T, et al. Olmesartan ameliorates a dietary rat model of non-alcoholic steatohepatitis through its pleiotropic effects. Eur J Pharmacol 2008;588:316–24.
12. Machado M, Marques-Vidal P, Cortez-Pinto H. Hepatic histology in obese patients undergoing bariatric surgery. J Hepatol 2006;45:600–6.
13. McCormack L, Petrowsky H, Jochum W, et al. Use of severely steatotic grafts in liver transplantation: A matched case control study. Ann Surg 2007;246:940–8.
14. McGovern BH, Ditelberg JS, Taylor LE, et al. Hepatic steatosis is associated with fibrosis, nucleoside analogue use, and hepatitis C virus genotype 3 infection in HIV-seropositive patients. CID 2006;43:365–72.
15. Nikeghbalian S, Nejatollahi SMR, Salahi H, et al. Does donor's fatty liver change impact on early mortality and outcome of liver transplantation. Transplant Proc 2007;39:1181–3.
16. Seo S, Maganti K, Khehra M, et al. De novo nonalcoholic liver disease after liver transplantation. Liver Transplant 2007;13:844–7.
17. Stravitz RT, Sanyal AJ. Drug-induced steatohepatitis. Clin Liver Dis 2003;7:435–51.
18. Szczepaniak LD, Nurenberg P, Leonard D, et al. Magnetic resonance spectroscopy to measure hepatic triglyceride content: Prevalence of hepatic steatosis in the general population. Am J Physiol Endocrinol Metab 2005;288:462–8.
19. Targher G, Bertolini L, Padovani R, et al. Prevalence of nonalcoholic fatty liver disease and its association with cardiovascular disease among type 2 diabetic patients. Diabetes Care 2007;30:1212–8.
20. Torres DM, Harrison SA. Diagnosis and therapy of nonalcoholic steatohepatitis. Gastroenterology 2008;134:1682–98.
21. Torres DM, Harrison SA. Insulin resistance in chronic hepatitis C, genotypes 1 and 4: The unfortunate reality. Hepatology 2008;47:2137–9.
22. Wanless IR, Lentz JS. Fatty liver hepatitis (steatohepatitis) and obesity: An autopsy study with analysis of risk factors. Hepatology 1990;12:1106–10.

# CHAPTER 29

# LIVER TRANSPLANTATION

*Miranda Y. Ku, MD, MPH, and James F. Trotter, MD*

*3mo MR*

## 1. What is the current basis for prioritizing patients for cadaveric transplantation?

Priority for liver transplantation is currently determined by the MELD (Model for End-stage Liver Disease) score, which incorporates serum creatinine (Cr), bilirubin (bili), and internationalized normalized ratio (INR) into the following mathematical equation predictive of 90-day survival:

$$\text{MELD score} = (0.957 \times \ln[\text{Cr(mg/dL)}] + 0.378 \times \ln[\text{bili(mg/dL)}] + 1.12 \times \ln[\text{INR}] + 0.643) \times 10$$

A MELD score predicts 90-day mortality, and therefore patients with high MELD scores have a higher priority for transplantation. Patients with a MELD score <9 have only a 2% 90-day mortality rate, whereas patients with a MELD score of ≥40 have a 71% mortality rate. Liver allocation based on MELD score differs in two major respects compared with the previous system:

- Subjective measures, such as degree of ascites and encephalopathy, are not included.
- Time on the waiting list plays a minor role, serving only to break ties between patients with the same score.

## 2. Why was the MELD score developed?

The two most important determinants under the previous allocation system were the Child-Turcotte-Pugh (CTP) score and waiting time. This system had two weaknesses—subjective clinical measures (ascites and encephalopathy) and inclusion of waiting time, which is a poor predictor of need for transplantation. As a result, the MELD score was developed to objectively prioritize the sickest patients for transplantation.

## 3. For patients with chronic liver disease, when is the appropriate time to refer for liver transplantation?

The decision to list a patient for transplantation ultimately rests on the judgment and experience of the physicians at the transplant center. In general, patients should be considered for listing if they have a MELD score ≥14 or life-threatening complications of end-stage liver disease, including ascites, encephalopathy, portal hypertensive bleeding, jaundice, significant weight loss, or hepatocellular carcinoma (HCC). Coexistent medical disorders such as coronary artery disease, chronic obstructive lung disease, cardiomyopathy, or pulmonary hypertension may jeopardize successful liver transplantation, especially in the elderly. Consequently, patients with comorbid conditions need to be evaluated to determine their candidacy for transplantation. There is no advantage gained by early listing of patients for liver transplantation, because waiting time no longer determines priority for transplantation.

*MELD ≥14*
*Complic.*
*B/Resp*

## 4. Which patients with HCC are considered and prioritized for transplantation?

Long-term survival for carefully selected patients with HCC is similar to that for patients undergoing transplantation for nonmalignant causes. The United Network for Organ Sharing (UNOS) requires careful staging of candidates with HCC to determine the extent of malignant disease. The extent of hepatic disease is assessed with abdominal computed tomography (CT), and chest CT (and bone scanning at some centers) is used to determine the presence of metastatic hepatoma. Patients who fulfill the Milan criteria (defined as one tumor ≤5 cm or ≤3 tumors of each <3 cm; no macrovascular involvement; and no radiographic evidence of extrahepatic disease) are awarded a high priority for transplantation with 22 points. A 10% increase is given to patients for every 3 months on the waiting list. In most centers, such patients are transplanted within a few months before HCC progresses. Liver transplant recipients fulfilling the Milan criteria have the same 3- to 4-year actuarial survival as patients without malignancy with, a 5-year survival of 75% to 85%.

Although controversial, recent studies have proposed expanding the current selection criteria for patients with HCC. For example, the UCSF (University of California at San Francisco) criteria include:

*5 : 3*
*6.5 : 4.5 → <8*

- Single tumor <6.5 cm
- Maximum three tumors with none >4.5 cm
- Cumulative tumor size <8 cm

Use of this set of criteria in liver allocation for HCC has been reported to have a 5-year post-transplantation survival rate of 75%. These criteria, however, are not currently used by UNOS to prioritize patients for transplantation.

## 5. What can be done to improve the availability of donor organs?

In 1998, the U.S. Department of Health and Human Services began a national organ and tissue donor initiative to increase donation rate, which has been historically low. The original initiative developed regulations to ensure collaboration between hospitals and organ procurement organizations in the event of brain death to identify potential donors, improved education and awareness of the need for donation, and funded research projects to ascertain effective interventions for increasing donation. Subsequent efforts increased the deceased-donor (DD) availability between 2000 and 2005 by 30%.

## 6. Given the high waiting list mortality, is living donor liver transplantation (LDLT) an option?

Yes. Approximately 10% of patients listed for liver transplantation in the United States die each year awaiting a suitable donor organ. LDLT was developed in response to the DD organ shortage and waiting list mortality. Adult-to-adult LDLT grew rapidly until 2001, when about 10% of all liver transplantations were performed with a living donor. Currently, living donor liver transplants constitute 3% of all transplantations. Most adult-to-adult LDLTs in the United States use the right hepatic lobe. A recent report found that transplant candidates who underwent LDLT have a significant survival advantage.

## 7. What are the advantages and disadvantages of LDLT?

The most important advantage of LDLT is a reduction in waiting time for the recipient. Once the recipient has been accepted as an acceptable candidate for LDLT and the donor is approved, surgery can occur within hours to days. An expedited transplantation may allow the surgery to occur prior to clinical decompensation, which could jeopardize the success of the surgery. Disadvantages of LDLT include risk to the donor (risk of death and morbidity). Finally, LDLT recipients may have more biliary complications than do recipients of cadaveric organs.

## 8. Who are potential recipients for LDLT?

The selection of appropriate recipients is an evolving process. The most appropriate recipients are ideal liver transplant candidates in urgent need of transplantation, mainly those at substantial risk of dying prior to DD transplantation, that is, decompensated liver disease and/or HCC. The LDLT recipient candidate undergoes the same evaluation as the DD recipient. There is controversy whether patients with stable chronic liver disease should be evaluated for LDLT, but many centers believe the risks to the donor outweigh the benefits to the recipients in these patients. Patients with multiple coexisting conditions, previous major abdominal surgery, or extensive mesenteric vein thrombosis have increased risk for postoperative complications and may not be suitable for LDLT.

## 9. List the diseases for which liver transplantation is performed.

### ACUTE LIVER FAILURE (8%): THE ABCs

- A: Acetaminophen, autoimmune hepatitis, *Amanita* mushroom toxin
- B: Hepatitis B
- C: Cryptogenic
- D: Drugs (acetaminophen, isoniazid, disulfiram, other)
- E: Esoterica (Wilson disease, Budd-Chiari)
- F: Fatty infiltration (Reye syndrome, acute fatty liver of pregnancy)

### CHRONIC LIVER DISEASE (82%)

- Chronic viral hepatitis (hepatitis C [HCV], hepatitis B)
- Alcoholic liver disease
- Cryptogenic cirrhosis
- Autoimmune hepatitis
- Primary biliary cirrhosis
- Primary sclerosing cholangitis
- Nonalcoholic steatohepatitis
- Budd-Chiari syndrome
- Drug-induced cirrhosis (methotrexate, amiodarone)
- Sarcoidosis
- Polycystic liver disease

### CONGENITAL/METABOLIC LIVER DISEASE (8%)

- Hemochromatosis
- Wilson's disease
- $\alpha_1$-Antitrypsin deficiency
- Cystic fibrosis
- Amyloidosis

# OTHER (2%)

- Hepatoblastoma
- Hemangioendothelioma
- Metastatic carcinoid tumor
- Retransplantation

**10. A 33-year-old man was diagnosed with acute hepatitis A 3 weeks ago. His jaundice has progressively worsened since then. Today, his wife found him to be mildly confused and brought him to the emergency department. What is the definition of acute liver failure (fulminant hepatic failure)?**

There are approximately 2500 cases of acute liver failure (ALF) in the United States each year. *Acute liver failure* is defined as acute hepatitis complicated by encephalopathy occurring within 8 weeks of disease onset in the absence of preexisting liver disease. Patients typically present with progressive lethargy and jaundice over several days. The most common causes of acute liver failure in the United States (in descending order) are acetaminophen (46%), indeterminate (15%), drug-induced (12%), hepatitis B (7%), hepatitis A (3%), and other (18%).

Because of the rapid progression of ALF, patients require prompt referral to a liver transplant center. Patients may progress from mild encephalopathy to full coma within a matter of hours. However, some patients recover spontaneously without orthotopic liver transplantation (OLT). Without transplantation, the majority of patients with acute hepatitis who progress to ALF will die. The two most common causes of death are cerebral edema and infection. Survival after transplantation for ALF ranges from 70% to 80% depending on the etiology. Prognostic schemes have been devised to identify patients with little to no chance of recovery so that emergency transplantation can be pursued. The King's College criteria were developed to try to identify patients with the highest risk of death without transplantation. These criteria may be used to help patients with ALF who would benefit from transplantation:

- Prothrombin time >100 seconds

Or any three of the following:   (3/5)

- Age <10 years or >40 years
- Etiology: non-A, non-B hepatitis; halothane; drug reaction
- Duration of jaundice before onset of encephalopathy >7 days
- Prothrombin time >50 seconds
- Serum bilirubin >18 mg/dL

**11. A 21-year-old woman is admitted following an overdose of acetaminophen. How do you determine whether she should be referred for liver transplantation?**

The most common cause of ALF is acetaminophen. Acute ingestion of acetaminophen may cause severe hepatic injury via the toxic metabolite *N*-acetyl-*p*-benzoquinoneimine, a metabolite of the cytochrome P450 system. Chronic alcohol ingestion may induce the cytochrome P450 system, which will reduce the amount of acetaminophen required to induce hepatotoxicity. Without treatment, an acetaminophen level above 300 µg/mL at 4 hours or above 45 µg/mL at 15 hours is associated with a 90% risk of hepatotoxicity. If patients present within 4 hours of ingestion, activated charcoal can reduce acetaminophen absorption. *N*-Acetylcysteine (Mucomyst), a glutathione precursor, remains the treatment of choice for acetaminophen-induced hepatotoxicity. Although more effective when given within 10 hours of ingestion, *N*-acetylcysteine can be given up to 24 hours after ingestion.

**12. Is human immunodeficiency virus (HIV) infection a contraindication to liver transplantation?**

No. While HIV infection was previously a contraindication to liver transplantation, the advent of highly active antiretroviral therapy (HAART) has altered the selection process for infected patients. The selection criteria for HIV patients are evolving but include:

- Patient on HAART treatment
- CD4 count ≥100 to 200 mm$^3$
- Absence of HIV-related infections or malignancies

In a recent published series, survival post transplantation in HIV-infected individuals was comparable to that of non-HIV patients. However, some HIV-infected liver transplant recipients suffer from very accelerated recurrent HCV.

**13. What conditions are considered contraindications to liver transplantation?**

The decision to perform a liver transplantation in a specific patient is based on the judgment and experience of the physicians at the transplant center.

## ABSOLUTE CONTRAINDICATIONS

- Extrahepatic malignancy (excluding squamous cell carcinoma of the skin)
- Active uncontrolled sepsis/infection
- Active alcohol or illicit drug use
- Psychosocial factors precluding recovery after transplantation
- Uncontrolled cardiopulmonary disease (coronary artery disease, congestive heart failure, valvular disease, pulmonary hypertension, restrictive lung disease, and severe chronic obstructive pulmonary disease)

## RELATIVE CONTRAINDICATIONS

- Advanced age (≥65 years old)
- Obesity
- Portal vein and/or mesenteric vein thrombosis
- Cholangiocarcinoma
- Psychiatric illness
- Poor social support
- HIV infection (see earlier discussion)

**14. A 45-year-old man with end-stage liver disease is evaluated for liver transplantation. Which features of the patient's psychosocial profile connote a good prognosis for continued abstinence from alcohol?**

For patients with a history of alcohol abuse, most centers require a period of abstinence (at least 6 to 12 months) and evaluation by a substance abuse professional prior to transplantation. Recognition of alcoholism by the patient and family members is especially important, and patients demonstrate this through adherence to an alcohol rehabilitation program. Features associated with a low rate of recidivism include absence of comorbid substance abuse, good social function, and absence of family history of alcohol abuse.

**15. Which factors measured in the recipient prior to transplantation correlate with reduced postoperative survival?**

Previous reports have suggested that clinical factors, including Child-Pugh class, are not good predictors of survival after transplantation. However, poor renal function prior to transplantation does predict poorer survival. Recipient hyponatremia was associated with a 3-month survival rate of 84% compared to 95% among individuals without pretransplantation hyponatremia. Advanced age, retransplantation, and extensive stage HCC are also associated with a worse outcome. HCV infection significantly impairs long-term patient and allograft survival due to recurrent HCV in the transplanted liver.

**16. Which immunosuppressants are used in liver transplantation? What are their mechanisms of action and side effects?**

See Table 29-1.

## Table 29-1. Mechanism of Action and Side Effects of Immunosuppressants

| DRUG | MECHANISM OF ACTION | TOXICITIES |
| --- | --- | --- |
| Tacrolimus | Calcineurin inhibitor: suppresses IL-2–dependent T-cell proliferation | Renal insufficiency, neurologic, diabetes mellitus, diarrhea |
| Cyclosporine | Same as tacrolimus | Hypertension, renal insufficiency, neurologic, hyperlipidemia, hirsutism |
| Azathioprine | Inhibits T- and B-cell proliferation by interfering with purine synthesis | Bone marrow depression, hepatotoxicity, dyspepsia |
| Mycophenolate mofetil Mycophenolic acid | Selective inhibition of T- and B-cell proliferation by interfering with purine synthesis | Bone marrow depression, diarrhea, dyspepsia |
| Corticosteroids | Cytokine inhibitor (IL-1, IL-2, IL-6, TNF, and IFNγ) | Diabetes mellitus, obesity, hypertension, osteopenia, infection, emotional lability |
| Sirolimus | Inhibition of the mammalian target of rapamycin (mTOR) decreasing B-cell and T-cell proliferation | Neutropenia, thrombocytopenia, pneumonitis, hyperlipidemia, hepatic artery thrombosis* |
| OKT3 | Blocks T-cell CD3 receptor, preventing stimulation by antigen | Cytokine release syndrome, pulmonary edema, increased risk of infections/lymphoproliferative disorders |
| Daclizumab/basiliximab/thymoglobulin | Monoclonal antibody that blocks IL-2 receptor inhibiting T-cell activation | Hypersensitivity reactions with basiliximab |

*Sirolimus is associated with a *black box warning* due to hepatic artery thrombosis.
IL, interleukin; TNF, tumor necrosis factor.

CNI + MMF/MPA/ AZA + cstds
TAC/CSA

### 17. What is the typical immunosuppressive regimen?

The specific immunosuppressive regimen varies from center to center. Current immunosuppressive therapy usually involves two or three agents to prevent allograft rejection in the immediate postoperative period. Typically, this involves a combination of a calcineurin inhibitor (CNI) such as tacrolimus (TAC) with one or more other agents. Currently, more than 90% of liver transplant recipients receive tacrolimus, and the remainder receive cyclosporine. A secondary agent, such as mycophenolate mofetil (MMF), mycophenolic acid (MPA), or azathioprine (AZA), is used along with a CNI. These agents operate through different mechanisms to increase the immunosuppressive effect while minimizing the nephrotoxic side effect of CNIs. Cyclosporine and tacrolimus prevent T-cell activation through inhibition of calcineurin, a calcium-dependent phosphatase involved in intracellular signal transduction. Azathioprine, MMF, and MPA prevent expansion of activated T and B cells. AZA is a purine analogue that becomes metabolized to its active compound, 6-mercaptopurine, and then inhibits DNA and RNA synthesis, particularly in rapidly proliferating T cells. MMF and MPA are noncompetitive inhibitors of an enzyme necessary for synthesis of guanine, a purine nucleotide.

Corticosteroids are used as first-line therapy in immunosuppression at many centers. However, there is increasing evidence that long-term maintenance corticosteroids may not be necessary to prevent rejection. Therefore, many liver transplant recipients are weaned completely off of corticosteroids within a few months after surgery. The most common regimen in the immediate postoperative period is TAC with MMF or MPA with a short course (weeks to months) of corticosteroids.

Liver allocation based on a MELD score has affected the administration of immunosuppression. Inclusion of creatinine as a determinant in MELD has increased the priority and number of liver transplant recipients with renal insufficiency. As a result, post-transplantation immunosuppressive regimens are configured to minimize nephrotoxicity. One strategy is to reduce or avoid tacrolimus exposure immediately after surgery. Many centers have introduced the use of rabbit antithymocyte globulin (rATG) as induction therapy. Another strategy is to reduce TAC exposure by increasing doses of MMF or MPA.

### 18. A liver transplant patient has just sustained a grand mal seizure 36 hours post transplantation. The cyclosporine level is within acceptable limits. The patient is in a postictal state but has no obvious focal neurologic deficits. Which factors contribute to an increased risk of seizures post transplantation?

Both cyclosporine and tacrolimus (FK506) are associated with neurotoxicity, including tremor, seizures, paresthesias, ataxia, and delirium. The neurologic side effects are usually reversible with a reduction in dosage or discontinuation of the drug.

### 19. A patient, 3 weeks post transplantation, receives erythromycin for atypical pneumonia. Does this drug affect immunosuppressive therapy?

Cyclosporine and tacrolimus are metabolized by the cytochrome P450-3A4 system. Medications that inhibit P450-3A4 will raise cyclosporine and tacrolimus levels and place the patient at risk for toxicity or overimmunosuppression. Medications that induce P450-3A4 will lower levels and increase the risk of rejection or require higher doses of the immunosuppressant. If these medications are necessary, dose adjustment and monitoring of cyclosporine and tacrolimus may be necessary. Medications that commonly interact with cyclosporine and tacrolimus include the following:

| Increase Cyclosporine/Tacrolimus Levels | Decrease Cyclosporine/Tacrolimus Levels |
| --- | --- |
| Erythromycin (inh CYP 3A4) | Phenytoin |
| Clarithromycin | Carbamazepine |
| Ketoconazole | Phenobarbital |
| Fluconazole | Rifampin |
| Itraconazole | |
| Verapamil | |
| Diltiazem | |
| Amiodarone | |

### 20. A patient who had an uncomplicated transplantation is noted to have rising liver enzyme levels on day 10 after transplantation. What is the differential diagnosis, and which tests should be obtained?

Elevated liver enzymes within the first 7 to 14 days after transplantation may be the first indication of a significant problem with the hepatic allograft. One of the most common causes of elevated liver enzymes is acute allograft rejection. Approximately 10% to 30% of liver transplant recipients experience acute cellular rejection within the first 3 months after transplantation. Early diagnosis is critical to ensure prompt initiation of immunosuppressive therapy (corticosteroid pulse or OKT3) to prevent graft loss. Liver biopsy remains the gold standard for the diagnosis of rejection. The differential includes thrombus of the hepatic artery or portal vein, biliary leak or stricture, cholangitis, drug toxicity, recurrent viral hepatitis, and opportunistic infection. In general, opportunistic infections and recurrent viral hepatitis appear later than day 10. Appropriate tests may include cyclosporine or tacrolimus level, hepatic Doppler ultrasound, cholangiogram, and liver biopsy. If these are unrevealing, infectious etiologies should be considered.

**21. A patient with cirrhosis from chronic hepatitis C undergoes liver transplantation. Ten days later his liver enzymes increase. What are the histologic findings of acute rejection versus post-transplantation hepatitis C on liver biopsy?**

The differentiation between recurrent hepatitis C and acute cellular rejection is one of the most problematic areas in clinical transplantation. In many cases, the histologic findings on the liver biopsy are inconclusive in differentiating these two disorders. The histologic features of acute cellular rejection include:

- Mixed cellular infiltrate (including eosinophils) in the portal triad
- Inflammation of the bile ducts presenting as either apoptosis or intraepithelial lymphocytes
- Endothelialitis of the central or portal veins

Recurrent hepatitis C can be difficult to distinguish from rejection. The histology may demonstrate a predominant lymphocytic infiltrate in the portal areas rather than the mixed cellular infiltrate of rejection. Other histologic findings of HCV include spotty parenchymal inflammation and vacuolization of the biliary epithelium.

**22. Describe the other post-transplantation complications manifested by elevated liver enzymes.**

Hepatic artery thrombosis remains a serious complication following transplantation. The clinical presentation may be variable but is usually associated with elevated transaminases. Other signs include decreased bile output, persistent elevation of the prothrombin time or bilirubin, and/or bacteremia. Cessation of hepatic artery blood flow preferentially causes ischemic damage to the biliary tree, resulting in breakdown of the biliary tree and development of bilomas, bile leaks, and eventually strictures. Early hepatic artery thrombosis may be amenable to interventional radiologic intervention but usually warrants reoperation. In hepatic artery thrombosis, retransplantation is usually required for successful long-term outcome.

In the early post-transplantation period, portal vein thrombosis may present with signs of graft dysfunction and require immediate revascularization or retransplantation. Late thrombosis may be well tolerated or lead to graft dysfunction and/or portal hypertension. Balloon angioplasty, stent placement, and thrombolytic infusion have been used to reestablish the portal circulation.

Biliary leaks or strictures may be asymptomatic but can also lead to jaundice, bacteremia, or sepsis. Biliary leaks can occur at the biliary anastomosis and within the liver as a result of bile duct destruction. Ischemic damage from hepatic artery thrombosis may be a contributing factor.

Medications may also cause elevated liver enzymes. A cholestatic pattern may occur with cyclosporine, tacrolimus, azathioprine, sulfa drugs, and various antibiotics. A hepatocellular pattern may occur with azathioprine, nonsteroidal anti-inflammatory drugs, and some antibiotics.

The most common opportunistic infection of the hepatic allograft is cytomegalovirus (CMV) infection, and the infection may present as elevated liver enzymes, fever, cytopenias, and/or lethargy. Tissue invasive disease may cause life-threatening complications when the liver, lungs, or gastrointestinal tract are involved. The most common time period for CMV disease is 4 to 12 weeks after transplantation. With generally lower levels of immunosuppression and effective prophylaxis, the occurrence of CMV disease in liver transplant recipients is decreasing to less than 5% at some centers.

Recurrent hepatic disease may also first present with abnormal liver enzymes. Almost all patients with hepatitis C will develop recurrence of hepatitis C infection. Most patients will have mild to moderate transaminase elevations and mild to moderate inflammation on biopsy. In a minority of patients, both hepatitis B and C infection may lead to fibrosing cholestatic hepatitis, which can lead to cirrhosis and graft loss during the first year. Recurrent disease may also occur with autoimmune hepatitis, primary biliary cirrhosis, and sclerosing cholangitis (Fig. 29-1).

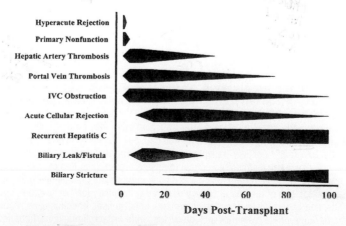

**Figure 29-1.** Post-transplantation complications and time of occurrence.

**23. A patient having early allograft rejection is treated with a 7-day course of OKT3 returns 1 week later with headache, mild fatigue, low-grade fever, and increased liver enzymes. Is this OKT3 toxicity?**

This is unlikely to be OKT3 toxicity. Reactions due to OKT3 toxicity are termed *first-dose syndrome* and can occur within 30 to 60 minutes of the first few doses. These include fever (70% to 100%), rigors (30%), flash pulmonary edema, bronchospasm, arthralgias, nausea, vomiting, and diarrhea (15% to 20%). One concern would be aseptic meningitis, which can present during or after OKT3 toxicity and can present with headache, fever, fatigue, and meningismus.

**24. If the patient does not have OKT3 toxicity, what is the most likely diagnosis?**

CMV is the most likely diagnosis (in the patient described in Question 23), which is a common infection following liver transplantation. It typically occurs 1 to 6 months after surgery. The greatest risk of recurrent CMV disease occurs in *mismatched* recipients who have never had CMV exposure (CMV IgG negative) and are receiving a graft from a CMV IgG-positive donor. The prophylactic regimen for CMV disease varies from center to center. Prophylaxis is usually administered to all mismatched recipients with oral ganciclovir or valganciclovir for up to 3 months after transplantation. However, IgG-negative recipients receiving a graft from an IgG-negative donor often receive no prophylaxis.

Signs of CMV infection include fever, malaise, leukopenia, thrombocytopenia, and organ involvement (hepatitis, gastroenteritis, pancreatitis, pneumonia, and retinitis). Viremia is detected by CMV DNA blood level and has gained wide acceptance as a diagnostic tool. In addition, the liver biopsy is diagnostic if the viral inclusions are present in the hepatic parenchyma or if the immunohistochemical stains are positive. With the advent of CMV viral assay testing, CMV IgM antibody testing has no role in the diagnosis of CMV disease in liver transplant recipients.

**25. What are the clinical, biochemical, and histologic features of chronic rejection?**

Chronic allograft rejection is generally characterized by an insidious but progressive rise in alkaline phosphatase and bilirubin. Patients are usually asymptomatic and synthetic function remains intact until the late stages. The pathogenesis of this syndrome remains unclear, but the evidence favors loss of bile ducts and the development of obliterative arteriopathy in the small hepatic arteries. Histological findings include a normal-appearing parenchyma with few mononuclear infiltrates in the portal areas but absence of bile ducts in almost all of the portal triads. Later in the course, patients develop strictures and dilations in the larger bile ducts resembling primary sclerosing cholangitis. In these cases, the clinical course may be complicated by recurrent attacks of biliary sepsis. The differential diagnosis at this stage includes hepatic artery thrombosis, CMV cholangitis, anastomotic strictures of the biliary tree, and recurrent primary sclerosing cholangitis.

Chronic rejection is currently very uncommon and usually occurs in liver transplant recipients who are noncompliant with their immunosuppressive therapy. The process frequently progresses to graft failure, but recent reports indicate that 20% to 30% of patients may respond to additional immunosuppressive therapy. Patients with progressive liver failure caused by chronic rejection may require evaluation for retransplantation.

**26. How often is it necessary to perform a second liver transplantation, and for what reasons are retransplantations performed?**

Fewer than 10% of the liver transplantations performed in the United States are retransplantations. Early retransplantations are usually performed for primary nonfunction and hepatic artery thrombosis. Improved surgical techniques have reduced the early retransplantation rate. Late retransplantations may occur for recurrence of the original disease or chronic rejection. Recurrent disease may occur with viral hepatitis, autoimmune hepatitis, primary sclerosing cholangitis, and, rarely, primary biliary cirrhosis.

**27. Describe the long-term metabolic complications that occur in the liver transplant recipient.**

Although patients experience a dramatic improvement in their quality of life following liver transplantation, they are at risk for complications associated with the use of immunosuppressive regimens. The most common metabolic complications include diabetes, hypertension, and renal insufficiency. Diabetes may occur following transplantation due to corticosteroids and in patients receiving calcineurin inhibitors. Hypertension is common with cyclosporine and tacrolimus and the associated renal insufficiency may exacerbate this problem. Hyperlipidemia also occurs following transplantation due to corticosteroids, sirolimus, and cyclosporine. Although metabolic complications may be ameliorated by a reduction in immunosuppression, persistent hyperlipidemia or diabetes requires aggressive treatment. All of these factors may place patients at greater risk for cardiovascular or cerebrovascular disease, and patients should receive counseling regarding appropriate diet, exercise, and smoking cessation. Renal insufficiency frequently occurs after liver transplantation and is more frequent in patients receiving cyclosporine than tacrolimus. Up to 28% of patients develop end-stage renal disease (ESRD) 10 years after transplantation. Other risk factors for developing ESRD include advanced age, hypertension, diabetes, hepatitis C, renal disease prior to liver transplantation, and postoperative acute renal failure (ARF).

Because of the frequency and severity of post-transplantation renal disease, most centers have instituted strategies to address this problem. The most common approach is to reduce or completely withdraw CNI (tacrolimus or cyclosporine) and replace or supplement the immunosuppressive regimen with an alternative agent without nephrotoxicity such as MMF, MPA, or sirolimus. However, there is no convincing evidence that this approach measurably affects patient/graft survival or ESRD.

Patients may be at risk for osteoporosis associated with corticosteroid use, particularly if they received significant steroids prior to transplantation. A low threshold for measurement of bone density prior to transplantation may be appropriate in high-risk populations such as patients with cholestatic liver disease. Patients at risk should consult with an endocrinologist for an assessment of appropriate therapy, which may include calcium, vitamin D supplementation, and other agents.

### 28. Are liver transplant recipients at increased risk to develop cancer?

Immunosuppression significantly increases the risk of malignancy and complicates approximately 2% of liver transplantations. The most common malignancy following liver transplantation is squamous cell carcinoma of the skin. Therefore, patients should avoid exposure to ultraviolet light and wear protective clothing and sunscreen if they participate in activities leading to sun exposure.

Post-transplantation lymphoproliferative disorder (PTLD) occurs in 1% of patients after liver transplantation. Most are large B-cell type non-Hodgkin's lymphoma caused by Epstein-Barr virus (EBV) infection in the setting of chronic immunosuppression. The two most important risk factors for PTLD are the degree of immunosuppression (including OKT3) and EBV donor mismatch (EBV IgG-negative recipient and EBV IgG-positive donor). The clinical presentation is variable and includes fever, lymphadenopathy, weight loss, and/or organ involvement. Extranodal involvement is common in the gastrointestinal tract, liver, lung, and bone marrow. Treatment is a marked reduction in immunosuppression and/or use of antiviral agents, which may result in complete resolution of disease. Referral for oncology consultation is also necessary for consideration of chemotherapy or radiation, which is required for many patients.

### 29. A liver transplant patient comes to the emergency department complaining of cough and shortness of breath. How does one suspect, diagnose, and treat *Pneumocystis jiroveci (carinii)* pneumonia?

*P. jiroveci* pneumonia (PCP), formerly known as *P. carinii*, is an opportunistic infection that can occur, although rarely, in post-transplantation patients. The clinical presentation can be variable, but typical symptoms include fever, shortness of breath, and nonproductive cough. If left untreated, PCP may have a rapid course to respiratory failure. As a result, patients typically receive prophylaxis with trimethoprim–sulfamethoxazole for up to 1 year following transplantation. Definitive diagnosis often requires bronchoscopy or bronchoalveolar lavage and should not delay treatment in the appropriate setting. With institution of prophylaxis and more conservative immunosuppressive regimens, the incidence of PCP at most transplant centers is less than 1%. Patients with a sulfa allergy may receive inhaled pentamidine as prophylaxis.

### 30. What factors contribute to metabolic bone disease after transplantation?

Chronic liver diseases, particularly cholestatic liver diseases, are associated with osteopenia. The pathogenesis was originally thought to be related to decreased bile salt flow and vitamin D malabsorption, but plasma vitamin D levels are normal. Instead, these patients appear to have inhibition of bone formation and low or normal bone resorption. Prior to transplantation, therefore, these patients may already have significant bone loss. Following transplantation, glucocorticoids worsen the condition and place the patients at risk for fractures. One study measured the bone density of 20 women with primary biliary cirrhosis. At 3 months after transplantation, their bone fell at a mean rate of 18.1% per year. The nadir in bone density appeared to occur within the first 6 months. As glucocorticoid use decreased, bone density improved and ultimately surpassed the pretransplantation density at 2 years.

### 31. A patient who underwent liver transplantation for cirrhosis due to hepatitis C returns with persistently elevated liver enzymes. Liver biopsy reveals chronic active hepatitis but no cirrhosis. Should he be treated with interferon α and/or ribavirin?

Virtually all patients who receive a liver transplant for hepatitis C will have recurrent infection, with 20% to 40% developing cirrhosis by the fifth postoperative year. Therefore, the survival of liver transplant recipients with recurrent HCV is reduced compared to patients who undergo liver transplantation for other indications. Diagnosis of recurrence requires the presence of HCV viremia and histology of recurrent HCV on liver biopsy. A small minority develop fibrosing cholestatic hepatitis, which may have an aggressive course and lead to graft loss within 1 year. Most patients will have mild to moderate elevations in transaminases and mild to moderate fibrosis on biopsy, and the optimal management of these patients is less clear.

The decision to treat HCV after transplantation is based largely on histology. Patients should undergo biopsies 6 to 12 months (or whenever liver function tests are elevated) after surgery to determine the extent of histologic injury. Patients with stage 2 or higher fibrosis are generally considered candidates for treatment with pegylated-interferon and ribavirin. Other factors must be considered prior to instituting therapy related to side effects of therapy such as psychological state, cytopenia, and physical recovery from transplantation. In addition, the side effect profile of PEG-interferon and ribavirin is substantially worse compared with non–transplant recipients. Furthermore, there is a low likelihood of achieving a sustained virologic response (SVR)—about 25% or half that of non–transplant recipients. The reasons for this low response rate include:

- Higher proportion of genotype 1 in liver recipients
- Virtually all liver recipients previously failed by interferon therapy
- Immunosuppression reduces effect of interferon
- Marginal renal function reduces total exposure to ribavirin
- Relatively high rate of treatment reduction and discontinuation

## 32. Is retransplantation for recurrent hepatitis C recommended?

The prevalence of HCV infection in patients undergoing retransplantation has significantly increased since 1990. As a result, HCV is the most common indication for liver transplantation in the United States. Because recurrent hepatitis C causes graft failure in an increasing number of patients, retransplantation is being considered more frequently. However, retransplantation for patients with graft failure caused by recurrent hepatitis C is controversial for two reasons:

- Long-term survival rates for retransplantation of recipients with graft failure due to HCV is only 50%.
- The critical shortage of DD livers forces clinicians to select patients with the best chance of survival after transplantation.

Therefore, most transplant centers will not offer retransplantation to patients with graft loss due to recurrent HCV or offer it on a very limited basis.

## BIBLIOGRAPHY

1. Beresford TP, Turcotte JG, Merion R, et al. A rational approach to liver transplantation for the alcoholic. Psychosomatics 1990;31:241–54.
2. Berg CL, Gillespie BW, Merion RM, et al. Improvement in survival associated with adult-to-adult living donor transplantation. Gastroenterology 2007;133:1806–13.
3. Curley S, Carlton B, Abdalla E. Liver transplantation for hepatocellular carcinoma. UpToDate 2003;11:1.
4. Eason JD, Loss GE, Blazek J, et al. Steroid-free liver transplantation using rabbit antithymocyte globulin induction: Results of a prospective randomized trial. Liver Transpl 2001;7:693–7.
5. Eastell R, Dickson ER, Hodgson SF, et al. Rates of vertebral bone loss before and after liver transplantation in women with primary biliary cirrhosis. Hepatology 1991;14:296–300.
6. Eckhoff DE, Pirsch JD, D'Alessandro AM, et al. Pretransplant status and patient survival following liver transplantation. Transplantation 1995;60:920–5.
7. El-Serag HB, Marrero JA, Rudolph L, et al. Diagnosis and treatment of hepatocellular carcinoma. Gastroenterology 2008;134:1752–63.
8. Forman LM, Lewis JD, Berlin JA, et al. The association between hepatitis C infection and survival after orthotopic liver transplantation. Gastroenterology 2002;122:889–96.
9. Foster PF, Fabrega F, Karademir S, et al. Prediction of abstinence from ethanol in alcoholic recipients following liver transplantation. Hepatology 1997;25:1469–77.
10. Fung J, Marcos A. Rapamycin: Friend, foe, or misunderstood? Liver Transpl 2003;9:469–72.
11. Ghobrial RM, Freise CE, Trotter JF, et al. Donor morbidity after living donation for liver transplantation. Gastroenterology 2008;135:468–76.
12. Golling M, Safer A, Kriesche B, et al. Transplant survival following liver transplant: A multivariate analysis. Transpl Proc 1998;30:3239–40.
13. González E, Rimola A, Navasa M, et al. Liver transplantation in patients with non-biliary cirrhosis: Prognostic value of preoperative factors. J Hepatol 1998;28:320–8.
14. Heard KJ. Acetylcysteine for acetaminophen poisoning. N Engl J Med 2008;359:285–92.
15. Hooks MA, Wade CS, Millikan WJ. Muromonab CD-3: A review of its pharmacology, pharmacokinetics, and clinical use in transplantation. Pharmacotherapy 1991;11:26–23.
16. Levitsky J, Singh N, Wagener MM, et al. A survey of CMV prevention strategies after liver transplantation. Am J Transpl 2008;8:158–61.
17. Londoño MC, Guevara M, Rimola A, et al. Hyponatremia impairs early posttransplantation outcome in patients with cirrhosis undergoing liver transplantation. Gastroenterology 2006;130:1135–43.
18. Makin AJ, Wendon J, Williams R. A 7-year experience of severe acetaminophen-induced hepatotoxicity (1987-1993). Gastroenterology 1995;109:1907–16.
19. McCashland T, Watt K, Lyden E, et al. Retransplantation for hepatitis C: Results of a U.S. multicenter retransplant study. Liver Transplantation 2007;13:1246–53.
20. Murray KF, Carithers RL. AASLD practice guidelines: Evaluation of the patient for liver transplantation. Hepatology 2005;41:1–26.
21. O'Grady JG, Alexander GJM, Hayllar KM, et al. Early indicators of prognosis in fulminant hepatic failure. Gastroenterology 1989;97:439–45.
22. Ojo AO, Held PJ, Port FK, et al. Chronic renal failure after transplantation of a nonrenal organ. N Engl J Med 2003;349:931–40.
23. Prottas JM, Batten HL. The willingness to give: The public and the supply of transplantable organs. J Health Polit Policy Law 1991;16:121–4.
24. Roland ME, Barin B, Carlson L, et al. HIV-infected liver and kidney transplant recipients: 1- And 3-year outcomes. Am J Transpl 2008;8:355–65.

25. Shah SA, Grant DR, McGilvray ID, et al. Biliary strictures in 130 consecutive right lobe living donor liver transplant recipients: Results of a Western center. Am J Transpl 2007;7:161–7.
26. Shapiro R, Young JB, Milford EL, et al. Immunosuppression: Evolution in practice and trends, 1993-2003. Am J Transplant. 2005;5:874–86.
27. Shiffman ML. Treating chronic hepatitis C virus after liver transplantation: Balancing the risks against the chance for success. Liver Transpl 2007;13:1088–91.
28. Trotter JF, Adam R, Lo CM, et al. Documented deaths of hepatic lobe donors for living donor liver transplantation. Liver Transpl 2006;12:1485–8.
29. Vale JA, Proudfoot AT. Paracetamol (acetaminophen) poisoning. Lancet 1995;346:547–52.
30. Wiesner RH, Batts KP, Krom RA. Evolving concepts in the diagnosis, pathogenesis, and treatment of chronic hepatic allograft rejection. Liver Transpl Surg 1999;5:388–400.
31. Wiesner R, Edwards E. Model for end-stage liver disease (MELD) and allocation of donor livers. Gastroenterology 2003;124:91–6.
32. Wong T, Devlin J, Rolando N, et al. Clinical characteristics affecting the outcome of liver retransplantation. Transplantation 1997;64:878–82.
33. Yao FY, Ferrell L, Bass NM, et al. Liver transplantation for hepatocellular carcinoma: Expansion of the tumor size does not adversely impact survival. Hepatology 2001;33:1394–403.

# ASCITES

*Carlos Guarner, MD, and Bruce A. Runyon, MD*

# CHAPTER 30

### 1. What are the most common causes of ascites?

Ascites is the accumulation of fluid within the peritoneal cavity. More than 80% of patients with ascites have decompensated chronic liver disease. However, it is important to know the other possible causes of ascites, because the treatment and prognosis may be quite different. Peritoneal carcinomatosis is the second most common cause of ascites, followed by alcoholic hepatitis, heart failure, fulminant or subacute hepatic failure, pancreatic disease, dialysis ascites, nephrotic syndrome, hepatic vein obstruction, chylous ascites, bile ascites, and miscellaneous disorders of the peritoneum.

### 2. Should a diagnostic tap be performed routinely on all patients with ascites at the time of admission to the hospital?

Ascites is readily diagnosed when large amounts of fluid are present in the peritoneal cavity. If clinical examination is not definitive in detecting or excluding ascites, ultrasonography may be helpful. In addition, ultrasonography may provide information about the cause of ascites, such as by documenting parenchymal liver disease, splenomegaly, and an enlarged portal vein. Abdominal tap may be performed easily and safely, and analysis of ascitic fluid provides useful data for differentiating causes of ascites. Prior to the era of prevention of infection by selective intestinal decontamination, up to 30% of patients with cirrhosis and ascites had ascitic fluid infection at the time of admission to the hospital or developed it during hospitalization. This infection is less common now but remains a preventable cause of death in these patients. As a rule, therefore, diagnostic abdominal tap should be performed routinely:

- In all patients with new-onset ascites and
- At the time of admission in patients with ascites

In addition, it should be repeated in patients whose clinical condition deteriorates during hospitalization, especially when they develop signs or symptoms of bacterial infection, hepatic encephalopathy, gastrointestinal hemorrhage, or deterioration of renal function. Patients with refractory ascites are currently submitted to repeated large-volume paracentesis in the outpatient clinic. Recent studies have demonstrated that the incidence of ascitic fluid infection or bacterascites is very low in these patients. Therefore, it seems reasonable to obtain a cell count and differential on all samples of ascitic fluid in the paracentesis clinic setting and to culture only samples of ascitic fluid of symptomatic outpatients and when the fluid is cloudy, consistent with an elevated cell count.

### 3. How should a diagnostic paracentesis be performed?

Although paracentesis is a simple and safe procedure, precautions should be taken to avoid complications. Paracentesis should be performed under sterile conditions. The abdomen should be cleaned and disinfected with an iodine or similar solution, and the physician should wear sterile gloves during the entire procedure. The needle should be inserted in an area that is dull to percussion. The midline between the umbilicus and symphysis pubis was the preferable site of needle insertion in the past. However, three factors have changed this philosophy:

- Frequency of therapeutic paracentesis
- Thickness of the panniculus in the midline in the obese patient
- Frequency of obesity in patients with cirrhosis

Now the left lower quadrant appears to be the best site for needle insertion. Because the panniculus is less thick in this area, the needle traverses less tissue. Occasionally even a 3.5-inch needle will not reach ascitic fluid in the midline in obese patients. Therapeutic taps in the lower quadrants drain more fluid than midline taps. Patients on lactulose tend to have a distended cecum. Therefore, the left lower quadrant is chosen over the right lower quadrant. A site is chosen in the left lower quadrant two finger-breadths (3 cm) cephalad from the anterior superior iliac spine and two finger-breadths medial to this landmark.

Scars should be avoided, because they are often sites of collateral vessels and adherent bowel. Between 30 and 50 mL of ascitic fluid should be withdrawn for analysis.

## 4. What tests should be routinely ordered on ascitic fluid?

Analysis of ascitic fluid is useful for the differential diagnosis of ascites. However, it is not necessary to order all tests on every specimen. The most important tests are cell count, bacterial culture, albumin, and total protein.

The *white blood cell count* is probably the single most important test performed on ascitic fluid, because it provides immediate information about possible bacterial infection. An absolute neutrophil count of 250 cells/mm$^3$ or greater (total white cell count or nucleated cell count × % polymorphonuclear cells [PMNs]) provides presumptive evidence of bacterial infection of ascitic fluid and warrants initiation of empirical antibiotics. An elevated white blood cell count with a predominance of lymphocytes strongly suggests peritoneal carcinomatosis or tuberculous peritonitis.

*Albumin* concentration of ascitic fluid allows calculation of the serum-ascites albumin gradient to classify specimens into high- or low-gradient categories (see Question 6).

Ascitic fluid should be cultured by inoculating *blood culture* bottles at the bedside. The sensitivity of this method is higher than that of the older technique (sending a tube or syringe of fluid to the lab) in detecting bacterial growth. Automated systems for bacterial growth culture such as BacT/ALERT provide an earlier microbiologic diagnosis of ascitic fluid infection (usually within 12 hours). Specific culture for tuberculosis should be ordered when tuberculous peritonitis is suspected on clinical grounds and the ascitic fluid white cell count is elevated with a predominance of lymphocytic cells.

*Total protein* concentration of ascitic fluid has been used to classify ascitic fluid into transudates and exudates. This classification is not particularly helpful, because greater than 30% of cirrhotic ascites samples are exudates. Nevertheless, total protein concentration of ascitic fluid should be ordered routinely, because it is useful for determining which patients are at high risk of developing spontaneous bacterial peritonitis (SBP) (total protein less than 1.0 g/dL) and for differentiating spontaneous from secondary bacterial peritonitis. Measurement of glucose and lactate dehydrogenase (LDH) in ascitic fluid also has been found to be helpful in making this distinction (see Question 11).

*Amylase activity* of ascitic fluid is markedly elevated in pancreatic ascites and gut perforation into ascites.

*Gram stain* of ascitic fluid usually demonstrates no bacteria in patients with cirrhosis and early SBP, but it may be helpful in identifying patients with gut perforation, in whom multiple types of bacteria are seen.

*Cytology* of ascitic fluid is useful in detecting malignant ascites when the peritoneum is involved with the malignant process. Unfortunately, ascitic fluid cytology is not useful in detecting hepatocellular carcinoma, which seldom metastasizes to the peritoneum.

*Other tests* proposed as helpful in detecting malignant ascites, such as fibronectin, cholesterol, ferritin, transferrin, lactate, ceruloplasmin, $\alpha_2$-microglobulin, $\alpha$1-antitrypsin, interleukin 8, and carcinoembryonic antigen, have limited, if any, value in ascitic fluid analysis.

## 5. Should a diagnostic thoracocentesis be performed in patients with cirrhosis and pleural hydrothorax?

*Hepatic hydrothorax* is defined as the accumulation of ascitic fluid in the pleural space in a patient with cirrhosis, in whom a cardiac, pulmonary, or pleural cause has been excluded. From 5% to 10% of cirrhotic patients with ascites develop hepatic hydrothorax, mainly in the right side (almost 70% of the cases), but it can also be in the left side and bilateral. In a recent study, almost 10% of cirrhotic patients admitted to the hospital with hepatic hydrothorax have a spontaneous bacterial empyema and 40% of these episodes were not associated with SBP. In consequence, a diagnostic thoracocentesis in cirrhotic patients with ascites could be useful to evaluate other causes of pleural effusion in selected patients and to diagnose spontaneous bacterial empyema in cirrhotic patients with a suspected bacterial infection and negative studies of urine, ascitic fluid, and blood specimens.

## 6. Why is it useful to measure serum-ascites albumin gradient?

Serum-ascites albumin gradient (SAAG) is more useful than the total protein concentration of ascitic fluid in the classification of ascites. This gradient is physiologically based on oncotic-hydrostatic balance and is related directly to portal pressure. The serum-ascites albumin gradient is calculated by subtracting the albumin concentration of ascitic fluid from the albumin concentration of serum obtained on the same day:

$$SAAG = albumin_{serum} - albumin_{ascites}$$

Patients with gradients of 1.1 g/dL or greater have portal hypertension, whereas patients with gradients less than 1.1 g/dL do not:

Serum–ascites albumin gradient     Serum–ascites albumin gradient

$\geq 1.1 g/dL$            $< 1.1 g/dL$

↓                 ↓

Portal hypertension     Normal portal pressure

## 7. What are the causes of high (i.e., ≥1.1 g/dL) serum-ascites albumin gradients?

The most common cause of a high serum-ascites albumin gradient is cirrhosis, but any cause of portal hypertension leads to a high gradient (e.g., alcoholic hepatitis, cardiac ascites, massive liver metastases, fulminant hepatic failure, Budd-Chiari syndrome, portal vein thrombosis, veno-occlusive disease, myxedema, fatty liver of pregnancy, *mixed ascites*). Mixed ascites is due to two different causes, including one that causes portal hypertension (e.g., cirrhosis and tuberculous peritonitis).

## 8. What are the causes of low (i.e., <1.1 g/dL) serum-ascites albumin gradients?

Low-gradient ascites is found in the absence of portal hypertension and is usually due to peritoneal disease. The most common cause is peritoneal carcinomatosis. Other causes are tuberculous peritonitis, pancreatic disease, biliary ascites, nephrotic syndrome, serositis, and bowel obstruction or infarction.

## 9. What are the variants of ascitic fluid infection?

Ascitic fluid infection can be spontaneous or secondary to an intra-abdominal, surgically treatable source of infection. More than 90% of ascitic fluid infections in cirrhotic patients are spontaneous. According to the characteristics of ascitic fluid culture and PMN count, four different variants of ascitic fluid infection have been described in cirrhotic patients:

1. *Spontaneous bacterial empyema* (SBP) is defined as an ascitic fluid infection with PMN count of 250 cells/mm$^3$ or greater and positive culture (usually for a single organism).
2. *Culture-negative neutrocytic ascites* (CNNA) is defined as an ascitic fluid PMN count of 250 cells/mm$^3$ or greater with a negative culture.
3. *Bacterascites* is defined as an ascitic fluid PMN count less than 250 cells/mm$^3$ with a positive culture for a single organism.
4. *Polymicrobial bacterascites* is defined as an ascitic fluid with PMN count less than 250 cells/mm$^3$ with a positive culture for more than one organism. This condition usually is caused by gut puncture by the needle during attempted paracentesis.

## 10. What is the diagnostic criterion of spontaneous bacterial empyema?

Current diagnostic criterion of spontaneous bacterial empyema is a positive pleural fluid with a pleural fluid PMN count greater than or equal to 250 cells/μL and the exclusion of parapneumonic infections. *Culture-negative spontaneous bacterial empyema* is defined when the patient has a negative pleural fluid culture and a PMN greater than or equal to 500 cells/μL without a parapneumonic infection.

## 11. How do you differentiate spontaneous from secondary peritonitis?

It is important to differentiate spontaneous from secondary peritonitis in cirrhotic patients, because treatment for SBP is medical, whereas treatment for secondary peritonitis is usually surgical. Although secondary peritonitis represents less than 10% of ascitic fluid infections, it should be considered in any patient with neutrocytic ascites. Analysis of ascitic fluid is helpful in differentiating the two entities. Secondary bacterial peritonitis should be suspected when ascitic fluid analysis shows two or three of the following criteria (Runyon criteria):

- Total protein greater than 1 g/dL
- Glucose less than 50 mg/dL
- Lactate dehydrogenase (LDH) greater than 225 mU/mL (or higher than the upper limit of normal for serum)

Most of the ascitic fluid cultures in such patients are polymicrobial, whereas in patients with SBP the infection is usually monomicrobial. Patients with suspected secondary peritonitis must be evaluated by emergency radiologic techniques to confirm and localize the possible visceral perforation. In patients with nonperforation secondary peritonitis, these criteria are not as useful; however, PMN cell count after 48 hours of treatment increases beyond the pretreatment value and ascitic fluid culture remains positive. Conversely, ascitic fluid PMN cell count decreases rapidly in appropriately treated patients with SBP, and ascitic fluid culture becomes negative. Determination of ascitic fluid carcinoembryonic antigen and alkaline phosphatase levels (greater than 5 ng/mL and/or greater than 240 U/L, respectively) may be helpful to diagnose secondary bacterial peritonitis due to occult intestinal perforation (higher specificity than Runyon criteria).

## 12. Who is at high risk of developing SBP?

- Patients with cirrhosis admitted to the hospital with gastrointestinal hemorrhage
- Patients with cirrhosis and ascitic fluid total protein less than 1.5 g/dL and advanced liver disease, especially those with high bilirubin (greater than 3.2 mg/dL) or low platelet count (less than 98,000 cells/mm$^3$), Child-Pugh of 9 or higher, hyponatremia (130 mEq/L or less), or renal dysfunction (serum creatinine 1.2 mg/dL or higher or blood urea nitrogen 25 mg/dL or higher)
- Patients with cirrhosis who have survived an episode of SBP
- Patients with fulminant hepatic failure

## 13. What is the pathogenesis of SBP?

Gram-negative bacteria are the most common causative agents isolated in bacterial infections in patients with cirrhosis. Therefore, it has been suggested that the gut may be the source of the bacteria. Direct passage of intestinal bacteria to portal blood or ascitic fluid has not been documented in patients with cirrhosis, if the gut mucosa has not lost its integrity. *Bacterial translocation*, defined as the passage of viable bacteria from gastrointestinal tract to mesenteric lymph nodes, has been demonstrated in an experimental model of rats with cirrhosis and ascites and in patients with cirrhosis who underwent laparotomy. In fact, genetic identity has been observed between bacteria isolated in the gut, mesenteric lymph nodes, and ascitic fluid in rats with cirrhosis. Intestinal bacterial overgrowth seems to be the main mechanism of bacterial translocation in cirrhotic rats. Reducing the quantity of intestinal flora has been shown to decrease the incidence of bacterial translocation and SBP. A recent experimental study observed that rats with cirrhosis and severe intestinal oxidative damage in the ileum and cecum have a higher incidence of bacterial translocation, suggesting a possible role of functional mucosal alterations in the pathogenesis of SBP. Several immune deficiencies, especially decreased activity of the reticuloendothelial system and low serum complement levels, lead to frequent and prolonged bacteremia in patients with cirrhosis and to colonization of body fluids, such as ascitic fluid. The development of a bacterial infection depends on the capacity of ascitic fluid to kill the bacteria. In vitro, the capacity of ascitic fluid to kill bacteria (i.e., opsonic activity) is related directly to total protein and C3 concentration of ascitic fluid. Patients with cirrhosis and low ascitic fluid opsonic activity have low C3, low total protein, and thus a higher incidence of SBP. In contrast, patients with high ascitic fluid opsonic activity have high C3 and high total protein; thus, bacterial colonization may resolve spontaneously.

## 14. What single test provides early information about possible ascitic fluid infection?

The decision to start empirical antibiotic treatment must be made as soon as possible, because the survival rate depends in part on early diagnosis and treatment. Gram stain is positive in only 5% to 10% of patients, and bacterial culture of ascitic fluid takes at least 12 hours to demonstrate growth. The ascitic fluid neutrophil count is highly sensitive in detecting bacterial infection of peritoneal fluid, and the result should be available in a matter of minutes. An absolute neutrophil count of 250 cells/mm$^3$ or greater warrants empiric antibiotic treatment. Ascitic fluid for cell count should be immediately injected into a tube containing an anticoagulant (i.e., *purple top* tube) to avoid clotting of the specimen. The laboratory should perform the cell count in less than 60 minutes, but this is unusual. Different studies have demonstrated that the use of urine *dipsticks* to detect neutrophils in ascitic fluid has a high sensitivity, specificity, and negative predictive value and reduces the time from paracentesis to a presumptive diagnosis of SBP from a few hours to as little as 90 seconds. Recently, a large series from 70 French hospitals reported a low sensitivity of the reagent strips and a high risk of false-negatives, especially in patients with SBP and PMN counts of 250 cells/mm$^3$ to 500 cells/mm$^3$. Therefore, a standard cell count and differential should be performed by the laboratory to confirm the results, but empirical antibiotics can be immediately started in patients with a positive urine dipstick. The use of reagent strips for the diagnosis of SBP could be especially important in those hospitals where ascitic fluid PMN count is not performed on an emergency basis.

## 15. What is the treatment of choice for suspected SBP?

A relatively broad-spectrum antibiotic combination, such as an aminoglycoside plus ampicillin, was routinely used in the past for treatment of suspected SBP. However, most patients with cirrhosis treated with an aminoglycoside developed nephrotoxicity, even if serum levels were controlled. Third-generation cephalosporins cover most of the flora responsible for SBP; they are more effective than the combination of ampicillin and aminoglycoside and lack nephrotoxicity. Cefotaxime or a similar cephalosporin should be started when SBP is suspected. Recently, it was demonstrated that 2.0 g of cefotaxime, given intravenously every 8 to 12 hours, is as effective as dosing every 6 hours. A short course of therapy (5 days) has been shown to be as effective as a long course (10 days). Amoxicillin-clavulanic acid, initially intravenously (1 to 0.2 g/8 hr) and then orally (500 to 125 mg/8 hr), has been shown to be as effective as cefotaxime but less expensive. Unfortunately, intravenous amoxicillin-clavulanic acid is not available in the United States. A short course of intravenous ciprofloxacin 200 mg/12 hr during 2 days followed by oral ciprofloxacin (500 mg/12 hr for 5 days) is also an effective treatment of SBP. Patients with uncomplicated SBP (i.e., those without shock, ileus, gastrointestinal hemorrhage, or hepatic encephalopathy) can be safely treated with oral ofloxacin (400 mg/12 hr). However, oral or intravenous quinolones should not be used as empiric treatment of patients on quinolone prophylaxis with suspected bacterial infection. These patients develop infections caused by gram-negative cocci or quinolone-resistant gram-negative bacilli. Empiric cefotaxime or amoxicillin-clavulanic acid is also effective in such patients. One recent study has shown that intravenous albumin administration, at a dose of 1.5 g/kg at the time of diagnosis of SBP and 1 g/kg on day 3 of treatment, reduces the incidence of renal impairment and death. Albumin should be considered, especially in patients with SBP and blood urea nitrogen (BUN) greater than 30 mg/dL and/or serum bilirubin greater than 4 mg/dL (Fig. 30-1).

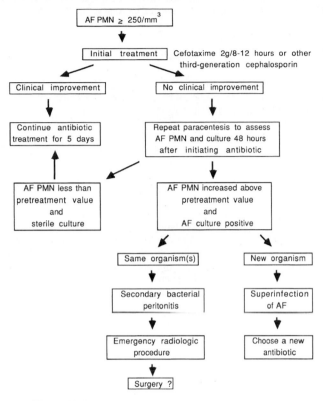

**Figure 30-1.** Management of spontaneous bacterial peritonitis.

## 16. When should antibiotic treatment be started in a patient with cirrhosis and suspected ascitic fluid infection?

Empirical antibiotic treatment must be started as soon as possible to improve survival rates. Therefore, it is important to perform routine bacterial cultures of ascitic fluid, blood, urine, and sputum as well as an ascitic fluid cell count and differential when a hospitalized patient with ascites develops clinical signs of possible infection (fever, abdominal pain, encephalopathy) or shows deterioration in clinical or laboratory parameters. In addition, ascitic fluid and urine should be analyzed when patients with cirrhosis and ascites are admitted to the hospital; about 20% are infected at this time. A high level of suspicion for bacterial infection is appropriate, because it is a reversible cause of deterioration and a frequent cause of death in patients with cirrhosis. Empirical antibiotics should be started immediately after performing cultures and ascitic fluid analysis whenever

- Bacterial infection is suspected based on abdominal pain or fever
- Ascitic fluid neutrophils are 250 cells/mm³ or higher

See Figure 30-1.

## 17. Should the PMN cell count in ascitic fluid be monitored during treatment of SBP?

Ascitic fluid culture becomes negative after a single 2 g dose of cefotaxime in 86% of patients with SBP. The neutrophil count also decreases rapidly to normal values during therapy in 90%. Superinfection or early recurrence after treatment with third-generation cephalosporins is uncommon. Repeat paracentesis is not necessary, if the setting (advanced cirrhosis) is typical, one organism is cultured, and the patient has the usual dramatic response to treatment. However, 2 or 3 days after starting antibiotic treatment, repeat paracentesis can be considered to confirm the decrease in PMNs in the fluid and sterility of the fluid.

## 18. Does bacterascites represent a real peritoneal infection? Should it be treated?

Studies have documented the short-term natural history of monomicrobial nonneutrocytic bacterascites. A repeat paracentesis of patients with bacterascites before starting antibiotic therapy showed that in 62% to 86%, the episode of bacterascites resolved spontaneously. Of interest, all patients who progressed to SBP had symptoms of bacterial infection at the time of the first tap. Such data demonstrate that bacterascites is a dynamic process; its evolution may depend on several factors, including systemic and ascitic fluid defenses as well as organism virulence. According to these studies, symptomatic patients with bacterascites should be treated with antibiotics. Asymptomatic patients need not receive antibiotic treatment but should be reevaluated with a second tap. If the PMN count is 250/mm$^3$ or greater, antibiotics should be started.

**19. What does the presence of bacterial DNA in blood and ascitic fluid represent in cirrhotic patients?**

New molecular biologic techniques have demonstrated the presence of bacterial DNA in blood and ascitic fluid in both patients and rats with cirrhosis and ascites. In approximately 30% of patients with cirrhosis and ascites, bacterial DNA can be detected despite a negative culture and normal PMN count in ascitic fluid. The presence of bacterial DNA represents episodes of bacterial translocation, as has been demonstrated in rats with cirrhosis. These patients have a systemic cytokine response similar to those observed in patients with SBP and its presence has been related to a poor survival. More information is required to recommend if these patients require antibiotic treatment or prophylaxis.

**20. Which subgroups of patients with liver disease should receive treatment to prevent bacterial infection?**

Because enteric aerobic gram-negative bacteria are the most frequent causative agents isolated in bacterial infections in cirrhosis and because bacterial translocation seems to be an important step in pathogenesis, inhibition of intestinal gram-negative bacteria should be an effective method of preventing bacterial infections. Patients with liver disease who are at high risk of developing bacterial infection and/or SBP should be considered for selective intestinal decontamination (SID). SID consists of the inhibition of the gram-negative flora of the gut with preservation of gram-positive cocci and anaerobic bacteria. Preservation of the anaerobes is important in preventing intestinal colonization, overgrowth, and subsequent translocation of pathogenic bacteria. Several trials have shown that SID with oral norfloxacin is highly effective in preventing bacterial infections and/or SBP in inpatients with cirrhosis and:

- Gastrointestinal hemorrhage (400 mg twice daily) or
- Low ascitic fluid protein (400 mg/day) and
- In patients with fulminant hepatic failure (400 mg/day)

Long-term antibiotic therapy has been used in preventing the first episode of SBP as well as recurrences. Long-term prophylactic treatment decreases the incidence of SBP in both conditions, but increases the appearance of quinolone-resistant bacteria and infections. Secondary prophylaxis is generally well accepted, especially in patients awaiting liver transplantation. Long-term primary prophylaxis has been evaluated in patients with advanced liver disease, such as those with low ascitic fluid total protein (less than 1.5 g/dL) and high serum bilirubin (greater than 3 mg/dL) or low platelet count (less than 98,000 cells/mm$^3$), hyponatremia (less than 130 mEq/L) or impaired renal function (serum creatinine level 1.2 mg/dL or greater, blood urea nitrogen level 25 mg/dL or greater). Primary prophylaxis with norfloxacin had a great impact in the clinical course of these patients, since it reduced the incidence of spontaneous bacterial peritonitis, the development of hepatorenal syndrome, and improved survival.

**21. Are there alternative prophylactic treatments to quinolones for preventing bacterial infections in cirrhosis?**

Prophylaxis with oral quinolones or trimethoprim-sulfamethoxazole promotes infections caused by quinolone-resistant gram-negative bacilli; this reduces the efficacy of the preventive treatment, especially in patients submitted to long-term prophylaxis. Therefore, it is very important to evaluate nonantibiotic drugs for preventing bacterial infections in cirrhosis. Several experimental studies in cirrhotic rats have demonstrated the efficacy of short-term prevention of bacterial translocation and SBP with different drugs, such as β-blockers, prokinetics, probiotics, antioxidants, and bile salts. Unfortunately, no clinical trials have been published demonstrating any effect of these drugs in patients with cirrhosis. A recent multicenter study has demonstrated that parenteral ceftriaxone (1 g/day for 7 days) is more effective than oral norfloxacin (400 mg twice daily) in preventing bacterial infections in patients with cirrhosis admitted to the hospital with gastrointestinal hemorrhage and severe liver disease. Parenteral ceftriaxone is an excellent alternative to oral norfloxacin but with a higher cost.

**22. What is the treatment of spontaneous bacterial empyema?**

Microbiological studies of pleural fluid have shown that gram-negative bacteria are present in almost 50% of patients with spontaneous bacterial empyema, the others being culture negative. Therefore, patients with spontaneous bacterial empyema should be treated with broad-spectrum antibiotics as in patients with SBP. Chest tube is not necessary and should be avoided. Patients surviving a spontaneous bacterial empyema should be evaluated for liver transplantation.

**23. Why is it important to know the sodium balance in patients with cirrhosis and ascites?**

Ascites formation in cirrhosis is due to renal retention of sodium and water. The aim of medical treatment of ascites in patients with cirrhosis is to mobilize the ascitic fluid by creating a net negative balance of sodium. This goal is accomplished by reducing sodium intake in the diet and increasing urinary sodium excretion. Therefore, knowledge of urinary excretion of sodium allows the clinician to plan initial treatment. In addition, urinary sodium excretion is an easily determined prognostic indicator. Patients with cirrhosis and a urinary sodium excretion less than 10 mEq/day have a 2-year survival rate of 20%, whereas those with sodium excretion greater than 10 mEq/day have a 2-year survival rate of 60%.

**24. Describe the initial treatment of patients with cirrhosis and ascites.**

Patients with cirrhosis and ascites should be treated initially by dietary sodium restriction (50 to 88 mEq/day) and diuretics. A more severe restriction of sodium intake may worsen anorexia and malnutrition. Water restriction is usually not necessary, if serum sodium concentration is greater than 120 mEq/L. In 15% to 20% of patients, a negative sodium balance may be obtained with dietary sodium restriction in the absence of diuretics. However, because 80% to 85% of patients need diuretics, it is reasonable to start diuretics in all patients. The initial dose of diuretics should be 100 mg of spironolactone and 40 mg of furosemide—both drugs are given orally in a single morning dose. If the body weight does not decrease or the urinary sodium excretion does not increase after 2 to 3 days of treatment, the dose of both diuretics should be progressively increased, usually in simultaneous increments of 100 mg/day and 40 mg/day, respectively. Serial monitoring of urinary sodium excretion and daily weight is the best way to determine the optimal dose of diuretics. Doses should be increased until a negative sodium balance is obtained (i.e., random or *spot* urinary sodium concentration >potassium concentration) with corresponding weight loss. The ceiling doses of spironolactone and furosemide are 400 mg and 160 mg per day, respectively. Once ascites has been mobilized, diuretic dosage should be adjusted individually to keep the patient free of ascites. Patients with tense ascites should be treated initially with a therapeutic paracentesis of 4 or more liters (Fig. 30-2).

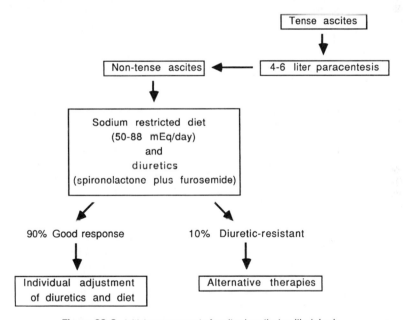

**Figure 30-2.** Initial management of ascites in patients with cirrhosis.

**25. What is refractory ascites?**

Refractory ascites is an inadequate response to sodium-restricted diet (less than 90 mmol/day) and high-dose diuretic treatment (400 mg/day spironolactone and 160 mg/day furosemide). This inadequate response is manifested by the absence of weight loss (less than 0.8 kg over 4 days) or the development of complications of diuretics, such as hepatic encephalopathy, renal impairment, hyponatremia, or hypokalemia or hyperkalemia. Excessive sodium intake, bacterial infection, occult gastrointestinal hemorrhage, and intake of prostaglandin inhibitors (e.g., aspirin or nonsteroidal anti-inflammatory drugs) should be excluded before labeling patients as refractory. Early ascites recurrence (within 4 weeks after initial mobilization) is considered also refractory ascites. Less than 10% of patients with cirrhosis are refractory to standard medical therapy. This small group should be evaluated for other therapeutic options, such as liver transplantation, chronic outpatient paracentesis (usually every 2 weeks), peritoneovenous shunt, or transjugular intrahepatic portosystemic stent-shunt (TIPS).

## 26. Which patients should be treated with large-volume paracentesis?

Large-volume paracentesis is an old but safe and effective procedure to mobilize ascitic fluid in cirrhotic patients. Interest in this procedure has been renewed in the past decade. Recently, it has been shown that therapeutic paracentesis not only is safe but also may have additional beneficial effects on the hemodynamic status of patients with tense ascites. However, repeated large-volume paracenteses cause depletion of proteins and, theoretically, may predispose to SBP. Therefore, therapeutic paracentesis should not be used as a routine treatment of all patients with cirrhosis and ascites and should be reserved for treating patients with tense and/or refractory ascites.

## 27. Should volume expanders be infused after large-volume paracentesis?

Plasma volume expansion after large-volume paracentesis is controversial. Volume expanders were introduced to avoid theoretical hemodynamic disturbances that may develop in patients with cirrhosis after therapeutic paracentesis of 5 or more liters of ascitic fluid. One study reported that patients receiving albumin infusion after large-volume paracentesis had less hyponatremia and azotemia than patients who did not receive albumin. However, albumin infusion did not decrease symptomatic complications or hospital readmissions or increase survival rates. Because albumin infusion is expensive, less costly volume expanders have been tried. Paracentesis-induced circulatory dysfunction, defined as an increase in plasma renin activity of more than 50% of the preparacentesis value to a level of more than 4 ng/mL/hr, is observed with a higher incidence in patients with cirrhosis not submitted to volume expansion or treated with nonalbumin expanders after a large-volume paracentesis. A study has observed that patients developing paracentesis-induced circulatory dysfunction have a worse long-term prognosis. A recent study has demonstrated that the incidence of paracentesis-induced circulatory dysfunction is similar in patients treated with albumin or saline (170 mL of 3.5% saline solution per liter of ascites removed at 999 mL/hr) after total paracentesis, when less than 6 L of ascitic fluid was evacuated. The cost of saline infusion was 100-fold less expensive than albumin infusion. These data suggest that repeated paracentesis of less than 6 L does not require albumin infusion and can be safely substituted with saline infusion. However, infusion of saline may lead to the recurrent, rapid need for another large-volume paracentesis. At this time, albumin should be viewed in patients submitted to a large-volume paracentesis of 6 L or more as optional until it is demonstrated that volume expansion after therapeutic paracentesis has a beneficial effect on morbidity or survival. More recent data have observed that an early decrease in systemic vascular resistances after total paracentesis is due to an increase in arterial vasodilation that may be related to an abrupt decrease in intra-abdominal pressure after fast paracentesis. These data suggest that hemodynamic disturbances after total paracentesis could be prevented by reducing the flow rate of ascites extraction, making volume expansion unnecessary. Two recent pilot studies have evaluated the role of an oral vasoconstrictor (midodrine) in the prevention of paracentesis-induced circulatory dysfunction compared with albumin infusion with opposite results. More data are required.

## 28. Is there currently any indication for peritoneovenous shunt?

Peritoneovenous shunt was introduced for the treatment of patients with cirrhosis and refractory ascites in 1974 by LeVeen and associates. After initial enthusiasm, many complications were reported and the enthusiasm decreased progressively. The number of complications is especially high in patients with severe hepatocellular insufficiency. Obstruction of the shunt, especially at the venous end despite the collocation of a titanium tip, is the main complication and requires the implantment of a new shunt. In addition, peritoneovenous shunt does not reduce mortality during the initial hospitalization and does not improve long-term survival in cirrhotic patients. Therefore, peritoneovenous shunts should be only considered in patients with cirrhosis and refractory ascites who are not candidates for liver transplantation or TIPS and in whom large-volume paracentesis is difficult.

## 29. Which patients with cirrhosis and ascites should be considered for TIPS?

TIPS is an interventional radiologic technique that consists of creating a fistula between a hepatic vein and a portal vein and then placing an expandable metal stent in the balloon-dilated fistula to maintain patency. This technique was introduced to treat patients with recurrent variceal hemorrhage by decreasing portal pressure. Initial results show that TIPS could be useful in the treatment of cirrhotic patients with refractory ascites. However, the incidence of shunt dysfunction is still quite high. Two recent trials performed in patients with refractory ascites have demonstrated that TIPS plus medical therapy is superior to medical therapy (diuretics plus total paracentesis when required) alone for the control of ascites but does not improve survival, length of hospitalization, and quality of life. The incidence of hepatic encephalopathy was higher in the TIPS group, but other complications of cirrhosis such as variceal hemorrhage or acute renal failure were similar in the two groups. In one study, the cost of the TIPS group was significantly higher than in the medical therapy group. These data suggest that TIPS should be reserved as second-line therapy or a bridge to liver transplantation, especially in those patients with relatively preserved liver function. An additional concern regarding TIPS is the high incidence of TIPS dysfunction that requires frequent ultrasound evaluations and reinterventions. The recent introduction of polytetrafluoroethylene (PTFE)-covered stents improves shunt patency and reduces the incidence of TIPS dysfunction and episodes of encephalopathy.

## 30. Which patients with cirrhosis and ascites should be evaluated for liver transplantation?

Ascites is the most frequent complication of patients with cirrhosis and usually is associated with a poor liver function based on Child-Pugh or MELD score. The probability of survival after the first onset of ascites has been estimated at 50% and 20% after 1 and 5 years of follow-up, respectively. The prognosis is even worse in patients with diuretic-resistant ascites; the 1-year survival rate is 25%. Because the 1-year survival rate after liver transplantation is greater than 75%, patients with cirrhosis who develop ascites should be considered for liver transplantation. Once the fluid becomes diuretic resistant, consideration for transplantation becomes even more urgent. However, some alcoholic patients with diuretic-resistant ascites may become diuretic sensitive after months of alcohol abstinence.

### 31. What is the treatment of hepatic hydrothorax?

The initial treatment of hepatic hydrothorax is the same as ascites, salt restriction, diuretics and large-volume paracentesis, if the patient has ascites. Therapeutic thoracocentesis has a high incidence of complications in patients with cirrhosis (10% develop pneumothorax) and should be avoided, if it is not necessary to relieve pulmonary symptoms. Patients with recurrent or refractory hepatic hydrothorax should be carefully evaluated. Thoracotomy and pleurodesis is usually ineffective. Thoracotomy and surgical repair of the diaphragmatic defects could be performed by using a videothoracoscope and could be useful for selected patients. Use of TIPS is under evaluation and could be a good option for patients with refractory hepatic hydrothorax and Child-Pugh score less than 12 and MELD score less than 18.

### 32. What is dilutional hyponatremia in patients with cirrhosis?

Dilutional hyponatremia is a frequent complication of cirrhosis associated with a high morbidity and mortality and poor prognosis. One-year probability of survival after developing dilutional hyponatremia was 25.6% in a recent study. *Dilutional hyponatremia* is defined as a serum sodium lower than 130 mEq/L in the presence of an expanded extracellular fluid volume, as indicated by the presence of ascites and/or edema. It is mainly due to a severe water renal retention secondary to an increased nonosmotic secretion of vasopressin.

### 33. What is the treatment of dilutional hyponatremia?

Traditional treatment of dilutional hyponatremia is fluid restriction (1 to 1.5 L/day) and discontinuation of diuretics, if the patient has symptoms such as encephalopathy or hyponatremia is extremely severe (less than 125 mEq/L). Recent investigations have demonstrated that vasopressin $V_2$ receptor antagonists (vaptans) are effective in improving serum sodium in the short and long term in patients with cirrhosis and hyponatremia despite diuretic treatment. Current ongoing studies are designed to evaluate if vaptans are also useful for the treatment of ascites and to reduce the frequency of paracentesis in patients with cirrhosis and refractory ascites.

### 34. What is the hepatorenal syndrome?

The hepatorenal syndrome occurs in patients with advanced liver failure and portal hypertension. It is a functional renal failure caused by intrarenal vasoconstriction due to arterial vasodilatation in the splanchnic circulation and severe reflex activation of the endogenous vasoconstrictive systems. According to clinical outcome, hepatorenal syndrome can be divided into two types:

- *Type I* is characterized by a rapid and progressive reduction of renal function defined by a doubling of the initial serum creatinine to a level greater than 2.5 mg/dL or a 50% reduction in the initial 24-hour creatinine clearance to a level less than 20 mL/min in less than 2 weeks. Clinical presentation is acute renal failure.
- In *type II*, renal failure does not have such a rapidly progressive course. These patients develop a clinical picture of refractory ascites.

### 35. What are the criteria of hepatorenal syndrome?

A recent meeting of the International Ascites Club has modified slightly the diagnostic criteria of hepatorenal syndrome:

1. Cirrhosis with ascites
2. Serum creatinine greater than 133 μmol/L (1.5 mg/dL).
3. No improvement in serum creatinine (decrease to a level of 133 μmol/L) after at least 2 days with diuretic withdrawal and volume expansion with albumin. The recommended dosage of albumin is 1 g/kg of body weight per day up to a maximum of 100 g/day.
4. Absence of shock
5. No current or recent treatment with nephrotoxic drugs
6. Absence of parenchymal kidney disease as indicated by proteinuria greater than 500 mg/day, microhematuria (greater than 50 red blood cells per high-power field), and/or abnormal renal ultrasonogram

### 36. Describe the treatment of patients with hepatorenal syndrome.

Liver transplantation is currently the treatment of choice in patients with hepatorenal syndrome. Unfortunately, patients with hepatorenal syndrome type I usually die before an organ is available. The mortality rate of untreated patients with hepatorenal syndrome type I is almost 100% in less than 2 months. Treatments such as hemodialysis, peritoneovenous shunt, albumin infusion, and dopamine infusion have been evaluated and found to be of only transient benefit or without benefit. Recent prospective but uncontrolled studies have shown that hepatorenal syndrome can be reversed by the administration of vasoconstrictive drugs, such as octreotide and midodrine, ornipressin, terlipressin, or norepinephrine, with albumin infusion or other volume expanders. Two recent randomized controlled trials have demonstrated that terlipressin associated with albumin infusion is an effective treatment in patients with hepatorenal syndrome type 1, improving renal function. However, probability of survival was not significantly increased in terlipressin group, but a beneficial effect on survival was observed in those patients responding to the therapy. These agents allow some patients to survive long enough to undergo liver transplantation. Therefore, terlipressin plus albumin should be considered for the management of patients with cirrhosis and hepatorenal syndrome type 1, particularly in patients who are candidates for liver transplantation. Terlipressin is administered as an intravenous bolus of 1 mg every 4 hours and increased to 2 mg every 4 hours after 3 days of treatment if a significant decrease in serum creatinine is not observed (at least 25% reduction). However, terlipressin is not available in the United States. In the United States, (1) octreotide and midodrine or (2) norepinephrine (if the patient is in intensive care and not taking oral medications) are options for treatment of hepatorenal syndrome. Octreotide is best given as a continuous infusion of 50 μg/hr but can be given subcutaneously starting with a dose of 100 μg followed in 8 hours by 200 μg, then 200 μg every 8 hours. Midodrine is given orally with a 7.5-mg dose followed in 8 hours by a 10-mg dose, then in 8 hours 12.5 mg, then 12.5 mg every 8 hours. The goal is to increase mean arterial blood pressure 15 mm Hg. Although the original publication did not include the use of greater than 12.5 mg, 15 mg every 8 hours can be used as needed. If systolic blood pressure rises above 140 mm Hg, the dose can be reduced. However, hypertension on this treatment is so rare that it calls into question the diagnosis of hepatorenal syndrome. Usually the systolic blood pressure is in the 70 to 80 mm Hg range in the setting of hepatorenal syndrome. Norepinephrine is administered by continuous infusion at an initial dosage of 0.1 μg/kg/min and increased every 4 hours by 0.05 μg/kg/min if mean arterial pressure does not increase at least 10 mm Hg. TIPS insertion seems to be another option for the temporary treatment of hepatorenal syndrome, especially in those patients with preserved liver function. More data are required.

### 37. Is it possible to prevent hepatorenal syndrome?

Short-term mortality of patients with hepatorenal syndrome type 1 is almost 100% in the following 2 months. A high proportion of episodes of type 1 hepatorenal syndrome have a precipitating factor. Therefore, prevention of this factor is probably the best treatment of type 1 hepatorenal syndrome. In one study, albumin infusion (1.5 g/kg body weight on the first day plus 1 g/kg body weight on the third day) decreased the incidence of hepatorenal syndrome type 1 from 33% to 10% and increased survival. This beneficial effect was especially observed in those patients with serum bilirubin higher than 4 mg/dL and serum creatinine higher than 1 mg/dL. Therefore, albumin infusion could be restricted to these patients. As commented, long-term primary prophylaxis of SBP with norfloxacin in cirrhotic patients with advanced liver disease decreased the 1-year probability of developing an hepatorenal syndrome from 41% to 28% and increased 1-year survival from 48% to 60%. More studies are required to evaluate groups at high risk of developing hepatorenal syndrome and its prevention.

## WEBSITE

http://www.aasld.org/

### BIBLIOGRAPHY

1. Alessandria C, Ottobrelli A, Debernardi-Venon W, et al. Noradrenalin vs terlipressin in patients with hepatorenal syndrome: A prospective, randomized, unblinded, pilot study. J Hepatol 2007;47:499–505.
2. Bureau C, Garcia-Pagan JC, Otal P, et al. Improved clinical outcome using polytetrafluoroethylene-coated stents for TIPS: Results of a randomized study. Gastroenterology 2004;126:469–75.
3. Castellote J, Lopez C, Gornals J, et al. Rapid diagnosis of spontaneous bacterial peritonitis by use of reagent strips. Hepatology 2003;37:893–6.
4. Chiva M, Guarner C, Peralta C, et al. Intestinal oxidative mucosal damage and bacterial translocation in cirrhotic rats. Eur J Gastroenterol Hepatol 2003;15:145–59.
5. Colla S, Vilaa MC, Molina L, et al. Mechanisms of early decrease in systemic vascular resistance after total paracentesis: Influence of flow rate of ascites extraction. Eur J Gastroenterol Hepatol 2004;16:347–53.
6. Duvoux C, Zanditenas D, Hezode C, et al. Effects of noradrenalin and albumin in patients with type I hepatorenal syndrome: A pilot study. Hepatology 2002;36:374–80.
7. Esrailian E, Pantangco ER, Kyulo NL, et al. Octreotide/midodrine therapy significantly improves renal function and 30-day survival in patients with type 1 hepatorenal syndrome. Dig Dis Sci 2007;52:742–8.
8. Evans LT, Kim WR, Poterucha JJ, et al. Spontaneous bacterial peritonitis in asymptomatic outpatients with cirrhotic ascites. Hepatology 2003;37:897–901.
9. Fernández J, Navasa M, Planas R, et al. Primary prophylaxis of spontaneous bacterial peritonitis delays hepatorenal syndrome and improves survival in cirrhosis. Gastroenterology 2007;133:818–24.
10. Fernández J, Ruiz del Arbol L, Gómez C, et al. Norfloxacin versus ceftriaxone in the prevention of bacterial infections in patients with advanced cirrhosis and hemorrhage. Gastroenterology 2006;131:1049–56.
11. Francés R, Benlloch S, Zapater P, et al. A sequential study of serum bacterial DNA in patients with advanced cirrhosis and ascites. Hepatology 2004;39:484–91.

12. Francés R, Zapater P, González-Navajas JM, et al. Bacterial DNA in patients with cirrhosis and non-infected ascites mimics the soluble immune response established in patients with spontaneous bacterial peritonitis. Hepatology 2008;47:978–85.
13. Gines P, Uriz J, Calahorra B, et al. Transjugular intrahepatic portosystemic shunting versus paracentesis plus albumin for refractory ascites in cirrhosis. Gastroenterology 2002;123:1834–47.
14. Gines P, Wong F, Watson H, et al. Effects of satavaptan, a selective vasopressin V2 receptor antagonist, on ascites and serum sodium in cirrhosis with hyponatremia: A randomized trial. Hepatology 2008;47:1–10.
15. Guarner C, González-Navajas JM, Sánchez E, et al. The detection of bacterial DNA in blood of rats with CCl4-induced cirrhosis represents episodes of bacterial translocation. Hepatology 2006;44:633–9.
16. Guarner C, Solá R, Soriano G, et al. Risk of a first community-acquired spontaneous bacterial peritonitis in cirrhotics with low ascitic fluid protein levels. Gastroenterology 1999;117:414–9.
17. Martín-Llahi M, Pépin MN, Guevara M, et al. Terlipressin and albumin vs albumin in patients with cirrhosis and hepatorenal syndrome: A randomized study. Gastroenterology 2008;134:1352–9.
18. Moore KP, Wong F, Gines P, et al. The management of ascites in cirrhosis: Report on the Consensus Conference of the International Ascites Club. Hepatology 2003;38:258–66.
19. Moreau R, Durand F, Poynard T, et al. Terlipressin in patients with cirrhosis and type I hepatorenal syndrome: A retrospective multicenter study. Gastroenterology 2002;123:923–30.
20. Nousbaum JB, Cadranel JF, Nahon P, et al. Diagnostic accuracy of the Multistix 8 SG reagent strip in diagnosis of spontaneous bacterial peritonitis. Hepatology 2007;45:1275–81.
21. Ortega R, Gines P, Uriz J, et al. Terlipressin therapy with and without albumin for patients with hepatorenal syndrome: Results of a prospective, nonrandomized study. Hepatology 2002;36:941–54.
22. Ortiz J, Soriano G, Coll P, et al. Early microbiologic diagnosis of spontaneous bacterial peritonitis with BacT/ALERT. J Hepatol 1997;26:839–44.
23. Planas R, Montoliu S, Balleste B, et al. Natural history of patients hospitalized for the management of cirrhotic ascites. Clin Gastroenterol Hepatol 2006;4:1385–94.
24. Ricart E, Soriano G, Novella MT, et al. Amoxicillin-clavulanic acid versus cefotaxime in the therapy of bacterial infections in cirrhotic patients. J Hepatol 2000;32:596–602.
25. Rimola A, Garcia-Tsao G, Navasa M, et al., International Ascites Club. Diagnosis, treatment and prophylaxis of spontaneous bacterial peritonitis: A consensus document. J Hepatol 2000;32:142–53.
26. Rossle M, Ochs A, Gulberg V, et al. A comparison of paracentesis and transjugular intrahepatic portosystemic shunting in patients with ascites. N Engl J Med 2000;342:1701–7.
27. Runyon BA, Canawati HN, Akriviadis EA. Optimization of ascitic fluid culture technique. Gastroenterology 1988;95:1351–5.
28. Runyon BA. Low-protein-concentration ascitic fluid is predisposed to spontaneous bacterial peritonitis. Gastroenterology 1986;191:1343–6.
29. Runyon BA. Management of adult patients with ascites caused by cirrhosis. Hepatology 1998;27:264–72.
30. Runyon BA, Montano AA, Akriviadis EA, et al. The serum-ascites albumin gradient is superior to the exudate-transudate concept in the differential diagnosis of ascites. Ann Intern Med 1992;117:215–20.
31. Sakai H, Sheer TA, Mendler M, et al. Choosing the location for non-image guided abdominal paracentesis. Liver Int 2005;25:984–6.
32. Salerno F, Corboc A, Ginés P, et al. Diagnosis, prevention and treatment of hepatorenal syndrome in cirrhosis. Gut 2007;56:1310–6.
33. Sanyal AJ, Boyer T, Garcia-Tsao G, et al. A randomized, prospective, double-blind, placebo-controlled trial of terlipressin for type 1 hepatorenal syndrome. Gastroenterology 2008;134:1360–8.
34. Sanyal AJ, Genning Ch, Reddy KR, et al. The North American Study for the Treatment of Refractory Ascites. Gastroenterology 2003;124:634–41.
35. Sola-Vera J, Miñana J, Ricart E, et al. Randomized trial comparing albumin and saline in the prevention of paracentesis-induced circulatory dysfunction in cirrhotic patients with ascites. Hepatology 2003;37:1147–53.
36. Such J, Runyon BA. Spontaneous bacterial peritonitis. Clin Infect Dis 1998;27:669–704.
37. Terg R, Cobas S, Fassio E, et al. Oral ciprofloxacin after a short course of intravenous ciprofloxacin in the treatment of spontaneous bacterial peritonitis: Results of a multicenter, randomized study. J Hepatol 2000;33:564–9.
38. Wu S, Lin OS, Chen Y, et al. Ascitic fluid carcinoembryonic antigen and alkaline phosphatase levels for the differentiation of primary from secondary bacterial peritonitis with intestinal perforation. J Hepatol 2001;34:215–21.
39. Xiol X, Guardiola J. Hepatic hydrothorax. Curr Opin Pulm Med 1998;4:239–42.

# LIVER ABSCESS

*Jorge L. Herrera, MD*

### 1. What are the two major categories of liver abscess?

The two types of liver abscess are pyogenic and amebic. Pyogenic abscesses usually arise from intra-abdominal infections, whereas amebic abscesses arise from colonic infection with invasive *Entamoeba histolytica*. This differentiation is important because diagnostic approach and management differ for the two conditions.

### 2. Describe the clinical features of pyogenic liver abscess.

Most patients are middle-aged or older, with a recent shift in age toward younger patients. The median age is 51 years. The condition is equally prevalent in both sexes. The clinical findings are nonspecific but may include fever, chills, right-upper-quadrant pain, malaise, and weight loss. Fever may be absent in up to 30% of cases. Abdominal pain is present in only 45% of cases. Only 37% present with the classic findings of fever and right-upper-quadrant tenderness, reinforcing the often nonspecific nature of signs and symptoms. In many patients, the clinical presentation may be dominated by the underlying cause, such as appendicitis, diverticulitis, or biliary disease.

Comorbidities are common, including diabetes mellitus, malignancy, alcoholism, cardiovascular disease, and chronic renal failure. The mean duration of symptoms before hospital admission is 26 days, with a range of 1 to 200 days and a median of 14 days.

### 3. What are the clinical features of amebic liver abscess?

Patients tend to be younger (30 to 40 years), are more often male, have more severe right-upper-quadrant pain, and are febrile in 85% of cases. A history of travel to endemic areas is common, although it may be remote. Prior symptoms suggestive of previous colonic amebiasis are present in only 5% to 15% of patients. Concurrent hepatic abscess and amebic dysentery are unusual. Approximately 80% of patients present with symptoms that develop quickly over 2 to 4 weeks. Involvement of the diaphragmatic surface of the liver may lead to right-sided pleural pain or referred shoulder pain.

### 4. What laboratory features are distinctive in patients with liver abscess?

Results of routine laboratory tests are not diagnostic for pyogenic or amebic liver abscess. Leukocytosis is often present but may be absent in a significant number of patients. Normochromic normocytic anemia is present in more than 70% of patients. Eosinophilia is characteristically absent in patients with amebic abscess. The erythrocyte sedimentation rate is invariably raised. Liver test abnormalities are not specific. More than 90% of patients have elevation of alkaline phosphatase (AP), but aspartate aminotransferase (AST), and alanine aminotransferase (ALT) are elevated to lesser degrees. If significant hyperbilirubinemia is present, the biliary tree is the likely source of the abscess; bilirubin levels are lowest in patients with cryptogenic liver abscess. Hypoalbuminemia is frequently described, and a level less than 2 g/dL carries a poor prognosis. Blood cultures are positive in 50% of patients with pyogenic abscess, and 75% to 90% of aspirates from the abscesses are positive for bacteria.

### 5. What are the most common sources of pyogenic liver abscess?

Biliary tract disease is the most common known source of pyogenic liver abscess, accounting for 35% of cases. In most cases the cause cannot be identified, and the disease is therefore termed cryptogenic. Most abscesses related to biliary disease result from cholangitis or acute cholecystitis. Malignant tumors of the pancreas, common bile duct, and ampulla account for 10% to 20% of hepatic abscesses originating in the biliary tree. Endoscopic or surgical intervention in the biliary tree also may result in hepatic abscess formation. Parasitic invasion of the biliary tree by roundworms or flukes can lead to biliary infection and hepatic abscess.

Another common source of pyogenic liver abscesses is intra-abdominal infections with bacterial seeding through the portal vein. Diverticulitis, Crohn's disease, ulcerative colitis, and bowel perforation account for 30% of pyogenic liver abscesses. Appendicitis is a rare cause of liver abscess except in older or immunocompromised patients, in whom the diagnosis of appendicitis may be delayed. About 15% of liver abscesses arise by direct extension from a contiguous source, such as a subphrenic abscess or empyema of the gallbladder. Pyogenic infection may be carried to the liver in hepatic arterial blood flow from distant localized infections, such as endocarditis or severe dental disease.

**Table 31-1.** Bacteriology of Pyogenic Liver Abscess

| GRAM-NEGATIVE AEROBES (50% TO 70%) | GRAM-POSITIVE AEROBES (25%) | ANAEROBES (40% TO 50%) |
| --- | --- | --- |
| *Escherichia coli* (35% to 45%) | *Streptococcus faecalis* | *Fusobacterium nucleatum* |
| *Klebsiella* sp. | β Streptococci | *Bacteroides* sp. |
| *Proteus* sp. | α Streptococci | *Bacteroides fragilis* |
| *Enterobacter* sp. | Staphylococci | *Peptostreptococcus* sp. |
| *Serratia* sp. | *Streptococcus milleri* | *Actinomyces* sp. |
| *Morganella* sp. | *Clostridium* sp. | |
| *Actinobacter* sp. | | |
| *Pseudomonas* sp. | | |

Adapted from Frey CF, Zhu Y, Suzuki M, Isaji S: Liver abscess. Surg Clin North Am 69:259–271, 1989.

**6. List the organisms that commonly cause pyogenic liver abscess.**

Gram-negative organisms are implicated in 50% to 70% cases. *Escherichia coli* is the most common aerobic gram-negative organism cultured. Aerobic gram-positive organisms account for approximately 25% of infections, and up to 50% of cases are caused by anaerobes. Recent reports suggest that aerobes are becoming a more common cause of abscess than anaerobes (Table 31-1).

**7. Do negative cultures from an abscess aspirate indicate a nonpyogenic abscess?**

No. Although most cultures are positive, a negative culture may reflect improper handling of the specimen or prior antibiotic therapy. Proper collection and culture techniques are of critical importance for growing anaerobic organisms. Culture material should be transported to the laboratory immediately in the syringe used for aspiration to avoid exposure to air. Never submit swabs for culture of liver abscess. Anaerobic organisms may require at least several days and up to 1 week or more for sufficient growth to establish a diagnosis. For this reason, a Gram stain of the aspirate is of paramount importance. A Gram stain that demonstrates organisms with no growth in cultures after 2 or 3 days suggests an anaerobic pathogen. All aspirated material should be cultured for aerobic, anaerobic, and microaerophilic organisms.

**8. What abnormalities can be detected on standard radiologic studies of patients with liver abscess?**

A chest radiograph may be abnormal in 50% to 80% of patients with liver abscess. Right-lower-lobe atelectasis, right pleural effusion, and an elevated right hemidiaphragm may be clues to the presence of a liver abscess. Perforation of a pyogenic liver abscess into the thoracic cavity may result in empyema. In plain abdominal films, air can be seen in the abscess cavities in 10% to 20% of cases. Gastric displacement due to enlargement of the liver also may be seen. These features are not sensitive for the diagnosis of liver abscess.

**9. Which imaging studies should be obtained in evaluating a suspected liver abscess?**

Ultrasonography has traditionally been considered the initial procedure of choice. It is noninvasive, readily available, and highly accurate, with a sensitivity of 80% to 90%. It is the preferred modality to distinguish cystic from solid lesions and in most patients is more accurate than computed tomography (CT) scanning for visualizing the biliary tree. Ultrasonography, however, is operator dependent, and its accuracy may be affected by the patient's habitus or overlying gas. Currently, with the increasing availability of helical CT with intravenous contrast, some consider it the initial procedure of choice. It is not operator dependent, it is more sensitive than ultrasound, and it aids in the identification of smaller abscesses that may be missed on ultrasound examination. CT scanning provides an assessment not only of the liver but also of the entire peritoneal cavity, which may provide information about the primary lesions causing the liver abscess.

Magnetic resonance imaging (MRI) does not add much to the sensitivity of CT scanning. Scintigraphy with technetium sulfur colloid is sensitive for detecting lesions greater than 2 cm in diameter. Gallium scanning may add to the sensitivity of technetium scanning, because pyogenic liver abscess avidly takes up gallium. Amebic abscesses, however, tend to concentrate gallium only in the periphery of the abscess cavity. In general, scintigraphy is the least helpful of the scanning modalities.

**10. What areas of the liver are usually affected by hepatic abscess?**

| Right lobe only | 60% of patients |
| Both lobes | 20% to 30% |
| Left lobe only | 5% to 20% |

11. **How can the location, size, and number of liver abscesses help to determine the source?**
   - *Pyogenic liver abscesses* arising from a biliary source tend to be multiple and of small size and involve both lobes of the liver. Septic emboli from the portal vein may be solitary and tend to be more common in the right lobe of the liver because most of the portal vein flow goes to the right lobe. Abscesses arising from a contiguous source tend to be solitary and localized to one lobe only.
   - *Amebic liver abscesses* tend to be solitary and large. Most commonly, they are located in the right lobe of the liver. The right lobe receives a major part of the venous drainage from the cecum and ascending colon, which are the parts of the bowel most commonly affected by amebiasis. Abscesses located in the dome of the liver or complicated by a bronchopleural fistula are typically amebic in origin.

12. **When should a hepatic abscess be aspirated?**
   Hepatic abscesses should be aspirated if they are thought to be pyogenic and not amebic. Patients with multiple abscesses, coexistent biliary disease, or an intra-abdominal inflammatory process are more likely to have pyogenic abscess. In such patients, aspiration under ultrasound guidance with Gram stain and culture helps to guide antibiotic selection. Aspiration of amebic abscesses should be considered under the following circumstances:

   - When pyogenic abscess or secondary infection of an amebic abscess cannot be excluded
   - When the patient does not respond to adequate therapy for amebic liver abscess
   - When the abscess is very large with risk of rupture and/or causes severe pain

13. **In what situation should an amebic liver abscess be treated by open surgical drainage?**
   When the amebic abscess is located in the left lobe of the liver and response to therapy is not dramatic within the first 24 to 48 hours, open surgical drainage should be performed. Complications of left-lobe amebic abscess, such as cardiac tamponade, are associated with high mortality and require prompt intervention to prevent their occurrence.

14. **Does aspiration of an amebic hepatic abscess yield diagnostic material in most patients?**
   No. Trophozoites are found in less than 20% of aspirates. Although classically the contents of amebic abscess are described as *anchovy paste* in appearance, in practice most aspirated material does not conform to this description. The contents of an amebic abscess are typically odorless. Foul-smelling aspirates or a positive Gram stain should suggest a pyogenic abscess or secondarily infected amebic abscess.

15. **How often is the biliary tree involved in patients with amebic liver abscess?**
   Bile is lethal to amebas; thus, infection of the gallbladder and bile ducts does not occur. In patients with a large amebic or pyogenic abscess, compression of the biliary system may result in jaundice, but cholangitis occurs only with secondary bacterial infection.

16. **How can the diagnosis of an amebic abscess be confirmed?**
   Amebic abscesses are best differentiated from pyogenic abscesses by serologic tests:

   | | |
   |---|---|
   | Hemagglutination (IHA) | Gel diffusion precipitin (GDP) |
   | Indirect immunofluorescence (IF) | Complement fixation (CF) |
   | Counterimmunoelectrophoresis (CIE) | Latex agglutination (LA) |
   | Immunoelectrophoresis (IEP) | Enzyme-linked immunosorbent assay (ELISA) |

   Serologic tests are positive only in patients with invasive amebiasis, such as hepatic abscess or amebic colitis. They are negative in asymptomatic carriers. With the exception of CF, these tests are highly sensitive (95% to 99%). The IHA is extremely sensitive, and a negative test excludes the diagnosis; a titer greater than 1:512 is present in almost all patients with invasive disease. IHA, however, remains positive for many years, and a positive titer may indicate prior infection. GDP titers usually become negative 6 months after the infection, and this is the test of choice for patients from endemic areas with prior exposure to amebiasis. A high GDP titer in a patient with hepatic abscess suggests an amebic abscess, even if the patient has a prior history of invasive amebiasis. In general, the choice of serologic tests depends on availability and epidemiologic considerations.

17. **Describe the treatment for pyogenic liver abscess.**
   For single abscess or several large abscesses, treatment consists of antibiotics and appropriate drainage. Drainage should be performed percutaneously whenever possible. The combination of percutaneous drainage with intravenous antibiotics results in a 76% cure rate, compared with 65% for antibiotic alone and 61% for surgery alone.

It is not clear whether percutaneous catheter drainage is superior to aspiration without catheter placement. Most centers favor catheter drainage over simple aspiration. Surgical drainage should be performed only if more conservative measures do not result in complete resolution or if surgery is needed to treat a primary intraabdominal lesion. For multiple microabscesses, antibiotic therapy and correction of the underlying biliary abnormality may suffice.

Antibiotic coverage involves a combination of antibiotics directed against anaerobes, gram-negative aerobes, and enterococci. Thus, the combination of an aminoglycoside or cephalosporin for aerobic gram-negative organisms, clindamycin or metronidazole for anaerobes, and penicillin or ampicillin for enterococci is commonly used. The antibiotic regimen may be altered as needed, depending on culture results or clinical response. Intravenous treatment should be continued for 14 days or longer if drains are still in place with a minimum of 4 weeks of therapy.

### 18. Describe the treatment for amebic liver abscess.

Metronidazole is the only drug active against the extraintestinal form of amebiasis. A dosage of 750 mg 3 times/day for 10 days is recommended. Even at this dose, metronidazole is somewhat less effective in the intestinal form of the disease; thus, a luminal amebicide such as iodoquinol (diiodohydroxyquin), paromomycin, or diloxanide furoate should be prescribed to eradicate the intestinal form and prevent recurrence. Uncomplicated amebic abscess should be managed conservatively with metronidazole. Needle aspiration should be considered for large (greater than 7 cm) abscesses and for patients who fail to respond after 7 days of metronidazole. Operative intervention should be performed only for complications or when conservative therapy fails.

### 19. List the potential complications of pyogenic liver abscess.

Untreated, pyogenic liver abscesses have a mortality rate of 100%. Other complications include rupture into the peritoneal cavity, which may form subphrenic, perihepatic, or subhepatic abscess, or peritonitis. Rupture into the pleural space may cause empyema. Rupture into the pericardial sac may result in pericarditis and pericardial tamponade. Metastatic septic emboli involving the lungs, brain, or eyes also may occur.

### 20. List the potential complications of amebic liver abscess.

The complications of amebic liver abscess are similar to those of pyogenic liver abscess. Rupture into the pleural space results in amebic empyema. Rupture into the lung parenchyma may produce a lung abscess or bronchopleural fistula. Pericardial extension occurs in 1% to 2% of patients and is associated with amebic abscesses in the left lobe of the liver. A serous pericardial effusion may indicate impending rupture. Constrictive pericarditis occasionally follows suppurative amebic pericarditis. Brain abscess from hematogenous spread of the infection also has been reported.

### 21. What is the prognosis for patients with liver abscess?

The prognosis depends on the rapidity of diagnosis and the underlying illness. Patients with amebic liver abscess generally do well with appropriate treatment; morbidity and mortality rates are 4.5% and 2.2%, respectively, in recent series. Response to treatment is prompt and dramatic. Healing of the abscess leads to residual scar tissue associated with subcapsular retraction. Occasionally, in patients with large abscess, a residual cavity surrounded by fibroconnective tissue may persist.

The mortality rate associated with pyogenic liver abscess has been reduced to 5% to 10% with prompt recognition and adequate antibiotic therapy; it is highest in patients with multiple abscesses. Mortality is highly dependent on the underlying disease process. Morbidity remains high at 50%, primarily because of the complexity of therapy and the need for prolonged drainage.

### 22. Is a vaccine against amebiasis feasible?

Gal/GalNAc-specific lectin is a recombinant antigen that provides protection in animal models to amebiasis. Human immunity is linked to intestinal IgA against the lectin. The clonal population structure of *E. histolytica* and, specifically, the high degree of sequence conservation of the Gal/GalNAc-specific lectin suggests that a vaccine could be broadly protective.

## WEBSITE

http://ww.aasld.org/

## BIBLIOGRAPHY

1. Akgun Y, Tacyildiz IH, Celik Y. Amebic liver abscess: Changing trends over 20 years. World J Surg 1999;23:102–6.
2. Block MA. Abscesses of the liver (other than amebic). In: Haubrich WS, Schaffner F, Berk JE, editors. Bockus Gastroenterology. 5th ed. Philadelphia: WB Saunders; 1995. pp. 2405–27.
3. Chen W, Chen CH, Chiu KL, et al. Clinical outcome and prognostic factors of patients with pyogenic liver abscess requiring intensive care. Crit Care Med 2008;36:1184–8.
4. Chou FF, Sheen-chen SM, Chen YS, et al. Single and multiple pyogenic liver abscesses: Clinical course, etiology and results of treatment. World J Surg 1997;21:384–9.
5. Chung RT, Friedman LS. Liver abscess and bacterial, parasitic, fungal and granulomatous liver disease. In: Sleisenger MH, Fordtran JS, editors. Gastrointestinal Disease: Pathophysiology, Diagnosis, Management. 7th ed. Philadelphia: WB Saunders; 2002. pp. 1343–73.
6. Derici H, Tansug T, Reyhan E, et al. Acute intraperitoneal rupture of hydatid cysts. World J Surg 2006;30:1879–83.
7. Haque R, Huston CD, Hughes M, et al. Amebiasis. N Engl J Med 2003;348:1565–73.
8. Ferraioli G, Garlaschelli A, Zanaboni D, et al. Percutaneous and surgical treatment of pyogenic liver abscesses: Observation over a 21-year period in 148 patients. Dig Liver Dis 2008;40:697–8.
9. Lederman ER, Crum NF. Pyogenic liver abscess with a focus on *Klebsiella pneumoniae* as a primary pathogen: An emerging disease with unique clinical characteristics. Am J Gastroenterol 2005;100:322–31.
10. Monroe LS. Gastrointestinal parasites. In: Haubrich WS, Schaffner F, Berk JE, editors. Bockus Gastroenterology. 5th ed. Philadelphia: WB Saunders; 1995. pp. 3123–34.
11. Ng FH, Wong WM, Wong BC, et al. Sequential intravenous/oral antibiotic vs. Continuous intravenous antibiotic in the treatment of pyogenic liver abscess. Aliment Pharmacol Ther 2002;16:1083–90.
12. Rajak CL, Gupta S, Jain S, et al. Percutaneous treatment of liver abscesses: Needle aspiration versus catheter drainage. Am J Roentgenol AJR 1998;170:1035–9.
13. Seeto RK, Rockey DC. Pyogenic liver abscess: Changes in etiology, management and outcome. Medicine 1996;75:99–113.
14. Tan YM, Chung AY, Chow PK, et al. An appraisal of surgical and percutaneous drainage for pyogenic liver abscesses larger than 5 cm. Ann Surg 2005;241:485–90.

# INHERITABLE FORMS OF LIVER DISEASE

Bruce R. Bacon, MD

# CHAPTER 32

## HEMOCHROMATOSIS

**1. How do we classify the various iron-loading disorders in humans?**

The usual way to classify iron-overload syndromes is to distinguish between hereditary hemochromatosis (HH), secondary iron overload, and parenteral iron overload.

- *Hereditary hemochromatosis* results in increased iron absorption from the gut, with preferential deposition of iron in the parenchymal cells of the liver, heart, pancreas, and other endocrine glands. Most HH (about 85% to 90%) is found in patients who are homozygous for the C282Y mutation found in *HFE*, the gene for hemochromatosis. Over the past several years, however, mutations in other genes have been found that can lead to iron overload. These include mutations in transferrin receptor-2 (TfR2), ferroportin, hemojuvelin, and hepcidin.
- In *secondary iron overload*, some other stimulus causes the gastrointestinal tract to absorb increased amounts of iron. Here, the increased absorption of iron is caused by an underlying disorder rather than by an inherited defect in regulation of iron absorption. Examples include various anemias due to ineffective erythropoiesis (e.g., thalassemia, aplastic anemia, red cell aplasia, and some patients with sickle cell anemia), chronic liver disease, and, rarely, excessive intake of medicinal iron.
- In *parenteral iron overload*, patients have received excessive amounts of iron as either red blood cell transfusions or iron-dextran given parenterally. In patients with severe hypoplastic anemias, red blood cell transfusion may be necessary. Over time, patients become significantly iron loaded. Unfortunately, some physicians give iron-dextran injections to patients with anemia that is not due to iron deficiency; such patients can become iron loaded. Parenteral iron overload is always iatrogenic and should be avoided or minimized. In patients who truly need repeated red blood cell transfusions (in the absence of blood loss), a chelation program with deferoxamine should be initiated to prevent toxic accumulation of excessive iron.

**2. What are neonatal iron overload and African iron overload?**

- *Neonatal iron overload* is a rare condition that is probably related to an immune-mediated intra-uterine hepatic defect. Infants are born with modest increases in hepatic iron and many patients do very poorly; liver transplantation can be lifesaving.
- *African iron overload*, previously called Bantu hemosiderosis, was thought to be a disorder in which excessive amounts of iron were ingested from alcoholic beverages brewed in iron drums. Recent studies have suggested that this disorder does have a genetic component in that about 45% to 50% of patients have mutations in ferroportin. Thus, African Americans may be at risk for developing iron overload from an inherited disease.

**3. How much iron is usually absorbed per day?**

A typical Western diet contains approximately 10 to 20 mg of iron, which usually is found in heme-containing compounds. Normal daily iron absorption is approximately 1 to 2 mg, representing about a 10% efficiency of absorption. Patients with iron deficiency, HH, or ineffective erythropoiesis absorb increased amounts of iron (up to 3 to 6 mg/day).

**4. Where is iron normally found in the body?**

The normal adult male contains about 4 g of total body iron, which is roughly divided between the 2.5 g of iron in the hemoglobin of circulating red blood cells, 1 g of iron in storage sites in the reticuloendothelial system of the spleen and bone marrow and the parenchymal and reticuloendothelial system of the liver, and 200 to 400 mg in the myoglobin of skeletal muscle. In addition, all cells contain some iron because mitochondria contain iron both in heme, which is the central portion of cytochromes involved in electron transport, and in iron sulfur clusters, which also are involved in electron transport. Iron is bound to transferrin in both the intravascular and extravascular compartments. Storage iron within cells is found in ferritin and, as this amount increases, in hemosiderin. Serum ferritin is proportional to total body iron stores in patients with iron deficiency or uncomplicated HH and is biochemically different from tissue ferritin.

## 5. Discuss the genetic defect in patients with HH.

In 1996, the gene responsible for hemochromatosis was identified and named *HFE*. *HFE* codes for a major histocompatibility complex (MHC) type 1–like protein that is membrane spanning with a short intracytoplasmic tail, a transmembrane region, and three extracellular alpha loops. A single missense mutation results in loss of a cysteine at amino acid position 282 with replacement by a tyrosine (C282Y), which leads to disruption of a disulfide bridge and thus to the lack of a critical fold in the alpha$_1$ loop. As a result, *HFE* fails to interact with $\beta_2$-microglobulin ($\beta_2$M), which is necessary to the function of MHC class 1 proteins.

In 1997, it was demonstrated that the *HFE*/$\beta_2$M complex binds to transferrin receptor and is necessary for transferrin receptor–mediated iron uptake into cells. This observation linked *HFE* with a protein of iron metabolism. C282Y homozygosity is found in approximately 85% to 90% of patients with hemochromatosis. A second mutation, whereby a histidine at amino acid position 63 is replaced by an aspartate (H63D), is common but less important in cellular iron homeostasis. Recently, a third mutation has been characterized whereby a serine is replaced by a cysteine at amino acid position 65 (S65C). Like H63D, S65C has little impact on iron loading unless it is present as a compound heterozygote with the C282Y mutation. Additional recent discoveries show that hepcidin, a 25–amino acid peptide, is found to be deficient in patients with hemochromatosis and is considered the iron regulatory hormone. Thus, in patients with *HFE* mutations and in those with mutations in TfR2, hemojuvelin, and hepcidin, there is a deficiency of hepcidin production by the liver. Hepcidin in normal amounts interferes with the activity of ferroportin at the basolateral surface of the enterocyte preventing iron absorption. Thus, when there is hepcidin deficiency, there is an increase in iron absorption despite the fact that individuals are in fact iron loaded.

## 6. What are the usual toxic manifestations of iron overload?

In chronic iron overload, an increase in oxidant stress results in lipid peroxidation to lipid-containing components of the cell, such as organelle membranes. This process causes organelle damage. Hepatocellular injury and/or death ensues with phagocytosis by Kupffer cells. Iron-loaded Kupffer cells become activated, producing profibrogenic cytokines such as transforming growth factor $\beta_1$ (TGF-$\beta$1), which, in turn, activates hepatic stellate cells. Hepatic stellate cells are responsible for increased collagen synthesis and hepatic fibrogenesis.

## 7. What are the most common symptoms in patients with HH?

Currently, most patients are identified by abnormal iron studies on routine screening chemistry panels or by screening family members of a known patient. When identified in this manner, patients typically have no symptoms or physical findings. Nonetheless, it is useful to be aware of the symptoms that patients with more established HH can exhibit. Typically, they are nonspecific and include fatigue, malaise, and lethargy. Other more organ-specific symptoms are arthralgias and symptoms related to complications of chronic liver disease, diabetes, and congestive heart failure.

## 8. Describe the most common physical findings in patients with HH.

The way in which patients come to medical attention determines whether they have physical findings. Currently, most patients at diagnosis have no symptoms and no findings. Thus, patients identified by screening tests have no abnormal physical findings. In contrast, physical findings in patients with advanced disease may include grayish or "bronzed" skin pigmentation, typically in sun-exposed areas; hepatomegaly with or without cirrhosis; arthropathy with swelling and tenderness over the second and third metacarpophalangeal joints; and other findings related to complications of chronic liver disease.

## 9. How is the diagnosis of hemochromatosis established?

Patients with abnormal iron studies on screening blood work, any of the symptoms and physical findings of hemochromatosis, or a positive family history of hemochromatosis should have blood studies of iron metabolism either repeated or performed for the first time. These studies include serum iron, total iron-binding capacity (TIBC) or transferrin, and serum ferritin. The transferrin saturation (TS) should be calculated from the ratio of iron to TIBC or transferrin. If the TS is greater than 45% or if the serum ferritin is elevated, hemochromatosis should be strongly considered, especially in patients without evidence of other liver disease (e.g., chronic viral hepatitis, alcoholic liver disease, nonalcoholic steatohepatitis) known to have abnormal iron studies in the absence of significant iron overload.

If iron studies are abnormal, mutation analysis of *HFE* should be performed. If patients are homozygous for the C282Y mutation or compound heterozygotes (C282Y/H63D) and younger than the age of 40 years or in those with normal liver enzymes (alanine aminotransferase and aspartate aminotransferase) and a ferritin level less than 1000 ng/mL, no further evaluation is necessary. Plans for therapeutic phlebotomy can be initiated. In patients older than the age of 40 years or with abnormal liver enzymes or markedly elevated ferritin (greater than 1000 ng/mL), the next step is to perform a percutaneous liver biopsy to obtain tissue for routine histology, including Perls' Prussian blue staining for storage iron and biochemical determination of hepatic iron concentration (HIC). The main purpose for performing a liver biopsy in these individuals is to determine the degree of fibrosis since increased fibrosis has been associated with markedly elevated ferritin levels and elevated liver enzymes. Also, biochemical determination of HIC can be obtained and then from the HIC, the HII can be calculated. Calculation of the HII was more important in the past than it is now that we have genetic testing.

**10. How commonly do abnormal iron studies occur in other types of liver disease?**

In various studies, approximately 30% to 50% of patients with chronic viral hepatitis, alcoholic liver disease, and nonalcoholic steatohepatitis have abnormal serum iron studies. Usually, the serum ferritin is abnormal. In general, an elevation in transferrin saturation is much more specific for HH. Thus, if the serum ferritin is elevated and the transferrin saturation is normal, another form of liver disease may be responsible. In contrast, if the serum ferritin is normal and the transferrin saturation is elevated, the likely diagnosis is hemochromatosis, particularly in young patients. Differentiation of HH in the presence of other liver diseases is now much easier with the use of genetic testing (*HFE* mutation analysis for C282Y and H63D).

**11. Is computed tomography (CT) or magnetic resonance imaging (MRI) useful in diagnosing hemochromatosis?**

In massively iron-loaded patients, CT and MRI show the liver to be white or black, respectively, consistent with the kinds of changes associated with increased iron deposition. In more subtle and earlier cases, overlap is tremendous, and imaging studies are not useful. Thus, in heavily iron-loaded patients, the diagnosis is usually apparent without imaging tests, and in mild or subtler cases, they are unhelpful. CT or MRI is useful only in the patient who is likely to have severe iron overload but for whom a liver biopsy is either unsafe or refused. Again, this problem is less common with the advent of genetic testing.

**12. On liver biopsy, what is the typical cellular and lobular distribution of iron in HH?**

In early HH in young people, iron is found entirely in hepatocytes in a periportal (zone 1) distribution. In heavier iron loading in older patients, iron is still predominantly hepatocellular, but some iron may be found in Kupffer cells and bile ductular cells. The periportal-to-pericentral (zone 1–to–zone 3) gradient is maintained but may be less distinct in more heavily loaded patients. When patients develop cirrhosis, the pattern is typically micronodular, and regenerative nodules may show less intense iron staining.

**13. How useful is HIC?**

Since genetic testing has become readily available, liver biopsy and determinations of HIC and HII are less important. Nonetheless, whenever a liver biopsy is performed in a patient with suspected HH, the quantitative HIC should be obtained. In symptomatic patients, HIC is typically greater than 10,000 µg/g. The iron concentration threshold for the development of fibrosis is approximately 22,000 µg/g. Lower iron concentrations can be found in cirrhotic HH with a coexistent toxin, such as alcohol or hepatitis C or B virus. Young people with early HH may have only moderate increases in HIC. In the past, discrepancies in HIC concentration with age were clarified by use of the HII.

**14. How is the HII used in diagnosing HH?**

The HII, introduced in 1986, is based on the observation that HIC increases progressively with age in patients with homozygous HH. In contrast, in patients with secondary iron overload or in heterozygotes, there is no progressive increase in iron over time. Therefore, the HII was thought to distinguish patients with homozygous HH from patients with secondary iron overload and heterozygotes. The HII is calculated by dividing the HIC (in µmol/g) by the patient's age (in years). A value greater than 1.9 was thought to be consistent with homozygous HH. With the advent of genetic testing, we have learned that many C282Y homozygotes do not have phenotypic expression to the degree that would cause an elevated HII and they will not have increased iron stores. Thus, the HII is no longer the gold standard for the diagnosis of HH. The HII is not useful in patients with parenteral iron overload.

**15. How do you treat a patient with HH?**

Treatment of HH is relatively straightforward and includes weekly or twice-weekly phlebotomy of 1 unit of whole blood. Each unit of blood contains about 200 to 250 mg of iron, depending on the hemoglobin. Therefore, a patient who presents with symptomatic HH and who has up to 20 g of excessive storage iron requires removal of over 80 units of blood, which takes close to 2 years at a rate of 1 unit of blood per week. Patients need to be aware that this treatment can be tedious and prolonged. Some patients cannot tolerate removal of 1 unit of blood per week, and occasionally schedules are adjusted to remove only ½ unit every other week. In contrast, in young patients who are only mildly iron-loaded, iron stores may be depleted quickly with only 10 to 20 phlebotomies. The goal of initial phlebotomy treatment is to reduce tissue iron stores, not to create iron deficiency. Once the ferritin is less than 50 ng/ml and the transferrin saturation is less than 50%, the majority of excessive iron stores have been successfully depleted, and most patients can go into a maintenance phlebotomy regimen (1 unit of blood removed every 2 to 3 months).

**16. What kind of a response to treatment can you expect?**

Many patients feel better after phlebotomy therapy has begun, even if they were asymptomatic before treatment. Energy level may improve, with less fatigue and less abdominal pain. Liver enzymes typically improve once iron stores have been depleted. Increased hepatic size diminishes. Cardiac function may improve, and about 50% of patients with glucose intolerance are more easily managed. Unfortunately, advanced cirrhosis, arthropathy, and hypogonadism do not improve with phlebotomy.

## 17. What is the prognosis for a patient with hemochromatosis?

Patients who are diagnosed and treated before the development of cirrhosis can expect a normal life span. The most common causes of death in hemochromatosis are complications of chronic liver disease and hepatocellular cancer. Patients who are diagnosed and treated early should not experience any of these complications.

## 18. Because hemochromatosis is an inherited disorder, what is my responsibility to family members once a patient has been identified?

Once a patient has been fully identified, all first-degree relatives should be offered screening with genetic testing (*HFE* mutation analysis for C282Y and H63D) and tests for transferrin saturation and ferritin. If genetic testing shows that the relative is a C282Y homozygote or a compound heterozygote (C282Y/H63D) and has abnormal iron studies, HH is confirmed. A liver biopsy may not be necessary. HLA studies are no longer performed.

## 19. Should general population screening be done to evaluate for hemochromatosis?

With the advent of genetic testing, it was suggested that HH may be a good disease for population screening. This was because genetic testing was available, phenotypic expression was easy to determine, there was a long latent period between diagnosis and disease manifestations, and treatment is effective and safe. Several large-scale population studies have been performed and demonstrate that about half of C282Y homozygotes have evidence of phenotypic expression with increased iron stores. Thus, interest in population screening has waned since many people would be identified with a genetic disorder who do not go on to develop iron overload.

# $\alpha_1$-ANTITRYPSIN DEFICIENCY

## 20. What is the function of $\alpha_1$-AT in healthy people?

$\alpha_1$-Antitrypsin ($\alpha_1$-AT) is a protease inhibitor synthesized in the liver. It is responsible for inhibiting trypsin, collagenase, elastase, and proteases of polymorphonuclear neutrophils. In patients deficient in $\alpha_1$-AT, the function of these proteases is unopposed. In the lung, this can lead to a progressive decrease in elastin and development of premature emphysema. The liver fails to secrete $\alpha_1$-AT, and aggregates of the defective protein are found, leading by unclear means to the development of cirrhosis. More than 75 different protease inhibitor (Pi) alleles have been identified. Pi MM is normal, and Pi ZZ results in the lowest levels of $\alpha_1$-AT.

## 21. How common is $\alpha_1$-AT deficiency?

$\alpha_1$-AT deficiency occurs in approximately 1 in 2000 people.

## 22. Where is the abnormal gene located?

The gene is located on chromosome 14 and results in a single amino acid substitution (replacement of glutamic acid by lysine at the 342 position), which causes a deficiency in sialic acid.

## 23. What is the nature of the defect that causes $\alpha_1$-AT deficiency?

$\alpha_1$-AT deficiency is a protein-secretory defect. Normally this protein is translocated into the lumen of the endoplasmic reticulum, interacts with chaperone proteins, folds properly, is transported to the Golgi complex, and then is exported out of the cell. In patients with $\alpha_1$-AT deficiency, the protein structure is abnormal because of the deficiency of sialic acid, and the proper folding in the endoplasmic reticulum occurs for only 10% to 20% of the molecules, with resultant failure to export via the Golgi complex and accumulation within the hepatocyte. In one detailed Swedish study, $\alpha_1$-AT deficiency of the Pi ZZ type caused cirrhosis in only about 12% of patients. Chronic obstructive pulmonary disease (COPD) was present in 75% of patients, and of these, 59% were classified as having primary emphysema. It is not known why some patients with low levels of $\alpha_1$-AT develop liver or lung disease and others do not.

## 24. Describe the common symptoms and physical findings of $\alpha_1$-AT deficiency.

Adults with liver involvement may have no symptoms until they develop signs and symptoms of chronic liver disease. Similarly, children may have no specific problems until they develop complications from chronic liver disease. In adults with lung disease, typical findings include premature emphysema, which can be markedly exacerbated by smoking.

## 25. How is the diagnosis of $\alpha_1$-AT deficiency established?

It is useful to order $\alpha_1$-AT levels and phenotype in all patients evaluated for chronic liver disease because no clinical presentation suggests the diagnosis (apart from premature emphysema). Certain heterozygous states can result in chronic liver disease; for example, SZ as well as ZZ patients can develop cirrhosis. MZ heterozygotes usually do not develop disease unless they have some other liver condition, such as alcoholic liver disease or chronic viral hepatitis. There are, however, occasional patients who have significant liver disease and no other abnormalities are identified other than MZ heterozygosity. Liver disease due to other causes may progress more rapidly.

**26. What histopathologic stain is used to diagnose $\alpha_1$-AT deficiency?**

Periodic acid–Schiff (PAS)–diastase. PAS stains both glycogen and $\alpha_1$-AT globules a dark, reddish-purple, and diastase digests the glycogen. Thus, when a PAS-diastase stain is used, the glycogen has been removed by the diastase, and the only positively staining globules are those due to $\alpha_1$-AT. In cirrhosis, these globules characteristically occur at the periphery of the nodules and can be seen in multiple sizes within the hepatocyte. Immunohistochemical staining also can be used to detect $\alpha_1$-AT globules, and electron microscopy can show characteristic globules trapped in the Golgi apparatus.

**27. How is $\alpha_1$-AT deficiency treated?**

The only treatment for $\alpha_1$-AT–related liver disease is symptomatic management of complications and liver transplantation. With liver transplantation, the phenotype becomes that of the transplanted liver.

**28. What is the prognosis for patients with $\alpha_1$-AT deficiency? Should family screening be performed?**

The prognosis depends entirely on the severity of the underlying lung or liver disease. Typically, patients who have lung disease do not have liver disease, and those who have liver disease do not have lung disease, although in some patients both organs are severely involved. In patients with decompensated cirrhosis, the prognosis relates largely to the availability of organs for liver transplantation. Patients with transplants typically do fine. Family screening should be performed with $\alpha_1$-AT levels and phenotype. This screening is largely for prognostic information; definitive therapy for liver disease, other than liver transplantation, is not available.

## WILSON DISEASE

**29. How common is Wilson disease?**

Wilson disease has an estimated prevalence of 1 in 30,000 people.

**30. Where is the Wilson disease gene located?**

The abnormal gene responsible for Wilson disease, an autosomal recessive disorder, is located on chromosome 13 and recently has been cloned. The gene has homology for the Menkes disease gene, which also results in a disorder of copper metabolism. The Wilson disease gene (called *ATP7B*) codes for a P-type adenosine triphosphatase, which is a membrane-spanning copper-transport protein. The exact location of this protein within hepatocytes is not definite, but it most likely causes a defect in transfer of hepatocellular lysosomal copper into bile. This defect results in the gradual accumulation of tissue copper with subsequent hepatotoxicity. Unfortunately, there are over 60 mutations in the Wilson disease gene, and genetic testing has limited usefulness.

**31. What is the usual age of onset of Wilson disease?**

Wilson disease is characteristically a disease of adolescents and young adults. Clinical manifestations have not been seen before the age of 5 years. By 15 years of age, almost one-half of the patients have some clinical manifestations of the disease. Rare cases of Wilson disease have been identified in patients in their 40s or 50s.

**32. Which organ systems are involved in Wilson disease?**

The liver is uniformly involved. All patients with neurologic abnormalities due to Wilson disease have liver involvement. Wilson disease also can affect the eyes, kidneys, joints, and red blood cells. Thus, patients can have cirrhosis, neurologic deficits with tremor and choreic movements, ophthalmologic manifestations such as Kayser-Fleischer rings, psychiatric problems, nephrolithiasis, arthropathy, and hemolytic anemia.

**33. What are the different types of hepatic manifestations in Wilson disease?**

The typical patient who presents with symptoms from Wilson disease already has cirrhosis. However, patients can present with chronic hepatitis, and in all young people with chronic hepatitis a serum ceruloplasmin level should be performed as a screening test for Wilson disease. Rarely, patients present with fulminant hepatic failure, which is uniformly fatal without successful liver transplantation. Finally, patients can present early in the disease with hepatic steatosis. As with chronic hepatitis, young patients with fatty liver should be screened for Wilson disease.

**34. How is the diagnosis of Wilson disease established?**

Initial evaluation should include measurement of serum ceruloplasmin and, if abnormal, a 24-hour urinary copper level. About 85% to 90% of patients have depressed serum ceruloplasmin levels, but a normal level does not rule out the disorder. If the ceruloplasmin is decreased or the 24-hour urinary copper level is elevated, a liver biopsy should be performed for histologic interpretation and quantitative copper determination. Histologic changes include hepatic steatosis, chronic hepatitis, or cirrhosis. Histochemical staining for copper with rhodamine is not particularly sensitive. Usually, in established Wilson disease, hepatic copper concentrations are greater than 250 μg/g (dry weight) and can be as high as 3000 μg/g. Although elevated hepatic copper concentrations can occur in other cholestatic liver diseases, the clinical presentation allows an easy differentiation between Wilson disease and primary biliary cirrhosis, extrahepatic biliary obstruction, and intrahepatic cholestasis of childhood.

## 35. What forms of treatment are available for patients with Wilson disease?

The mainstay of treatment has been the copper-chelating drug D-penicillamine. Because D-penicillamine is frequently associated with side effects, trientine also has been used. Trientine is equally efficacious and probably has fewer side effects. Maintenance therapy with dietary zinc supplementation also has been used. Neurologic disorders can improve with therapy. Patients who present with complications of chronic liver disease or with fulminant hepatic failure should be quickly considered for orthotopic liver transplantation.

## 36. Is it necessary to perform family screening in Wilson disease?

Wilson disease is an autosomal recessive disorder, and all first-degree relatives of the patient should be screened. If the ceruloplasmin level is reduced, a 24-hour urinary copper level should be obtained, followed by a liver biopsy for histology and quantitative copper determination. Genetic testing can be valuable for family screening if genotyping has been done on the proband and is available to family members.

## 37. Compare Wilson disease and HH.

Both disorders involve abnormal metal metabolism and are inherited as autosomal recessive disorders. The mechanism of tissue damage is probably related to metal-induced oxidant stress for both disorders. In HH, the gene is on chromosome 6, whereas in Wilson disease the abnormal gene is on chromosome 13. HH occurs in approximately 1 in 250 people, but Wilson disease occurs in only about 1 in 30,000. The inherited defect in HH causes an increased absorption of iron by the intestine, with the liver a passive recipient of the excessive iron; in contrast, the inherited defect in Wilson disease is in the liver, resulting in decreased hepatic excretion of copper with excessive deposition and subsequent toxicity. Although the liver is affected in both Wilson disease and HH, the other affected organs are quite variable. In hemochromatosis, the heart, pancreas, joints, skin, and endocrine organs are affected; in Wilson disease, the brain, eyes, red blood cells, kidneys, and bone are affected. Both disorders are fully treatable if diagnosis is made promptly before the development of end-stage complications.

## WEBSITE

http://www.aasld.org

## BIBLIOGRAPHY

1. Bacon BR. Genetic, metabolic, and infiltrative diseases affecting the liver. In: Fauci AS, Braunwald E, Kasper DL, et al, editors. Harrison's Principles of Internal Medicine. 17th ed. New York: McGraw-Hill; 2008. pp. 1980–3.
2. Bacon BR, Britton RS. Clinical penetrance of hereditary hemochromatosis. N Engl J Med 2008;358:291–2.
3. Bacon BR, Olynyk JK, Brunt EM, et al. HFE genotype in patients with hemochromatosis and other liver diseases. Ann Intern Med 1999;130:953–62.
4. Bacon BR, Powell LW, Adams PC, et al. Molecular medicine and hemochromatosis: At the crossroads. Gastroenterology 1999;116:193–207.
5. Bassett ML, Halliday JW, Powell LW. Value of hepatic iron measurements in early hemochromatosis and determination of the critical iron level associated with fibrosis. Hepatology 1986;6:24–9.
6. Crystal RG. $\alpha_1$-Antitrypsin deficiency, emphysema, and liver disease: Genetics and strategies for therapy. J Clin Invest 1990;85:1343–52.
7. Edwards CQ, Griffen LM, Goldgar D, et al. Prevalence of hemochromatosis among 11,065 presumably healthy blood donors. N Engl J Med 1988;318:1355–62.
8. Eriksson S, Calson J, Veley R. Risk of cirrhosis and primary liver cancer in alpha1-antitrypsin deficiency. N Engl J Med 1986;314:736–9.
9. Feder JN, Gnirke A, Thomas W. A novel MHC class I-like gene is mutated in patients with hereditary haemochromatosis. Nat Genet 1996;13:399–408.
10. Fleming RE, Bacon BR. Orchestration of iron homeostasis. N Engl J Med 2005;352:1741–4.
11. Hill GM, Brewer GJ, Prasad AS, et al. Treatment of Wilson disease with zinc. I: Oral zinc therapy regimens. Hepatology 1987;7:522–8.
12. Hodges JR, Millward-Sadler GH, Barbatis C, et al. Heterozygous MZ alpha1-antitrypsin deficiency in adults with chronic active hepatitis and cryptogenic cirrhosis. N Engl J Med 1981;304:557–60.
13. Larsson C. Natural history and life expectancy in severe alpha1-antitrypsin deficiency, Pi Z. Acta Med Scand 1978;204:345–51.
14. Niederau C, Fischer R, Sonnenberg A, et al. Survival and causes of death in cirrhotic and noncirrhotic patients with primary hemochromatosis. N Engl J Med 1985;313:1256–62.
15. Perlmutter DH. The cellular basis for liver injury in $\alpha_1$-antitrypsin deficiency. Hepatology 1991;13:172–85.
16. Scheinberg IH, Jaffe ME, Sternlieb I. The use of trientine in preventing the effects of interrupting penicillamine therapy in Wilson disease. N Engl J Med 1987;317:209–13.
17. Schilsky ML. Identification of the Wilson disease gene: Clues for disease pathogenesis and the potential for molecular diagnosis. Hepatology 1994;20:529–33.
18. Sternlieb I. Perspectives on Wilson disease. Hepatology 1990;12:1234–9.
19. Stremmel W, Meyerrose KW, Niederau C, et al. Wilson disease: Clinical presentation, treatment, and survival. Ann Intern Med 1991;15:720–6.

# LIVER HISTOPATHOLOGY

Janet K. Stephens, MD, PhD, and
George H. Warren, MD

CHAPTER 33

## LIVER MICROANATOMY AND INJURY PATTERNS

### 1. Explain the role of liver biopsy.

Liver biopsies play an important role in patient care. They can confirm or advance a diagnosis, guide additional studies, help to evaluate therapeutic efficacy, and gauge prognosis. The liver biopsy must be of adequate size and contain an appropriate number of portal tracts and central veins to allow proper assessment. However, the liver has a limited pattern of pathologic response to injury, especially for inflammatory diseases and, as in other organs, the biopsy represents a static look at an ongoing dynamic process.

### 2. Many liver biopsy reports say that the basic architecture is intact and then list a string of abnormalities. What is the basic architecture?

Histologically, the liver has three functional components: hepatocytes, central veins and sinusoids, and portal tracts (triads). The basic liver architecture is formed by cords of hepatocytes, which, in adults, are one cell-layer thick. The cords are separated by vascular sinusoids lined by endothelial cells and Kupffer cells; the latter are part of the reticuloendothelial system and have macrophage function. Central veins, also called terminal hepatic venules, collect the circulating blood after it percolates through the sinusoids and then carry the blood to larger hepatic veins. Distributed at regular intervals are portal tracts, which contain interlobular bile ducts, small hepatic arteries, small portal veins, and fibrous stroma with scant numbers of mononuclear cells. The row of hepatocytes immediately adjacent to the portal tract is termed the limiting plate.

### 3. What are the geographic differences in pathology between portions of hepatic acini?

The functional unit of the liver is represented by hepatic acini, which are three-dimensional units built around a central axis containing a portal tract and its blood vessels. From the portal area, plates of hepatocytes radiate out toward central veins, located at the periphery of the acinus. The acinus can be divided into three zones: zone 1 is closest to the portal tracts, zone 3 is closest to the central veins, and zone 2 lies between. A gradient exists between zone 1 and zone 3; zone 1 is the best supplied with oxygen and nutrients.

### 4. What is meant by distortion of the hepatic architecture?

Usually, it indicates fibrosis and perhaps formation of regenerative nodules of hepatocytes. These changes can alter the relationships of central veins, portal tracts, and hepatic cords.

### 5. How are degrees of fibrosis designated?

The pathologist indicates how much fibrosis is present (using a trichrome stain to identify collagen) and its pattern of distribution—that is, whether portal tracts and central veins are connected by scar (bridging fibrosis) and whether the scarring has altered the architecture into nodules of hepatocytes (cirrhosis).

### 6. What criteria are used to define the presence of cirrhosis?

Cirrhosis is the end stage of all chronic liver disease. By definition, it is a process that diffusely involves the liver with progressive fibrosis, resulting in the formation of nodules. Therefore, focal scarring, even if significant and associated with nodules, is not cirrhosis because the process is not diffuse.

### 7. Can cirrhosis be diagnosed on a needle biopsy specimen?

Not always. Micronodular cirrhosis (nodules 3 mm or less), which may develop as a result of ethanol injury, biliary tract disease, or hemochromatosis, is usually uniform throughout the liver, and nodules may be identified on a needle specimen. Macronodular cirrhosis (nodules greater than 3 mm), due most commonly to chronic viral hepatitis, is less uniform. One sometimes sees relatively sparse fibrosis in a needle specimen, with some fairly normal lobules noted, even when cirrhosis is suspected clinically. By nature of the biopsy technique, the softer lobular tissue may come out in the needle more easily than the fibrous tissue, or the needle may pass through large nodules and appear relatively uninvolved histologically. The end result is that scarring can be underrepresented.

**8. What types of liver cell injury are seen on needle specimens? What causes each type?**

It may be difficult to determine a specific etiology for liver injury seen on needle biopsy, because both hepatocytes and bile ducts have a limited pattern of response. Histopathologic features may overlap in many disease processes (Table 33-1).

**Table 33-1.** Types of Liver Cell Injury

| TYPE OF INJURY | CAUSES |
| --- | --- |
| Fatty change | Ethanol, fatty liver disease, obesity, diabetes, drugs |
| Councilman bodies | Viral hepatitis, drugs, toxins, ischemia (acidophilic bodies) |
| Mallory bodies (hyaline) | Ethanol, obesity, diabetes, drugs, Wilson disease, biliary tract disease, hepatocellular carcinoma |
| Hydropic change | Viral hepatitis, drugs, cholestasis, fatty liver disease (ballooning degeneration) |
| Cholestasis | Duct obstruction or injury, drugs, viral hepatitis |
| Interlobular duct injury | Primary biliary cirrhosis, primary sclerosing cholangitis, hepatitis C |
| Piecemeal necrosis | Viral hepatitis, primary biliary cirrhosis, drugs, Wilson disease |
| Increased iron stores | Hemochromatosis, transfusions, hemolysis |
| Granulomas | Sarcoid, infections (tuberculosis, fungi), drugs |

## FATTY CHANGE AND STEATOHEPATITIS

**9. Injury from either acute or chronic ethanol ingestion is one of the most common insults to the liver. Describe the major characteristics of mild and severe injury.**

Alcoholic liver disease results in a spectrum of changes, including fatty liver, alcoholic hepatitis, and alcoholic cirrhosis. In fatty liver, as the name implies, the hepatocytes contain globules of fat, usually larger than and compressing the hepatocyte nucleus (referred to as macrovesicular steatosis). Initially, this change occurs around central veins but may extend to involve the entire acinus. Biopsies from patients with alcoholic hepatitis may also show fatty change. In addition, hepatocytes are swollen, with areas of necrosis, associated with acute inflammation (polymorphs, polymorphonuclear neutrophils [PMNs]). Hepatocytes may contain perinuclear Mallory bodies, which represent aggregates of the intermediate filament cytokeratin. Alcoholic cirrhosis, which is micronodular, may have superimposed fatty change and/or hepatitis (Fig. 33-1).

**10. What are Mallory bodies?**

Mallory bodies (Mallory hyaline) are irregular, ropelike eosinophilic intracytoplasmic strings that represent aggregates of cytokeratin intermediate filaments (cytokeratins 8 and 18). The cytokeratins form a filamentous support network within the hepatocytes. Cellular damage due, for example, to hepatocyte ballooning degeneration, can cause the keratins to misfold and aggregate. Mallory bodies may be found in alcoholic and nonalcoholic steatohepatitis, and Wilson disease, cholestatic conditions such as primary biliary cirrhosis (PBC) and with certain drugs, such as amiodarone. Although the fat and neutrophils can resolve relatively quickly after alcohol abstinence, hyaline can take up to 6 weeks to disappear.

**11. How does scarring progress with alcohol injury?**

Many patients with ethanol injury show initial scarring around central veins with delicate, spider- web–like fibrosis along the sinusoids. Eventually, bridging fibrosis connects central veins and portal tracts and adjacent portal tracts. When cirrhosis is fully developed, most of the native central veins have been obliterated.

**12. Is alcoholic cirrhosis micronodular or macronodular?**

Micronodular, because the scarring is relatively uniform throughout the liver. These small, *micro*nodules have become subdivided by the portal-central bridging fibrosis. With complete alcohol abstinence, the nodules can regenerate to

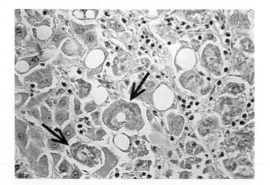

**Figure 33-1.** Photomicrograph showing alcoholic hepatitis with prominent hyaline (hematoxylin-eosin stain).

a size larger than 3 mm, but the central veins are decreased in number and the nodules lack multiple portal tracts. One sees usually central veins and portal tracts in some nodules of macronodular cirrhosis (e.g., those from viral hepatitis).

**13. Sometimes a biopsy shows *alcoholic hepatitis*, but the patient denies drinking ethanol. Is the pathologist's diagnosis incorrect, or is there a differential diagnosis for alcoholic hepatitis?**

It is clear that similar patterns of injury can be seen in nonalcoholics, especially in the setting of diabetes and obesity, referred to as nonalcoholic steatohepatitis (NASH) or nonalcoholic fatty liver disease. This represents a significant form of chronic liver disease in both adults and children, with a spectrum ranging from indolent to end-stage liver disease. It may be an underlying cause of cryptogenic cirrhosis and has been reported to recur in allograft livers. Other conditions associated with NASH include acute starvation, accelerated weight loss, intestinal bypass, disorders of lipid metabolism (i.e., abetalipoproteinemia, hyperlipidemia, lipodystrophy), and various drugs (i.e., amiodarone, perhexiline, tamoxifen, synthetic estrogens, nifedipine, corticosteroids). Careful clinicopathologic correlation is required to determine the cause. Liver biopsy evaluation allows the degree of steatosis, inflammation, and fibrosis to be graded and staged.

## VIRAL HEPATITIS

**14. How can a liver biopsy help in patients with viral hepatitis?**

A biopsy is helpful in assessing the amount of inflammatory activity (grade), its chronicity, and the degree of irreversible fibrosis or cirrhosis (stage). It can help to predict and evaluate response to medication. It is also useful in determining the presence of a second process, in addition to viral hepatitis.

**15. When, if ever, is a biopsy ordered for patients with hepatitis A? With hepatitis B and C?**

Because hepatitis A does not cause chronic liver disease, biopsy is rarely needed. Biopsies may be performed to distinguish severe cholestasis in hepatitis A from large duct obstruction or to determine whether bridging necrosis or the rare fulminant necrosis is present. Usually, if a patient has IgM anti–hepatitis A, there is no need for biopsy. Hepatitis B, hepatitis B and D coinfection, and hepatitis C can cause chronic hepatitis leading to cirrhosis, in addition to acute and/or fulminant disease. Liver biopsy helps to determine the severity of liver injury due to inflammatory activity and fibrosis. The histologic features may help to determine both treatment and prognosis.

**16. Does chronic hepatitis have unique histopathologic features?**

No. Chronic hepatitis is a clinical and pathologic syndrome that may have a variety of causes. It is a chronic necroinflammatory process in which hepatocytes are preferentially injured compared with bile ducts. In addition to viral infection, chronic hepatitis may be autoimmune or drug related. Histologic features of chronic cholestatic disease, including PBC, primary sclerosing cholangitis (PSC), and autoimmune cholangitis, as well as metabolic diseases including Wilson disease and $\alpha_1$-antitrypsin deficiency, may overlap with those of chronic hepatitis.

**17. What features are typical of chronic hepatitis?**

Although parenchymal inflammation predominates in acute hepatitis, chronic hepatitis is usually associated with varying degrees of portal and periportal inflammation, parenchymal hepatitis, and fibrosis. The inflammatory cell infiltrate is typically mononuclear and includes lymphocytes, plasma cells, and macrophages. Once the inflammatory infiltrate crosses the limiting plate, it is usually associated with local hepatocyte damage, piecemeal necrosis, and inflammation, also termed *interface hepatitis*. Lobular inflammation is accompanied by some hepatocellular necrosis (acidophilic or Councilman bodies). With time, chronic hepatitis leads to progressive fibrosis and, without treatment, to cirrhosis. The fibrosis begins in portal areas, extends to periportal areas, and begins bridging to other portal tracts and central veins.

**18. How is chronic hepatitis graded and staged?**

Various systems are used to evaluate chronic hepatitis, the simplest of which was proposed by Batts and Ludwig. A 4-point grading system is used for both inflammatory activity and degree of fibrosis:

### INFLAMMATORY ACTIVITY

- Grade 1: Minimal patchy, piecemeal necrosis, and lobular inflammation/necrosis
- Grade 2: Mild portal inflammation with piecemeal necrosis involving some or all portal tracts with focal hepatocellular damage
- Grade 3: Moderate piecemeal necrosis involving all portal tracts with increased hepatocellular damage
- Grade 4: Severe portal inflammation with piecemeal necrosis; bridging fibrosis and diffuse hepatocellular damage may be present

## FIBROSIS

- Stage 1: Portal fibrosis (fibrous portal expansion)
- Stage 2: Periportal fibrosis (periportal fibrosis with rare portal-portal septa)
- Stage 3: Septal fibrosis (fibrous septa with architectural distortion)
- Stage 4: Cirrhosis

*Example*: A liver biopsy from a patient with hepatitis C (Fig. 33-2) shows mild portal inflammation with piecemeal necrosis in most of the portal tracts and periportal expansion with a few fibrous septa. This corresponds to chronic hepatitis C with mild activity (grade 2 of 4) and portal and focal bridging fibrosis (stage 2 of 4).

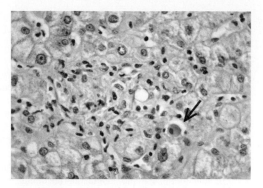

**Figure 33-2.** Photomicrograph showing chronic hepatitis C with portal inflammation and interface hepatitis, including an acidiphil body (*arrow*), with periportal and focal bridging fibrosis (hematoxylin-eosin stain).

### 19. What features in the liver biopsy help to predict etiology?

Biopsies from patients with chronic hepatitis B may show some of the changes described previously, as well as a *ground-glass* change to the cell cytoplasm. This change reflects accumulation of hepatitis B surface antigen within the endoplasmic reticulum of the hepatocytes. Chronic hepatitis C may be associated with prominent lymphoid aggregates within portal tracts, sometimes including germinal centers and, occasionally, bile duct damage, although not to the degree seen in primary biliary disorders. In addition, biopsies may show focal, nonzonal macrovesicular steatosis. The inflammatory infiltrate in patients with autoimmune hepatitis shows typically a predominance of plasma cells.

### 20. Can chronic viral hepatitis be confused with other injuries?

Autoimmune hepatitis looks quite similar to chronic viral hepatitis, but plasma cells are more prominent in autoimmune injury, and various confirmatory serologic tests are available including autoantibody levels to smooth muscle (SMA), nuclear proteins (ANA), liver/kidney microsome type I (anti-LKM), and soluble liver antigen/liver pancreas (anti-SLA/LP). Some drug injuries, PBC, PSC, and other disorders can pose difficult diagnostic problems. Some cases of $\alpha_1$-antitrypsin deficiency show piecemeal necrosis, but a periodic acid–Schiff–diastase stain will highlight the diagnostic magenta colored cytoplasmic globules in hepatocytes, representing the retention of the abnormal enzyme within the rough endoplasmic reticulum.

## CHOLESTASIS

### 21. In patients with acute or chronic cholestasis, can the liver biopsy distinguish among the various differential diagnoses?

Sometimes. Diagnosing cholestasis requires evaluation of the many causes in a systematic fashion. Is the cholestasis a result of increased production of bilirubin, decreased excretion of bilirubin, or liver cell injury? Hemolysis usually causes only mild hyperbilirubinemia. Extrahepatic obstruction is diagnosed typically by tests other than liver biopsy. Therefore, cases coming to liver biopsy are the difficult ones to solve; clinical and radiologic findings have solved the easy cases. The pathologist must ask whether the specimen shows associated inflammation or noninflammatory, "bland" cholestasis. The pathologist must also look for clues that suggest large duct obstruction or interlobular duct inflammatory injury. Subtle lesions in the head of the pancreas and ampulla of Vater can be missed. A stone may be missed. Other questions include the following:

- Does the patient have hepatitis?
- Has viral injury been excluded?
- What are the patient's toxic exposures at work, home, or play?
- Has every drug been sought and disclosed?
- Have granulomatous causes been excluded?

## DRUG INJURY

### 22. What histologic changes suggest drug- or toxin-related liver injury?

Three findings should make a pathologist press the clinician to *find the drug*:

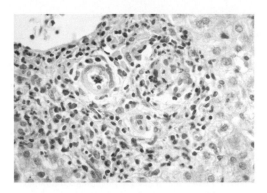

**Figure 33-3.** Photomicrograph showing drug-induced hepatitis with prominent eosinophils (hematoxylin-eosin stain).

1. *Significant fatty change,* which most often is related to toxic ethanol injury.
2. A liver biopsy that shows features of a *hypersensitivity reaction.* Such cases may resemble viral hepatitis but with an abundance of eosinophils. Eosinophils may also be present nonspecifically with viral hepatitis, connective tissue disorders, and some neoplasms (usually an infiltrate of Hodgkin disease). However, when eosinophils are a striking feature, the clinician should search for a drug, a toxin, or even a nutritional supplement (Fig. 33-3). Granulomas may also be part of the inflammatory reaction in drug injury.
3. A liver that looks like it is recovering from a point-in-time injury, with *numerous liver cell mitotic figures.* These findings suggest that a single or short episode of drug or toxin exposure may be to blame.

## BILE DUCT DISORDERS

### 23. In a patient with large duct obstruction, conjugated hyperbilirubinemia, an ultrasound showing bile duct stones, and clinical cholangitis, what would a biopsy show?

In this clinical situation, it is unusual that a liver biopsy would be necessary. If done, such a biopsy could show centrilobular cholestasis, portal tract edema, and neutrophils within portal tract stroma as well as bile duct epithelium and lumens. One needs to remember that neutrophils within edematous portal stroma are a feature of large duct obstruction, even when frank cholangitis is not present.

### 24. When is PBC diagnosed?

PBC is chronic progressive cholestatic liver disease that occurs in middle-aged patients, usually women, and is often associated with other autoimmune diseases. Patients may present with jaundice and pruritus. Laboratory testing reveals an elevated serum anti–mitochondrial antibody (AMA) as well as increased alkaline phosphatase, bilirubin, and γ-glutamyl transpeptidase.

### 25. How is PBC staged?

The histologic staging of PBC takes into account the degree of bile duct damage and fibrosis.

- *Stage 1* (early disease) is characterized by damage to septal and larger interlobular bile ducts, reflected by biliary epithelial damage with infiltration of the duct by lymphocytes, plasma cells, eosinophils, and rare polymorphs. The inflammatory infiltrate may include granulomas and lymphoid follicles (florid duct lesion; Fig. 33-4). At this point, the process is confined within the portal tract.
- In *Stage 2* disease, the inflammatory process extends beyond the portal tract, and changes of interface hepatitis (piecemeal necrosis) may be seen. Bile ducts begin to disappear and proliferation of bile ductules (cholangioles) may also be present along the edges of the portal tracts. These changes are associated with features of chronic cholestasis, including feathery degeneration within the cytoplasm of hepatocytes, accumulation of bile pigment, periportal accumulation of copper (not generalized as in Wilson disease), and, occasionally, Mallory bodies.

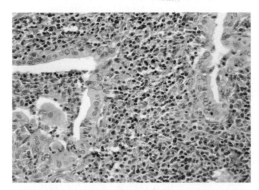

**Figure 33-4.** Photomicrograph showing primary biliary cirrhosis, with a florid duct lesion (hematoxylin-eosin stain).

- *Stage 3* is associated with increasing fibrosis and bridging between portal areas, with decreased amounts of inflammation.
- *Stage 4* represents *biliary* (micronodular) cirrhosis.

### 26. What are the histologic features of PSC?

PSC shares many clinical biochemical and pathologic features with PBC, although it can affect both intrahepatic **and** extrahepatic ducts. PSC is strongly associated with inflammatory bowel disease, particularly ulcerative colitis. Patients may present with increased alkaline phosphatase and positive perinuclear antineutrophil cytoplasmic antibodies (pANCAs). The classic lesion of PSC is *onionskin* or concentric periductular fibrosis, with damage to the ductal epithelium.

### 27. How is PSC staged?

Like PBC, PSC is staged according to bile duct changes and fibrosis.

- *Stage 1* (early disease) is associated with bile duct damage and inflammation and is largely confined within portal tracts.
- In *Stage 2* disease, the fibroinflammatory process is periportal.
- In *Stage 3* bridging fibrosis is present and bile ducts are decreased in numbers.
- *Stage 4* represents end-stage disease (cirrhosis).

### 28. What are the most common biopsy findings in patients with PSC?

The onionskin lesion is seen rarely on percutaneous biopsy. The most common findings on biopsy, in early-stage disease, are nonspecific fibrosis with inflammation of portal tracts and paucity of normal bile ducts. In addition, in patients with extrahepatic disease, it may be hard to separate intrahepatic PSC from the superimposed effects of extrahepatic obstruction. Obstruction causes proliferation and dilatation of interlobular ducts and an increased number of periportal PMNs. A major goal of the biopsy interpretation is to consider PSC and then to suggest endoscopic retrograde cholangiopancreatography (ERCP) to confirm the diagnosis.

## GRANULOMATOUS INFLAMMATION

### 29. What is a granuloma?

A granuloma is a sharply (or fairly sharply) defined aggregate of histiocytes.

### 30. How common are granulomas in liver biopsies?

Most systemic granulomatous diseases involve the liver to some extent. Granulomas may be identified in 10% of routine liver biopsies, probably in relation to the liver's large population of phagocytic cells, including Kupffer cells.

### 31. What causes granulomas in the liver?

The differential list is long and varied. Tuberculosis and sarcoidosis are the most common causes. Other infectious agents include bacteria (brucellosis, nocardiosis, tularemia, Q fever [*Coxiella burnetii*], spirochetes), various fungi, protozoa, and viruses (cytomegalovirus, Epstein-Barr virus). Noninfectious causes, in addition to sarcoidosis, include PBC, drug reaction, extrahepatic inflammatory disease (chronic granulomatous disease of childhood, chronic inflammatory bowel disease, rheumatoid arthritis), neoplasms (Hodgkin disease), and foreign substances (talc, mineral oil).

### 32. In patients with fever of unknown origin, do negative stains for fungi and acid-fast bacilli exclude infection?

Not at all. Cultures for these organisms are more sensitive than special histologic stains. If infection is a possibility, a core of liver should be submitted with sterile precautions and without fixative to the microbiology laboratory. In addition, tissue in formalin should be sent to the surgical pathology laboratory for microscopic sections. Tissue may also be sent for molecular analysis to determine whether an infectious agent is present.

### 33. What are the different types of granulomas? Is the distinction of diagnostic use?

- *Epithelioid granulomas* are nodular aggregates of plump macrophages, often associated with multinucleated giant cells, lymphocytes, and plasma cells. They are typically seen in sarcoidosis. The presence of central caseating necrosis suggests or tuberculosis.
- *Fibrin-ring granulomas* are formed by a fibrin band encircling a lipid droplet, with associated inflammation. They were first described with Q fever but may also be seen after infection with cytomegalovirus or Epstein-Barr virus as well as with drug (allopurinol) toxicity and in association with systemic lupus erythematosus.
- *Lipogranulomas* are composed of lipid deposits and vacuolated macrophages. They are formed in the presence of exogenous or endogenous fat accumulation.
- *Microgranulomas* are composed of small, round clusters of plump Kupffer cells. They are a relatively nonspecific finding.

### 34. How often are liver granulomas secondary to a drug reaction?

Perhaps one third of granulomatous liver reactions are caused by drugs, including sulphonamides, allopurinol, phenylbutazone, carbamazepine, procainamide, diphenylhydantoin, quinidine, isoniazid, and sulfanilamide.

## INHERITED LIVER DISEASE

### 35. What is hematochromatosis?

Hemochromatosis is an autosomal recessive disorder that leads to massive deposits of iron in many organs, including liver, pancreas, heart, joints, and skin. The gene responsible for hereditary hemochromatosis, *HFE,* is located on chromosome 6. The two most common (missense) mutations are C282Y (present in up to 80% of cases) and H63D. Untreated, hemochromatosis leads to the development of micronodular cirrhosis. Liver biopsies may be relatively normal or show bridging fibrosis or even micronodular cirrhosis. Hepatocyte iron is deposited in a graded fashion, from periportal areas to central veins, and can be scored on a 4-point system. In genetic hemochromatosis, hepatocytes and biliary epithelium both contain increased stainable iron.

## 36. Is a liver biopsy necessary to diagnosis genetic hemachromatosis?

Prior to the availability of genetic testing, the diagnosis of hemochromatosis was established with liver biopsy and quantitative iron determination. In general, young patients accumulate less iron than older patients, and menstruating women will have less iron than men of the same age. Quantitative iron testing allowed determination of the hepatic iron index (HII):

$$[\text{Hepatic iron concentration (mg/g liver dry wt)/age/55.8}]$$

Patients with genetic homozygous hemochromatosis characteristically would show an HII greater than 1.9, whereas patients with other causes of iron overload, including chronic alcoholic liver disease, showed an HII less than 1.9. With the availability of genetic testing for the C282Y and/or H63D mutations, liver biopsy is more often reserved for evaluation of clinical status or complications (i.e., degree of fibrosis, development of hepatocellular carcinoma) rather than for primary diagnosis. A biopsy can also help determine if other disease processes are present, such as hepatitis C or fatty liver disease.

## 37. What disorders are problematic in the clinical differential diagnosis of hemochromatosis?

The list of disorders associated with increased hepatic iron is long. The pattern of distribution of the iron in the liver may be of some help in establishing the diagnosis:

### PREDOMINANTLY HEPATOCELLULAR DISTRIBUTION

- Genetic hemochromatosis
- Alcoholic liver disease
- Porphyria cutanea tarda

### DISTRIBUTED PREDOMINANTLY IN KUPFFER CELLS

- Multiple transfusions
- Hemolytic anemias

### MIXED HEPATOCELLULAR AND KUPFFER CELL DISTRIBUTION

- Megaloblastic anemia
- Anemia secondary to chronic infection

## 38. What is Wilson disease? Can liver biopsy help to establish the diagnosis?

Wilson disease is an autosomal recessive disorder of copper metabolism, characterized by excessive accumulation of copper in the liver and other organs. The gene for Wilson disease has been localized to chromosome 13 (13q14-q21) and codes for a P-type adenosine triphosphatase (ATPase) responsible for copper transport. More than 280 mutations of this gene have been identified. Genetic evaluation is difficult because most patients are compound heterozygotes, possessing one copy each of two different mutations. The disease can show a range of appearances on liver biopsy, depending to some extent on the patient's age. In children and young adolescents, the most common appearance may be fatty change. In older adolescents and young adults, a liver biopsy may show chronic hepatitis with piecemeal necrosis. Adults tend to show cirrhosis, and Mallory bodies may be part of this change. In either adolescents or adults, confluent necrosis leading to fulminant hepatic failure may follow.

## 39. What other tests are helpful in patients with Wilson disease?

Quantitative copper testing of the liver is useful. In patients with Wilson disease, levels are typically greater than 250 mg/g dry weight liver (normal level, 38 mg/g). The levels may be much higher in the absence of cirrhosis. Conditions associated with chronic cholestasis (PBC, PSC) also have elevated liver copper levels (range, 150 to 350 mg/g). Other helpful measurements include serum ceruloplasmin (less than 20 mg/dL in patients with Wilson disease; normal levels, 23 to 50 mg/dL) and 24-hour urinary copper (greater than 100 mg/dL; normal, less than 30 mg/dL).

## 40. What are the features of $\alpha_1$-antitrypsin ($\alpha_1$-AT) deficiency on liver biopsy?

$\alpha_1$-AT is the major circulating inhibitor of serine proteases (Pi). Its primary target is the potent elastase found in PMNs. It thus acts to protect tissues against injury during active, acute inflammation. It is a 52-kDa glycoprotein synthesized in the liver under the control of codominant alleles at a locus on the long arm of chromosome 14. These genes are highly polymorphic, with more than 75 known alleles. Many of the Pi variants are associated with fairly normal serum concentrations and function and thus are of little clinical significance. However, a few result in low circulating levels of $\alpha_1$-AT (i.e., PiZZ) and are of pathologic significance. Liver biopsies from affected patients demonstrate classic PAS-positive, diastase-resistant globules within periportal hepatocytes. Portal fibrosis and chronic hepatitis may also be present. Liver cell dysplasia may be seen, and patients older than age 50, especially men, are at risk of developing hepatocellular carcinoma.

**41. Is the presence of PAS-positive, diastase-resistant globules diagnostic for $\alpha_1$-AT deficiency?**

No. Various inflammatory conditions may be associated with overproduction of the enzyme, as may congestion or hypoxia. Clinical correlation with electrophoretic analysis is required.

## NEOPLASMS

**42. Discuss the role of liver biopsy in diagnosing metastatic neoplasms.**

First, an adequate sample of the neoplasm must be obtained. Biopsy can confirm metastasis to the liver from a known primary tumor. Some biopsies show a tumor that is probably metastatic but for which no primary tumor is known. In such cases, various immunohistochemical stains can be performed on biopsy tissue and help to guide further workup.

**43. Discuss the role of biopsy in diagnosing primary liver tumors.**

Hepatocellular carcinoma can be diagnosed on needle core biopsies performed under radiologic guidance. High-grade hepatocellular carcinomas are usually straightforward, but low-grade hepatocellular carcinomas can be difficult to distinguish from normal tissue or a regenerative nodule in the setting of cirrhosis (Fig. 33-5). Intrahepatic cholangiocarcinoma is typically a well- to moderately differentiated adenocarcinoma. On a core biopsy, it may be difficult to distinguish from a metastatic process. Immunohistochemical stains may help, along with careful clinical and radiologic correlation. Liver cell adenomas in women taking oral contraceptives may show characteristic features, but, occasionally, well-differentiated hepatocellular carcinomas can resemble liver cell adenomas. Focal nodular hyperplasia is a localized lobulated nodule of hyperplastic liver cells surrounding a central scar. This condition can be confused with macronodular cirrhosis on a needle biopsy specimen (or even a wedge biopsy specimen). Definitive classification may require excision of the nodule.

**44. Can the clinical laboratory help in classifying tumors?**

Marked elevation of serum alpha-fetoprotein levels in hepatocellular carcinomas or similar markers for other tumors can be a great help.

## TRANSPLANTATION

**45. Describe the role of liver biopsy in the evaluation of transplant recipients with abnormal liver function tests (LFTs) in the early postoperative period.**

Liver transplantation is a well-accepted treatment for patients with advanced liver disease that is unresponsive to conventional therapy. In the first few weeks and months after transplantation, the major causes of abnormal LFTs include preservation injury, acute rejection, opportunistic infections (e.g., cytomegalovirus, hepatitis), vascular compromise, and/or biliary stricture. Of these, acute allograft rejection is the most common and results from direct alloantigenic stimulation of recipient T cells by donor dendritic cells (antigen-presenting cells). The effector T cells can then preferentially injure biliary epithelial cells of both interlobular and septal bile ducts as well as endothelial cells of intrahepatic arteries and veins. Hepatocytes and sinusoidal lining cells are not prime targets.

**46. What are the main histologic features of acute rejection?**

Acute rejection is characterized by mixed, predominantly mononuclear cells infiltrates within portal tracts. The inflammatory infiltrates include lymphocytes, macrophages, plasma cells, PMNs, and eosinophils. The inflammatory cells typically infiltrate bile duct epithelium and are associated with bile duct damage. Subendothelial inflammation (endothelialitis), which may involve both portal and central veins and even the hepatic artery, is also a feature. These histologic features can be scored semiquantitatively. The most common grading system is the Banff schema, a consensus document proposed by an international panel of pathologists and liver transplant physicians. The Banff schema uses two components. The first is a global assessment of the overall rejection grade (indeterminate to severe). The second

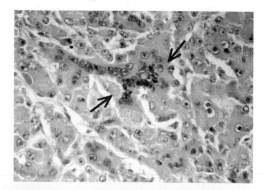

**Figure 33-5.** Photomicrograph showing hepatocellular carcinoma with prominent giant cell (*arrows*) (hematoxylin-eosin stain).

component involves scoring the three main features of acute allograft rejection on a scale of 0 (absent) to 3 (severe) to product an overall rejection activity index (RAI).

**47. What criteria help to distinguish recurrent hepatitis C after transplantation from allograft rejection?**

Hepatitis C (HCV) recurs in virtually all patients transplanted for that disease. The distinction of recurrent hepatitis from acute allograft rejection can be difficult. There are three main phases to recurrent HCV:

- The first is *graft reinfection* (0 to 2 months post-transplant). HCV-related inflammation is rarely seen at this time. Liver biopsies may show mild lobular disarray, occasional necrotic hepatocytes (acidophil bodies), and fatty change.
- The second stage is *established graft infection* (2 to 4 months), which is characterized by features of acute hepatitis including lobular disarray, ballooning degeneration of hepatocytes, acidophil bodes, and Kupffer cell prominence. Varying degrees of portal tract inflammation may also be present.
- The third stage is *progressive liver damage* (greater than 6 months), which shows features more typical of *chronic* HCV infection. This includes mononuclear portal infiltrates with interface hepatitis. Bile duct damage, although it may occur, is focal and mild. Up to half of patients will have histologic evidence after 1 year.

**48. Describe the role of liver biopsy in the evaluation of abnormal LFTs in the first year after transplantation (and beyond).**

Common causes of abnormal LFTs in the first year after transplantation include acute rejection (usually caused by inadequate immunosuppression), opportunistic infection, recurrent viral hepatitis, chronic rejection, steatohepatitis, and various recurrent diseases (e.g., PBC, PSC, autoimmune hepatitis). Chronic rejection occurs as a consequence of repeated episodes of acute rejection that are unresponsive to immunosuppression. The main histologic abnormalities are loss of small bile ducts (*ductopenic* rejection) and/or obliterative vasculopathy (affecting large and medium-sized arteries). The former can be diagnosed by liver biopsy, whereas the latter may require examination of the explanted liver. Chronic ductopenic rejection is characterized classically by bile duct loss in more than 50% of portal tracts, in either a single biopsy or a series of biopsies. It is probably irreversible. Unlike acute allograft rejection, the degree of bile duct damage is typically out of proportion to the degree of inflammation.

**49. How can a liver biopsy help in the evaluation of a bone marrow transplant recipient with elevated LFTs?**

Complications of bone marrow transplantation include veno-occlusive disease (VOD) and graft-versus-host disease (GVHD). VOD leads to liver dysfunction and is due to the use of high-dose cytoreductive therapy. It develops within 1 to 4 weeks after transplantation. On biopsy, it is characterized by occlusion of central veins, sinusoidal fibrosis, and pericentral hepatocyte necrosis. Acute GVHD develops within 6 weeks after transplantation and affects the skin, gastrointestinal tract, and liver. It is characterized by degenerative bile duct lesions with some degree of mononuclear inflammation. Cholestasis may be present. Chronic GVHD is a multiorgan process that develops 80 to 400 days after transplantation and is often preceded by acute GVHD. The changes in the liver are similar to those in acute disease, but the ducts show more prominent changes and are likely to be reduced in number or destroyed. A prominent periportal mononuclear infiltrate, or even piecemeal necrosis, may be seen.

## WEBSITES

http://tpis.upmc.com/TPIShome/

http://www.afip.org/Departments/HepGastr_dept/index.html

http://www.gastroatlas.com/

http://www.pathology2.jhu.edu/liver/

http://www-medlib.med.utah.edu/WebPath/GIHTML/GIIDX.html

http://www-medlib.med.utah.edu/WebPath/LIVEHTML/LIVERIDX.html

http://www-medlib.med.utah.edu/WebPath/ORGAN.html#2

### BIBLIOGRAPHY

1. Alvarez F, Berg PA, Biandin FB, et al. International Autoimmune Hepatitis Group Report: Review of criteria for diagnosis of autoimmune hepatitis. J Hepatol 1999;31:929–38.
2. Anonymous. Update of the International Banff Schema for Liver Allograft Rejection: Working recommendations for the histopathologic staging and reporting of chronic rejection. Hepatology 2000;31:792–9.

3. Brunt EM. Pathology of fatty liver disease. Mod Pathol 2007;20:S40–8.
4. Burt AD, Portmann BC, Ferrell LD. Development, structure and function of the liver. In: MacSween's Pathology of the liver. 5th ed. New York: Churchill Livingstone, Elsevier; 2007.
5. Chahal P, Levy C, Litzow MR, et al. Utility of liver biopsy in bone marrow transplant patient. J Gastroenterol Hepatol 2008;l23:222–5.
6. Crawford AR, Lin XZ, Crawford JM. The normal adult human liver biopsy: A quantitative reference standard. Hepatology 1998;28:323–31.
7. Bedossa P, Poynard T. An algorithm for the grading of activity in chronic hepatitis C. The METAVIR Cooperative Study Group. Hepatology 1996;24:289–93.
8. Dam-Larsen S, Franzmann MB, Christoffersen P, et al. Histological characteristics and prognosis in patients with fatty liver. Gastroenterology 2005;40:460–7.
9. Demetris AJ, Adams D, Bellamy C, et al. Update of the International Banff Schema for Liver Allograft Rejection: Working recommendations for the histopathologic staging and reporting of chronic rejection. An international panel. Hepatology 2000;31:792–9.
10. Demetris AJ, Eghtesad B, Marcos A, et al. Recurrent hepatitis C in liver allografts: Prospective assessment of diagnostic accuracy, identification of pitfalls and observations about pathogenesis. Am J Surg Pathol 2004;28:658–69.
11. Goodman ZD. Drug hepatotoxicity. Clin Liver Dis 2002;6:381–97.
12. Hamilton SR, Aaltonen LA. World Health Organization Classification of Tumors. Pathology and genetics of tumors of the digestive system. Lyon: IARC Press; 2000. pp. 157–202.
13. Ishak KG, Goodman ZD, Stocker JT. Tumors of the liver and intrahepatic bile ducts. In: Atlas of Tumor Pathology, Third Series, Fascicle 31. Washington: Armed Forces Institute of Pathology; 2001. 356 pages.
14. Kleiner DE, Brunt EM, Van Natta M, et al. Design and validation of a histological scoring system for nonalcoholic fatty liver disease. Hepatology 2005;41:1313–21.
15. Knodell R, Ishak, Black W, et al. Formulation and application of a numerical scoring system for assessing histological activity in asymptomatic chronic active hepatitis. Hepatology 1981;1:431–5.
16. Larrey D. Hepatoxicity of herbal remedies. J Hepatol 1997;26:47–51.
17. Lefkowitch JH. Hepatic granulomas. J Hepatol 1999;30:40–5.
18. Poupon R. Autoimmune overlapping syndromes. Clin Liver Dis 2003;7:865–78.
19. Rousselet MC, Michalak S, Dupre F, et al. Sources of variability in histological scoring of chronic viral hepatitis. Hepatology 2005;41:256.
20. Schiano T, Azeem S, Bodian C, et al. Importance of specimen size in accurate needle liver biopsy evaluation of patients with chronic hepatitis C. Clin Gastroenterol Hepatol 2005;3:930–35.
21. Stickel F, Egerer G, Seitz HK. Hepatoxicity of botanicals. Publ Health Nutr 2000;3:113–24.
22. Valla DC, Benhamou HP. Hepatic granulomas and hepatic sarcoidosis. Clin Liver Dis 2000;4:269–85.

# CHAPTER 34

# HEPATOBILIARY CYSTIC DISEASE

*Randall E. Lee, MD, FACP*

**1. Describe the five major classes and subtypes of congenital bile duct cysts (Fig. 34-1)**

**Type Ia:** cystic extrahepatic bile duct dilation*
**Type Ib:** segmental extrahepatic bile duct dilation
**Type Ic:** fusiform, diffuse or cylindrical bile duct dilation*
**Type II:** extrahepatic duct diverticula
**Type III:** choledochocele
**Type IVa:** multiple intrahepatic and extrahepatic duct cysts*
**Type IVb:** multiple extrahepatic duct cysts
**Type V:** intrahepatic duct cysts

**2. Describe the typical clinical presentation of a bile duct cyst.**

The classic clinical presentation of a bile duct cyst is the triad of abdominal pain, jaundice, and abdominal mass. Infants and children manifest this symptom triad more than adults. Often, only one or two of these symptoms are present at any one time. Other presenting symptoms include cholangitis and pancreatitis. Bile duct cysts may also be incidental findings.

**3. Compare the main features of Caroli disease and Caroli syndrome**

Initially described by Caroli in 1958, both entities are characterized by congenital cystic dilations of the intrahepatic bile ducts. The extrahepatic bile ducts are not affected. The biliary dilations may affect the entire liver, or be isolated to one

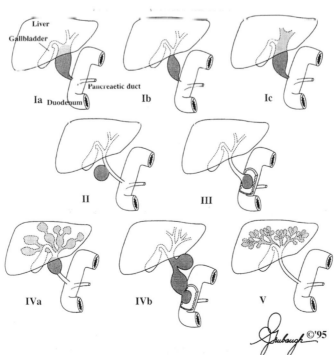

**Figure 34-1.** Classification of bile duct cysts.

*Usually associated with an anomalous pancreatobiliary junction (APBJ).

lobe. In the rare *Caroli disease*, these cystic intrahepatic biliary dilations predispose to bile stasis leading to recurrent intrahepatic calculi and cholangitis.

In the more common *Caroli syndrome,* the cystic intrahepatic biliary dilations are associated with congenital hepatic fibrosis. Consequently, in addition to the symptoms stemming from bile stasis, patients with Caroli syndrome often have manifestations of portal hypertension, such as splenomegaly, ascites, and variceal bleeding.

Treatment of patients with either entity must be individualized. Such patients may benefit from various combinations of surgical, endoscopic, and oral dissolution therapy for biliary stones, partial hepatic resection, or liver transplantation.

## 4. What is the incidence of malignancy within a congenital bile duct cyst?

The reported incidence of malignancy within a congenital bile duct cyst ranges from 10% to 30%, although this may be an overestimation since the true incidence of bile duct cyst disease is unknown. The risk of malignancy appears to increase with the age of the patient at presentation. Malignancy has been reported in all types of bile duct cysts, including Type III (choledochocele).

## 5. Describe the preferred treatment for patients with bile duct cyst disease.

The preferred treatment is complete surgical excision of the cyst with hepatoenterostomy rather than cystenterostomy and internal drainage. Complete excision significantly reduces, but does not eliminate, the risks of developing bile duct malignancy, strictures, and cholangitis. Patients with symptomatic intrahepatic bile duct cyst disease may need the affected lobe resected, or be considered for liver transplantation.

## 6. What is the role of cholangiopancreatography in patients with bile duct cyst disease?

Patients with extrahepatic bile duct cysts have an increased incidence of anomalous pancreaticobiliary junction. Cholangiopancreatography—percutaneously, endoscopically, or intraoperatively—allows definitive identification of the pancreatic duct insertion, which may be important to the planning of excision. In addition, cholangiography can distinguish multiple intrahepatic bile duct cysts from multiple hepatic cysts, which appear similar on computed tomography (CT). Magnetic resonance cholangiopancreatography (MRCP) is not as good as direct cholangiopancreatography for characterizing the pancreatobiliary junction but has less risk. Endoscopic retrograde cholangiopancreatography (ERCP) should be performed with caution in patients with suspected Caroli disease or Caroli syndrome because of the increased risk of recurrent cholangitis and sepsis. Nevertheless, therapeutic ERCP remains a useful tool for the management of acute cholangitis due to bile duct stones.

## 7. Provide a differential diagnosis for a cystic hepatic lesion.

- Simple liver cyst
- Polycystic liver disease
- Echinococcal cyst
- Neoplastic

## 8. What is the significance of a simple hepatic cyst?

Simple hepatic cysts (often called solitary hepatic cysts) are benign fluid collections usually surrounded by a thin columnar epithelium. They frequently are noted as an incidental finding on diagnostic imaging examinations. Simple hepatic cysts are not associated with cystic disease in other organs, and there is no genetic transmission. Many, but not all, simple hepatic cysts are solitary, and most are asymptomatic. Cyst-related symptoms include abdominal pain, increasing abdominal girth, and obstructive jaundice. Laparoscopic surgical unroofing of the simple cyst is the first line definitive therapy if symptoms develop.

## 9. Describe the ultrasonographic, CT, and magnetic resonance imaging (MRI) characteristics of a simple hepatic cyst

On ultrasound examinations, a simple hepatic cyst has no internal echoes, a smooth margin with the surrounding parenchyma, and no appreciable wall. The absence of any of these characteristics should make one suspect a complication, such as a cyst infection, or another diagnosis, such as hydatid cyst or biliary cyst disease.

A simple hepatic cyst appears on CT as a thin-walled lesion that does not enhance with iodinated intravenous contrast agents. The density of the lesion is that of water. On MRI, a simple hepatic cyst is a homogeneous, very-low-intensity lesion on T1-weighted scans and a discrete high-intensity lesion on T2-weighted scans.

These imaging characteristics, as well as a stable appearance over time, are diagnostic for a simple uncomplicated hepatic cyst that does not require treatment.

## 10. What disease commonly is associated with polycystic liver disease (PLD)?

PLD is characterized by numerous cysts scattered throughout the liver parenchyma. Most commonly it is associated with autosomal dominant polycystic kidney disease (ADPKD), a common inherited disorder that causes about 10% of all end-stage kidney disease requiring dialysis. More than 75% of all patients with ADPKD also have polycystic liver disease. There are also strong associations between ADPKD and intracranial saccular aneurysms (berry aneurysms), mitral valve prolapse, and colonic diverticula. Most families affected by ADPKD have a genetic defect located on chromosome 16 (*ADPKD1*) or chromosome 4 (*ADPKD2*).

Polycystic liver disease also is manifest in the rare autosomal dominant polycystic liver disease (ADPLD) that is caused by a mutation in the gene on chromosome 19 that encodes for the protein hepatocystin. Patients with ADPLD have no kidney disease but also may have an increased risk for intracranial aneurysms.

Some authors recommend that patients with polycystic liver disease of either type should be screened for intracranial aneurysms by either magnetic resonance or computed tomography angiography.

## 11. What are the risk factors for polycystic liver disease in patients with ADPKD?

Polycystic liver disease is the most common extrarenal manifestation of ADPKD. The presence and severity of polycystic liver disease in patients with ADPKD increase with age, female gender, number and frequency of pregnancies, and severity of renal disease. Massive polycystic liver disease associated with ADPKD has only been reported in women.

## 12. Describe the clinical manifestations of complicated polycystic liver disease

The common complications of polycystic liver disease usually are related to mass effect. Compression of adjacent structures by large cysts may be manifest by chronic pain, anorexia, dyspnea, or obstructive jaundice. Liver cyst infection rarely occurs but is associated with significant morbidity. Clinical clues to the presence of a cyst infection include fever, right-upper-quadrant abdominal pain, and leukocytosis. A definitive diagnosis of cyst infection usually requires percutaneous CT or ultrasound-guided fine-needle aspiration, but determining just which cyst is infected may be problematic.

## 13. How does the presence of liver cysts affect hepatic function?

Hepatic function usually is not affected by liver cysts. In the absence of complications, the serum aminotransferase, bilirubin, and alkaline phosphatase levels typically are within normal range or only slightly elevated. In patients with ADPKD, serum chemistry abnormalities generally reflect the degree of renal dysfunction.

## 14. What are the treatment options for patients with symptomatic polycystic liver disease?

Symptomatic liver cysts may be treated either percutaneously or surgically. Simple ultrasound- or CT-guided percutaneous aspiration results in rapid reaccumulation of the cyst fluid. The rate of cyst recurrence is greatly reduced by instilling a sclerosing agent, such as absolute ethanol, at the time of aspiration. Patients treated in this manner may experience a low-grade fever and transient pain as well as ethanol intoxication. Percutaneous sclerosis of a liver cyst is contraindicated when the cyst communicates with either the biliary system or peritoneal cavity.

Infected cysts do not resolve with systemic antibiotic therapy alone. Administration of antibiotics should be combined with either percutaneous or surgical drainage. Patients with intractable pain or anorexia due to massive polycystic hepatomegaly may be candidates for either isolated orthotopic liver transplant or combined liver and kidney transplant if they are dialysis dependent.

## 15. What is echinococcosis?

Echinococcosis is a parasitic infection caused by the tapeworm *Echinococcus*. There are four known species of *Echinococcus* that cause human disease:

- *E. granulosus* (cystic echinococcosis)
- *E. oligarthus*
- *E. vogeli* (polycystic echinococcosis)
- *E. multilocularis* (alveolar echinococcosis)

*E. oligarthus* and *E vogeli* are found in Central and South America. *E. multilocularis* is found throughout the planet's arctic regions including Alaska. *E. granulosus* has a worldwide distribution. The cystic and polycystic types of echinococcosis both form large fluid-filled cysts that do not invade adjacent tissue. In contrast, alveolar echinococcosis is characterized by exogenous budding, local tissue infiltration, and metastatic spread.

### 16. Describe the usual life cycle of *E. granulosus.*

*E. granulosus* is the small tapeworm responsible for cystic echinococcosis. The adult worm is only 2 to 8 mm long and consists of a scolex with suckers and a coronet of hooklets, followed by three or four body segments called proglottids. The last proglottid typically is gravid with hundreds of eggs. Each egg measures only about 0.03 mm in diameter. The adult worm lives in the intestinal lumen of the definitive host, usually a predator such as a dog or fox. Eggs discharged from the gravid proglottid segment leave the definitive host in the feces. The eggs are ingested through contaminated food or water by intermediate hosts such as sheep, cattle, goats, and pigs. Ingested eggs hatch in the duodenum, and the larvae penetrate the intestinal mucosa to be carried by the circulatory system to the capillary beds of distant organs. As a defense mechanism, the intermediate host lays down layers of connective tissue around each larva, thus forming the hydatid cyst. New scolices bud from the inner wall of the cyst. Over time, daughter cysts may form within the original cyst. When infected viscera are eaten by a predator, the scolices develop into adult worms.

### 17. Where and how does *E. granulosus* infect humans?

Human infection by *E. granulosus* is the most common of the *Echinococcus* zoonoses and occurs throughout the world. It is a significant public health problem in Central and South America, China, Mediterranean and Middle East countries, eastern Europe, and the Russian Federation. Most human cystic echinococcosis cases in the United States occur in immigrants from these regions. Cystic echinococcosis is estimated to have a global cost of over US$4 billion per year in human disability and economic losses to livestock. Human infections occur most commonly in sheep- and cattle-raising areas where dogs assist in herding. The dogs eat infected viscera and excrete infective eggs in their feces. Humans usually are infected as intermediate hosts when they ingest feces/egg-contaminated food or water or allow infected dogs to lick them in the mouth. Over one-half of all human infections involve the liver. Additional common sites for echinococcal cysts are the lungs, spleen, kidneys, heart, bones, and brain (Fig. 34-2).

### 18. Describe the typical clinical presentation of hepatic cystic echinococcosis

Patients unsuspectingly harbor the infection for years until they present with a palpable abdominal mass or other symptoms. The hydatid cyst diameter usually increases by 1 to 5 cm per year. The symptoms of hepatic cystic echinococcosis are related primarily to the mass effect of the slowly enlarging cyst: abdominal pain from the stretching hepatic capsule, jaundice from compression of the bile duct, or portal hypertension from portal vein obstruction. Approximately 20% of patients have cysts that rupture into the biliary tree and may have symptoms similar to those of choledocholithiasis or cholangitis. Rupture of a cyst into the peritoneal cavity may cause an intense antigenic response, resulting in eosinophilia, bronchial spasm, or anaphylactic shock.

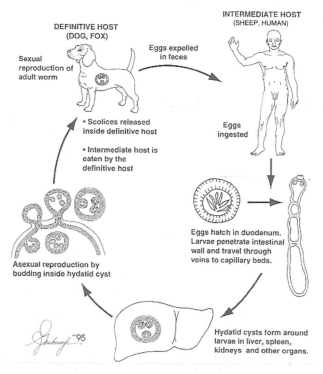

Life cycle of *Echinococcus granulosus.*

**Figure 34-2.** Life cycle of *Echinococcus granulosus.*

## 19. How is cystic echinococcosis diagnosed?

Confirming a diagnosis of cystic echinococcosis usually requires a combination of diagnostic imaging and serologic tests. CT scans may show the hydatid cyst as a sharply defined, low-density lesion with spokelike septations. The presence of a calcified rim of daughter cysts greatly enhances the specificity of the CT findings. When imaged by ultrasound, the hydatid cyst appears as a complex mass with multiple internal echoes from debris and septations. Enzyme-linked immunosorbent assay or indirect hemagglutinin serologic assays for echinococcal antibodies are positive in about 85% to 90% of patients. Recovery of scolices from a suspected hydatid cyst by percutaneous needle aspiration is diagnostic, but this technique must be used with caution because of the risk of spilling scolices into the peritoneal cavity.

## 20. What are the treatment options for hepatic cystic echinococcosis?

The optimal treatment of hepatic cystic echinococcosis depends on the local expertise and the characteristics of the individual patient. Surgical cyst resection generally is the preferred method of therapy for large or infected cysts. Percutaneous cyst drainage and irrigation with a scolicidal agent (Puncture, Aspiration, Injection, Reaspiration [PAIR]) is a safe and effective alternative therapy for those with uncomplicated cysts or for patients who are not surgical candidates. Chemotherapy with albendazole in the peritreatment period reduces the recurrence rate of both techniques. Pretreatment ERCP helps to rule out cyst communication with the biliary or pancreatic duct systems. Persistent postoperative biliary fistulas may be diagnosed and treated by ERCP with endoscopic sphincterotomy.

## 21. What hepatobiliary cystic neoplasm with malignant potential can be mistaken for a simple cyst, polycystic liver disease, or a hydatid cyst?

Hepatobiliary cystadenoma is an uncommon neoplasm that may be mistaken for other hepatobiliary cystic diseases. Generally found as incidental findings on abdominal imaging examinations, a hepatobiliary cystadenoma typically has thick irregular walls and internal septations, distinguishing it from a simple cyst. If symptomatic at presentation, patients most commonly complain of abdominal pain. Other common symptoms include jaundice and anorexia. Lined with biliary epithelium, these cystic lesions have a high potential for transformation to cystadenocarcinoma and the treatment of choice is surgical resection of the entire neoplasm.

## BIBLIOGRAPHY

1. Bayraktar Y. Clinical characteristics of Caroli's disease. World J Gastroenterol 2007;13:1930–3.
2. Bayraktar Y. Clinical characteristics of Caroli's syndrome. World J Gastroenterol 2007;13:1934–7.
3. Budke CM, Deplazes P, Torgerson PR. Global socioeconomic impact of cystic echinococcosis. Emerg Infect Dis 2006;12:296–303.
4. Gabow PA. Autosomal dominant polycystic kidney disease. N Engl J Med 1993;329:332–42.
5. Garcea G, Pattenden CJ, Stephenson J, et al. Nine-year single-center experience with nonparasitic liver cysts: Diagnosis and management. Dig Dis Sci 2007;52:185.
6. Habib S, Shakil O, Couto OF, et al. Caroli's disease and orthotopic liver transplantation. Liver Transpl 2006;12:416.
7. Kassahun WT, Kahn T, Wittekind C, et al. Caroli's disease: Liver resection and liver transplantation. Experience in 33 patients. Surgery 2005;138:888.
8. Mabrut JY, Partensky C, Jaeck D, et al. Congenital intrahepatic bile duct dilation is a potentially curable disease: Long-term results of a multi-institutional study. Ann Surg 2007;246:236.
9. Millwala F, Segev DL, Thuluvath PJ. Caroli's diseases and outcomes after liver transplantation. Liver Transpl 2008,14.11.
10. Park DH, Kim MH, Lee SK, et al. Can MRCP replace the diagnostic role of ERCP for patients with choledochal cysts?. Gastrointest Endosc 2005;62:360.
11. Russell RT, Pinson CW. Surgical management of polycystic liver disease. World J Gastroenterol 2007;13:5052–9.
12. Soreide K, Soreide JA. Bile duct cyst as precursor to biliary tract cancer. Ann Surg Oncol 2007;14:1200.
13. Tappe D, Stich A, Frosch M. Emergence of polycystic neotropical echinococcosis. Emerg Infect Dis 2008;14:292–7.
14. Thomas KT, Welch D, Trueblood A, et al. Effective treatment of biliary cystadenoma. Ann Surg 2005;241:769–75.
15. Todani T, Watanabe Y, Narusue M, et al. Congenital bile duct cysts: Classification, operative procedures, and review of thirty-seven cases including cancer arising from choledochal cyst. Am J Surg 1977;134:263–9.
16. Ulrich F, Pratschke J, Pascher A, et al. Long-term outcome of liver resection and transplantation for Caroli's disease and syndrome. Ann Surg 2008;247:357.

# CHAPTER 35

# GALLBLADDER: STONES, SLUDGE, AND POLYPS

Cynthia W. Ko, MD, MS, and
Sum P. Lee, MD, PhD

### 1. How common are gallstones in Western populations?

In studies performed in the United States and Italy, about 10% to 20% of adults have gallstones. In the United States, the age-standardized prevalence of gallstones is similar for non-Hispanic white and Mexican American men (8.6% and 8.9%, respectively) men but lower in non-Hispanic black men (5.3%). In women, the age-adjusted prevalence of gallstones was 26.7% for Mexican Americans, 16.6% for non-Hispanic whites (16.6%), and 13.9% for non-Hispanic blacks (13.9%).

### 2. What is the natural history of asymptomatic and symptomatic gallstones?

Between 60% to 80% of all gallstones are asymptomatic at a given time. The risk of developing symptoms or complications from asymptomatic gallstones is 2% to 4% per year. However, once gallstones manifest clinically, the risk of symptoms problems is relatively high. Uncomplicated biliary colic generally precedes development of more serious complications such as acute cholecystitis or biliary obstruction.

### 3. What are the risk factors for gallstones?

- Gallstones are more common with increasing age, body mass index, and central obesity.
- Women are twice as likely as men to develop gallstones. Native Americans and Hispanics have a higher prevalence of gallstones than do non-Hispanic whites or African Americans.
- Men and women with low levels of recreational physical activity are at higher risk for cholecystectomy.
- Diets high in carbohydrates and especially simple sugars, low in vegetable proteins, and low in fiber are associated with symptomatic gallstones.

### 4. What are the symptoms of biliary colic?

Biliary colic is characterized by severe, episodic pain in the epigastrium or right upper quadrant. Pain sometimes occurs following a large meal but may occur without any precipitating events. The interval between attacks of biliary colic is unpredictable. Nonspecific dyspeptic symptoms, such as ill-defined abdominal discomfort, nausea, vomiting, or fatty food intolerance, are not characteristic of biliary tract disease. Cholecystectomy performed for nonspecific dyspeptic complaints will usually not relieve these symptoms.

### 5. What are the three principal factors involved in gallstone formation?

- *Cholesterol supersaturation*—amount of cholesterol secreted by the liver into bile exceeds the carrying capacity of bile acids and phospholipids in bile
- *Accelerated nucleation*—precipitation of cholesterol crystals from supersaturated bile. Certain proteins, most importantly mucin, may accelerate precipitation of cholesterol crystals
- *Gallbladder hypomotility*—gallbladder stasis alters bile composition and allows crystals to precipitate

### 6. Name some drugs, medical conditions, or medical therapy associated with gallstone/sludge formation

- Biliary sludge and stones form commonly during pregnancy. Gallstones are also more common in patients with diabetes mellitus, ileal Crohn's disease, or spinal cord injury.
- Total parenteral nutrition (TPN) and fasting cause gallbladder stasis and promote sludge and stone formation.
- The antibiotic ceftriaxone is excreted into bile. It may precipitate with calcium and form sludge or stones in the gallbladder.
- Progestins, oral contraceptives, and octreotide (somatostatin) impair gallbladder emptying and promote sludge and stone formation.
- Medications, including thiazide diuretics and estrogen replacement therapy, may increase the risk of symptomatic gallstones.

### 7. What is biliary sludge?

Biliary sludge is composed of microscopic precipitates of cholesterol or calcium bilirubinate. On ultrasonography, sludge appears as low-amplitude echoes without postacoustic shadows that layer with gravity (Fig. 35-1). It can also

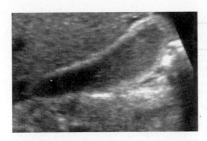

**Figure 35-1.** Ultrasonography showing biliary sludge. Microscopic crystals in the gallbladder generate low-amplitude echoes without postacoustic shadowing.

be diagnosed by microscopic examination of a fresh sample of gallbladder bile. In certain clinical situations, sludge may evolve into gallstones. It may also disappear spontaneously. Sludge is thought to represent the earliest stages of gallstone formation.

### 8. Can gallbladder sludge cause symptoms or complications?

Yes. Passage of sludge of the gallbladder into the cystic duct and common bile duct can cause symptoms identical to those caused by gallstones. Sludge is associated with biliary colic, pancreatitis, cholangitis, and cholecystitis. Biliary sludge can be found in a large proportion of patients with *idiopathic* pancreatitis.

### 9. What is the risk of gallstones in the obese? Why are gallstones more common with obesity?

The prevalence of gallstones relative to nonobese women is increased 2-fold in women with a body mass index greater than $30 \text{kg/m}^2$ and 7-fold in women with a body mass index greater than $45 \text{kg/m}^2$. The incidence of new gallstones in obese women is estimated at 2% to 3% per year, with approximately two thirds of these stones being asymptomatic. Gallstones are highly associated with intra-abdominal adiposity. In the obese, there is marked cholesterol supersaturation of bile. Obesity is also associated with gallbladder hypomotility. Both these factors may predispose to gallstone formation. Gallstone prevalence increases with insulin resistance, which is more common in the obese.

### 10. Why is rapid weight loss a risk factor for development of gallstones? Can such gallstones be prevented?

About 25% of obese patients undergoing rapid weight loss develop gallstones. During rapid weight loss through dieting or bariatric surgery, cholesterol is mobilized from adipose tissue and secreted into bile. Prolonged fasting leads to supersaturation of bile with cholesterol, increased mucin production, and decreased gallbladder motility, all of which promote gallstone formation. Both aspirin and ursodeoxycholic acid may prevent stone formation during rapid weight loss. Some experts advocate prophylactic cholecystectomy in obese patients undergoing bariatric surgery, although this practice remains controversial.

### 11. How do yellow, black, and brown biliary stones differ clinically?

- *Yellow stones* are almost pure cholesterol monohydrate. They account for more than 80% of gallstones in Western populations, and are associated with obesity and insulin resistance. A key pathogenic factor is hypersecretion of cholesterol into bile by the liver.
- *Brown stones* are more common in Asian populations and are associated with colonization of bile by bacteria and/or parasites. Brown stones have a soft, claylike consistency and are found in the intrahepatic and extrahepatic ducts but not the gallbladder. They are more common among Asian populations and may present as acute pyogenic cholangitis.
- *Black stones* are associated with chronic hemolysis, long-term total parenteral nutrition, and cirrhosis. They form in the gallbladder from bilirubin precipitation and are usually quite soft; however, they may contain some calcium salts and be radiopaque. They rarely cause obstruction.

### 12. Discuss complications from the migration of gallstones

Large gallstones occasionally erode through the gallbladder wall into the gastrointestinal tract, where they may cause obstruction. Most frequently, the stones impact in a normal ileum. This *gallstone ileus* is the second most common cause of small bowel obstruction in adults without prior surgery. Stones escaping the small bowel may impact in the colon if it is narrowed by previous diverticular disease. Plain films frequently demonstrate air in the gallbladder or biliary tree. In patients with a bowel obstruction and air in the biliary tree, gallstone ileus should be suspected. Rarely, stones may enter the stomach by way of a fistula and obstruct the pylorus (*Bouveret syndrome*). Cholecystocolonic fistulas also may occur, leading in some cases to diarrhea provoked by the entry of bile salts into the colon.

### 13. What causes acute cholecystitis in patients with gallstones?

Stones may impact in the neck of the gallbladder or cystic duct, resulting in distention and inflammation of the gallbladder wall (cholecystitis). Cultures of bile during the early phase of the disease are usually sterile. Secondary bacterial infection and even gangrene may ensue after prolonged obstruction.

### 14. What are the symptoms of acute cholecystitis? How should patients with acute cholecystitis be treated?

Patients with acute cholecystitis typically have epigastric or right upper quadrant abdominal pain lasting longer than 3 hours. Low-grade fevers and vomiting are common. *Murphy's sign*, an inspiratory pause during palpation of the right upper quadrant, may be present. On ultrasound, patients will have a thickened gallbladder wall with pericholecystic fluid. Hepatobiliary scintigraphy will show absence of gallbladder filling, reflecting obstruction of the cystic duct. Patients with acute cholecystitis should be hospitalized and given intravenous fluids and antibiotics, then undergo cholecystectomy if they are adequate operative candidates. Most evidence favors early cholecystectomy (within 7 days), which is associated with shorter hospital stays and similar incidence of conversion to open cholecystectomy compared with delayed treatment (1 to 2 months). Patients may develop recurrent biliary tract symptoms if cholecystectomy is delayed.

### 15. Should patients with asymptomatic stones be treated? What is the treatment of choice for patients with symptomatic stones?

The risk of developing gallstone-related symptoms is not great (2% to 4% per year). In patients with gallbladder stones, complications usually occur after development of uncomplicated biliary colic, so there is no advantage to prophylactic cholecystectomy. Once complications develop, laparoscopic cholecystectomy is the treatment of choice, with a mortality rate of 0.1% to 0.2%. Patients with common bile duct stones, even if asymptomatic, are at higher risk for complications, and should be advised to undergo cholecystectomy and stone extraction. Depending on local expertise, common bile duct stones may be removed at the time of surgery or with endoscopic retrograde cholangiopancreatography (ERCP).

### 16. What treatment options are available for patients who do not want to undergo cholecystectomy?

Because laparoscopic cholecystectomy is generally safe and effective, it is the preferred method of treatment in patients who are adequate surgical patients. In selected patients, stones may be treated with dissolution therapy. Common bile duct stones may be removed endoscopically. The risk of recurrent gallstones is high with either nonoperative treatment method.

### 17. Who is a candidate for oral bile acid dissolution therapy?

*Oral bile acid dissolution therapy*, usually with ursodeoxycholic acid, is limited to patients with small stones (usually less than 1 cm) that are composed of cholesterol and are not calcified. The cystic duct must be patent. Oral dissolution therapy is slow, costly, and limited by frequent recurrence of stones.

### 18. What nonsurgical methods are available for stone removal or destruction?

- *Endoscopic sphincterotomy* and *stone extraction* remain the nonsurgical procedure of choice for removal of common bile duct stones.
- Large common bile duct stones may be crushed with an endoscopically placed mechanical lithotriptor prior to removal.
- For gallbladder stones, *extracorporeal shock wave lithotripsy* has been used with some success, although this procedure is rarely performed clinically. This procedure is most likely to be successful with small, single stones. Lithotripsy is frequently combined with oral bile acid therapy to maximize dissolution rates. A functioning gallbladder is necessary to expel the fragments into the duodenum during the months after therapy, but biliary colic frequently occurs with lithotripsy as stone fragments pass.

### 19. How accurate is ultrasonography for detection of cholecystolithiasis? Of choledocholithiasis?

Gallbladder stones can be diagnosed by ultrasonography with a sensitivity and specificity of over 90%, where they appear as high-amplitude echoes with postacoustic shadowing (Fig. 35-2). Sludge usually can be seen as movable echogenic material without shadowing. Transabdominal sonography is the radiologic procedure of choice for diagnosing gallbladder disease. Unfortunately, the sensitivity of transabdominal ultrasound drops to about 30% to 40% for detection of stones within the common duct. Common bile duct stones may be suspected in appropriate clinical situations if dilated intrahepatic and common ducts are visualized.

### 20. What is the role of magnetic resonance cholangiopancreatography in diagnosing common bile duct stones?

Magnetic resonance cholangiopancreatography (MRCP) has high sensitivity (greater than 90%) and specificity (greater

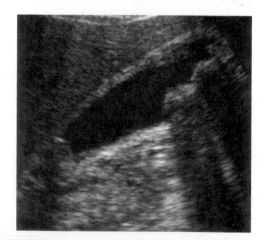

**Figure 35-2.** Ultrasonography showing gallstones. Stones appear as high-amplitude echoes within the gallbladder with postacoustic shadows.

*US Sn 30-40*

than 97%) for diagnosing common bile duct stones compared with ERCP. It is a useful test for the noninvasive diagnosis of common bile duct stones.

*CBD Stones   MRCP Sn 90 Sp 97   EUS Sn 98 Sp 98*

**21. What is the role of endoscopic ultrasonography in diagnosing common bile duct stones?**

Endoscopic ultrasonography (EUS) has a high sensitivity (greater than 98%) and specificity (greater than 98%) for common bile duct stones compared with more invasive methods such as ERCP or surgical cholangiography. It is a useful, less invasive test than ERCP to diagnose common bile duct stones. The choice of EUS or MRCP for noninvasive diagnosis of common bile duct stones depends on local availability, expertise, and costs.

**22. A 65-year-old woman undergoes transabdominal ultrasonography due to postprandial abdominal pain. A 1-cm polyp is found in the gallbladder. What is the differential diagnosis?**

Polypoid lesions of the gallbladder wall include cholesterol polyps (the most common type), inflammatory polyps, adenomas, adenocarcinoma, and metastatic disease, particularly melanoma. The differentiation of neoplastic and benign lesions is a primary problem. Malignant lesions are more likely to be sessile and larger than 1 cm. Computed tomography (CT) or EUS may help in this differential diagnosis. In appropriate candidates with polyps greater than 1 cm, cholecystectomy is recommended due to the potential for malignancy. Smaller polyps may be followed by ultrasound, looking for a change in size or the appearance of new polyps.

*<1cm US*
*>1cm/sessile CCY*

**23. What is a porcelain gallbladder?**

A porcelain gallbladder is characterized by intramural calcification of the gallbladder wall. The diagnosis can be made by plain abdominal radiography or abdominal CT. Prophylactic cholecystectomy is recommended to prevent development of carcinoma, which may occur in over 20% of cases.

*porcelain 20% risk*

**24. What is Mirizzi syndrome?**

Mirizzi syndrome occurs when a stone becomes impacted in the neck of the gallbladder or cystic duct, causing extrinsic compression of the common bile duct. The diagnosis should be considered in patients with cholecystitis who have higher than usual bilirubin levels (greater than 5 mg/dL) or dilation of the intrahepatic or common hepatic duct but *not* the common bile duct.

*Acute Cholecysty + ↑↑ Bili or dil'd IHBq common hepatic NOT CBD*

**25. What is the clinical significance of a low gallbladder ejection fraction?** *EF< 35%*

*Gallbladder dysmotility* is defined as a gallbladder ejection fraction less than 35%. It is often suspected in patients with biliary-type pain who do not have gallstones on ultrasonography. Gallbladder dysmotility may be diagnosed by hepatobiliary scintigraphy with cholecystokinin infusion. Management of patients with gallbladder dysmotility is controversial. Symptoms of biliary-type pain will resolve in 25% to 40% without treatment. In patients who undergo cholecystectomy, symptoms do not uniformly resolve, suggesting that another disorder may be responsible for the symptoms. Thus, further work needs to be done to understand the clinical significance of biliary dysmotility, and in particular the effectiveness of cholecystectomy in treating this disorder.

*CCK scintig*
*Bil dysmotil (∅GS, EF<35%)*

**26. Describe the clinical manifestations and treatment of acute acalculous cholecystitis**

Acute acalculous cholecystitis usually occurs in older patients who are critically ill. Symptoms frequently associated with gallstone-related cholecystitis are often absent, and patients may present only with fevers. Complications can develop rapidly, and 50% to 70% of patients may develop gangrene, empyema, or perforation of the gallbladder. The most useful diagnostic test is transabdominal ultrasound. Hepatobiliary scintigraphy is limited by frequent false-positive results. Management should include supportive treatment with antibiotic coverage of anaerobic and gram-negative bacteria. Gallbladder decompression by percutaneous cholecystostomy tube placement is often effective.

*fever*
*US   Abx*
*P-C tube.*

**BIBLIOGRAPHY**

1. Attili AF, De Santis A, Capri R, et al. The natural history of gallstones: The GREPCO experience. Hepatology 1995;21:655–60.
2. Barie PS, Fischer E. Acute acalculous cholecystitis. J Am Coll Surg 1995;180:232–44.
3. Bingener J, Richards ML, Schwesinger WH, et al. Laparoscopic cholecystectomy for biliary dyskinesia: Correlation of preoperative cholecystokinin cholescintigraphy results with postoperative outcome. Surg Endosc 2004;18:802–6.
4. Boerma D, Rauws EA, Keulemans YC, et al. Wait-and-see policy or laparoscopic cholecystectomy after endoscopic sphincterotomy for bile-duct stones: A randomised trial. Lancet 2002;360:761–5.
5. Buscarini E, Tansini P, Vallisa D, et al. EUS for suspected choledocholithiasis: Do benefits outweigh costs? A prospective, controlled study. Gastrointest Endosc 2003;57:510–8.
6. Cano N, Cicero F, Ranieri F, et al. Ultrasonographic study of gallbladder motility during total parental nutrition. Gastroenterology 1986;91:313–7.

7. Carr-Locke DL. Therapeutic role of ERCP in the management of suspected common bile duct stones. Gastrointest Endosc 2002;56:S170–4.
8. Cirillo DJ, Wallace RB, Rodabough RJ, et al. Effect of estrogen therapy on gallbladder disease. JAMA 2005;293:330–9.
9. Diehl AK. Epidemiology and natural history of gallstone disease. Gastroenterol Clin North Am 1991;20:1–19.
10. Everhart JE, Khare M, Hill M, et al. Prevalence and ethnic differences in gallbladder disease in the United States. Gastroenterology 1999;117:632–9.
11. Gracie WA, Ransohoff DF. The natural history of silent gallstones. N Engl J Med 1982;307:798–800.
12. Gurusamy KJ, Samraj L. Early vs. delayed cholecystectomy for acute cholecystitis. Cochrane Database Syst Rev 2006;4: CD005440.
13. Ko CW, Beresford AA, Schulte SJ, et al. Incidence, natural history, and risk factors for biliary sludge and stones during pregnancy. Hepatology 2005;41:359–65.
14. Ko CW, Sekijima JH, Lee SP. Biliary sludge. Ann Intern Med 1999;130:301–11.
15. Lai PB, Kwong KJ, Leung KL, et al. Randomized trial of early versus delayed laparoscopic cholecystectomy for acute cholecystitis. Br J Surg 1998;85:764–7.
16. Lee SP, Nicholls JF, Park HZ. Biliary sludge as a cause of acute pancreatitis. N Engl J Med 1992;326:589–93.
17. Leitzmann MF, Rimm EB, Willett WC, et al. Recreational physical activity and the risk of cholecystectomy in women. N Engl J Med 1999;341:777–84.
18. Leitzmann MF, Tsai CJ, Stampfer MJ, et al. Thiazide diuretics and the risk of gallbladder disease requiring surgery in women. Arch Intern Med 2005;165:567–73.
19. Maclure KM, Hayes KC, Colditz GA. Weight, diet, and the risk of symptomatic gallstones in middle-aged women. N Engl J Med 1989;321:563–9.
20. Patel NA, Lamb JJ, Hogle NJ, et al. Therapeutic efficacy of laparoscopic cholecystectomy in the treatment of biliary dyskinesia. Am J Surg 2004;187:209–12.
21. Prat F, Amouyal G, Amouyal P, et al. Prospective controlled study of endoscopic ultrasonography and endoscopic retrograde cholangiography in patients with suspected common-bile duct lithiasis. Lancet 1996;347:75–9.
22. Romagnuolo J, Bardou M, Rahme E, et al. Magnetic resonance cholangiopancreatography: A meta-analysis of test performance in suspected biliary disease. Ann Inern Med 2003;139:547–57.
23. Rome Group for Epidemiology and Prevention of Cholelithiasis (GREPCO). Prevalence of gallstone disease in an Italian adult female population. Am J Epidemiol 1984;119:796–805.
24. Ruhl CE, Everhart JE. Association of diabetes, serum insulin, and C-peptide with gallbladder disease. Hepatology 2000;31:299–303.
25. Shiffman ML, Kaplan GD, Brinkman-Kaplan V, et al. Prophylaxis against gallstone formation with ursodeoxycholic acid in patients participating in a very-low-calorie diet program. Ann Intern Med 1995;122:899–905.
26. Shiffman ML, Sugerman HJ, Kellum JM, et al. Gallstone formation after rapid weight loss: A prospective study in patients undergoing gastric bypass surgery of morbid obesity. Am J Gastroenterol 1991;86:1000–5.
27. Stampfer MJ, Maclure KM, Colditz GA, et al. Risk of symptomatic gallstones in women with severe obesity. Am J Clin Nutr 1992;55:652–8.
28. Syngal S, Coakley EH, Willett WC, et al. Long-term weight patterns and risk for cholecystectomy in women. Ann Intern Med 1999;130:471–7.
29. Terzi C, Sokmen S, Seckin S, et al. Polypoid lesions of the gallbladder: Report of 100 cases with special reference to operative indications. Surgery 2000;127:622–7.
30. Tint GS, Salen G, Colalillo A, et al. Ursodeoxycholic acid: A safe and effective agent for dissolving gallstones. Ann Intern Med 1982;97:351–6.
31. Tsai CJ, Leitzmann MF, Willett WC, et al. Dietary protein and the risk of cholecystectomy in a cohort of US women: The Nurses' Health Study. Am J Epidemiol 2004;160:11–8.
32. Tsai CJ, Leitzmann MF, Willett WC, et al. Glycemic load, glycemic index, and carbohydrate intake in relation to risk of cholecystectomy in women. Gastroenterology 2005;129:105–12.
33. Tsai CJ, Leitzmann MF, Willett WC, et al. Long-term intake of dietary fiber and decreased risk of cholecystectomy in women. Am J Gastroenterol 2004;99:1364–70.
34. Tsai CJ, Leitzmann MF, Willett WC, et al. Prospective study of abdominal adiposity and gallstone disease in US men. Am J Clin Nutr 2004;80:38–44.
35. Wudel LJ, Wright JK, Debelak JP, et al. Prevention of gallstone formation in morbidly obese patients undergoing rapid weight loss: Results of a randomized controlled pilot study. J Surg Res 2002;102:50–6.

# SPHINCTER OF ODDI DYSFUNCTION

# CHAPTER 36

*Erik Springer, MD, and*
*Raj J. Shah, MD*

### 1. What is the sphincter of Oddi?

The sphincter of Oddi is a fibromuscular sheath that encircles the terminal portion of the common bile duct, main pancreatic duct (Wirsung), and common channel in the second portion of the duodenum. It is made up of smooth muscle. Three interconnected sphincters exist: choledochus, pancreaticus, and ampullae Fig. 36-1. Ruggero Oddi, as a medical student, published the early morphologic observations of the sphincter in 1887.

### 2. How does the sphincter of Oddi function?

- Regulates bile and pancreatic juice into the duodenum
- Reduces duodenal reflux into the pancreatic and biliary ducts
- Contracts tonically during the interdigestive period to promote gallbladder filling
- Contracts phasically in the digestive period to promote flow of bile into the duodenum.

Its activity is increased by cholinergic stimulation. Endogenous substances also control the sphincter. Motilin increases the intensity of sphincter contractions. Cholecystokinin (CCK) is induced by food intake and stimulates contraction of the gallbladder and relaxation of the sphincter. Vasoactive intestinal peptide (VIP) and nitric oxide promote sphincter relaxation.

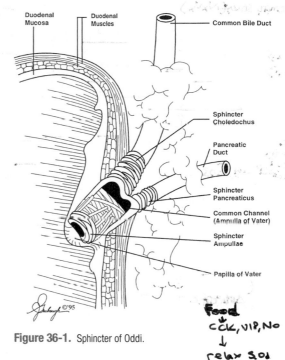

**Figure 36-1.** Sphincter of Oddi.

### 3. What is sphincter of Oddi dysfunction (SOD)?

SOD is a benign disorder characterized by a functional or structural obstruction at the level of the sphincter of Oddi. It is suspected in patients presenting with upper abdominal pain suggestive of a biliary or pancreatic origin. Objective measures such as transient elevations in liver or pancreatic enzymes and ductal dilation on noninvasive imaging are sought to support the clinical suspicion.

### 4. Describe the pathophysiology of SOD.

There are two abnormalities that can lead to SOD, and both may be present in a single patient. One is a primary motor abnormality of the sphincter termed *biliary dyskinesia* or *spasm* (elevated pressure). The other is fibrosis or inflammation, most likely from recurrent passage of biliary stones/microlithiasis. Symptoms may be more pronounced following cholecystectomy due to the loss of the ability to decompress elevated biliary pressure when the gallbladder distends. Further, it has been postulated that cholecystectomy may sever neuroinhibitory pathways that normally cause sphincter relaxation in response to increased biliary pressure. However, SOD is also identified in patients with an intact gallbladder.

### 5. Name typical symptoms of SOD.

Symptoms can be either biliary or pancreatic in nature. Pain is located in the epigastrium or right upper quadrant with radiation to the back or the right infrascapular region and may be meal related. It is episodic or continuous with periodic exacerbations. Symptoms compatible with irritable bowel syndrome or nonulcer dyspepsia often coexist. Another manifestation is *idiopathic* acute pancreatitis as a result of sphincter hypertension. Other structural abnormalities such as costochondritis, ulcer, gastroesophageal reflux disease, malignancy, biliary stones, and chronic pancreatitis must be ruled out before the diagnosis of SOD is pursued.

**6. Who is at risk for SOD?**

*[handwritten: 30-50F 1y. post CCY]*

Woman in their third through fifth decades of life are at risk; the female predominance is as high as 90%. Symptoms often become apparent after cholecystectomy (hence the older term *post-cholecystectomy syndrome*), but in many cases patients will have had empiric cholecystectomy for pain that was thought to originate from the gallbladder.

**7. How common is SOD?**

The incidence in patients who have undergone cholecystectomy has been estimated to be approximately 1%.

**8. What diagnostic evaluation should be considered in a patient presenting with symptoms suggestive of SOD?**

*[handwritten: H&P, PC/LFTS, US/CT, +/- DGD, 24hPH, +/- g.empty studies (Nxvx)]*

A thorough history and physical exam will often determine which diagnostic testing is required prior to pursuing a diagnosis of SOD. The physical exam during a flare of pain often reveals a non–toxic-appearing patient with tenderness in the epigastrium or right upper quadrant. Hepatic enzymes and pancreatic enzymes should be obtained during or soon after any flare of pain. Imaging with ultrasound or computed tomography (CT) is performed to exclude cholelithiasis, chronic pancreatitis, or other intra-abdominal pathology. If nausea and vomiting is a predominant feature, then gastric emptying studies can be considered. If dyspeptic or reflux-type symptoms are apparent, then a 24-hour esophageal pH study or upper endoscopy is reasonable.

**9. Are there noninvasive tests that may be used to diagnose SOD?**

*[handwritten: CCK us scintig]*

In general, these tests are not definitive but may be used to suggest a diagnosis of SOD. Provocation studies involve a stimulus with a fatty meal or CCK and ultrasound imaging to assess for an abnormal increase of the bile duct diameter (greater than 2 mm). The Nardi provocation test involves the administration of morphine and neostigmine to increase sphincter pressure and pancreatic secretion, respectively, and is considered positive if pain or elevation in hepatic enzymes occurs. Hepatobiliary scintigraphy uses a technetium-99 m–labeled dye that is hepatically excreted and assesses for delayed biliary drainage. Secretin is used to evaluate for outflow obstruction in the pancreatic duct by assessing pancreatic duct diameter with transabdominal ultrasound or magnetic resonance cholangiopancreatography (MRCP). In general, if there is a sustained dilation (longer than 30 minutes), the test is considered positive. Secretin-stimulated MRCP has been

*[handwritten: SOD 2 secretin MRCP pre ERCP not S2/3]*

used in identifying patients with suspected SOD Type II (see later for SOD classifications) who are likely to benefit from sphincterotomy but insensitive to predict abnormal manometry in those with suspected SOD Type III.

**10. When should you consider endoscopic retrograde cholangiopancreatography (ERCP) with sphincter of Oddi manometry (SOM)?**

SOM should be considered in those patients with symptoms that are significantly disrupting the patient's quality of life, when an alternative diagnosis is not identified, and after failed therapeutic medication trials. Since there is often an overlap with dysmotility or irritable bowel syndrome–type symptoms, antispasmodics and low-dose antidepressants/selective serotonin reuptake inhibitor (SSRIs) should initially be tried. Narcotic-requiring pain may suggest a need for manometric studies; however, these medications interfere with accurate pressure measurements. Ideally, manometry should be performed prior to patients becoming narcotic dependent.

*[handwritten: Antispastic]*

**11. How is SOM performed, and what manometric criteria define SOD?**

Deep cannulation of the biliary or pancreatic duct is required during ERCP. SOM is most commonly performed using a water perfusion, aspirating catheter. A microtransducer solid state manometry catheter is also available, which eliminates volume loading of the pancreatic ductal system. In one small study, a comparison between the two catheter systems demonstrated a reduction in post-ERCP pancreatitis using the microtransducer catheter. Either system requires the catheter be attached to external transducers as the recordings are displayed and recorded on a computer monitor or paper strip. Prior to performing pull-through measurements across the sphincter, a duodenal baseline is obtained. The major criterion for SOD is defined as a mean basal pressure increase of 35 or 40 mm Hg [or greater] (upper limits of normal for the solid state or perfusion catheter systems, respectively) above the duodenal baseline for a 30-second duration, on two separate pull-throughs, and across both proximal and distal leads. Less-established criteria assess basal ductal pressure, phasic sphincter contractile frequency and amplitude, and phasic contractile duration.

**12. Which medications can interfere with SOM pressure measurements?**

Narcotics and smooth muscle relaxants should be held prior to the procedure. During the ERCP, narcotic analgesia and antimotility agents (i.e., glucagon) should be avoided. Benzodiazepines or propofol are predominantly used, as they do not appear to affect sphincter pressure. One study has shown, however, that meperidine had no effect on the basal sphincter pressure. Nevertheless, it is still generally avoided or limited to 1 mg/kg.

**13. What are the possible complications of ERCP with SOM?**

These are similar to ERCP performed for other indications and include post-ERCP pancreatitis (PEP), cholangitis, perforation, bleeding, and sedation- or anesthesia-related adverse events. Suspected SOD is an independent risk factor for the development of PEP and ranges from 15% to 30%.

Factors that increase PEP include difficult cannulation, number of pancreatic duct injections, female gender, and a prior episode of pancreatitis or PEP.

## 14. In multivariate analysis, have any preprocedural pharmacologic agents been shown to help reduce post-ERCP pancreatitis in patients with suspected SOD?

Well-designed studies utilizing gabexate, allopurinol, corticosteroids, and octreotide have failed to show efficacy. However, a meta-analysis of four randomized controlled trials using rectally administered nonsteroidal anti-inflammatory drugs (NSAIDs) did seem to reduce PEP risk but further multicenter studies are required before widespread application.

## 15. What is the Milwaukee classification?

The standard categorization of SOD is the Milwaukee classification (also known as Geenan-Hogan) generally applied in the postcholecystectomy patient. Classification is performed before SOM and is predictive of the frequency of abnormal SOM and symptomatic response to sphincterotomy. Currently, the Modified Milwaukee criteria (less stringent than the original Milwaukee criteria) are used. Abnormal laboratory values during an episode of pain should normalize in the absence of pain to be consistent with transient outflow obstruction and SOD. The schemes are similar for both biliary and pancreatic types (Tables 36-1 and 36-2).

**Table 36-1.** Modified Milwaukee Classification: Biliary

| Type I | Biliary type pain, ALT/AST/Alk Phos >1.1× ULN, bile duct > 10 mm |
| Type II | Biliary type pain and either ALT/AST/Alk Phos >1.1× ULN or bile duct > 10 mm |
| Type III | Biliary type pain only |

ALT, alanine aminotransferase; AST, aspartate aminotransferase; Alk Phos, alkaline phosphatase; ULN, upper limit of normal.

**Table 36-2.** Modified Milwaukee Classification: Pancreatic

| Type I | Pancreatic type pain, and amylase/lipase >ULN and dilated pancreatic duct* |
| Type II | Pancreatic type pain and either amylase/lipase >ULN or dilated pancreatic duct* |
| Type III | Pancreatic type pain only |

*Pancreatic duct >6mm in the head and >5mm in the body of the pancreas
ULN, upper limit of normal

Table 36-3 displays the results of studies in which patients were stratified into SOD types before SOM. The right column gives the percentage of those who had biliary sphincter hypertension. In general, it is thought that patients with SOD Type I or II are more likely to have a structural outflow obstruction (i.e., stenosis) versus SOD Type III patients, who are more likely to have a functional problem with the sphincter.

**Table 36-3.** Percentage of Patients in SOD Patients (Types I,II,III) with Elevated Basal Sphincter Pressure

| SUSPECTED BILIARY SOD TYPE | ELEVATED BASAL SPHINCTER PRESSURE |
| --- | --- |
| I | >90% |
| II | 55% to 65% |
| III | 25% to 60% |

From: Sherman S . What is the role of ERCP in the setting of abdominal pain of pancreatic or biliary origin (suspected sphincter of Oddi dysfunction)? Gastrointest Endosc 2002;56 (Suppl):S258–66.
Silverman WB, Slivka A, Rabinovitz M, et al. Hybrid classification of sphincter of Oddi dysfunction based on simplified Milwaukee criteria. Dig Dis Sci 2001;46:278–81.

## 16. Does normal SOM on one occasion rule out SOD?

No, SOD has been documented in patients with persistent symptoms who have previously had normal sphincter pressures.

## 17. Are there medicines to treat SOD?

SOD, especially milder cases, can be treated medically. A low-fat diet to decrease pancreaticobiliary stimulation may improve symptoms. The improvement, however, can also be related to concomitant upper intestinal tract dysmotility as fat increases gastric emptying time. Pharmacologic therapy has also been investigated. Medications that decrease the pressure of the sphincter (such as calcium channel blockers and nitrates) have been shown to reduce symptoms in some patients. However, treatment is often hampered by side effects. Antispasmodic agents may be useful as well.

### 18. How is SOD treated endoscopically?

The standard endoscopic treatment for SOD is sphincterotomy. Manometry is deferred in patients with Type I SOD because of the high clinical response rate. In SOD Type II and III patients, manometry should be performed to document either biliary or pancreatic sphincter hypertension. Only those with sphincter hypertension are expected to have benefit from sphincterotomy.

### 19. What is the clinical response rate of sphincterotomy for treatment of SOD?

It is dependent on the initial SOD classification. There is a higher response in patients with SOD Type I. If benefit is achieved, improvement is generally long term (years) in the absence of restenosis of the sphincterotomy (Table 36-4).

**Table 36-4.** Response Rate of Sphincterotomy

| SOD TYPE | PAIN RELIEF FROM SPHINCTEROTOMY IF SOM IS ABNORMAL | PAIN RELIEF FROM SPHINCTEROTOMY IF SOM IS NORMAL |
| --- | --- | --- |
| I | >90% | >90% |
| II | 85% | 35% |
| III | 55% to 65% | <10% |

SOD, sphincter of Oddi dysfunction; SOM, sphincter of Oddi manometry.

### 20. Can pharmacologic agents cause clinical SOD?

Yes. Among the most notable substances are opiates. Increased pressure in the biliary duct has been documented following administration of fentanyl and morphine. Some patients will experience biliary-type pain following use of these agents. In addition, SOD has been documented in a series of male opium addicts. It is theorized that long-term opium use leads to sphincter hypertension and sustained dysfunction.

### 21. During manometry, which segment (biliary or pancreatic) should be studied?

In general, the segment that is studied is based on objective parameters such as biochemical abnormalities or imaging. In Type III cases, biliary sphincterotomy for elevated pressures is the usual initial intervention reserving pancreatic manometry for those patients who fail to respond. In the case of recurrent idiopathic pancreatitis, if biliary manometry were normal, then one would proceed with pancreatic manometry. Others advocate measuring both sphincters during the same procedure since there may be up to a 40% discordance of abnormal pressures between the two sphincters.

### 22. In SOD patients, when should the pancreatic duct be stented?

In patients undergoing biliary sphincterotomy for SOD, prophylactic pancreatic stenting in the setting of pancreatic sphincter hypertension reduces the incidence of PEP compared to those who did not receive a stent (7% versus 26%). Further, stenting reduces PEP in patients with suspected SOD and normal biductal manometry results (2.4% versus 9.0%). Pancreatic duct stenting should also be performed in patients undergoing pancreatic sphincterotomy and considered in those with a history of PEP. A meta-analysis of studies that compared stenting versus no stenting and included patients at a high risk of developing PEP showed a reduction in pancreatitis rates (5.8% versus 15.5%; odds ratio, 3.2; 95% confidence interval, 1.6 to 6.4) with the use of pancreatic stents. In general, however, endoscopist discretion and expertise are required in determining the appropriateness of pancreatic stenting as technical factors may prevent its placement and patients who have a failed attempt at pancreatic stenting are at a higher risk for developing PEP.

### 23. Why do some patients with documented SOD not respond to biliary sphincter ablation?

Abnormal manometry in a symptomatic patient does not prove a cause-effect relationship. It may be a consequence (i.e., chronic narcotic use or chronic pancreatitis) rather than an etiology of disease. One controlled study suggested that somatosensory hypersensitivity of peripheral nociceptive neurons at the referred pain area (e.g., right upper quadrant) in patients with biliary SOD may explain persistent pain. Other potential reasons for a lack of response include an incomplete sphincterotomy, restenosis, concomitant pancreatic sphincter hypertension, underlying chronic pancreatitis, or a disease unrelated to the biliary or pancreatic system.

## WEBSITES

http://www.joplink.net/prev/200211/05.html

http://www.vhjoe.org/Volume5Issue2/5-2-4.htm

### BIBLIOGRAPHY

1. Aymerich RR, Prakash C, Aliperti G. Sphincter of Oddi manometry: Is it necessary to measure both biliary and pancreatic sphincter pressures? Gastrointest Endosc 2000;52:183–6.
2. Corazziari E, Shaffer EA, Hogan WJ, et al. Functional disorders of the biliary tract and pancreas. Gut 1999;45(Suppl. 2):II48–54.
3. Coyle WJ, Pinau BC, Tarnasky PR, et al. Evaluation of unexplained acute and acute recurrent pancreatitis using endoscopic retrograde cholangiopancreatography, sphincter of Oddi manometry and endoscopic ultrasound. Endoscopy 2002;34:617–23.
4. Craig AG, Peter D, Saccone GTP, et al. Scintigraphy versus manometry in patients with suspected biliary sphincter of Oddi dysfunction. Gut 2003;52:352–7.
5. Elmunzer BJ, Waljee AK, Elta GH, et al. A meta-analysis of rectal NSAIDs in the prevention of post-ERCP pancreatitis. Gut 2008;57:1262–7.
6. Elta GH, Barnett JL. Meperidine need not be proscribed during sphincter of Oddi manometry. Gastrointest Endosc 1994;40:7–9.
7. Eversman D, Fogel EL, Rusche R, et al. Frequency of abnormal pancreatic and biliary sphincter manometry compared with clinical suspicion of sphincter of Oddi dysfunction. Gastrointest Endosc 1999;50:637–41.
8. Fazel A, Quadri A, Catalano MF, et al. Does a pancreatic duct stent prevent post-ERCP pancreatitis? A prospective randomized study. Gastrointest Endosc 2003;57:291–4.
9. Freeman ML. Pancreatic stents for prevention of post-endoscopic retrograde cholangiopancreatography pancreatitis. Clin Gastroenterol Hepatol 2007;5:1354–65.
10. Freeman ML, DiSario JA, Nelson DB, et al. Risk factors for post-ERCP pancreatitis: A prospective, multicenter study. Gastrointest Endosc 2001;54:425 34.
11. Frenz MB, Wehrmann T. Solid state biliary manometry catheter: Impact on diagnosis and post-study pancreatitis. Curr Gastroenterol Rep 2007;9:171–4.
12. Goff JS. Effect of propofol on human sphincter of Oddi. Dig Dis Sci 1995;40:2364–7.
13. Kurucsai G, Joó I, Fejes R, et al. Somatosensory hypersensitivity in the referred pain area in patients with chronic biliary pain and a sphincter of Oddi dysfunction: New aspects of an almost forgotten pathogenetic mechanism. Am J Gastroenterol 2008;103:2717–25.
14. Linder JD, Geels W, Wilcox CM. Prevalence of sphincter of Oddi dysfunction: Can results from specialized centers be generalized? Dig Dis Sci 2002;47:2411–5.
15. MoLoughlin MT, Mitchell RM. Sphincter of Oddi dysfunction and pancreatitis. World J Gastroenterol 2007;13:6333–43.
16. Mousavi S, Toussy J, Zahmatkesh M. Opium addiction as a new risk factor of sphincter of Oddi dysfunction. Med Sci Monit 2007;13:CR528–31.
17. Park S, Watkins JL, Fogel EL, et al. Long-term outcome of endoscopic dual pancreatobiliary sphincterotomy in patients with manometry-documented sphincter of Oddi dysfunction and normal pancreatogram. Gastrointest Endosc 2003;57:481–91.
18. Pereira SP, Gillams A, Sgouros SN, et al. Prospective comparison of secretin-stimulated magnetic resonance cholangiopancreatography with manometry in the diagnosis of sphincter of Oddi dysfunction types II and III. Gut 2007;56:809–13.
19. Rosenblatt ML, Catalano MF, Alcocer E, et al. Comparison of sphincter of Oddi manometry, fatty meal sonography, and hepatobiliary scintigraphy in the diagnosis of sphincter of Oddi dysfunction. Gastrointest Endosc 2001;54:697–704.
20. Saad AM, Fogel EL, McHenry L, et al. Pancreatic duct stent placement prevents post-ERCP pancreatitis in patients with suspected sphincter of Oddi dysfunction but normal manometry results. Gastrointest Endosc 2008;67:255–61.
21. Sharma SS. Sphincter of Oddi dysfunction in patients addicted to opium: An unrecognized entity. Gastrointest Endosc 2002;55:427–30.
22. Sherman S. What is the role of ERCP in the setting of abdominal pain of pancreatic or biliary origin (suspected sphincter of Oddi dysfunction)? Gastrointest Endosc 2002;56(Suppl):S258–66.
23. Sherman S, Lehman GA. Sphincter of Oddi dysfunction: Diagnosis and treatment. J Pancreas 2001;2:382–400.
24. Silverman WB, Slivka A, Rabinovitz M, et al. Hybrid classification of sphincter of Oddi dysfunction based on simplified Milwaukee criteria. Dig Dis Sci 2001;46:278–81.
25. Singh P, Das A, Isenberg G, et al. Does prophylactic stent placement reduce the risk of post-ERCP acute pancreatitis? A meta-analysis of controlled trials. Gastrointest Endosc 2004;60:544–50.
26. Tarnasky PR, Palesch YY, Cunningham JT, et al. Pancreatic stenting prevents pancreatitis after biliary sphincterotomy in patients with sphincter of Oddi dysfunction. Gastroenterology 1998;115:1518–24.
27. Toouli J, Roberts-Thomson IC, Kellow J, et al. Manometry based randomized trial of endoscopic sphincterotomy for sphincter of Oddi dysfunction. Gut 2000;46:98–102.
28. Varadarajulu S, Hawes RH, Cotton PB. Determination of sphincter of Oddi dysfunction in patients with prior normal manometry. Gastrointest Endosc 2003;58:341–4.
29. Wehrman T, Stergiou N, Schmitt T, et al. Reduced risk for pancreatitis after endoscopic microtransducer manometry of the sphincter of Oddi: A randomized comparison with the perfusion manometry technique. Endoscopy 2003;35:472–7.

# CHAPTER 37

# ACUTE PANCREATITIS

*Henrique J. Fernandez, MD, and*
*Jamie S. Barkin, MD, MACP, MACG*

## 1. What are the causes of acute pancreatitis (AP)?

- *Obstruction:* gallstones, microlithiasis (biliary sludge), ampullary or pancreatic tumors, papillary stenosis, worms or foreign bodies obstructing the ampulla, sphincter of Oddi dysfunction, choledochocele, duodenal diverticula, and possibly pancreas divisum
- *Toxins:* alcohol (ethyl alcohol, methyl alcohol), scorpion venom, organophosphate insecticides, drugs (which cause 1% to 2% of cases of AP).
- *Trauma:* accidental blunt trauma to abdomen, iatrogenic (endoscopic retrograde cholangiopancreatography [ERCP], postoperative trauma)
- *Metabolic abnormalities:* hypertriglyceridemia, hypercalcemia
- *Inherited conditions:* cystic fibrosis, hereditary pancreatitis
- *Infectious:* parasitic, viral, and bacterial
- *Vascular:* ischemia (after heart surgery), atherosclerotic emboli, vasculitis (systemic lupus erythematosus, polyarteritis nodosa)
- *Miscellaneous:* peptic ulcer disease, Crohn's disease, Reye syndrome, hypothermia
- *Idiopathic*

## 2. What are the most common causes of AP?

Gallstones and alcohol are the most common causes of AP in the United States and worldwide. During the past 20 years, the age-standardized rate for the incidence of pancreatitis has been 16 per 100,000 people/year in men and 10.2 per 100,000 people/year in women.

Alcohol-induced pancreatitis is the more common cause in men, accounting for approximately 50% of the cases (worldwide incidence of 7.9 per 100,000 people), followed by gallstone pancreatitis with 25% of the cases (worldwide incidence of 3.5 per 100,000 people).

In women, gallstone pancreatitis is the most common cause, accounting for 50% of the cases (worldwide incidence of 4.8 per 100,000 people/year), followed by idiopathic and alcohol-induced pancreatitis.

Idiopathic AP, a diagnosis of exclusion, ranks as the third most common cause of AP in men (worldwide incidence of 3.8 per 100,000 people/year) and second most common cause in women (worldwide incidence of 1.9 per 100,000 people/year). Approximately 10% of idiopathic cases are secondary to microlithiasis when followed with abdominal ultrasound or other type of imaging study. Previous studies showed a higher incidence of microlithiasis ranging from 50% to 75% of the idiopathic cases. Therefore, in patients with recurrent idiopathic pancreatitis, elective cholecystectomy can be considered.

## 3. Which drugs have been reported to cause AP?

Drug-induced pancreatitis can occur immediately upon initiation of the drug or be delayed by months; it must be considered as an etiology of AP in all patients.

Studies have classified the drugs depending on their published weight of evidence and the clinical presentation of the pancreatitis after the patient has been exposed to the agent. This classification is as follows:

- Class 1—drugs with positive rechallenge (1A: excluding other causes for pancreatitis; 1B: not excluding other causes of acute pancreatitis, for example, alcohol)
- Class 2—drugs with more than four cases reported in the literature
- Classes 3 and 4—no consistent data to relate the drug to AP.

Unfortunately; this is strictly a classification without hard scientific evidence of cause and effect (Box 37-1).

**Box 37-1.** Drug-Induced Pancreatitis Classification

**Class 1a**: α-Methyldopa, arabinoside, azodisalicylate, bezafibrate, cannabis, carbimazole, codeine, cytosine, dapsone, enalapril, furosemide, isoniazid, mesalamine, metronidazole, pentamidine, pravastatin, procainamide, pyritinol, simvastatin, stibogluconate, sulfamethoxazole, sulindac, tetracycline, and valproic acid

**Class 1b**: All *trans*–retinoic acid, amiodarone, azathioprine, clomiphene, dexamethasone, ifosfamide, lamivudine, losartan, lynestrenol–methoxyethinylestradiol, 6-mercaptopurine, meglumine, methimazole, nelfinavir, norethindronate/mestranol, omeprazole, Premarin, sulfamethazole, trimethoprim–sulfamethazole

**Class 2**: Acetaminophen, chlorothiazide, clozapine, DDI, erythromycin, estrogen, L-asparaginase, pegaspargase, propofol, and tamoxifen

A pneumonic on the drugs that cause acute pancreatitis is "**NO IDEA**"

    **N**: NSAIDs: sulindac, salicylates

    **O**: Other: valproate

    **I**: Inflammatory bowel disease medications (sulfasalizine, 5-ASA)

      Immunosuppressant (L-asparaginase, azathioprine, 6-mercaptopurine)

    **D**: Diuretics (furosemide, thiazides)

    **E**: Estrogens

    **A**: Antibiotics (metronidazole, sulfonamides, tetracycline, nitrofurantoin, stibogluconate)

      Acquired immunodeficiency syndrome (AIDS) (didanosine, pentamidine)

### 4. How is pregnancy associated with AP?

AP in pregnancy is a rare condition. Cholithiasis or microlithiasis is present in 50% to 90% of the cases. Other causes include hyperlipidemia and medications. Most episodes occur after the second trimester and have a favorable overall prognosis. In patients with biliary acute pancreatitis who were managed conservatively, the recurrence rate was up to 50% versus no recurrence in those with biliary AP who underwent cholecystectomy. Therefore, these patients should undergo cholecystectomy after delivery if the patient can safely wait.

### 5. Which infectious agents have been implicated in causing AP?

- *Viruses:* mumps, coxsackievirus, cytomegalovirus, and varicella-zoster, herpes simplex, Epstein-Barr, hepatitis A, and hepatitis B
- *Bacteria: Mycoplasma, legionella, leptospira, salmonella, Mycobacterium tuberculosum,* brucellosis
- *Fungi: Aspergillus, Candida albicans*
- *Parasites: Toxoplasma, Cryptosporidium, Ascaris, Clonorchis sinensis*

### 6. How do parasitic infections caused by *C. sinensis* and *Ascaris lumbricoides* cause AP?

These parasitic infections cause biliary-pancreatic obstruction. They cause AP by blocking the main pancreatic duct and obstructing drainage of pancreatic secretions.

### 7. Is there an increased incidence of AP in patients with AIDS?

Yes. Up to 10% of patients with human immunodeficiency virus (HIV) infection/AIDS develop AP. The cause is usually multifactorial, with drug and infections being the most common. The likely drugs include didanosine and pentamidine. The most likely infections causing AP are cytomegalovirus, *Cryptosporidium,* and *Toxoplasma.*

### 8. How does penetrating or blunt trauma cause AP?

Penetrating trauma results from any foreign body causing damage to the pancreas and disrupting its duct system or parenchyma (e.g., gunshot or stab wounds).

However, the most common cause of trauma that results in pancreatitis is blunt trauma, caused by compression of the pancreas against the spine. This is commonly caused by motor vehicle accidents with compression of the pancreas by the steering wheel or seat belt and is usually seen in adults. Bicycle handle bar injury causes pancreatic trauma in children.

Trauma causing AP can range from mild to severe injury, and the latter may include transection of the gland. Nonrupture of the pancreatic duct causes AP, whereas acute rupture of the pancreatic duct may result in pancreatic ascites or pancreatic duct strictures and chronic pancreatitis.

### 9. What is pancreas divisum? Is it associated with an increased incidence of recurrent AP?

Pancreas divisum is a common (7% in whites, rare in blacks or Asians) congenital anomaly of the pancreatic ducts. It occurs when the embryologic pancreatic ducts, dorsal and ventral, have failed to fuse into one pancreatic duct. Each of the ducts then has a separate duodenal draining site, with the ventral duct draining into the major papilla and the dorsal duct draining into its own/accessory papilla (minor papilla). Patients with pancreas divisum have the majority of the exocrine pancreas drain through an accessory pancreatic duct and through an accessory papilla, prompting pressures to build up. This congenital anomaly in a majority of patients is asymptomatic, whereas it is associated with AP in 10% of patients. It is unclear if this is a cause-and-effect situation; if there are obstructive changes in the dorsal pancreatic duct with dilation, then cause and effect is more likely. A small minority of patients (approximately 5%) with pancreas divisum develop AP.

## 10. What is the relationship between hypertriglyceridemia and AP?

Hypertriglyceridemia can cause AP in up to 3% of patients. It is a more common cause than hypercalcemia. Serum triglyceride levels greater than 800 mg/dL are usually needed to induce an episode of AP. These levels need to be determined when patients are on their usual medications and eating a regular diet. Treatment options are diet and lipid-lowering agents to reduce recurrence after the initial AP episode has resolved. Even patients undergoing pancreas transplantation with history of hyperlipidemia have a high incidence of AP after transplantation.

## 11. What is the relationship between hypercalcemia and AP?

Any cause of hypercalcemia (hyperparathyroidism) can increase the risk of having an episode of AP. There is a 10-fold increased risk of AP in patients with primary hyperparathyroidism compared with the normal population. Possible mechanisms are the calcium activation of the trypsinogen to trypsin in the pancreas and/or calcification and stone formation in the pancreatic duct with resulting obstruction.

## 12. How is the diagnosis of AP made?

The diagnosis of AP is based on clinical assessment, biochemical analysis, and radiologic evaluation.

Clinically AP is characterized by abdominal pain; 40% to 70% of patients have pain radiating to their backs, which is associated with nausea and vomiting. Up to 30% to 40% of patients do not present with the classic clinical presentation of pain or their pain presentation was hidden by other clinical symptoms like coma or multiorgan system failure.

Laboratory data for diagnosis of AP include at least a 3-fold elevation in serum amylase and/or lipase. Other pancreatic enzymes tested in the serum and/or the urine can be used for diagnosis; however, these tests are not widely available. These tests include pancreatic isoamylase, phospholipase $A_2$, elastase 1, and trypsinogen-2.

The role of imaging is in patients in whom the diagnosis of AP is not clinically apparent by history or laboratory findings. Computed tomography (CT) of the abdomen with contrast after the patient has been hydrated is used to determine pancreatic inflammation and severity of the disease and is able to exclude other sources of pathology or any complication. Either abdomen CT with pancreas protocol or magnetic resonance imaging (MRI) with gadolinium is accurate in imaging the pancreas and determining if pancreatitis is present and its severity. These imaging studies are usually done after 5 days, to see if necrosis is present in the appropriate clinical setting to determine if CT-guided aspiration is appropriate in an attempt to diagnose pancreatic infection and may on occasion be used to determine the extent of the disease. In critical ill patients, CT of the abdomen is less difficult to perform and is preferred over MRI.

## 13. How does serum amylase compare to serum lipase in the diagnosis of AP?

Serum amylase typically increases within 6 to 12 hours of AP onset and gradually declines over the first week. Conversely, serum lipase increases within 24 hours of AP onset and remains elevated in the serum for a longer period than serum amylase, thereby making its sensitivity higher compared with serum amylase. Serum amylase levels may be falsely elevated in several nonpancreatic conditions (see Question 14). Total serum amylase is 40% from pancreatic origin and 60% from extrapancreatic sources. Therefore, some studies have shown superior specificity of serum lipase compared with serum amylase in the diagnosis of AP. Fractionation of elevated serum amylase into pancreatic-type isoamylase and salivary-type isoamylase may help in the diagnosis of AP and exclude a pancreatic source.

## 14. What are the causes of hyperamylasemia and hyperlipasemia?

### HYPERAMYLASEMIA

- Acute pancreatitis
- Diseases that mimic AP: pancreatic pseudocyst, chronic pancreatitis, pancreatic carcinoma, biliary tract disease, intestinal obstruction or pseudoobstruction, acute appendicitis, ectopic pregnancy
- Other: renal failure, parotitis, macroamylasemia, ovarian cyst or cystic neoplasm, lung cancer, HIV infection

*HYPERLIPASEMIA*

- Acute pancreatitis
- Diseases that mimic AP: pancreatic pseudocyst, chronic pancreatitis, pancreatic carcinoma, biliary tract disease, intestinal obstruction or pseudoobstruction, acute appendicitis
- Other: renal failure

## 15. What are macroamylasemia and macrolipasemia?
In these pathologies, the lipase and/or the amylase are bound to serum immunoglobulin, which results in a higher molecular mass that is not easily excreted by the kidney compared to the normal size amylase and lipase molecule. This poor clearance results in increased levels of these serum enzymes. Diagnosis is made by measuring the levels of amylase and/or lipase in the serum as well as in the urine. In macroamylasemia and macrolipasemia, the serum levels are elevated but the urine levels are low and there is a low amylase-lipase–creatinine clearance ratio (usually ACR less than 1%).

Conditions associated with macroamylasemia and macrolipasemia include celiac sprue, inflammatory bowel disease, and malignancies such as lymphomas and rheumatologic diseases (connective tissue diseases).

## 16. What cause of AP should be suspected in patients who present with normal serum amylase levels?
The prevalence of patients with normal serum amylase levels who have AP is between 20% and 30%. This occurs in patients in whom diagnosis is delayed, in those with alcohol-related pancreatitis, and in those with hypertriglyceridemia. Serum amylase has a shorter serum half-life than lipase; therefore, check serum lipase if serum amylase levels are normal. Alcoholic pancreatitis can result with pancreatic atrophy and normal serum levels with acute inflammation. One mechanism of normal amylase in AP caused by hypertriglyceridemia is the result of interference in the measurement of serum amylase levels by the triglycerides. It is unclear if diluting the serum sample allows for true values of serum amylase, but when performed, there may be an elevated reading. To consider hypertriglyceridemia as a cause of AP, the levels should be greater than 800 mg/dL.

## 17. Does the magnitude of hyperamylasemia or hyperlipasemia correlate with the severity of AP?
No, the levels of amylase and/or lipase do not correlate with the severity of AP or its prognosis.

## 18. What is the most reliable serum marker for diagnosing biliary AP?
Serum alanine transaminase (ALT) elevations of more than 2-fold of normal in patients older than 50 years has a sensitivity of 74% and specificity of 84% in predicting the biliary origin of AP. Other markers such as elevated bilirubin, alkaline phosphatase, and amylase:lipase ratios are not specific in predicting the biliary source of AP.

## 19. How is AP classified?
The Atlanta classification divides AP into mild and severe disease.

- **Mild AP** has been defined as minimal organ dysfunction and is associated with a self-limited course.
- **Severe AP** consists of organ failure (see later for criteria) and/or local pancreatic complications such as pseudocyst or necrotizing pancreatitis. The level of severity and survival can be predicted by clinical scores (see Question 20) including Ranson score criteria and APACHE II (Acute Physiology and Chronic Health Evaluation) score.

A classification using radiologic images (Balthazar CT-enhanced scoring system) differentiates AP in interstitial pancreatitis and necrotizing pancreatitis. In general, interstitial pancreatitis (interstitial edema and inflammation) is associated with mild disease with a mortality rate of approximately of 1%. Conversely, necrotizing pancreatitis (focal/diffuse necrosis) is associated with severe disease, needing more intensive management and having a mortality rate of 10% in patients with aseptic necrosis and up to 30% in patients with infected necrosis.

The Atlanta symposium defined *organ failure* as:

- Shock (systolic blood pressure [SBP] less than 90 mm Hg)
- Pulmonary insufficiency ($Pao_2$ less than 60 mm Hg)
- Renal failure (serum creatinine greater than 2 mg/dL)
- Gastrointestinal bleeding (greater than 500 mL of blood loss in 24 hours)

**20. What prognostic scoring systems are used to assess the severity of AP?**

The most widely used clinical prognostic scores include Ranson criteria, Glasgow prognostic criteria, APACHE II classification system, and Balthazar CT-enhanced scoring system.

- *Ranson criteria:* Consists of 11 indices measured at two time stages (admission and at 48 hours after admission). Limitation of these criteria is that the measurements are taken in a timely fashion and therefore results are not available for 48 hours. This has a very high false-positive rate, with a sensitivity of 75%, specificity of 77%, positive predictive value of 49%, and negative predictive value of 91%. The score obtained with each criterion correlates with mortality (score: ≤3, 5% mortality; 3–5, 10% mortality; ≥6, more than 60% mortality and more complications from AP) (Table 37-1).
- *Glasgow prognostic criteria:* These criteria reduces the 11 indices used in Ranson's criteria to 8. It is used to obtain the prognosis of gallstone-induced AP. The limitations of this criteria are that it uses SI units (not used in the United States) and is solely determined after 48 hours of admission (Box 37-2).
- *APACHE II classification system:* This scoring system can be used at any time after admission. This score uses age, acute physiologic parameters, and chronic health status to get a final prognostic score. A score of 8 or higher is associated with a high mortality. It is cumbersome to use and is mostly found at specific websites that provide the score after the parameters are submitted. It has an accuracy of approximately 90% (Box 37-3).
- Patients with pancreatitis and poor outcome usually have *SIRS (systemic inflammatory response syndrome).* SIRS consists of the following and can be determined anytime during the patient's admission:
- *Heart rate*—greater than 90 beats/min
- *Temperature* —greater than 38° C or less than 36° C
- *Respiratory rate*—greater than 20 breaths/min or $Paco_2$ less than 32 mm Hg
- *White blood cell count*—greater than 12,000 cells/μL or less than 4000 cells/μL or greater than 10% band forms
- *Balthazar CT-enhanced scoring system:* This score system is based on the *radiologic CT findings* of inflammation, presence of collections, and degree of necrosis. The presence of pancreatic necrosis predicted a more severe outcome (major complication, longer hospitalization, and/or death). A CT severity index of less than 2 is associated with a low morbidity and mortality. On the other hand, a score of greater than 5 is 17 times more likely to predict prolonged hospitalization and 10 times more likely to predict surgical debridement of the necrosis, and the patient is 8 times more likely to die (Table 37-2).

**Table 37-1.** Ranson Criteria

| AT ADMISSION | WITHIN 48 HOURS OF ADMISSION |
|---|---|
| Age >55 years | Hct decrease >10% |
| WBC >16,000/mm³ | Serum Ca level <8 mg/dL |
| Glucose >200 mg/dL | Fluid sequestration of >6 L |
| Serum LDH >350 IU/L | BUN increased >5 mg/dL |
| AST >250 IU/L | $Pao_2$ <60 mm Hg<br>Base deficit of >4 mmol/L |

WBC, white blood cells; LDH, lactate dehydrogenase; AST, aspartate aminotransferase; Hct, hematocrit; Ca, calcium; BUN, blood urea nitrogen; $Pao_2$, partial pressure of oxygen in arterial blood.

**Box 37-2.** Simplified Glasgow Criteria

Age >55 ybears
WBC >15,000/mm³
Glucose >180 mg/dL
Serum LDH >600 IU/L
Serum Ca level <8 mg/dL
$Pao_2$ <60 mm Hg
BUN >45 mg/dL
Albumin <3.2 mg/dL

WBC, white blood cells; LDH, lactate dehydrogenase; Ca, calcium; BUN, blood urea nitrogen; $Pao_2$, partial pressure of oxygen in arterial blood.

**Box 37-3.** Apache II Classification System

**Age**: ≥45 years assigns ascending points to age 75 (6 points maximum)
**Acute Physiology Score**: Points assigned for abnormal values (50 points maximum)
    Vital signs
    ABGs
    Serum electrolytes
    GCS score (15 minus actual GCS score)
**Chronic Health Score**: Points assigned for severe organ system dysfunction or immunocompromised patient.
    Heart: New York Heart Association functional Class IV
    Lungs: Severe chronic obstructive, restrictive or vascular disease.
    Liver: Cirrhosis, portal hypertension, encephalopathy/coma
    Kidney: Chronic dialysis
    Immunocompromised: Leukemia, lymphoma, AIDS, or immunosuppressive therapy

ABGs, arterial blood gases; GCS, Glasgow Coma Scale.

**Table 37-2.** Balthazar Computed Tomography Severity Index

| Grade of Acute Pancreatitis | | Points |
|---|---|---|
| A | Normal pancreas | 0 |
| B | Enlargement of the pancreas | 1 |
| C to B+ Pancreatic inflammation | | 2 |
| D to C+ Single fluid collection | | 3 |
| E to C+ Multiple fluid collection and/or presence of gas | | 4 |
| **Percentage of Necrosis** | | |
| No necrosis (0%) | | 0 |
| <30% of the pancreas | | 2 |
| 30% to 50% of the pancreas | | 4 |
| >50% of the pancreas | | 6 |

Grade of AP (0 to 4) + Percentage of necrosis (0 to 6) = computed tomography severity index (0–10)

## 21. What is the role of serum markers in assessing the severity of AP?

Several serum markers can in theory be used for prognosis and enable us to distinguish between mild and severe pancreatitis; however, data are very limited. These markers are trypsinogen activation peptide, polymorphonuclear leukocyte elastase, interleukin 6, interleukin 1β, interleukin 8, tumor necrosis factor, platelet activation factor, procalcitonin, antithrombin III, substance P, C-reactive protein, and hematocrit (hemoconcentration). Only two of these at present are clinically useful.

C-reactive protein has been used in Europe with good levels of accuracy in predicting severe pancreatitis at 48 hours of admission but not at admission.

Several studies suggest that hematocrit levels ≥ 44 (hemoconcentration) at admission and failure to decrease in 24 hours may be predictive of necrotizing AP and organ failure. This is especially useful when combined with an elevated blood urea nitrogen (BUN) on admission. Both should decrease with adequate hydration.

## 22. What are other prognostic indicators in AP?

Mortality during the first week of AP results from SIRS (see Question 20).

An additional prognostic factor is elevated body mass index (BMI). Obese individuals tend to have severe AP with increased associated morbidity and mortality compared with nonobese patients.

## 23. What are the major systemic complications of AP?

- *Respiratory failure:* due to acute respiratory distress syndrome (ARDS) and found in 20% of patients with acute severe pancreatitis. Exudate pleural effusion, left more frequent than right, may occur, with diagnosis made by the finding of high amylase levels in the pleural fluid more than in the serum.
- *Renal failure:* due to renal hypoperfusion, leading to acute tubular necrosis (ATN)
- *Shock:* due to third spacing of fluids, peripheral vasodilatation, and depressed left ventricular function

- *Hyperglycemia:* caused by insulin deficiency due to islet cell necrosis and/or hyperglucagonemia
- *Disseminated intravascular coagulation:* antithrombin III value of 69% at admission was the best cutoff value to predict fatal outcome, having a sensitivity of 81% and specificity of 86%.
- *Fat necrosis:* suggested by the finding of tender red nodules on the skin (subcutaneous tissue). This is caused by elevated circulating lipase that can also affect peritoneum, mediastinum, bone, pericardium, pleura, and joints; the latter can mimic acute arthritis.
- *Retinopathy (Purtscher's):* very rare complication due to occlusion of the posterior retinal artery with aggregated granulocytes.
- *Encephalopathy:* manifested by several stages from agitation and disorientation to hallucinations and coma.

## 24. When is infection of pancreatic necrosis suspected?

Infection of pancreatic necrosis usually occurs 5 to 14 days after the onset of the disease. It should be suspected if the patient, despite having aggressive supportive care, does not have clinical improvement. Its hallmark is ongoing fever, leukocytosis, and worsening abdominal pain. In this case, CT with contrast is the ideal choice to diagnose and localize the area of necrosis. If necrosis is confirmed, CT-guided percutaneous aspiration can provide information regarding aseptic versus septic fluid, and the patient is treated accordingly to the organism obtained. The presence of gas bubbles within the pancreas or in the retroperitoneum suggests the presence of pancreatic necrosis already infected.

## 25. What is the most common organism isolated in infected pancreatic necrosis?

Infected pancreatic necrosis is usually caused by a single organism (80%). The infection results from bacterial translocation of intestinal flora via hematogenous, biliary, and lymphatic spread with colonization of the pancreatic necrotic tissue. The organisms most commonly isolated are *Escherichia coli* (50%), *Enterococcus* spp., *Staphylococcus* spp., *Klebsiella* spp., *Proteus* spp., *Pseudomonas* spp., *Streptococcus faecalis,* and *Bacteroides* spp. (and, rarely, *Candida* spp.).

Medical treatment depends on stability of the patient. If the patient is unstable, then debridement is the therapy of choice—this is the usual clinical situation. However, if the patient is stable, then adjusting the antibiotic coverage depending on the sensitivity from the aspirate is an alternative initial management decision.

## 26. How is AP treated?

Treatment of AP depends of the severity of the disease and development of complications.

- ***Mild*** AP is treated with general supportive care that consists of intravenous hydration. Fluid resuscitation is the foundation of care and should be started at a rate of 150 to 200 mL/hr, depending on the volume status of the patient. Intravenous analgesia is used for pain control, and if a prolonged period (longer than 7 days) of no oral intake is expected, nutritional support is necessary. Fluid resuscitation should be given to maintain adequate urinary output and can be crystalloid (preferred), colloids, transfusion of packed red blood cells (if hematocrit decreases to less than 25 g/dL), and albumin if levels are greater than 2 g/dL. Nasogastric tube can be placed in cases of ileus and/or nausea and vomiting. In mild AP, there is no role for prophylactic antibiotics.
- ***Severe*** AP has a higher morbidity and mortality. Thus, supportive care should be given in a monitored setting (intensive care unit), and special attention if given to the development of systemic complications and to restoring and monitoring volume status. In the case of pancreatic necrosis, there is no final consensus regarding the use of prophylactic antibiotics. The latest double-blind trials have shown no benefit in the use of prophylactic antibiotics. Prophylactic antibiotics may promote the development of resistant organisms and/or fungal superinfection. Therefore, suspect the development of infected necrosis.

  Sterile necrosis calls for drainage if symptomatic and/or increasing in size.

  If this necrotic tissue becomes infected, the standard approach has been surgical debridement. Regarding the timing of debridement, postpone the procedure 30 days after the onset of the pancreatitis, if the patient is stable. This approach was associated with less mortality but more long-term antibiotic use, fungal pancreatic infection, and antibiotic-resistant bacteria (see Question 25).

## 27. When and via what route should nutritional support be initiated in patients with AP?

Resumption of enteral nutrition should be the goal in the treatment of acute pancreatitis. It should be started as soon as the patient is able to eat and does not have nausea, vomiting, or evidence of abdominal ileus. In mild acute pancreatitis, there is no role for parenteral feeding or nasojejunal enteral feeds, because patients tend to start oral intake within 1 week after onset of the disease. If oral feeding is predicted not to resume for a period of more than 7 days, parenteral nutrition versus nasojejunal enteral tube feedings are recommended. Total parenteral nutrition (TPN) is associated with line infections and increased bowel permeability. There is strong evidence that using enteral nutrition is more beneficial, preserves the bowel function and integrity and reduces bacterial translocation (decreasing pancreatic infection). This can be given via nasojejunal tube feeds. In addition, the costs of enteral nutrition are less expensive than those of TPN. The delivery of elemental or semielemental formulas into the duodenum has been shown to decrease pancreatic stimuli by 50%. Also, a small randomized study showed no difference in morbidity and mortality between nasogastric delivery of nutrition (low-fat semielemental formula) versus nasojejunal delivery.

**28. When should ERCP be performed in biliary AP?**
ERCP with sphincterotomy should be performed emergently after admission when:

- There is evidence of acute cholangitis in the setting of acute biliary pancreatitis.
- There is evidence of a persistent common bile duct (CBD) stone shown by radiologic or clinical features as persistent jaundice, elevated liver function tests, and/or dilated CBD on abdominal ultrasound. The best clinical predictor to show persistent CBD stone is an elevated serum total bilirubin level of greater than 1.35 on hospital day 2 (sensitivity, 90%; specificity, 63%).
- Some authors believe that patients with biliary pancreatitis that is severe or predicted to be severe (controversial) should undergo ERCP.

The routine use of prelaparoscopic ERCP for *presumed* biliary pancreatitis is not justified. In this case, preoperative magnetic resonance cholangiopancreatography (MRCP) or endoscopic ultrasound is indicated.

Patients without elevated liver function tests or evidence of a stone preoperatively should have an intraoperative cholangiogram at the time of laparoscopic cholecystectomy with bile duct exploration if needed. If a stone cannot be removed, postoperative ERCP is indicated.

**29. Should patients undergo a cholecystectomy after an episode of biliary AP?**
Yes, there is a 20% risk of recurrent biliary complications as acute pancreatitis, cholecystitis, or cholangitis within 6 to 8 weeks of the initial episode of biliary AP. These recurrent complications were associated with increased hospital stay.

**30. How soon should a cholecystectomy be performed after an attack of biliary AP?**
It is well established that cholecystectomy within 1 week after the first episode of biliary AP prevents further biliary complications and decreases hospital stay.

In patients with mild biliary pancreatitis, laparoscopic cholecystectomy is considered safe within the first week. Studies have shown that discharging the patient home to undergo an elective laparoscopic cholecystectomy results in 20% of those patients experiencing adverse events that require readmission before the scheduled surgery and that usually the surgery is done 6 weeks after the initial episode of AP.

In the case of severe biliary AP, laparoscopic cholecystectomy should be delayed until after 1 week of initial episode, allowing the patient to recover from the acute episode.

In patients with comorbid diseases who are unable to undergo cholecystectomy, an endoscopic sphincterotomy may be a good choice to prevent further episodes of biliary AP.

**31. Should patients with coexisting alcoholism and cholelithiasis undergo cholecystectomy to prevent further attacks of AP?**
No, cholecystectomy does not prevent further attacks of AP in patients with coexisting alcoholism; in these patients, the disease follows the alcohol-related pancreatitis pattern. Even stopping alcohol intake has unknown effects. However, if the serum markers suggest stone passage, an elective cholecystectomy with liver biopsy and intraoperatory cholangiogram should be considered.

**32. What are acute pancreatic fluid collections?**
Acute fluid collections are accumulation of fluid due to pancreatic inflammation. They occur in up to 57% of patients having an episode of severe AP. They do not have communication with any pancreatic duct and lack a clear wall of confinement. Their pancreatic enzyme content level is low, and most of them improve spontaneously within 6 weeks with conservative management. A minority of these fluids can develop a true nonepithelialized capsule progressing to a pseudocyst formation.

**33. What are pseudocysts?**
Pseudocysts are pancreatic fluid collections that are high in pancreatic enzyme content, associated with pancreatic duct disruption and communicate initially with the pancreatic duct. They usually develop between 4 to 6 weeks from the onset of AP. Their capsule lacks an epithelial lining (hence, their name). They may occur in any part of the pancreas but most commonly are located at the body-tail of the pancreas.

## 34. When should a pseudocyst be suspected?

A pseudocyst should be suspected when there is

- No improvement of AP
- The patient has persistent elevation in amylase/lipase levels
- Development of an epigastric mass after the onset of AP
- Persistent abdominal pain

## 35. What are the indications for pseudocyst drainage?

Indications for pseudocyst drainage are

- Symptomatic (pain and/or abdominal bloating)
- Progressive enlargement
- Presence of complications (infected, hemorrhagic, pancreatic ascites, extrinsic abdominal compression on organs, and subsequent obstruction)
- Suspected malignancy

## 36. How are pancreatic pseudocysts drained?

Pseudocysts that meet criteria for drainage can be treated radiologically, endoscopically, or surgically, depending on location, size, experience of the physician performing the procedure, and relationship with the pancreatic ducts.

- *Asymptomatic pseudocysts* or small ones (less than 6 cm) generally are treated conservatively and followed with abdominal ultrasound.
- *Surgical drainage* is the gold standard.
- *Radiologic drainage* can be done via CT-guided percutaneous catheter drainage. This procedure is mostly reserved for high-risk patient who cannot undergo surgery or who have an immature pseudocyst or infected pseudocysts.
- *Endoscopic* drainage can be performed with the support of endoscopic ultrasound when the pseudocyst is adherent to the stomach or the duodenum. It can be done by creating a cystogastrostomy or a cystoduodenostomy or by insertion of a stent via the ampulla through the pancreatic duct (PD) into the pseudocyst cavity.

## 37. What are possible complications of an untreated pancreatic pseudocyst?

- *Infection:* Diagnosis made by pseudocyst aspiration and may be treated with drainage
- *Pancreatic ascites:* Leakage of the pseudocyst contents or pancreatic duct into the abdominal cavity. ERCP and analysis of ascitic fluid (high amylase and high protein) may be diagnostic, and placement of a stent into the pancreatic duct is a treatment choice, combined with the use of octreotide; nothing per mouth and total parenteral nutrition improve the outcome. If this fails, surgical approach should be considered.
- *Fistula formation:* Usually occurs after external drainage of the pseudocysts
- *Rupture:* Secondary to a rupture of the pseudocyst into the abdominal or thoracic cavities. Manifesting as acute abdomen or pleural effusion. Surgical approach is the treatment of choice.
- *Bleeding:* It is the most life threatening of the complications. It occurs when the pseudocyst erodes into an adjacent vessel (pseudoaneurysm), blood becomes confined in the cyst versus spontaneous drainage to the gut via the pancreatic duct or a fistula formation. This condition should be suspected in patients with AP and gastrointestinal bleed or acute nonexplained decrease in the hematocrit with abdominal pain. This can be diagnosed by abdomen CT and should be treated with embolization of the vessel.
- *Obstruction:* Pseudocysts can cause obstruction of (1) the biliary system (the head of the pancreas, the CBD), (2) vessels (inferior vena cava, portal vein), (3) intestinal duodenal obstruction, and (4) urinary system obstruction.
- *Jaundice:* May be due to the pseudocyst occluding the CBD

## 38. What is a pancreatic abscess?

A pancreatic abscess is a collection of pus in the pancreas that is contained to an epithelium-lined cavity, originally formed from necrotic tissue or an infected pseudocyst. It is a complication that occurs 4 to 6 weeks after the onset of AP.

It needs to be treated with drainage, usually via surgery.

## BIBLIOGRAPHY

1. Arvanitakis M, Dehaye M, De Maertelaere V, et al. Computed tomography and magnetic resonance imaging in the assessment of acute pancreatitis. Gastroenterology 2004;126:715–23.
2. Badalow N, Baradarian R, Iswara K, et al. Drug induced pancreatitis: An evidence-based review. Clin Gastroenterol Hepatol 2007;5:648–61 quiz 644.

3. Balthazar EJ. CT diagnosis and staging of acute pancreatitis. Radiol Clin North Am 1989;27:19–37.
4. Banks PA, Freeman ML. Practice guidelines in acute pancreatitis. Am J Gastroenterol 2006;101:2379–400.
5. Besselink MG, Verwer TJ, Schoenmaeckers EJ, et al. Timing of surgical intervention in necrotizing pancreatitis. Arch Surg 2007;142:1194–201.
6. Brown A, Orav J, Banks PA. Hemoconcentration is an early marker for organ failure and necrotizing pancreatitis. Pancreas 2000;20:367–72.
7. Dellinger RP, Tellado JM, Soto NE, et al. Early antibiotic treatment for severe acute necrotizing pancreatitis: Randomized double blind, placebo-controlled study. Ann Surg 2007;245:674–83.
8. Eatock FC, Chong P, Menezes N, et al. A randomized study of early nasogastric versus nasojejunal feeding in severe acute pancreatitis. Am J Gastroenterol 2005;100:432–9.
9. Felderbauer P, Karakas E, Fendrich V, et al. Pancreatitis risk in primary hyperparathyroidism: Relation to mutations in the SPINK1 trypsin inhibitor (N34S) and the cystic fibrosis gene. Am J Gastroenterol 2008;103(2):368–74.
10. Fosmark C, Baillie J. AGA Institute technical review on acute pancreatitis. Gastroenterology 2007;132(5):2022–44.
11. Galasso PJ, Litin SC, O'Brien JF. The macroenzymes: A clinical review. Mayo Clin Proc 1993;68:349–54.
12. Garg PK, Tandon RK, Madan K. Is biliary microlithiasis a significant cause of idiopathic recurrent acute pancreatitis? A long-term follow up study. Clin Gastroenterol Hepatol 2007;5:75–9.
13. Grochowiecki T, Szmidt J, Galazka Z, et al. Do high levels of serum triglycerides in pancreas graft recipients before transplantation promote graft pancreatitis? Transplant Proc 2003;35:2339–40.
14. Hernandez A, Petrov MS, Brooks DC, et al. Acute pancreatitis and pregnancy: A 10 year single center experience. J Gastrointest Surg 2007;11:1623–7.
15. Isenmann R, Runzi M, Kron M, et al. German antibiotics in severe acute pancreatitis study group. Prophylactic antibiotic treatment in patients with predicted severe acute pancreatitis: A placebo-control double blind trial. Gastroenterology 2004;126:997–1004.
16. Kingsnorth A, O'Reilly D. Acute pancreatitis. BMJ 2006;332:1072–6.
17. Lankisch PG, Karimi M, Bruns A, et al. Time trends in incidence of acute pancreatitis in Luneburg: A population-based study. In:Presented at the 38th annual meeting of the American Pancreatic Association. Chicago, IL; 2007.
18. Lankisch PG, Lowenfels AB, Maisonneuve P. What is the risk of alcoholic pancreatitis in heavy drinkers? Pancreas 2002;25:411–2.
19. Levy P, Boruchowicz A, Hastier P, et al. Diagnostic criteria in predicting a biliary origin of acute pancreatitis in the era of endoscopic ultrasound: Multicentre prospective evaluation of 213 patients. Pancreatology 2005;5:450–6.
20. Maeda K, Hirota M, Ichihara A, et al. Applicability of disseminated intravascular coagulation parameters in the assessment of the severity of acute pancreatitis. Pancreas 2006;32:87–92.
21. Marik PE, Zaloga GP. Meta-analysis of parenteral nutrition versus enteral nutrition in patients with acute pancreatitis. Br Med J 2004;328:1407.
22. Matos C, Bali MA, Delhaye M, et al. Magnetic resonance imaging in the detection of pancreatitis and pancreatic neoplasms. Best Pract Res Clin Gastroenterol 2006;20:157–78.
23. McCullough L, Sutherland F, Preshaw R, et al. Gallstone pancreatitis: Does discharge the patient and readmission for cholecystectomy affect outcome? J Hepatobiliary Pancreat Surg 2003;5:96–9.
24. Mofidi R, Duff MD, Wigmore SJ, et al. Association between early systemic inflammatory response, severity of multiorgan dysfunction and death in acute pancreatitis. Br J Surg 2006;93:738–44.
25. O'Keefe SJ, Lee RB, Anderson FP, et al. Physiological effects of enteral and parenteral feeding on pancreatobiliary secretion in humans. Am J Physiol 2005;289:G181–7.
26. Oria A, Cimmino D, Ocampo C, et al. Early endoscopic intervention versus early conservative management in patients with acute gallstone pancreatitis and biliopancreatic obstruction. A randomized clinical trial. Ann Surg 2007;245:10–7.
27. Pamuklar E, Semelka RC. MR imaging of the pancreas. Magn Reson Imaging Clin N Am 2005;13:313–30.
28. Rana SS, Bhasin DK, Nanda M, et al. Parasitic infestations of the biliary tract. Curr Gastroenterol Rep 2007;9:156–64.
29. Rettally C, Skarda S, Garza MA, et al. The usefulness of laboratory tests in the early assessment of severity of acute pancreatitis. Crit Rev Clin Lab Sci 2003;40:117–49.
30. Schiphorst AH, Besselink MG, Boerma D, et al. Timing of cholecystectomy after endoscopic sphincterotomy for common bile duct stones. Surg Endosc 2008.
31. sphincterotomy VK, Howden CW. Metaanalysis of randomized controlled trials of endoscopic retrograde cholangiography and endoscopic sphincterotomy for the treatment of acute biliary pancreatitis. Am J Gastroenterol 1999;94:3211–4.
32. Urbach DR, Khajanchee YS, Jobe BA, et al. Cost-effective management of common bile duct stones: A decision analysis of the use of endoscopic retrograde cholangiopancreatography (ERCP) intraoperative cholangiography, and laparoscopic bile duct exploration. Surg Endosc 2001;15:4–13.
33. Werner J, Feuerback S, Uhl W, et al. Management of acute pancreatitis: From surgery to interventional intensive care. Gut 2005;54:426–36.
34. Whitcomb D. Acute pancreatitis. N Engl J Med 2006;354:2142–50.
35. Working Party of the British Society of Gastroenterology, Association of Surgeons of Great Britain and Ireland, Pancreatic Society of Great Britain and Ireland, Association of Upper GI Surgeons of Great Britain and Ireland. UK guidelines for the management of acute pancreatitis. Gut 2005;54(Suppl. 3):iii1–9.
36. Yadav D, Agarwal N, Pitchmoni CS. A critical evaluation laboratory tests in acute pancreatitis. Am J Gastroenterol 2002;97:1309–18.
37. Yadav D, Pitchumoni CS. Issues in hyperlipidemic pancreatitis. J Clin Gastroenterol 2003;36:54–62.

# CHRONIC PANCREATITIS

*Henrique J. Fernandez, MD, and*
*Jamie S. Barkin, MD, MACP, MACG*

## 1. What classification system is used for chronic pancreatitis (CP)?

Chronic pancreatitis (CP) is a continuous irreversible inflammatory and fibrotic condition that leads to impairment of exocrine and endocrine function of the organ. The most used classification of CP is the Marseilles-Rome classification modified by Sarles; this classification divides CP into four groups based on epidemiology, molecular biology, and morphology (Table 38-1).

## 2. What is the most common cause of CP in adults?

In Western societies, alcohol abuse is the most common cause of CP, accounting for approximately two-thirds of the causes in most of the retrospective data. A prospective study performed in Denmark and limited to patients with alcohol pancreatitis, showed an annual incidence of 8.2 cases per year per 100,000 population and a prevalence of 27.4 cases per year per 100,000 population. A Japanese retrospective study showed an annual prevalence of 28.5 cases per 100,000 population with a male:female ratio of 3.5:1. This limited epidemiologic information is due to the wide geographic variation and the different habits of the population, with variations in individual sensitivity to alcohol. It has been shown that at least 5 years of alcohol intake exceeding 150 g/day is needed to develop CP. Multiple cofactors may be involved in the development of CP such as high fat/protein diet, multivitamin and antioxidant deficiency, and genetic predisposition.

## 3. What are other causes of CP?

- Autoimmune
- Metabolic due to hyperparathyroidism (hypercalcemia) or hypertriglyceridemia
- Nutritional/tropical
- Obstructive due to strictures (trauma or previous episodes of pancreatitis) or malignancies
- Genetic including hereditary pancreatitis and cystic fibrosis
- Idiopathic

## 4. What is autoimmune pancreatitis?

This is the most recently described form of CP. It is also known as sclerosing pancreatitis, lymphoplasmacytic pancreatitis, or idiopathic tumefactive chronic pancreatitis. It is characterized by the presence of autoantibodies, increased serum immunoglobulin levels, elevated Ig4 levels in the serum, and a response to administration of

**Table 38-1.** Marseilles-Rome Classification

| TYPE | CHARACTERISTICS | EXAMPLE |
|---|---|---|
| Calcifying CP (lithogenic) | Irregular fibrosis<br>Intraductal protein plugs<br>Intraductal stones<br>Ductal injury | Most cases belong to this group<br>Leading cause:<br>Alcohol abuse |
| Obstructive CP | Glandular changes<br>Uniform fibrosis<br>Ductal dilation<br>Acinar atrophy<br>Improvement with pancreatic duct obstruction removal | Common cases:<br>Benign ductal stricture<br>Intraductal tumor |
| Inflammatory CP | Mononuclear cell infiltration<br>Exocrine parenchymal destruction<br>Diffuse fibrosis<br>Atrophy | Associated disorders/autoimmune diseases:<br>Primary sclerosing cholangitis<br>Sjögren's syndrome, Autoimmune pancreatitis |
| Asymptomatic pancreatic fibrosis | Silent diffuse perilobular fibrosis | Idiopathic senile CP |

CP, chronic pancreatitis.
Modified by Sarles.

corticosteroids. Patient normally presents with an abdominal mass and jaundice with complaints of abdominal pain. Imaging shows a diffuse or focal enlargement of the pancreas with pancreatic duct stricture. Pathology reports show lymphoplasmacytic infiltrate. This type of CP has been associated with other autoimmune disorders such as primary sclerosing cholangitis, autoimmune hepatitis, primary biliary cirrhosis, Sjögren syndrome, and scleroderma.

### 5. What is tropical or nutritional pancreatitis?

Tropical pancreatitis is the most common form of CP of unknown etiology that affects persons in areas of India and countries near the equator such as Indonesia, Brazil, and Africa. In some patients a mutation in the *SPINKI* gene has been found. It presents in children and young adults with abdominal pain, severe malnutrition, dilated pancreatic duct with large duct calculi, and exocrine-endocrine insufficiency with development of diabetes mellitus.

### 6. What is obstructive CP?

Any type of obstruction of the pancreatic duct either malignant or benign can lead to CP. Causes include strictures from trauma, calcific stones, papillary stenosis, pseudocysts, pancreas divisum, and malignant tumors. Removing the obstruction can reverse some of the pancreatic damage and preserve organ function.

### 7. What is hereditary pancreatitis?

Hereditary pancreatitis is an autosomal dominant disorder with a high penetrance in the range of 80% that accounts for less than 1% of all cases of CP. It affects both sexes equally, presents as episodes of recurrent acute pancreatitis in children aged 10 to 12 years who then develop CP. Patients with this condition have the predisposition of developing pancreatic cancer with an approximate incidence of 40% by age 70. Genetic testing for trypsinogen gene mutations are specific for hereditary pancreatitis, with the condition found in the long arm of chromosome 7. The most common mutation is the R122H substitution mutation. These genetic studies should be offered to young patients with recurrent pancreatitis, especially those with a family history of pancreatic disease.

### 8. How is cystic fibrosis associated with CP?

Cystic fibrosis (CF) is the most common autosomal recessive defect in white patients. Patients with CF besides the sinopulmonary disease commonly have exocrine pancreatic insufficiency in the range of 85%. CF is due to mutations in the cystic fibrosis transmembrane conductance regulator (*CFTR*) gene. The *CFTR* gene causes decreased and defective acinar and ductular pancreatic secretions, resulting in pancreatic duct obstruction and acinar cell destruction with posterior fibrosis and pancreatitis.

### 9. What is idiopathic CP?

These are the cases that cannot be related to alcohol abuse or other conditions previously described. It accounts for 10% to 30% of cases of CP.

### 10. What is the most common presenting symptom of CP?

Abdominal pain is the most common symptom occurring in up to 80% of the patients. The pain is described as epigastric that radiates to the back, dull, constant, that worsens 15 to 30 minutes after meals and improves with sitting or leaning forward, and frequently is associated with nausea and vomiting.

### 11. What are the causes of weight loss in patients with CP?

These include:

- Pancreatic exocrine insufficiency with malabsorption of proteins, carbohydrates, and fat (needs to have more than 90% of nonfunctioning pancreas)
- Uncontrolled diabetes mellitus
- Decreased caloric intake due to fear of increasing abdominal pain (sitophobia)
- Early satiety due to delayed gastric emptying or gastric outlet obstruction-duodenal obstruction.

### 12. Is steatorrhea an early symptom of CP?

No, steatorrhea occurs when more than 90% of the exocrine function is impaired or insufficient. It signifies advanced disease. It occurs before protein deficiency since lipolysis decreases faster than proteolysis. It manifests as foul-smelling, greasy, loose stools, and liposoluble vitamin deficiency (A, D, E, K).

### 13. Is diabetes mellitus an early manifestation of CP?

No, diabetes mellitus occurs late in the course of CP. Up to 70% of patients with CP will develop diabetes mellitus. Those with chronic calcifying disease are more likely to develop diabetes compared with those with noncalcifying disease patients. Diabetes is caused by the destruction of the insulin-producing beta cell by the CP, which also destroys the alpha cells that produce glucagon; these patients have hyperglycemia with frequent episodes of hypoglycemia. Patients with diabetes caused by CP suffer retinopathy and neuropathy at same levels compared with other types of diabetes. On the other hand, diabetic ketoacidosis and nephropathy are uncommon.

### 14. Are measurements of serum pancreatic enzymes helpful in the diagnosis of CP?

Pancreatic fibrosis results in destruction of the acinar cell with subsequent decreased production of amylase and lipase. These enzymes are not helpful in the diagnosis of CP. Levels may be elevated, normal, or decreased despite clinical symptoms of pain. There is no sensitive or specific test for the diagnosis of CP; however, low levels of trypsinogen or fecal elastase may suggest CP.

### 15. What do elevated levels of bilirubin and alkaline phosphatase suggest in the patient with CP?

Elevated levels of bilirubin and/or alkaline phosphatase in the setting of CP suggest biliary obstruction due to compression of the intrapancreatic portion of the bile duct secondary to fibrosis, pancreatic mass or carcinoma, and edema of the organ. Also, elevated enzymes can be due to alcohol intake or other hepatotoxic drugs.

### 16. What specialized test directly measures pancreatic exocrine function?

Pancreatic exocrine secretions are high in bicarbonate. The *secretin stimulation test*, with or without the administration of cholecystokinin (CCK) measures the volume of these pancreatic secretions and the concentration of bicarbonate after the injection of secretin. This is an invasive test needing placement of a duodenal catheter (Dreiling tube) to collect the secretions. This test, due to its complexity, is not widely available and it has a sensitivity of 75% to 95%. It is more sensitive for diagnosis of advanced disease (Table 38-2).

### 17. What conditions may be associated with a false-positive secretin stimulation test?

Primary diabetes mellitus, celiac sprue, cirrhosis, Billroth II gastrectomy, and in the recovery phase of an episode of acute pancreatitis.

### 18. What indirect tests of pancreatic exocrine function are used?

Indirect tests measure pancreatic enzymes in the serum and stool or any metabolites of the enzymes in serum, urine, or breath after an orally administered compound. Because these studies measure the level of pancreatic maldigestion, the more advanced the disease, the more sensitive will be the measurement. Exocrine function is impaired after 90% of the organ is impaired and these studies are not sensitive in early pancreatic disease.

Some of the studies are:

- *Serum trypsinogen*: very low (20 ng/mL) in patients with advanced CP and steatorrhea
- *Fecal chymotrypsin*
- *Fecal elastase*: more stable and easier to use than the chymotrypsin stool test
- *Olein test*
- *Fecal fat determination*: quantitative 72-hour fecal test. Collected after the patient follows a diet for 3 days that contains 100 g/day of fat.
- *Measurements of metabolites in the urine*: Pancreolauryl test or bentiromide test, no longer available in the United States

### 19. Are plain abdominal radiographs helpful in the diagnosis of CP?

Yes, the finding of diffuse pancreatic calcifications in plain abdominal radiographs is specific for CP. It is seen in 30% to 40% of the patients with CP. Calcifications are not seen in early stages of the disease, so abdominal radiograph usefulness is mostly in advanced disease.

### 20. What other imaging modalities are used in the diagnosis of CP?

- Transabdominal ultrasound (US)
- Computed tomography (CT)
- Magnetic resonance imaging (MRI)

**Table 38-2.** Secretin Stimulation Test

| BICARBONATE LEVEL | RESULTS |
| --- | --- |
| <50 mEq/L | Consistent with chronic pancreatitis |
| 50 to 75 mEq/L | Indeterminate |
| >75 mEq/L | Normal |

All three studies are able to show pancreatic duct dilation, calcifications, pancreatic duct filling defects, and pseudocysts. US has a sensitivity of 60% to 70% and a specificity of 80% to 90%. CT has 10% to 20% more sensitivity than US with similar specificity. MRI shows more detail in the evaluation of the pancreatic duct.

**21. What is the role of endoscopic retrograde cholangiopancreatography (ERCP) in the diagnosis of CP?**

ERCP is the test of choice to visualize abnormalities in the pancreatic duct in patients with moderate-advanced CP. It is consider the gold standard in evaluating the pancreas with a sensitivity of 90% and a specificity of 100%. However, it is an invasive and risky procedure (complications of 5% and mortality of 0.1%). With the development of new technology, such as the magnetic retrograde cholangiopancreatography (MRCP), the role of ERCP has been limited to a therapeutic role. Findings on ERCP suggestive of CP include the characteristic *chain of lakes* beading of the main pancreatic duct, ecstatic side branches, and intraductal filling defects. Also, it can be useful in differentiating CP from pancreatic adenocarcinoma, with adenocarcinoma showing a dominant stricture and CP showing ductular changes with multiple areas of stenosis, dilation, irregular branching ducts, and intraductal calculi. In autoimmune pancreatitis, the main pancreatic duct is narrowed with areas of stenosis.

**22. What is the Cambridge Grading system of CP based on ERCP findings?**

See Table 38-3.

**23. What is the role of endoscopic ultrasound (EUS) in the diagnosis of CP?**

EUS allows excellent visualization of the pancreatic duct and the parenchyma. CP can be diagnosed based on abnormal ductal findings and/or abnormal parenchymal findings (see Question 24). A minimum of three criteria are needed to diagnose CP. Studies comparing ERCP with EUS have shown good correlation of the findings in patients with CP. In mild CP, EUS may show abnormalities not seen in the ERCP or functional testing.

**24. What are the EUS criteria for the diagnosis of CP?**

See Table 38-4.

**25. What is the role of MRCP in the diagnosis of CP?**

MRCP is an excellent initial study for the evaluation of CP, because it is a noninvasive test and evaluates both pancreatic parenchyma and ducts. Studies have shown good correlation with the ductular findings obtained in MRCP with those obtained in ERCP. MRCP visualizes ductular anatomy when a stricture is present and therefore is able to identify cysts not connected with the ductular system. Its limitations are the inability to evaluate areas where the pancreatic duct is small (pancreatic tail or side branches).

**Table 38-3.** Cambridge Grading System of Chronic Pancreatitis on ERCP

| GRADE | PANCREATIC DUCT | SIDE BRANCHES |
|---|---|---|
| Normal | Normal | Normal |
| Equivocal | Normal | <3 Abnormal |
| Mild | Normal | ≥3 Abnormal |
| Moderate | Abnormal | ≥3 Abnormal |
| Marked | Abnormal + one or more of the following:<br>• Large cavity (>10 mm)<br>• Ductal obstruction<br>• Severe duct dilation or irregularities<br>• Intraductal filling defects or calculi | ≥3 Abnormal |

ERCP, endoscopic retrograde cholangiopancreatography.

**Table 38-4.** Chronic Pancreatitis (Endoscopic Ultrasound Criteria)

| | |
|---|---|
| Ductal findings | Dilated main duct<br>Dilated side branches<br>Duct irregularities<br>Hyperechoic duct margins<br>Stones/calcifications |
| Parenchymal findings | Hyperechoic foci<br>Hyperechoic strands<br>Gland lobularity<br>Cystic cavities |

The more findings, the more likely is the accuracy of diagnosis of chronic pancreatitis.

### 26. What is the most common complication of CP?

The most common complication of CP is the development of pseudocysts, which occurs in approximately 25% of patients. Pseudocysts should be suspected in patients with stable CP who have:

* Persistent abdominal or back pain
* Development of an epigastric mass that may cause obstructive symptoms, such as nausea, vomiting, and jaundice

Pseudocysts can be:

* Acute (resolution within 6 weeks) or
* Chronic (no self-resolution and persisting for longer than 6 weeks)

### 27. How are pseudocysts treated?

Asymptomatic pseudocysts or ones (less than 6 cm) that are not increasing in size are generally treated conservatively and followed with abdominal ultrasound. Pseudocysts that meet criteria for drainage can be treated radiologically, endoscopically or surgically, depending on location, size, experience of the physician performing the procedure, and relationship with the pancreatic ducts.

*Surgery:* It is the gold standard. It is done in patients who have had:

* Failure with percutaneous or endoscopic drainage (increases morbidity)
* Multiple or large pseudocysts
* High risk for complications as fistulas or bleeding or pseudocysts near the ampulla or pancreatic duct obstruction
* High suspicion for malignancy

*Radiology:* Can be done via percutaneous catheter drainage, this procedure is mostly reserved for high-risk patient who cannot undergo surgery, for immature pseudocyst, and for infected pseudocysts.

*Endoscopic drainage* can be performed with the support of EUS when the pseudocyst is adherent to the stomach or the duodenum. It can be done by creating a cystogastrostomy or a cystoduodenostomy or with the insertion of a stent via the ampulla through the pancreatic duct into the pseudocyst cavity.

### 28. What are other complications of CP?

* *Distal common bile duct (CBD) obstruction:* occurs in 5% to 10% of patients with CP. Compression of the intrapancreatic portion of the CBD at the head of the pancreas by edema, fibrosis, or pseudocyst causes jaundice, pain, dilated ducts, and potentially cholangitis. If untreated, it can lead to biliary cirrhosis.
* *Duodenal obstruction:* occurs in 5% of patients with CP. External compression of the duodenum by the pancreas causes nausea, vomiting, weight loss, gastric outlet obstruction and post-prandial gastric fullness.
* *External pancreatic fistulas:* occurs after surgical or percutaneous drainage of a pseudocyst
* *Internal pancreatic fistulas:* occurs spontaneously after pancreatic duct rupture or pseudocyst leakage
* *Pseudoaneurysms:* pseudocyst erosion into the splenic vein
* *Splenic vein thrombosis:* due to pancreatic inflammation or pseudocyst obstruction in the pancreas with subsequent gastric varices formation
* *Pancreatic adenocarcinoma:* Patients with CP have a lifetime predisposition to pancreatic cancer of 4%.

### 29. How is distal CBD obstruction diagnosed and treated?

Distal CBD obstruction should be suspected in the setting of CP with elevated alkaline phosphatase, as an early finding. Subsequently, jaundice and/or ascending cholangitis may occur. They are caused by inflammation, fibrosis, or pseudocyst formation at the head of the pancreas. Imaging studies such as ERCP or MRCP may demonstrate narrowing of the distal CBD in form of gradual tapering, bird beak stenosis or hourglass stricture.

Treatment options: In the case of no complications (cholangitis, secondary biliary cirrhosis), observe the patients for less than 2 months with serial liver function tests (LFTs). If any complication or persistent elevated LFTs are seen, surgical decompression is warranted. Endoscopic biliary stent may provide temporary relief but needs to be frequently exchanged due to stent blockage or migration. For younger patients, surgical biliary bypass with cholecystojejunostomy or choledochojejunostomy is preferred. If pseudocyst is the cause of the biliary obstruction, surgical biliary decompression may be combined with cystojejunostomy.

### 30. How is duodenal obstruction diagnosed and treated?

Duodenal obstruction is suspected in the setting of early satiety and postprandial abdominal bloating or diagnosis of gastric outlet obstruction. It is best diagnosed by upper gastrointestinal series. Treatment includes initial supportive therapy; however, persistent obstruction warrants surgical approach, usually gastrojejunostomy. If biliary obstruction is also present, biliary bypass is performed and may be combined with pancreatojejunostomy, if persistent pain resulting from pancreatic duct obstruction is present. If the patient is not a good surgical candidate, placement of a duodenal stent is an option.

### 31. How are pancreatic fistulas treated?

The general approach for the treatment of pancreatic fistulas includes reducing pancreatic secretions with somatostatin analog (octreotide 50 to 200 µg subcutaneously every 8 hours), and keeping the pancreas at rest by remaining nothing per mouth and total parenteral nutrition. This approach takes several weeks, and sometimes a more invasive intervention is needed.

Other approaches are ERCP placement of a pancreatic duct stent if the site of the pancreatic fistula is easily identified or surgical decompression or resection if there is persistence of the fistula after medical treatment.

If pancreatic ascites or pancreatic pleural effusion develops, large volume paracentesis with diuretics or thoracentesis with diuretics, respectively, may be an additional type of treatment.

### 32. How is pancreatic ascites or pancreatic pleural effusion diagnosed?

The diagnosis is made by examining the fluid obtained from the paracentesis or thoracentesis, which typically has an elevated concentration of amylase (>1000 IU/L).

### 33. Why does the presence of gastric varices in the absence of esophageal varices suggest CP?

The splenic vein travels above the body and tail of the pancreas. Chronic inflammation with CP may lead to splenic vein thrombosis. Splenic vein thrombosis leads to intrasplenic vein hypertension, splenomegaly, and collateral formation of gastric varices through the short gastric veins. Massive gastrointestinal bleed may occur from these short gastric varices. Splenectomy is the treatment of choice if bleeding persists.

### 34. Are signs of fat-soluble vitamin deficiencies highly suggestive of CP?

No, although absorption of fat-soluble vitamins (A, D, E, and K) is decreased in CP, clinical manifestations of deficiency of these vitamins are uncommon.

### 35. Are patients with CP predisposed to nephrolithiasis?

Yes, patients with steatorrhea have high concentrations of long-chain fatty acids in the colon that bind to intraluminal calcium by formation of insoluble calcium soaps. With less calcium in the lumen to bind with oxalate, more oxalate is absorbed, which increases concentration in the blood stream and subsequently in the kidney, producing oxaluria and nephrolithiasis.

### 36. How should hyperoxaluria be treated in patients with CP?

Hyperoxaluria is treated with pancreatic enzymes replacement, low-oxalate diet, diet with low concentration of long-chain triglycerides, and increased intake of calcium (3 g/day) or aluminum in the form of antacids (3.5 g/day)

### 37. Can patients with CP develop vitamin $B_{12}$ malabsorption?

Yes, pancreatic proteases usually destroy cobalamin binding proteins and allow the $B_{12}$ to bind to the intrinsic factor. In pancreatic insufficiency, vitamin $B_{12}$ instead of binding to intrinsic factor, competitively binds to the cobalamin binding protein, which decreases the absorption of the vitamin in the terminal ileum. Vitamin $B_{12}$ malabsorption can occur in 40% of the patients with CP due to lack of pancreatic proteases. The treatment of choice is pancreatic enzyme supplementation.

### 38. How is steatorrhea from CP treated?

Steatorrhea occurs when less than 10% of the exocrine pancreas is functional. The main therapeutic modality in the treatment of steatorrhea is pancreatic enzyme replacement.

Pancreatic enzymes replacement consists of lipase to prevent fat and other pancreatic enzymes malabsorption. The initial starting dose is 30,000 IU or more with each meal. It can be given 10,000 IU before meals and 20,000 IU during the meal to ensure adequate mixing or with and after meals or snacks. Pancreatic enzymes tend to be inactivated by acid. They are available in two forms: nonenteric (easily inactivated by gastric acid, appropriate for achlorhydric and Billroth II patients) and enteric-coated form, which improves effectiveness in the presence of gastric acid.

Dietary modifications are a last resort and consist, first, of restricting fat intake usually to less than 20 g/day and giving medium-chain triglycerides (MCT), which do not need lipase, and/or biliary salts for its degradation and subsequent absorption. These MCTs are given after unsuccessful treatment with restricting fat intake and pancreatic enzymes.

### 39. What are nonsurgical modalities of pain control in CP?

Abdominal pain is the most common symptom of CP. It is important to initially consider lifestyle modifications as alcohol and smoking cessation, small low-fat meals, and the usage of nonnarcotic analgesics. In the case that these measures do not work, a step-up approach is usually needed.

With persistent abdominal pain, the approach can be divided between medical treatment and surgical treatment (to be discussed in Question 41).

Medical treatment for persistent pain includes:

- *Pancreatic enzyme supplement* may decrease abdominal pain by diminishing the stimulation of the pancreas and decreasing the abdominal distention and diarrhea associated with malassimilation. In the case of chronic pain, the best form of pancreatic enzymes is the one with high protease content and noncoated instead of high lipase and enteric-coated form used for steatorrhea.
- *Somatostatin* at a dose of 200 μg subcutaneously every 8 hours may also reduce the pain of CP. However, it has not been shown to be effective in a randomized control study.
- *Narcotic analgesics* may be needed in patients with inadequate control with previous measures; however, significant drug addiction is a significant risk if pain persists.
- *Celiac plexus blockage* by alcohol or steroids has limited results of decreasing pain and lasts between 2 and 6 months and repeated sessions are required.

### 40. Does endoscopy have a role in pain control in CP?

Endoscopy may have a role in the management of pain in CP in patients with a ductal obstruction by a dominant stricture or an obstructing stone in the head of the pancreas. No randomized study with good statistical power has been done to show effectiveness of endoscopic management of pain in CP. Some small studies have shown that endoscopic sphincterotomy with pancreatic stricture dilation and pancreatic duct stent placement relieves recurrent pain associated with CP. Other studies have shown pain improvement after removal of pancreatic stones with pancreatic duct sphincterotomy, extracorporeal lithotripsy, and stone extraction.

### 41. What is the role of surgery in pain control in CP?

The role of surgery is reserved for those patients with persistent pain despite medical treatment. The role of surgery is to decompress the pressure inside of the pancreas. They are technically difficult procedures; however, pain relief can be achieved in 80% of the patients.

There are several surgical modalities commonly used:

- Lateral pancreatojejunostomy (modified Puestow procedure), preferred in patients with distal duct obstruction in the head of the pancreas
- Pancreatoduodenectomy with pylorus preservation or with antrectomy *Whipple procedure* in patients with diffuse glandular disease
- Partial resection of the pancreas, preferred for patients with localized small duct disease usually in the tail of the pancreas
- Duodenum-preserving pancreatic head resection, similar indication as Whipple procedure

Multiple studies have shown that organ-preserving surgeries are better in achieving pain control likely due to less extensive (advanced) disease, but there is no change between procedures regarding preservation of endocrine and exocrine function. Despite surgery, the progression of pancreatitis continues. Several studies have shown that surgical approach is superior to endoscopic therapy for relief of pain.

## WEBSITES

http://www.pancreas.org

http://www.pancreas.org/physicians/physicians_diseaseinfo.html

# BIBLIOGRAPHY

1. Applebaum SE, O'Connell JA, Aston CE, et al. Motivations and concerns of patients with access to genetic testing for hereditary pancreatitis. Am J Gastroenterol 2001;96:1610–7.
2. Barkin JS, Reiner DK, Deutch E. Sandostatin for control of catheter drainage of pancreatic pseudocyst. Pancreas 1991;16:245–8.
3. Bhutani M. Endoscopic ultrasound in pancreatic diseases: Indications, limitations, and the future. Gastroenterol Clin North Am 1999;28:747–70.
4. Brown A, Hughes M, Tenner S, et al. Does pancreatic enzyme supplementation reduce pain in patients with chronic pancreatitis? A meta-analysis. Am J Gastroenterol 1997;92:2032–5.
5. Catalano MF, Lahoti S, Geenen JE, et al. Prospective evaluation of endoscopic ultrasonography, endoscopic retrograde pancreatography, and secretin test in the diagnosis of chronic pancreatitis. Gastrointest Endosc 1998;48:11–7.
6. Choudari CP, Lehman GA, Sherman S. Pancreatitis and cystic fibrosis gene mutations. Gastroenterol Clin North Am 1999;28:543–9.
7. Chowdhury RS, Forsmark CE. Review article: Pancreatic function testing. Aliment Pharmacol Ther 2003;17:733.
8. Cohn JA, Friedman KJ, Noone PG, et al. Relation between mutations of the cystic fibrosis gene and idiopathic pancreatitis. N Engl J Med 1998;339:653–8.
9. Copenhagen Pancreatic Study: An interim report from a prospective multicenter study. Scand J Gastroenterol 1981;16:305.
10. Creighton J, Lyall R, Wilson DI, et al. Mutations in the cationic trypsinogen in patients with chronic pancreatitis. Lancet 1999;354:42–3.
11. Greenberger NJ. Enzymatic therapy in patients with chronic pancreatitis. Gastroenterol Clin North Am 1999;28:687–93.
12. Gress F, Schmitt C, Sherman S, et al. Endoscopic ultrasound-guided celiac plexus block for managing abdominal pain associated with chronic pancreatitis: A prospective single center experience. Am J Gastroenterol 2001;96:409–16.
13. Hamano H, Kawa S, Horiuchi A, et al. High serum IgG concentrations in patients with sclerosing pancreatitis. N Engl J Med 2001;344:732–8.
14. Kloppel G, Luttges J, Lohr M, et al. Autoimmune pancreatitis: Pathological, clinical, and immunological features. Pancreas 2003;27:14.
15. Kozarek RA, Ball TJ, Patterson DJ, et al. Endoscopic pancreatic duct sphincterotomy: Indications, technique, and analysis of results. Gastrointest Endosc 1994;40:592–8.
16. Kozarek RA, Jiranek GC, Traverso LW. Endoscopic treatment of pancreatic ascites. Am J Surg 1994;168:223–6.
17. Lin Y, Tamakoshi A, Matsuno S, et al. Nationwide epidemiological survey of chronic pancreatitis in Japan. J Gastroenterol 2000;35:136.
18. Lowenfels AB, Maisonneuve P, Lankisch PG. Chronic pancreatitis and other risk factors for pancreatic cancer. Gastroenterol Clin North Am 1999;28:673–85.
19. Malka D, Hammel P, Sauvanet A, et al. Risk factors for diabetes mellitus in chronic pancreatitis. Gastroenterology 2000;119:1324.
20. Rebours V, Boutron-Rualt MC, Schnee M, et al. Risk of pancreatic adenocarcinoma in patients with hereditary pancreatitis: A national exhaustive series. Am J Gastroenterol 2008;103:111.
21. Sarles H, Adler G, et al. The pancreatitis classification of Marseilles - Rome 1988. Scandinavian J Gastroenterol 1989;24:641–2.
22. Schneider A, Suman A, Rossi L, et al. SPINK1/PSTI mutations are associated with tropical pancreatitis and type II diabetes mellitus in Bangladesh. Gastroenterology 2002;123:1026.
23. Scolapio JS, Malhi-Chowla N, Ukleja A. Nutritional supplementation in patients with acute and chronic pancreatitis. Gastroenterol Clin North Am 1999;28:695–707.
24. Shea JC, Bishop MD, Parker EM, et al. An enteral therapy containing medium-chain triglycerides and hydrolysed peptides reduces postprandial pain associated with chronic pancreatitis. Pancreatology 2003;3:36–40.
25. Smits ME, Badiga SM, Rauws EA, et al. Long-term results of pancreatic stents in chronic pancreatitis. Gastrointest Endosc 1995;42:461–7.
26. Sossenheimer MJ, Aston CE, Preston RA, et al. Clinical characteristic of hereditary pancreatitis in a large family, based on high risk haplotype. Am J Gastroenterol 1997;92:1113–6.
27. Strate T, Bachmann K, Busch P, et al. Resection vs drainage in treatment of chronic pancreatitis: Long term results of a randomized trial. Gastroenterology 2008;134:1406–11.
28. Whitcomb C, Preston RA, Aston CE, et al. A gene of hereditary pancreatitis maps to long arm of chromosome 7q35. Gastroenterology 1996;110:1975.
29. Whitcomb DC. The spectrum of complications of hereditary pancreatitis: Is this model for future gene therapy? Gastroenterol Clin North Am 1999;28:525–41.
30. Yoshida K, Toki F, Takeuchi T, et al. Chronic pancreatitis caused by an autoimmune abnormality: Proposal of the concept of autoimmune pancreatitis. Dig Dis Sci 1995;40:1561–8.

# CHAPTER 39

# PANCREATIC CANCER

*Sergey V. Kantsevoy, MD, PhD, and*
*Peter R. McNally, DO*

**1. How common is pancreatic cancer (PC) and what are the most common types of malignant tumors?**

PC is the second most common gastrointestinal malignancy with 37,170 cases diagnosed in the United States in 2007. Almost 90% of PCs are adenocarcinoma arising from ductular epithelium. About 5% of PCs originate from the pancreatic islet cells. Other rare types of PC include sarcomas, lymphomas, and cystadenocarcinomas.

**2. What are the common symptoms of PC, and where are the tumors usually located?**

Patients with PC usually present with abdominal pain, frequently radiating to the back; weight loss; nausea; anorexia; generalized weakness; and easy fatigability. It is rare for PC to present prior to 45 years and it is more common in men (1.3:1 men-to-women ratio). Most PCs originate in the head of the pancreas (HOP), and obstruction of the bile duct may cause jaundice, leading to earlier presentation. Jaundice may never develop or develop late in patients with a tumor in the body or tail of the pancreas; in such patients, jaundice usually indicates the presence of liver metastases (Table 39-1).

**Table 39-1.** Pancreatic Cancer

| LOCATION | PREVALANCE | AVERAGE SIZE |
| --- | --- | --- |
| Head of pancreas (HOP) | 60% to 70% | 2.5 to 3.0 cm |
| Body of pancreas | 5% to 15% | |
| Tail of pancreas (TOP) | 10% to 15% | 5.0 to 7.0 cm |

**3. What is the Courvoisier sign?**

A palpable, distended gallbladder in the right upper quadrant in a patient with jaundice is called the Courvoisier sign. Usually it results from a malignant bile duct obstruction such as PC with complete obstruction of the distal common bile duct and accumulation of bile in the gallbladder. This finding is not specific for PC. Patients with distal cholangiocarcinoma or an ampullary mass may also present with Courvoisier sign.

**4. What is the survival rate for patients with PC?**

Less than 20% of patients with PC are alive 1 year after diagnosis and less than 3% survive longer than 5 years. Surgical resection of the tumor is the only curative treatment. At the time of diagnosis, 40% of patients already have locally advanced disease, and more than 40% have visceral metastasis. The stage of the disease at presentation (localized tumor less than 3 cm) and the surgeon's ability to remove the tumor completely are the most important determinants of treatment outcome and long-term survival.

**5. What are the identifiable risk factors for PC?**

Smoking is the most important environmental risk factor for PC that is increased further in those with homozygous deletions of the gene for glutathione *S*-transferase T1 (*GSTT1*). Cessation of smoking diminishes the risk for PC after 15 years of abstinence. The second most important environmental factor associated with PC appears to be dietary influences. High intake of fat and meat is linked to neoplasia, while a protective effect is ascribed to fresh fruits and vegetables. Extensive studies have failed to prove a definitive link between coffee or alcohol intake and development of PC. Predisposing environmental hazards include oil refining, paper manufacturing, and chemical manufacturing. Recent studies indicate persons without a familial history of diabetes that develop such, after the age of 50 years, are at an increased risk for PC. Hereditary pancreatitis comprises a small fraction of the cases of PC, but the autosomal dominant abnormality in trypsinogen increases the risk for PC by age 70 to greater than 40%. Nonhereditary forms of chronic pancreatitis have an increased risk for PC, estimated to be about 2% per decade, independent of the type of pancreatitis (Fig. 39-1).

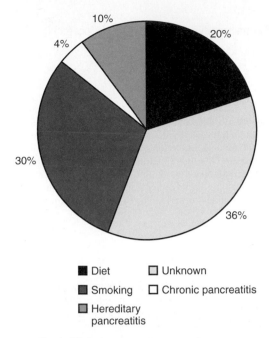

- ■ Diet
- ■ Smoking
- ■ Hereditary pancreatitis
- □ Unknown
- □ Chronic pancreatitis

**Figure 39-1.** Risk factors for pancreatic cancer.

## 6. What genetic alterations have been identified to be associated with increased risk for PC?

Our understanding of the genetic alterations associated with increased risk for the development of pancreatic neoplasia continues to grow. Although identification of more than one first-degree relative with PC carries a substantial risk for development of PC, the precise genetic link for this remains unknown. Hereditary pancreatitis and the tryptase enzymatic defect carry a potent risk for pancreatic neoplasia by the age of 70 years of greater than 40%. Peutz-Jeghers syndrome (PJS) is an autosomal dominant polyposis syndrome, where hamartomatous polyps are found throughout gastrointestinal tract, but neoplasia risk is greatest outside the gastrointestinal lumen (i.e., in the thyroid, breast, gonads, and especially the pancreas). The familial atypical multiple mole melanoma (FAMMM) is characterized by greater than 50 dysplastic nevi and malignant melanomas in two or more first- or second-degree relatives. Other conditions associated with increased risk for PC are listed in Table 39-2.

**Table 39-2.** Conditions or Disorders Associated With Increased Risk for Pancreatic Neoplasm

| CONDITION | GENETIC DEFECT | INCREASED RISK BY FOLD | RISK BY AGE 70 YR |
|---|---|---|---|
| No history | None | 1 | 0.5% |
| One FDR with PC | ? | 2.3 | 1.15% |
| HBOC | BRAC1 | 2.0 | 1% |
| | BRAC2 | 3.5 to 10 | 5% |
| Cystic fibrosis | CFTR | ? | <5% |
| FAMMM/MPCS | P16 (CDKN2A) | 20 to 34 | 17% |
| Three FDRs with PC | ? | 32 | 16% |
| HP | PRSS1, SPINK1 | 50 to 80 | 40% |
| PJS | STK11/LKB1 | 132 | 30% to 60% |

FDR, first-degree relative; PC, pancreatic cancer; HBOC, hereditary breast and ovarian cancer; FAMMM, familial multiple mole melanoma pancreatic carcinoma; MPCS, melanoma pancreatic carcinoma syndrome; HP, hereditary pancreatitis; PJS, Peutz-Jeghers syndrome.

## 7. What are the available serum markers for early detection of PC?

Several serum tumor markers have been shown to correlate with the presence of PC. The most widely used is the carbohydrate antigen CA 19-9; unfortunately, this marker can be elevated in a number of benign inflammatory disorders of the pancreas, biliary disease, and other intestinal tumors. Using a cutoff of greater than 200 U/mL improves the sensitivity to 97% and specificity to 98% to correctly discriminate the presence of PC. Other tumor makers being used or under research for detection of PC are listed in Table 39-3.

**Table 39-3.** Serum Tumor Markers Used in Pancreatic Cancer

| SERUM MARKER | SENSITIVITY | SPECIFICITY |
|---|---|---|
| CA 19-9 | 70% to 90% | 90% |
| CEA | 16% to 92% | 49% to 93% |
| CA 50 | 65% to 90% | 58% to 73% |
| CA 125 | 45% to 60% | 76% to 86% |
| TIMP-1 | 60% to 99% | 50% to 90% |

TIMP-1, tissue inhibitor metalloproteinase 1.

## 8. Are there precursor lesions to PC?

Yes. Careful molecular analysis has lead to the identification and characterization of three precursor lesions for PC:

- Intraductular papillary mucinous neoplasms (IPMNs)
- Mucinous cystic neoplasms (MCNs)
- Pancreatic intraepithelial neoplasms (PanIN)

The common features of each of these lesions are further outlined in Table 39-4. Although characterization of these precursor lesions has been an advance in our understanding of pancreatic neoplasia, management decisions based on identification of these lesions remain difficult. Most would recommend that MCNs be resected completely and examined carefully for small foci of invasive carcinoma. Large (>3 cm) IPMNs should be resected, particularly when they contain a mural nodule or are associated with a dilated pancreatic duct. PanIN lesions are too small to be detected with current imaging modalities, but improvements in imaging techniques and better understanding of the molecular alterations in PanIN may allow for early detection in asymptomatic persons in the future.

## 9. What imaging modalities are used to diagnose PC?

Transabdominal ultrasound is usually the first diagnostic test. Its sensitivity in the detection of pancreatic tumors is around 70%. Computed tomography (CT) and magnetic resonance imaging (MRI) are more sensitive than transabdominal ultrasound, especially for detection of regional and distal metastases. Endoscopic ultrasonography with fine needle aspiration is the most accurate (sensitivity: 77% to 100%) diagnostic modality to detect small tumors and to evaluate the local spread of tumor into surrounding organs and blood vessels. Endoscopic retrograde cholangiopancreatography (ERCP) is sensitive (78% to 95%) and specific (88% to 95%) for PC and frequently is used to perform palliative drainage of the biliary ducts.

## 10. What is the *double-duct sign* in patients with PC?

The double-duct sign, noted on ERCP, demonstrates the presence of stenosis of the common bile duct and pancreatic duct in the head of the pancreas. In patients with obstructive jaundice or a pancreatic mass, the double-duct sign has a specificity of 85% in predicting PC.

## 11. Are there high-risk groups for the development of PC that may benefit from CT and or EUS screening?

Yes. A recent prospective screening of asymptomatic individuals with a strong family history of PC or PJS using CT and endoscopic ultrasonography (EUS) suggest a beneficial utility for this proactive approach.

Listed below are the high-risk groups that should be considered for PC screening at Centers of Excellence with devoted expertise in this area:

- Individuals with hereditary polyposis (HP)
- Individuals with PJS
- Individuals with more than two first-degree relatives with PC
- Individuals with more than three relatives with PC independent of degree
- CDKN2a mutation carriers of a family with melanoma pancreatic carcinoma syndrome (MPCS)
- BRCA2a mutation carriers with at least one PC case in first- or second-degree relative

**Table 39-4.** Common Features of Pancreatic Precursor Lesions for Pancreatic Cancer

| TYPE OF PRECURSOR LESION | AGE | GENDER | CYST-TO-DUCT COMMUNI-CATION | CYST SIZE (CM) | LOCATION | MUCIN FROM AMPULLA | MULTIPLICITY |
|---|---|---|---|---|---|---|---|
| MCNs | 40 to 50 | ♀ >> ♂ | Usually not connected | 1 to 3 | Tail of pancreas | No | Rare |
| IPMNs | 60s | ♂ >> ♀ | Always | <1 | Head > tail of pancreas | Yes | 20% to 30% |
| PanIN | ↑ With age | ♀ = ♂ | N/A | Microscopic | Head > tail of pancreas | No | Often |

IPMN, intraductular papillary mucinous neoplasm; MCN, mucinous cystic neoplasm; PanIN, pancreatic intraepithelial neoplasm.

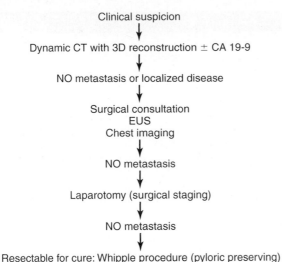

Clinical suspicion

↓

Dynamic CT with 3D reconstruction ± CA 19-9

↓

NO metastasis or localized disease

↓

Surgical consultation
EUS
Chest imaging

↓

NO metastasis

↓

Laparotomy (surgical staging)

↓

NO metastasis

↓

Resectable for cure: Whipple procedure (pyloric preserving)

**Figure 39-2.** Pancreatic staging algorithm.

## 12. What are the new staging modalities for PC?

A stepwise staging approach for PC is shown in Figure 39-2. CT is considered the best first test for staging PC. New three-dimensional CT imaging has been shown to improve estimation of vascular involvement. EUS plus FNA is helpful in obtaining diagnostic tissue and complementary for evaluation of vascular and lymph node staging. Positron emission tomography (PET) or FDG-PET scanning may be superior to conventional imaging techniques in detecting lesions smaller than 2 cm in size, and the use of FDG-PET scanning is growing. Several studies suggest that the incidence of CT-occult metastases ranges between 5% and 15%. This has led some centers to perform diagnostic laparoscopy in all patients who have potentially resectable PC, whereas some centers perform diagnostic laparoscopy only in patients believed to be at higher risk for having CT-occult metastases (e.g., presence of ascites, large primary tumor, markedly elevated CA19-9 level). Please see Chapters 68, 69, 70, and 73 for detailed discussion and illustration of these techniques in the evaluation and management of PC.

## 13. What are the common biochemical abnormalities in patients with PC?

Patients with biliary tract obstruction can present with elevated serum bilirubin and alkaline phosphatase (obstructive pattern). Serum amylase is elevated in only 5% of patients.

## 14. Is chemotherapy effective for patients with advanced PC?

Traditional chemotherapy with 5-fluorouracil has an overall response rate below 10% with no effect on quality of life or survival. Gemcitabine, which in one study demonstrated improvement in disease-related symptoms and survival in advanced PC, is now under clinical evaluation as a single agent and in combination with 5-fluorouracil and cisplatin.

## 15. What is the median survival after the diagnosis of advanced PC?

PC has the poorest prognosis among gastrointestinal tumors. It is the fifth leading cause of death in the United States. The median survival of patients with advanced pancreatic carcinoma is approximately 4 months.

## 16. Describe the role of celiac blockade in patients with PC.

Celiac blockade (chemical splanchnectomy) is an injection of 50% alcohol on each side of the aorta at the level of the celiac axis. This procedure has been shown prospectively to improve preexisting pain significantly and to delay onset of pain in asymptomatic patients. Celiac blockade can be done at laparotomy, under radiologic guidance, or at the time of endoscopic ultrasound.

## 17. What is a Whipple resection?

Whipple resection (pancreaticoduodenectomy) is the most common surgical procedure for resectable cancer located in the head of the pancreas. It involves a partial gastrectomy (resection of the antrum), cholecystectomy, and removal of the distal common bile duct, duodenum, head of the pancreas, proximal jejunum, and regional lymphatic nodes. The procedure usually includes pancreaticojejunostomy, hepaticojejunostomy, and gastrojejunostomy.

## 18. What surgical procedures are used for cancer in the body and tail of the pancreas?

Surgical resection usually consists of distal pancreatectomy and splenectomy. This operation is technically easier than the Whipple procedure.

## 19. When do patients with PC need palliative procedures?

Patients with unresectable cancer in the head of the pancreas can develop obstructive jaundice, pruritus, or cholangitis. These conditions can be palliated by endoscopic placement of plastic or self-expanding metal stents (Wallstent). If endoscopic stent placement is not possible, transhepatic transcutaneous stents can be inserted by an interventional radiologist. When placement of stents by an endoscopist or radiologist fails, bypass surgical procedure (cholecystojejunostomy or hepaticojejunostomy) may be indicated. In patients with duodenal obstruction by a large pancreatic mass, endoscopy with palliative placement of an expandable stent into the duodenum is indicated to relieve the obstruction. If endoscopy is not possible, surgical bypass procedure (gastrojejunostomy) may be performed.

## WEBSITES

http://daveproject.org/ViewFilms.cfm?Film_id=50

www.nccn.org

www.vhjoe.com

### BIBLIOGRAPHY

1. Brand RE, Lynch HT. Genotype/phenotype of familial pancreatic cancer. Endocrinol Metab Clin North Am 2006;35:405–15.
2. Brentnall TA. Management strategies for patients with hereditary pancreatic cancer. Curr Treat Options Oncol 2005;6:437–45.
3. Brugge WR, Lauwers GY, Shani D, et al. Cystic neoplasms of the pancreas. N Engl J Med 2004;351:1218–26.
4. Canto MI, Goggins M, Hruban RH, et al. Screening for early pancreatic neoplasia in high-risk individuals: A prospective controlled study. Clin Gastroenterol Hepatol 2006;4:766–81.
5. Croce CM. Oncogenes and cancer. N Engl J Med 2008;358:502–11.
6. Dewitt J, Devereaux BM, Lehman GA, et al. Comparison of endoscopic ultrasound and computed tomography for the preoperative evaluation of pancreatic cancer: A systematic review. Clin Gastroenterol Hepatol 2006;4:717–25.
7. Gardner TB, Chari ST. Autoimmune pancreatitis. Gastroenterol Clin North Am 2008;37:439–60.
8. Habbe N, Langer P, Sina-Frey M, et al. Familial pancreatic cancer syndromes. Endocrinol Metab Clin North Am 2006;35:417–30.
9. Hurban RH, Maitra A, Kern SE, et al. Precursors to pancreatic cancer. Gastroenterol Clin North Am 2007;36:831–49.
10. Koopmann J, Rosenzweig CN, Zhang Z, et al. Serum markers in patients with resectable pancreatic adenocarcinoma: Macrophage inhibitory cytokine 1 versus CA19-9. Clin Cancer Res 2006;12:442–6.
11. Liu RC, Traverso LW. Diagnostic laparoscopy improves staging of pancreatic cancer deemed locally unresectable by computed tomography. Surg Endosc 2005;19:638–42.
12. Maemura K, Takao S, Shinchi H, et al. Role of positron emission tomography in decisions on treatment strategies for pancreatic cancer. J Hepatobiliary Pancreat Surg 2006;13:435–41.
13. Michl P, Pauls S, Gress TM. Evidence-based diagnosis and staging of pancreatic cancer. Best Pract Res Clin Gastroenterol 2006;20:227–51.
14. Pakzad F, Groves AM, Ell PJ. The role of positron emission tomography in the management of pancreatic cancer. Semin Nucl Med 2006;36:248–56.
15. Pappas S, Ferderle MP, Lokshin AE, et al. Early detection and staging of adenocarcinoma of the pancreas. Gastroenterol Clin North Am 2007;413–29.
16. Soriano A, Castells A, Ayuso C, et al. Preoperative staging and tumor resectability assessment of pancreatic cancer: Prospective study comparing endoscopic ultrasonography, helical computed tomography, magnetic resonance imaging, and angiography. Am J Gastroenterol 2004;99:492–501.

# CYSTIC DISEASE OF THE PANCREAS

*Randall E. Lee, MD, FACP*

# CHAPTER 40

## 1. Provide a differential diagnosis for a cystic pancreatic lesion.

- Pancreatic pseudocyst (about 75% to 90% of cystic pancreatic lesions)
- Cystic neoplasm
  - Primary cystic neoplasm (about 10% of cystic pancreatic lesions):
    - Serous cystadenoma
    - Mucinous cystic neoplasm (MCN)
    - Intraductal papillary mucinous neoplasm (IPMN)
  - Solid neoplasm with cystic degeneration:
    - Pancreatic ductal adenocarcinoma
    - Pancreatic metastasis (ovarian adenocarcinoma most common)
    - Solid pseudopapillary neoplasm (SPN)
    - Islet cell neoplasms
- Retention cyst

## 2. What is the difference between a true pancreatic cyst and a pancreatic pseudocyst?

A true pancreatic cyst has an epithelial cell lining. A pancreatic pseudocyst is lined only by inflammatory tissue; it has no epithelium. True pancreatic cysts account for only 10% to 15% of all cystic lesions of the pancreas.

## 3. Define an *acute fluid collection*.

An acute fluid collection is a collection of enzyme-rich pancreatic juice occurring within 48 hours in the course of acute pancreatitis. It is located in or near the pancreas, does not have a well-defined wall, and generally requires only observation.

## 4. Define an *acute pancreatic pseudocyst*.

An acute pancreatic pseudocyst is a collection of pancreatic juice enclosed by a wall of nonepithelialized granulation tissue that arises due to acute pancreatitis. It requires at least 4 weeks to form and contains no significant solid debris.

## 5. Define a *chronic pancreatic pseudocyst*.

A chronic pancreatic pseudocyst is a collection of pancreatic juice enclosed by a wall of fibrous or granulation tissue. It arises from pancreatic duct leaks due to pancreatic duct stones or strictures associated with chronic pancreatitis.

## 6. Describe the typical clinical presentation of a pancreatic pseudocyst.

Formation of a pancreatic pseudocyst should be suspected if a patient with acute pancreatitis develops any of the following:

- Failure of acute pancreatitis symptoms to resolve after about 7 to 10 days
- Recurrence of acute pancreatitis symptoms after initial improvement
- Epigastric abdominal mass
- Persistently elevated serum amylase
- Obstructive jaundice

## 7. What criteria suggest that a pseudocyst will not resolve spontaneously?

A pancreatic pseudocyst has a low probability of spontaneous resolution if there is concurrent evidence of chronic pancreatitis, such as pancreatic calcifications, or if the pseudocyst is a consequence of traumatic pancreatitis. The strict criteria of drainage required for a pseudocyst whose diameter is greater than 6 cm or that persists for longer than 6 weeks are no longer accepted as absolute.

## 8. When should a pseudocyst be drained?

A pseudocyst should be drained if it causes symptoms, increases in size, shows evidence of infection, causes critical compression of an adjacent structure such as the bile duct, or is complicated by internal hemorrhage. Asymptomatic pseudocysts may be observed carefully, regardless of size or duration.

**9. Compare the three methods for draining a pancreatic pseudocyst.**

- *Surgical drainage* is the procedure of choice for patients in whom a cystic neoplasm cannot be ruled out. An intraoperative biopsy of the cyst wall can confirm the presence or absence of a malignant epithelial cell lining. Surgical drainage also is indicated for patients who have multiple or recurrent pseudocysts or concurrent pancreatic duct stricture. Surgical drainage of a thin-walled pseudocyst should be delayed for 4 to 6 weeks. This delay allows thickening and maturation of the pseudocyst wall, thus increasing the holding power of sutures.
- *Percutaneous catheter drainage* is preferred for high-risk patients with symptomatic thin-walled or expanding pseudocysts or infected pseudocysts. This method should not be used in patients who have a main pancreatic duct stricture because of the high risk of creating a pancreaticocutaneous fistula.
- *Endoscopic drainage* may be considered for selected patients. The outcome of endoscopic drainage is highly dependent on the skill and expertise of the endoscopist. In actual practice, the choice of drainage procedure usually depends on the skills and resources available, as well as the individual patient characteristics.

**10. What criteria suggest that a pancreatic pseudocyst may undergo successful endoscopic drainage?**

- Endoscopic retrograde cholangiopancreatography (ERCP) demonstrates a communication between the pseudocyst and the main pancreatic duct.
- The pseudocyst impinges on and is adherent to the wall of the stomach or duodenum, creating an endoluminal bulge. Imaging with endoscopic ultrasonography (EUS) and computed tomography (CT) is recommended to confirm close contact between the pseudocyst and adjacent gastric or duodenal wall, to avoid puncturing large submucosal blood vessels, to rule out the presence of a pseudoaneurysm, and to help distinguish a true pseudocyst from a cystic neoplasm.
- Endoscopic drainage is more likely to be successful with chronic pseudocysts (about 90%) compared with acute pseudocysts (about 70%). A pseudocyst with a wall greater than 1 cm thick is a poor candidate for endoscopic drainage because of the difficulty in puncturing the pseudocyst wall.

**11. Describe a pancreatic abscess.**

A pancreatic abscess is a circumscribed intra-abdominal collection of pus containing little or no pancreatic necrosis caused by acute pancreatitis or pancreatic trauma. A pancreatic abscess may appear as an ill-defined, nonenhancing fluid collection of mixed densities. Unfortunately, this CT appearance may be confused with a noninfected pseudocyst. The presence of gas within the cystic area strongly suggests infection by gas-forming organisms.

**12. What clinical criteria suggest the development of a pancreatic abscess?**

A pancreatic abscess typically develops from secondary bacterial infection of necrotic pancreatic tissue during an episode of acute pancreatitis. The abscess often causes temperatures greater than 38.5 °C, leukocytosis greater than 10,000 cells/mm$^3$, and increasing abdominal pain. All of these signs also may be found in noninfected patients with severe pancreatitis. Percutaneous needle aspiration of the area and Gram stain of the fluid may help to confirm the diagnosis of pancreatic abscess.

**13. Define *hemosuccus pancreaticus.***

Hemosuccus pancreaticus describes the rare phenomenon of major bleeding into the main pancreatic duct from a pseudoaneurysm. Massive gastrointestinal or intra-abdominal bleeding from pseudocyst erosion into a pancreatic or peripancreatic blood vessel occurs in about 5% to 10% of patients with pseudocysts. Patients with hemosuccus pancreaticus form a subset of this group. Clinical signs suggestive of pseudoaneurysm hemorrhage include an enlarging pulsatile abdominal mass with or without a bruit, recurrent gastrointestinal bleeding, and increasing abdominal pain. For patients suspected of having pseudoaneurysm hemorrhage, obtain a bolus contrast helical CT scan to confirm the diagnosis, followed by angiography for further localization and embolization or immediate surgical exploration.

**14. When should you suspect that a cystic pancreatic lesion is not a pseudocyst?**

Consider an alternate diagnosis if a *pseudocyst* is not associated with convincing historical, clinical, or diagnostic imaging evidence of pancreatitis or pancreatic trauma. Conversely, a history of pancreatitis does NOT rule out a cystic pancreatic neoplasm.

**15. What is a serous cystadenoma?**

A serous cystadenoma (SCA) is a cystic pancreatic neoplasm characterized by numerous cysts filled with a glycogen-rich, low-viscosity serous fluid and lined by flat or cuboidal epithelium. Imaging with CT, EUS, or magnetic resonance imaging (MRI) classically shows a honeycomb of small cysts with a sunburst calcification in a central scar. SCAs grow slowly and more than 99% of reported cases are benign. Conservative observation may be appropriate for an elderly or high-surgical risk patient. Complete surgical resection is indicated if the patient is symptomatic or if the diagnosis is uncertain.

The usual presenting symptoms of SCAs are nonspecific gastrointestinal complaints such as nausea, vomiting, abdominal pain, and weight loss, or an abdominal mass. Up to one third may be discovered incidentally during autopsy or abdominal imaging. SCAs are found most commonly in middle-aged women.

### 16. What disease commonly manifests by retinal and central nervous system (CNS) hemangioblastomas, renal cell carcinoma, pheochromocytoma, and pancreatic cysts?

Von Hippel–Lindau (VHL) disease is an autosomal dominant disorder caused by mutation and deletion of the VHL tumor suppressor gene on chromosome 3p25-26. Affected individuals develop an assortment of cysts and malignancies in multiple organs over their lifetime. The most common manifestations of VHL are retinal and CNS hemangioblastomas, renal cell carcinoma, and pancreatic cysts. Patients with VHL also have an increased risk for pancreatic serous cystadenomas, and neuroendocrine tumors, but do not have an increased risk for pancreatic carcinoma. An evaluation for VHL is recommended for patients who have a VHL-associated lesion and a family history of VHL-associated lesions, or any individual with two or more VHL-associated lesions.

### 17. Describe the characteristics of an MCN.

MCN is a cystic pancreatic neoplasm characterized by large cysts filled with mucin and lined by a columnar epithelium. Many MCNs have an ovarian-like stroma surrounding the epithelial cells. MCNs typically form in the pancreas tail or body and are much more common in women than in men. The most frequent presenting symptoms are epigastric pain and an enlarging abdominal mass. Obstructive jaundice is rare. Radiologic images usually show larger and less numerous cysts compared with serous cystadenomas. ERCP/MRCP (magnetic resonance cholangiopancreatography) generally shows no communication between the pancreatic ducts and the neoplasm.

A single MCN may contain both benign and malignant epithelium. Most clinicians consider all MCNs as potentially malignant. The treatment of choice is complete surgical resection with highly detailed histologic examination. The 2- and 5-year survival rate for patients with invasive mucinous cystadenocarcinoma is about 65% and 30%, respectively, which is much higher than that for patients with pancreatic ductal adenocarcinoma.

### 18. What is an IPMN? How does it differ from a MCN?

An IPMN is a pancreatic neoplasm that originates within the duct system and may appear cystic because of duct dilations. IPMNs are classified as either branch-duct type or main-duct type. The main-duct type IPMN frequently arises in the pancreas head and is more likely to undergo malignant transformation. Unlike MCNs, IPMNs afflict both genders equally and tend to arise in the head of the pancreas. An ovarian-like stroma is not found around the epithelial cells. An IPMN may be found in an elderly patient who has recurrent pancreatitis. Obstructive jaundice, abdominal pain, and weight loss also are common presenting symptoms. ERCP/MRCP confirms direct communication between the pancreatic ducts and the neoplasm. The finding of mucin extruding from the ampulla of Vater is considered highly specific for an IPMN.

### 19. How does the surgical management of an IPMN differ from that of a MCN?

Most experts recommend resection of any MCN because of the high risk of malignancy. The cystic areas of a MCN usually define the margins of the neoplasm. Careful preoperative imaging studies usually can localize an MCN and allow for a segmental pancreatic resection. In contrast, an asymptomatic branch-duct IPMN with cysts less than 3 cm and without mural nodules may be managed conservatively. All main-duct IPMNs should be considered for resection. Unlike MCNs the cystic areas surrounding an IPMN may extend beyond the margins of the actual neoplasm, resulting in imprecise preoperative localization. Adding to the localization difficulty is the tendency of IPMNs to spread microscopically along the pancreatic duct. Hence, an initial partial pancreatectomy may require extension to total pancreatectomy based upon the intraoperative frozen section and pancreatoscopy findings.

### 20. What is the utility of EUS in the evaluation of a cystic pancreatic lesion?

EUS imaging alone may add some incremental diagnostic information to the usual battery of transabdominal ultrasound, contrast-enhanced CT, and MRI. Similarly, EUS-guided fine needle aspiration (EUS-FNA) and microbiopsy of cystic pancreatic lesions may assist the diagnosis, but is useful only if the information would significantly change the management plan, such as resection versus no resection. The utility of cyst fluid analysis for tumor markers is not yet proven. EUS-FNA carries the risk of intraperitoneal tumor seeding, infection, and pancreatitis.

### 21. What conditions are most commonly associated with a pancreatic retention cyst?

Pancreatic retention cysts are dilated areas of the pancreatic duct that result from an obstruction of the duct. Retention cysts usually are less than 1 cm in diameter and commonly are associated with chronic pancreatitis, advanced cystic fibrosis, or a duct-obstructing carcinoma.

## WEBSITES

www.gastroatlas.com (pancreas)

www.pancreas.com

www.vhl.org

## BIBLIOGRAPHY

1. Banks PA, Freeman ML. The Practice Parameters Committee of the American College of Gastroenterology: Practice guidelines in acute pancreatitis. Am J Gastroenterol 2006;101:2379–400.
2. Crippa S, Salvia R, Warshaw AL, et al. Mucinous cystic neoplasm of the pancreas is not an aggressive entity: Lessons from 163 resected patients. Ann Surg 2008;247:571–9.
3. Das A, Wells CD, Nguyen CC. Incidental cystic neoplasms of pancreas: What is the optimal interval of imaging surveillance? Am J Gastroenterol 2008;103:1657–62.
4. Jacobson BC, Baron TH, Adler DG, et al. ASGE guideline: The role of endoscopy in the diagnosis and the management of cystic lesions and inflammatory fluid collections of the pancreas. Gastrointest Endosc 2005;61:363–70.
5. Khalid A, Brugge W. ACG practice guidelines for the diagnosis and management of neoplastic pancreatic cysts. Am J Gastroenterol 2007;102:2339–49.
6. Oh H, Kim M, Hwang C, et al. Cystic lesions of the pancreas: Challenging issues in clinical practice. Am J Gastroenterol 2008;103:229–39.
7. Serikawa M, Sasaki T, Fujimoto Y, et al. Management of intraductal papillary mucinous neoplasm of the pancreas: Treatment strategy based on morphologic classification. J Clin Gastroenterol 2006;40:856–92.
8. Shuin T, Yamasaki I, Tamura K, et al. Von Hippel-Lindau disease: Molecular pathological basis, clinical criteria, genetic testing, clinical features of tumors and treatment. Jpn J Clin Oncol 2006;36:337–43.
9. Tanaka M, Chari S, Adsay V, et al. International consensus guidelines for management of intraductal papillary mucinous neoplasms and mucinous cystic neoplasms of the pancreas. Pancreatology 2006;6:17–32.
10. Tseng JF, Warshaw Al, Sahani DV, et al. Serous cystadenoma of the pancreas: Tumor growth rates and recommendations for treatment. Ann Surg 2005;242:413–9.

# CHAPTER 41

# CELIAC DISEASE, TROPICAL SPRUE, WHIPPLE DISEASE, LYMPHANGIECTASIA, IMMUNOPROLIFERATIVE SMALL INTESTINAL DISEASE, AND NONSTEROIDAL ANTI-INFLAMMATORY DRUGS

*Francis Amoo, MD, Di Zhao, MD, and Ingram M. Roberts, MD*

### 1. What is the best screening test for fat malabsorption?

Microscopic examination of stool using Sudan stain to detect fat is the best screening test for fat malabsorption. This test has a 100% sensitivity and 96% specificity. A stool sample is smeared on a microscope slide and mixed with ethanolic Sudan III and glacial acetic acid. The slide is covered, heated just until boiling, and then examined for the presence of fatty acid globules. The presence of more than 100 globules greater than 6 μm in diameter per high-powered field (×430) indicates a definite increase in fecal fat excretion. The number of globules correlates well with the quantitative amount of fecal fat present.

### 2. What is the best quantitative test for fat malabsorption?

The 72-hour stool fat collection. The patient is given a diet consisting of 100 g of fat per day. Stool is collected, usually for 72 hours. The normal coefficient for absorption is approximately 93% of ingested fat. Consequently, if 100 g of fat is digested, 7 g or less of fat should appear in stool over a 24-hour period. If greater than 7 g of fecal fat is present, steatorrhea secondary to malabsorption is confirmed.

### 3. Under what physiologic conditions is fecal fat excretion increased?

- Diet high in fiber (greater than 100 g/day)
- Ingestion of solid-form dietary fat (e.g., whole peanuts)
- In the neonatal period, when intraluminal levels of pancreatic lipase and bile salts are low
- When olestra is consumed

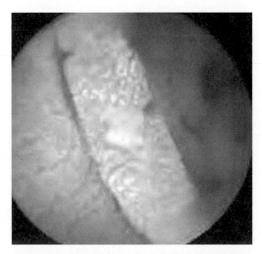

**Figure 41-1.** Ulceration in celiac disease seen by capsule endoscopy.

### 4. What is the gluten-sensitive enteropathy (GSE) panel?

A panel of serologic tests used to detect celiac disease. Three antibodies are directed against the connective tissue (reticulin-like structures) or surface component of smooth muscle fibrils (Fig. 41-1):

- A-EmA: anti–endomysial antibody (IgA)

A-EmA has 100% specificity for celiac disease, whereas its sensitivity is 85% and 90%, respectively, for untreated adult and childhood celiac disease. It can persist in low titers in 10% to 25% of patients on a gluten-free diet, despite normal histology.

- AGA: anti–gliadin antibody (IgG or pooled Ig)

AGA has fairly good sensitivity (68% to 76%), but it also may be found in 10% to 20% of patients with other diseases that affect the small intestinal mucosa. AGA is a helpful test in monitoring GSE, because it always becomes negative with the regrowth of jejunal villi in celiac patients after a gluten-free diet.

- R1-ARA: anti–reticulin antibody (IgA)

RI-ARA has a higher specificity than AGA in celiac children but a relatively low sensitivity (less than 40% to 50%). Patients with IgA deficiency and celiac disease may have a negative anti–endomysial antibody.

## 5. What is tissue transglutaminase?
Recently, tissue transglutaminase has been touted as the most sensitive and specific marker for celiac disease. Tissue transglutaminase is believed to be the autoantigen to which the endomysial antibodies react. Studies have shown that specificity for antitransglutaminase is comparable to that for anti–endomysial antibodies; however, some investigators have observed that the antibody to transglutaminase is a more sensitive test, detecting 98% to 100% of patients with celiac sprue.

## 6. Name the conditions to consider in previously responsive patients with celiac sprue who begin to deteriorate (Fig. 41-2)
- *Noncompliance* with gluten-free diet is the most common cause of deterioration in a previously responsive patient.
- *Lymphoma* is the most common malignancy complicating celiac disease, especially that of mucosal T-cell origin. Diagnosis of lymphoma requires a high index of suspicion because onset can be insidious or abrupt, and the histologic appearance can be indistinguishable from that of celiac sprue. A careful search for lymphoma is needed in patients with celiac sprue who do not respond to gluten withdrawal and patients with recurrent weight loss and malabsorption despite strict adherence to a gluten-free diet. Computed tomography (CT) scan and exploratory laparotomy may be necessary to establish the diagnosis.
- *Refractory sprue* has clinical features and mucosal lesions indistinguishable from celiac sprue, but patients do not respond to a gluten-free diet, either at the onset of diagnosis or after becoming refractory to dietary therapy. Some patients may respond to corticosteroids or other immunosuppressive drugs, such as azathioprine, cyclophosphamide, or cyclosporine. Other patients do not respond to any treatment and face a dismal prognosis. The absence of Paneth cells on small bowel biopsy is a poor prognostic sign.
- *Collagenous sprue* is a subset of refractory sprue characterized by the progressive development of a thick band of collagen-like material beneath the basement membrane of epithelial cells. It is usually refractory to all forms of treatment other than parenteral alimentation.

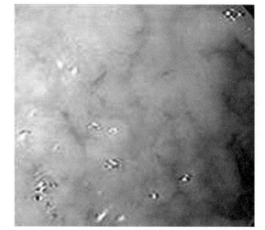

**Figure 41-2.** Nodular mucosa in celiac disease seen by capsule endoscopy.

## 7. What are the hepatic manifestations of celiac sprue, and how are they managed?
Asymptomatic elevation of liver function tests, predominantly aminotransferases, can be seen in up to 42% of celiac patients. Strict adherence to a gluten-free diet will lead to a reduction in aminotransferase levels in the majority of individuals. Failure of liver function test improvement despite treatment with a gluten-free diet, should prompt consideration of coexistent forms of autoimmune liver disease such as autoimmune hepatitis, primary biliary cirrhosis, or primary sclerosing cholangitis.

## 8. Describe the manifestations of Whipple disease
Whipple disease is a chronic systemic illness with various potential manifestations. The most common presentation includes:

- Weight loss (90%)
- Diarrhea (greater than 70%)
- Arthralgias (greater than 70%)

Arthralgias may exist for many years before the diagnosis of Whipple disease. Cardiac involvement includes congestive heart failure, pericarditis, and valvular heart disease (30%). Lymphadenopathy and hyperpigmentation are frequent findings on physical examination. Hematochezia is rare, but occult bleeding has been detected in up to 80% of patients with Whipple disease. The most common central nervous system manifestations (5%) are dementia, ocular disturbances, meningoencephalitis, and cerebellar symptoms, including ataxia and mild clonus. Endoscopic findings may show a pale, shaggy mucosa in the duodenum and jejunum with erythema, ulceration and friability.

9. **What is the differential diagnosis of a macrophage infiltrate of the small bowel lamina propria?**
   - *Whipple disease:* inclusions are rounded or sickle-shaped.
   - *Mycobacterium avium-intracellulare:* inclusions contain acid-fast bacilli. This condition is commonly seen in acquired immunodeficiency syndrome (AIDS) patients with small bowel involvement.
   - *Histoplasmosis or cryptococcosis:* inclusions contain large, round, encapsulated organisms.
   - *Macroglobulinemia:* no inclusions are seen, and there are only faintly staining, homogeneously periodic acid–Schiff (PAS)-positive macrophages.
   - *Miscellaneous disease:* PAS-positive macrophages are frequently present in the normal gastric and rectal mucosa and may contain lipids or mucin, respectively.

10. **What causes Whipple disease?**
    *Tropheryma whippelii* causes the disease in humans but has been cultured only recently. The organism was identified by direct amplification of a 16S-rRNA sequence from a microbial pathogen in tissue. According to phylogenetic analysis, this bacterium is a gram-positive actinomycete that is not closely related to any known genus. Prolonged treatment with antibiotics (up to 6 months) is often required to eradicate the organism. Measurements of *T. whippelii* DNA concentration in tissue by polymerase chain reaction is the most sensitive marker of patient response to antibiotic therapy. Of interest, *T. whippelii* DNA has been found in the small intestine of asymptomatic patients, suggesting that host factors play a role in disease penetration, just as in *Helicobacter pylori* infection.

11. **What are the complications of the enteropathy induced by nonsteroidal anti-inflammatory drugs (NSAIDs)?**
    NSAID-induced enteropathy is associated with intestinal bleeding, protein loss, ileal dysfunction, and malabsorption. There is no close relationship between upper endoscopic findings and evidence of intestinal bleeding among NSAID-treated patients, even when blood loss has led to iron-deficiency anemia. Chronic blood loss and protein loss seem to occur from the inflammatory site. Protein loss can result in significant hypoalbuminemia. Ileal dysfunction can lead to bile acid malabsorption and, in rare cases, mild vitamin $B_{12}$ malabsorption. Mefenamic acid (Postel) and sulindac (Clinoril) have been implicated as causes of severe malabsorption with subtotal villus atrophy that resembles celiac disease.

12. **Does scleroderma produce any manifestations in the small bowel?**
    Patients with scleroderma may have small bowel dysfunction due to absent cycling of the normal contractile pattern, known as the migrating motor complex. Small bowel motility studies reveal markedly diminished amplitude in all phasic pressure waves. This finding may manifest clinically as intestinal pseudo-obstruction and bacterial overgrowth. Patients may suffer from nausea, vomiting, abdominal pain, diarrhea, and malabsorption. Small bowel radiographic series may show megaduodenum and dilated loops of jejunum.

13. **How does octreotide affect intestinal motility and bacterial overgrowth in scleroderma?**
    Octreotide evokes alternating phase-1 and phase-3 activity in normal people and patients with scleroderma. In patients with scleroderma, these complexes propagate at the same velocity and have two-thirds the amplitude of spontaneous complexes in normal people. This effect is independent of motilin because octreotide inhibits motilin release. Octreotide may retard gastric antral motility, unlike erythromycin, which markedly stimulates gastric antral motor activity.

14. **Describe the different forms of lymphangiectasia.**
    - *Congenital intestinal lymphangiectasia* (Milroy disease) results from a malformation of the lymphatic system. Many areas in the body can be affected. Patients with congenital disease may present at any time from childhood to adulthood and usually have asymmetric lymphedema.
    - *Secondary lymphangiectasia* results from a disease that blocks intestinal lymph drainage. Causes of secondary lymphangiectasia include extensive abdominal or retroperitoneal carcinoma, lymphoma, retroperitoneal fibrosis, chronic pancreatitis, mesenteric tuberculosis or sarcoidosis, Crohn's disease, chronic congestive heart failure, and even constrictive pericarditis.

15. **What are the clinical manifestations of abetalipoproteinemia?**
    Abetalipoproteinemia is an autosomal recessive condition characterized by the inability to form chylomicrons and very-low-density lipoprotein particles by the enterocytes because of abnormal apoprotein B. Most patients have severe fat malabsorption and retardation and rarely survive the third decade. The largest series of patients has been studied at the National Institutes of Health.

16. **What are the different clinical presentations of eosinophilic gastroenteritis?**
    Eosinophilic gastroenteritis is characterized by eosinophilic infiltration in the gastrointestinal tract. Clinical features and severity depend on the layer and location of involvement. Mucosal involvement leads to protein-losing enteropathy,

fecal blood loss, and malabsorption. Involvement of the muscle layer often causes obstruction of gastric or small bowel. Subserosal involvement causes ascites, pleural effusion, or, on occasion, pericarditis.

### 17. How are patients with eosinophilic gastroenteritis treated?

The mainstay of treatment for eosinophilic gastroenteritis is corticosteroids, even though no controlled trials have been performed. The recommended dosage of prednisone is usually 20 to 40 mg/day for treatment of the initial episode and relapses, with 5 to 10 mg/day for maintenance. Some patients respond to a short course of treatment but may suffer relapse. Others may require long-term maintenance therapy. The course of disease may wax and wane in severity but is rarely life threatening. The therapeutic effect of oral sodium cromoglycate is controversial. Trial elimination diets have occasionally been successful, but relapse is common.

### 18. What are the common causes of diarrhea in a patient with Crohn's disease and ileal resection?

- *Ileal resection less than 100 cm:* bile salt diarrhea. Normally, conjugated bile acids are reabsorbed in the ileum. When less than 100 cm ileum is resected, bile acids pass into the colon, causing direct irritation of the colonic epithelium and net water secretion by the colon. Bile-salt diarrhea is typically watery, may not start until a normal diet is resumed after surgery, is precipitated by a meal (typically after breakfast when a large amount of bile is stored in the gallbladder), and does not lead to weight loss. Patients benefit from an empirical trial of cholestyramine, a bile acid–binding agent.
- *Ileal resection greater than 100 cm:* steatorrhea. When greater than 100 cm of ileum is lost to surgical resection or disease, the daily loss of bile acids exceeds the ability of the liver to synthesize new bile acids; hence, the total circulation bile acid pool is diminished. Bile acid deficiency leads to impaired intraluminal micellar fat absorption or steatorrhea. Patients benefit from a low-fat diet or supplement of medium-chain triglycerides. The diminished circulating pool of bile acids also promotes formation of cholesterol gallstones.

### 19. Where are the endemic areas for tropical sprue?

Tropical sprue is endemic in Puerto Rico, Cuba, the Dominican Republic, and Haiti but not in Jamaica or the other West Indies islands. It is found in Central America, Venezuela, and Colombia. Sprue is common in the Indian subcontinent and Far East, although little information is available from China. Sprue has been reported among several visitors to countries in the Middle East. It is rare in Africa, although the occurrence of sprue among populations living in the central and southern parts is now well established.

### 20. How is tropical sprue treated?

The most effective therapy for tropical sprue in returning travelers or expatriates is a combination of folic acid and tetracycline. Folic acid should be given in a dosage of 5 mg/day orally and tetracycline in a dosage of 250 mg 4 times/day. Vitamin $B_{12}$ should be given parenterally, in addition to the above combination, if a deficiency of this vitamin is discovered. Treatment should be continued for at least several months or until intestinal function returns to normal. Treatment with folic acid alone may be effective in reversing small bowel abnormalities or even in curing the acute illness but not in curing the chronic form. On the other hand, long-term treatment with tetracycline alone may result in cure of both acute and chronic forms of sprue.

### 21. How is bacterial overgrowth diagnosed?

The gold standard for the diagnosis of bacterial overgrowth is demonstration of increased concentrations of bacteria (greater than $10^5$ colony-forming units/mL) in fluid obtained from the intestine during duodenal or jejunal intubation. If quantitative culture of the small bowel aspirate is not possible, the diagnosis can be made with various breath tests. With the lactulose-hydrogen breath test, a rise in breath hydrogen level of 12 ppm from baseline values is taken as diagnostic of bacterial overgrowth; some investigators have suggested that the lactulose hydrogen breath test may be used to diagnose bacterial overgrowth, however, this remains controversial. The $^{14}C$-glycocholate and $^{14}C$-D-xylose breath tests detect the release of the radiolabeled carbon dioxide as the result of bacterial deconjugation of bile acid and metabolism of xylose. Normalization of the Schilling test after treatment with antibiotics is highly suggestive of bacterial overgrowth.

### 22. What is the mechanism of hyperoxaluria in short bowel syndrome?

Normally, intraluminal calcium binds to oxalate and prevents intestinal absorption of oxalate. With short bowel syndrome, malabsorption of fat leads to excessive luminal free fatty acids, which bind to calcium, allowing oxalate to pass unbound and become available for absorption. Excessive luminal free fatty acids and bile acids appear to increase colonic permeability to oxalate, further increasing its absorption. Therefore, hyperoxaluria appears to depend on the presence of an intact colon. To prevent calcium oxalate nephrolithiasis in patients with bowel disease, a low-oxalate and low-fat diet should be recommended.

### 23. What is immunoproliferative small intestinal disease (IPSID)?

Also known as alpha heavy-chain disease, IPSID is a type of lymphoma composed of dense lymphoplasmacytic mucosal infiltrate that secretes an abnormal alpha-heavy chain protein. The disease usually affects the small intestine from the second part of the duodenum distally into the jejunum. It presents in young adults and is usually associated with poor socioeconomic conditions in the Mediterranean region and many developing nations.

### 24. What causes IPSID and how is it treated?

Although its exact etiology is unclear, early-stage IPSID has been linked to a bacterial origin. Recently, investigators have established an association between IPSID and *Campylobacter jejuni* with use of polymerase chain reaction and DNA sequencing techniques. Early-stage disease frequently responds to tetracycline or other broad-spectrum antibiotic treatment and may result in complete remission. IPSID that has progressed to high-grade lymphoma may respond systemic combination chemotherapy.

### 25. What are the most common clinical manifestations of IPSID?

- Abdominal pain
- Diarrhea
- Malabsorption
- Weight loss
- Growth retardation
- Paraproteinemia with overproduction of heavy chain of IgA

### 26. What is video capsule endoscopy, and what are the indications/contraindications for its use?

Video capsule endoscopy uses a noninvasive *pill-sized* digital imaging system that the patient swallows after an overnight fast. As the capsule travels the gastrointestinal (GI) tract, images are sent by radiofrequency to a recorder belt worn by the patient. After 8 hours, the belt is removed, and the images are downloaded and processed on a computer workstation. The capsule is single use and eventually excreted with bowel movements. Indications for use are obscure GI bleeding in adults, diagnostic evaluation of Crohn's disease, and assessment of disease activity, surveillance of inherited polyposis syndromes, workup of suspected small bowel tumors, and detection of drug-induced small bowel injury. Contraindications include gastroparesis, advanced dementia, swallowing disorders, known stricture or partial/intermittent small bowel obstruction, and patients with defibrillators/pacemakers. The main disadvantage of the capsule is that it does not allow tissue sampling or therapeutic intervention.

## WEBSITES

http://www.celiac.org

http://www.vhjoe.com

http://www.vhjoe.org/Volume6Issue2/6-2-7.htm

### BIBLIOGRAPHY

1. Akbulut H, Soykan I, Yakaryilmaz F, et al. Five-year results of the treatment of 23 patients with immunoproliferative small intestinal disease: A Turkish experience. Cancer 1997;80:8–14.
2. Balasekaran R, Porter JL, Santa Ana CA, et al. Positive results on tests for steatorrhea in persons consuming olestra potato chips. Ann Intern Med 2000;132:279–82.
3. Bardella MT, Fraquelli M, Quatrini M, et al. Prevalence of hypertransaminasemia in adult celiac patients and effect of gluten-free diet. Hepatology 1995;22:833–6.
4. Bjarnason I, Hayllar J, Macpherson AJ, et al. Side effects of nonsteroidal antiinflammatory drugs on the small and large intestine in humans. Gastroenterology 1993;104:1832–47.
5. Bratten JR, Spanier J, Jones MP. Lactulose breath testing does not discriminate patients with irritable bowel syndrome from healthy controls. Am J Gastroenterol 2008;103:958–63.
6. Dray X, Vahedi K, Lavergne-Slove A, et al. Mycobacterium avium duodenal infection mimicking Whipple's disease in a patient with AIDS. Endoscopy 2007;39:E296–7.
7. Eliakim R. Video capsule endoscopy of the small bowel. Curr Opin Gastroenterol 2008;24:159–63.
8. Fernollar F, Puechat X, Raoult D. Whipple's disease. N Engl J Med 2007;356:55–66.
9. Fleming JL, Wiesner RH, Shorter RG. Whipple's disease: Clinical, biochemical, and histopathologic features and assessment of treatment in 29 patients. Mayo Clin Proc 1988;63:539–51.
10. Hofmann AF, Poley R. Role of bile acid malabsorption in pathogenesis of diarrhea and steatorrhea in patients with ileal resection: I. Response to cholestyramine or replacement of dietary long chain triglyceride by medium chain triglyceride. Gastroenterology 1972;62:918–34.
11. Klipstein FA. Tropical sprue in travelers and expatriates living abroad. Gastroenterology 1981;80:590–600.
12. Lecuit M, Abachin E, Martin A, et al. Immunoproliferative small intestinal disease associated with *Campylobacter jejuni*. N Engl J Med 2004;350:239–48.

13. Marth T, Schneider T. Whipple disease. Curr Opin Gastroenterol 2008;24:141–8.
14. McNally PR. Literature review. Virt Hum J Endosc 2007;6.
15. Ramzan NN, Loftus Jr E, Burgart LJ. Diagnosis and monitoring of Whipple disease by polymerase chain reaction. Ann Intern Med 1997;126:520–7.
16. Raoult D, Birg ML, La Scola B. Cultivation of the bacillus of Whipple's disease. N Engl J Med 2000;342:620–5.
17. Relman DA, Schmidt TM, MacDermott RP, et al. Identification of the uncultured bacillus of Whipple's disease. N Engl J Med 1992;327:293–301.
18. Roberts IM. Workup of the patient with malabsorption. Postgrad Med 1987;81:32–42.
19. Rondonotti E, Spada C, Cave D, et al. Video capsule enteroscopy in the diagnosis of celiac disease: A multicenter study. Am J Gastroenterol 2007;102:1624–31.
20. Soudah HC, Hasler WL, Owyang C. Effect of octreotide on intestinal motility and bacterial overgrowth in scleroderma. N Engl J Med 1991;325:1461–7.
21. Sblattero D, Berti I, Trevisol C, et al. Human recombinant tissue transglutaminase ELISA: An innovative diagnostic test for celiac disease. Am J Gastroenterol 2000;95:1253–7.
22. Seissler J, Boms S, Wohlrab U, et al. Antibodies to human recombinant tissue transglutaminase measured by radioligand assay: Evidence for high diagnostic sensitivity for celiac disease. Horm Metab Res 1999;31:375–9.
23. Sollid LM. Molecular basis of celiac disease. Annu Rev Immunol 2000;18:53–81.
24. Street S, Donoghue HD, Neild GH. Tropheryma whippelii DNA in saliva of healthy people [letter]. Lancet 1999;354:1178–9.
25. Talley NJ, Shorter RG, Phillips SF, et al. Eosinophilic gastroenteritis: A clinicopathological study of patients with disease of the mucosa, muscle layer, and subserosal tissues. Gut 1990;31:54–8.
26. Trier JS. Celiac sprue. N Engl J Med 1991;325:1709–19.
27. Volta U, Molinaro N, Fusconi M, et al. IgA antiendomysial antibody test: A step forward in celiac disease screening. Dig Dis Sci 1991;36:752–6.
28. Yamada T, Alpers DH, Owyang C, et al. Textbook of Gastroenterology. 2nd ed Philadelphia, JB: Lippincott; 1995.

# CROHN'S DISEASE

Bret A. Lashner, MD, and
Aaron Brzezinski, MD

# CHAPTER 42

## DIAGNOSIS

### 1. What are the usual symptoms and signs suggestive of Crohn's disease?

The symptoms of Crohn's disease are determined by the site and type of involvement (i.e., inflammatory, stenotic, or fistulizing). The most common site of involvement is ileocolitis. These patients present with diarrhea, abdominal pain that is usually insidious, in the right lower quadrant, frequently triggered or aggravated after meals, and may be associated with a tender, inflammatory mass in the right lower quadrant and weight loss. The diarrhea is usually nonbloody, and this may be one of the clues in clinical history that helps differentiate Crohn's disease from ulcerative colitis, where bloody diarrhea is almost universal. Patients frequently have fever, weight loss, perianal fistulas and/or fissures, and extraintestinal manifestations such as aphthous stomatitis, arthritis, and erythema nodosum. Patients with isolated colonic disease usually present with diarrhea, abdominal pain, and weight loss.

Perianal skin tags are very common and at times mistaken for external hemorrhoids, and it is not until these are excised and the course is complicated by a nonhealing wound that the diagnosis of Crohn's disease is entertained. At times, the main symptoms are related to perianal fistulae and/or abscess, even though most of these patients have other areas of involvement by Crohn's disease. Gastroduodenal Crohn's disease is less common and can mimic complicated peptic ulcer disease with abdominal pain, early gastric satiety, or symptoms of duodenal obstruction.

Patients can present with mild, moderate, or severe disease. This is a clinical judgment based on the severity of diarrhea, abdominal pain, the presence or absence of dehydration, anemia, malnutrition, and tachycardia. The Crohn's Disease Activity Index (CDAI) combines weighted scores of clinical and laboratory variables to estimate disease severity. CDAI scores of less than 150 indicate a clinical remission and scores over 450 indicate severely active disease. For a very helpful online CDAI calculator, please refer to http://www.ibdjohn.com/cdai/.

### 2. How Is the diagnosis of Crohn's disease established?

The diagnosis of Crohn's disease is established by history, physical examination, endoscopy, biopsies, radiographs, and laboratory tests. Crohn's disease presents most commonly between ages 15 and 25. The diagnosis should be suspected in patients with chronic diarrhea, finding characteristic intestinal ulcerations and excluding alternative diagnoses. The ulcerations of Crohn's disease may be aphthoid (Fig. 42-1) but also could be deep and serpiginous along the longitudinal axis of the bowel (Fig. 42-2). Skip areas, cobblestoning, and rectal sparing are characteristic findings. Air contrast barium enema, small bowel series with or without a peroral pneumocolon, computed tomography (CT) enterography, or colonoscopy each may demonstrate these typical lesions. On a small bowel series, Crohn's disease often leads to separation of bowel loops, a narrowed and ulcerated terminal ileum, and in advanced cases the so-called *string sign* (Fig. 42-3). The biopsies of involved areas have architectural distortion and a chronic inflammatory infiltrate, and in about 10% to 30% of cases of Crohn's colitis there are noncaseating granulomas that usually are diagnostic. Typical lesions of Crohn's disease also may be seen in the upper gastrointestinal tract. The inflammation is localized in the ileocecal region in approximately 50% of cases, the small bowel in approximately 25% of cases, the colon in 20% of cases, and the upper gastrointestinal tract or perirectum in 5% of cases.

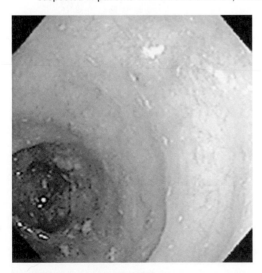

**Figure 42-1.** Aphthoid ulcers in a patient with Crohn's colitis.

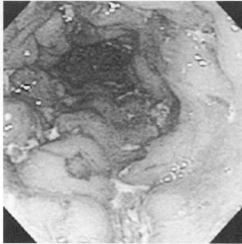

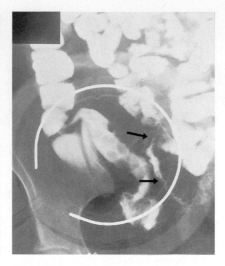

**Figure 42-2.** Deep, serpiginous ulcers of Crohn's disease.

**Figure 42-3.** *String sign* from a small bowel series in a patient with Crohn's disease.

### 3. Which diseases can mimic the symptoms and signs of Crohn's disease?

The differential diagnosis of Crohn's disease is long. The most common mimics of Crohn's colitis are ulcerative colitis, ischemic colitis, diverticulitis, or colorectal cancer. For Crohn's ileitis, infection with *Yersinia enterocolitica* or *Mycobacterium tuberculosis* may mimic disease. In immunosuppressed patients, viral infections such as cytomegalovirus (CMV) can mimic Crohn's disease. Other important diseases in the differential diagnosis of Crohn's disease include the irritable bowel syndrome, intestinal lymphoma, celiac sprue, radiation enteropathy, and nonsteroidal anti-inflammatory drug–induced enteropathy.

### 4. What serologic tests can help established the diagnosis?

Clinical, endoscopic, and histological findings can establish the diagnosis and differentiate between Crohn's disease and ulcerative colitis in 85% to 90% of patients (Table 42-1). In the remaining 10% to 15% of patients with *indeterminate*

**Table 42-1.** Some Distinguishing Features of Ulcerative Colitis and Crohn's Disease

|  | ULCERATIVE COLITIS | CROHN'S DISEASE |
| --- | --- | --- |
| Rectal bleeding | Usual | Sometimes |
| Abdominal mass | Rare | Often |
| Abdominal pain | Sometimes | Often |
| Perianal disease | Extremely rare | 5% to 10% |
| Upper gastrointestinal symptoms | Never | Occasional |
| Cigarette smoking | Very rare | Common |
| Malnutrition | Sometimes | Common |
| Low-grade fever | Sometimes | Often |
| Rectal disease | Usual | Sometimes |
| Continuous disease | Usual | Sometimes |
| Granulomas | Never | 10% |
| Crypt abscesses | Common | Rare |
| Discrete ulcers | Rare | Common |
| Aphthoid ulcers | Rare | Common |
| Cobblestone lesions | Never | Common |
| Skip lesions | Rare | Common |
| Ileal involvement | Rare, backwash ileitis | Usual |
| Fistulas | Never | Common |
| Cancer | Rare | Very rare |
| Microscopic skip lesions | Rare | Common |
| Transmural inflammation | Never | Common |

colitis, serologic testing can be helpful. A positive anti–*Saccharomyces cerevisiae* antibody (ASCA) and a negative perinuclear antineutrophil cytoplasmic antibody (pANCA) are most consistent with Crohn's disease, while the converse is consistent with ulcerative colitis.

## ETIOLOGY

### 5. Is cigarette smoking associated with Crohn's disease?

Yes, Crohn's disease is more common among cigarette smokers, and continued smoking is associated with early recurrence, more severe complications, and a higher likelihood for repeat surgery. All are associated with cigarette smoking. Patients with Crohn's disease *must quit smoking*!

### 6. What infectious agents might be responsible for Crohn's disease?

*Mycobacterium avium paratuberculosis (MAP)* causes Johne disease, a granulomatous inflammation of the terminal ileum and other parts of the intestine, in ruminants. In a small number of patients with Crohn's disease, in situ hybridization and culture of resected specimens have found *MAP* and other atypical mycobacteria. However, a causal relationship has not been determined, and treatment of such infections is effective only in a few patients. Other infectious agents, such as the measles virus or the measles vaccine, have been proposed, but the evidence is inconclusive and an etiologic association has not established. It is possible that an infectious agent or cellular material from an infectious agent triggers an abnormal immune response by the innate intestinal immune system.

### 7. Is there a genetic predisposition for developing Crohn's disease?

The principal theory on the pathogenesis of Crohn's disease is that in a genetically predisposed individual, an environmental agent (i.e., infection, dietary substance that enters the bloodstream through a permeable intestine, or nicotine) triggers an uncontrolled inflammatory response. The incidence of Crohn's disease can be at least 10 per 100,000 in the certain populations. Crohn's disease occurs in more than one first- or second-degree family member in approximately 20% of cases. Children whose parent has Crohn's disease have a lifetime risk of less than 3% of developing Crohn's disease. Spouses of patients with Crohn's disease rarely develop Crohn's disease. The genetic predisposition occurs from a number of important genetic mutations in key regulatory proteins of intestinal inflammation. Studies of genetic linkages among kindreds with inflammatory bowel disease led to the discovery of the *NOD-2/CARD-15* mutation in chromosome 16 (*IBD-1*). Depending on the population studied, this mutation can be seen in as many as 30% of patients with Crohn's disease; however, it is also seen in non–Crohn's disease patients, and in Japan, this mutation is only rarely seen in patients with Crohn's disease. In the European and American Caucasian population, the presence of this mutation appears to predict stenotic disease involving the terminal ileum. Mutations in the interleukin-23 receptor (*IL-23R*) gene on chromosome 1 have been shown to be protective for Crohn's disease development.

## NATURAL HISTORY

### 8. Is mortality increased in patients with Crohn's disease?

Patients with Crohn's disease, in general, do not have an increased mortality compared with age- and sex-matched controls. Some complications of Crohn's disease, such as malignancy, short bowel syndrome, hypercoagulable state, and primary sclerosing cholangitis, do have an increased mortality. Fortunately, these complications are rare.

### 9. Are there factors that predict a flare-up of Crohn's disease activity?

Cigarette smoking is the most important clinical risk factor for symptomatic recurrence. Smokers have a recurrence at least twice as high as nonsmokers. The effect of oral contraceptive use on recurrence rate is controversial. While oral contraceptive use is not associated with an increased recurrence rate, there is a synergistic effect between smoking and oral contraceptive use; the combined effects are greater than the sum of the individual effects. Other important risk factors for symptomatic recurrence are intestinal infections or nonsteroidal anti-inflammatory drug use.

### 10. Does behavior of disease predict its natural history?

According to its behavior, Crohn's disease has been classified as either inflammatory, stricturing, or fistulizing disease. Inflammatory-type disease is characterized by intestinal ulcerations and the main symptoms are diarrhea, abdominal pain, an inflammatory mass, and when it is severely active fever and weight loss. Inflammatory-type disease responds best to anti-inflammatory therapy, particularly corticosteroids and infliximab, but recurrence is the rule rather than the exception. The natural history of inflammatory-type disease is aggressive with early recurrence. Stricturing-type disease, on the other hand, has a more indolent course that does not respond well to anti-inflammatory therapy. While all Crohn's disease begins as inflammation, the predominant pathology in patients with stricturing disease is extensive fibrosis in the lamina propria. Surgery is the best therapeutic option in patients with stricturing disease, and the need for a second surgery is lower than with other types of Crohn's disease. Fistulizing-type disease is characterized by enterocutaneous and/or enteroenteric fistulas. Fistulas occur in areas of inflammation and often originate in a segment of bowel proximal to a stricture. Following successful medical or surgical therapy for fistulas, recurrence is common. Most patients with inflammatory or fistulizing disease will benefit from maintenance medical therapy to minimize the risk for recurrence.

### 11.  Do patients with Crohn's disease have an excess cancer risk?

Small bowel cancer in Crohn's disease is a rarely reported phenomenon; less than 100 cases have been reported in the literature. Epidemiologic studies, though, have suggested that the relative risk of small bowel cancer in Crohn's disease is greatly elevated. Small bowel cancer in Crohn's disease follows the same distribution as Crohn's disease (ileum > jejunum > duodenum), which is exactly opposite to the distribution of sporadic small bowel cancer. Excluded loops and chronic fistulas also are risk factors for small bowel cancer in Crohn's disease. Like in ulcerative colitis, colorectal cancer is increased in patients with extensive colonic Crohn's disease. Colorectal cancer in Crohn's disease occurs near areas of inflammation. However, since the premalignant lesion of dysplasia is not as widespread, when present, in the colon of patients with Crohn's disease as it is in patients with ulcerative colitis, cancer surveillance colonoscopy is less likely to be effective in decreasing mortality.

### 12.  What are the extraintestinal manifestations of Crohn's disease?

The extraintestinal manifestations of Crohn's disease are similar to those seen in ulcerative colitis. A polyarticular nondeforming arthritis is the most common extraintestinal manifestation, occurring in about 20% of patients; the arthritis responds to treatment of bowel symptoms. Primary sclerosing cholangitis is less common in patients with Crohn's disease than in ulcerative colitis patients; it follows a course independent of disease activity, and does not respond to anti-inflammatory therapy directed to the bowel, including surgery. Erythema nodosum, pyoderma gangrenosum, iritis, uveitis, pancreatitis, nephrolithiasis, cholelithiasis, amyloidosis, osteoporosis, and ankylosing spondylitis are all extraintestinal manifestations of Crohn's disease. Nephrolithiasis most often is from oxalate stones. Patients with Crohn's disease with fat malabsorption have preferential binding of luminal calcium to fatty acids rather than oxalate and the subsequent increased absorption of dietary oxalate with stone formation.

## TREATMENT

### 13.  Which 5-aminosalicylic acid preparations are effective in treating Crohn's disease patients?

5-Aminosalicylic acid (5-ASA) agents have been used for many years to treat inflammatory bowel disease, mostly ulcerative colitis, patients. The response to 5-ASA in Crohn's disease in induction and maintenance of remission is less than in ulcerative colitis. 5-ASA is a topical agent and not a systemic medication; therefore, it needs to be delivered to the site of inflammation. Sulfasalazine requires bacterial cleavage of the diazo bond between sulfapyridine and 5-ASA for the 5-ASA to have a local anti-inflammatory effect. Since bacteria are only present in sufficient numbers in the large bowel, sulfasalazine is effective only in patients with Crohn's colitis. Other oral 5-ASA compounds that are used for colonic disease include Asacol, which is 5-ASA coated with a compound that dissolves at pH 7 (terminal ileum); Dipentum, which is two molecules of 5-ASA bound by a diazo bond; and Colazal, which is 5-ASA delivered in a proform by a carrier. Pentasa is 5-ASA coated with ethylcellulose beads, which dissolve and release 5-ASA throughout the small and large bowel, and Lialda, which is 5-ASA imbedded into a metallomultimatrix that ensures sustained delivery throughout the colon with once-daily dosing. Theoretically, Pentasa should be most effective in patients with extensive small bowel disease. 5-ASA is also available in the form of suppositories or enemas for patients with proctitis or involvement up to the sigmoid colon. 5-ASA agents are used only in patients with mildly to moderately active disease, their role in maintenance of remission of Crohn's disease is debatable.

### 14.  Should steroids be used in Crohn's disease?

Steroids are effective in treating inflammatory-type Crohn's disease. Long-term use is not recommended, though, due to the many serious adverse effects such as osteoporosis, diabetes, and cataracts, just to name a few. Steroids are not effective in stricturing Crohn's disease and actually may worsen patients with fistulas, especially if localized infection is not adequately drained.

Budesonide is a very potent steroid with a very high rate first-pass metabolism, 85% to 90%. Therefore, the systemic side effects are greatly diminished but not entirely eliminated. The preparation available in the United States delivers the medication in the distal ileum and cecum in patients who have not had small bowel resection. In Canada, budesonide is also available as an enema. Budesonide has been effective for induction of remission in patients with moderately active Crohn's disease and has been approved for maintenance of remission. It is advisable to prescribe supplemental calcium and vitamin D to patients taking steroids, regardless of the route of administration.

### 15.  What is the role for immunosuppressive therapy in Crohn's disease?

Both azathioprine and 6-mercaptopurine are commonly used in patients with Crohn's disease. Both are purine analogs that interfere with DNA synthesis of rapidly dividing cells such as lymphocytes and macrophages. Because these drugs do not have a clinical effect for 2 to 3 months, or longer, these drugs are primarily used in maintaining remission in inflammatory-type and fistulizing-type Crohn's disease, and can be given for 4 years or longer. Important adverse effects include pancreatitis, allergy, and leukopenia. White blood cell counts and liver function tests need to be checked on a periodic basis. There are two main strategies to start these medications; traditionally, the medication was started at a low dose and the dose was increased according to the speed at which the white blood cells decreased. Since the thiopurine methyltransferase (TPMT) enzyme activity can be measured, the preferred option is to start the dose predicted according to body weight to those patients with a normal enzyme level activity, at a reduced dose for patients with intermediate TPMT enzyme activity, and to explore alternative therapies in patients with low or absent TPMT activity. Whatever regimen one chooses, it is very important to monitor liver tests and the white blood cells on a regular basis. Nonresponders can have levels of the active metabolite, 6-thioguanine (6-TG), measured to see if the lack of response is due to lack of adherence to a medical regimen (6-TG level of 0), underdosing (6-TG level of less than 230 pmol/$8 \times 10^8$ red blood cells), or true lack of response (6-TG level greater than 230 pmol/$8 \times 10^8$ red blood cells).

## 16. Which biologic therapies are effective for patients with Crohn's disease?

Infliximab (Remicade) is an IgG1 chimeric mouse-human antibody to tumor necrosis factor (TNF) that, when infused intravenously, binds to soluble TNF and to the TNF on surface membranes of inflammatory cells, causing complement fixation and cell lysis. It has been approved for use in inflammatory-type Crohn's disease (a single infusion of 5 mg/kg) and fistulizing Crohn's disease (three infusions of 5 mg/kg) as well as for long-term maintenance therapy. In randomized clinical trials, 48% of patients with inflammatory-type disease and 55% of patients with fistulizing disease achieved complete remission, figures significantly higher than for placebo-treated patients. Side effects during the infusion such as nausea, headache, and pharyngitis can be attenuated with slowing the infusion.

Since its approval by the U.S. Food and Drug Administration in 1998, there has been a great deal of experience gained with the use of Infliximab. We have learned that the long-term response rate is 60% to 70% and that, with continued use every 8 weeks, patients often maintain remission. Tuberculosis, opportunistic infections, and, to a lesser extent, malignancies have been the main complications of its use, and the analysis of 500 patients at the Mayo Clinic revealed a 1% mortality rate among patients receiving Infliximab. With chronic use, patients may form anti-infliximab antibodies, which may decrease its effectiveness, in which case higher doses or more frequent infusions are required. When a long period elapses between infusions, there is a higher risk of immediate- or delayed-infusion reactions that precludes its subsequent use.

Adalimumab (Humira) is a fully human anti-TNF antibody that is approved for induction and maintenance therapy for Crohn's disease. It is given as a 40 mg subcutaneous injection every 2 weeks after a loading dose of 160 mg at week 0 and 80 mg at week 2. Its effectiveness and toxicities are very similar to those of infliximab with the exception of lower antibody formation to adalimumab. Certolizumab (Cimzia) is a pegylated Fab fragment of a humanized anti-TNF antibody. Its effectiveness and toxicity are similar to those of infliximab and adalimumab, and it is given as a monthly subcutaneous injection. Natalizumab (Tysabri), an anti-integrin antibody, is another biologic agent approved for use in Crohn's disease. Its effectiveness appears to be similar to that of other biologic agents, and rate of opportunistic infections may be lower. Natalizumab was associated with a case of progressive multifocal leukoencephalopathy (PML) in a patient with Crohn's disease in a clinical trial (as well as additional cases in multiple sclerosis patients), causing its use to be restricted to patients enrolled in an international registry.

## 17. Which medications are effective in maintaining remission?

Patients who have a high risk of recurrence following a medically or surgically induced remission should be considered for maintenance medications. Smokers, patients who have had more than one surgery, and patients with inflammatory-type or fistulizing disease have the highest risk of recurrence. Long-term therapy with azathioprine or 6-mercaptopurine has the best maintenance effects. Methotrexate is effective in some patients and can be used in patients who either fail treatment with azathioprine or 6-mercaptopurine or who have side effects precluding the use of these agents. 5-ASA agents have a lesser maintenance effect. Budesonide is approved for maintenance, as are infliximab, adalimumab, certolizumab, and natalizumab.

## 18. What are the indications for surgery in Crohn's disease?

The adage *a chance to cut is a chance to cure* does not apply to Crohn's disease since surgery is not a cure for Crohn's disease. The main goal of surgery is to treat the most important problem while preserving as much bowel as possible. Wide resection margins are not associated with decreased recurrence and should be avoided. The indications for surgery include active inflammatory-type disease refractory to medical therapy, prednisone dependence, intestinal strictures, fistulas, abscesses, growth retardation, bleeding, perforation, severe anorectal disease, dysplasia, and cancer. Besides resection and abscess drainage, there is considerable experience with stricture-plasty (opening a stricture without removing bowel) and advancement flap surgery (removing a perirectal fistula by advancing normal mucosa over the internal os). A close working relationship between the internist/gastroenterologist and colorectal surgeon is extremely important for controlling disease and decreasing morbidity.

**19. What therapeutic regimen is most often effective for stricturing-type Crohn's disease?**

Usually, stricturing-type Crohn's disease will require surgery. Anti-inflammatory therapy is not likely to relieve symptoms. The goals of surgery are to relieve symptoms and preserve bowel length. The surgery offered need not be a resection, though. Stricureplasties of strictured segments of small bowel or anastomosis can provide long-term relief of obstructive symptoms. In the most common type of strictureplasty, an incision is made on the longitudinal axis of a short stricture that is sutured along a perpendicular. Prior to performing a strictureplasty, the surgeon will send a frozen section to rule out carcinoma at the site of the stricture. In some patients, endoscopic balloon dilatation at the site of an ileocolic anastomosis relieves symptoms, delaying the need for surgery. There is no evidence that steroid injection into the anastomotic site at the time of balloon dilation is effective.

**20. What therapeutic regimen is most often effective for inflammatory-type Crohn's disease?**

Inflammatory-type Crohn's disease should respond to anti-inflammatory agents. 5-ASA agents usually are tried first due to the limited toxicity; however, their efficacy is limited. Antibiotics such as ciprofloxacin or metronidazole are effective, particularly in patients with colonic and perianal disease. Steroids or infliximab is usually tried next due to the relatively rapid onset of action. Azathioprine/6-mercaptopurine and methotrexate are usually reserved for steroid-dependent inflammatory disease and for maintenance of remission. All of the available biologic agents—infliximab, adalimumab, certolizumab, and natalizumab—are indicated for inflammatory-type Crohn's disease. These agents should be used as monotherapy (i.e., without immunosuppressive therapy) to limit potential toxicity.

**21. What therapeutic regimen is most often effective for fistulizing Crohn's disease?**

An assessment of the degree of mucosal activity is an important determinant of therapy for fistulizing Crohn's disease. When active disease is present, anti-inflammatory therapy with 5-ASA agents, azathioprine, 6-mercaptopurine, or biologic agents could be extremely helpful. In perianal fistulas, combined medical and surgical treatment is usually required. Sepsis should be adequately drained and placement of noncutting Seton sutures can facilitate continued drainage and promote healing (Fig. 42-4). Antibiotics, azathioprine, 6-mercaptopurine, or infliximab is usually beneficial. If the mucosal disease is quiescent, then surgical therapy with an advancement flap procedure may be appropriate.

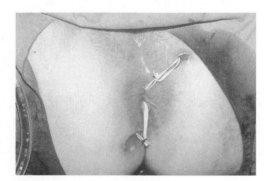

**Figure 42-4.** Seton sutures placed in the perineum.

**22. When should nutritional support be used in patients with Crohn's disease?**

Nutritional support can be used as primary or adjuvant therapy for Crohn's disease. Interestingly, bowel rest and total parenteral nutrition (TPN) will greatly improve most patients with inflammatory-type or fistulizing-type disease. Enteral nutrition is almost as effective as steroids in inducing remission in inflammatory-type Crohn's disease—it has much fewer side effects but it takes longer to induce remission. Unfortunately, when food is introduced, symptoms and signs of active disease quickly return. Nutritional support also is effective in children with Crohn's disease and growth retardation. Due to the expense and morbidity of TPN, long-term TPN should be reserved for patients with a short bowel syndrome or extensive small bowel disease or in patients who need nutritional support and in whom enteral nutrition is not tolerated.

## WEBSITE

http://www.ibdjohn.com/cdai/

**BIBLIOGRAPHY**

1. Brant SR, Picco MF, Achkar JP, et al. Defining complex contributions of NOD2/CARD15 gene mutations, age at onset, and tobacco use in Crohn's disease phenotypes. Inflamm Bowel Dis 2003;9:281–9.
2. Bousvaros A, Antonioli DA, Colletti RB, et al. Differentiating ulcerative colitis from Crohn's disease in children and young adults: Report of a working group of the North American Society for Pediatric Gastroenterology, Hepatology, and Nutrition and the Crohn and Colitis Foundation of America. J Pediatr Gastroenterol Nutr 2007;44:653–74.
3. Columbel JF, Loftus EV, Tremaine WJ, et al. The safety profile of infliximab in patients with Crohn's disease: The Mayo Clinic experience in 500 patients. Gastroenterology 2004;126:19–31.

4. Colombel JF, Sandborn WJ, Rutgeerts P, et al. Adalimumab for maintenance of clinical response and remission in patients with Crohn's disease: The CHARM trial. Gastroenterology 2007;132:52–65.
5. Cosnes J, Cattan S, Blain A, et al. Long-term evolution of disease behavior of Crohn's disease. Inflamm Bowel Dis 2002;8:244–50.
6. Dubinsky MC, Lamothe S, Yang HY, et al. Pharmacogenomics and metabolite measurement for 6-mercaptopurine therapy in inflammatory bowel disease. Gastroenterology 2000;118:705–13.
7. Dubinsky MC, Wang D, Picornell Y, et al. IL-23 receptor (IL-23R) gene protects against pediatric Crohn's disease. Inflamm Bowel Dis 2007;13:511–5.
8. Fazio VW, Marchetti F, Church JM, et al. Effect of resection margins on recurrence of Crohn's disease of the small bowel: A randomized controlled trial. Ann Surg 1996;224:563–71.
9. Feagan BG, Fedorak RN, Irvine EJ, et al. A comparison of methotrexate with placebo for the maintenance of remission in Crohn's disease. North American Crohn Study Group Investigators. N Engl J Med 2000;342:1627–32.
10. Hugot JP, Chamaillard M, Zouali H, et al. Association of NOD2 leucine-rich repeat variants with susceptibility to Crohn's disease. Nature 2001;411:599–603.
11. Munkholm P, Langholz E, Davidsen M, et al. Intestinal cancer risk and mortality in patients with Crohn's disease. Gastroenterology 1993;105:1716–23.
12. Ogura Y, Bonen DK, Inohara N, et al. A frameshift mutation in NOD2 is associated with susceptibility to Crohn's disease. Nature 2001;411:603–6.
13. Present DH, Rutgeerts P, Targan S, et al. Infliximab for the treatment of fistulas in patients with Crohn's disease. N Engl J Med 1999;340:1398–405.
14. Ruemmele FM, Targan SR, Levy G, et al. Diagnostic accuracy of serological assays in pediatric inflammatory bowel disease. Gastroenterology 1998;115:822–9.
15. Schreiber S, Khaliq-Kareemi M, Lawrance IC, et al. Maintenance therapy with certolizumab pegol for Crohn's disease. N Engl J Med 2007;357:239–50.
16. Silverstein MD, Loftus EV, Sandborn WJ, et al. Clinical course and costs of care for Crohn's disease: Markov model analysis of a population-based cohort. Gastroenterology 1999;117:49–57.
17. Targan SR, Feagan BG, Fedorak RN, et al. Natalizumab for the treatment of active Crohn's disease: Results of the ENCORE Trial. Gastroenterology 2007;132:1672–83.
18. Targan SR, Hoenir SB, Van Deventer SCH, et al. A short-term study of chimeric monoclonal antibody cA2 to TNF-alpha for Crohn's disease. N Engl J Med 1997;337:1029–35.
19. Timmer A, Sutherland LR, Martin F, et al. Oral contraceptive use and smoking are risk factors for relapse in Crohn's disease. Gastroenterology 1998;114:1143–50.
20. Valentine JF, Sninsky CA. Prevention and treatment of osteoporosis in patients with inflammatory bowel disease. Am J Gastroenterol 1999;94:878–83.

# 43 CHAPTER

# ULCERATIVE COLITIS

*Ramona O. Rajapakse, MD, and*
*Burton I. Korelitz, MD*

### 1. What is ulcerative colitis (UC)?
UC is a chronic inflammatory disease of the colon. It is distinct from Crohn's disease of the colon in that the inflammation is restricted mostly to the mucosa and involves only the colon. The rectal segment is almost always involved, whereas in Crohn's disease of the colon, the rectum is usually spared.

### 2. Define *backwash ileitis*.
*Backwash ileitis* refers to unusual cases of UC that involve the terminal ileum. The endoscopic, histologic, and radiologic appearance of backwash ileitis is the same as that of UC. When deep linear ulcers and strictures are seen in the ileum, Crohn's ileitis is the more likely diagnosis.

### 3. What is indeterminate colitis?
As more information is gathered about the pathogenesis of UC and Crohn's disease, the distinction between them at times can be unclear. In about 7% of patients, when the inflammatory process is limited to the colon (no ileal involvement), the endoscopic, histologic, or radiologic findings are insufficiently distinct to separate the two diseases. The colitis is then referred to as indeterminate. Other patients carry the diagnosis of UC for many years until a change in signs and symptoms, consistent with Crohn's disease, influences a change in diagnosis. In some patients the diagnosis of Crohn's disease of the colon is recognized only after colectomy and the development of recurrent ileitis in the ileostomy or ileoanal pouch performed for what was thought to be UC.

### 4. Why is it important to distinguish between UC and Crohn's disease?
Medical treatment of the two diseases overlaps, but, UC is curable by total colectomy, while Crohn's disease can never be considered cured by resection. Therefore, the correct diagnosis is of the utmost importance.

### 5. What causes UC?
The cause is unknown. The greatest risk factor is a positive family history. Approximately 15% of patients with inflammatory bowel disease (IBD) have a first-degree relative with the disease, but the familial association is less in UC than in Crohn's disease. Similarly, the incidence of IBD in first-degree relatives of patients with IBD is 30 to 100 times higher than in the general population. The cause technically remains unknown, although research has clarified that there are genetic, environmental, and immunologic contributions. The exact genetic link for UC has not been identified. Dietary antigens and bacteria have been proposed as possible triggers, but no evidence supports these theories. The incidence of UC is significantly higher in nonsmokers than in smokers and higher still in ex-smokers than in nonsmokers, supporting a protective effect of smoking. Whether this protective effect is secondary to nicotine or other constituents of cigarettes has not been fully established.

### 6. Who gets UC?
In most patients, UC has its onset in the second or third decades of life. However, there may be a second peak in the fifth or sixth decades, although this peak may be false because of other types of colitis that mimic UC. The disease has been described in all nationalities and ethnic groups but is more common in whites than in nonwhites. It is also more common in Jews than non-Jews. The hereditary link is supported by population-based studies.

### 7. What are the signs and symptoms of UC?
The predominant symptom at onset of UC is diarrhea with or without blood in the stool. If inflammation is confined to the rectum (proctitis), blood may be seen on the surface of the stool; other symptoms include tenesmus, urgency, rectal pain, and passage of mucus without diarrhea.

Other distributions of UC are proctosigmoiditis; left-sided disease, which extends more proximal to the descending colon, splenic flexure, or distal transverse colon; and universal colitis, which involves any length proximal to the mid-transverse colon and often the entire colon. The inflammation is almost always confluent in distribution and almost always involves the rectum when it is untreated with medication by enema.

More extensive colitis may be accompanied by systemic symptoms such as weight loss and malaise in addition to bloody diarrhea. Although pain is not a dominant feature, patients may complain of crampy abdominal discomfort relieved by a bowel movement and may have abdominal tenderness, usually localized to the left lower quadrant. Occasionally patients may present with constipation secondary to rectal spasm; accompanying rectal discharge might be disclosed on careful history. Although patients may present with extraintestinal manifestations before bowel symptoms, more often they parallel the severity of the primary bowel disease.

## 8. How are patients with UC classified?

Truelove and Witts divided patients into those with severe, moderate, and mild disease based on symptoms, physical findings, and laboratory values. We add to this list the severity of endoscopic and radiologic appearances. A plain film of the abdomen showing any degree of dilation of the colon or ulceration and edema of the mucosa outlined by air (even if not dilated) is indicative of a severe attack. Although endoscopic appearance does not always correlate well with clinical symptoms, the presence of severe mucosal disease indicates the need for more aggressive management (Table 43-1).

**Table 43-1.** Clinical Guide for Severity of Ulcerative Colitis

| | |
|---|---|
| **Mild** | Fewer than 4 stools daily, with or without blood, with no systemic disturbance and a normal erythrocyte sedimentation rate (ESR) |
| **Moderate** | More than 4 stools daily but with minimal systemic disturbance |
| **Severe** | More than 6 stools daily with blood and systemic disturbance as shown by fever, tachycardia, anemia, or ESR > 30 |

## 9. How are the extraintestinal manifestations of UC classified?

Although UC involves primarily the bowel, it may be associated with manifestations in other organs. These manifestations are divided into those that coincide with the activity of bowel disease and those that occur independently of bowel disease (Table 43-2).

**Table 43-2.** Extracolonic Manifestations of Ulcerative Colitis

| EXTRACOLONIC MANIFESTATION | COINCIDES WITH COLITIS ACTIVITY |
|---|---|
| Colitic arthritis | Yes |
| Ankylosing spondylitis | No |
| Pyoderma gangrenosum | Yes |
| Erythema nodosum | Yes |
| Primary sclerosing cholangitis | No |
| Uveitis | Often, but not always |
| Episcleritis | Often, not always |

## 10. What is colitic arthritis?

Colitic arthritis is a migratory arthritis affecting the knees, hips, ankles, wrists, and elbows. Usually the joint involvement is asymmetrical, not bilateral. It responds well to corticosteroids.

## 11. Describe the association between UC and ankylosing spondylitis.

Although ankylosing spondylitis is more commonly associated with Crohn's disease than UC, patients with UC have a 30-fold increased risk of developing ankylosing spondylitis, which does not parallel disease activity. Many patients with early sacroiliitis alone are asymptomatic, and the diagnosis is made on radiographs.

## 12. Discuss the hepatic complications of UC.

Hepatic complications include fatty liver, pericholangitis, chronic active hepatitis, cirrhosis, and primary sclerosing cholangitis. Although most patients with sclerosing cholangitis have UC, only a minority of patients with UC develop sclerosing cholangitis. It is usually suspected with the finding of an abnormally elevated alkaline phosphatase or γ-glutamyl transferase (GGTP) enzyme. Sclerosing cholangitis is sometimes improved with ursodeoxycholic acid therapy (Actigall). Patients with sclerosing cholangitis and UC have a higher risk of developing colon cancer than those without. In addition, they are also at risk of developing cholangiocarcinoma. Cholestyramine may help in alleviating the pruritus associated with the disease, but the only cure is liver transplantation.

### 13. What are the ocular complications of UC?

Ocular complications include uveitis, iritis, and episcleritis. Uveitis causes eye pain, photophobia, and blurred vision and requires prompt intervention to prevent permanent visual impairment. It usually responds to topical steroids but sometimes systemic steroids are required.

### 14. Describe the association between UC and thromboembolic events.

Patients with IBD are at increased risk of thromboembolic events, most commonly deep venous thrombosis of the lower extremities. After a search for other causes of a hypercoagulable state, patients should receive standard therapy for the thrombosis.

### 15. How do I evaluate a patient with UC?

The management of UC depends on the severity and location of disease activity, which are best assessed by a careful clinical history, with emphasis on the duration and severity of symptoms, and physical examination, followed by endoscopic evaluation to determine the extent and severity of mucosal involvement. Although flexible sigmoidoscopy may indicate the severity of the disease, full colonoscopy is essential to determine the extent as well as the full severity. A history of recent travel, antibiotic or NSAID use should be sought. Laboratory evaluations should include a CBC, chemistries, and stool studies for c/s, ova and parasites and C. difficile. All of the above should provide an indication of severity and extent of disease (i.e. proctitis, left sided or pancolitis) which will impact upon choice of therapy. See Table 43-1. A plain radiograph of the abdomen should be performed in flat and upright positions if the disease is severe in order to recognize depth of ulceration and early or advanced toxic megacolon, which may be suspected by the presence of tympany in any of the segments of the abdomen. Anti–*Saccharomyces cerevisiae* antibody (ASCA) and a negative perinuclear antineutrophil cytoplasmic antibody (pANCA) have no role in the primary diagnosis of UC but may be useful in differentiating between UC and Crohn's colitis. If disease severity is mild to moderate, medical therapy may be commenced on an out-patient basis. However if the disease is severe by all the criteria outlined above, hospital admission should be considered.

### 16. What are 5-ASA products?

Sulfasalazine, the first 5-ASA product, has been used successfully for many years in the treatment of mild-to-moderate UC. It is linked to sulfapyridine by a diazo bond that is cleaved by colonic bacteria. The active moiety is the 5-ASA. The side effects most commonly caused by sulfasalazine include nausea, vomiting, fever, and a rash, all of which are attributable primarily to the sulfapyridine, which is only a carrier. It also may cause agranulocytosis, autoimmune hemolytic anemia, folic acid deficiency, and infertility secondary to changes in sperm count and morphology. Newer preparations that contain only 5-ASA (mesalamine) are carried through or released in the small bowel. Mesalamine is currently available as a 4-g, 60 ml enema (Rowasa), as a suppository, and in oral formulations (Asacol, Pentasa, Dipentum, Colazal, Lialda) (Table 43-3).

**Table 43-3.** 5-ASA Products

| 5-ASA | CARRIER MOLECULE | RELEASE | SITE OF ACTIVITY |
|---|---|---|---|
| Asacol | Eudragit-S | pH > 7.0 | Terminal ileum and colon |
| Pentasa | Ethylcellulose beads, time release | pH > 6.0 | Small bowel and colon |
| Olsalazine | Azo bond | Bacteria | Colon (ileum with bacterial overgrowth) |
| Sulfasalazine | Sulfapyridine | Bacteria | Colon (ileum with bacterial overgrowth) |
| Lialda | Matrix | Colon | Colon |
| Colazal | Di-Azo bond | Colon | Colon |
| Dipentum | Dimer | Left colon | Left colon |

### 17. How do I treat proctitis and proctosigmoiditis?

For mild-to-moderate ulcerative proctitis, topical therapy may suffice. If disease is limited to the anorectal region, a Canasa suppository can be used once or twice daily. Hydrocortisone foam (Cortifoam) or hydrocortisone enemas (Cortenema) also may be used either alone or in alternation with the 5-ASA product. For proctosigmoiditis, the mesalamine enema, used alone or in alternation with a hydrocortisone enema, is effective. Only the mesalamine enema, not the Cortenema, has maintenance value. The patient must lie on the left side for at least 20 minutes after introducing the enema to ensure adequate delivery to the affected area. In some instances when tenesmus is severe, the enema is better introduced in the knee-chest position, taking advantage of the downhill gravity. Occasionally oral therapy may work better than enemas or suppositories; in other cases, a combination is required.

### 18. How do I treat an exacerbation of UC?

When the disease extends more proximally, oral therapies are required in addition to, or instead of, topical therapy. Choice of oral 5-ASA product is determined by the extent of involvement. Pentasa (4 g), Asacol (3.2 g), Colazal (6.75 g), or Lialda can be used for universal colitis and Dipentum (1 g) for left-sided colitis. The dose of Asacol may be titrated within the limits of tolerability to a maximum of 4.8 gm/day. It is not yet known whether still higher doses of any of the three would have increased efficacy. If the disease fails to resolve with 5-ASA therapy or is moderately severe at presentation, a short course of oral corticosteroids should be prescribed to bring the disease under control. The maximal effective oral dose of prednisone is 60 mg daily. The dose may be tapered to 40 mg/day after 2 to 7 days, if the disease is brought under control. The formula for further tapering of prednisone is individualized. The 5-ASA drugs should be given concurrently with prednisone. Prednisone and other corticosteroids are not maintenance drugs.

### 19. What should I do if the disease is severe?

Severe disease requires admission to hospital for intravenous corticosteroids and fluids. Patients should be monitored carefully by serial physical examination, lab tests, and plain radiographs of the abdomen. Severe UC may progress to toxic megacolon and/or perforation. It is treated with intravenous corticosteroids, antibiotics, a small bowel tube attached to suction, log rolling from side to side and to the supine and prone positions, and sometimes by rectal tube. If these maneuvers are not successful, subtotal colectomy should be considered, preferably before a perforation occurs. If the colon is dilated and the mucosal surface is ragged on abdominal films, a surgical colleague should be involved in management decisions.

If there is no response to intravenous corticosteroids, consideration should be given to the use of intravenous cyclosporine, Infliximab or surgery depending on the urgency of the clinical situation and local experience in management of this most severe complication. Rapid deterioration in clinical condition warrants early surgical intervention with ileostomy and subtotal colectomy. If there is time for a trial of cyclosporine, it should be administered only by physicians with extensive experience in its use. It is administered at a dose of 4 mg/kg/day intravenously by continuous infusion, with close monitoring of blood pressure, renal function, electrolytes, and drug blood levels. Cyclosporine should not be initiated if the serum cholesterol is low because it increases the risk of seizures. Bactrim is administered concurrently to prevent *Pneumocystis carinii* pneumonia. Failure to respond within 3 days portends a poor prognosis for medical therapy. There is emerging data that Infliximab may be useful in severe UC as it is in severe Crohn's disease when intravenous steroids have failed. It has the advantage of having less short-term toxicity than cyclosporine and of being useful for maintenance therapy. Early medical intervention in expert hands can significantly reduce the number of severely ill patients who go to surgery.

### 20. Define *toxic megacolon*.

*Toxic megacolon* is defined as a severe attack of colitis with total or segmental dilation of the colon (diameter of transverse colon usually greater than 5 to 6 cm). It can be recognized by plain radiographs showing the colon to be outlined by air (not after endoscopy) even with a diameter less than 5 cm. Megacolon is considered toxic if two or more of the following criteria are positive in addition to the colon persistently outlined by air:

- Tachycardia with a pulse rate greater than 100 beats/min
- Temperature greater than 101.5 °F
- Leukocytosis greater than 10,000 cells/mm$^3$
- Hypoalbuminemia less than 3.0 g/dL

### 21. How do I prevent a relapse?

Maintenance therapy should be initiated at the same time or soon after acute-phase therapy. For mild-to-moderate disease, a 5-ASA product may be all that is necessary. In our experience this will be true in only 20% to 30% of patients. For more severe or recurrent disease, an immunosuppressive medication such as 6-mercaptopurine (6-MP)/azathioprine or Infliximab (anti-TNF) is more effective. 6-MP should be started at a dose of 50 mg/day, and the patient should be followed carefully with weekly blood counts for the first 3 weeks and less often thereafter. If the initial dose is tolerated well and the white cell count is normal, the dose may be gradually increased if clinically warranted. Early toxic reactions to these medications include leukopenia, pancreatitis (3%), hepatitis, rash, and fever. The occurrence of pancreatitis or hepatitis usually precludes further use of the same drug. Patients with allergic-type reactions may be carefully desensitized to the causative medication or its alternative (6-MP versus AZA). High levels of the 6-MP metabolites 6-MMP (6-methylmercaptopurine) and 6-TG (6-thioguanine) or low levels of thiopurine methyltransferase (TPMT) may predict which patients will develop toxicity.

Infliximab, an established anti-TNF for Crohn's disease, is now U.S. Food and Drug Administration approved for the treatment of UC. Induction therapy consists of infusions of 5 mg/kg IV at weeks 0, 2, and 6 followed by maintenance infusions every 2 months. The maintenance dose is 5mg/kg IV. If the patient has breakthrough symptoms before 2 months, serum infliximab levels as well as antibodies to the chimeric component (HACA) may be checked. The dose of infliximab maybe  increased to 7.5mg/kg or 10mg/kg with or without premedication with benadryl, tylenol or steroids depending on the presence or absence of antibodies. There is some concern that combination therapy with 6-MP/AZA and Infliximab may increase the risk of infections and lymphomas in this patient population. Until further data are available, combination versus solo therapy should be decided based on the severity and fragility of disease as well as patient and physician preference.

## 22. Are there adjunctive therapies for UC?

Probiotics are defined as live microbial feed that have benefit to the human host. The most widely studied probiotic is VSL#3, which is a combination of *Lactobacillus, Bifidobacterium*, and *Streptococcus*. VSL#3 has been shown to reduce the incidence of the first episode of pouchitis if used immediately after total proctocolectomy and ileal-pouch anal anastomosis. It may also be useful in maintenance therapy for pouchitis after remission has been achieved with antibiotics. The evidence for benefit in active or chronic UC is less convincing but it may be useful as an adjunctive therapy.

Omega-3 capsules in high doses may also be useful in chronic UC by providing the short chain fatty acids that are trophic to colonocytes. Multivitamins are not necessary if the patient is eating a well-balanced diet. Oral iron supplements may cause constipation and distension. Oral potassium supplements may be irritating to the gastrointestinal tract, and magnesium supplements cause diarrhea, which is undesirable.

## 23. How often should patients have surveillance colonoscopy?

The current recommendations are as follows: for patients with left-sided colitis, surveillance should begin after 15 years from the onset of colitis. For patients with universal colitis, surveillance should begin after 8 years of colitis. Three biopsy specimens should be obtained every 10 cm throughout the colon. The likelihood of detecting dysplasia in flat mucosa increases with the number of random biopsies taken. To achieve a greater than 90% detection rate, more than 33 biopsies should be taken. In addition, any strictured, raised, polypoid areas or those with unusual shapes or textures should be biopsied. Surveillance colonoscopy should be repeated annually for universal disease, perhaps less often for left-sided disease. The variables which influence the risk of dysplasia and colon cancer are duration of disease, extent of disease, and severity (chronicity) of disease.

Newer techniques such as chromoendoscopy and narrow band imaging (NBI) allow better visualization of abnormal mucosa. Although these techniques allow targeted biopsies, their role in routine surveillance of UC has yet to be determined.

## 24. What should be done if a polyp or dysplasia is found?

Obvious polyps should be removed and the area surrounding the polyp biopsied. If the area is free of premalignant changes (indicating an adenomatous polyp), nothing further need be done except for the usual surveillance. However, if dysplasia is found, colectomy is the treatment of choice. Dysplasia is a premalignant lesion classified as high grade, low grade, or indefinite. Although everyone agrees that high-grade dysplasia anywhere in the colon warrants proctocolectomy, there is less consensus about the management of low-grade dysplasia. The diagnosis of low-grade dysplasia can be challenged when the biopsy samples are taken from areas of marked inflammation. Intensive treatment of the disease may lead to the recognition that the diagnosis of dysplasia was not accurate. Biopsy samples should be taken preferably from flat mucosa without inflammation. If a recommendation of colectomy depends on the diagnosis of dysplasia, a second expert gastrointestinal pathologist should review the biopsy slides before the final decision is made.

It has been our experience that when dysplasia or cancer involves the rectal segment, an ileostomy with colectomy should be favored over an ileal pouch-anal anastomosis.

## 25. Is surveillance effective?

Studies have shown that as many as 42% of patients with UC who are found to have high-grade dysplasia either already have cancer or develop it within a short time. The presence of low-grade dysplasia is also predictive of cancer: 19% of patients develop cancer of the colon or may even have cancer at the time of diagnosis. The finding of no dysplasia is predictive of a good short-term outcome. Outcome and case-controlled studies have shown that cancer in patients in a surveillance program is detected at an earlier and therefore more favorable stage. Patients who undergo screening have improved survival rates and lower cancer-related mortality rates.

## 26. Is there a role for chemoprevention in UC?

There is increasing evidence that long-term mesalamine use may reduce the risk of colon cancer in these patients. The mechanism may be secondary to inhibition of cell growth and proliferation via inhibition of prostaglandins and lipoxygenases or via activation of apoptosis. Ursodeoxycholic acid may also be useful in reducing colon cancer risk, especially in the sub population of patients with primary sclerosing cholangitis.

Further studies are required to clarify these issues. It is likely that maintenance therapy is effective mainly by suppressing inflammation and that surveillance biopsies are as important for recognizing microscopic inflammation as they are for recognizing dysplasia.

### 27. Is diet important in the management of UC?

No evidence suggests that any one diet is beneficial in patients with UC. Apart from the advice that patients with lactose intolerance should avoid lactose-containing food, no dietary restrictions are necessary.

### 28. Does stress exacerbate UC?

No studies to date support any role for psychological stresses, personality types, or overt psychiatric illness in the causation or exacerbation of UC. However, an anxiolytic agent or an antidepressant may be helpful if chronic illness leads to depression.

Sometimes the addition of an anxiolytic agent or an antidepressant may be the final step required to bring UC under control.

As with any chronic illness, the approach to management should be multifaceted with expert medical and surgical teams, a psychopharmacologist, and knowledgeable ancillary staff.

### 29. How does menstruation affect UC?

Scattered information supplements our experience that the symptoms of both UC and Crohn's disease are aggravated or provoked coincidentally with the premenstrual period and in some cases throughout menstruation. Occasionally a 2- to 3-day course of steroids is warranted.

### 30. Do patients with UC have problems with fertility and pregnancy?

In considering the effects of UC on pregnancy and vice versa, two aspects are important: the effect of the disease itself and the effect of the medications used to treat the disease. Well-controlled disease appears to have no deleterious effects on fertility or pregnancy. However, if the disease is active at any time during pregnancy, the incidence of fetal loss may be increased. It is therefore important to maintain control of the disease before and during pregnancy.

Mesalamine (5-ASA) has a long record of safety in pregnancy. Corticosteroids have also proven to be safe during pregnancy. With regard to the immunosuppressants 6-MP and azathioprine, data from the transplant literature suggest safety during pregnancy. One study concerning UC and Crohn's disease treated with immunosuppressives concluded that they are safe and need not be discontinued for pregnancy. In our experience, however, these medications may cause fetal loss when used by women before pregnancy and an increased incidence of congenital abnormalities and spontaneous abortions when used by men within 3 months of conception. We therefore suggest that patients should discontinue these drugs, if clinically feasible, at least 3 months before planned conception. If a woman is in remission, immunosuppressives may be stopped without expectation of early recurrence. If the disease is active, pregnancy should be postponed. Sulfasalazine causes defects in sperm morphology and motility. It should be replaced with one of the newer 5-ASA products in male patients who are contemplating starting a family.

### 31. What medications are contraindicated in patients with UC?

Evidence suggests that nonsteroidal anti-inflammatory drugs (NSAIDs) may precipitate exacerbations of the disease and in some cases may even be implicated in the onset of disease. The NSAIDs in common use include aspirin, ibuprofen, and naproxen. These drugs should be avoided in patients with UC.

Anticoagulant therapy with warfarin may lead to increased bleeding in patients with active disease and bloody diarrhea. Ironically, heparin therapy has been reported to improve disease activity in some patients. Although heparin therapy is not the standard of care, it may be useful when anticoagulation is required for patients with active UC. Opioid derivatives should be avoided if possible in patients with any type of colitis because of their propensity to cause toxic dilatation of the colon.

### 32. What are the surgical options for management of UC?

When medical management fails or complications such as perforation or dysplasia occur, subtotal colectomy with ileostomy or ileoanal pouch is the procedure of choice. Many patients are frightened by the prospect of having an ileostomy, but education can do much to alleviate their fears. Fortunately, a large number of patients with ileostomies become accustomed to them and continue to lead normal lives.

The ileoanal pouch is a possible alternative. It consists of a double loop of ileum that is fashioned into a pouch and stapled to the rectal stump and stripped of its mucosa, thereby preserving the anal sphincter. Disadvantages of the pouch include recurrent inflammation or pouchitis, frequent bowel movements, nocturnal incontinence, and the continued need for surveillance endoscopy. Pouchitis responds well to metronidazole, Cipro, or Bismuth, alone or in combination. These drugs can be used to treat the acute illness and also as maintenance therapy to prevent recurrence. Probiotics may also be used (see earlier). In some cases, 5-ASA products, steroids, or maintenance immunosuppressive medications may be required. Refractory pouchitis may require excision of the pouch and substitution of an ileostomy at a later date.

## WEBSITES

http://www.ccfa.org

http://www.niddk.nih.gov

## BIBLIOGRAPHY

1. Adler DJ, Korelitz BI. The therapeutic efficacy of 6-mercaptopurine in refractory ulcerative colitis. Am J Gastroenterol 1990;85:717–22.
2. Francella A, Dyan A, Bodian C, et al. The safety of 6-mercaptopurine for childbearing patients with inflammatory bowel disease: A retrospective cohort study. Gastroenterology 2003;124:9–17.
3. Lichtiger S, Present DH, Kornbluth A, et al. Cyclosporine in severe ulcerative colitis refractory to steroid therapy. N Engl J Med 1994;330:1841–5.
4. Marshall JK, Irvine EJ. Rectal aminosalicylate therapy for distal ulcerative colitis: A meta-analysis. Aliment Pharmacol Ther 1995;9:293–300.
5. Orholm M, Munkholm P, Langholz E, et al. Familial occurrence of inflammatory bowel disease. N Engl J Med 1991;324:84–8.
6. Pemberton JH, Kelly KA, Beart RW, et al. Ileal pouch-anal anastomosis for chronic ulcerative colitis: Long-term results. Ann Surg 1987;206:504–13.
7. Rajapakse RO, Korelitz BI, Zlatanic J, et al. Outcome of pregnancies when fathers are treated with 6-mercaptopurine for inflammatory bowel disease. Am J Gastroenterol 2000;95:684–8.
8. Sandborn WJ. Pouchitis following ileal pouch-anal anastomosis: Definition, pathogenesis and treatment. Gastroenterology 1994;107:1856–60.
9. Sutherland LR, May GR, Shaffer EA. Sulfasalazine revisited: A meta-analysis of 5-aminosalicylic acid in the treatment of ulcerative colitis. Ann Intern Med 1993;118:340–9.
10. Truelove SC, Witts LJ. Cortisone in ulcerative colitis: Final report on a therapeutic trial. BMJ 1955;2:1041–8.
11. Winawer SJ, Fletcher RH, Miller L, et al. Colorectal cancer screening: Clinical guidelines and rationale. Gastroenterology 1997;112:594–642.
12. Woolrich AJ, DaSilva MD, Korelitz BI. Surveillance in the routine management of ulcerative colitis: Predictive value of low-grade dysplasia. Gastroenterology 1992;103:431–8.
13. Zlatanic J, Korelitz BI, Rajapakse R, et al. Complications of pregnancy and child development after cessation of treatment with 6-mercaptopurine for inflammatory bowel disease. J Clin Gastroenterol 2003;36:303–9.

# EOSINOPHILIC GASTROENTERITIS

Seth A. Gross, MD, and
Sami R. Achem, MD, FACP, FACG, AGAF

**CHAPTER 44**

### 1. How is eosinophilic gastroenteritis (EGE) defined?

EGE is a rare condition produced by intense infiltration of eosinophils of one or more organs of the gastrointestinal (GI) tract. It is defined by having GI symptoms, eosinophilic infiltration in at least one or more areas of the GI tract, absence of eosinophilic involvement in organs outside the GI tract, and no evidence of a parasitic infection. Peripheral eosinophilia can be absent in *up to 20% of cases*. Patients with this condition can present with eosinophilic esophagitis, gastritis, enteritis, proctocolitis, and other unusual presentations such as pancreatitis, obstructive jaundice, and/or ascites.

### 2. What is the incidence of EGE?

This disease is uncommon, so it is difficult to estimate its true incidence. There are few series of published cases in the literature, and those available usually comprise less than 50 patients. The rarity of this condition can be illustrated by two reports: a Mayo Clinic–based study that found only 40 cases during a 30-year period and a study from China, describing only 15 patients in an 18-year period. Most of the cases occur in whites with a slight male predominance. The disease is often diagnosed in the third to fifth decade of life but can affect any age group. Studies from different parts of the world suggest that it is a disorder that spares no ethnic group.

### 3. What is the etiology of EGE?

The etiology and pathogenesis of the disease are poorly understood. Similar to other allergic diseases, EGE involves a Th-2 cytokine (interleukin [IL]-3, IL-5, and IL-13) and chemokine inflammatory response. It has been proposed that an imbalance in the T-cell paradigm leads to increased cytokine production resulting in IgE synthesis and eosinophilia. Eosinophils function as antigen presenting cells and mediate inflammation by releasing preformed granular proteins: eosinophil cationic protein (ECP), eosinophil-derived neurotoxin (EDN), eosinophil peroxidase, and major basic protein (MBP). Eosinophils also secrete Th-2–type proinflammatory cytokines, such as IL-3, IL-4, IL-5, IL-18, transforming growth factor, and lipid mediators that are cytotoxic to human intestinal epithelium. It is unknown what precipitating factor(s), such as antigen exposure, lead to chemoattraction of eosinophils to the GI tract. The recent development of a lymphopenic rat model of EGE may help advance the understanding of the pathogenesis of this disorder. Patients with EGE may report a history of eczema, food or seasonal allergies, asthma, atopy, and hay fever, suggesting a component of a hypersensitivity response. A familial susceptibility has also been reported in about 10% of patients with EGE.

### 4. What are the clinical features of EGE?

The clinical presentation of EGE is often nonspecific and frequently tends to imitate other more common disorders, such as functional digestive diseases or inflammatory bowel disease. The spectrum of symptoms ranges from often vague, nonspecific complaints to dramatic complications such as gastric outlet obstruction, acute abdomen, perforated viscous, small bowel obstruction, pancreatitis, obstructive jaundice, and unexplained ascites.

It is not rare for patients to experience a protracted course of waxing and waning symptoms before a definitive diagnosis is made. The most common presenting complaint is abdominal pain (two-thirds of patients), followed by nausea, vomiting, and diarrhea. Other manifestations include weight loss, abdominal distention, diarrhea, anorexia, ascites, dysphagia, edema, malabsorption, melena, perforation of the digestive tract, jaundice, and pyloric stenosis.

### 5. What is the Klein classification for EGE?

EGE has been classified by Klein and colleagues based on the site of infiltration of the different layers of the GI tract (mucosal, submucosal, and serosal involvement). The clinical symptoms associated with EGE are often dependent on the layer and site of the gastrointestinal tract involved.

### 6. Why does EGE have so many different clinical faces?

The eosinophilic infiltration of the affected organs and the depth of the inflammatory infiltration of the intestinal wall layers and of the surrounding visceral structures determine the clinical manifestations.

- *Mucosal eosinophilic infiltration*: Eosinophilic involvement limited to the mucosa is the most common subtype of EGE reported in 25% to 100% of cases. The typical histologic changes of EGE demonstrate eosinophilic infiltration of the mucosa and submucosa and are shown in Figure 44-1, A and B. The presentation for this subtype is often nonspecific with clinical complaints including nausea, vomiting, abdominal pain, gastrointestinal bleeding, diarrhea, anemia, protein-losing enteropathy, and weight loss. Intestinal eosinophilic mucositis can be complicated by malabsorption with weight loss, protein-losing enteropathy, chronic intestinal blood loss (iron deficiency), recurrent gastroduodenal ulcer disease, eosinophilic colitis, or acute intestinal bleeding.
- *Inflammation of the intestinal muscle layer*: Muscle layer involvement occurs in approximately 13% to 70% of the cases and results in a rigid gut with symptoms of dysmotility (i.e., dysphagia, food impaction, and esophageal stricture); see Figures 44-2, 44-3, and 44-4. Gastric involvement may result in vomiting and abdominal pain with obstruction of the gastric outlet; small intestine infiltration may cause obstruction and/or bacterial overgrowth. Recurrent acute cholangitis or pancreatitis can present in patients with ampullary infiltration, presumably due to ampullary stenosis (Fig. 44-5).

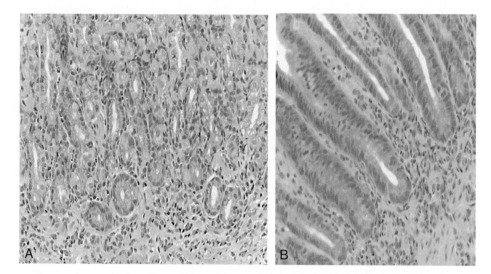

**Figure 44-1.** *A,* Endoscopic biopsy (hematoxylin and eosin, ×20) from the gastric antrum: Histopathology shows the eosinophilic mucosal and submucosal infiltration. *B,* Endoscopic biopsy (hematoxylin and eosin, ×20) from the duodenum: Histopathology shows the typical eosinophilic inflammatory infiltration of the mucosa and submucosa.

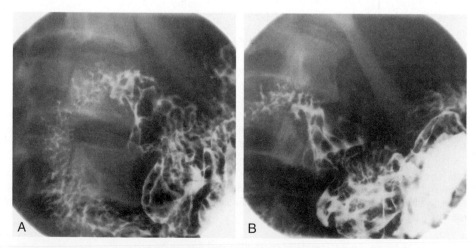

**Figure 44-2.** *A,* Barium double contrast: Cobblestone pattern is a typical sign of thickened mucosal folds. This patient has gastric and duodenal eosinophilic gastroenteritis. *B,* Barium double contrast of the gastric antrum and duodenum: Roughened mucosal folds are typical in eosinophilic gastroenteritis.

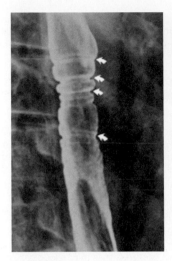 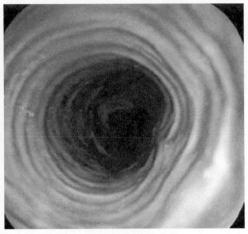

**Figure 44-3.** Barium swallow demonstrating multiple rings in the proximal esophagus.

**Figure 44-4.** Endoscopy demonstrating multiple concentric rings or *coiled spring* appearance of the esophagus in eosinophilic esophagitis.

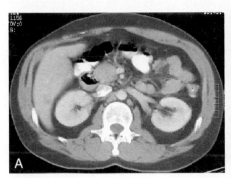 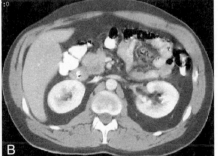

**Figure 44-5.** *A,* Early pancreatitis in duodenal eosinophilic gastroenteritis. *B,* Early pancreatitis in eosinophilic gastroenteritis. Duodenal wall thickening.

- *Subserosal/serosal inflammation:* Subserosal/serosal inflammation presents in approximately 12% to 40% of cases as eosinophilic peritonitis, ascites, severe bloating, or an inflammatory tumor with bowel obstruction. Ascitic eosinophil counts can reach greater than 80%. The subserosal involvement often is accompanied by muscular infiltration that can be visualized by abdominal ultrasound, computed tomography (CT), or magnetic resonance imaging (MRI). On occasion, even extraintestinal involvement with pleural effusions has been reported.

## 7. Is there an increase in the recognition of cases of eosinophilic infiltration of the GI tract?

There has been increased incidence of eosinophilic esophagitis likely related to improved recognition. The classic presentation would be a young man with a recurrent dysphagia and/or episodes of food impaction. Other symptoms have also included reflux-like symptoms not responding to double-dose proton pump inhibitor therapy. Endoscopic signs include a ringed esophagus, furrows, and white spec-lesions. This entity was originally described extensively in children, but many recent reports have clearly shown that it affects adults. too.

## 8. What is hypereosinophilia syndrome (HES)?

HES is an idiopathic condition associated with peripheral eosinophilia greater than 1500 cells/μL, gastroenteritis lasting for longer than 6 consecutive months, and evidence of eosinophil-induced organ damage, where other causes of hypereosinophilia, such as allergic, parasitic, and malignant disorders, have been excluded. HES can involve organs outside of the GI tract, including the skin, heart, brain, lungs, and kidney. HES has recently been reclassified as either a myeloproliferative or lymphocytic disorder, suggesting a hematologic origin. The prevalence of this disorder is unknown. It tends to affect more frequently young to middle-aged patients with a 4:1 male predominance. The tyrosine kinase inhibitor imatinib offers a new therapeutic option for about 90% of these patients.

## 9. What is the differential diagnosis of EGE?

Patients with eosinophils on intestinal biopsy, or any form of inflammation with peripheral eosinophilia should be evaluated for the possibility of EGE. There are, however, many other diseases that can produce similar findings (Tables 44-1 and 44-2).

**Table 44-1.** Causes of Gastrointestinal Symptoms and Increased Intestinal Eosinophils

| DISORDER | CLINICAL TIPS |
| --- | --- |
| Irritable bowel syndrome (IBS) | Peripheral eosinophilia is absent in 20% of the patients with eosinophilic gastroenteritis, which can lead to confusion with IBS and reinforces the need to examine mucosa biopsies to look for eosinophilic gastroenteritis (EGE). Careful review of the colonic histology can usually distinguish IBS by its lack of mucosal eosinophils. |
| Gastroesophageal reflux disease (GERD) | May mimic eosinophilic esophagitis. Patients may complain of intermittent dysphagia and reflux-like symptoms. Esophageal biopsies may also reveal increased number of eosinophils in both disorders adding further confusion, but when eosinophils number >20/hpf, eosinophilic esophagitis is more likely. Patient with reflux-like symptoms that do not improve with a double-dose proton pump inhibitor (PPI) trial for at least 6 weeks should be considered for esophagogastroduodenoscopy (EGD), and esophageal biopsy sample should be carefully examined for eosinophils, even if examination is macroscopically normal. |
| Medications | Interferon, gemfibrozil, enalapril, carbamazapine, clofazimine, and cotrimoxazole |
| *Helicobacter pylori* | Patients with *H. pylori* gastritis may have diffuse intestinal eosinophilia, but the significance of this finding simultaneously occurring in patients with *H. pylori* is still unknown. |
| Intestinal parasites | *Ancylostoma* (hookworm), *Anisakis; Ascaris, Capillaria, Isospora belli* (immunocompromised patients), pinworm (*Enterobious vermicularis*), strongyloides, *Toxocara, Trichura, Trichinella* are common examples. These infections may be diagnosed by using concentration methods in several fresh stool samples (sedimentation methods after fixation with ethyl-acetate formalin for ova and cysts; or polyvinyl alcohol fixatives for protozoan trophozoites). Complementary diagnostic tests include serologic tests and biopsies of the digestive tract. |
| Cytomegalovirus | Single report in an immunocompetent child presenting with protein losing enteropathy and having complete resolution without specific therapy in a 4-week period |
| Inflammatory bowel disease (IBD) | Collagenous colitis can be associated with eosinophilic infiltration of the colon, but has a characteristic distinctive collagen band in the submucosa. Ulcerative colitis and Crohn's disease are rarely associated with peripheral eosinophilia |
| Food allergies | Milk, gluten; may need to consider a formal allergy evaluation including skin prick test, CAP–fluorescent enzyme immunoassay (CAP-FEIA). |
| Celiac disease | Celiac disease is associated with small intestinal infiltration by inflammatory cells including eosinophils. The serologic findings (IgA antibodies to gliadin, endomysium, and tissue transglutaminase), the response to a gluten-free diet with resolution of the symptoms and the small intestinal villous atrophy will support the diagnosis |
| Hypereosinophilia syndrome (HES) | Eosinophilia >1500 cells/μL, gastroenteritis lasting for longer than 6 consecutive months and evidence of eosinophil-induced organ damage |

**Table 44-2.** Forms of Vasculitis Associated With Gastrointestinal Symptoms and Increased Intestinal Eosinophils

| SYSTEMIC VASCULITIS | CLINICAL TIPS |
| --- | --- |
| CTD: scleroderma, dermatomyositis, and polymyositis | Can be found with mucosal and muscular eosinophilic/basophilic infiltration accompanied by peripheral blood eosinophilia. Serologic tests for autoantibodies and biopsies will lead to the proper diagnosis. |
| Churg-Strauss syndrome | Granulomatous vasculitis syndrome with eosinophilia. Other organs such as the kidneys, heart, and colon can be involved. Asthma as the cardinal feature often precedes vasculitis up to 10 years. |
| Polyarteritis nordosum | May have considerable variability of manifestations due to the varying involvement of kidneys, lungs, skin, joints, and nervous system and abdominal pain. There is a perivascular infiltration with a variable eosinophilic component. |
| Eosinophilic fascitis | Also known as diffuse fasciitis with eosinophilia or Shulman syndrome is a rare connective tissue disorder characterized by swelling, thickening, and induration of the skin. It tends to cause limitation of movement, rapidly progressing to joint contractures as a result of fascial inflammation and fibrosis. There is symmetric skin induration, edema of the extremities and joint contractures leading to immobility. The most common sites of involvement include neck, extremities and trunk. Laboratory findings include eosinophilia of up to 30%, hypergammaglobulinemia, and an elevated erythrocyte sedimentation rate. |

*Continued*

**Table 44-2** Forms of Vasculitis Associated With Gastrointestinal Symptoms and Increased Intestinal Eosinophils—Cont'd

| SYSTEMIC VASCULITIS | CLINICAL TIPS |
| --- | --- |
| Eosinophilic granuloma or histiocytosis X | Rare and typically presents with multisystem involvement (liver, spleen, lung, bone marrow, lymph nodes, brain). Occasionally, there is isolated involvement of the intestinal tract. Biopsies of these organs can be distinguished from eosinophilic gastroenteritis by the characteristic staining patterns of Langerhans cells. |
| Inflammatory fibroid polyps | Most often are found in the gastric antrum (70%; and 20% in the small bowel) and are not accompanied by peripheral eosinophilia. They present with symptoms of bowel obstruction. The typical histopathology allows the differentiation from eosinophilic gastroenteritis: arborizing capillaries concentrically surrounded by spindle cells (fibroblasts or endothelial cells) and a variable eosinophilic infiltrate. |
| GI malignancies | Can present with peripheral blood eosinophilia. Examples are gastric, colonic, pancreatic tumors, hematologic malignancies such as Hodgkin lymphoma, mycosis fungoides, chronic myelogenous leukemia, or extra intestinal adenocarcinomas of the lung/ ovary/ or uterus can also occur with peripheral eosinophilia. |
| Organ Transplant | Patients who have under gone solid organ transplant can develop intestinal eosinophilia secondary immunosuppression causing an imbalance of Th-1/Th-2 lymphocytes. Intestinal eosinophilia has been seen in patients on an immunosuppression regimen using tacrolimus. |

## 10. What are possible radiographic features of EGE?

Gastric retention or small intestinal hypomotility can be demonstrated by barium studies. Double-contrast barium enema or enteroclysis can show mucosal thickening with a cobblestone or sawtooth silhouette, nodular filling defects, or coarse folds in the small intestine. EGE can mimic regional enteritis (Crohn's disease). Eosinophilic esophagitis presents with circumferential rings or a feline esophagus appearance (see Fig. 44-4). Muscle layer disease presents with stiffened and narrowed tubular gut strictures, complicated by obstruction of the esophagus, gastric outlet, duodenum, jejunum, ileum, or colon. CT or MRI can reveal duodenal, jejunoileal, or colonic wall thickening, inflammatory tumors, or ascites.

## 11. What are rational steps to diagnose EGE?

### HISTORY AND PHYSICAL EXAM

- Pertinent questions include food allergies, signs of atopic disease such as wheezing and eczema, rhinitis, and signs of malnutrition such as edema, anemia, and failure to thrive.
- Consider a formal allergy evaluation including skin prick test, CAP-fluorescent enzyme immunoassay (CAP-FEIA), formerly known as radioallergosorbent test (RAST), which detects antigen IgE antibody. Food challenge to a few selected foods (milk, soy, egg, wheat, nuts, fish). Patch test has not been studied in EGE.

### LABORATORY STUDIES

- Exclude parasitic intestinal disease by duodenal aspirates and three stool samples.
- Obtain appropriate serologic tests to exclude parasitic infestation.
- Endoscopy
  - Esophagus: typical findings of eosinophilic esophagitis include concentric rings, furrows, and white specs/nodules.
  - Other sites of the digestive tract: Findings may vary from a normal appearing mucosa to thickening of folds, nodules, friability, erythema, erosions, and ulcers.
  - Always obtain *multiple* tissue samples during endoscopy
- *Histopathology* remains the diagnostic hallmark of the disease. However, the specific criteria (i.e., the number of eosinophils) required for the diagnosis remains a subject of debate. Useful clues include eosinophilic infiltration through the wall depth including the epithelium and crypts, eosinophilic aggregates or abscess, and eosinophilic degranulation.
- When endoscopic biopsy samples are taken, it is recommended that large and deep biopsy samples (due to inflammation sparing the mucosal layer) be retrieved from up to 10 different locations including the stomach and the small bowel (patchy distribution with sampling error may lead to nondiagnostic biopsies in up to 20%). It is also recommended that endoscopic biopsy samples be taken from mucosa with both abnormal and normal appearance. Although not often involved, colonic or ileal biopsies can prove diagnostic. In deep muscular or peritoneal disease, the diagnosis is sometimes only found in the surgical resection specimen or in the *full-thickness surgical biopsy (open or laparoscopic surgery)*. Eosinophilic duodenitis with involvement of the duodenal papilla (Vater) can manifest as pancreatitis or cholangitis.

## 12. What should be excluded in patients with suspected EGE?

- Drug-induced eosinophilia: aspirin, gold therapy, gemfibrozil, clofazimine, L-tryptophan, enalapril
- Intestinal parasites
- Irritable bowel disease (IBD) or collagenous colitis
- Collagen-vascular disease: Polyarteritis nodosa (PAN), systemic lupus erythematosus (SLE), systemic sclerosis, dermatomyositis, Churg-Strauss
- Malignant infiltration
- Lymphoma: Sezary T-cell and intestinal lymphomas, chronic myelogenous leukemia, Hodgkin disease

## 13. What are other treatment modalities for EGE?

Current treatment strategies are based on small studies. There are insufficient data derived from well-designed controlled trials to offer treatment recommendations.

### DIET THERAPY CONSISTS OF EITHER ELIMINATION DIETS OR ELEMENTAL DIETS

- Elemental diets are used for patients with multiple food allergies. However, these diets have not been critically evaluated in EGE. They are expensive and difficult to follow due to taste. They should not be used for longer than 6 to 8 weeks.
- Elimination diets (six food elimination diets [milk, soy, eggs, fish, wheat, nuts]) have been effective in eosinophilic esophagitis (mostly studied in children), and may be applicable to EGE, but this regimen has not been studied critically in EGE. In responders, a new food may be introduced every 5 to 7 days.

### PHARMACOLOGIC THERAPY

- *Steroids* are indicated for patients who fail or decline dietary therapy or those with severe presentations. Usual dosage is 1 to 2 mg kg/d for at least a month. This is tapered over 2 to 3 months. Most patients do not require maintenance therapy; however, a small number will require 2 to 3 months of corticosteroid therapy for symptoms to resolve. Patients who relapse, who are unable to taper steroids, or who have steroid-related side effects require a steroid-sparing option. Budesonide is effective for those with ileocolonic disease.
- Cases of eosinophilic esophagitis have clinically and histologically responded to *fluticasone* propionate MDI that is *swallowed*, *NOT inhaled*. Recently, *oral budesonide* has also been reported to be effective for the treatment of eosinophilic esophagitis in children.
- One report documented effectiveness of *non–enteric-coated budesonide* (formula of water-soluble tablets produced for rectal enema dissolutions) in gastric transmural EGE with ascites.
- Severe diseases should be treated with *parenteral methylprednisolone* (bolus of 125 mg followed by 0.5 mg/kg/day b.i.d.). Even in severe duodenal obstruction, a parenteral glucocorticoid therapeutic trial is recommended before surgery is considered.
- Recurrences occur in up to 40% and can be treated with *repeat short courses of prednisone. Topical corticosteroids* have been reported to be effective.

### NONGLUCOCORTICOID IMMUNE-MODULATOR THERAPIES AND FUTURE THERAPIES

- *Montelukast:* a leukotriene-1 receptor antagonist has been used with mixed results in small studies
- Suplatast tosilate: a leukotriene inhibitor is not available in the United States
- *Cromoglycate sodium* and *ketotifen:* These mast cell stabilizers have been used in selected cases with some success, larger studies are required.
- Anti–interleukin-5 (mepolizumab): A small number of patients have been treated with monoclonal antibody against IL-5 with encouraging results for hypereosinophilia syndrome and eosinophilic esophagitis.
- *Anti-IgE therapy (omalizumab):* This is a humanized anti-IgE monoclonal antibody found to be effective in treating allergic asthma and rhinitis. It was shown to decrease the absolute eosinophil count and IgE levels and improve symptoms in a small study of nine patients.

## 14. What is the natural history of EGE?

EGE is considered a chronic relapsing condition. The true natural history has yet to be defined; therefore, close follow-up of these patients is recommended. Larger prospective studies are needed to better define the natural history of the disease as well as assess the success of the current available therapies.

## WEBSITES

http://dave1.mgh.harvard.edu/media/presentations/Goldfinger_2_16_06_EosEsop/Goldfinger_2_16_06_EosEsop.swf

http://www.vhjoe.com

### BIBLIOGRAPHY

1. Chen MJ, Chu CH, Lin SC, et al. Eosinophilic gastroenteritis: Clinical experience with 15 patients. World J Gastroenterol 2003;9:2813–6.
2. Cousins L, Graham M, Tooze R, et al. Eosinophilic bowel disease controlled by the BB rat-derived lymphopenia/Gimap5 gene. Gastroenterology 2006;131:1475–85.
3. Foroughi S, Foster B, Kim N, et al. Anti-IgE treatment of eosinophil-associated gastrointestinal disorders. J Allergy Clin Immunol 2007;120:594–601.
4. Furuta GT, Liacouras CA, Collins MH, et al. Eosinophilic esophagitis in children and adults: A systematic review and consensus recommendations for diagnosis and treatment. Gastroenterology 2007;133:1342–63.
5. Garrett JK, Jameson SC, Thomson B, et al. Anti-interleukin-5 (mepolizumab) therapy for hypereosinophilic syndromes. J Allergy Clin Immunol 2004;113:115–9.
6. Kelly KJ. Eosinophilic gastroenteritis. J Pediatr Gastroenterol Nutr 2000;30(Suppl.):S28–35.
7. Khan S. Eosinophilic gastroenteritis. Best Pract Res Clin Gastroenterol 2005;19:177–98.
8. Khan S, Orenstein SR. Eosinophilic gastroenteritis. Gastroenterol Clin North Am 2008;37:333–48, v.
9. Klein NC, Hargrove RL, Sleissenger MH, et al. Eosinophilic gastroenteritis. Medicine (Baltimore) 1970;49:299–319.
10. Mendez-Sanchez N, Chavez-Tapia NC, Vazquez-Elizondo G, et al. Eosinophilic gastroenteritis: A review. Dig Dis Sci 2007;52:2904–11.
11. Mishra A, Hogan SP, Brandt EB, et al. An etiological role for aeroallergens and eosinophils in experimental esophagitis. J Clin Invest 2001;107:83–90.
12. Mishra A, Rothenberg ME. Intratracheal IL-13 induces eosinophilic esophagitis by an IL-5, eotaxin-1, and STAT6-dependent mechanism. Gastroenterology 2003;125:1419–27.
13. Roufosse F, Cogan E, Goldman M. Recent advances in pathogenesis and management of hypereosinophilic syndromes. Allergy 2004;59:673–89.
14. Roufosse FE, Goldman M, Cogan E. Hypereosinophilic syndromes. Orphanet J Rare Dis 2007;2:37.
15. Stein ML, Collins MH, Villanueva JM, et al. Anti-IL-5 (mepolizumab) therapy for eosinophilic esophagitis. J Allergy Clin Immunol 2006;118:1312–9.
16. Talley NJ, Shorter RG, Phillips SF, et al. Eosinophilic gastroenteritis: A clinic pathological study of patients with disease of the mucosa, muscle layer, and subserosal tissues. Gut 1990;31:54–8.
17. Venkataraman S, Ramakrishna BS, Mathan M, et al. Eosinophilic gastroenteritis—An Indian experience. Indian J Gastroenterol 1998;17:148–9.
18. von Wattenwyl F, Zimmermann A, Netzer P. Synchronous first manifestation of an idiopathic eosinophilic gastroenteritis and bronchial asthma. Eur J Gastroenterol Hepatol 2001;13:721–5.

# BACTERIAL OVERGROWTH

Travis J. Rutland, MD, and
Jack A. DiPalma, MD

**1. Define *bacterial overgrowth*.**

Small intestinal bacterial overgrowth (SIBO) is defined as greater than $10^5$ CFU/mL of bacteria in the proximal small bowel or greater than $10^3$ CFU/mL of isolates routinely found in colonic flora.

**2. What is the usual bacterial presence in the gastrointestinal tract?**

Stomach $<10^4$/mL

Jejunum $<10^5$/mL

Ileum $<10^6$ /mL

Colon $<10^{10}$/mL

The type of species that colonize the small intestine is changed in bacterial overgrowth. In health, small bowel bacteria resemble oropharyngeal flora with gram-positive, aerobic organisms. In overgrowth, bacteria are mostly gram-negative, including *Escherichia coli;* anaerobic bacteria, including *Clostridia* and *Bacteroides* spp., also predominate.

**3. What are the natural protective mechanisms against SIBO?**

- Gastric acid
- Bile acid
- Pancreatic enzyme activity
- Small intestinal motility (migrating motor complex)
- Ileocecal valve

**4. What factors influence small intestinal bacterial proliferation?**

- Structural lesions
- Motility
- Excessive bacterial load
- Deficiency in host defenses

**5. What kind of structural lesions predispose to overgrowth?**

Obstruction to outflow of luminal contents can occur at the site of surgical anastomosis or with webs, adhesions, or strictures. Surgical diversions and blind loops or neoreservoirs, such as the continent ileostomy, predispose to small intestinal bacterial overgrowth. The jejunoileal bypass, once a popular surgical procedure for morbid obesity, created a long segment of diverted bowel and was often complicated by overgrowth. Diverticula and duplications are frequently colonized with colonic-type bacteria, leading to overgrowth. There is an increased prevalence of SIBO in disorders that may result in intestinal failure. There is a frequent association of SIBO and Crohn's disease, especially among those who have undergone surgery.

**6. How do motility disorders cause overgrowth?**

Delayed transit of intestinal contents results in stasis. Overgrowth complicates intestinal pseudo-obstruction syndromes. The intestinal *housekeeper* migratory motor complex, when disrupted, is associated with bacterial overgrowth. Paralytic ileus results in bacterial proliferation. SIBO has been identified in 62.5% of patients with scleroderma in previous studies.

**7. How can an excessive bacterial load be delivered to the small bowel?**

Absence or incompetence of the ileocecal valve and enteric fistula can deliver bacteria to the small bowel in amounts that exceed clearing capacity.

**8. Which impairments of host defenses are important?**

- Acid suppression by surgery or medications
- Hypochlorhydric disorders such as pernicious anemia
- Immune deficiencies, particularly absence of secretory immunoglobulin A (IgA)
- Undernutrition, which can decrease gastric acidity and immune function

9. **What conditions are associated with small intestinal bacterial overgrowth?**

### REDUCED GASTRIC ACID

- Pernicious anemia
- Atrophic gastritis
- Gastric surgery
- Medications (H2 receptor antagonists, proton pump inhibitors)
- Neoreservoirs

### STRUCTURAL ABNORMALITIES

- Small bowel diverticula
- Adhesions
- Surgical anastomosis and diversions
- Fistulas (coloenteric, gastrocolic)
- Strictures
- Absent or incompetent ileocecal valves
- Webs
- Neoreservoirs

### DYSMOTILITY SYNDROMES

- Diabetes
- Acute enteric infection
- Scleroderma
- Intestinal pseudo-obstruction syndromes

10. **What are the other risk factors for bacterial overgrowth?**
Evidence indicates that overgrowth with colonic-type bacteria should be considered in patients older than 75 years of age with chronic diarrhea, anorexia, or nausea, even if they have no apparent predisposition. Dysmotility is probably responsible. Additional data suggest that overgrowth may cause diarrhea or abdominal pain in children, especially those younger than 2 years. Recent data implicate bacterial overgrowth in some patients with irritable bowel syndrome.

11. **What are the symptoms of overgrowth?**
Clinical manifestations vary. Diarrhea, anorexia, nausea, weight loss, and anemia are cardinal symptoms, but the nature of the small bowel abnormality influences the presentation. Patients obstructed by stricture may have bloating and pain. Overgrowth in small intestinal diverticula may present insidiously with metabolic derangements. The eventual clinical consequence of overgrowth, regardless of cause, is steatorrhea, leading to weight loss. Malabsorption results in hypocalcemic disorders, night blindness, vitamin K deficiency, and osteomalacia. Cobalamin deficiency is common with severe overgrowth.

12. **Why do patients with bacterial overgrowth develop anemia?**
Anemia may be megaloblastic and macrocytic as a result of cobalamin deficiency. Microcytic anemia due to iron deficiency results mainly from blood loss, not bacterial overgrowth. Anaerobic bacteria compete for uptake of cobalamin–intrinsic factor complex. Whereas luminal bacteria consume cobalamin, folic acid is a product of bacterial substrate fermentation. Thus, an important clinical observation in small intestinal bacterial overgrowth is the finding of low $B_{12}$ and high folate levels.

13. **What other micronutrient deficiencies are clinically important?**
In addition to iron and cobalamin deficiencies, other micronutrient deficiencies include deficiencies of water-soluble vitamins (e.g., thiamin and nicotinamide) and decreased absorption of fat-soluble vitamins (vitamins A, D, E, and K). Trace element malabsorption has not been carefully studied in overgrowth syndromes.

14. **What is the association between SIBO and sepsis?**
The possible contribution of SIBO to bacterial translocation and resultant sepsis is important in intestinal failure. In these patients, sepsis is a major cause of morbidity and mortality. There is increased intestinal permeability and impaired host immune defense in patients with SIBO.

### 15. How is bacterial overgrowth diagnosed?

Small intestinal bacterial overgrowth is confirmed by the demonstration of elevated numbers of small bowel bacteria colonies and the replacement of oropharyngeal with predominantly colonic organisms. Because small bowel intubation and aspiration for microbial analysis are cumbersome, overgrowth is considered in patients with predisposing factors and appropriate history. Indirect testing may help to substantiate the diagnosis.

### 16. What indirect testing can be used?

See Table 45-1.

| Table 45-1. Diagnosis of Small Intestinal Bacterial Overgrowth | |
| --- | --- |
| History | Prior surgery, medical conditions such as osteomalacia, night blindness, easy bruisibility, tetany |
| Examination | Systemic disease: weight loss and malabsorption |
| Laboratory values | Hemoglobin (decreased), mean corpuscular volume (increased), vitamin $B_{12}$ (decreased), folic acid (increased), fecal fat (increased) |
| Tests | Schilling test with intrinsic factor (decreased), $^{14}$C-glycocholic acid (increased), $^{14}$C-D-xylose (decreased), hydrogen testing with glucose or lactulose, jejunal aspirate for bacterial colony counts and strain identification |

### 17. What are the limitations of testing?

- *Jejunal intubation* for aspiration with bacterial colony counts and stain identification can provide a definitive diagnosis by showing jejunal counts greater than $10^5$ with colonic organisms. There is a risk of potential contamination by oropharyngeal bacteria during small bowel intubation. Additionally, bacterial overgrowth can be patchy and thus missed by a single aspiration. Because the test is cumbersome, some clinicians rely on indirect testing. Jejunal intubation can be performed endoscopically, and protected catheters can be used to obtain more reliable aspirates.
- *Radiolabeled breath tests* using glycocholic acid or xylose have been used for diagnosis of overgrowth. Glycocholic acid is released by bacterial deconjugation of radiolabeled bile acids. Xylose is catabolized by gram-negative aerobes and is absorbed in the proximal small bowel.
- *Fasting breath hydrogen* is elevated in overgrowth patients, and early rises after glucose or lactulose challenge reflect small bowel fermentation of the substrate by abnormal concentrations of bacteria. The diagnosis is established when the exhaled breath $H_2$ level increases by more than 10 parts per million greater than baseline on two consecutive samplings, or if the fasting breath hydrogen level exceeds 20 parts per million. Double peaks (SIBO and colonic peaks) have been previously thought to represent abnormal lactulose breath tests, but these results may occur from rapid orocecal transit, resulting in the premature delivery of fermentable substrate to the colonic bacteria. The reliability of breath testing has been criticized in patients with intestinal failure because of rapid transit. In patients with short-bowel syndrome or intestinal failure, it is recommended to combine lactulose breath testing with scintigraphy. This increases specificity to 100%, but sensitivity remains low at 38.9%. Additionally, approximately 15% to 27% of the population does not generate hydrogen post lactulose ingestion but instead produces methane. The measurement of hydrogen quantification alone with significantly underestimate the prevalence of SIBO in this population. Combining measurements of hydrogen and methane gas will permit the detection of those who harbor *Methanobrevibacter smithii*.

In general, *scintigraphic* and *hydrogen breath tests* are attractive alternatives to intubation tests for bacterial overgrowth. Hydrogen testing, although simple, inexpensive, and nonradioactive, does not have sufficient sensitivity or specificity.

### 18. What about other testing methods?

Quantification of urinary excretion of indican, drug metabolites, and conjugated *para*-aminobenzoic acid do not distinguish overgrowth from other types of malabsorption. An alternative approach to consider is a therapeutic trial of antibiotics. Most patients with SIBO show a symptomatic response within 1 week of initiation of therapy.

### 19. What is the treatment for bacterial overgrowth?

#### I. CORRECTION OF THE UNDERLYING CONDITION

- Surgery
- Prokinetic agents

## II. NUTRITION

- Lactose-free, low-residue diet
- Increase calories
- Micronutrient supplementation ($B^{12}$, fat-soluble vitamins, trace elements)

## III. ANTIBIOTICS

## IV. PROBIOTICS

## V. PROKINETIC AGENTS

### 20. What are the antibiotic agents used in the treatment of SIBO?

- Amoxicillin–clavulanic acid (500 mg 3 times daily)
- Ciprofloxacin (250 mg twice daily)
- Chloramphenicol (250 mg 4 times daily)
- Doxycycline (100 mg twice daily)
- Metronidazole (250 mg 3 times daily)
- Neomycin (500 mg 4 times daily)
- Norfloxacin (800 mg daily)
- Tetracycline (250 mg 4 times daily)
- Trimethoprim–sulfamethoxazole (1 DS tablet twice daily)
- Rifaximin (1200 mg daily) (Divided TID)

### 21. Do prokinetic agents help?

Surgery is often impractical or unacceptable, and prokinetic agents are tried to relieve stasis and improve outflow of small intestinal contents. However, standard stimulatory agents are not very effective. The long-acting somatostatin analog octreotide has been shown to stimulate motility in normal subjects and patients with scleroderma. It reduces overgrowth and improves symptoms in scleroderma.

### 22. How long should overgrowth be treated with antibiotics?

The objective of antibiotic therapy is not to eradicate the bacterial flora but rather to modify the bacterial milieu in a manner that results in symptomatic improvement. In general, a 7- to 10-day course of antibiotics may improve symptoms for several months in 46% to 90% of patients and results in negative breath tests in 20% to 75%. Other patients may require extended therapy, continuous courses, or rotating antibiotic regimens. Prolonged antibiotic therapy poses significant risk, including resistance and enterocolitis.

### 23. What about probiotics?

Studies have shown several potential mechanisms of action for probiotics; however, well-conducted clinical trials demonstrating benefit have not been performed. The most widely available probiotics are lactic acid bacteria and nonpathogenic yeasts. *Saccharomyces boulardi* is a probiotic used in the treatment of pseudomembranous colitis that has stated efficacy for bacterial overgrowth in children. Because antibiotics have potential side effects, probiotic therapy is attractive. A recent study in adults, however, showed no efficacy of *S. boulardi* in the treatment of overgrowth.

## BIBLIOGRAPHY

1. Ahar A, Flourie B, Rambaud JC, et al. Antibiotic efficacy in small intestinal bacterial overgrowth-related chronic diarrhea: A cross-over, randomized trial. Gastroenterology 1999;117:794–7.
2. de Boissieu D, Chaussain M, Badoual J, et al. Small-bowel bacterial overgrowth in children with chronic diarrhea, abdominal pain, or both. J Pediatr 1996;128:203–7.
3. Kumar A, Forsmark CE, Toskes PP. The response of small bowel bacterial overgrowth to treatment: Effects of coexisting conditions. Gastroenterology 1996;110:A340.
4. Lauritano EC, Gabrielli M, Lupascu A, et al. Rifaximin dose-finding study for the treatment of small intestinal bacterial overgrowth. Aliment Pharmacol Ther 2005;22:31–5.
5. Melcher EA, Levitt MD, Slavin JL. Methane production and bowel function parameters in healthy subjects on low and high fiber diets. Nutr Cancer 1991;16:85–92.
6. Pimentel M, Lin HC. Eradication of small bowel bacterial overgrowth reduces symptoms of irritable bowel syndrome. Am J Gastroenterol 2000;95:3503–6.
7. Quigley EM, Quera R. Small intestinal bacterial overgrowth: Roles of antibiotics, prebiotics, and probiotics. Gastroenterology 2006;130:S78–S90.
8. Riordan SM, McIver CJ, Wakefield D, et al. Small intestinal bacterial overgrowth in the symptomatic elderly. Am J Gastroenterol 1997;92:47–51.
9. Riordan SM, McIver CK, Walker BM, et al. The lactulose breath hydrogen test and small intestinal bacterial overgrowth. Am J Gastroenterol 1996;91:1795–803.
10. Rose S, Young MA, Reynolds JC. Gastrointestinal manifestations of scleroderma. Gastroenterol Clin North Am 1998;27:563–94.

11. Scarpellini E, Gabrielli M, Lauritano CE, et al. High dosage rifaximin for the treatment of small intestinal bacterial overgrowth. Aliment Pharmacol Ther 2007;25:781–6.
12. Shanahan F. The host-microbe interface within the gut. Best Pract Res Clin Gastroenterol 2002;16:915–31.
13. Sherman PM. Bacterial overgrowth. In: Yamada T, editor. Textbook of Gastroenterology. Philadelphia: JB Lippincott; 1991. pp. 1530–9.
14. Soudah HC, Hasler WL, Owyang C. Effect of octreotide on intestinal motility and bacterial overgrowth in scleroderma. N Engl J Med 1991;325:1461–7.
15. Toskes PP, Kumar A. Enteric bacterial flora and bacterial overgrowth syndrome. In: Feldman M, editor. Sleisenger and Fordtran's Gastrointestinal and Liver Disease. 6th ed Philadelphia: WB Saunders; 1998. pp. 1523–35.

# COLORECTAL CANCER AND COLON CANCER SCREENING

Stephen P. Laird, MD, MS, and
Neil W. Toribara, MD, PhD

CHAPTER 46

### 1. What is colorectal cancer (CRC)?

CRC includes both colon and rectal cancer. Over 95% of the primary cancers arising in the large bowel are adenocarcinomas; the remainder are lymphomas, malignant carcinoids, leiomyosarcomas, and Kaposi sarcomas. Several variants of adenocarcinomas have been described. These include *signet-ring carcinomas, mucinous* or *colloid carcinomas,* and *scirrhous carcinomas.* As a general rule, poorly differentiated adenocarcinomas tend to be more aggressive, metastasize earlier, and have a poorer prognosis than well-differentiated tumors.

### 2. How does the pathophysiology of rectal cancer differ from cancer elsewhere in the colon?

The rectum is relatively immobile, lacks a serosal covering, and is located largely behind the peritoneal reflection, surrounded by perirectal fat. As a result, rectal cancers more commonly spread contiguously via direct extension into local structures, whereas colon cancer more commonly spreads via lymphatics and hematogenously. Thus, rectal cancers that have spread beyond the mucosa are treated with surgery and adjuvant radiation with or without chemotherapy, whereas colon cancers are treated with surgery and chemotherapy rather than radiation. Some evidence such as distribution of malignancies within the colon in hereditary nonpolyposis colorectal cancer (HNPCC) and differing cellular surface markers also suggests that biological differences may play a role.

### 3. How common is colorectal cancer?

Cancer is the second leading cause of death in the United States (after cardiovascular disease), and CRC is the second leading cause of death from malignancies (after lung cancer). The lifetime risk of developing CRC is 1 in 18 (5.5%) in women and 1 in 17 (5.9%) in men and is influenced by hereditary and lifestyle factors. The incidence is estimated at 147,000 new cases per year, with an estimated 49,960 deaths in 2008. The incidence of CRC peaked in the mid 1980s and has slowly declined since that time, reflecting the effects of increased availability of colonoscopy, gradual acceptance of CRC screening, and the lag time between polyp formation and malignant transformation.

### 4. Do the genetic defects leading to sporadic CRC differ from those in genetic syndromes associated with colon cancer?

Yes. It appears that all CRC develops from previously normal mucosa by an accumulation of genetic abnormalities, although the methods by which these abnormalities accumulate differ. In most sporadic CRC and familial adenomatous polyposis (FAP) syndrome, genetic abnormalities accumulate via loss of large pieces of DNA, known as loss of heterozygosity (LOH). The most common acquisition sequence of genetic abnormalities is thought to be *APC, ras, p53,* and *DCC,* although the order of allelic deletion is not as important as the cumulative loss of DNA or LOH. There is some evidence for a distinct hyperplastic polyp-serrated adenoma-carcinoma pathway having a genetic signature distinct from the more common tubular adenoma pathway described earlier. Translating this knowledge into a practical stool-based DNA test, in which DNA isolated from a stool sample is tested for a panel of mutations in genes commonly involved in colonic carcinogenesis, has proved to be difficult, although efforts are still ongoing. In HNPCC and a small minority of sporadic CRCs, the abnormalities accrue through accumulation of point mutations, which cannot be corrected because of defects in the DNA repair system.

### 5. Describe the natural sequence from colon adenoma to colon cancer.

In one of the major milestones in gastroenterology, the 2004 National Polyp Study showed that removal of colonic adenomas during colonoscopy prevented subsequent development of colorectal cancer, showing that colonic adenomas are a vital step, which can be interrupted, in the carcinogenic progression of sporadic CRC. The prevalence curves for adenomas and colorectal cancers parallel each other, with the adenoma curve shifted 5 to 10 years earlier than carcinomas. This suggests that the time needed for an adenoma to develop into cancer is 5 to 10 years, thus giving a significant window of time to discover and remove premalignant lesions. There is accumulating evidence that there is a second pathway to the development of CRC in which some hyperplastic polyps (previously thought to be benign lesions without malignant potential) may develop into serrated adenomas, which are adenomas with a distinct histology and probably a distinct array of genetic abnormalities (*BRAF* mutations, extensive DNA methylation, and microsatellite instability). These serrated adenomas have a potential for malignant transformation equal to or perhaps greater than tubular adenomas.

### 6. How prevalent are colonic adenomas among the U.S. population?

The prevalence of adenomatous polyps appears to be highly dependent on the population studied. Two colonoscopic studies in asymptomatic populations have reported rates of 23% to 25% prevalence in male and female patients between the ages of 50 and 82 years. Two other studies involving only men in Department of Veterans Affairs Medical Centers had prevalence rates of approximately 40% and small studies have suggested prevalences of 50% or greater in some populations.

### 7. Where in the colon are polyps most commonly located?

Autopsy series have shown a relatively even distribution of adenomas throughout the colon, although larger polyps have a distal predominance, as expected from the distribution of CRCs. Recently, there has been an increased interest in *flat* or *nonpolypoid* neoplasms whose prevalence may be as high 10%. These are more difficult to detect during standard endoscopy and, in the case of sessile serrated adenomas, which have both a predominant right colon distribution and malignant potential, may be significant contributors to missed or interval cancers (CRCs arising between screening or surveillance colonoscopies).

### 8. Give the mean age of onset and describe the anatomic distribution of CRC.

True sporadic CRCs occur at a mean age of 69; approximately 60% are distal to the splenic flexure (thus theoretically within the reach of a flexible sigmoidoscope). However, some studies have suggested that older patients and blacks appear to have an increased proportion of CRCs in the right colon.

### 9. How are malignant polyps defined? How are they clinically managed?

Pathologists prefer the term *severe dysplasia* for adenomas with a focus of carcinoma in situ or intramucosal carcinoma, because complete endoscopic removal is curative. The term *malignant polyp* is reserved for the approximately 5% of adenomas in which a focus of carcinoma has invaded beyond the muscularis mucosa into the submucosa, where lymphatic spread with metastasis is possible. A malignant polyp has at least one of the following characteristics:

- Poorly differentiated cancer
- Invasion of veins or lymphatics
- Extension of the carcinoma to less than 2 mm of the margin
- Invasion of submucosa of the bowel wall

When malignant polyps are found, consideration should be given to early re-endoscopy and/or local surgical resection. Endoscopic removal of a malignant polyp is associated with a 10% to 25% relapse rate.

### 10. How is colon cancer staged, and how does this affect prognosis?

Although the overall 5-year survival is about 62% in the United States, there are significant differences among ethnic groups. Although histology and syndromes (HNPCC colorectal cancers have a better prognosis stage for stage than sporadic CRCs) have some effect, the best single determinant of prognosis is stage at diagnosis. The two most widely used staging methods are the Duke's and TNM (tumor, node, metastasis) systems. Both give essentially equivalent information for prognostic purposes. The Duke's system is simpler and still widely used by gastroenterologists and surgeons, whereas TNM staging is used more widely among oncologists and pathologists (Table 46-1).

**Table 46-1.** Duke's Classification Versus Tumor, Node, Metastasis (TMN) Staging

| DUKE'S CLASSIFICATION* | 5-YEAR SURVIVAL (%) | TMN STAGING† | | 5-YEAR SURVIVAL (%) |
|---|---|---|---|---|
| | | Stage 0 Carcinoma in situ | Tis N0 M0 | 100 |
| Stage A Limited to mucosa | 95 to 100 | Stage I Tumor invades submucosa Tumor invades muscularis propria | T1 N0 M0 T2 N0 M0 | 95 80 |
| Stage B1 Into muscularis propria Stage B2 Through serosa | 80 to 85 75 | Stage II Tumor invades through muscularis propria into serosa or pericolonic/perirectal tissue Tumor perforates or directly invades other organs | T3 N0 M0 T4 N0 M0 | |

*Continued*

**Table 46-1** Duke's Classification Versus Tumor, Node, Metastasis (TMN) Staging—Cont'd

| DUKE'S CLASSIFICATION* | 5-YEAR SURVIVAL (%) | TMN STAGING† | | 5-YEAR SURVIVAL (%) |
|---|---|---|---|---|
| Stage C1 1 to 4 regional nodes positive Stage C2 >4 regional nodes positive | 65 42 | Stage III Any perforation with nodal metastases N1: 1 to 3 nodes N2: ≥4 nodes N3: Any lymph node along named vascular trunk | TX N1 M0 TX N2 M0 TX N3 M0 | |
| Stage D‡ Distant metastases | 5 | Stage IV Any invasion of bowel wall with or without lymph node metastases but with evidence of distant metastases | TX NX M1 | |

*Gastrointestinal Study Group Modification.
†American Joint Committee on Cancer.
‡Included only in the Turnbull modification of Duke's classification.

### 11. Describe the workup for CRC after the initial diagnosis.

Surgical removal of the cancer remains the only curative therapy. Before surgery, visualization of the entire bowel, preferably by full colonoscopy, is indicated to exclude synchronous lesions (either adenomas or cancers) that may influence the operation. Preoperative laboratory tests should include complete blood count, blood chemistry panel-20, and carcinoembryonic antigen (CEA). If the CEA level is elevated at the time of diagnosis (approximately 60% of cases), it provides a convenient method for assessing effectiveness of the surgery and detecting early recurrences. Preoperative abdominal computed tomography (CT) scan and chest radiograph are useful in looking for metastatic disease. In rectal cancers, preoperative staging with transrectal ultrasound helps to determine the utility of adjunct radiation therapy.

### 12. What surgical margins are recommended?

Most surgeons attempt to include at least 5 cm on either side of the tumor within the resection block, although margins as small as 2 cm may be acceptable in the distal rectum to preserve sphincter function.

### 13. Describe the recommended schedule of colonoscopic follow-up after surgery.

If a preoperative colonoscopy clears the remainder of the colon of polyps or synchronous malignancy and the surgical margins are tumor free, colonoscopy before 1 to 3 years after resection is probably not indicated. The risk for developing metachronous neoplasms in a post malignancy resection patient is about the same as for a patient with an adenoma of unfavorable histology; therefore, intervals between colonoscopic screening exams should be similar, every 3 to 5 years.

### 14. Are there any effective blood tests to screen for CRC?

Serum tests to diagnose CRC are limited by the inherent problem that markers produced by malignant cells are hardest to detect in the early, small tumors that have the best prognosis. To date, no putative serum markers of CRC have sufficient sensitivity or specificity to warrant use as primary screening modalities. CEA, the most widely used CRC tumor marker, is therefore useful only to assess efficacy of surgery or monitoring for recurrences in cancers already known to be CEA positive. Even this use has been challenged by those who believe that the clinical benefit of diagnosing recurrences is minimal. (Caveat: Because CEA is excreted in the bile, elevated levels may be difficult to interpret in the presence of biliary obstruction or hepatic dysfunction.) A reasonable surveillance approach in CEA-positive tumors is to check CEA levels every 2 months for the first 6 months, every 4 months for up to 2 years, and then every 6 months for up to 5 years.

### 15. List the risk factors for developing CRC.

Age, diet, environment, personal history of colonic neoplasm, family history of colonic neoplasm, familial colon cancer syndromes, and inflammatory bowel disease.

### 16. What is the effect of age on the risk of developing CRC?

The risk of developing CRC increases with age, starting at about age 40 and roughly doubling with each decade. Below age 40, the incidence of CRC is less than 6 in 100,000; however, by age 80 the incidence is approximately 500 per 100,000 in men and 400 per 100,000 in women. Because over 90% of colorectal cancers occur after age 50, most screening programs have arbitrarily chosen this as a starting age.

### 17. Discuss the effect of diet on the risk for developing CRC.

Diet is thought to account for the major differences in the incidence rates of CRC worldwide. Although epidemiologic studies and animal models suggest that a high-fat, low-fiber diet (typical of Western nations) increases the risk of developing CRC, prospective trials of low-fat, high-fiber diets have shown no significant effect. Similarly, other micronutrients, such as folate, reducing agents (vitamins C and E), beta-carotene, and eicosanoids, showed promise in experimental conditions but either failed to yield positive results in controlled trials or still are under investigation. Calcium supplementation is the only dietary intervention that has shown a positive, albeit modest, effect in humans, using adenomas as a surrogate marker for the development of CRC.

**18. Do environmental factors increase the risk for developing CRC?**

The risk of developing CRC is directly related to environmental factors. This effect is evident in comparing the rates of CRC in populations emigrating from a region with a low rate to a region with a high rate. For example, the incidence of colon cancer in the Japanese (low incidence) emigrating to the United States (high incidence) led to a 10-fold increase in incidence over a single generation, much too fast to be a selection phenomenon. In general, the United States and Western European nations have a higher rate of CRC than developing nations.

**19. Which adenoma features are associated with a greater malignant potential?**

Adenomatous polyps are considered premalignant lesions, but the actual risk of neoplastic transformation is unknown. Large size, villous architecture, and dysplasia are features of adenomas that have a higher risk of developing a carcinoma within a given polyp. Some researchers believe that serrated adenomas may have an increased rate and risk of malignant transformation, although there is insufficient evidence to state this definitively.

**20. What are the recommendations for CRC screening in people at average risk for CRC?**

Men and women at average risk should be offered screening for CRC and adenomatous polyps at age 50 years. Options for CRC screening include:

- Fecal occult blood test (FOBT)
- Flexible sigmoidoscopy
- FOBT and flexible sigmoidoscopy
- Colonoscopy

Stool DNA testing and CT colonography are two methods that appear to have a great deal of promise, although their utility in everyday clinical practice has yet to be defined. It is important to differentiate between screening modalities that are primarily effective at detecting CRCs, those that can detect both cancers and their precursor lesions, and those that can detect CRCs and identify and remove polyps. Each approach has its advantages and disadvantages, and each person should make an informed decision regarding their preference.

**21. Give the current guidelines for surveillance colonoscopy in patients with a history of adenomatous polyps.**

A periodic surveillance program should be customized according to adequacy of the preparation and endoscopic findings.

| Colonoscopy Findings | Next Colonoscopy |
| --- | --- |
| One or two tubular adenomas | 5 years |
| Large sessile (>2 cm) adenoma | 3 to 6 months |
| Inadequate colon preparation | Repeat within 3 to 6 months |
| Large (>1 cm) adenoma, villous histology, or dysplasia | 3 years |

**22. Who is considered to be at increased risk for developing CRC?**

People at increased risk are defined as those individuals who have a personal history of CRC or an adenomatous polyp, a predisposing illness for CRC such as inflammatory bowel disease (IBD), a first-degree relative (parent, sibling, child) with CRC or an adenomatous polyp, or a gene carrier for familial colon cancer syndromes. The risk of developing CRC is increased approximately 2-fold if a first-degree relative has been diagnosed with CRC over age 65. The younger the age at which the relative was diagnosed, the higher is the risk. The risk also rises if more than one first-degree relative has been diagnosed with CRC. Perhaps more significant, the same risk seems to apply if first-degree relatives were found to have adenomatous polyps. Evidence suggests a slightly increased risk (approximately 1.5-fold) if third-degree relatives (e.g., cousins) have been diagnosed with CRC.

**23. Which method of CRC screening is recommended for individuals at increased risk of developing CRC?**

Colonoscopy is the only recommended screening modality in this patient population.

## 24. List the familial colon cancer syndromes.
- FAP and Gardner's syndrome (FAP with extracolonic manifestations)
- Hamartomatous polyp syndromes: Peutz-Jeghers syndrome (PJS) and juvenile polyposis syndrome (JPS)
- HNPCC

## 25. What tests are available for hereditary CRC?
Diagnosis of an APC germline mutation is based on one of several DNA-based tests:

- Sequencing of the entire genome (95% sensitive)
- Combination of confirmation strand gel electrophoresis screening and protein truncation testing (80% to 90% sensitive)
- Protein truncation alone (80% sensitive)
- Linkage analysis (98% sensitive in most families with the FAP mutation)

There are more than 228 germline mutations and more than 47 polymorphisms in the seven MMR genes associated with HNPCC. These multiple mutations have limited the development of inexpensive diagnostic assays for HNPCC and diagnosis is now based on direct DNA sequencing.

Patients with JPS and their family members are appropriate candidates for genetic testing for germline mutations MAD4 and BMP1A using direct DNA sequencing.

The only clearly identified gene mutation in PJS is *STK11/LKB1*, which leads to 40% to 60% of cases and can be diagnosed by mutation analysis of *STK11*.

Candidate mutations associated with common familial colon cancer have not been characterized well enough to warrant routine genetic testing (Table 46-2).

**Table 46-2.** Features of Colon Cancer Syndromes

| FEATURES | SPORADIC CRC | HNPCC | FAP | ATTENUATED FAP | JPS | PJS |
|---|---|---|---|---|---|---|
| Average age of CRC (yr) | 69 | 44 | 39 | 49 | 34 | 40 |
| Incidence | Lifetime 1:18 (F) 1:17 (M) | 1:2000 | 1:10,000 | 1:9000 | 1:100,000 | 1:200,000 |
| Colon polyps | Few polyps | Few polyps, proximal distribution | >100 polyps in teens | ≈30 polyps with proximal distribution | ≈100s in colon, scattered elsewhere in GI tract | >2 P-J polyps in GI tract |
| Gene abnormality | Multiple | MLH1, MSH2, MSH6, PMS2, PMS1 | APC (>90%), ? MYH (≈5%) | APC (>90%), ? MYH (≈5%) | MADH4/ SMA4 and BMPRIA (53%) | STK11/ LKB1 (≈55%) |
| Mode of inheritance | ? | Autosomal dominant | Autosomal dominant | Autosomal dominant | Autosomal dominant | Autosomal dominant |

CRC, colorectal cancer; HNPCC, hereditary nonpolyposis colorectal cancer; FAP, familial adenomatous polyposis; JPS, juvenile polyposis syndrome; PJS, Peutz-Jeghers syndrome.

## 26. What is the recommended surveillance for people with a family history of CRC who do not fit the genetic profiles?
- People with a first-degree relative with CRC or adenomatous polyp diagnosed at age younger than 60 years or two first-degree relatives with CRC diagnosed at any age should have a screening colonoscopy starting at age 40 years or 10 years younger than the earliest diagnosis in the family (whichever is first), and repeated every 5 years.
- People with a first-degree relative with CRC or adenomatous polyp diagnosed at age older than 60 years or two second-degree relatives (grandparent, aunt, or uncle) with CRC should be screened as average-risk persons but beginning at age 40 years.
- People with one second-degree relative with CRC should be screened as average risk.

## 27. How do FAP and Gardner syndrome increase the risk of CRC?

FAP and Gardner syndrome are inherited in an autosomal dominant manner with their phenotypic expression dependent on the location of the mutation in their *APC* gene. Their fully expressed forms are characterized by the development of hundreds to thousands of colonic adenomas. One hundred percent of patients expressing this phenotype develop CRC without colectomy. Most patients begin developing adenomas in their teens, and screening in families with a known proband should start at that time. One third of FAP cases arise as de novo mutations. The increased risk of CRC is thought to be due to the sheer number of adenomatous polyps; each polyp has the same risk of malignant transformation as an *ordinary* sporadic adenoma.

## 28. How are FAP and Gardner syndrome diagnosed?

The *APC* gene is responsible for both FAP and Gardner syndrome. Most disease-causing mutations result in premature stop codons, which give rise to truncated proteins. Commercial tests are available to detect truncated proteins and to directly sequence the gene. The results can be used for accurate screening of affected kindreds. Members of FAP kindreds who have not developed adenomas by age 40 have not inherited the polyposis phenotype. The position of the mutation gives rise to the phenotype of the FAP. For example, mutations in the extreme beginning or end of the *APC* gene can cause an attenuated form of FAP, which is characterized by fewer adenomas (1 to 100) with a right-sided predominance.

## 29. In addition to colonoscopy, what other tests should be considered in FAP?

Patients with FAP are at increased risk of extracolonic tumors, including thyroid cancer, pancreatic cancer, duodenal and ampullary cancer, and gastric cancer; therefore, periodic thyroid function tests, liver function tests, and upper gastrointestinal tract screening with both forward and side-viewing endoscopes are recommended.

## 30. What is the role of NSAIDs in treating FAP?

Both sulindac and celecoxib decrease the number of adenomas in patients with FAP, but neither is associated with complete regression. Therefore, chemoprevention cannot replace prophylactic colectomy, although the timing of the colectomy may be delayed.

## 31. How do hamartomatous polyp syndromes affect the risk of developing CRC?

Along with PJS and JPS, the differential diagnosis includes Cowden disease and the Bannayan-Ruvalcaba-Riley syndrome. Phenotypic features of hamartomatous syndromes display considerable overlap. Emerging understanding of the germline mutations may provide more accurate distinctions between these. Hamartomatous polyp syndromes appear to be associated with a slightly increased risk of developing CRC, although nowhere near the risk associated with APC syndromes.

## 32. What is HNPCC?

HNPCC is an autosomal dominant inherited disease in which colon cancer is caused by inactivation of one of the proteins involved in DNA proofreading (usually hMSH2 or hMLH1) leading to early onset of colon cancers and extracolonic cancers (e.g., endometrial, ovarian, gastric, urinary tract, renal cell, biliary, and gallbladder). Colon cancer arises from discrete adenomas, which rapidly accumulate point mutations, resulting in a markedly accelerated progression from adenoma to carcinoma. Because the term *nonpolyposis* is misleading and the recognition that some members of these kindreds may develop cancers other than CRC, there has been a trend toward calling this entity by its original designation, *Lynch syndrome*.

## 33. How is HNPCC diagnosed?

Diagnosis is based on either the Amsterdam criteria, the Amsterdam criteria II, or the Bethesda guidelines. The more stringent Amsterdam criteria increase the chances of finding a germline mutation in either *MSH2* or *MLH1* to 25% to 86%. The Bethesda guidelines are more sensitive but less specific than the Amsterdam criteria. Interestingly, there are a significant number of families fitting the Amsterdam criteria who do not appear to have abnormalities in the mismatch repair genes. These families should be screened endoscopically as outlined in the following section (Table 46-3 and Box 46-1).

### Table 46-3. Amsterdam Criteria

| AMSTERDAM CRITERIA* | AMSTERDAM CRITERIA II |
|---|---|
| 1. One member diagnosed with CRC before age 50 years | 1. At least three affected relatives with an HNPCC-associated cancer |
| 2. Two affected generations | 2. One of whom is an FDR of the other two |
| 3. Three affected relatives, one of them a FDR of the other two | 3. At least two successive generations |
| 4. Exclude FAP | 4. One member diagnosed with CRC before age 50 years |
| 5. Pathologic confirmation | 5. Exclude FAP |
| | 6. Pathologic confirmation |

CRC, colorectal cancer; FAP, familial adenomatous polyposis; FDR, first-degree relative; HNPCC, hereditary nonpolyposis colorectal cancer.
*All criteria must be met.

---

**Box 46-1.** Revised Bethesda Guidelines

(Meeting any listed feature is sufficient to proceed with testing for microsatellite instability.)
1. Colorectal cancer diagnosed in a patient who is younger than 50 years of age
2. Presence of synchronous, metachronous colorectal or other HNPCC-associated tumors[1] regardless of age
3. Colorectal cancer with the MSI-H histology diagnosed in a patient who is younger than 60 years old[2]
4. Colorectal cancer diagnosed in one or more first-degree relatives with an HNPCC-related tumor, with one of the cancers being diagnosed younger than age 50 years.
5. Colorectal cancer diagnosed in two or more first-or second-degree relatives with HNPCC-related tumors, regardless of age.

[1]Colorectal, endometrial, stomach, ovarian, pancreas, ureter and renal pelvis, biliary tract, and brain (usually glioblastoma as seen in Turcot syndrome) tumors, sebaceous gland adenomas and keratoacanthomas in Muir-Torre syndrome, and carcinoma of the small bowel.
[2]MSI-H (microsatellite instability-high tumors) refers to changes in two or more of the five NCI-recommended panels of microsatellite markers; histology features include presence of tumor-infiltrating lymphocytes, Crohn-like lymphocytic reaction, mucinous/signet ring differentiation, or medullary growth pattern.

## 34. Outline the screening recommendation for patients with HNPCC.

Screening with colonoscopy for all members of the family should begin at age 20 to 25 years, repeated semiannually until age 40, and then yearly thereafter. Some individuals with known mutations may elect to have a subtotal colectomy before developing malignancies.

## 35. What is MYH-associated polyposis (MAP)?

MYH polyposis is a recently described autosomal recessive polyposis syndrome that is phenotypically similar to attenuated APC (15 to 500 adenomas) but does not have an *APC* germline mutation. This biallelic germline mutation causes nucleotide transversion G:C → T:A in the *APC* gene. MYH is a protein that acts synergistically with two other proteins, OGG1 and MTH1, in the base excision repair pathway to repair DNA replication errors caused by oxidative stress. These mutations have been demonstrated in both adenomas and carcinomas. It is unknown what percentage of patients with polyposis syndrome have this mutation.

## 36. What is microsatellite instability (MSI)?

Microsatellites are short repeated DNA sequences (up to 10 nucleotides in length) that are susceptible to somatic mutation by misalignment. Ordinarily, this mismatch in the number of repeats is repaired by the DNA proofreading complex (which includes *MSH2, MLH1, MSH6, MLH3, PMS1,* and *PMS2,* the so-called mismatch repair genes). When this complex is inactivated (usually by changes in *MSH2* or *MLH1*), mismatched bases, including the commonly occurring microsatellite repeat misalignments, cannot be repaired, leading to a rapid accumulation of genome-wide mutations. MSI is observed in approximately 85% of HNPCC colon cancers and 15% of sporadic colon cancers. As MSI is thought to be common in the malignant transformation of serrated but not tubular adenomas, the former lesions may be responsible for many of the MSI-positive sporadic cancers. The commonly accepted method for detecting MSI is by using a standard panel of five microsatellites, with abnormalities in two or more constituting the MSI-high (MSI-H) phenotype commonly associated with HNPCC. It appears that MSI-positive CRCs have a better prognosis stage-for-stage compared with microsatellite stable cancers; however, they may not respond as well to 5-FU–based chemotherapy. This argues for MSI testing becoming a routine part of the workup for newly diagnosed CRC cases.

## 37. How does inflammatory bowel disease (IBD) affect the risk of developing CRC?

Patients with chronic IBD have an increased risk of developing colorectal cancer, particularly those with chronic ulcerative colitis (CUC). Please see Chapter 43 for colonoscopy screening recommendations in ulcerative colitis.

## 38. Which two clinical conditions should raise suspicion for the presence of colon cancer?

An unexplained iron deficiency anemia or sepsis with *Streptococcus bovis* as the pathogen should trigger investigation for colorectal cancer.

## 39. Is FOBT effective in detecting colon polyps and cancer?

Yes. Even in the absence of iron deficiency anemia, FOBT has been shown to decrease mortality by 15% to 30% in three large randomized, controlled trials using guaiac-based methods. Immunologic methods for testing human hemoglobin have shown some promise for increasing specificity but have not been widely used because of increased cost. Only large polyps (greater than 1.5 cm in diameter) and cancers bleed enough to be detected routinely by FOBT. Thus, although FOBT screening can reduce mortality from CRC by discovering malignancies at earlier, curable stages, it is considerably less effective in detecting adenomas, whose removal prior to malignant transformation is a much more cost-effective strategy.

**40. Does a program of periodic sigmoidoscopy decrease mortality from CRC?**

Yes. The magnitude of this decrease is determined by a number of factors, including distribution of CRCs, extent of the exam, predictive value of the procedure for lesions beyond the extent of the exam, and number of patients undergoing screening. Colonoscopic studies have shown that patients with adenomas within the reach of the flexible sigmoidoscope have an increased risk of significant lesions (large adenomas, adenomas with villous histology, and cancers) in the proximal colon and should have a full colonoscopy. With this strategy, one can detect approximately 80% of significant lesions with an examination to the splenic flexure and two thirds of significant lesions if only the descending colon is reached. However, the same data suggest that one half of significant lesions in the proximal colon have no sentinel lesions within the reach of a flexible sigmoidoscope and would be missed during screening.

**41. What is the sensitivity and specificity of an air contrast barium enema?**

Carefully performed, air contrast barium enemas have sensitivities and specificities in the 90% range; however, in most centers the figures are considerably lower, perhaps because modern ultrasound-, CT-, or MRI-based procedures have become more fashionable.

**42. How effective is CT colonography (CTC) as a screening test?**

Also known as *virtual colonoscopy*, CTC is an evolving technology for CRC screening. The problem to date with CTC as a screening option was the variability of the earlier multicenter trial results. Unpublished data from the 2005 National CT Colonography Trial (ACRIN 6664) showed 90% sensitivity and 86% specificity for adenomas larger than 1 cm. For smaller polyps of 6 mm or larger, the sensitivity and specificity were 78% and 88%, respectively. These preliminary results suggest CTC may be a viable option for CRC screening in selected populations (incomplete or failed colonoscopy, high risk for sedation, patient preference if at average risk for CRC). Nevertheless, this would suggest a 14% false-positive rate resulting in inappropriate referral for colonoscopy. Additional data from the ACRIN 6664 trial should answer questions regarding patient preferences and cost-effectiveness of CTC compared to optical colonoscopy (OC). Ultimately, cost-effectiveness will hinge on how smaller polyps are managed. The American College of Radiology (ACR) recommends polyps of 5 mm or smaller not be reported at all and that patients with two polyps of 6 to 9 mm be offered the option of CTC follow-up in 3 years or OC with polypectomy. Many are concerned this could lead to the underdiagnosis of important colonic adenoma findings with delayed surveillance, as well as a concern regarding the ethics of incomplete disclosure with patients. In one study of 6000 consecutive polyps found on OC, 12% of polyps 5 to 10 mm had advanced histology and 1% were cancerous. In another retrospective study using the new ACR guidelines, one-third of all patients with high-risk findings (3% of total patients) with a recommended surveillance interval of 3 years would have been told after CTC that they are normal and to come back in 5 to 10 years. CTC has poorer sensitivity than colonoscopy in the detection of flat or depressed lesions. Flat polyps have been reported to be significantly more likely to contain high-grade dysplasia than protuberant polyps. How this affects the overall acceptance of CTC as a viable screening modality remains to be seen.

**43. Can CRC be prevented with medicines (chemoprevention)?**

Because we cannot prevent CRCs by elimination of causative factors, the possibility of chemoprevention has generated considerable enthusiasm. NSAIDs, including sulindac and aspirin, have shown promise in both experimental models and epidemiologic studies. Recent studies have shown protective effects; however, maximum efficacy requires higher doses (more than 14 tablets/wk), which markedly increase the risk of gastrointestinal tract toxicity and potential bleeding. Aspirin use for adenoma prevention at present can only be recommended for those at increased risk for adenoma formation who have no history of ulcer disease or stroke. Sulindac decreases the number and size of adenomas in patients with FAP but does not completely prevent progression to cancer. Its efficacy in sporadic adenomas is unclear, although preliminary results of a trial using a combination of sulindac and DMFO (dimethylfluoroornithine) have shown significant promise at doses that may lower the potential gastrointestinal tract toxicity. Selective cyclooxygenase-2 inhibitors, which have a much lower gastrointestinal toxicity profile, are more effective than sulindac for FAP. Randomized, double-blind prospective studies have shown both rofecoxib and celecoxib to be effective at also decreasing sporadic adenoma recurrence, although only the latter is currently available.

**BIBLIOGRAPHY**

1. AGA Institute Position on CT Colonography. Gastroenterology 2006;131:1627–8.
2. Banerjee S, Van Dam J. CT Colonography for colon cancer screening. Gastrointest Endosc 2006;63:121–33.
3. Bresalier RS. Malignant neoplasms of the large intestine. In: Feldman M, Friedman LS, Brandt L, editors. Sleisenger and Fordtran's Gastrointestinal and Liver Disease. Philadelphia: WB Saunders; 2006. pp. 2760–810.
4. Butterly LF, Chase MP, Pohl H, et al. Prevalence of clinically important histology in small adenomas. Clin Gastroenterol Hepatol 2006;4:343–8.
5. Cole BF, Baron JA, Sandler RS, et al. Folic acid for the prevention of colorectal adenomas: A randomized clinical trial. JAMA 2007;297:2351–9.
6. Cotton PB, Durkalski VL, Benoit CP, et al. Computed tomographic colonography (virtual colonoscopy): A multicenter comparison with standard colonoscopy for detection of colorectal neoplasia. JAMA 2004;291:1713–9.

7. Das D, Arber N, Jankowski J. Chemoprevention of colorectal cancer. Digestion 2007;76:51–67.
8. East JE, Saunders BP, Jass JR. Sporadic and syndromic hyperplastic polyps and serrated adenomas of the colon: Classification, molecular genetics, natural history, and clinical management. Gastroenterol Clin N Am 2008;37:25–46.
9. Jemal A, Siegel R, Ward E, et al. Cancer statistics, 2008. CA Cancer J Clin 2008;58:71–96.
10. Johnson CD, Harmsen W, Wilson L, et al. Prospective blinded evaluation of computed tomographic colonoscopy for screen detection of colorectal polyps. Gastro 2003;125:311–9.
11. Levin B, Lieberman DA, McFarland B, et al. Screening and surveillance for the early detection of colorectal cancer and adenomatous polyps 2008: A joint guideline for the American Cancer Society, the U.S. Multi-Society Task Force on Colorectal Cancer, and the American College of Radiology. Gastroenterology 2008;134:1570–95.
12. Lieberman DA, Weiss DG, Bond JH, et al. Use of colonoscopy to screen asymptomatic adults for colorectal cancer. Veterans Affairs Cooperative Study Group 380. N Engl J Med 2000;343:162–8.
13. Lieberman D, Moravec M, Holub J, et al. Polyp size and advanced histology in patients undergoing colonoscopy screening: Implications for CT colonography. Gastroenterology 2008;135:1100–5.
14. Lynch HT, de la Chapelle A. Hereditary colorectal cancer. N Engl J Med 2003;348:919–32.
15. Mavranezouli I, East JE, Taylor SA. CT colonography and cost-effectiveness. Eur Radiol 2008;18:2485–97.
16. Oono Y, Fu K, Nakamura H, et al. Progression of a sessile serrated adenoma to an early invasive cancer within 8 months. Dig Dis Sci 2008;54:906–9.
17. Pickhardt PJ, Choi JR, Inku H, et al. Computed tomographic virtual colonoscopy to screen for colorectal neoplasia in asymptomatic adults. N Engl J Med 2003;349:2191–200.
18. Pineau BC, Paskett ED, Chen GJ, et al. Virtual colonoscopy using oral contrast compared with colonoscopy for the detection of patients with colorectal polyps. Gastro 2003;125:304–10.
19. Ransohoff DF, Sandler RS. Screening for colorectal cancer. N Engl J Med 2002;346:40–4.
20. Rockey DC, Georgsson MA. Mass screening with CT colonography. Clin Gastroenterol Hepatol 2005;3:S37–41.
21. Rustgi A. Hereditary gastrointestinal polyposis and non polyposis syndromes. N Engl J Med 1994;331:1694–702.
22. Sandler RS, Halabi JA, Baron, et al. A randomized trial of aspirin to prevent colorectal adenomas in patients with previous colorectal cancer. N Engl J Med 2003;348:883–90.
23. Soetikno RM, Kaltenbach T, Rouse RV, et al. Prevalence of nonpolypoid (flat and depressed) colorectal neoplasms in asymptomatic and symptomatic adults. JAMA 2008;299:1027–35.
24. Tuma R. Drugs to prevent colon cancer show promise, but hurdles remain for chemoprevention. J Natl Cancer Inst 2008;400:764–6.
25. Umar A, Boland CR, Terdiman JP, et al. Revised Bethesda Guidelines for hereditary nonpolyposis colorectal cancer (Lynch syndrome) and microsatellite instability. J Natl Cancer Inst 2004;96:261–8.
26. Vasen HF, Moslein G, Alonso A, et al. Guidelines for the clinical management of familial adenomatous polyposis (FAP). Gut 2008;57:704–13.
27. Vijan S, Hwang I, Inadomi J, et al. The cost effectiveness of CT colonography in screening for colorectal neoplasia. Am J Gastroenterol 2007;102:380–90.
28. Winawer SJ, Zauber AG, Gerdes H, et al. Risk of colorectal cancer in the families of patients with adenomatous polyps. N Engl J Med 1996;334:82–7.

# CONSTIPATION AND FECAL INCONTINENCE

*Christina Tennyson, MD, and*
*Suzanne Rose, MD, MSEd*

### 1. What is constipation?

While difficult to define precisely, patients may consider any one of these symptoms as a sufficient description of constipation: infrequent bowel movements, painful passage of stool, hard consistency of stool, or difficulty in evacuating stool. Population studies reveal that 5% to 30% of the population experiences constipation and that its prevalence increases with age. Women outnumber men by 2:1. The Rome III committee developed the criteria indicated in Table 47-1.

---

**Table 47-1.** Rome III Criteria

**Chronic Constipation***

Chronic constipation must include ≥2 of the following:

| | |
|---|---|
| In at least 25% of defecations: | Straining |
| In at least 25% of defecations: | Lumpy or hard stools |
| In at least 25% of defecations: | Sensation of incomplete evacuation |
| In at least 25% of defecations: | Sensation of anorectal obstruction/blockage |
| In at least 25% of defecations: | Manual maneuvers to facilitate |
| <3 bowel movements per week | |

AND the following criteria must be met:
  Loose stools are rarely present (excluding the use of laxatives)
  Insufficient criteria to establish a diagnosis of irritable bowel syndrome (IBS)

**Functional Defecation Disorders***

Must meet the criteria for functional constipation
At least two of the following must be present during repeated attempts to defecate:
- Impaired evacuation (based on balloon expulsion test or imaging test)
- Inappropriate contraction of the pelvic floor muscles (i.e., anal sphincter or puborectalis) or less than 20% relaxation of the basal resting sphincter pressure as seen on manometry, imaging, or EMG
- Inadequate propulsive forces as determined by manometry or imaging

Adapted from Longstreth, et al: Gastroenterology 130:1480, 2006.
Adapted from Bharucha, et al: Gastroenterology 130:1510, 2006.
*Criteria fulfilled for 3 or more months with onset of symptoms at least 6 months prior to diagnosis.

---

### 2. Describe the normal mechanism of stool passage:

Continence is maintained via the pelvic floor muscles, including the internal and external anal sphincters and puborectalis muscle. The internal anal sphincter (IAS) is under autonomic control via the enteric nervous system; it is tonically contracted and contributes the majority of the resting pressure (80%) in the anal canal. The external anal sphincter (EAS) is a striated muscle, innervated by the pudendal nerve, and it is partially contracted at rest. Contraction of the EAS is stimulated by rising external pressures (erect posture, coughing) via a spinal reflex. The puborectalis muscle forms a U-shaped sling around the anorectal junction and maintains an approximately 90-degree angle between the rectum and anal canal. This muscular configuration forms a physical obstruction and, under normal conditions, prevents the involuntary passage of solid stool. The puborectalis is a striated muscle and can voluntarily contract to further narrow the anorectal angle.

When stool or flatus distends the rectum, a reflex relaxation of the IAS occurs, called the sampling reflex. Rectal contents contact the anal mucosa and, if liquid or solid feces is detected, the EAS contracts to prevent soiling.

Defecation results from coordinated contraction and relaxation of both smooth and striated muscles. Stretch receptors in the rectum sense fecal material and initiate a spinal reflex arc called the rectoanal inhibitory reflex (RAIR). This stimulates inhibitory nerves and leads to relaxation of the IAS. The striated muscles of the pelvic floor (puborectalis and pubococcygeus) relax, and there is movement of the pelvic floor complex downward. The rectoanal angle is then opened from approximately 90 to 130 degrees, and the anal canal is stretched in the anteroposterior direction by flexure of the hips in the sitting or squatting position. As the EAS relaxes, the passage of stool can occur, facilitated by rectal smooth muscle contraction. This is often accompanied by concomitant diaphragmatic and abdominal muscular contraction, resulting in expulsion of the rectal contents.

### 3. What are the major causes of constipation?

There are primary causes and secondary causes of constipation. Primary refers to constipation with no external known cause or physical abnormality or condition, and it is usually a result of a problem in the gastrointestinal tract, with regard to the function of the intestine.

*Primary* etiologies include irritable bowel syndrome (IBS), pelvic floor disorders, colonic inertia, and chronic constipation.

*Secondary* causes of constipation are due to problems influencing bowel habits due to another problem. Examples of secondary constipation are listed in Table 47-2.

**Table 47-2.** Secondary Causes of Chronic Constipation

| | |
|---|---|
| Metabolic disorders | Hypothyroidism, diabetes mellitus, hypercalcemia |
| Collagen vascular diseases | Scleroderma |
| Inherited muscular disorders | Familial visceral myopathy |
| Neoplastic processes | Colorectal cancer, ovarian cancer |
| Nonenteric neurologic disorders | Parkinson disease, spinal cord injury, multiple sclerosis |
| Medications | Opiates, antacids (calcium and aluminum), anticholinergics, anticonvulsants, antidepressants, parkinsonian agents, diuretics, iron, antihypertensive agents, calcium channel blockers |

### 4. Describe the workup for constipation.

A thorough patient history should focus on defining the symptoms, identifying the duration of constipation, and assessing for the presence of alarm signs and symptoms, such as blood per rectum, weight loss, anemia, risk factors for colon cancer, and signs of systemic illnesses. Direct questioning about medical history, diet and exercise, prescription and over-the-counter medications should be included in this history. The Bristol Stool Form Scale, which assesses stool consistency and form, is helpful in the evaluation of constipation. Stool form may serve as a predictor of transit time, and change in form may correlate with change in transit time. The scale ranges from Type 1 stool (hard lumps) to Type 7 (entirely liquid, with no solid pieces).

A physical examination, including an abdominal exam, detailed digital rectal exam, and neurologic assessment, should be performed. A detailed rectal exam begins with a visual inspection of the anorectal area for hemorrhoids, fissures, or skin changes. By gently touching the perineal skin with a piece of cotton, a reflex contraction of the EAS, known as the *anal wink*, can be elicited. A digital rectal examination may identify stool, an impaction, blood, or a stricture. An assessment of resting tone may be performed by inserting the examining finger; the strength of the external sphincter may be assessed by asking the patient to squeeze. After allowing resting tone to be restored, the patient should be asked to bear down, allowing the examiner to appreciate perineal descent and the ability of the sphincter complex to relax. A limited laboratory analysis of thyroid-stimulating hormone and calcium may be performed to exclude metabolic disorders. Colonoscopy should be performed in patients older than age 50 for colorectal cancer screening (or earlier as per guidelines depending on risk stratification) but cannot be endorsed in all patients who present with constipation. The ACG task force guidelines have concluded that for patients without alarm symptoms, empiric treatment may be initiated without a diagnostic workup. Colonoscopy for colon cancer screening should be considered as a separate issue.

### 5. What tests are used in the evaluation of chronic constipation?

In patients who are refractory to therapy, testing may help to define the problem and to provide appropriate therapy. Table 47-3 describes the various tests that are at the physician's disposal and what information may be learned from performing them. In addition to those tests listed in the table, assessment of colonic transit is being studied with a wireless capsule (SmartPill Corporation) with promising preliminary results.

**Table 47-3.** Workup of Refractory Constipation

| STUDY | HOW PERFORMED AND INFORMATION OBTAINED |
|---|---|
| Colon marker study | • The patient swallows a capsule or series of capsules containing radiopaque plastic rings.<br>• Abdominal radiograph taken on subsequent day(s) according to one of several protocols.<br>• Number and distribution of the rings are evaluated to determine if transit is normal or delayed. |

*Continued*

**Table 47-3** Workup of Refractory Constipation—Cont'd

| STUDY | HOW PERFORMED AND INFORMATION OBTAINED |
|---|---|
| Scintigraphy | • Ingestion of radiolabeled material<br>• Patient followed for up to 3 to 5 days to determine transit times throughout the GI tract. |
| Anorectal manometry (and EMG) | • Pressure-recording catheter is passed across the anal sphincter<br>• Assessments of resting and squeeze pressures made.<br>• With balloon distention within the rectum, rectal sensory thresholds and internal anal sphincter relaxation assessed.<br>• Can be combined with surface EMG studies of the pelvic floor muscles and external anal sphincter to diagnose entities such as anorectal dyssynergia or anismus |
| Balloon Expulsion Study | • The patient inserts either a silicone-filled stool-like device or a balloon filled with water into the rectum.<br>• Patient is asked to expel the balloon (with privacy).<br>• Most normal subjects will be able to expel the device within a minute. Dyssynergia should be suspected if the device cannot be expelled within 3 minutes. |
| Defecography (or MR defecography) | • Placement of barium paste or contrast into the rectum<br>• Videoradiography taken before and during evacuation of rectal contents<br>• Assesses the completeness of rectal expulsion, evaluates for anatomic abnormalities of the rectum (rectocele), prolapse, or pelvic floor dysfunction<br>• Similar information may be obtained by doing a functional MRI study of the pelvis. |
| Colon manometry | • Clinical investigation tool using probes with recorders to measure colonic contractions over time<br>• Measurements recorded with regard to response to meals, sleep, time awake or stressors |

### 6. How can primary constipation be further defined?

Based on assessment of colonic and anorectal function, primary chronic constipation can be divided into several major classes:

- Impaired colonic transit
- Normal colonic transit with anorectal dysfunction due to impaired rectoanal inhibitory reflex or physiologic abnormalities (i.e., Hirschsprung or short segment Hirschsprung)
- Constipation-predominant IBS
- Pelvic floor dysfunction
- Idiopathic normal transit constipation

### 7. What causes impaired colonic transit? How is it diagnosed?

Delayed colonic transit may occur in isolated segments of the colon, in the entire colon, or as part of a diffuse gastrointestinal (GI) motility disorder. Colonic inertia describes a dysfunction of propulsive forces of the colon. Studies with radiopaque markers reveal persistence of markers throughout the left and right colon 5 to 7 days after ingestion, while other tests of upper GI motility are normal. Scintigraphic studies (and where available, manometric studies) may also be performed to evaluate colonic transit. Colonic inertia is more commonly seen in women than men, and when it is severe and *in selected cases*, it may be treated with surgery (subtotal colectomy).

### 8. What causes impaired rectoanal inhibitory reflex? How is it diagnosed?

An impaired rectoanal inhibitory reflex (RAIR) is found in 8% to 10% of adults with severe idiopathic constipation. In children, it often is seen in conjunction with aganglioniosis of the colon (Hirschsprung disease). Adults may have a similar condition called short-segment Hirschsprung disease. Aganglioniosis occurs within a very short segment of the distal colon, but ganglia are present in full-thickness biopsies of the remaining colon. With balloon distention on anal manometry, the IAS fails to relax and the rectoanal inhibitory reflex is lost. Although uncommon, it is important to consider this syndrome, especially in young adults with long-standing severe constipation, because a surgical solution often provides good symptomatic response.

### 9. What is dyschezia?

Dyschezia means difficulty in defecating. Various physiologic abnormalities may lead to dyschezia. The symptom of dyschezia may indicate pelvic floor dysfunction.

### 10. What is anorectal dyssyngergia?

Dysfunction of the pelvic musculature, also termed anismus, spastic pelvic floor syndrome, or anorectal dyssynergia, can cause functional rectal obstruction. It consists of one of the following: impaired relaxation during a defecatory effort secondary to spasticity of the levator ani, failure of perineal descent, an abnormally angulated rectoanal axis, or a combination of these factors that leads to functional obstruction of the anal outlet, terminating defecation. Often there appears to be abnormal coordination of the various muscles involved in defecation. In approximately two thirds of patients, dyssynergia is an acquired behavioral problem. A significant number of patients with dyssynergia may also have delayed transit. Biofeedback may ameliorate the condition.

## 11. What other physiologic abnormalities may lead to anorectal dysfunction, and how are they diagnosed?

- *Impaired rectal sensation* leads to a decreased motor response and a decrease in the urge to defecate, as determined by balloon distention studies of the rectum.
- *Megarectum* is often seen in patients with a longstanding history of fecal impactions and can be evident in children and in physically or mentally impaired elderly patients. Occasionally, megarectum is associated with neurologic disease, such as lumbosacral spinal cord lesions. Increased rectal compliance, diminished rectal sensation, and impaired IAS relaxation are noted on manometry.
- In a *rectocele*, rectal contents are directed away from the anal canal and toward the vagina during increased abdominal pressure, leading to incomplete evacuation and retention of feces in the pouch. Defecography (or MR defecography) remains the test of choice for diagnosing a rectocele since it is often not detected via endoscopy and barium enema. Clinically, the patient may report a need or urge to insert a finger in the vagina (i.e., digitation) in order to facilitate defecation.

## 12. How is constipation due to irritable bowel syndrome diagnosed?

Constipation-predominant IBS is diagnosed clinically. Usually it is seen in young or middle-aged adults, predominantly women. Constipation is noted along with abdominal pain, bloating, flatulence, straining, or incomplete evacuation. Patients with idiopathic constipation do not commonly have abdominal pain (see Chapter 62). The symptom of abdominal pain is the key to differentiating between IBS and chronic constipation.

## 13. Describe the general management of constipation.

Primary care physicians manage most patients who complain of constipation. Reassurance is beneficial to those who are concerned about irregularities in daily or weekly stool patterns. Dietary modifications, such as increasing fiber, may increase weekly bowel movements. Increased exercise may accelerate colonic transit time, but evidence is limited. Other lifestyle modifications may include increased fluid intake and encouraging dedicated bathroom time. A change or substitution of constipating medications may allow resumption of normal bowel pattern. See Table 47-4 for medical treatment options.

**Table 47-4.** Medical Therapy for Chronic Constipation

| MEDICATION | EXAMPLES | MECHANISM OF ACTION |
|---|---|---|
| Bulk-forming laxatives, dietary fiber | Psyllium<br>Wheat bran<br>Calcium polycarbophil<br>Methylcellulose | Increase stool weight, accelerate transit |
| Osmotic laxatives | Lactulose<br>PEG 3350<br>Sorbitol<br>Magnesium hydroxide | Agents cause water retention in the lumen |
| Stool softeners | Docusate | Affect surface qualities allowing water to interact with the stool, resulting in soft stool |
| Stimulant laxatives | Bisacodyl<br>Senna<br>Cascara | Stimulate nerve endings to promote intestinal contractions; may have inhibitory effect on water absorption |
| Suppositories, enemas | Glycerine suppository<br>Bisacodyl suppository<br>Sodium phosphate enemas | Stimulate rectum and promote defecation |
| Probiotics | *Bifidobacterium animalis*<br>*Lactobacillus casei* | Use may alter intestinal flora with improvement of symptoms |
| Chloride channel activator | Lubiprostone | Activates type 2 chloride channels in the small intestine to promote fluid secretion and enhanced motility |

## 14. Describe the proper use of dietary fiber.

Bulk-forming laxatives and dietary fiber often benefit patients with mild, chronic constipation and can be initiated once fecal impaction and obstruction have been ruled out. Patients should be encouraged to increase daily consumption of dietary fiber with a goal of 20 to 35 g/day. The starting dose for these agents should be low and gradually increased over 2 to 3 weeks to minimize bloating and flatulence. Psyllium, derived from plant husks, has a very high water-binding capacity, and it is generally administered in a powdered form mixed with water, 1 to 3 times/day. Wheat fiber may be mixed with food. Methylcellulose, a synthetic compound taken in either liquid or tablet form, is not absorbed and is generally not degraded by colonic bacteria. Patients should be counseled to drink adequate fluids. Increased fiber may make some patients' symptoms worse and, in those patients with megarectum or with colonic inertia, it may prove more beneficial to limit the amount of bulk by following a low-residue diet.

### 15. How do osmotic laxatives work?

Osmotic laxatives increase the water content of stools by trapping solute, inhibiting absorption, and stimulating intestinal secretion. Lactulose and sorbitol are nondigestible disaccharides providing osmotically active solutes. They are well tolerated but may lead to increased colonic gas production and abdominal distention. Magnesium and phosphate sulfates are poorly absorbed in the intestines and, through osmotic action, often lead to passage of liquid stool. They should not be used in patients who have renal impairment, because hypermagnesemia and hyperphosphatemia have been reported. Polyethylene glycol (PEG), a nonabsorbable polymer, can be used for chronic constipation.

### 16. How do cathartics work, and are stool softeners effective?

Cathartics stimulate intestinal motor activity and cause secretion of electrolytes. Anthranoids (aloe, cascara, and senna) are glycosides derived from plants; they are converted by bacteria in the colon to active forms that increase propulsive waves in the colon, leading to passage of stool. Anthraquinones are synthetic derivatives that also exert some action on the small intestine. Polyphenols (bisacodyl and sodium picosulfate) act via similar mechanisms. The safety of both classes for long-term daily use is not yet determined. Melanosis coli, a pigmentation of the colon noted in long-term users of laxatives, generally affects the proximal more than the distal colon and may persist for years after termination of laxative use. Melanosis coli is of no known medical consequence.

Docusate sodium, a detergent widely used as a stool softener, stimulates mild fluid secretion by the small intestine and colon but has little effect on stool volume or colonic motility. Although widely used, there is little evidence to support its use in the treatment of constipation.

### 17. What is lubiprostone, and how does it work?

Lubiprostone is a bicyclic fatty acid derivative that activates type II chloride channels in the small intestinal epithelial cells. It causes secretion of chloride into the intestinal lumen, resulting in an increase of water and sodium into the lumen. Lubiprostone leads to an increase of fluid in the gastrointestinal lumen, possibly promoting enhanced motility and softer stool. It increases the number of spontaneous bowel movements and has not been found to cause electrolyte abnormalities. Lubiprostone is now U.S. Food and Drug Administration approved for both chronic constipation and for IBS with constipation. (Please note that there are two different approved doses for the two conditions.)

### 18. Is surgery ever indicated for constipation?

Surgical treatment for constipation should be reserved for highly selected patients, such as those with Hirschsprung disease. In highly selected patients with disabling constipation due to proven colonic inertia, a subtotal colectomy with ileorectal anastomosis can provide good results. It is important to rule out a pan GI dysmotility syndrome or a systemic disorder prior to considering surgery. It should be noted that there are also surgical techniques being studied for the treatment of pelvic floor dysfunction.

### 19. Are there other treatments for constipation?

There is promising data that probiotics may improve symptoms in patients with constipation and may enhance colonic transit.

Patients diagnosed with dyssynergic defecation may benefit from biofeedback and bowel retraining. There are reports in the literature using galvanic stimulation and botulinum toxin for this condition. Alternative treatments for constipation such as herbal remedies, acupuncture, and abdominal massage have been pursued by many patients. Unfortunately, there are little data with regard to these types of treatments, and they should be considered in light of the potential risks and benefits.

### 20. What is fecal incontinence? Who is generally affected?

Fecal incontinence *in adults* is the involuntary loss of stool. In population-based studies involving all ages, the prevalence of incontinence ranges from 2% to 14%. This number may underestimate the problem because many patients are hesitant to report this embarrassing symptom to their physicians. In geriatric patients, the prevalence is even higher: 10% to 17% of nursing home residents and 13% to 47% of hospitalized elderly patients report incontinence. Women develop incontinence more often than men. Incontinence can have a profound impact on quality of life.

## 21. Describe the pathophysiology of fecal incontinence.

Normal functioning requires an intact neuromuscular system, the ability to sense impending defecation, to differentiate between gas, liquid, and solid, and the motivation to maintain continence. The major abnormalities of continence mechanisms involve impairments in rectal sensation, abnormal rectal compliance, and anal sphincter dysfunction, secondary to muscle dysfunction or interruption and nerve damage.

Impaired proprioception in the levator ani, puborectalis, and sphincters can decrease the ability to sense rectal filling, leading to the loss of the normal *warning* of imminent defecation. The IAS relaxes before the patient senses rectal distention, leading to incontinence. Longstanding diabetics may develop sensory abnormalities from neuropathy with similar consequences.

Changes in rectal compliance can lead to incontinence. The rectum has elastic properties that allow it to maintain low intraluminal pressure in response to increasing volumes. If compliance is diminished, smaller volumes may lead to increased intraluminal pressures and incontinence, often associated with urgency and frequency. A reduced compliance may result from inflammation or fibrosis, as seen with inflammatory bowel disease or radiation proctitis. Conversely, incontinence also may result from increased rectal compliance and diminished sensation, as in fecal impaction and megarectum. In these cases, intact involuntary pathways relax the IAS before the patient senses rectal distention, with resultant incontinence from *overflow* diarrhea.

Myopathic damage from disruption of the anal sphincters and sacral neuropathic disorders can diminish the high-pressure zone necessary to maintain continence, leading to soiling. Some patients suffer from early muscle fatigue which can lead to incontinence. Rarely, massive diarrhea may overwhelm the normal continence mechanism.

## 22. What are the risk factors associated with incontinence?

Risk factors include:

- Gender (females experience a greater incidence)
- Advancing age
- Neurologic disease
- Increased body mass
- Decreased activity
- Depression and diabetes

See Table 47-5 for causes of incontinence.

**Table 47-5.** Causes of Fecal Incontinence

| CAUSE | EXAMPLES |
| --- | --- |
| Anatomic defects/anal sphincter weakness or disruption | Obstetric injury, status post surgery (e.g., sphincterotomy for anal fissure) |
| Congenital disorders | Spina bifida |
| Diarrheal disorders | Inflammatory bowel disease Malabsorption syndromes Radiation injury |
| Collagen vascular disease | Scleroderma |
| Neurologic disorders | Diabetes mellitus Multiple sclerosis Cerebrovascular accident Dementia |
| Overflow incontinence | Fecal impaction |

## 23. Describe the workup for incontinence.

A good history and physical exam are vital. The history should include general information about frequency, duration, and pattern of soilage; symptoms of diarrhea, constipation (e.g. megarectum), urgency, or straining; and dietary intake. Prior anorectal surgery or trauma, diabetes mellitus or thyroid disease, neurologic events or illness, and progressive dementia may contribute to incontinence. A thorough obstetric history includes information about all deliveries, use of forceps for delivery, length of second stage of labor, and history of episiotomy or significant perineal lacerations that may have affected the perineal floor. Finally, a comprehensive medication history must be obtained, including direct inquiry about over-the-counter medications, laxatives, and dietary substitutes such as sorbitol.

The physical exam must include careful inspection of the perineum, looking for scars, obvious lacerations, fissures, and hemorrhoids. A digital rectal exam must be performed to detect distal rectal masses and/or fecal impaction. The resting tone and squeeze pressures of the anal sphincter should be noted, and the strength of puborectalis contraction assessed. Neurologic evaluation should include a mental status examination, assessment of sacral reflexes (anal wink), checking the integrity of the spinal pathway, and evaluation of perineal sensation. Visualization of the anus with anoscopy and/or via retroflex view during an endoscopic evaluation, as indicated, should complete the exam. In patients with diarrhea, stool studies should be considered to exclude an infectious etiology.

### 24. What specialized tests are available for the evaluation of incontinence?

Table 47-6 identifies the tests that may be ordered to determine the precise cause of incontinence.

**Table 47-6.** Tests for the Evaluation of Fecal Incontinence

| STUDY | HOW PERFORMED AND INFORMATION OBTAINED |
| --- | --- |
| Anorectal manometry | • Balloon catheters to test the function of the sphincters<br>• Enables measurement of the resting tone of the internal anal sphincter (IAS), squeeze pressure of the external anal sphincter (EAS), and functional length of the high-pressure zone created by the sphincters.<br>• Rectal sensation and rectal compliance may also be measured. |
| Anal endosonography | • Placement of an ultrasound probe in anal canal<br>• Quick and easy evaluation of the structural integrity of the anal sphincters: IAS and EAS. |
| Electromyography (EMG) of the sphincters and/or puborectalis | • Performed with surface electrodes or needles.<br>• Allows for detection of denervation, conduction defects, and abnormalities in striated muscle function.<br>• This test may serve both a diagnostic and therapeutic function. |
| Pudendal nerve terminal latency (PNTL) | • Stimulation of the right and/or left pudendal nerves at the ischial tuberosities and measuring the time to detect a contraction of the EAS.<br>• A normal PNTL is approximately 2.0 msec.<br>• A prolonged PNTML may be seen in patients with obstetric injury, neurogenic incontinence, and rectal prolapse. |
| Defecography or magnetic resonance (MR) defecography | • Defecography evaluates the anatomy and change in pelvic floor muscle position with defecation.<br>• Abnormalities often missed in endoscopic evaluation of the rectum, such as prolapse, perineal descent, and intussusception, are often detected with defecography.<br>• MR defecography is becoming more widely available and may assess similar information. |

### 25. What is medical therapy for incontinence?

One first proceeds by correcting all modifiable factors to decrease stool frequency and improve consistency. Dietary changes, such as limiting sorbitol, lactose, and fructose ingestion and increasing dietary fiber, may firm the stool, allowing better rectal sensation and enhancing sphincter function. Over-the-counter medications that may cause diarrhea (e.g., magnesium-containing antacids) should be eliminated. Loperamide or diphenoxylate may be helpful in reducing stool frequency. Anal plugs have been evaluated, mostly in Europe, and may be helpful in some patients but there is a high level of intolerability to this form of treatment. A gel form of phenylephrine, a selective $\alpha_1$-adrenergic agonist, may improve anal sphincter tone when applied.

Other nonsurgical options have focused on mechanisms to tighten the anal canal; they have included perianal injections of fat, collagen, or synthetic gel. Radiofrequency electrical energy has been applied to achieve a tightening effect, as well. In addition, several studies have shown improvement in symptoms of incontinence in patients who have been treated with sacral nerve stimulation.

### 26. What is biofeedback and how is it used to treat incontinence?

Biofeedback is a method used to treat incontinence by training the abdominal and pelvic floor muscles. It is usually performed by a therapist, and it may be helpful to patients with anal sphincter weakness or decreased rectal sensation who have structurally normal sphincters. Patients can be taught to recognize rectal distention and to increase the EAS pressure in response to balloon distention. In order for biofeedback to be effective, the patient must be able to understand the process, be sufficiently motivated, have some rectal sensation, and be able to generate a squeeze pressure through voluntary control of the EAS. Outcomes vary based on individual patient characteristics.

## 27. What are surgical options for treating incontinence?

Operative resuspension of rectal prolapse restores continence in up to two thirds of patients. Various surgical procedures have been used including apposition techniques, plication procedures, muscle transfer surgeries, artificial sphincter, and colostomy. Repair of sphincteric defects, with removal of scar tissue and direct apposition of the sphincters, successfully relieves incontinence in approximately 50% of patients. Posterior sphincter plication can be used to treat patients with anatomically intact sphincters that function poorly. The outcome of anterior repair after obstetric injury has been studied, but has shown deterioration over time, with more disappointing outcomes for those with prolonged pudendal latencies. Other techniques, such as anal encirclement with a wire or a Silastic ring to tighten the anal canal mechanically, have been used, but frequent complications occur. Dynamic graciloplasty requires electrical stimulation of the gracilis muscle after it has been surgically transposed around the anal canal. Newer techniques using artificial sphincters are currently under study. Antegrade colonic irrigation via appendicostomy or cecostomy is a technique that has been used mostly in children but there is some experience with the adult patient. The strategy is to apply large volume enemas via the stoma to keep the colon clear of stool. Colostomy has been reserved for immobile patients suffering from recurrent bacteremia secondary to skin breakdown with fecal contamination of decubitus ulcers.

## WEBSITE

www.fda.gov/Drugs/DrugSafety/PostmarketDrugSafetyInformationforPatientsandProviders/ucm103223.htm

## BIBLIOGRAPHY

1. Andrews CN, Bharucha AE. The etiology, assessment, and treatment of fecal incontinence. Nat Clin Pract Gastroenterol Hepatol 2005;2:516–25.
2. Bellicini N, Molloy PJ, Caushaj P, et al. Fecal incontinence: A review. Dig Dis Sci 2008;53:41–6.
3. Bharucha AE, Wald A, Enck P, et al. Functional anorectal disorders. Gastroenterology 2006;130:1510–8.
4. Brandt LJ, Prather CM, Quigley EM, et al. Systematic review on the management of chronic constipation in North America. Am J Gastroenterol 2005;100(Suppl. 1):S5–S21.
5. Brown SR, Nelson RL. Surgery for faecal incontinence in adults. Cochrane Database Syst Rev 2007;2: CD001757.
6. Byrne CM, Solomon MJ, Young JM, et al. Biofeedback for fecal incontinence: Short-term outcomes of 513 consecutive patients and predictors of successful treatment. Dis Colon Rectum 2007;50:417–27.
7. Cooper ZR, Rose S. Fecal incontinence: A clinical approach. Mount Sinai J Med 2000;67:96–105.
8. DiPalma JA, Cleveland MV, McGowan J, et al. A randomized, multicenter, placebo-controlled trial of polyethylene glycol laxative for chronic treatment of chronic constipation. Am J Gastroenterol 2007;102:1436–41.
9. Dudding TC, Vaizey CJ, Kamm MA. Obstetric anal sphincter injury: Incidence, risk factors, and management. Ann Surg 2008;247:224–37.
10. Ganeshan A, Anderson EM, Upponi S, et al. Imaging of obstructed defecation. Clin Radiol 2008;63:18–26.
11. Hawes SK, Ahmad A. Fecal incontinence: A woman's view. Am J Gastroenterol 2006;101(Suppl.):S610–7.
12. Heymen S, Scarlett Y, Jones K, et al. Randomized, controlled trial shows biofeedback to be superior to alternative treatments for patients with pelvic floor dyssynergia-type constipation. Dis Colon Rectum 2007;50:428–41.
13. Jonkers D, Stockbrügger R. Review article: Probiotics in gastrointestinal and liver diseases. Aliment Pharmacol Ther 2007;26(Suppl. 2):133–48.
14. Koebnick C, Wagner I, Leitzmann P, et al. Probiotic beverage containing *Lactobacillus casei Shirota* improves gastrointestinal symptoms in patients with chronic constipation. Can J Gastroenterol 2003;17:655–9.
15. Lacy BE, Levy LC. Lubiprostone: A chloride channel activator. J Clin Gastroenterol 2007;41:345–51.
16. Landefeld CS, Bowers BJ, Feld AD, et al. National Institutes of Health state-of-the-science conference statement: Prevention of fecal and urinary incontinence in adults. Ann Intern Med 2008;148:449–58.
17. Lewis SJ, Heaton KW. Stool form scale as a useful guide to intestinal transit time. Scand J Gastroenterol 1997;32:920–4.
18. Locke GR 3rd, Pemberton JH, Phillips SF. American Gastroenterological Association medical position statement: Guidelines on constipation. Gastroenterology 2000;119:1761–6.
19. Longstreth GF, Thompson WG, Chey WD, et al. Functional bowel disorders. Gastroenterology 2006;130:1480–91.
20. Mowatt G, Glazener C, Jarrett M. Sacral nerve stimulation for faecal incontinence and constipation in adults. Cochrane Database Syst Rev 2007;CD004464.
21. Norton C, Thomas L, Hill J; Guideline Development Group. Management of faecal incontinence in adults: Summary of NICE guidance. BMJ 2007;334:1370–1.
22. Person B, Kaidar-Person O, Wexner SD. Novel approaches in the treatment of fecal incontinence. Surg Clin North Am 2006;86:969–86.
23. Picard C, Fioramonti J, Francois A, et al. Review article: Bifidobacteria as probiotic agents—physiological effects and clinical benefits. Aliment Pharmacol Ther 2005;22:495–512.
24. Ramkumar D, Rao SS. Efficacy and safety of traditional medical therapies for chronic constipation: Systematic review. Am J Gastroenterol 2005;100:936–71.
25. Rao SS. Constipation: Evaluation and treatment of colonic and anorectal motility disorders. Gastroenterol Clin N Am 2007;36:687–711.
26. Rao SS, Seaton K, Miller M, et al. Randomized controlled trial of biofeedback, sham feedback, and standard therapy for dyssynergic defecation. Clin Gastroenterol Hepatol 2007;5:331–8.
27. Tan JJ, Chan M, Tjandra JJ. Evolving therapy for fecal incontinence. Dis Colon Rectum 2007;50:1950–67.
28. Wald A. Clinical practice. Fecal incontinence in adults. N Engl J Med 2007;356:1648–55.
29. Wheeler TL 2nd, Richter HE. Delivery method, anal sphincter tears and fecal incontinence: New information on a persistent problem. Curr Opin Obstet Gynecol 2007;19:474–9.

# DIVERTICULITIS

*Matthew R. Quallick, MD, and*
*Stephen R. Freeman, MD*

### 1. What is a diverticulum? What type are colonic diverticula?

A diverticulum is a circumscribed pouch or sac that either occurs naturally or is created by herniation of a lining mucous membrane through a muscular defect of a tubular organ. Typical colonic diverticula are false or pulsion diverticulum with only the mucosa and submucosa herniating through the muscle layers of the colon. True diverticula containing all layers of the bowel wall do occur in the colon and are congenital.

### 2. How common is diverticular disease? What are the most frequent complications?

Diverticulosis is known to increase with age, with prevalence rates of 5% by age 40, 30% by age 60, and 65% by age 85 in Western societies. However, there are no recent population based studies in the last 30 years in the United States. Most (70%) remain asymptomatic, 15% to 25% develop diverticulitis, and 5% to 15% develop bleeding.

### 3. How do diverticula develop? Who is at risk for developing diverticulosis?

Although the specific cause is unknown, development of diverticula likely involves mechanical, environmental, and lifestyle factors. Etiologic factors include increased luminal pressure, long intestinal transit time, small stool volume, lack of dietary fiber, age-related factors, and hypersegmentation. Decreased dietary fiber in the colonic lumen leads to decreased stool volume and increasing segmentation during peristalsis.

Contributing factors include age older than 50, obesity, sedentary lifestyle, corticosteroids, NSAIDs, smoking, alcohol use, and polycystic kidney disease.

### 4. What is hypersegmentation?

*Segmentation* is the motility process in which proximal and distal segmental muscular contractions separate the lumen into isolated chambers. In diverticulosis, this process is believed to be exaggerated, leading to herniation of the mucosa at four constant points of weakness in the colonic wall where the vasa recta penetrate the circular muscle layer. The diverticula, therefore, tend to develop in rows between the mesenteric and lateral teniae coli. This concept is based partly on the principles of the law of LaPlace. This law states that colonic wall pressure is proportional to wall tension and inversely proportional to the radius of the colon. This helps explain, in part, why the sigmoid colon with its smaller diameter is at higher risk of developing diverticula.

### 5. What is myochosis?

*Myochosis* is thickening of the circular and longitudinal (teniae) muscular layers of the colon, shortening of the teniae, and luminal narrowing and usually grossly seen in people with sigmoid diverticulosis. The thickening shortens the teniae leading to a narrowing of the sigmoid colon allowing obliteration of the lumen and segmentation of the colon. This thickening occurs without hypertrophy or hyperplasia of the smooth muscle. Histologically, the teniae have excess elastin deposition.

### 6. Where are diverticula located?

In Western societies, 95% of diverticula are located in sigmoid and distal descending colon. Sixty-five percent are isolated to sigmoid colon, 24% involve other areas to a lesser degree, and 7% are equally dispersed throughout the colon. Only 3% to 4% of cases spare the sigmoid colon. In Asian populations, diverticula are more common in the right colon demonstrating that other factors (genetic and environmental) must be important in this site-specific pathogenesis. As these cultures adopt Western diets, the incidence of diverticulosis and left-sided diverticula increases.

### 7. How does diverticulitis develop?

The exact pathophysiology is unknown at this time. The prevailing theory is that the narrow neck of the diverticulum becomes obstructed by fecal material. This eventually leads to bacterial overgrowth and resulting distention of the pseudodiverticulum and culminating in focal ischemia. It is the tissue ischemia that results in micro or free perforation.

**8. How should symptomatic diverticulosis be managed?**

Most clinicians encourage a high-fiber diet, regardless of the presence or absence of symptoms, despite the lack of data to support this advice. Abdominal pain is thought to be related to spasm or distention of the colon, probably a factor in the pathogenesis of diverticulosis. Although no therapy has been proven to be effective, a high-fiber diet and antispasmodics are often recommended. New studies have suggested a possible benefit of nonabsorbable antibiotics (Rifaximin), mesalamine, and probiotics, but the data at this time are not conclusive. Advice to avoid foods containing seeds and nuts has no scientific foundation and eliminates many nutritious and high-fiber foods.

**9. What is diverticular or segmental colitis?**

An association exists between lumenal mucosal inflammation, most commonly in the sigmoid colon, and diverticular disease, whether or not the inflammation is within or around diverticula. The pathogenesis is unclear but likely multifactorial. Clinical symptoms, such as rectal bleeding, left-sided abdominal pain, and endoscopic findings, are varied. Histologic changes vary widely and include changes similar to inflammatory bowel disease (IBD). Treatment is similar to IBD, with fiber, antibiotics, and/or aminosalicylates. Whether this is an autonomous disorder is still debated.

**10. What are the common signs and symptoms of early diverticulitis?**

The most common symptoms are abrupt onset of abdominal pain and an alteration in bowel pattern. Early acute diverticulitis is characterized by circumscribed abdominal pain and tenderness. The usual location of the pain is the left lower quadrant, but because diverticula, and hence diverticulitis, can develop at any site, inflammation may mimic other conditions. For example, transverse colon diverticulitis may mimic peptic ulcer disease, and right colon diverticulitis may mimic acute appendicitis. Signs of inflammation, such as fever and elevated white blood count, help to distinguish diverticulitis from the spasm of irritable bowel syndrome.

**11. What are the signs and symptoms of severe diverticulitis?**

As the disease progresses in severity, localized abscess and phlegmonous reaction may develop. In addition to pain and tenderness, a mass may develop. Systemic signs of infection become more pronounced (i.e., fever and leukocytosis). In elderly or immunocompromised patients and patients taking corticosteroids, abdominal exam and usual signs are unreliable. Therefore, a high index of suspicion and use of imaging studies, such as a computed tomography (CT) scan, are important to avoid significant delay in diagnosis and increased operative mortality.

Obstipation has long been taught as a symptom of diverticulitis, but, in fact, diarrhea is not uncommon. Rectal bleeding is not a symptom of diverticulitis.

**12. What is the Hinchey classification system? How does it predict outcome?**

The Hinchey classification system is a strictly anatomic means of categorizing the severity of an acute episode of diverticulitis.

- Stage 1: small pericolic or mesenteric abscess
- Stage 2: larger abscess extending into the pelvis
- Stage 3: rupture of a diverticular abscess leading to purulent peritonitis
- Stage 4: free-rupture (rupture of a diverticulum that is not inflamed or obstructed. This results in fecal material being released directly into the peritoneum or fecal peritonitis).

Mortality for stages 1 and 2, less than 5%; stage 3, 13%; and stage 4, 43%. This classification system does not consider the underlying patient characteristics.

**13. What is the natural history of diverticulitis?**

Most initial presentations of diverticulitis are uncomplicated (75%). Of these cases, 85% are effectively managed medically. After successful medical management of the first episode:

- One third remain asymptomatic.
- One third have episodic discomfort without frank diverticulitis.
- One third have a second episode.

With a second attack of diverticulitis, the morbidity increases from 25% to 50% and mortality from 1.3% to 5%, to 5% to 10%.

Initial presentations of diverticulitis complicated by abscess usually require surgery (90% to 95%). A recurrence of diverticulitis after surgery is seen in 2% to 11% of cases.

**14. List the common complications of diverticulitis.**

Fistula, abscess, obstruction (from edema or compression due to abscess), stricture, and peritonitis from perforation.

**15. Between what organs do fistulous communications develop?**

Bowel, urinary bladder, skin, pelvic floor, and vagina may be involved in fistulous disease associated with diverticulitis.

- The most common is *colovesicular fistula* (colon to urinary bladder), which is seen almost exclusively in men or in women with a prior hysterectomy. Pneumaturia is a pathognomonic sign of this fistula. Another clue is recurrent urinary tract infections, especially involving multiple organisms.
- *Colovaginal fistulas* occur almost exclusively in women with prior hysterectomies. The differential diagnosis includes Crohn's disease, previous pelvic irradiation, gynecologic surgery, and pelvic abscess from any cause. The diagnosis is suspected in the proper setting (recent diverticulitis) with the presence of vaginal symptoms: vaginal discharge, severe vaginitis, flatus vaginalis, and feculent discharge.

**16. What techniques are used to diagnose and localize fistulas?**

Demonstration of a colovesicular fistula is often difficult. Reflux of contrast through the fistula via contrast enema or cystogram confirms the diagnosis, but such reflux is seen in a minority of patients. Cystoscopy and endoscopy are not very sensitive means of demonstrating the fistula. Identification of a colovaginal fistula can also be difficult. Barium enema, oral charcoal, vaginography, methylene blue installation into the vagina and/or colon, and combined vaginoscopy and colonoscopy are various means of attempting to localize the fistula. Treatment is surgical resection of the diseased section of bowel.

**17. How is a diverticular stricture differentiated from strictures of other causes?**

The signs favoring a diverticular stricture are the presence of diverticula in the region of the colonic stricture, the suggestion of an extraluminal mass contributing to the stricture, and intramural or extraluminal extravasation of contrast. The length of the stricture is helpful.

- *Malignant strictures* are usually less than 3 cm in length and associated with abrupt shoulders at either end.
- *Diverticular strictures* are longer (3 to 6 cm) with smoother contours. Strictures between 6 and 10 cm are more likely to be due to *Crohn's disease* or *ischemia*. Location of the stricture may be helpful. For example, the splenic flexure is an uncommon site for diverticulitis but a common site for ischemia.

**18. Which drugs are known to exacerbate diverticulitis?**

- *Corticosteroids* in high doses have been associated with development of acute diverticulitis. A cause-and-effect relationship is debatable, but inhibition of epithelial cell renewal has been hypothesized. Clearly, high-dose steroids may mask the usual signs and symptoms of diverticulitis, leading to a delay in diagnosis and more serious disease.
- *Nonsteroidal anti-inflammatory drugs* also have been associated with more severe diverticulitis. The masking of early signs and symptoms has been hypothesized as the most likely reason.

**19. What imaging modalities are available to diagnose diverticulitis? What is the role of each?**

- *CT* is the test of choice for the diagnosis of simple and complicated diverticulitis, with a sensitivity of 90% to 95% and a specificity of 72% for diverticulitis. CT offers the added advantage of providing extraluminal information and helps to identify patients with nondiverticular causes for their symptoms, including ischemic colitis, mesenteric thrombosis, tubo-ovarian abscess, appendicitis, and pancreatitis.
- *Ultrasonography* of the abdomen and pelvis has a sensitivity and specificity of 84% and 80%, respectively.
- *Contrast enema* and *colonoscopy* are generally discouraged when diverticulitis is severe or abscess is suspected due to the increased risk of perforation (Table 48-1). Complete evaluation of the colon with either barium enema or colonoscopy should be performed once the acute episode has resolved (about 6 weeks later) to rule out colorectal carcinoma or inflammatory bowel disease.

**20. How is mild diverticulitis defined and treated?**

Mild diverticulitis should be suspected in patients with appropriately localized abdominal pain (usually in the left lower quadrant) with associated fever and/or leukocytosis. Patients with mild diverticulitis are nontoxic and able to take food and fluids orally without vomiting. Keep in mind the qualifying factors (see Table 48-1). Treatment of mild disease is generally performed on an outpatient basis. Diet is commonly modified to include only clear liquids or a low-residue diet for 2 to 4 days (but switch to a high-residue diet following resolution of symptoms). After complete resolution of the acute event, the entire colon should be evaluated, if not already recently done, to determine the extent of disease and exclude other diagnostic considerations (i.e., colon carcinoma). Colonoscopy is the preferred method of evaluation; however, barium enema with flexible sigmoidoscopy or CT colonography may be a reasonable alternative.

## Table 48-1. Diagnostic Approach for Acute Diverticulitis

**History and Physical Examination**

Usually more than 60 years old
Left lower quadrant tenderness and unremitting abdominal pain
Fever
Leukocytosis

**Differential Diagnosis**

| ELDERLY PATIENTS | MIDDLE-AGED AND YOUNG PATIENTS | OTHER |
|---|---|---|
| Ischemia | Appendicitis | Amebiasis |
| Carcinoma | Salpingitis | Collagen vascular disease |
| Volvulus | Inflammatory bowel disease | Infectious colitis |
| Obstruction | Penetrating ulcer | Postirradiation proctosigmoiditis |
| Penetrating ulcer | Urosepsis | Prostatitis |
| Nephrolithiasis/urosepsis | Pancreatitis | Irritable bowel syndrome |

**Qualifiers**

Extremes of age (more virulent)
Asian ancestry (right-sided symptoms)
Corticosteroids
Immunosuppression
Chronic renal failure (abdominal examination insensitive)

**Evaluations**

- *Plain x-rays:* Good initial first step. May show ileus, obstruction, mass effect, ischemia, perforation
- *CT scan:* Very helpful in staging the degree of complications and evaluating for other diseases. Should be considered in all cases of diverticulitis with a palpable mass or clinical toxicity, failure of medical therapy, orthopedic complications, and corticosteroid use.
- *Ultrasound:* Can be a safe and helpful noninvasive test to evaluate acute diverticulitis. Over 20% of exams are suboptimal because of intestinal gas; highly operator-dependent.
- *Contrast enema:* For mild-to-moderate cases when the diagnosis is in doubt, water-soluble contrast exam is safe and helpful; otherwise, delay the exam for 6 to 8 weeks.
- *Endoscopy:* Acute diverticulitis is a relative contraindication to endoscopy; must exclude perforation first. Examine only when the diagnosis is in doubt (rectal bleeding, anemia) to exclude ischemic bowel, Crohn's disease, carcinoma, and other possibilities.

Modified from Freeman SR, McNally PR: Diverticulitis. Med Clin North Am 77:1152, 1993.

### 21. What antibiotic regimen is appropriate for moderately severe disease? How is treatment otherwise different?

Antibiotics are usually given intravenously, most often on an inpatient basis. If present, abscess drainage is required and can be performed percutaneously under CT guidance. Many antibiotic regimens are appropriate (see Table 48-2). One goal for more severe disease is adequate coverage of *Pseudomonas aeruginosa*. Resistance of *Bacteroides fragilis* group microorganisms to cefoxitin or cefotetan precludes their selection as a single antibiotic choice. Aminoglycoside based regimens have fallen out of favor because of their associated toxicity profile (ototoxicity and nephrotoxicity) and the availability of less toxic alternatives that have demonstrated equal efficacy.

### 22. How is the management of severely ill patients different?

Severely ill patients usually are toxic with signs of peritonitis. The main difference in treatment compared to patients with less serious disease is the threshold for surgery. In toxic patients, an imaging study, such as a CT scan, may be helpful in directing treatment, but early surgery is most likely to result in a favorable outcome and rarely necessitates prior diagnostic studies.

### 23. What are the indications and goals for surgery?

Emergent surgery should be performed for diffuse peritonitis, frank perforation, large (greater than 4 cm) contained abscess that cannot be drained percutaneously, sepsis, and lack of clinical improvement or worsening despite 3 days of conservative management. Chronic diverticulitis can lead to complications, such as strictures, stenosis, and fistulas, all of which may require surgical intervention. Similarly, those individuals with recurrent episodes of *moderate* and *severe* acute diverticulitis may benefit from elective surgery to prevent further attacks, but this should be taken on a case-by-case basis. The traditional recommendation of elective colectomy for all patients with two episodes of diverticulitis or first episode at age younger than 50 years has fallen out of favor and should no longer be routine practice. The exception would be immunocompromised patients who benefit from elective colectomy following a single episode

**Table 48-2.** A Guide to Antimicrobial Therapy in Acute Diverticulitis

| MODIFYING CIRCUMSTANCES | CAUSE | FIRST CHOICE | ALTERNATIVE | COMMENTS |
|---|---|---|---|---|
| Mild, nonperforating, with no high-risk factors | Aerobes<br>*Escherichia coli*<br>*Klebsiella* spp.<br>Streptococci<br>*Proteus* spp.<br>*Enterobacter* spp.<br>Anaerobes<br>*Bacteroides fragilis*<br>Peptostreptococci<br>Peptococci<br>*Clostridium* spp. | 1. TMP/SMX* + metronidazole OR<br>2. Ciprofloxacin + metronidazole | 1. Cephalexin for TMP/SMX* or Ciprofloxacin<br>2. Clindamycin for metronidazole OR<br>3. Amoxicillin-clavulanic acid | Outpatient, oral |
| Moderately ill, possible local abscess, ± high-risk factors | Same, including *Pseudomonas Aeruginosa* | 1. Ampicillin-sulbactam<br>2. Ticarcillin-clavulanate<br>3. Imipenem-cilastatin<br>4. Ertapenem | 1. Ciprofloxacin + metronidazole<br>2. Second-generation ceph** + metronidazole | Inpatient, IV + CT (catheter drainage of abscess) Consider surgery |
| Severely ill, toxic, peritonitis | Same, including *Pseudomonas Aeruginosa* | Same | Same + third or fourth-generation Ceph*** + metronidazole | Inpatient, IV + CT Consider early surgery |

Modified from Freeman SR, McNally PR: Diverticulitis. Med Clin North Am 77:1161, 1993.
*TMP/SMX, trimethoprim-sulfamethoxazole.
**Cefazolin or cefuroxime.
***Cefotaxime, ceftriaxone, ceftizoxime, ceftazidime, cefepime.

of diverticulitis given the typically more advanced disease at presentation, lower response to medical management, and worse outcomes with emergent surgery. The goals of emergent surgery are primarily to adequately drain the infected area, to remove the affected region of colon (generally at least the entire sigmoid), and, finally, to restore bowel continuity, although all of these objectives may not be met at the time of the initial operation. Goals of elective surgery are much the same but should be accomplished in a single operation and may also include repair of fistulas if present.

**24. What operations are available in the management of diverticulitis?**
Surgery requiring abscess drainage and fecal diversion may be done in one, two, or, in rare cases, three stages (see Fig. 48-1) and is based on a classification that assesses the degree of peritoneal contamination and determines the advisability of performing a primary anastomosis. Factors to be considered include risk of breakdown at the anastomosis based on nutritional status, appearance of tissues, and extent of contamination.

In the past decade, laparoscopic surgery has become applicable to an increasingly wider range of problems. This attractive technique has been used successfully for complicated diverticulitis. Several series demonstrate equal safety and effectiveness with laparoscopic surgery compared to the conventional approach of open laparotomy. The advantages of the laparoscopic approach include decreased morbidity, shorter hospitalization, less pain and fewer complications. As a result of these benefits, the laparoscopic approach will likely soon become the procedure of choice for stage 1 and 2 disease, but the approach for more severe cases may continue to be an open procedure.

- *Single operation*—ideal; thorough preoperative bowel preparation allowed; surgery is elective; diseased bowel is resected and the remaining colon is anastomosed to maintain normal continuity. Examples of appropriate clinical scenarios include chronic obstruction, intractable pain, or recurrent episodes of medically responsive diverticulitis.
- *Two-stage procedure*—bowel preparation cannot be performed beforehand-usually for medically unresponsive disease. A diverting colostomy is created and the diseased bowel segment is removed. Later (3 to 6 months), a second operation is performed to reestablish bowel continuity. The two-stage procedure is the procedure of choice for perforated diverticulitis.
- *Three-stage procedure*—outdated and rarely if ever indicated: it has a higher mortality rate of 12% to 32% vs 1% to 12% compared to the two-stage procedure as well as higher morbidity. The initial operation is simple drainage of the pericolonic abscess and creation of a diverting colostomy. A second operation in 2 to 8 weeks is performed for resection of the diseased bowel with reanastomosis to maintain bowel continuity and preservation of the colostomy to protect the anastomosis. A third surgery is performed in 2 to 4 weeks to take down the colostomy (Fig. 48-1).

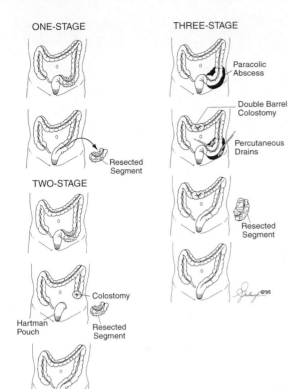

**Figure 48-1.** Surgical options for treating complicated diverticulitis. One-stage surgery includes resection of diseased bowel and reanastomosis to reestablish normal bowel continuity. Two-stage surgery for more complicated disease involves fecal diversion via a proximal colostomy and resection of the diseased segment. The distal segment of the colon can be oversewn (Hartman pouch) or brought out as a mucous fistula. This is currently the most frequently performed operation for diverticulitis complicated by abscess. The first step in three-stage surgery involves fecal diversion and simple drainage of the involved area. Later, the involved area is resected at a second operation and a reanastomosis of the segment is performed, leaving the suture line protected by diverting colostomy. At a third surgery, the colostomy is taken down and bowel continuity is reestablished. (From Freeman SR, McNally PR: Diverticulitis. Med Clin North Am 77:1161, 1993.)

## WEBSITES

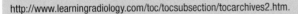

http://www.learningradiology.com/toc/tocsubsection/tocarchives2.htm.

http://www.radiologyassistant.nl/en/42d54f75d111d.

http://www.ssat.com/cgi-bin/divert.cgi.

## BIBLIOGRAPHY

1. Bordeianou L, Hodin R. Controversies in the surgical management of sigmoid diverticulitis. J Gastrointest Surg 2007;11:542–8.
2. Bretagnol F, Pautrat K, Mor C, et al. Emergency laparoscopic management of perforated sigmoid diverticulitis: A promising alternative to more radical procedures. J Am Coll Surg 2008;2006:654–7.
3. Chautems RC, Ambrosetti P, Ludwig A, et al. Long term follow-up after first acute episode of sigmoid diverticulitis: Is surgery mandatory? A prospective study of 118 patients. Dis Colon Rectum 2002;45:962–6.
4. Domiquez EP, Sweeney JF, Choi YU. Diagnosis and management of diverticulitis and appendicitis. Gastroenterol Clin N Am 2006;35:367–91.
5. Dwivedi A, Chahin F, Agrawal S, et al. Laparoscopic colectomy vs. open colectomy for sigmoid diverticular disease. Dis Colon Rectum 2002;45:1309–14.
6. Freeman SR, McNally PR. Diverticulitis. Med Clin North Am 1993;77:1149–67.
7. Jacobs DO. Diverticulitis. N Engl J Med 2007;357:2057–66.
8. Klein S, Mayer L, Present DH, et al. Extraintestinal manifestations in patients with diverticulitis. Ann Intern Med 1988;108:700–2.
9. Lorimer JW, Doumit G. Comorbidity is a major determinant of severity in acute diverticulitis. Am J Surg 2007;193:681–5.
10. Ludeman L, Shepard NA. What is diverticular colitis? Pathology 2002;34:568–72.
11. Petruzziello L, Iacopini F, Bulajic M, et al. Review article: Uncomplicated diverticular disease of the colon. Aliment Pharmacol Ther 2006;23:1379–91.
12. Schechter S, Mulvey J, Eisenstat TE. Management of uncomplicated acute diverticulitis: Results of a survey. Dis Colon Rectum 1999;42:470–5 discussion, 475–476.
13. Solomkin JS, Mazuski JE, Baron EJ, et al. Guidelines for the selection of anti-infective agents for complicated intra-abdominal infections. CID 2003;37:997–1005.
14. Young-Fadok TM, Sarr MG. Diverticular disease of the colon. In: Yamada T, editor. The Textbook of Gastroenterology. 4th ed. Philadelphia: Lippincott; 2003. pp. 1843–63.
15. Wong WD, Wexner SD, Lowry A, et al. Practice parameters for the treatment of sigmoid diverticulitis-supporting documentation. The Standards Task Force, American Society of Colon and Rectal Surgeons. Dis Colon Rectum 2000;43:290–7.

# CHAPTER 49

# DISEASES OF THE APPENDIX

*Kevin Rothchild, MD, and*
*Jonathan A. Schoen, MD*

**1. Describe the anatomy and function of the human appendix.**

The vermiform (Latin for *wormlike*) appendix is usually 6 to 9 cm in length, arising from the convergence of the three taenia coli at the base of the cecum. It is now considered an immunologic organ that participates actively in the secretion of immunoglobulins, particularly IgA. Some theorize that the appendix may also act as a *safehouse* for normal intestinal flora during periods of acute infection.

**2. What is the presumed etiology of appendicitis?**

Fecaliths or hypertrophied lymphoid tissue, causing obstruction of the lumen, are the dominant etiologic factors. Fecaliths are found in about 90% of cases of gangrenous, ruptured appendicitis. The luminal obstruction causes distention of the appendix from both continued mucosal secretion and resident bacterial overgrowth. Ultimately, venous pressure is exceeded and areas of wall infarction with bacterial invasion occur.

**3. What are the signs and symptoms of appendicitis?**

Acute appendiceal distention initially stimulates visceral afferent pain fibers, producing vague, dull, diffuse pain in the mid-abdomen (periumbilical) or lower epigastrium. Low-grade fever, anorexia, nausea, and vomiting may occur after the onset of pain. The inflammatory process soon involves the serosa of the appendix and, in turn, the parietal peritoneum, producing the characteristic shift in pain to the right lower quadrant.

**4. What are the laboratory findings?**

Mild leukocytosis (10,000 to 18,000/mm$^3$) is usually present with early, uncomplicated appendicitis. C-reactive protein is elevated as well, with a sensitivity of 93% and a specificity of 80%.

**5. Where and what is the McBurney point?**

Charles McBurney was an American surgeon born in 1845. He presented his treatise on the area of greatest abdominal pain during appendicitis in 1899. His point of maximal tenderness is located over an area at the distal two-thirds along an axis drawn from the umbilicus to the anterior superior iliac spine.

**6. What are the psoas and obturator signs?**

Irritation of the retroperitoneal psoas muscle (pain on right hip extension) or internal obturator muscle (pain on internal rotation of the flexed right hip) by an inflamed retrocecal appendix.

**7. What is the Rovsing sign?**

Palpation of the left lower quadrant leads commonly to right lower quadrant pain in acute appendicitis.

**8. The peak incidence of acute appendicitis occurs in what age group?**

Ages 15 to 19 years.

**9. The risk of perforation of the appendix is highest in what age groups?**

Although the overall incidence is not as common as in the teen years, appendiceal perforation is higher in children (younger than 5 years) and the elderly, in some series approaching rates of 75%. Those with diabetes and immunosuppressed patients are also at risk for higher complication rates overall.

**10. What is the surgical mortality rate for nonperforated appendicitis? Perforated appendicitis?**

Less than 0.1% for nonperforated and as high as 3% for perforated appendicitis. In the elderly, the mortality rate for perforated appendicitis can be as high as 15%.

**11. List the differential diagnosis for right lower quadrant pain both in women and in children.**

The list is considerably longer for women than for men. It includes ectopic pregnancy, tubo-ovarian abscess, pelvic inflammatory disease, mittelschmerz, ovarian torsion, incarcerated hernia, Crohn's stricture or abscess, diverticulitis, Meckel diverticulitis, typhlitis, carcinoid tumor, infectious colitis, cholecystitis, and peptic ulcer disease. Valentino sign is pain secondary to gastric or biliary fluid collecting in the right lower quadrant from perforated duodenal ulcer. In children, gastroenteritis, mesenteric adenitis, and terminal ileitis commonly mimic appendicitis. Etiology is usually viral but can also be secondary to *Yersinia enterocolitica* infection.

**12. What is a Meckel's diverticulum?**

A congenital omphalomesenteric mucosal remnant that may contain ectopic gastric mucosa. Located on the antimesenteric side of the ileum, it generally adheres to the rule of 2s: found in 2% of the population, 2 feet from the ileocecal valve, and 2% will develop diverticulitis.

**13. What is an acceptable incidence rate for negative appendectomy? Has this rate changed with the increasing use of ultrasound and computed tomography (CT) scanning?**

A negative exploration rate of 10% to 15% is within acceptable standards of surgical care. Interestingly, a large study showed that despite a surge in the use of CT and ultrasound in emergency rooms, and despite the reported 95% rate of sensitivity/specificity, the actual rate of negative appendectomy has remained unchanged.

**14. In older patients (older than 50 years), what condition may be indistinguishable from acute appendicitis?**

Acute diverticulitis of either a redundant sigmoid colon or the cecum itself may present with right lower quadrant pain, fever, and leukocytosis. It is also important to rule out perforated cecal cancer in this setting.

**15. What features of pelvis inflammatory disease (PID) can help distinguish it from appendicitis?**

High fever, cervical motion tenderness (chandelier sign), cervical discharge, pain related to menses, and tendency for bilateral pain can often differentiate PID from appendicitis.

**16. What is the most common malignant tumor of the appendix? Describe its management.**

Carcinoid is the most common tumor of the appendix, and the appendix is the most common site of carcinoid tumors. Most large series report an incidence of 0.2 to 0.3 in appendectomy specimens. Appendectomy is all that is required in distal tumors that are less than 2 cm in size. If the tumor is greater than 2 cm or it has extension into the mesoappendix or cecum, formal right hemicolectomy is appropriate. Palliative resection of the presumed appendiceal primary is indicated in the presence of metastatic disease.

A *mucocele* is the second most commonly encountered tumor of the appendix, in which a distended appendix is secondary to obstruction of the appendiceal orifice by mucoid material. Cysts smaller than 2 cm are almost always benign, while larger tumors may harbor malignancy. Rupture of these cysts may spread epithelial cells in mucoid fluid throughout the peritoneum, or pseudomyxoma peritonei of appendiceal origin.

**17. What is the proper treatment for late/perforated appendicitis that presents as an abscess?**

Radiology-guided drainage (usually CT guided) is indicated in the presence of an established abscess, provided that the patient has no evidence of diffuse peritonitis or uncontrolled sepsis. Although delayed (after 6 to 8 weeks) appendectomy is not always required, rates of recurrent appendicitis can approach 20%, so many surgeons prefer to operate in an elective setting.

**18. What is the most common complication after appendectomy?**

Wound infection. In the setting of perforation or abscess, the wound edges can be left open as a delayed primary closure to prevent this complication. The laparoscopic approach has reduced this complication significantly.

**19. In what patient population is ultrasound particularly helpful in making the diagnosis of acute appendicitis?**

Ultrasound can be particularly helpful in the pediatric as well as pregnant patients, in which CT scan is usually avoided. In addition, it is helpful to delineate any gynecologic abnormalities. A noncompressible, distended (larger than 8 mm), painful tubular structure on ultrasound predicts appendicitis, with reported sensitivity of 84% to 94% and specificity of 92%.

### 20. What other imaging modality is often used (and abused)?

CT scanning has a quoted sensitivity of 90% to 100% and up to a 97% specificity. Even with these results, CT scanning has never been proved to reduce the rates of negative appendectomy or perforated appendicitis. Nothing should replace the clinical decision-making of the examining physician, which includes deciding whether imaging studies are even warranted.

### 21. When is laparoscopic appendectomy appropriate?

Laparoscopic appendectomy was first reported in 1983, and its use has increased steadily since. Although a bias may exist toward the use of laparoscopy with less advanced appendicitis, mortality and length of stay are similar or improved. Cosmesis, postoperative pain, and wound infection rates are also improved. In addition, laparoscopy allows visualization of the entire abdomen in women, the obese, or equivocal clinical situations. There has been concern raised about increased intra-abdominal abscess rates after laparoscopic appendectomy; however, the data is inconclusive.

### 22. During an abdominal exploration for right lower quadrant pain, is removal of a normal appendix appropriate in patients with Crohn's disease?

Yes. If the base of the appendix and the surrounding area of the cecum are free of disease, an appendectomy should still be performed in the setting of Crohn's disease. If an enterocutaneous fistula develops postoperatively, it almost always results from diseased terminal ileum rather than the appendiceal stump.

### 23. Is an appendectomy during pregnancy a safe procedure?

Acute appendicitis is the most frequently encountered extrauterine disease requiring surgery during pregnancy. The appendix shifts superiorly above the right iliac crest by the fourth month of pregnancy. Abdominal tenderness is less localized because the inflamed appendix is no longer near the parietal peritoneum. These factors along with the leukocytosis of pregnancy can make the clinical diagnosis more difficult. Fetal demise increases from 5% in simple appendicitis to 28% if there is perforation; therefore, early intervention is the rule if appendicitis is suspected.

### 24. If an ovarian tumor is discovered during laparoscopic or open exploration, what steps should be taken?

The normal appendix should be removed after obtaining peritoneal washings, which are studied for tumor cytology. The ovarian mass itself should not be touched or biopsied. Ovarian cancer is staged with a strictly performed technique and should be done at a later procedure.

### 25. Does nonoperative therapy have any role in treating acute appendicitis?

Treating appendicitis with antibiotics alone is not common practice in North America. European studies have shown some success; however, they have documented high recurrence rates (up to 40%) and high costs of delivery. Delayed appendectomy is more often seen after resolution of contained abscess or inflammation by antibiotics (with or without catheter drainage) in patients after perforation.

### 26. What is a Mitrofanoff procedure?

A Mitrofanoff appendicovesicostomy is a procedure preformed to obviate the need for urethral catheterization in those with neurogenic bladder (such as patients with spina bifida). The appendix is removed from its attachments to the cecum while maintaining its blood supply; then one end is sutured to the urinary bladder and the other end is sutured to the skin to form a stoma, usually near the umbilicus.

## BIBLIOGRAPHY

1. Affleck DG, Handrahan DL, Egger MJ, et al. The laparoscopic management of appendicitis and cholelithiasis in pregnancy. Am J Surg 1999;178:523–9.
2. Bollinger RR, Barbas AS, Bush EL, et al. Biofilms in the large bowel suggest an apparent function of the human vermiform appendix. J Theor Biol 2007;8:32.
3. Carr NJ. The pathology of acute appendicitis. Ann Diagn Pathol 2000;4:46–58.
4. Collins DC. 71,000 Human appendix specimens. A final report summarizing 40 years of study. Am J Proctol 1963;14:365–81.
5. Flum D, Morris A. Misdiagnosis of appendicitis and the use of diagnostic imaging. J Am Coll Surg 2005;6:933–9.
6. Martin JP, Connor PD, Charles K. Meckel's diverticulum. Am Fam Physician 2000;61:1037–42.
7. McBurney C. Experience with early operative interference in cases of disease of the vermiform appendix. N Y Med J 1889;50:676–84.
8. McGory ML, Maggard MA, Kang H, et al. Malignancies of the appendix: Beyond case series reports. Dis Colon Rectum 2005;48:2264–71.
9. Meakins JL. Appendectomy and appendicitis. Can J Surg 1999;42:90.
10. Mingin GC, Baskin LS. Surgical management of the neurogenic bladder and bowel. Int Braz J Urol 2003;29:53–61.
11. Nguyen N, Zainabadi K, Mavandadi S, et al. Trends in utilization and outcomes of laparoscopic versus open appendectomy. Am J Surg 188 2004;6:813–20.
12. Semm K. Endoscopic appendectomy. Endoscopy 1983;15:59–64.
13. Temple LK, Litwin DE, McLeod RS. A meta-analysis of laparoscopic versus open appendectomy in patients suspected of having acute appendicitis. Can J Surg 1999;42:377–83.

# COLITIS: PSEUDOMEMBRANOUS, MICROSCOPIC, AND RADIATION

# CHAPTER 50

*Jill M. Watanabe, MD, MPH, and*
*Christina M. Surawicz, MD*

## PSEUDOMEMBRANOUS COLITIS

### 1. What is *Clostridium difficile?*

First isolated in 1935 and named by its difficult isolation from the feces of infants, *Bacillus difficile* is an anaerobic, gram-positive, spore-forming, toxin-producing bacteria. By the 1970s, this bacillus was renamed *Clostridium difficile* and its toxins were implicated as a major cause of antibiotic-associated diarrhea and as the cause of pseudomembranous colitis (PMC). *C. difficile* infection (CDI) has historically been precipitated by the use of broad-spectrum antibiotics, which disrupt the normal fecal flora, promoting *C. difficile* overgrowth, but sporadic cases can occur. Although many patients with *C. difficile* infections are asymptomatic carriers, patients with CDI can experience a spectrum of symptoms, ranging from a self-limited course of diarrhea to PMC. Severe cases of CDI can cause ileus and toxic megacolon, necessitating surgery and admission to the intensive care unit (ICU) and can result in death.

### 2. How is CDI defined?

Although 20% to 30% of persons who take antibiotics develop diarrhea, only 10% to 20% of these cases are caused by *C. difficile*. Most patients with CDI experience abdominal pain and cramping with fever and leukocytosis. In severe cases, CDI is associated with a leukemoid reaction (white blood cells >25,000 to 30,000 leukocytes/mm$^3$), severe hypoalbuminemia, and shock. CDI has been defined as three or more unformed or watery stools for 1 to 2 days with associated *C. difficile* toxin in stool or by culturing the toxigenic *C. difficile* organism. CDI can also be diagnosed with the recognition of PMC at endoscopy, surgery, or autopsy or by histopathology.

### 3. What causes PMC?

PMC is due to overgrowth of *C. difficile*, which causes disease by the production of two toxins: A and B. *C. difficile* strains that do not produce toxins are not pathogenic. Toxin B is more toxic than toxin A; *C. difficile* strains that produce toxin B but not toxin A can cause CDI. Toxins A and B cause mucosal damage and inflammation of the colon by disrupting the actin cytoskeleton of the intestinal epithelial cells while triggering an inflammatory cascade. In 20% to 30% of cases, PMC is limited to the proximal colon.

### 4. What are the risk factors for CDI?

The risk factors for *C. difficile* disease include antibiotic exposure, hospitalization (especially surgical patients, ICU patients, and posttransplant patients), and advanced age. Other risk factors include invasive procedures (especially gastrointestinal procedures), renal failure, cancer chemotherapy, and residence in a nursing home. Recently, there have been reports of severe CDI in previously low-risk populations such as pregnant women. Some cases have resulted in severe disease and death. Hospital settings remain an important reservoir, in part, because the spores of the anaerobic bacillus, *C. difficile*, can survive for many years. As many as 20% to 30% of hospitalized patients are colonized with *C. difficile* and two-thirds of these infected hospitalized patients have historically been asymptomatic carriers.

### 5. Which antibiotics are most commonly implicated?

Clindamycin and cephalosporins (especially third-generation) have been most commonly associated with CDI in the past, followed by expanded-spectrum penicillins; more recently, fluoroquinolones have been implicated as a significant risk factor. Of note, CDI can occur with any antibiotic, even single-dose preoperative antibiotics and, paradoxically, by antibiotics that are used to treat this condition.

### 6. Why do some people develop *C. difficile* diarrhea while others are simply colonized?

Studies of patients with *C. difficile* colonization have shown that serum levels of IgG antibody against toxin A have been associated with protection from disease expression and prevention of recurrences. The risk of developing CDI is decreased in hospitalized patients already colonized with *C. difficile*.

**7. How has the epidemiology of CDI changed over the past decade?**

Since the early 2000s, the morbidity and mortality of CDI have been increasing with epidemics reported in the United States, Canada, and Europe. The Centers for Disease Control and Prevention (CDC) has reported an increase in hospital billings attributed to CDI. There were 82,000 reported cases of CDI in 1996, 178,000 reported cases in 2003, and 250,000 reported cases in 2005. There is also evidence to suggest the severity of CDI is increasing; *C. difficile*–related mortality by listing on death certificates in the United States rose from 5.7 deaths per million in 1999 to 23.7 deaths per million in 2004. In addition to these epidemics of severe cases of CDI, CDI has been reported among patients in the community previously thought to be at very low risk to acquire CDI. Over the past decade, case reports of community-acquired CDI (CA-CDI) have been reported among younger patients, peripartum women, and patients taking proton pump inhibitors, often in the absence of antibiotic exposure.

**8. What accounts for the changing epidemiology of CDIs?**

The changing epidemiology of *C. difficile* has been attributed, in part, to the evolution of a hypervirulent strain, designated BI/NAP1/027 (restriction-endonuclease analysis group BI, North American Pulsed Field type 1, polymerase chain reaction ribotype 027). This strain is not a new strain (first isolated in 1984), but over time, this strain has demonstrated increasing resistance to fluoroquinolones. The BI/NAP1/027 strain has also been associated with an increasing rate of treatment failure as well as an increasing rate of CDI recurrence. This epidemic strain has not been implicated in the cases of CA-CDI.

**9. What possible factors mediate the hypervirulence of the BI/NAP1/027 strain?**

The fluoroquinolones-resistant B1/NAP1/027 strains have been associated with higher concentrations of both toxins A and B in vitro. The B1/NAP1/027 strain also carries two genes of interest. The first gene, *tcdC*, has an 18–base pair deletion; this mutation renders the *tcdC* gene ineffective in inhibiting the production of toxins A and B. The second gene encodes a binary toxin, *C. difficile* toxin (CDT), similar to iota toxin found in *Clostridium perfringens*. The binary toxin is not fully understood, but is known to cause fluid accumulation in rabbit ileal loops.

**10. How is the diagnosis of CDI made?**

The diagnosis of CDI is challenged by the fact that the best and most sensitive tests have the slowest turnaround time. Most labs now use enzyme immunoassays to detect toxin A or toxins A and B. However, these tests are imperfect and false-negative tests can be reported. In the setting of high clinical suspicion and negative test results, serial testing and empiric therapy may be necessary (Table 50-1).

**Table 50-1.** Diagnosis of *Clostridium difficile* Colitis

| DIAGNOSTIC TEST | ACCURACY | COMMENTS |
| --- | --- | --- |
| Tissue cytotoxin B assay | Sensitivity ≈94% to 100% | Gold standard (detects up to 10 pg toxin), but expensive, requires technical expertise |
| | Specificity ≈90% to 100% | Results not ready for 24 to 48 hr |
| Enzyme immunoassays | | |
| Toxin A | Sensitivity 60% to 95% Specificity ≈75% to 100% | Most widely used test, quick (2 hours) and less expensive |
| Toxins A and B | Sensitivity ≈79% to 80% Specificity ≈98% | Detects toxin A–/B+ strains Toxin B is more potent than toxin A and can cause disease in the absence of toxin A |
| Stool cultures | Sensitivity ≈90% to 100% Specificity ≈84% to 100% | Carriers test positive, results unavailable for 72 hours Does not distinguish nonpathogenic vs. pathogenic strains |
| Endoscopy | Sensitivity ≈50% Specificity ≈100% | 2-hour test, sensitivity low, but the presence of pseudomembranous colitis is diagnostic |

**11. What are the typical findings on colonoscopy?**

Colonoscopy may be normal or show nonspecific colitis. With severe disease, the colon mucosa has creamy white-yellow plaques (pseudomembranes). Histologic studies show that the pseudomembrane usually arises from a point of superficial ulceration, accompanied by acute and chronic inflammation of the lamina propria. The pseudomembrane is composed of fibrin, mucin, debris of sloughed mucosal epithelial cells, and polymorphonuclear cells.

**12. What are the hallmarks of severe CDI?**

Severe CDI is associated with fever, leukocytosis, hypoalbuminemia, shock, and high levels of C-reactive protein. Severe colitis can result in toxic megacolon and progress to colonic perforation and death by multiorgan failure.

**13. When is treatment indicated? What antibiotics are used?**

The first step is to discontinue the implicated antibiotics. About 20% of cases, which are mild, resolve spontaneously. Treatment to eradicate *C. difficile* should be given in all but the mildest cases. Clinical suspicion should prompt empiric treatment in patients with severe illness while awaiting test results. Oral vancomycin is the only U.S. Food and Drug Administration–approved treatment for CDI, but metronidazole has been first line in the past because its low cost and the concern that oral vancomycin use might promote vancomycin-resistant enterococci in the colon. Historically, the efficacy of metronidazole has been equal to that of vancomycin; however, reports of metronidazole treatment failure rates have been increasing to as high as 22% to 38% over the past several years. In severe cases of CDI, the use of oral vancomycin is recommended because of its faster efficacy and higher cure rates (97% versus 76%). Typical treatment courses are 10 to 14 days. Pancolectomy is necessary in patients who do not respond to therapy and develop toxic megacolon with rising levels of serum lactate (Table 50-2).

**Table 50-2.** Treatment for *Clostridium difficile* Disease

| CDI | DRUG/DOSE | COMMENT |
|---|---|---|
| Mild-moderate | Metronidazole 250 mg PO 4 times daily | Inexpensive, avoid in pregnancy and with breastfeeding |
| | Metronidazole 500 mg PO 3 times daily | |
| | Vancomycin 125 mg PO 4 times daily | Switch to vancomycin if no response to metronidazole in 72 hours |
| Severe | Vancomycin 125 to 250 mg PO 4 times daily | |
| | Vancomycin enemas, 500 mg 4 times daily | |
| Complicated | Metronidazole IV | Patients with ileus, recent abdominal surgery, unable to take orally |
| | Vancomycin 500 mg 4 times daily | Patients who can tolerate orally |
| | Vancomycin enemas, 500 mg 4 times daily | |

**14. When should you expect a response to treatment?**

Usually within 3 to 5 days.

**15. What other treatment options are under development and investigation?**

Bacitracin, fusidic acid, nitazoxanide, rifampicin, and teicoplanin have been shown to be effective in treating CDI, but they are not superior to vancomycin or metronidazole. Other treatment options under investigation include toxin binding polymers (e.g., tolevamer), a *C. difficile* vaccine, and monoclonal antibodies directed against toxins A and B.

**16. What should you do if symptoms recur after therapy?**

Although most patients respond to therapy, approximately 22% to 26% have recurrent symptoms after stopping the antibiotics. One recurrence makes further recurrences even more likely (up to 40%). Patients with recurrent *C. difficile* disease need retreatment, with either metronidazole or vancomycin in standard doses followed by 2 to 3 weeks of pulsed antibiotic treatment at lower doses. Management of repeated relapses include courses of higher-dose oral vancomycin, followed by pulsed/tapering doses of vancomycin as well as the use of probiotic agents, such as the nonpathogenic yeast *Saccharomyces boulardii* or the bacteria *Lactobacillus GG*. Fecal transplants from healthy donors can also be considered in refractory cases.

**17. How can we control *C. difficile* epidemics in hospitals?**

Prevention of CDI involves the judicious use of antibiotics as well as vigilant environmental control. Once diagnosed, patients with CDI should be isolated in rooms with personal bathrooms until their diarrhea resolves. Contact precautions should be initiated; *C. difficile* spores have been cultured from patient bathrooms, bedpans, stethoscopes, and blood pressure cuffs. Once patients depart from their isolation rooms, these rooms should be cleansed with a 10% bleach solution. *Clostridia* spores are not vulnerable to alcohol; handwashing with soap and water and use of disposable equipment and vinyl gloves may help prevent the transmission of *C. difficile* in health care settings.

## MICROSCOPIC COLITIS

**18. What is microscopic colitis (MC)?**

MC is a clinical syndrome characterized by chronic watery diarrhea, grossly normal appearing colonic mucosa, and abnormal histologic features. The first case was reported in 1976 when a woman with chronic diarrhea and a normal endoscopic gastrointestinal (GI) evaluation was found to have an abnormal colorectal biopsy. This patient's biopsy sample revealed a thickened subepithelial collagen band and a slight increase in lymphocytes in the lamina propria. This entity was thus named collagenous colitis (CC). Subsequent biopsy samples identified similar findings in other patients with chronic diarrhea but without the thickened collagen band. This clinical entity was named lymphocytic colitis (LC) and was first recognized in 1989. Since the first case reports, MC has become more widely recognized and may account for 10% to 20% of patients with chronic watery diarrhea. Curiously, patients who carry the diagnosis of LC or CC can subsequently be diagnosed with the other condition at another point in time. To date, it is unclear whether CC and LC are distinct clinical entities or represent the spectrum of one disease.

**19. What are the features of CC and LC?**

See Table 50-3.

**Table 50-3.** Features of Collagenous Colitis and Lymphocytic Colitis

| FEATURE | COLLAGENOUS COLITIS | LYMPHOCYTIC COLITIS |
|---|---|---|
| Gender incidence (female:male) | 7.5:1 | 2:1 |
| Mean age onset | 51 years | 43 years |
| Histology | | |
| Increased intraepithelial lymphocytes, >20/100 absorptive cells | Yes | Yes |
| Increased lymphocytes and plasma cells in lamina propria | Yes | Yes |
| Surface epithelial flattening or detachment | Yes | Yes |
| Subepithelial collagen band, >10 μm | Yes | No |

**20. What are the clinical features of MC?**

The most common clinical symptoms are diarrhea (95%), weight loss (91%), abdominal pain (40%), urgency (29%), and nocturnal diarrhea (22%). These symptoms can be severe in some patients.

**21. How do you distinguish MC from patients with irritable bowel syndrome (IBS)?**

The gold standard is colorectal biopsy, which will be normal in patients with IBS. There is considerable overlap of symptoms between MC and IBS. Studies have shown that as many as 33% of patients with biopsy-proved CC or LC will have a prior diagnosis of IBS and that as many as half of the patients diagnosed with MC will also meet the diagnostic criteria for IBS.

**22. Are there any laboratory tests or imaging studies that can help establish the diagnosis of MC?**

Laboratory tests and radiographic imaging are generally nondiagnostic. Fecal leukocytes may be present, but stool cultures are typically negative. C-reactive protein levels and the erythrocyte sedimentation rates may be elevated; anemia may be present. Barium enema and colonoscopy results typically are normal but can show subtle mucosal change.

**23. How common is MC?**

Studies from the United States, Europe, and Canada over the past 30 years show an incidence of CC at 0.6 to 6.2 per 100,000 people and an incidence of LC at 0.5 to 12.9 per 100,000 people. Overall, the incidence of MC has been increasing since the 1980s, but it is not known whether this increase is due to an increasing awareness and improved diagnosis of MC or whether the disease has become more common.

**24. Which parts of the colon are most commonly affected?**

MC involves the colon discontinuously, and the patchy involvement of the normal appearing colon necessitates a minimum of four biopsy samples to establish the diagnosis of MC. In one prior study, the highest yield was from biopsies of the transverse colon. Most cases can be diagnosed by biopsy samples taken within the range of flexible sigmoidoscopy; colonoscopy with biopsy of the right colon may be necessary to detect 10% of patients with isolated right-sided histopathology.

**25. What agents are associated with the pathogenesis of MC?**

Nonsteroidal anti-inflammatory drugs (NSAIDs) are thought to be an important pathogenic factor, although their role in this association is unknown. A case-control study showed that patients with CC were 3 times more likely to take NSAIDs. LC has been associated with the use of sertraline. Other potential medications associated with the development of MC include acarbose, lansoprazole, ranitidine, and ticlopidine.

**26. What are the associated conditions?**

A wide variety of associated conditions are found in case reports, including rheumatologic conditions (thyroid disease, celiac disease, diabetes, rheumatoid arthritis, and asthma/allergies) in up to 40% to 50% of patients with MC.

**27. What is the natural history of MC?**

The natural history is not known, but in one study, 505 of patients with MC experienced resolution of their symptoms after 3 years. However, as many as 30% of patients treated for MC experience persistent diarrhea 10 years after diagnosis. There is no increased risk of malignancy associated with MC.

**28. What are the treatment options?**

Initially, patients with MC can make dietary changes (avoid caffeine, alcohol, and dairy products) and stop the medications that have been associated with MC. Some patients do well on antidiarrheals (loperamide) or cholestyramine alone. Meta-analysis has shown that budesonide (9 mg daily) for 6 to 8 weeks has been effective in decreasing symptoms in 81% of patients with CC; however, symptoms often recur (61% to 80%) with the cessation of budesonide and patients often require slow subsequent tapers. Budesonide has also been shown to be effective in treating LC. Bismuth subsalicylate and sulfasalazine/mesalamine have also shown efficacy in the treatment of MC. Some patients require stronger immunosuppressants such as methotrexate or azathioprine. In rare cases, patients with severe and unresponsive disease may require surgery.

*Bud 9 x6w*

# RADIATION COLITIS

**29. Which part of the gastrointestinal tract is most commonly injured by radiation?**

Injury to the colon can occur with radiation treatment of rectal, cervical, uterine, prostate, urinary bladder and testicular cancer. The small bowel is protected by peristaltic movement into and out of the field of radiation and has a lower risk of injury than the colon. The relatively immobile colon, especially the rectosigmoid colon, is highly susceptible to radiation injury. Implants deliver smaller amounts of focused radiation and cause less damage to the colon than external beam radiation. Tumors that require higher doses of radiation, such as pelvic tumors, are associated with a greater risk of damage to the colon.

**30. What can be done to prevent radiation damage?**

Radiation damage can be reduced by limiting the dosage and area of exposure while shielding adjacent tissues.

**31. What symptoms are associated with irradiation?**

The initial symptoms of radiation exposure are nausea and vomiting. Diarrhea typically develops 5 days later. Loss of mucosal defenses increases the patient's risk of developing sepsis. Acute radiation injury to the colon typically occurs within 6 weeks and is manifested by diarrhea, tenesmus, and, rarely, bleeding. These symptoms are self-limited and typically resolve in 2 to 6 months without therapy. Chronic symptoms of radiation colitis and proctitis (or chronic radiation proctopathy) can occur nearly a year following radiation therapy but can be delayed by decades after the initial radiation exposure. The primary symptoms associated with chronic injury to the colon and rectum include diarrhea, obstructed defecation, rectal pain, and rectal bleeding.

*Acute N/V*
*<6w*
*chr 1yr+ bleedy, pain, dx*

**32. What are effects of localized radiation to the colon?**

Colonoscopy may be normal or may show telangectasias or friable mucosa. Early or acute changes include microscopic damage to mucosal and vascular epithelial cells. One typical histologic feature is the presence of atypical fibroblasts. Late changes commonly involve fibrosis with obliterative endarteritis resulting in chronic ischemia, stricture formation, and bleeding.

**33. How can radiation colitis and proctitis be managed?**

There are limited data on the appropriate treatment for radiation colitis and proctitis. Medications used to treat radiation colitis and proctitis include oral and topical sucralfate, oral and topical steroids, 5-ASA compounds, sulfasalazine, hyperbaric oxygen, and antibiotics (metronidazole).

**34. What are the endoscopic therapies for chronic bleeding?**

Argon laser photocoagulation, heater probe, and bipolar cautery have been used to treat localized bleeding from telangiectasias. Formaldehyde application has been used in patients with significant bleeding. Patients should be transfused with blood as needed and take oral iron.

## 35. How are chronic radiation-induced bowel strictures managed?

Patients with obstructive symptoms may benefit from the use of stool softeners. Dilation of the strictures may be necessary. Patients with long or angulated strictures may benefit from surgery as these lesions are more likely to perforate with dilating procedures.

## BIBLIOGRAPHY

1. Babb RR. Radiation proctitis: A review. Am J Gastroenterol 1996;91:1309–11.
2. Bartlett JG. Clinical practice. Antibiotic-associated diarrhea. N Engl J Med 2002;346:334–9.
3. Bartlett JG. Historical perspectives on studies of *Clostridium difficile* and *C. difficile* infection. Clin Infect Dis 2008;46(Suppl. 1):S4–11.
4. Bartlett JG. Narrative review: The new epidemic of *Clostridium difficile*-associated enteric disease. Ann Intern Med 2006;145:758–64.
5. Berthrong M. Pathologic changes secondary to radiation. World J Surg 1986;10:155–70.
6. Blossom DB, McDonald LC. The challenges posed by reemerging *Clostridium difficile* infection. Clin Infect Dis 2007;45:222–7.
7. Chande N, McDonald JW, Macdonald JK. Interventions for treating collagenous colitis. Cochrane Database Syst Rev 2008; CD003575.
8. Chande N, McDonald JW, Macdonald JK. Interventions for treating lymphocytic colitis. Cochrane Database Syst Rev 2008; CD006096.
9. Chen SW, Liang JA, Yang SN, et al. Radiation injury to intestine following hysterectomy and adjuvant radiotherapy for cervical cancer. Gynecol Oncol 2004;95:208–14.
10. Freeman HJ. Collagenous mucosal inflammatory diseases of the gastrointestinal tract. Gastroenterology 2005;129:338–50.
11. Gerding, DN. (2008) "Clostridium difficile: surveillance and diagnosis." CDC link: <http://wwwlrmei/CDI010>
12. Hookman P, Barkin JS. Review: *Clostridium difficile*-associated disorders/diarrhea and *Clostridium difficile* colitis: The emergence of a more virulent era. Dig Dis Sci 2007;52:1071–5.
13. Kochhar R, Sriram PV, Sharma SC, et al. Natural history of late radiation proctosigmoiditis treated with topical sucralfate suspension. Dig Dis Sci 1999;44:973–8.
14. Kuipers EJ, Surawicz CM. *Clostridium difficile* infection. Lancet 2008;371:1486–8.
15. Kyne L, Warny M, Qamar A, et al. Association between antibody response to toxin A and protection against recurrent *Clostridium difficile* diarrhoea. Lancet 2001;357:189–93.
16. Limsui D, Pardi DS, Camilleri M, et al. Symptomatic overlap between irritable bowel syndrome and microscopic colitis. Inflamm Bowel Dis 2007;13:175–81.
17. Madisch A, Miehlke S, Lindner M, et al. Clinical course of collagenous colitis over a period of 10 years. Z Gastroenterol 2006;44:971–4.
18. McDonald LC, Killgore GE, Thompson A, et al. An epidemic, toxin gene-variant strain of *Clostridium difficile*. N Engl J Med 2005;353:2433–41.
19. McFarland LV. Update on the changing epidemiology of *Clostridium difficile*-associated disease. Nat Clin Pract Gastroenterol Hepatol 2008;5:40–8.
20. Nielsen OH, Vainer B, Rask-Madsen J. Non-IBD and noninfectious colitis. Nat Clin Pract Gastroenterol Hepatol 2008;5:28–39.
21. Nyhlin N, Bohr J, Eriksson S, et al. Microscopic colitis: A common and an easily overlooked cause of chronic diarrhoea. Eur J Intern Med 2008;19:181–6.
22. Razavi B, Apisarnthanarak A, Mundy LM. *Clostridium difficile:* Emergence of hypervirulence and fluoroquinolone resistance. Infection 2007;35:300–7.
23. Shen EP, Surawicz CM. The changing face of *Clostridium difficile:* What treatment options remain? Am J Gastroenterol 2007;102:2789–92.
24. Shiraishi M, Hiroyasu S, Ishimine T, et al. Radiation enterocolitis: Overview of the past 15 years. World J Surg 1998;22:491–3.
25. Sunenshine RH, McDonald LC. *Clostridium difficile*-associated disease: New challenges from an established pathogen. Cleve Clin J Med 2006;73:187–97.
26. Surawicz CM. Probiotics, antibiotic-associated diarrhoea and *Clostridium difficile* diarrhoea in humans. Best Pract Res Clin Gastroenterol 2003;17:775–83.
27. Surawicz CM. Treatment of recurrent *Clostridium difficile*-associated disease. Nat Clin Pract Gastroenterol Hepatol 2004;1:32–8.
28. Tsujinaka S, Baig MK, Gornev R, et al. Formalin instillation for hemorrhagic radiation proctitis. Surg Innov 2005;12:123–8.

# UPPER GASTROINTESTINAL TRACT HEMORRHAGE

John S. Goff, MD

CHAPTER 51

**1. What are the signs and symptoms of upper gastrointestinal (UGI) bleeding?**

Hematemesis can vary from material that looks like coffee grounds (blood darkened from acid exposure) to massive amounts of bright red blood. Melena (black, tarry stool) is usually found in patients with an upper source, but it may be seen in patients with a right colon bleed and slow transit. Brisker UGI bleeding will result in maroon to red blood. It is likely that the source of bleeding is not from the UGI tract if it is bright red per rectum and not associated with orthostatic blood pressure changes or syncope.

**2. What historic facts will help with determining the source of UGI bleeding?**

Aspirin, other nonsteroidal anti-inflammatory drugs (NSAIDs), alcohol, or cigarettes are risk factors for gastric and duodenal lesions. Physical stress (trauma, central nervous system injury, burns) is a common cause of UGI bleeding, especially from gastritis. A history of heartburn and abdominal pain prior to onset of the bleeding suggests esophagitis and/or ulcer. A history of liver disease or suspected liver disease because of heavy alcohol use should alert one to the possibility of bleeding from varices or portal hypertensive gastropathy. Vomiting prior to bleeding suggests a Mallory-Weiss tear as the possible cause of the bleeding. Inquiring about previous bleeding episodes is often useful. Also, a history of an abdominal aortic aneurysm repair could suggest an enteric vascular fistula.

**3. How can the amount of acute blood lost be estimated clinically?**

The acute loss of 500 mL of blood will not result in detectable physiologic changes; however, loss of 1000 mL will produce orthostatic changes of 10 to 20 mm Hg in systolic blood pressure and a pulse rise of 20 beats/minute or more. Loss of 2000 mL or more of blood will produce shock.

**4. How might one distinguish an UGI bleed from a lower GI bleed in a patient who presents with blood per rectum?**

The most obvious factor that points to an UGI source is finding a positive gastric aspirate for blood. Black stool per rectum (melena) suggests UGI bleeding, but it can be seen in some patients with cecal bleeding. Pepto-Bismol also produces black stool because of the bismuth contained in the product. Red blood per rectum is not likely to be from an upper source if there is no associated syncope or orthostatic blood pressure changes. The presence of risk factors for UGI bleeding may be of some help (alcohol use, smoking, NSAID use, prior UGI bleed, UGI symptoms), but NSAIDs can cause colonic or small bowel ulcers in some patients.

**5. What are the first steps in managing a patient with UGI bleeding?**

The first step in management is to establish intravenous access with one or two, if the patient is having a major bleed, large-bore catheters. Volume replacement should be initiated, and vasopressors are used if the patient is hypotensive and does not respond promptly to fluid resuscitation. Blood tests (hematocrit [Hct], platelet count, prothrombin time, partial thromboplastin time) are run on blood obtained at the time of achieving intravenous access. A nasogastric tube, preferably of moderate to large size (>11 Fr), is placed next followed by consultation with the gastroenterology and surgery services. Unstable patients and those with comorbidities or advanced age and ongoing bleeding need to be placed in the intensive care unit.

**6. How does one interpret the Hct values in a patient with acute UGI bleeding?**

The Hct will fall over time as there is replacement of lost volume from extravascular fluid. In about 2 hours, approximately 25% of the final fall will be achieved and approximately 50% will occur in 8 hours. The final Hct value will be seen at 72 hours after the initial acute loss of blood. Obviously, this timetable will be accelerated if the patient is given intravenous fluid.

**7. Why place a nasogastric (NG) tube?**

The major reasons for placing a NG tube are to help determine the source of bleeding and to determine if the patient is still bleeding. The finding of red blood when the NG tube is placed is associated with increased mortality rates, increased number of complications, and higher blood transfusion requirements. A secondary benefit is the clearing of blood from the stomach to aid in performing an urgent upper endoscopy (esophagogastroduodenoscopy [EGD]). There should be no worry about causing increased bleeding in patients with known liver disease when passing an NG tube. Note: Approximately 15% of patients with UGI bleed without bloody or coffee ground material in the NG aspirate are found to have *stigmata* considered high risk to rebleed at endoscopy.

## 8. What types of fluid should be used for resuscitation and when?

The fluid of choice for initial resuscitation is crystalloid (normal saline or lactated Ringer's). Packed red blood cells are the blood product of choice. Type specific or universal donor blood can be given if the patient needs urgent replacement due to massive and ongoing losses. In elderly patients, the Hct should be kept around 30 to help avoid cardiac complications. Fresh frozen plasma (FFP) is to be considered if the patient is still bleeding and the international normalized ratio (INR) is greater than 1.5. Platelets are to be used if the count is less than 50,000 and there is ongoing bleeding.

## 9. Does every patient with UGI bleeding need to be hospitalized in the intensive care unit or even hospitalized?

Patients are best treated by triaging them according to their risk factors for further bleeding. This means that some can go home the same day as they present and others will need to go to the intensive care unit. The Rockall and Blatchford scores are two simple and clinically useful risk stratification tools used for UGI hemorrhage (Tables 51-1 and 51-2). The Rockall score has been successfully used to achieve such triage, but it has been called into question as to whether it can adequately predict rebleeding outcomes versus mortality outcomes. Risk factors for increased mortality associated with an acute UGI bleed are age greater than 65 years, comorbid illness, shock, and continued bleeding in the hospital. APACHE II score greater than 11, esophageal varices, and stigmata or recent bleeding at endoscopy are also predictors of a poor outcome. Patients with none of these risk factors and a clean-based, nonbleeding ulcer, mild gastritis, or low-grade esophagitis can be considered for discharge to home from the emergency department or the GI lab (Box 51-1).

## 10. What are the common causes of UGI bleeding? And uncommon causes?

Duodenal ulcers are the most common cause of acute UGI bleeding (30%) followed by gastric erosions (27%), gastric ulcers (22%), esophagitis (11%), duodenitis (10%), varices (5%), and Mallory-Weiss tears (5%). More unusual causes include (in no particular order) Dieulafoy ulcers (Fig. 51-1), GAVE (gastric antral vascular ectasia), cancer, portal hypertensive gastropathy, angiodysplasia, aortoenteric fistula, and hemobilia.

## 11. What are the endoscopic stigmata of bleeding peptic ulcer? How do they help stratify risk for rebleeding and mortality?

There are many endoscopy scoring systems used to describe and classify bleeding peptic ulcer disease. The Forrest Criteria is one that uses simple endoscopic description of the duodenal ulcer to predict risk of rebleeding and mortality (Table 51-3). A recent review of management of bleeding peptic ulcers recommended a tiered approach to level of care based on endoscopic stigmata (Table 51-4).

### Table 51-1. Rockall Score

| VARIABLE | POINTS MAXIMUM 11 |
|---|:---:|
| Age (yr) | |
| <60 | 0 |
| 60 to 79 | 1 |
| ≥80 | 2 |
| Shock | |
| Heart rate >100 beats/min | 1 |
| Systolic blood pressure <100 mm Hg | 2 |
| Coexisting illness: ischemic heart disease, congestive, heart failure, renal failure, hepatic failure, metastatic, cancer, other major illness | 2 |
| Endoscopic diagnosis | |
| No lesion observed, Mallory-Weiss tear | 0 |
| Peptic ulcer, erosive disease, esophagitis | 1 |
| Cancer of upper GI tract | 2 |
| Endoscopic stigmata of recent hemorrhage | |
| Clean base ulcer, flat pigmented spot | 0 |
| Blood in upper GI tract, active bleeding, visible vessel, clot | 2 |

GI, gastrointestinal.
The *clinical Rockall* score includes age, shock, and coexisting illness. The *complete Rockall* score includes clinical Rockall score plus endoscopic score. Patients with a clinical Rockall score of 0 or a complete Rockall score of ≤2 are considered low risk for rebleeding or death.
Adapted from Rockall TA, Logan RF, Devlin HB, et al: Risk assessment after acute upper gastrointestinal haemorrhage, Gut 38:316–321, 1996; and Rockall TA, Logan RF, Devlin HB, et al: Lancet 347:1138–1140, 1996.

## Table 51-2  Blatchford Score

| CLINICAL PARAMETERS AT PRESENTATION | POINTS MAXIMUM 23 |
|---|---|
| Systolic blood pressure (mm Hg) | |
| 100 to 109 | 1 |
| 90 to 99 | 2 |
| <90 | 3 |
| Blood urea nitrogen (mg/dL) | |
| 18 to 22 | 2 |
| 22 to 28 | 3 |
| 28 to 69 | 4 |
| >70 | 6 |
| Hemoglobin for ♂ (g/dL) | |
| 12.0 to 12.9 | 1 |
| 10.0 to 11.9 | 3 |
| <10.0 | 6 |
| Hemoglobin for ♀ (g/dL) | |
| 10.0 to 11.9 | 1 |
| <10 | 6 |
| Other variables at presentation | |
| Pulse >100 | 1 |
| Melena | 1 |
| Syncope | 2 |
| Hepatic disease | 2 |
| Cardiac failure | 2 |

Data from Blatchford O, Murray WR, Blatchford M: A risk score to predict need for treatment for upper gastrointestinal haemorrhage. Lancet 356:1318–1321, 2000.

---

**Box 51-1.** Low-Risk Selection Criteria for Early Discharge or Outpatient Management

Patients with nonvariceal, UGI bleed with *low risk selection criteria* may be considered for abbreviated hospital stay or outpatient treatment.
- Age less than 60 years
- Absence of hemodynamic instability
  - Pulse less than 100 bpm
  - Systolic BP greater than 100 mm Hg
  - No postural changes in pulse greater than 20 bpm
  - No postural change in systolic BP greater than 20 mm Hg
or
- Achieve hemodynamic stability within 3 hours from initial evaluation
- Hemoglobin greater than 8 to 10 g/dL
- Normal coagulation parameters
- Onset of bleeding outside the hospital
- EGD shows clean-based ulcer or no obvious bleeding
- Adequate social support at home with the ability to return to the hospital promptly

From Gralnek IM, et al. N Engl J Med 2008;359:928–937.

---

**Table 51-3.** Bleeding Peptic Ulcer Endoscopic Stigmata and Risk for Rebleeding and Mortality

| FORREST CLASSIFICATION | DESCRIPTION OF ENDOSCOPIC STIGMATA | EST. REBLEEDING RATE (%) | EST. MORTALITY (%) |
|---|---|---|---|
| IA | Spurting blood | >90 | 11 |
| IB | Oozing blood | 80 | |
| IIA | Nonbleeding visible vessel (raised, three-dimensional) | 40 to 60 | 11 |
| II-B | Adherent clot (must remove and characterize) | 20 to 30 | 7 |
| IIC | Pigmented spot (flat vessel) | 10 | 3 |
| III | Clean-based ulcer | 5 | 2 |

Adapted from Laine L, Peterson WL: Medical progress: Bleeding peptic ulcer. N Engl J Med 331:717–727, 1994; and Esrailian E, Gralnek IM: Non-variceal UGI bleeding: Epidemiology and diagnosis. Gastrointest Clin N Am 34:589–605, 2005.

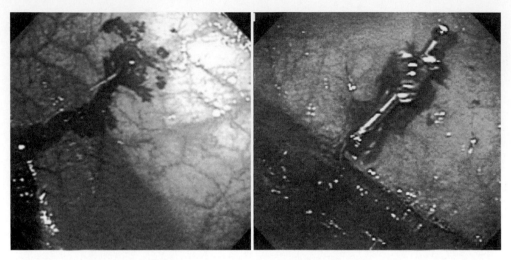

**Figure 51-1.** Endoscopic view of a spurting Dieulafoy ulcer (*ulcer* is a misnomer because there is no ulcer, just a bleeding artery), before and after hemoclip application.

**Table 51-4.** Management of UGI Bleed from Peptic Ulcer Based on EGD Findings

| CLINICAL RISK | EGD FINDINGS | MANAGEMENT |
|---|---|---|
| High | Forrest grade IA, IB, or IIA | i. Endoscopic hemostasis<br>ii. Admit the patient to a monitored bed or ICU setting<br>iii. Start intravenous PPI (80-mg bolus dose plus continuous infusion at 8 mg/hr) for 72 hours; no role for $H_2$ blocker, somatostatin, or octreotide<br>iv. Clear liquid diet 6 hours after endoscopy in stable patients<br>v. Transition to oral PPI after 72 hours of intravenous therapy<br>vi. Perform testing for *Helicobacter pylori*; initiate treatment if positive |
| High | Forrest grade IIB | i. Endoscopic hemostasis (only if bleeding or visible vessel beneath clot)<br>ii. Admit the patient to a monitored bed or ICU setting<br>iii. Start intravenous PPI (80-mg bolus dose plus continuous infusion at 8 mg/hr) for 72 hours; no role for $H_2$ blocker, somatostatin, or octreotide<br>iv. Clear liquid diet 6 hours after endoscopy in stable patients<br>v. Transition to oral PPI after 72 hours of intravenous therapy<br>vi. Perform testing for *H. pylori*; initiate treatment if positive |
| Low | Forrest IIc or III | i. No need for endoscopic hemostasis.<br>ii. Early hospital discharge after endoscopy if the patient has an otherwise low clinical risk and safe home environment<br>iii. Oral PPI<br>iv. Initiate oral intake with a regular diet 6 hours after endoscopy<br>v. Perform testing for *H. pylori*; initiate treatment if the result is positive |

EDG, esophagogastroduodenoscopy; UGI, upper gastrointestinal; PPI, proton pump inhibitor.
Adapted from Gralnek IM, Barkun AN, Bardou M: Current concepts: Management of acute bleeding from a peptic ulcer. N Engl J Med 359:928–937, 2008.

### 12. What is the role of NSAIDs in UGI bleeding?

There is an overall 2.7-fold increase in the relative risk for any gastrointestinal (GI) complication associated with the use of NSAIDs. If the patient is older than 50 years, the risk increase is 5.6. If the patient has a history of a prior GI bleed, the relative risk increase is 4.8, which is similar to the increase related to concomitant corticosteroid use. The increased relative risk is 12.7 for patients using NSAIDs and anticoagulants. There is a 6-fold increased risk of GI bleeding in patients taking NSAIDs who also have *Helicobacter pylori* infection.

### 13. How can one preventing bleeding in patients taking NSAIDs?

Misoprostol, given along with the NSAIDs, will prevent bleeding complication, while $H_2$ receptor antagonists will not. Proton pump inhibitors have been shown to decrease the ulcer/bleed risk by 4-fold. COX-2 selective prostaglandin inhibitors, such as Celebrex, are associated with significantly fewer ulcers than the traditional NSAIDs.

14. **What are the possible sources of bleeding in a patient with cirrhosis who presents with UGI bleeding?**

One must remember that having cirrhosis means there is only a 50% chance that the patient is bleeding from varices. The most common nonvariceal source of bleeding in such patients is gastric erosions ($\approx$50%), followed by Mallory-Weiss tears (15%), duodenal and gastric ulcers (13.8% each), and esophagitis (11%). Portal hypertensive gastropathy (PHG) is also a nonvariceal source of bleeding in cirrhotic patients, but it is related to portal pressure, unlike the other cited sources.

15. **How does one diagnose bleeding from a varix?**

The easiest way to confirm that varices are the source of bleeding is to see active bleeding coming from a varix. The next best criterion is seeing a fibrin/platelet plug on a varix. The weakest criterion is finding no other identifiable source in the setting of a moderate to large volume bleed. Endoscopic ultrasound (EUS) may be helpful in differentiating large gastric folds from gastric varices.

16. **Which patients need endoscopy and when?**

Ideally, all patients with UGI bleeding need an EGD, but this is only beneficial if the results of the EGD will affect patient management. Management changes include endoscopic therapy and triage that would result in shorter or no hospital stay (see Table 51-4). Patients older than 60 years, patients with liver disease, those with active bleeding, and those who rebleed are in clinical situations that have been shown to benefit from EGD because they often lead to therapeutic interventions that positively affect the patient's outcome.

17. **What techniques are available to the endoscopist for controlling active bleeding?**

The endoscopist usually relies heavily on cautery to control bleeding noted at the time of EGD. Modalities available include monopolar probes, bipolar probes, heater probes, the argon plasma coagulator, and Nd:YAG lasers. There are various pros and cons to the use of each of these, but they are all effective in controlling bleeding and preventing rebleeding except the monopolar technique. Frequently, epinephrine (1:10,000) is used to slow or stop the bleeding, which allows for more directed definitive treatment. Epinephrine alone is not as effective. Sclerosants (alcohol, ethanolamine, and others) injected into the bleeding site have been used alone with some success. Using endoscopically placed clips to clamp off small bleeding vessels in many types of bleeding lesions is very effective for controlling the bleeding (Fig. 51-2).

18. **What nonendoscopic therapies can be used to stop variceal bleeding?**

The addition of intravenous infusions of octreotide will lower portal pressure and can thus prevent rebleeding during the initial hospitalization. Vasopressin can be used to decrease portal pressure, but significant side effects are common. The Sengstaken-Blakemore tube, preferably with the Minnesota modification (a suction port above the esophageal balloon), is still a reasonable method for gaining control of a patient with massive bleeding from varices. Should medical or endoscopic therapy be ineffective, shunt surgery or a transjugular intrahepatic portosystemic shunt (TIPS) procedure will need to be considered depending on what is available in the community.

19. **What endoscopic therapy is available to control variceal hemorrhage?**

Sclerotherapy (ES) and rubber band ligation (EVL) are the main methods for controlling variceal bleeding via an endoscope. Both are reported to control active bleeding in up to 90% of cases. Rebleeding is less with EVL than ES (26% versus 44%). Patient mortality is reduced with use of endoscopic methods for treating varices. Mortality is less with EVL than with ES (24% versus 31%). There are fewer complications with EVL (11% versus 25%) and it takes fewer sessions to obliterate a patient's varices with EVL (3.7 versus 4.9 sessions). Endoloops have been occasionally used to treat varices, especially in the cardia.

20. **What are the special considerations that need to be addressed in patients with cirrhosis who have acute UGI bleeding?**

There is a higher likelihood of the patient having a serious coagulopathy that will need to be corrected. The patient is more prone to mental confusion from encephalopathy or alcohol withdrawal, which increases the risk of aspiration with its associated increase in mortality. Encephalopathy-related complications can be prevented by early endotracheal intubation and aggressive use of lactulose. Prophylactic antibiotics will prevent complications and reduce mortality. Quinolones alone or in combination with Augmentin (amoxicillin–clavulanate) have been used successfully.

21. **What is a visible vessel, and what is its significance?**

A visible vessel is the exposed side of a small vessel at the base of an ulcer. It may contain a fibrin/platelet plug or have an adherent clot over it. The finding is significant because of the increased risk for rebleeding. Those with an associated

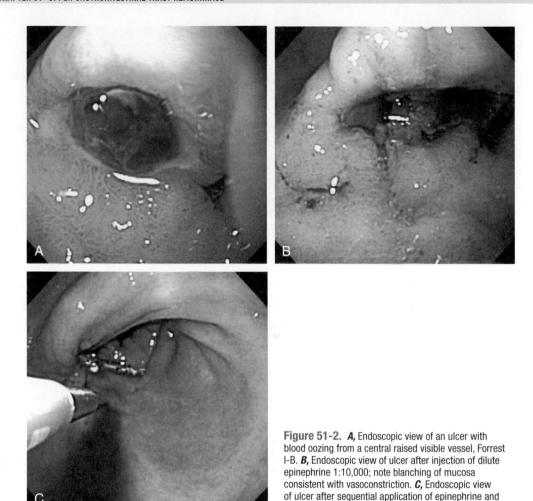

**Figure 51-2.** *A,* Endoscopic view of an ulcer with blood oozing from a central raised visible vessel, Forrest I-B. *B,* Endoscopic view of ulcer after injection of dilute epinephrine 1:10,000; note blanching of mucosa consistent with vasoconstriction. *C,* Endoscopic view of ulcer after sequential application of epinephrine and hemoclips. (Courtesy P. R. McNally, DO.)

adherent clot have a rebleed rate of 20% to 30%, while true visible vessels have rebleeding rates of about 50%. If the vessel is seen to be spurting at the time of endoscopy, there is a 90% chance it will rebleed. If the ulcer only has a red dot in its base, the rebleeding rate is around 10%. The rebleeding rate for an ulcer with a clean base is less than 5%. Endoscopic intervention will significantly lower these rebleeding rates (Fig. 51-2).

**22. Is there a role for other diagnostic tests when evaluating patients with UGI bleeding?**
Radiolabeled red blood cell scans are not usually helpful for defining an UGI bleeding source unless it is beyond the reach of an endoscope. Barium studies have no place in the management or diagnosis of acute UGI bleeding. Angiography can be used to define an active bleeding site (the site needs to be bleeding at a rate of at least 0.5 mL/min.) and to possibly treat it with either a selective vasopressin infusion or embolization of the feeding blood vessel. Patients with ulcerative lesions in the stomach or duodenum need to be tested for *H. pylori.*

**23. Which medications, if any, can be used to reduce rebleeding from UGI tract ulcers?**
Many studies have looked at intravenous $H_2$ receptor antagonists for prevention of rebleeding. Meta-analysis of these studies has shown that there is only marginal, if any, benefit. Intravenous omeprazole and pantoprazole have been shown to reduce rebleeding in several studies. There is limited evidence that intravenous octreotide can reduce the rebleeding rate of nonportal hypertensive sources of UGI tract bleeding. Factor replacement therapy may be needed for patients with specific clotting deficiencies. Fresh frozen plasma, recombinant factor VIIa (Novo-Seven), and desmopressin (DDAVP) can be useful in various situations.

**24. When and who should be treated with surgery for continued nonvariceal UGI bleeding?**

Patients older than 60 years and patients with significant comorbid illness need to be considered for surgery earlier due to the increased likelihood of a poor outcome with prolonged bleeding and multiple transfusions. Patients who have failed at least one attempt at endoscopic therapy, and certainly after two, need to go to surgery for rebleeding.

Giant ulcers (larger than 2 cm) are unlikely to be manageable with endoscopic methods, as are ulcers with bleeding from major arteries (larger than 2 mm).

**25. What medications are used for patients who go home after a bleeding episode?**

The main treatment after bleeding is acid suppression. Thus, patients need $H_2$ receptor antagonists or proton pump inhibitors. The latter are generally better at healing because of greater acid suppression. Antibiotics are added if the patient was found to be positive for *H. pylori*. Iron supplementation orally is indicated for replacement if the patient had a major bleed. Beta-blockers, possibly in conjunction with long-acting nitrates, should be considered for maintenance therapy in patients with bleeding due to portal hypertension. The selective COX-2 inhibitors should be substituted for standard NSAIDs in patients who need therapy for arthritic conditions.

**26. When and what should patients receive by mouth after an UGI bleed?**

Traditionally, patients are started on clear liquids once they have had an endoscopic evaluation or after several hours of observation during which there seems to be no more signs and symptoms of further bleeding. Solid food is reintroduced in 24 to 48 hours. However, there is some evidence that this delay until refeeding approach may not be necessary, but if there is a substantial risk of rebleeding, it would be best that there was no solid food in the stomach to deal with at the time of endoscopic or surgical intervention.

**27. When should patients be sent home after a UGI bleed?**

There is little need for prolonged hospital observation after a mild to moderate UGI bleed. Elderly patients who have required blood transfusions need to be observed for a day or two after their last sign of bleeding or transfusion.

**28. What should patients avoid once they have had a UGI bleed?**

Patients need to be instructed to avoid all alcohol after having an acute UGI bleed. Smoking should be discouraged, as should the use of caffeine-containing beverages, especially on an empty stomach or in large quantities. NSAIDs are not to be used unless accompanied by a drug that blocks their effect on GI bleeding, such as Cytotec (misoprostol) or a proton pump inhibitor.

**29. How and when should patients be followed up after their episode of UGI bleeding?**

An office visit is scheduled in 2 to 4 weeks to reinforce the use of treatment medications and to make long-term plans. A blood count is done to be sure the patient is responding appropriately to therapy. Patients need to be seen promptly if there are any signs of bleeding or return of their peptic symptoms. Endoscopy should be repeated in patients with major GI bleeding and no antecedent symptoms of peptic disease to confirm healing at 1 to 2 months after their bleed. Gastric ulcers need to be followed to complete endoscopic healing to be sure there is no cancer present. Patients with varices are seen for repeat ES or EVL within 7 to 10 days of their first treatment and then every 2 to 4 weeks until the varices are eradicated.

## WEBSITES

http://arthritis-research.com/content/7/S4/S14

http://www.mayoclinicproceedings.com/inside.asp?a=1&ref=8306a2

http://www.residentandstaff.com/issues/articles/2005-09_01.asp

https://daveproject.org/ViewPresentation.cfm?film_id=652&CFID=712504&CFTOKEN=78756655

## BIBLIOGRAPHY

1. Aljebreen AM, Fallone CA, Barkun AN. Nasogastric aspirate predicts high-risk endoscopic lesions in patients with acute upper-GI bleeding. Gastrointest Endosc 2004;59:172–8.
2. Church NI, Dallal HJ, Masson J, et al. Validity of the Rockall scoring system after endoscopic therapy for bleeding peptic ulcer: A prospective cohort study. Gastrointest Endosc 2006;63:606–12.

3. Das A, Wong RC. Prediction of outcome of acute GI hemorrhage: A review of risk scores and predictive modals. Gastrointest Endosc 2004;60:85–93.
4. Gralnek IM, Barkun AN, Bardou M. Current Concepts: Management of acute bleeding from a peptic ulcer. N Engl J Med 2008;359:928–37.
5. Huang JQ, Sridhan S, Hunt RH. Role of H. pylori infection and non-steroidal anti-inflammatory drugs in peptic ulcer disease: A meta-analysis. Lancet 2002;359:14–22.
6. Imperiale TF, Dominitz JA, Provenzale DT, et al. Predicting poor outcome from acute upper gastrointestinal hemorrhage. Arch Intern Med 2007;167:1291–6.
7. Khuroo MS, Yattoo GN, Javid G, et al. A comparison of omeprazole and placebo for bleeding peptic ulcers. N Engl J Med 1997;336:1054–8.
8. Lau JY, Leung WK, Wu JC, et al. Omeprazole before endoscopy in patients with gastrointestinal bleeding. N Engl J Med 2007;356:1631–16340.
9. Lau JYW, Sung JJY, Lam YH, et al. Endoscopic treatment compared with surgery in patients with recurrent bleeding after initial endoscopic control of bleeding ulcers. N Engl J Med 1999;340:751–6.
10. Lee JG, Turnipseed S, Romano PS, et al. Endoscopy-based triage significantly reduces hospitalization rates and costs of treating upper gastrointestinal bleeding. A randomized controlled trial. Gastrointest Endosc 1999;50:755–61.
11. Levine JE, Leontiadis GI, Sharma VK, et al. Meta-analysis: The efficacy of intravenous H2-receptor antagonists in bleeding peptic ulcer disease. Aliment Pharmacol Ther 2002;16:1137–42.
12. Lin HJ, Lo WC, Lee FY, et al. A prospective randomized comparative trial showing that omeprazole prevents rebleeding in patients with bleeding peptic ulcer after successful endoscopic therapy. Arch Int Med 1998;158:54–9.
13. Stiegmann GV, Goff JS, Michalitz-Onody PA, et al. Endoscopic sclerotherapy as compared with endoscopic variceal ligation for bleeding esophageal varices. N Engl J Med 1992;326:1527–32.

# LOWER GASTROINTESTINAL TRACT BLEEDING

*Maj. John Boger, MD, and*
*LTC J. David Horwhat, MD, FACG*

# CHAPTER 52

### 1. Define *lower gastrointestinal bleeding* (LGIB).

Any bleeding distal to the ligament of Treitz is considered LGIB. Due to differences in diagnostic evaluation, presentation, and therapy, many clinicians consider small intestinal and colonic bleeding as different entities.

### 2. How common is LGIB?

The annual incidence ranges between 20 and 30 per 100,000 population.

### 3. What populations are at increased risk?

Male sex and advanced age are important risk factors. The incidence increases with age with a 200-fold increased incidence between the third to ninth decades of life.

### 4. How does the risk of LGIB compare to that of upper GI bleed (UGIB)?

LGIB is one-fifth as common as UGIB.

### 5. What is the mortality associated with LGIB?

Mortality in most studies ranges from 2% to 5%. Patients developing LGIB during hospitalization have up to a 23% risk of death.

### 6. How is history important in assessing a patient with LGIB?

- *Onset*: Did symptoms start months ago with associated diarrhea or that day with a difficult-to-pass, hard, and constipated bowel movement?
- *Volume and consistency of bleeding:* Clots of blood on formed stool suggest an anorectal source. Squirts of blood with defecation suggest internal hemorrhoids as the source of bleeding. Repeated rectal bleeding of large volumes over a short time suggests arterial bleeding as can be seen with a diverticular or an angiodysplastic cause.
- *Symptoms:* Associated abdominal pain is uncommon with diverticular and vascular ectasia LGIB and may suggest UGIB from ulcer or intestinal ischemia. Acute or chronic diarrhea may suggest Crohn's disease or infectious or ulcerative colitis. Chronic abdominal pain with large meals may be a sign of intestinal ischemia.
- *Medical history:* Prior history of ulcer disease, cirrhosis, use or prescription of aspirin, nonsteroidal anti-inflammatory drugs (NSAIDs), or blood thinners. History of aortic aneurysm may suggest aortoenteric fistulas. Recent colonoscopy may indicate postpolypectomy bleeding. Prior radiation therapy for cervical or prostate carcinoma suggests angiodysplasia.

### 7. What can help differentiate between an upper and a lower source of bleeding?

#### SUGGESTION OF *UGI* SOURCE

- History: ulcer or chronic liver disease, use of aspirin or NSAIDs
- Symptoms: nausea, vomiting, or hematemesis
- Nasogastric (NG) aspirate: identification of blood or "*coffee grounds*" material
- Serum blood urea nitrogen (BUN)-to-creatinine ratio *greater than* 33 is highly suggestive

#### SUGGESTION OF *LGI* SOURCE

- Absence of UGI symptoms or risk factors
- NG aspirate positive for bile but negative for blood

### 8. What are the first steps taken in the management of a patient with significant LGIB?

1. Stabilize and resuscitate.
2. Place at least one large-bore IV line (lactated Ringer or normal saline)
3. Evaluate hemodynamic status: blood pressure, pulse, orthostatic vital signs if stable
4. Supplement oxygen by nasal cannula.
5. Order lab tests: complete blood count (CBC), electrolytes, international normalized ratio (INR), and type and screen for packed red blood cells (RBCs).
6. Get electrocardiogram for those with known arteriosclerotic heart disease (ASHD) or older than 50 years.
7. Physical examination:

   - Ear, nose, and throat (ENT) examination for telangiectasias or pigmented macules may indicate Osler-Weber-Rendu disease, Peutz-Jeghers syndrome, or vascular ectasia in the gut.
   - Cardiac auscultation for aortic stenosis (Heyde syndrome) is perhaps associated with vascular ectasia of the gastrointestinal (GI) tract and acquired type IIA von Willebrand syndrome.
   - Abdominal examination should assess for bowel sounds, abdominal bruit, tenderness, masses, and surgical scars. Hepatosplenomegaly, ascites, and/or caput medusae may indicate chronic liver disease with portal hypertension, suggesting an esophageal, gastric, or colonic variceal bleed.
   - Cutaneous purpura or petechiae suggest a coagulopathy, and spider angiomata or jaundice may be another indicator of chronic liver disease.
   - Joint hypermobility, swelling, or deformity may indicate a connective tissue disorder and possible use of aspirin or NSAIDs.
   - Digital rectal exam is *mandatory* for all patients with LGIB to evaluate for prolapsed internal hemorrhoids or masses and to characterize the color and consistency of blood/stool in the rectal vault.

### 9. How can continued or recurrent LGIB be determined?

This determination can be challenging. Frequent monitoring of the patient's hematocrit should be performed. However, early in presentation, the hematocrit is likely to underestimate the degree of blood loss due to volume contraction. On the other hand, through dilutional effects from crystalloid hydration, the hematocrit may be seen to decrease—even in the absence of ongoing active bleeding. This decrease may not represent continued hemorrhage. Hemodynamic parameters should be monitored for signs of worsening volume depletion especially in the setting of adequate volume resuscitation.

### 10. What are the causes of most common causes of LGIB?

See Figure 52-1 and Table 52-1.

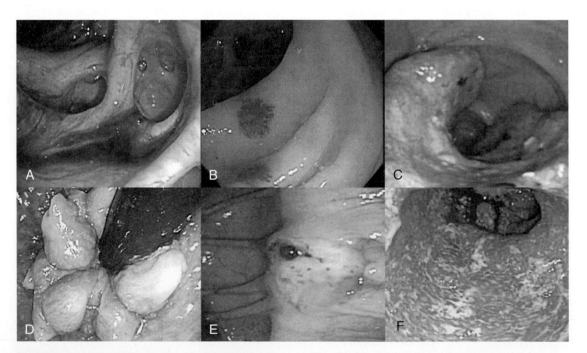

**Figure 52-1.** **A,** Diverticulosis. **B,** Angiodysplasia. **C,** Colonic adenocarcinoma. **D,** Internal hemorrhoids. **E,** Polypectomy site with stigmata of recent bleeding. **F,** Ulcerative colitis.

**Table 52-1.** Common Causes of Lower Gastrointestinal Bleeding

| ETIOLOGY | ESTIMATED PERCENTAGE |
| --- | --- |
| Diverticulosis | 30 |
| Colitis | 15 |
| Cancer/polyp | 13 |
| Angiodysplasia | 10 |
| Anorectal | 11 |
| Small bowel | 6 |
| No site | 8 |
| Upper gastrointestinal source | 8 |

### 11. Do NSAIDs increase the risk of LGIB?

Several case-control studies show a 2- to 3-fold increase in LGIB with a variety of different NSAIDs. One large study in patients with rheumatoid arthritis that compared naproxen with rofecoxib demonstrated that the use of COX-2–selective inhibitors may decrease this rate by 54%.

### 12. What types of colitis are associated with LGI bleeding?

Ischemia → Crohn's disease → Ulcerative colitis

LGIB caused by segmental colitis usually indicates an ischemic etiology.

### 13. Do all colonic vascular ectasias or angiodysplasia cause LGIB?

No. Angiodysplasia are commonly found in the colon during cancer screening examinations. They are more common among the elderly. Most (75%) of the bleeding vascular ectasias are found in the right colon. Endoscopic treatment of bleeding ectasias with injection, laser, or thermal techniques has been shown to be effective. One should be cautious with any endoscopic treatment of these lesions, especially in the thin-walled right colon.

### 14. How is postpolypectomy LGIB best managed?

Postpolypectomy bleeding is the cause of 2% to 5% of all acute LGIB. Most bleeding occurs at a mean of 5 days after polypectomy. The majority of patients have been receiving NSAIDs/aspirin or anticoagulants. Endoscopic treatment has been shown to be successful in 95% of cases.

### 15. What diagnostic modalities are available for localization of colonic bleeding?

- Colonoscopy
- Technetium-99 m–labeled red cell scintigraphy
- Selective angiography

### 16. What role does urgent colonoscopy have in the diagnosis of LGIB?

Ileocolonoscopy, following a rapid polyethylene glycol bowel purge, is the diagnostic method of choice for LGIB. This can establish a diagnosis in 74% to 90% of cases.

### 17. Discuss how nuclear medicine scintigraphy and angiography are used in the diagnosis and treatment of LGIB.

Both represent second-line tests following a nondiagnostic lower endoscopy—especially in the setting of ongoing bleeding. Both require active bleeding to manifest a positive result. Scintigraphy is noninvasive and can detect a bleeding rate as slow as 0.1 to 0.5 mL/min. The blush seen with scintigraphy (Figure 52-2) may remain difficult to localize; hence, the test's accuracy ranges from 75% to 97%. In comparison, angiography requires a slightly brisker rate of bleeding (0.5 to 1 mL/min) to demonstrate a positive result. The advantages of angiography's high specificity (near 100%) and ability to permit therapeutic embolization (Figure 52-3) are balanced by its higher risk of complications (2% to 4% overall), including contrast nephropathy, groin hematoma, and vascular perforation. Some centers advocate using scintigraphy to establish ongoing bleeding and to guide angiography for therapeutic intent.

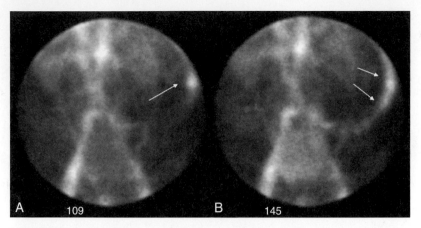

**Figure 52-2. A,** Technetium-99 m–labeled red cell scintigraphy with splenic fixture hemorrhage over time (**B**) as it tracks into the sigmoid. (Courtesy of Maj. Kevin Schlegel, DO.)

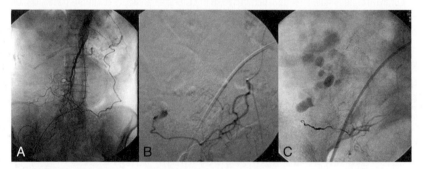

**Figure 52-3. A,** Angiography of superior mesenteric artery (SMA) with evidence of bleeding (*circle, bottom left*). **B,** Subselective angiography of ileocolic artery with (**C**) deployed coils for embolization. [Courtesy of LTC(P) Kenneth H. Cho, MD.]

## 18. What is the natural history of LGI bleeding from diverticulosis?
- Bleeding is a complication of 17% of patients with colonic diverticular disease.
- About 80% of patients stop bleeding spontaneously.
  - ○ 70% will not rebleed and will not require further treatment.
  - ○ 30% will rebleed and require treatment.
- About 60% of those requiring more than 4 units of blood transfused within a 24-hour period require surgery.

## 19. What endoscopic methods are available for hemostasis?
Diverticular bleeding can be treated with submucosal injections of dilute epinephrine and/or with contact electrocautery devices. Using suction to evert a diverticulum followed by band ligation has also been safely used. Angiodysplasias can be treated with contact electrocautery or with argon plasma coagulation, a noncontact monopolar current conducted via argon gas. Visible vessels and postpolypectomy bleeding can be managed with electrocautery and/or metallic endoscopically deployed clips.

## 20. What are the more common causes of small intestinal bleeding?
Ulceration (NSAIDs, Crohn), angiodysplasias, and cancer.

## 21. What diagnostic modalities are available for small intestinal bleeding?
- Double-balloon endoscopy
- Video capsule endoscopy
- Barium small bowel follow-through
- Conventional and magnetic resonance enteroclysis

## 22. How does double-balloon endoscopy (DBE) compare with video capsule endoscopy?
A 2007 meta-analysis shows similar diagnostic rates for GI bleeding. Capsule endoscopy has been shown to be an excellent tool to predict success in finding a lesion with DBE. Additionally, capsule endoscopy is very useful in determining whether an oral or anal approach with DBE will be more likely to find the lesion in question. They both have differing risks and advantages (Table 52-2).

**Table 52-2.** Comparison of Double-Balloon Endoscopy and Video Capsule Endoscopy

| DOUBLE-BALLOON ENDOSCOPY | VIDEO CAPSULE ENDOSCOPY |
| --- | --- |
| Ability to obtain biopsies | Inability to obtain biopsies |
| Ability to deliver endoscopic therapy | No sedation required |
| Superior localization | Decreased localization |
| Better resolution and camera control | Decreased picture resolution |
| Higher rates of complications | Lower complication rates |

### 23. What is the role of surgery in LGIB?

It is good practice to have surgical consultation in cases of GI hemorrhage. When there is massive hemorrhage with hemodynamic instability or recurrent bleeding despite other attempted therapies, surgery for definitive therapy may become necessary. An accurate diagnosis is vital because postoperative morbidity and mortality are dependent on localization of bleeding before surgery.

## WEBSITES

http://arthritis-research.com/content/7/S4/S14

http://brighamrad.harvard.edu/Cases/bwh/hcache/126/full.html

http://www.mayoclinicproceedings.com/inside.asp?a=1&ref=8306a2

http://www.residentandstaff.com/issues/articles/2005-09_01.asp

http://www.uhrad.com/intarc/int005.htm

### BIBLIOGRAPHY

1. Bauditz J, Lochs H. Angiogenesis and vascular malformations: Antiangiogenic drugs for treatment of gastrointestinal bleeding. World J Gastroenterol 2007;13:5979–84.
2. Bokhari M, Vernava A, Ure T, et al. Diverticular hemorrhage in the elderly—Is it well tolerated? Dis Colon Rectum 1996;39:191–5.
3. Chen X, Ran Z, Tong J. A meta-analysis of the yield of capsule endoscopy compared to double-balloon enteroscopy in patients with small bowel diseases. World J Gastroenterol 2007;13:4372–8.
4. Fidler J. MR imaging of the small bowel. Radiol Clin North Am 2007;45:317–31.
5. Green B, Rockey D. Lower gastrointestinal bleeding—Management. Gastroenterol Clin North Am 2005;34:665–78.
6. Junquera F, Saperas E, Videla S, et al. Long-term efficacy of octreotide in prevention of recurrent bleeding from gastrointestinal angiodysplasia. Am J Gastroenterol 2007;102:254–60.
7. Laine L, Connors LG, Reicin A, et al. Serious lower gastrointestinal clinical events with nonselective NSAID or Coxib use. Gastroenterology 2003;124:288–92.
8. Laine L, Smith R, Min K, et al. Systemic review: The lower gastrointestinal adverse effects of non-steroidal anti-inflammatory drugs. Aliment Pharmacol Ther 2006;24:751–67.
9. Longstreth G. Epidemiology and outcome of patients hospitalized with acute lower gastrointestinal hemorrhage: a population-based study. Am J Gastroenterol 1997;92:419–24.
10. Strate L. Lower GI bleeding: Epidemiology and diagnosis. Gastroenterol Clin North Am 2005;34:643–64.
11. Yoshie K, Fujita Y, Moriya A, et al. Octreotide for severe acute bleeding from portal hypertensive colopathy: A case report. Eur J Gastroenterol Hepatol 2001;13:1111–3.
12. Zhi F, Yue H, Jiang B, et al. Diagnostic value of double balloon enteroscopy for small-intestinal disease: Experience from China. Gastrointest Endosc 2007;66(Suppl. 3):S19–21.

# OCCULT AND OBSCURE GASTROINTESTINAL BLEEDING

*John S. Goff, MD*

**1. What is occult gastrointestinal (GI) bleeding?**

Bleeding that is not visible or hidden and is manifested by positive fecal occult blood (FOB) testing or iron deficiency anemia.

**2. What physical examination findings might provide a clue about the source of bleeding?**

Facial or oral telangiectasia can suggest hereditary telangiectasia (Osler-Weber-Rendu syndrome). Acanthosis nigricans in the axilla suggests possible malignancy. Perioral pigments spots are associated with Peutz-Jeghers syndrome (hereditary hamartomatous polyposis. See Figure 53-1. Purpura or ecchymoses implies a possible bleeding disorder.

**3. What tests are used to identify patients with occult GI bleeding, and which are the best?**

There are basically two methods for assessing occult blood in the stool. The old standard method uses guaiac fecal occult blood (FOB), and the newer products use immunochemical methods (iFOB). Both tests are designed to have high sensitivity and lower specificity to try to avoid false-negative results. The accumulating data have shown the iFOB to be much more sensitive (50% to 200% more) for detecting cancers and adenomas, but the false-positive rate also increases.

**4. What are the factors that influence the results of FOB testing besides bleeding from the GI tract?**

Pseudoperoxidase in various foods can result in a false-positive FOB test. The foods that can produce this unwanted situation are rare red meat, raw broccoli, turnips, cauliflower, radishes, cantaloupe, and parsnips. Rehydrating hemoccult cards will also produce more false-positive results. A false-negative result can be caused by vitamin C ingestion and delayed development of the card (more than 6 days). Iron ingestion probably does not cause false-positive results. There is some controversy over whether a stool specimen collected at digit rectal examination is more prone to produce false-positive results. Published studies seem to support the validity of a specimen collected at rectal examination.

**5. What is the proper procedure for FOB testing?**

For about 3 days before testing, the patient should avoid the items listed in Question 4. The patient should also avoid aspirin and nonsteroidal anti-inflammatory drugs. A sample of stool from three separate movements should be collected. The cards need to be developed within 7 days and should not be rehydrated.

**6. How much blood is needed to cause a positive FOB test?**

As little as 2 mL of blood in the GI tract can produce a positive FOB test.

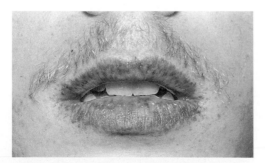

**Figure 53-1.** Perioral hyperpigmentation seen with Peutz-Jeghers syndrome.

**7. Who should be electively tested for occult blood and how often?**

All patients 50 years or older should have annual FOB testing unless they have had a normal colonoscopic examination within the past 5 to 10 years. Colonoscopy is now considered the preferred screening test for colon polyps and cancer.

**8. What can be expected to be found at colonoscopy in a patient older than 50 years who is FOB negative? Who is FOB positive?**

Those who are FOB negative have a cancer find rate at colonoscopy of 0.5% to 3% with a polyp find rate of 7% to 35%. These numbers change to 7% to 17% for cancer and 20% to 43% for polyps in those who are FOB positive.

### 9. How should a patient with a positive FOB test be evaluated?

The patient needs a full colonoscopy and, if negative, should be considered for evaluation of the upper GI tract with endoscopy (esophagogastroduodenoscopy [EGD]). The yield for EGD is increased by about 50% (13% versus 27%) if the patient is also iron deficient. Barium radiographs can be substituted, but the sensitivity for detecting causes of the positive FOB will be less. The primary utility of using a barium study in this setting is possibly to evaluate the small bowel.

### 10. What are some of the signs and symptoms of iron deficiency anemia?

Symptoms of iron deficiency include fatigue, tachycardia, pica (eating clay and other objects), and pagophagia (eating ice). Physical signs of iron deficiency are rare—they include cheilitis, glossitis, and koilonychia. Laboratory findings include high platelet counts, microcytosis, elevated total iron binding capacity, and low ferritin values. Microcytosis can also be seen with thalassemia, anemia of chronic disease, and sideroblastic anemia.

### 11. How should a patient with a positive FOB and iron deficiency anemia be initially evaluated?

If the patient has no GI symptoms, which is most common, the evaluation should start with a colonoscopy. If the colon is normal, an upper endoscopy (EGD) with biopsies of the second and third portion of the duodenum to look for sprue (celiac disease) is the next test. If both endoscopies are negative and the patient does not have sprue, a small bowel radiograph can be performed, but capsule endoscopy (CE) is much more sensitive and specific for small bowel lesions.

### 12. What tests would you do in a patient with iron deficiency (microcytic) anemia who does not respond to iron or has recurrence after an initial negative evaluation?

The first thing to consider would be repeat the upper and lower endoscopies. Small bowel endoscopy would be the next step in evaluating these patients, especially if not previously done. The choices are push enteroscopy, Sonde enteroscopy, CE, and double or single balloon enteroscopy. Of these it would appear that CE is the screening test of choice, but it has no ability to provide any therapeutic intervention and some lesions can be missed. Balloon-assisted enteroscopy has the potential to reach the farthest into the small bowel of the non-CE techniques and one can perform biopsies or do therapeutic interventions with these endoscopes. Consultation with a hematologist to consider bone marrow production problems might also be considered.

### 13. How would the evaluation be different if the patient was only iron deficient?

The initial emphasis would be on diagnosing sprue (celiac disease), non-GI tract sources of blood loss (e.g., menstrual bleeding, urinary tract), nutritional factors, and an evaluation for infectious causes (hookworm, strongyloidosis, ascariasis) if the patient is younger than 50 years. If the patient is older than 50 years, a full GI tract evaluation is needed.

### 14. What is the yield for combined colonoscopy and EGD in patients who are FOB positive with or without iron deficiency?

Lesions can be found in 48% to 71% of such patients. Colonoscopy will be positive in 20% to 30%, with 5% to 11% having cancer. EGD will be positive in 29% to 56% of cases. Synchronous lesions are found in 1% to 10% of patients.

### 15. How is sprue (celiac disease) diagnosed?

The best way to diagnose celiac disease is to demonstrate flattened small bowel villi in association with submucosal inflammation. The biopsies are usually obtained with EGD-directed duodenal biopsies. Serologic testing can also be useful and is particularly helpful for following these patients after treatment with a gluten-free diet as the antibody titers will fall. The most useful antibody tests are IgA level and, IgA tissue transglutaminase antibodies (TTA). A positive antibody test should always be confirmed with a small bowel biopsy and visa versa. Relatives of patients with sprue should be screened by testing for antigliaden antibodies or TTA. Genetic testing looking for *HLA DQ2* or *DQ\** can be helpful in sorting out complicated cases. See Chapter 41.

### 16. What is meant by obscure GI bleeding?

Clinically observable bleeding with a negative standard evaluation including such tests as an upper GI series, barium enema, EGD, and colonoscopy defines obscure GI bleeding.

### 17. What endoscopic tests are available for evaluating a patient with obscure GI bleeding, and how useful are they?

Repeat standard upper and lower endoscopy has a total yield of about 35% (29% upper, 6% lower). Enteroscopy with a long scope or balloon-assisted scope, which has a yield of 30% to 75%, is also helpful in evaluating the small bowel. CE is a noninvasive method for evaluating the entire small bowel. The yield for a source of obscure or occult bleeding with CE is 5% to 70%. Intraoperative endoscopy is moderately risky and is very invasive. The yield is high for finding a bleeding site (70% to 100%), and any lesion found can then be easily dealt with.

## 18. What radiologic tests are available for evaluating a patient with obscure GI bleeding, and how useful are they?

Small bowel evaluation with enteroclysis is preferred over a small bowel follow-through because of the increased yield (0% to 20% versus 0% to 6%). There has been increasing use of computed tomography enteroclysis to diagnose small bowel pathology. Radiolabeled–red blood cell scanning should be used for instances when it is thought the patient might be actively bleeding. If confirmed, then the radiologist can proceed to an urgent angiogram. Elective angiography may have yields up to 40%, but the data in this area are limited. Pharmacologically altering the patient's coagulation system to enhance angiography is not to be encouraged because of the high risk and poor yield. Meckel scans are useful in the young but are rarely useful in the middle-aged to elderly patient.

## 19. How would you sequence an evaluation of a patient with obscure GI bleeding?

The first step is to try to catch the patient in the act of bleeding. When there are obvious findings of hematemesis or hematochezia, one should try to obtain a radiolabeled–red blood cell scan to confirm continued active bleeding. A positive scan may help localize the bleeding to a specific part of the GI tract and will indicate that it would be a good time to perform an angiogram to better define the type and site of bleeding. If the patient does not have such acute bleeding episodes, the sequence for evaluation would start with repeating the upper and lower endoscopies, followed by small bowel enteroclysis, CE, small bowel balloon endoscopy, and then elective angiography. A last resort, but the best diagnostic and therapeutic procedure, would be intraoperative endoscopy.

## 20. Angiodysplasia (vascular malformations) are a common cause of obscure GI bleeding. How are these treated?

Endoscopic cautery (laser, bipolar, heater probe, argon plasma coagulation) is effective for reducing the blood requirements in these patients if the lesions can be reached with the endoscope. Angiographic embolization is useful if a feeding vessel can be selectively cannulated. Surgery may be useful for a localized lesion that is not otherwise accessible. Treatment for multiple vascular malformations (hereditary [Osler-Weber-Rendu] or nonhereditary) is use of estrogen-progesterone combinations, or, in difficult cases, long-acting octreotide may be helpful. Patients need to avoid NSAIDs and anticoagulants.

## 21. What other lesions are found to be a cause of obscure GI bleeding?

Cameron erosions (associated with large hiatal hernias (Figure 53-2), portal hypertensive gastropathy (Figure 53-3), GAVE (gastric antral vascular ectasia [*watermelon stomach*] (Figure 53-4), Crohn's disease, nonesophageal varices, tumors (lymphoma, leiomyoma, carcinoid, others), diverticula (particularly Meckel diverticulum in younger patients), small bowel or colonic ulcers, Dieulafoy ulcers, amyloidosis, and hemorrhoids.

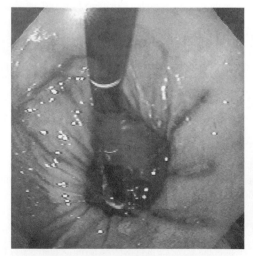

**Figure 53-2.** Endoscopic photograph of Cameron's (riding) erosions associated with large hiatal hernia. Here linear erosions can be seen running perpendicular to the impression of the diaphragmatic hiatus on the proximal stomach. (Courtesy of Peter McNally, DO.)

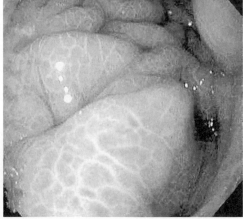

**Figure 53-3.** Endoscopic photograph of portal hypertensive gastropathy. (Courtesy of Mark Powis, MD.)

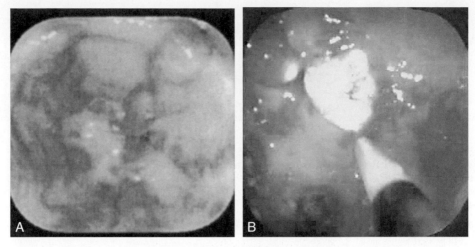

**Figure 53-4.** **A,** Endoscopic photograph of gastric antral vascular ectasia (GAVE) or watermelon stomach. **B,** Endoscopic photograph of GAVE after BiCAP therapy. (Courtesy of Mark Powis, MD.)

## WEBSITES

http://daveproject.org/SearchResults.cfm?portal=presentation&module=cjc

http://www.gastroatlas.com/

http://www.givenimaging.com/

http://www.vhjoe.org/Volume3Issue4/3-4-3.htm;

## BIBLIOGRAPHY

1. Allison JE, Tekawa IS, Ranson CJ, et al. A comparison of fecal occult-blood tests for colorectal cancer. N Engl J Med 1996;334:155–9.
2. Cave DR, Cooley JS. Intraoperative enteroscopy. Indications and techniques. Gastrointest Endosc Clin N Am 1996;6:793–802.
3. Chen YK, Gladden DR, Kestenbaum DJ, et al. Is there a role of upper gastrointestinal endoscopy in the evaluation of patients with occult-positive stool and negative colonoscopy? Am J Gastroenterol 1993;88:2026–9.
4. Costemagna G, Shah SK, Ricclono ME, et al. A prospective trial comparing small bowel radiographs and video capsule endoscopy for suspected small bowel disease. Gastroenterology 2002;123:994–1005.
5. de Leusse A, Vahedi L, Edery J, et al. Capsule endoscopy or push enteroscopy for first-line exploration of obscure gastrointestinal bleeding? Gastroenterology 2007;132:855–62.
6. Eli C, Remke S, May A, et al. The first prospective controlled trial comparing wireless capsule endoscopy to push enteroscopy in chronic gastrointestinal bleeding. Endoscopy 2002;43:685–9.
7. Filippone A, Cianci R, Milano A, et al. Obscure gastrointestinal bleeding and small bowel pathology: Comparison between wireless capsule endoscopy and multidetector-row CT enteroclysis. Abdom Imaging 2008;33:398–406.
8. Guittet L, Bouvier V, Mariotte N, et al. Comparison of a guaiac based and an immunochemical fecal occult blood test in screening for colorectal cancer in a general average risk population. Gut 2007;56:210–4.
9. Kepczyk T, Kadakia SC. Prospective evaluation of the gastrointestinal tract in patients with iron deficiency anemia. Dig Dis Sci 1995;40:1283–9.
10. Levin B, Lieberman DA, McFarland B, et al. Screening and surveillance for the early detection of colorectal cancer and adenomatous polyps 2008: A joint guideline from the American Cancer Society, the US Multi-Society Task Force on Colorectal Cancer, and the American College of Radiology. Gastroenterology 2008;134:1570–95.
11. Raju GS, Gerson L, Das A, et al. American Gastroenterological Association (AGA) Institute medical position statement on obscure gastrointestinal bleeding. Gastroenterology 2007;133:1694–717.
12. Rockey DC, Koch J, Cello JP, et al. Relative frequency of upper gastrointestinal and colonic lesions in patients with positive fecal occult-blood tests. N Engl J Med 1998;339:153–9.
13. Rossini FP, Arrigoni A, Pennazio M. Octreotide in the management of bleeding due to angiodysplasia of the small intestine. Am J Gastroenterol 1993;88:1424–8.
14. Tsujikawa T, Saitoh Y, Andoh A, et al. Novel single-balloon enteroscopy for diagnosis and treatment of the small intestine: Preliminary experiences. Endoscopy 2008;40:11–5.
15. Winawer SJ, Stewart ET, Zauber AG, et al. A comparison of colonoscopy and double-contrast barium enema for surveillance after polypectomy. N Engl J Med 2000;342:1766–72.

# 54 CHAPTER — EVALUATION OF ACUTE ABDOMINAL PAIN

Peter R. McNally, DO, and
James E. Cremins, MD

## 1. Provide a useful clinical definition of an *acute abdomen*.

This clinical scenario is characterized by severe pain, often of rapid onset, that prevents bodily movement. When patients experience symptoms of pain for longer than 6 hours, surgical intervention is usually necessary.

## 2. What are the four types of stimuli for abdominal pain?

1. Stretching or tension
2. Inflammation
3. Ischemia
4. Neoplasms

## 3. What are the three categories of abdominal pain (Fig. 54-1)?

1. *Visceral pain* occurs when noxious stimuli affect an abdominal viscus. The pain is usually dull (cramping, gnawing, or burning) and poorly localized to the ventral midline because the innervation to most viscera is multisegmental. Secondary autonomic effects such as diaphoresis, restlessness, nausea, vomiting, and pallor are common.
2. *Parietal pain* occurs when noxious stimuli irritate the parietal peritoneum. The pain is more intense and more precisely localized to the site of the lesion. Parietal pain is likely to be aggravated by coughing or movement.
3. *Referred pain* is experienced in areas remote from the site of injury. The remote site of pain referral is supplied by the same neurosegment as the involved organ; for example, gallbladder pain may be referred to the right scapula and pancreatic pain may radiate to the midback.

## 4. How does the character of the abdominal pain help in the evaluation?

See Table 54-1.

## 5. What are the important components of the physical examination for patients with acute abdominal pain?

- *General status:* Is the patient hemodynamically unstable? Does he or she need immediate hemodynamic resuscitation and emergent laparotomy (e.g., ruptured spleen, hepatic tumor, aneurysm, ectopic pregnancy, or mesenteric apoplexy)?
- *Inspection:* Visually evaluate for distention, hernias, scars, and hyperperistalsis.
- *Auscultation:* Hyperperistalsis suggests obstruction; absence of peristalsis (no bowel sounds heard over 3 minutes) suggests peritonitis (silent abdomen); bruits suggest presence of an aneurysm.
- *Percussion:* Tympany suggests either intraluminal or free abdominal air.
- *Palpation:* Start the examination away from the area of tenderness and be gentle. Abdominal pain with voluntary coughing suggests peritoneal signs. Deeply palpating the abdomen only diminishes patient trust and cooperation. The enlarged gallbladder will be missed on aggressive, deep palpation. Inspiratory arrest during light palpation of the right hypochondrium suggests gallbladder pain (Murphy sign). Localized pain suggests localized peritonitis (e.g., appendicitis, cholecystitis, diverticulitis). Classic findings on the abdominal examination of visceral ischemia or infarction are characteristically disproportionate to the degree of abdominal pain.

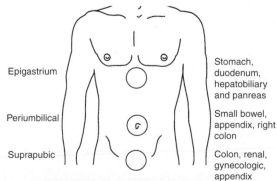

**Figure 54-1.** Location of visceral pain.

- *Pelvic and rectal exam:* These exams should be done in *all* patients with abdominal pain. A painful examination may be the only sign of pelvic appendicitis, diverticulitis, or tubo-ovarian pathology. Bimanual examination is critical to exclude an obstetric or a gynecologic cause.
- *Iliopsoas test:* With the legs fully extended in a supine position, the patient is requested to raise the legs unilaterally. Pain occurs when the right psoas muscle is inflamed (e.g., appendicitis).
- *Obturator test:* This test is performed by flexing the patient's thigh at right angle to the trunk and then rotating the leg externally. Inflammation of the obturator internus muscle causes pain (e.g., tubo-ovarian abscess or pelvic appendicitis).

**Table 54-1.** Classification of Pain by the Rate of Development

| | |
|---|---|
| Explosive and excruciating (instantaneous) | Myocardial infarction<br>Perforated ulcer<br>Ruptured aneurysm<br>Biliary or renal colic (passage of a stone) |
| Rapid, severe, and constant (over minutes) | Acute pancreatitis<br>Complete bowel obstruction<br>Mesenteric thrombus |
| Gradual and steady pain (over hours) | Acute cholecystitis<br>Diverticulitis<br>Acute appendicitis |
| Intermittent and colicky pain (over hours) | Early subacute pancreatitis<br>Mechanical small bowel obstruction |

6. **Which laboratory tests should be obtained in patients with acute abdominal pain?**
   Although laboratory tests are helpful in confirming the evolution of a disease process, they are frequently not helpful in localizing the cause of abdominal pain.

   - *Complete blood count (CBC).* Elevation of the white blood cell count suggests inflammation; however, absence of leukocytosis may be unhelpful early in the course of disease. A low hematocrit with a normal mean corpuscular volume (MCV) suggests acute blood loss, whereas a low hematocrit with a low MCV suggests iron deficiency from chronic gastrointestinal (GI) blood loss or malabsorption.
   - *Amylase elevations* (greater than500 IU) suggest pancreatitis but are not specific. Lipase enzyme elevations are more specific for pancreatic origin.
   - *Liver enzyme elevations* may be suggestive of hepatobiliary causes of pain. Elevations of aspartate or alanine aminotransferase suggest hepatocyte injury. Alkaline phosphatase or gamma glutamine transferase (GGT) elevations suggest canalicular or biliary injury. Total bilirubin elevations greater than 3 mg/dL suggest common bile duct obstruction or associated intrahepatic cholestasis.
   - *Evidence of pyuria* on urinalysis suggests urinary tract infection but also may be seen in nephrolithiasis or even pelvic appendicitis.
   - *Chemistry analysis* can be helpful in the global assessment of patient health, hyperglycemia, acidosis, and electrolyte disturbances.
   - *Pregnancy tests* (beta human chorionic gonadotropin) should be ordered for all premenopausal women.
   - *Stool examination* for occult blood is necessary.
   - *Electrocardiography* is performed for all patients with possible myocardial infarction or older than 50 years.

7. **Which radiologic tests should be ordered to evaluate the patient with acute abdominal pain?**
   The selection of tests depends on the likelihood of the pretest clinical diagnosis and the ability of the radiologic test to confirm clinical suspicion.

   - *Plain radiographs* of the abdomen are quick and readily available and can be done at the bedside. They reliably detect bowel obstruction and viscus perforation. Occasionally, they may suggest stone disease (one third of gallbladder stones and two thirds of renal stones are calcified) or ruptured aortic aneurysm (separation of aortic wall calcium and mass effect). Free intra-abdominal air is best detected with the patient in the left lateral decubitus position for 10 minutes. See Chapter 70.
   - *Ultrasound* of the abdomen is quick and noninvasive and can be performed at the bedside. The disadvantages of ultrasound include variable operator expertise and suboptimal examination in the obese or gaseous abdomen. Ultrasound is excellent for evaluating the gallbladder, bile ducts, liver, kidneys, appendix, and pelvic organs. See Chapter 70.
   - *Computed tomography (CT)* of the abdomen provides a detailed view of the anatomy. Oral and intravenous contrast agents are usually required. CT has become an extension of the physical examination and the single most helpful radiologic examination of the patient with acute abdominal pain. CT provides the best evaluation of the pancreas but often lacks spatial resolution to identify biliary stone disease. See Chapter 70.
   - *Hepatoiminodiacetic (HIDA) scan* is the most accurate test for acute cholecystitis. See Chapter 71.

8. **Pain referred to the abdomen can be confusing. What are the common extra-abdominal causes of referred abdominal pain?**
   - *Thoracic:* pneumonia, pulmonary embolism, pneumothorax, myocardial infarction or ischemia, esophageal spasm, or perforation
   - *Neurogenic:* tabes dorsalis, radicular pain (spinal cord compression from tumor, abscess, compression, or varicella zoster infection)

- *Metabolic:* uremia, porphyria, acute adrenal insufficiency
- *Hematologic:* sickle cell anemia, hemolytic anemia, Henoch-Schönlein purpura
- *Toxins:* insect bites (scorpion bite–induced pancreatitis), lead poisoning

9. **List the common causes of acute abdominal pain in gravid women.**
   - Appendicitis
   - Ovarian cysts complicated by torsion, rupture, and hemorrhage
   - Ectopic pregnancy
   - Gallbladder problems

10. **When the appendix is found to be entirely normal during a laparotomy performed for presumed appendicitis in a gravid woman, should the appendix be removed?**
    No. Removal of the normal appendix triples the risk of fetal loss.

11. **What is the most common cause of acute abdominal pain in elderly patients?**
    Biliary tract disease is responsible for 25% of all cases of acute abdominal pain in elderly patients requiring hospitalization. Bowel obstruction and incarcerated hernia are the next most common, followed by appendicitis.

12. **What symptoms are helpful in evaluating for appendicitis?**
    It is decidedly uncommon for acute appendicitis to present with nausea, vomiting, or diarrhea before abdominal pain. Usually acute appendicitis is heralded by pain and often followed by anorexia, nausea, and sometimes single-episode vomiting. Acute appendicitis should be first on the differential diagnosis list in any patient with acute abdominal pain without a prior history of appendectomy. A simple scoring system of clinical parameters and laboratory tests, the Alvarado Score, has been validated to be very predictive of acute appendicitis (Table 54-2).

13. **Discuss atypical forms of appendicitis.**
    When the appendix is retrocecal or retroileal in location, the inflamed appendix is often shielded from the anterior abdomen. The pain is often less pronounced, and localizing signs on physical examination are uncommon. Symptoms and signs of appendicitis in elderly patients are subtle. Pain is often minimal, fever is only mild, and leukocytosis is unreliable. A high index of suspicion is essential.

14. **Describe the ultrasound findings of acute appendicitis.**
    The appendix appears as a round target with an anechoic lumen, surrounded by a hypoechoic and thickened (greater than 2 mm) appendiceal wall. This finding with reproduction of pain under the transducer has a diagnostic accuracy of 95% and a negative predictive value of 97%. Although ultrasound evaluation for appendicitis has the advantage of bedside portability and lack of radiation, CT has been shown to have superior sensitivity, accuracy, and negative predictive value (96% versus 76%, 94% versus 83%, and 94% versus 76%, respectively).

15. **When laparotomy is performed for presumed appendicitis, what is the acceptable false-negative rate? How often is another cause identified in this setting?**
    A false-negative laparotomy rate of 10% to 20% is reported. In roughly 30% of these cases, some other cause of abdominal pain is identified, such as mesenteric lymphadenitis, Meckel diverticulum, cecal diverticulitis, pelvic inflammatory disease, ectopic pregnancy, or ileitis.

**Table 54-2.** Alvarado Score

| SYMPTOM | SCORE |
|---|---|
| Migration of pain | 1 |
| Anorexia | 1 |
| Raised temperature, >37.3° C | 1 |
| Rebound pain | 1 |
| Tenderness in the right iliac fossa | 2 |
| Nausea, vomiting | 1 |
| Differential white blood cell count >75% PMNs | 1 |
| Elevated leukocyte count | 2 |
| Total | 10 |

PMNs, polymorphonuclear leukocytes.
Alvarado score greater than 7 predictive of appendicitis: sensitivity of 95% and specificity 46%, with positive predictive value of 87% (95% confidence interval, 74% to 99%) and negative predictive value of 72.4% (95% confidence interval, 61% to 83%).

16. **What is the single best test to evaluate patients infected with human immunodeficiency virus (HIV) infection who complain of acute abdominal pain?**
Because of the variety of causes of abdominal pain in such patients, it has been argued that CT scan is the single best test.

17. **What are the cardinal features of a ruptured tubal pregnancy?**
    - Amenorrhea (missed period or scant menses)
    - Abdominal and pelvic pain
    - Unilateral, tender adnexal mass
    - Signs of blood loss

18. **What are the characteristics of acute intestinal obstruction?**
    - Nausea and vomiting
    - Failure to expel flatus
    - Prior abdominal surgery or presence of hernia
    - Peristaltic pain (colicky pain—every 10 minutes for jejunal obstruction and every 30 minutes for ileal obstruction)

19. **List the clinical characteristics of large bowel obstruction.**
    - Most patients are older than 50 years of age.
    - Lower abdominal cramping pain is gradual in onset.
    - Abdominal distention is a prominent feature.
    - Dilated loops of bowel with haustra distinguish the colon from the small bowel.
    - Sigmoidoscopy or single-column barium enema is important.
    - Causes include obstructing neoplasm and cecal or sigmoid volvulus.

20. **List the clinical characteristics of diverticulitis.**
    - Age older than 50 years
    - Localized left lower abdominal pain (often for several days' duration)
    - Palpable mass in left lower quadrant
    - Low-grade fever and leukocytosis (note 45% may have normal white blood cell count)

    Right-sided diverticulitis occurs in only 1.5% of patients in Western countries but is more common among Asians. Up to 75% of these patients present with right lower quadrant pain, often misdiagnosed as acute appendicitis.

21. **What are the characteristic CT findings of diverticulitis?**
    - Increased soft tissue density within pericolic fat, secondary to inflammation (98%)
    - Colonic diverticuli (84%)
    - Bowel wall thickening (70%)
    - Soft tissue masses representing phlegmon and pericolic fluid collections, representing abscesses (35%)
    - Sensitivity, specificity, and positive and negative predictive values are 97%, 100%, 100%, and 98%.

    Note: In 10% of patients, diverticulitis cannot be distinguished from carcinoma and a *gentle and cautious* endoscopic examination may need to be performed.

22. **List the clinical hallmarks of acute cholecystitis.**
    - Patients often give a history of prior episodes of milder abdominal pain.
    - Abdominal pain usually arises after a meal, especially in the evening after a large meal.
    - Pain typically crescendos over 20 to 30 minutes and then plateaus.
    - Pain lasting longer than 1 to 2 hours is usually accompanied by gallbladder wall inflammation.
    - Associated nausea occurs in 90% of patients; vomiting may follow onset of pain in 50% to 80%.
    - Radiation of pain to the back is common; pain radiates to the right scapula in 10% of cases.
    - Low-grade fever is common.
    - Right hypochondrium tenderness is generally present. Inspiratory arrest during gentle palpation of the right upper quadrant (Murphy sign) suggests acute cholecystitis.
    - Diagnostic tests include HIDA scan or ultrasound.

23. **What is the differential diagnosis of acute cholecystitis?**
    - Liver: alcoholic hepatitis, liver metastasis, Fitz-Hugh-Curtis syndrome, congestive hepatopathy
    - Pancreas: pancreatitis, pseudocyst

- GI tract: peptic ulcer disease with or without perforation, acute appendicitis (retrocecal)
- Kidney: pyelonephritis, renal colic
- Lung: pneumonia, pulmonary embolism, emphysema
- Heart: myocardial infarction, pericarditis
- Pre-eruptive varicella zoster

## 24. When should a patient undergo surgery for an acute abdomen?

When, in the judgment of the surgeon, a problem will be identifiable or treatable by surgical intervention. There is no substitute for good surgical judgment and intuition.

## 25. What conditions can result in an acute abdomen in HIV-infected patients?

Patients with HIV can have any of the usual causes of an acute abdomen; all non–HIV-specific diagnoses must be considered. Perforation is most often due to cytomegalovirus (CMV) infection in the distal small bowel or colon; this is the most common cause of the acute abdomen in late-stage HIV infection. CMV infection of the vascular endothelial cells leads to mucosal ischemic ulceration and perforation. HIV-associated lymphoma and Kaposi sarcoma also can lead to perforation, but this finding is rare. Acquired immunodeficiency syndrome (AIDS) cholangiopathy, papillitis, and drug-induced pancreatitis (e.g., pentamidine, sulfamethoxazole-trimethoprim [Bactrim], didanosine, ritonavir) are unique causes of abdominal pain in HIV-infected patients.

## 26. Are patients with systemic lupus erythematosus (SLE) at increased risk for intra-abdominal catastrophe?

Approximately 2% of patients with SLE develop lupus vasculitis, one of the most devastating complications of SLE. The fatality rate is greater than 50%. Small vessels of the bowel wall are affected, leading to ulceration, hemorrhage, perforation, and infarction.

## 27. How common are severe GI manifestations of polyarteritis nodosa (PAN)?

PAN is a vasculitis that may have visceral involvement. GI bleeding from intestinal ischemia is seen in 6% of cases, bowel perforation in 5%, and bowel infarction in 1.4%. Acalculous cholecystitis occurs in up to 17% because of direct vasculitic involvement of the gallbladder.

## 28. What causes of acute abdominal pain should be considered in illicit drug users?

Intravenous and smoked cocaine has been reported to cause acute mesenteric ischemia or *crack belly*. Endocarditis in parenteral drug abusers may be associated with mesenteric emboli and bowel infarction.

## WEBSITES

www.mc.vanderbilt.edu/surgery/trauma/egs/

www.cardinalglennon.com/Documents/Appendicitis%20and$20Abdominal%20Pain%207.09.pdf

## BIBLIOGRAPHY

1. Alvarado A. A practical score for the early diagnosis of acute appendicitis. Ann Emerg Med 1986;15:557–64.
2. Baker JB, Mandavia D, Swadron SP. Diagnosis of diverticulitis by bedside ultrasound in the emergency department. J Emerg Med 2006;30:327.
3. Bonkovsky HL, Siao P, Roig Z, et al. Case 20–2008: A 57-year-old women with abdominal pain and weakness after gastric bypass surgery. N Engl J Med 2008;358:2813–25.
4. Bundy DG, Byerley JS, Liles AE, et al. Does this child have appendicitis? JAMA 2007;298:438–51.
5. Denizbasi A, Unluer EE. The role of the emergency medical resident using the Alvarado Score in the diagnosis of acute appendicitis compared with the general surgery resident. Eur J Emerg Med 2003;10:296–301.
6. Dobbins C, Defontgalland D, Duthie G, et al. The relationship of obesity to the complications of diverticular disease. Colorectal Dis 2006;8:37.
7. Ghosheh B, Salameh JR. Laparoscopic approach to acute small bowel obstruction: review of 1061 cases. Surg Endosc 2007;21:1945–9.
8. Goh V, Halligan S, Taylor SA, et al. Differentiation between diverticulitis and colorectal cancer: Quantitative CT perfusion measurements versus morphologic criteria—Initial experience. Radiology 2007;242:456.
9. Humes DJ, Simpson J. Acute appendicitis: Clinical review. Br J Med 2006;333:530–4.
10. Lyon C, Clark DC. Diagnosis of acute abdominal pain in older patients. Am Fam Physician 2006;74:1537.
11. McKay R, Shepherd J. The use of the clinical scoring system by Alvarado in the decision to perform computed tomography for acute appendicitis in the ED. Am J Emerg Med 2007;25:489–93.
12. Paulson EK, Kalady MF, Pappas TN. Suspected appendicitis. N Engl J Med 2003;348:236–42.
13. Pearigen P. Unusual causes of abdominal pain. Emerg Med Clin North Am 1996;14:593.

14. Pickuth D, Heywang-Kobrunner SH, Spielmann RP. Suspected acute appendicitis: Is ultrasonography or computed tomography the preferred technique? Eur J Surg 2000;166:315–9.

15. Silen W. Cope's Early Diagnosis of the Acute Abdomen. Oxford: Oxford University Press; 1990.

16. Strasberg SM. Acute calculous cholecystitis. N Engl J Med 2008;358:2804–11.

17. Terasawa T, Blackmore C, Bent S, et al. Systematic review: Computed tomography and ultrasonography to detect acute appendicitis in adults and adolescents. Ann Intern Med 2004;141:537–46.

18. Wang LT, Prentiss KA, Simon JZ, et al. The use of the white blood cell count and left shift in the diagnosis of appendicitis in children. Pediatr Emerg Care 2007;23:69–76.

19. Westrom L, Mardh PA. Epidemiology and etiology and prognosis of acute salpingitis: A study of 1457 laparoscopically verified cases. In: Hobson D, Holmes KK, editors. Nongonococcal Urethritis and Related Diseases. Washington, DC: American Society of Microbiology; 1997. p. 84.

20. Zaidi E, Daly B. CT and clinical features of acute diverticulitis in an urban U.S. population: Rising frequency in young, obese adults. AJR Am J Roentgenol 2006;187:689.

# EVALUATION OF ACUTE DIARRHEA

*Kent C. Holtzmuller, MD*

**1. What is the definition of *acute diarrhea?***
*Diarrhea* is defined as the passage of an increased number of stools of less-than-normal form and consistency. Acute diarrhea refers to acute onset of symptoms of less than 14 to 30 days' duration. Diarrhea lasting longer than 1 month is considered chronic. The severity of acute diarrhea can be defined as *mild,* where no change in daily activities is noted; *moderate,* where a change in daily activities is required but the patient is able to function; and *severe,* where the patient is disabled by the symptoms.

**2. What is the impact of acute diarrhea in the United States and worldwide?**
American adults average about one episode of acute diarrhea annually. Acute diarrhea is one of the most common medical conditions seen by primary care practitioners. In the United States, approximately 1 million hospital admissions and 6000 deaths per year are attributed to acute diarrhea, and in most, an etiology is not identified. Worldwide, diarrhea-related diseases are among the most common causes of morbidity and mortality and, for children younger than 4 years, the most common cause of death.

**3. Who should undergo medical evaluation for acute diarrhea?**
Most cases of acute diarrhea are self-limited and require no medical evaluation. Nearly half of the cases last for less than 1 day. Evaluation should be reserved for patients with evidence of systemic toxicity (dehydration, bloody diarrhea, fever, severe abdominal pain), diarrhea of more than 48 hours' duration, and elderly or immunocompromised patients.

**4. What are the most common causes of acute bloody diarrhea?**
Infectious dysentery, inflammatory bowel disease (ulcerative colitis and Crohn's disease), and ischemic colitis.

**5. What is *dysentery?***
Dysentery is a disease process characterized by diarrhea that contains blood and polymorphonuclear cells. Dysentery results when an organism causes an inflammatory reaction, either by direct invasion of the colonic/ileal epithelium or by producing a toxin that causes cellular death and tissue damage. Symptoms associated with dysentery may include abdominal pain and cramping, tenesmus (painful urgency to evacuate stool), fever, and dehydration.

**6. Name the common causes of infectious dysentery in the United States**
*Campylobacter* and *Salmonella* spp. are the principal causes of dysentery in the United States. *Shigella* sp. and certain strains of *Escherichia coli* (specifically O157:H7) are less common. Rarer causes include *Yersinia, Entamoeba, Aeromonas,* and *Plesiomonas* spp.

**7. What is the significance of stool leukocytes (white blood cells) and how are they detected?**
The presence of fecal leukocytes helps to distinguish inflammatory from noninflammatory diarrhea. Normally, leukocytes are not present in stool. Fecal leukocytes are usually found in infectious diarrhea caused by *Campylobacter, Salmonella, Shigella,* and *Yersinia* spp.; *Clostridium difficile;* enterohemorrhagic and enteroinvasive strains of *E. coli;* and *Aeromonas* sp. In cases of ischemic colitis and inflammatory bowel disease, fecal leukocytes are the result of mucosal bleeding. Diarrhea secondary to toxigenic bacteria (e.g., enterotoxigenic *E. coli* [ETEC], *Vibrio cholerae*), viruses, and small bowel protozoa (e.g., *Giardia* sp.) do not contain stool leukocytes. The presence of white blood cells (WBCs) in the stool can be assayed by microscopic examination of the stool or by means of an immunoassay for the neutrophil marker lactoferrin. The sensitivity of fecal lactoferrin and microscopy for fecal WBCs is 92% and 72%, respectively.

**8. If 100 random patients with acute diarrhea underwent evaluation with stool cultures, how many would be positive? Which patients with acute diarrhea should be evaluated with a stool culture?**
Published studies show the diagnostic yield of stool cultures to be 1.5% to 5.6%. This percentage range can be increased if tested patients are selected carefully. A stool culture should be obtained from patients with dysentery

symptoms, persistent diarrhea (beyond 3 to 5 days) or from patients who are immunocompromised. Patients with dysentery symptoms are much more likely than the other two groups to have a positive stool culture. The rate of positive stool culture in patients hospitalized with dysentery is 40% to 60%.

**9. Which patients with acute diarrhea should be evaluated with an endoscopic examination?**
Generally, a flexible sigmoidoscopy or colonoscopy is not needed for the evaluation of acute diarrhea. Most cases of acute diarrhea are self-limited, and endoscopic exam findings add usually little information to the history, physical exam, and stool tests. However, patients with prolonged symptoms or those suspected to have pseudomembranous colitis, ischemic colitis, or inflammatory bowel disease should be considered for endoscopic evaluation.

**10. By what mechanisms do toxigenic organisms produce diarrhea?**
The toxins produced by organisms can be classified into two categories: cytotonic and cytotoxic. Cytotonic toxins cause a watery diarrhea by activation of intracellular enzymes, which cause net fluid secretion into the intestinal lumen. Examples of cytotonic toxins include those produced by *V. cholerae* and enterotoxigenic strains of *E. coli*. Cytotoxic toxins cause structural injury to the intestinal mucosa, which, in turn, causes inflammation and mucosal bleeding. Enterohemorrhagic *E. coli* produces a cytotoxic toxin (*Shiga*-like toxin).

**11. Which *Campylobacter* sp. are implicated as causes of dysentery? How is *Campylobacter* transmitted?**
*C. jejuni* accounts for 98% of reported *Campylobacter* isolates and is the most common cause of bacterial gastroenteritis in industrialized nations. The less common isolates are *C. fetus* and *C. fecalis*. Direct contact with fecal matter from infected persons or animals and ingestion of contaminated food or water have been implicated in the transmission of *Campylobacter* infection.

**12. Describe the clinical and endoscopic features of *Campylobacter* diarrhea**
The incubation period from ingestion until onset of symptoms is 1 to 7 days. Symptoms include diarrhea (often bloody), abdominal pain (can be confused with appendicitis on occasion), malaise, headache, and fever (sometimes high). With or without antibiotic therapy, most patients recover within 5 to 7 days. However, diarrhea can persist for 2 to 3 weeks and relapse may occur. The rectosigmoidoscopic findings of *Campylobacter* diarrhea may be indistinguishable from those of ulcerative colitis or Crohn's disease. The identification of comma-shaped, gram-negative bacteria on stool Gram stain suggests the diagnosis of *Campylobacter* infection. A rare, extraintestinal complication of *Campylobacter* infection is Guillain-Barré syndrome. Up to a third of Guillain-Barré cases in the United States are caused by *Campylobacter* infection.

**13. How are *Salmonella* organisms classified?**
*Salmonella* sp. are gram-negative, aerobic, and facultative anaerobic bacteria of the Enterobacteriaceae family. Using O and H antigens, 2500 different serotypes have been identified. The term "nontyphoidal salmonellosis" is used to denote disease caused by serotypes other than *S. typhi S. enteriditis* and *S. yphimurium* are the serotypes most commonly isolated in the United States.

**14. How is *Salmonella* infection acquired?**
Infection can be acquired by ingesting food contaminated with *Salmonella* or through contact with infected animals (includes reptiles). Ingestion of raw or poorly cooked animal products such as chicken, beef, and eggs can lead to infection. Cooking a meat thoroughly will kill the bacterium. Recent outbreaks have also been attributed to vegetables and unpasteurized milk. *Salmonella* is the leading cause of mortality from foodborne illness.

**15. List the types of illnesses that can be caused by *Salmonella***
- Acute gastroenteritis (The degree of colonic involvement determines the extent of the dysentery-like symptoms. Symptoms of fever, abdominal pain, and diarrhea occur 12 to 72 hours after infection. Illness is generally self-limited and resolves within 5 to 7 days.)
- Bacteremia (with or without gastrointestinal [GI] involvement)
- Localized infection (Bacteremia can result in localized nonintestinal infections—e.g., bone, joints, meninges. Predisposing conditions for localized infection include abdominal aortic aneurysm, prosthetic heart valve, vascular grafts, and orthopedic hardware.)
- Typhoidal or enteric fever
- Asymptomatic carrier states (more common in older age, in women [3:1], and in people with biliary disease)

**16. What is typhoid fever?**
Typhoid fever is a clinical syndrome characterized by marked hectic fever, persistent bacteremia, hepatosplenomegaly, and abdominal pain. The illness can be caused by any serotype of *Salmonella* but results most commonly from *S. typhi* and less commonly from *S. paratyphi*. Because humans are the only known reservoir of *S. typhi*, transmission is primarily by the fecal-oral route. The illness usually lasts for 3 to 5 weeks. Up to 90% of patients experience a *rose*

*spot* rash on the upper anterior trunk within the first or second week of illness. Although diarrhea is unusual, ulceration of Peyer patches in the intestinal wall may cause hemorrhage or perforation. A number of vaccines are successful against typhoid. Typhoid fever is rare in the United States and, when it occurs, is usually seen in international travelers.

## 17. How is *Salmonella* infection treated?

Nontyphoid *Salmonella* gastroenteritis is generally self-limited. A *Cochrane Database Systematic Review* showed that antibiotic therapy only increases the carrier rate. Antibiotics are *only* indicated for those at risk for increased morbidity:

- Infants up to 2 months of age
- Elderly persons
- Immunocompromised persons
- Persons with sickle-cell disease
- Persons with prosthetic grafts and valves
- Persons with extraintestinal findings

Treatment for those at-risk patients should last 2 to 5 days or until the patient is afebrile.

Typhoid fever (*S. typhi*) is best treated with antibiotics for 5 to 7 days for uncomplicated cases and up to 10 to 14 days for a severe infection. Unfortunately, antibiotic resistance is rapidly emerging (fluoroquinolones, 42%; trimethoprim-sulfamethoxazole (TMP-SMX), chloramphenicol, ampicillin, streptomycin, and sulfisoxazole, 12% to 13%).

## 18. Describe the characteristics of *Shigella* infection. How is it treated?

*Shigella* sp. is a gram-negative rod and member of the family Enterobacteriaceae. Most (90% to 95%) infections are caused by one of four species: *S. sonnei* (most common in the United States), *S. flexneri*, *S. dysenteriae*, and *S. boydii*. There are no nonhuman hosts for this organism. The organism is highly infectious, having a fecal-oral route of transmission. Infection can occur with the ingestion of as few as 10 to 100 organisms. Intestinal damage results primarily from direct invasion of the organism into the colonic epithelium and, to a lesser extent, from the production of an enterotoxin. The *Shigella* toxin is composed of an A subunit, which is catalytic, and a B subunit, which is responsible for binding. Stool volume is typically low and the diarrhea may be bloody, mucoid, or watery. The endoscopic appearance of shigellosis shows intense involvement of the rectosigmoid with variable proximal involvement. Approximately 15% of cases present with pancolitis. In children, *Shigella* infection has been associated with seizures. Antimicrobial therapy is recommended for all cases of shigellosis: a fluoroquinolone may be used or, if susceptible, trimethoprim-sulfamethoxazole or ampicillin.

## 19. What diarrheogenic illnesses are caused by *E. coli*?

*E. coli* belongs to the family Enterobacteriaceae, a facultative anaerobic, gram-negative bacteria. The organisms are common inhabitants of the human GI tract, and most strains do not have the virulence factors necessary to cause disease. The primary pathogenic strains of *E. coli* and the syndromes that they cause are listed next.

- *Enterotoxigenic E. coli* (ETEC) accounts for most cases of travelers' diarrhea but is relatively rare in the United States. Fecal-oral transmission through the ingestion of contaminated food or water is the primary means of spread. Disease is produced by the adherence of ETEC to the mucosa, followed by the production of toxins (heat-labile *cholera-like* toxins). Invasion of the mucosa does not occur. The illness is usually self-limited, lasting 3 to 5 days. Symptoms include watery diarrhea and abdominal cramping. Occasionally associated with this illness is low-grade fever and, rarely, bloody diarrhea.
- *Enteropathogenic E. coli* (EPEC) lacks invasive properties. Disease results from its enteroadherent properties. Illness caused by EPEC affects primarily young children (younger than age 3 years) and must be considered as a probable cause of nursery and pediatric outbreaks of diarrhea. Profuse watery diarrhea, which may become chronic, is the usual presentation. As with ETEC-caused illnesses, those caused by EPEC rarely result in bloody diarrhea.
- *Enteroinvasive E. coli* (EIEC) can invade the intestinal mucosa and cause acute dysentery. EIEC strains share characteristics with *Shigella* sp. and are not commonly found in the United States. Infants under age 1 are most susceptible to EIEC strains in developed countries.
- *Enteroaggregative E. coli* (EAEC) was identified in the 1980s and is responsible for diarrhea in children in developing countries, prolonged diarrhea in HIV infection in developing countries, and travelers' diarrhea.
- *Shiga-toxin E. coli* (STEC; also known as *enterohemorrhagic E. coli* [EHEC]) has a number of serotypes, but *E. coli* O157:H7 is the most important. *E. coli* O157:H7 is acquired primarily from the ingestion of contaminated beef, although outbreaks have also been associated with contaminated water, raw milk, unpasteurized juices, and person-to-person transmission among household members. Drinking water contaminated with farm waste has been implicated in several recent large outbreaks. The typical clinical presentation begins with severe abdominal cramps and watery diarrhea followed by rapid progression to bloody diarrhea. The organism is not invasive but produces a *Shiga*-like toxin, which is cytotoxic to vascular endothelium. The disease can cause hemolytic uremic syndrome and

thrombotic thrombocytopenia purpura (less than 10% of cases). The very young and very old are the most susceptible to fatal complications. The most common cause of acute renal failure in North American children is O157:H7 infection. This is the *only E. coli* species that will be tested when a stool culture is referred to a lab. Typically, the lab does not evaluate for ETEC, EPEC, EIEC, and EAEC.

## 20. What is the therapy for O157:H7-induced diarrhea?

Antibiotic therapy for O157:H7 should be avoided. Early therapy with antibiotics has been implicated in the development of hemolytic uremia syndrome. Supportive care, correction of fluid and electrolyte disturbances, and hemodialysis for acute renal failure are the mainstays of therapy. Antimotility agents should be avoided.

## 21. Describe the clinical presentation of infection with *Yersinia enterocolitica.*

The most common presentation includes diarrhea, abdominal pain, and low-grade fever. Microscopic examination of the stool usually shows red and white blood cells. Approximately 25% of the cases are grossly bloody. The clinical presentation of children and young adults may resemble that of appendicitis (right lower quadrant abdominal pain and tenderness, fever, and leukocytosis). Findings at surgery show mesenteric lymphadenitis and terminal ileitis. On rare occasions, a patient may progress to fulminant enterocolitis with intestinal perforation, peritonitis, and hemorrhage. Pharyngitis is common in children with *Y. enterocolitica* infection and is seen in up to 10% of adult cases. Patients with iron overload (hemochromatosis) are more susceptible to yersinial sepsis. Postinfectious manifestations of reactive arthritis, erythema nodosum, Reiter syndrome, thyroiditis, myocarditis, and glomerulonephritis have been reported.

## 22. Which organisms are associated with seafood-induced diarrhea?

*Vibrio parahaemolyticus* and *Vibrio vulnificus*, all members of the **Vibrio** genus, are halophilic organisms (i.e., it grows only in media containing salt) that have been isolated in fish, crustaceans, and shellfish. The diarrhea is characteristically watery, but bloody diarrhea may be seen in up to 15% of patients. Patients with liver disease have a high rate of mortality if infected with *V. vulnificus*. Other causes of seafood-induced diarrhea include norovirus, *Plesiomonas shigelloides*, *Campylobacter,* scromboid fish poisoning (fish contains high levels of histamine and heat stable amines), and ciguatera fish poisoning (toxin found in reef fish produced from a dinoflagellate).

## 23. What parasites cause bloody diarrhea?

*Entamoeba histolytica, Balantidium coli, Dientamoeba fragilis,* and *Schistosoma* spp. The most common cause of parasitic dysentery in the United States is amebiasis (*E. histolytica*). Although parasitic dysentery is uncommon in the United States, it is a significant cause of morbidity and mortality worldwide.

## 24. Who is at risk for amebiasis? What are the potential complications of amebic dysentery?

Travelers to and immigrants from endemic areas, institutionalized patients, and homosexual men. Complications include liver abscess, toxic megacolon, intestinal perforation, peritonitis, intussusception, obstruction, and ameboma (mass of granulation tissue in the terminal ileum/right colon. Amoebic dysentery should be considered in any patient who has persistent travelers' diarrhea (longer than 2 weeks).

## 25. Which laboratory studies are useful in the diagnosis of amebic dysentery?

- Microscopic examination of the stool for cysts and/or trophozoites or a colon ulcer biopsy yields positive results in only 50% of cases.
- Monoclonal antibody–based EIA stool assays for *E. histolytica* antigens have a sensitivity of 95%.
- Detection of circulating antibodies to *E. histolytica* by the indirect hemagglutination (IHAA) test. Approximately 80% to 90% of patients with amebic dysentery have a positive IHAA serology. A positive IHAA test in a patient with presumptive inflammatory bowel disease should raise the possibility of amebiasis.

## 26. Describe the treatment of amebic dysentery. What are the potential side effects?

Acute amebic dysentery is treated with metronidazole, 500 to 750 mg three times a day for 5 to 10 days, followed by an agent to treat intraluminal cysts such as iodoquinol 650 mg three times a day for 20 days. Consumption of alcohol during metronidazole therapy may induce an Antabuse effect (e.g., abdominal cramps, nausea, emesis, headache, flushing). Peripheral neuropathy is a potentially severe and chronic side effect of metronidazole. Other possible symptoms include a metallic taste and GI distress manifested by nausea, flatus, and diarrhea. Metronidazole is teratogenic and should not be taken during the first trimester of pregnancy.

## 27. Which parasites typically cause nonbloody diarrhea? What are the risks for acquisition?

*Giardia, Cryptosporidiosis,* and *Cyclospora* spp. typically cause self-limited nonbloody diarrhea. Contaminated water is the primary source for community outbreaks. *Giardia* sp. is a frequent culprit after consumption of water from mountainous lakes and streams. The lack of secretory IgA correlates with chronic giardiasis. *Cyclospora* sp. should be considered in travelers from Nepal. *Cyclospora* infection has also been implicated from imported fruit. Cryptosporidiosis is a significant cause of HIV-related diarrhea.

## 28. What is the most common cause of hospital-acquired diarrhea?

The number one cause of hospital-acquired diarrhea is *C. difficile* infection. It is rare that another bacterial agent is the cause of diarrhea in patients, unless part of a foodborne or waterborne outbreak.

Noninfectious causes of hospital-acquired diarrhea include enteral nutrition and hyperosmolar liquid medications (which commonly contain sorbitol). Other medications that can cause diarrhea include antacids, magnesium supplements, antibiotics, antineoplastics, cholinergics, theophylline, and prostaglandins.

For more information on pseudomembranous colitis (PMC), the reader is referred to Chapter 50.

## 29. List the risk factors and therapy for infectious dysentery

See Table 55-1.

## 30. The use of empiric antibiotics in the treatment of acute diarrhea is potentially detrimental in what ways?

Antibiotic therapy in patients with O157:H7 can precipitate the hemolytic uremia syndrome and, in patients with *Salmonella,* can prolong the chronic carrier state and increase relapse. Most patients with acute diarrhea do not require antibiotic therapy. Bacterial resistance is a significant problem in treating the bacterial organisms that cause diarrhea. Many of the diarrhea-causative bacterial organisms are resistant to the penicillins, tetracycline, and TMP-SMX. On the average, significant resistance is noted approximately 10 years following the introduction of an antibiotic.

## 31. Are antimotility agents contraindicated in patients with dysentery?

Historically, treatment of dysentery with antimotility agents, such as diphenoxylate-atropine (Lomotil) and loperamide (Imodium), has been contraindicated. It was believed that reduced intestinal motility would worsen dysentery by slowing pathogen clearance. Recent studies of patients with shigellosis dysentery who were given a combination of loperamide and antibiotic therapy had a shortened duration of diarrhea without adverse effects. Antimotility agents continue to be contraindicated in children with dysentery because of recurrent adverse case reports.

**Table 55-1.** Risk Factors and Therapy for Infectious Dysentery

| ORGANISM | RISK FACTORS/RESERVOIRS | THERAPY |
|---|---|---|
| *Aeromonas* spp.* | Contaminated water Fluoquinolone | TMP/SMX |
| *Campylobacter* spp.* | Contaminated food, water, raw milk, infected animals and humans Azithromycin | Erythromycin Fluroquinolone |
| *Salmonella* spp.* (nontyphoidal) | Food (milk, eggs, poultry, meats), water, infected humans | Fluroquinolone TMP-SMX, ceftraxone |
| *Shigella* spp.* | Food, water, infected humans TMP/SMX | Fluroquinolone |
| *Escherichia coli* | Beef, raw milk, untreated water, | Supportive care |
| Enterohemorrhagic *E. coli*\* | Contaminated food and water | Rifaximin |
| Enterotoxigenic *E. coli*\* | Contaminated food and water | Fluoquinolone |
| *Aeromonas* spp.* | Untreated water, shellfish | TMP-SMX |
| *Plesiomonas* spp. | Water, seafood, chicken | TMP-SMX |
| *Yersinia* spp.* | Food (milk products, tofu), water | TMP-SMX Ceftriaxone (severe) |
| *Entamoeba histolytica* | Travel to endemic areas (food, water, fruit) | Metronidazole |
| *Clostridium difficile* | Antibiotic use, hospitalization, chemotherapy | Metronidazole Vancomycin Cholestyramine |

TMP-SMX, trimethroprim-sulfamethoxazole.
*Mild-to-moderate symptoms do not require antibiotic therapy.

**32. Several members of a family develop nausea, emesis, and watery diarrhea 2 to 6 hours after a picnic. Food at the picnic included ham, rice, and custard pie. What type of bacteria is likely to be the cause?**

Enterotoxin-producing bacteria must be considered because the symptoms began soon after ingestion of the food. Two enterotoxin-producing bacteria that cause symptoms with such a short incubation are *Staphylococcus aureus* and *Bacillus cereus*. Coagulase-positive strains of *S. aureus* are responsible for many cases of food poisoning in the United States. *S. aureus* enterotoxin is heat-stable. The incubation period from ingestion to symptoms (nausea, emesis, abdominal cramping, and diarrhea) is approximately 3 hours (range, 1 to 6 hours). *S. aureus* favors growth in foods with high sugar content (e.g., custard) and high salt intake (e.g., ham). Recovery is generally complete in 24 to 48 hours. *B. cereus* is a spore-forming, gram-positive rod that produces a diarrheogenic, heat-labile enterotoxin. Vomiting can occur within 2 hours of ingestion of contaminated food. Almost all persons with *B. cereus* develop diarrhea. Meat and rice are the most common food vehicles for infection. *Clostridium perfringens* also produces an enterotoxin. However, the time of onset of symptoms is usually 8 to 16 hours after ingestion of contaminated food.

**33. What are the common causes and incidence of travelers' diarrhea?**

More than 80% of these cases are secondary to a bacterial pathogen. *E. coli* (ETEC and EAEC strains are most common), *Campylobacter, Salmonella*, and *Shigella* spp. account for most cases of travelers' diarrhea. The rate of illness in high-risk areas (Latin America, Southern Asia, and Africa) is 30% to 40%; in intermediate-risk areas (Caribbean islands, Middle East, China, and Russia), 15% to 20%; and in low-risk areas (United States, northern Europe, Australia, and Japan), less than 10%.

**34. How can one avoid travelers' diarrhea?**

*Safe* foods include steaming hot food and beverages, acidic foods such as citrus, dry foods, foods with high sugar content such as syrups and jellies, and carbonated drinks. Bottled, uncarbonated water is not always safe. Avoid uncooked vegetables and unpeeled fruits. Also consume only safe foods on airplanes that are departing from high-risk areas. Chemoprophylaxis with bismuth salicylate (2 tablets with meals and at bedtime) or with the poorly absorbed (less than 0.4%) antibiotic rifaximin (200 mg twice a day) is effective in reducing diarrhea. Probiotics have also been shown to be efficacious although less so than bismuth or rifaximin. Chemoprophylaxis should be given to persons with prior gastric surgery, those taking acid-blocking medicines ($H_2$ blockers and proton pump inhibitors), or those who are debilitated and immunosuppressed. Travelers who cannot risk or afford a short illness while traveling may opt for chemoprophylaxis.

**35. Describe the treatment of travelers' diarrhea**

Fluid replacement is the initial and primary therapy for any diarrhea. Bismuth subsalicylate is effective for mild diarrhea although large doses are required. Rifaximin (200 mg three times daily) is effective for treatment of moderate to severe illness. Ciprofloxacin and azithromycin are also effective in reducing symptoms. Ciprofloxacin-resistant strains of *Campylobacter* are common in parts of the developing world. Antimotility drugs can be used alone or with antibiotic therapy in adults but should be avoided in children.

**36. What is cholera?**

Cholera is a severe diarrheal disorder caused by *V. cholerae*, a gram-negative, comma-shaped bacteria. The illness is characterized by massive watery stool output, at times in excess of 1 L/hr. Dehydration, hypovolemic shock, and death occur rapidly if fluid replacement is not provided. The cholera organisms colonize the upper small bowel and release an enterotoxin that binds to and activates mucosal cyclic adenosine monophosphate (cAMP), which, in turn, activates chloride channels in mucosal crypts and leads to the massive secretory diarrhea. A second toxin, called the zonula occludens toxin (ZOT), increases intestinal permeability. The intestinal mucosa is not altered by the organism.

**37. How is cholera treated?**

Fluid replacement with either intravenous fluids or oral rehydration solution is the mainstay of therapy. A 2-day course of tetracycline is also beneficial.

**38. What is oral rehydration solution? How does it work?**

Oral rehydration solution (ORS) is composed primarily of water, salt, and glucose (1 L of purified water combined with 20 g of glucose, 3.5 g of sodium chloride, 2.5 g of sodium bicarbonate, and 1.5 g of potassium chloride). Glucose enhances sodium and water absorption across the small bowel villi, even in the presence of cholera enterotoxin. Rice starch can be substituted for glucose.

**39. What is a BRAT diet?**

BRAT stands for bananas, rice, applesauce, and toast. This diet, with its avoidance of dairy products, because a transient lactase deficiency may occur, is often recommended to patients with gastroenteritis and diarrhea.

**40. What viruses cause acute diarrhea?**

Acute viral gastroenteritis can be caused by caliciviruses (norovirus, Sapporo viruses), rotaviruses, enteric adenoviruses, coronavirus, and astrovirus. Rotavirus is a common cause of acute diarrhea in patients younger than 2 years. Norovirus (formally Norwalk-like virus) can cause widespread community outbreaks that affect persons of all ages. Fecal-oral transmission has been implicated as the transmission route for viral gastroenteritis. Raw shellfish has been implicated in outbreaks of Norovirus infection. Norovirus is likely the most common cause of foodborne illness.

**41. What are the clinical features of rotavirus gastroenteritis? What tests are available for diagnosis?**

The clinical presentation of rotavirus can range from an asymptomatic carrier state to severe dehydration that can lead to death. Children under the age of 2 are at greatest risk for infection. Following a 1- to 3-day incubation period, the rotavirus illness is characterized by vomiting and diarrhea for 5 to 7 days. Rotavirus accounts for 25% of cases of acute diarrhea among U.S. children. Rotavirus is more prevalent during cooler months. Adults can develop mild infection with rotavirus. Commercial immunoassays are available to detect rotavirus in the stool.

**42. You are on your honeymoon cruise, and 25% (300 people) of the ship's occupants are afflicted with acute gastroenteritis. What is the most likely causative agent?**

The most likely agent is a norovirus. Noroviruses are single-stranded RNA viruses in the family Caliciviridae. Most nonbacterial gastroenteritis illnesses are caused by norovirus.

**43. A 42-year-old woman is experiencing lower abdominal cramping, bloating, and intermittent diarrhea 6 months following an episode of dysentery that she experienced during a trip to Mexico. What are the possible mechanisms of her illness?**

Her diagnosis is most likely postinfectious irritable bowel syndrome (PI-IBS). Up to 30% of patients with IBS had the onset of their symptoms following an acute diarrheal illness. It has been estimated that 4% to 10% of patients with travelers' diarrhea experience PI-IBS. This disorder occurs more frequently in women. The differential diagnosis also includes parasitic infection, unmasking of celiac disease, and new-onset inflammatory bowel disease.

**44. What is Reiter's syndrome? Which enteric infections are associated with its development?**

Reiter syndrome is a triad of arthritis, urethritis, and conjunctivitis. Infections with *Salmonella* spp., *Shigella* spp., *C. jejuni*, and *Y. enterocolitica* have been associated with this syndrome. Approximately 80% of patients affected by Reiter syndrome are *HLA-B27* antigen–positive. The male-to-female ratio is 9:1.

**45. What is toxic megacolon? What are its risk factors?**

Toxic megacolon is a complication of colitis manifested by acute dilatation of the colon, with associated fever, tachycardia, leukocytosis, anemia, and postural hypotension. Transmural inflammation interferes with colonic motility, leading to colonic dilation and risk for perforation. Severe idiopathic panulcerative colitis carries the highest risk for toxic megacolon, but it may occur with any severe colitis (e.g., amebiasis, shigellosis, STEC, *C. difficile*, and *Campylobacter* spp.). Performance of barium enema or colonoscopy or the administration of antimotility agents (loperamide, diphenoxylate, anticholinergics, or opiates) in patients with severe colitis may precipitate toxic megacolon.

**46. How does one differentiate between acute infectious dysentery and acute onset of inflammatory bowel disease as the cause of bloody diarrhea?**

The clinical symptoms and endoscopic findings of the colon are often similar in the two diagnoses. When evaluating a patient with bloody diarrhea, the clinician must use historic data, assess the patient's potential risk factors (e.g., travel and antibiotic use history) and associated symptoms, and evaluate endoscopic appearance, radiologic findings, and laboratory data to narrow the differential. Many of the infectious dysentery illnesses are self-limited in nature. Dysenteric illnesses that do not spontaneously resolve and are culture-negative should undergo investigation for inflammatory bowel disease. Inflammatory bowel disease should be considered in patients with any additional findings, such as oral apthous ulcers, sacroileitis, spinal or peripheral arthropathy, perianal or cutaneous fistulas, a palpable abdominal mass, erythema nodosum, or erythema gangrenosum.

**47. How is acute bacterial dysentery differentiated from acute onset of ischemic colitis?**

The degree of bloody diarrhea is variable in patients with ischemic colitis, and it may be difficult to distinguish between the two diseases. Clinically, the patient with ischemic colitis complains of sudden-onset abdominal pain, and an acute abdominal series may show *thumbprinting* of the colonic mucosa.

Flexible sigmoidoscopy is the mainstay of diagnosis for ischemic colitis. The rectum is usually spared because of its collateral blood flow. Above the rectum, the mucosa becomes friable and edematous, and there may be hemorrhagic areas and ulcerations resembling those of Crohn's disease. Angiography is not generally helpful in the evaluation of ischemic colitis; ischemic colitis is a small-vessel disease (nonocclusive) compared with mesenteric midgut ischemia of the small bowel, which involves thrombosis or embolism in the superior mesenteric artery (occlusive). A barium enema is contraindicated in patients with suspected ischemic colitis, because colonic expansion during barium instillation may promote further ischemia.

## WEBSITE

http://www.cdc.gov/foodnet/

## BIBLIOGRAPHY

1. Bresee J, Widdowson M, Monroe S, et al. Foodborne viral gastroenteritis: challenges and opportunities. Clin Infect Dis 2002;35:748–53.
2. Centers for Disease Control and Prevention (CDC). *Shigella flexneri* serotype 3 infections among men who have sex with men—Chicago, Illinois, 2003–2004. MMWR Morb Mortal Wkly Rep 2005;54:820–2.
3. Chang HG, Tserenpuntsag B, Kacica M, et al. Hemolytic uremic syndrome incidence in New York. Emerg Infect Dis 2004;10:928–31.
4. Dupont HL, Jiang ZD, Belkind-Gerson J. Treatment of travelers diarrhea: randomized trial comparing rifaximin, rifaximin plus loperamide, and loperamide alone. Clin Gastroenterol Hepatol 2007;5:451–6.
5. Engberg J, Neimann J, Nielsen EM, et al. Quinolone-resistant *Campylobacter* infections: risk factors and clinical consequences. Emerg Infect Dis 2004;10:1056–63.
6. Gillespie IA, O'Brien SJ, Adak GK, et al. Campylobacter Sentinel Surveillance Scheme Collaborators: point source outbreaks of *Campylobacter jejuni* infection: are they more common than we think and what might cause them?. Epidemiol Infect 2003;130:367–75.
7. Goodgame RA. Bayesian approach to acute infectious diarrhea in adults. Gastroenterol Clin N Am 2006;35:249–73.
8. Gopal R, Ozerek A, Jeanes A. Rational protocols for testing faeces in the investigation of sporadic hospital-acquired diarrhoea. J Hosp Infect 2001;47:79–83.
9. House HR. Travel related infections. Emerg Med Clin North Am 2008;26:499–516.
10. Hsu RB, Chen RJ, Chu SH. Nontyphoid *Salmonella* bacteremia in patients with liver cirrhosis. Am J Med Sci 2005;329:234–7.
11. Kennedy M, Villar R, Vugia DJ, et al. Emerging Infections Program FoodNet Working Group: hospitalizations and deaths due to *Salmonella* infections, FoodNet, 1990–1999. Clin Infect Dis 2004;38(Suppl. 3):S142–8.
12. Khan WA, Bennish ML, Seas C, et al. Randomised controlled comparison of single-dose ciprofloxacin and doxycycline for cholera caused by *Vibrio cholerae* 01 or 0139. Lancet 1996;348:296–300.
13. Kimura AC, Johnson K, Palumbo MS, et al. Multistate shigellosis outbreak and commercially prepared food. U.S. Emerg Infect Dis 2004;10:1147–9.
14. Kristiansen MA, Sandvang D, Rasmussen TB. In vivo development of quinolone resistance in *Salmonella enterica* serotype Typhimurium DT104. J Clin Microbiol 2003;41:4462–4.
15. Kuusi M, Nuorti JP, Maunula L. A prolonged outbreak of Norwalk-like calicivirus (NLV) gastroenteritis in a rehabilitation centre due to environmental contamination. Epidemiol Infect 2002;129:133–8.
16. Lecuit M, Abachin E, Martin A, et al. Immunoproliferative small intestinal disease associated with *Campylobacter jejuni*. N Engl J Med 2004;350:239–48.
17. Ochoa TJ, Cleary TG. Epidemiology and spectrum of disease of *Escherichia coli* 0157. Curr Opin Infect Dis 2003;16:259–63.
18. Poutanen SM, Simor AE. *Clostridium difficile*-associated diarrhea in adults. CMAJ 2004;171:51–8.
19. Riddle MS, Sanders JW, Putnam SD, et al. Incidence, etiology, and impact of diarrhea among long-term travelers (U.S. military and similar populations): a systematic review. Am J Trop Med Hyg 2006;74:891–900.
20. Safdar N, Said A, Gangnon RE, et al. Risk of hemolytic uremic syndrome after antibiotic treatment of *Escherichia coli* 0157:H7 enteritis: a meta-analysis. JAMA 2002;288:996–1001.
21. Steffen R, Acar J, Walker E, et al. Cholera: assessing the risk to travellers and identifying methods of protection. Travel Med Infect Dis 2003;1:80–8.

# CHRONIC DIARRHEA

*Lawrence R. Schiller, MD*

**1. Define *chronic diarrhea*.**

Diarrhea is defined as an increase in the frequency and fluidity of stools. For most patients, diarrhea means the passage of loose stools. Although loose stools are often accompanied by an increase in the frequency of bowel movements, most patients do not classify frequent passage of formed stools as diarrhea. Because stool consistency is difficult to quantitate, many investigators use frequency of defecation as a quantitative criterion for diarrhea. By this standard, passage of more than two bowel movements per day is considered abnormal (Table 56-1). Some authors also incorporate stool weight in the definition of diarrhea. Normal stool weight averages approximately 80 g/day in women and 100 g/day in men. The upper limit of normal stool weight (calculated as the mean plus 2 standard deviations) is approximately 200 g/day. Normal stool weight depends on dietary intake, and some patients on high-fiber diets exceed 200 g/day without reporting that they are having diarrhea. Thus, stool weight by itself is an imperfect criterion for diarrhea.

**2. What other disorder may be described as *diarrhea*?**

Occasionally patients with fecal incontinence describe that problem as diarrhea, even when stools are formed. Physicians must be careful to distinguish fecal incontinence from diarrhea, because incontinence is usually due to problems with the muscles and nerves regulating continence and not just to passage of unusually voluminous or liquid stools.

**3. What is the basic mechanism of all diarrheal diseases?**

Diarrhea is due to the incomplete absorption of fluid from luminal contents. Normal stools are approximately 75% water and 25% solids. Normal fecal water output is approximately 60 to 80 mL per day. An increase of fecal water output of 50 to 100 mL is sufficient to cause loosening of the stool. This volume represents approximately 1% of the fluid load entering the upper intestine each day; thus, malabsorption of only 1% to 2% of fluid entering the intestine may be sufficient to cause diarrhea (Figure 56-1).

**4. What pathologic processes can cause diarrhea?**

Excessive stool water is due to the presence of some solute that osmotically obligates water retention within the lumen. This solute can be some poorly absorbed, osmotically active substance, such as magnesium ions, or can be an accumulation of ordinary electrolytes, such as sodium or potassium, that normally are absorbed easily by the intestine. When excess stool water is due to ingestion of a poorly absorbed substance, the diarrhea is called *osmotic diarrhea*. Examples of this include lactose malabsorption and diarrhea induced by osmotic laxatives. When the excessive stool water is due to the presence of extra electrolytes due to reduction of electrolyte absorption or stimulation of electrolyte secretion, the diarrhea is known as *secretory diarrhea*. Causes of secretory diarrhea include infection, particularly infections that produce toxins that reduce intestinal fluid electrolyte absorption; reduction of mucosal surface area due to disease or surgery; absence of an ion transport mechanism; inflammation of the mucosa; ingestion of drugs or poisons; endogenous secretagogues such as bile acids; dysfunction due to abnormal regulation by nerves and hormones; and tumors producing circulating secretagogues.

**TABLE 56-1.** Criteria for Diagnosis of Diarrhea

| CRITERION | NORMAL RANGE | DIARRHEA, IF: |
|---|---|---|
| Increased stool frequency | 2 to 14 stools per week | >2 stools per day |
| More liquid stool consistency | Soft—formed stools | Loose—unformed |
| Increased stool weight | | |
|   Men | 0 to 240 g/24 hr | >240 g/24 hr |
|   Women | 0 to 180 g/24 hr | >180 g/24 hr |

**Figure 56-1.** Fluid loads through the intestine. Each day approximately 9 to 10L of fluid pass into the jejunum. This consists of approximately 2L of ingested food and drink, 1.5L of saliva, 2.5L of gastric juice, 1.5L of bile, and 2.5L of pancreatic juice. The jejunum absorbs most of this load as nutrients are taken up, and the ileum absorbs most of the rest. The colon absorbs more than 90% of the fluid load reaching it, leaving only 1% of the original fluid entering the jejunum excreted in stool. Substantial fluid malabsorption in the small bowel can overwhelm colonic absorptive capacity and may result in diarrhea. Less severe disruption of colonic absorption can lead to diarrhea because of the lack of any more distal absorbing segment. A reduction of absorptive efficiency of only 1% for the total intestine can result in diarrhea.

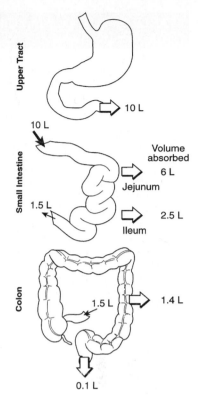

## 5. List three classifications of diarrheal diseases.

Because the symptom of diarrhea has such a broad differential diagnosis, it is useful to classify the type of diarrhea to restrict the differential diagnosis to a more manageable number of conditions. Several schemes have been proposed, three of which can be useful clinically:

1. Differentiate between acute and chronic diarrheal diseases. Most cases of acute diarrhea are due to infections, which are typically self-limited and which will run their courses over a few weeks. Diarrheas that last longer than this are probably due to some other mechanism. For practical purposes, a duration of 4 weeks can be used to differentiate acute and chronic diarrheas.
2. Categorize the diarrhea by epidemiologic characteristics (see Question 6).
3. Divide diarrheal diseases by the characteristics of the stools produced. In this scheme, diarrheas are classified as watery, inflammatory, and fatty (see Questions 7 through 10). These distinctions are based on the gross characteristics of the stool and laboratory testing when appropriate. Watery stools are typically runny and lack blood, pus, or fat. Watery diarrhea is subdivided into secretory and osmotic types, depending on stool electrolyte concentrations. Fatty stools have an excess of fat, which can be shown by qualitative testing with the Sudan stain or by quantitative analysis of a timed stool collection for fat. Inflammatory diarrheas typically contain blood or pus. If not grossly evident, these characteristics can be detected by a fecal occult blood test or by staining the stool for neutrophils. Classifying diarrheas by stool characteristics enables the physician to sort quickly through more likely and less likely diagnoses (Table 56-2). This scheme is thus very useful in chronic diarrheas in which construction of a reasonable differential diagnosis can lead to more appropriate testing and more rapid diagnosis.

## 6. What are the likely causes of diarrhea, according to epidemiologic characteristics?

### TRAVELERS

- Bacterial infection (mostly acute)
- Protozoal infection (e.g., amebiasis, giardiasis)
- Tropical sprue

### EPIDEMICS/OUTBREAKS

- Bacterial infection
- Viral infection (e.g., rotavirus)
- Protozoal infections (e.g., cryptosporidiosis)
- Brainerd diarrhea (epidemic idiopathic secretory diarrhea)

### PATIENTS WITH ACQUIRED IMMUNODEFICIENCY SYNDROME (AIDS)

- Opportunistic infections (e.g., cryptosporidiosis, cytomegalovirus, herpes, *Mycobacterium avium* complex)
- Drug side effect
- Lymphoma

### INSTITUTIONALIZED PATIENTS

- *Clostridium difficile* toxin–mediated colitis
- Food poisoning

**TABLE 56-2.** Tests for Evaluation of Systemic Diseases Associated With Chronic Secretory Diarrhea

| CATEGORY | CONDITION | DIAGNOSTIC TESTS |
|---|---|---|
| Endocrine diseases | Hyperthyroidism | Thyroid-stimulating hormone, $T_4$ |
| | Addison disease | ACTH-stimulation test, cortisol |
| | Panhypopituitarism | ACTH-stimulation test, TSH |
| | Diabetes mellitus | Blood glucose, glycosylated hemoglobin |
| Endocrine tumor syndromes | MEN-1 (Wermer syndrome) | |
| | Hyperparathyroidism | Parathormone |
| | Pancreatic endocrine tumors | Gastrin, VIP, insulin, glucagon |
| | Pituitary tumors | Prolactin, growth hormone, ACTH |
| | (Also may have adrenal cortical tumors, thyroid adenomas) | |
| | MEN-2a (Sipple syndrome) | |
| | Medullary thyroid cancer | Calcitonin |
| | Pheochromocytoma | Urine metanephrine |
| | Hyperparathyroidism | Parathormone |
| | MEN-2b (same as MEN-2a + neuromas, Marfanoid phenotype) | |
| Hematologic diseases | Leukemia, lymphoma | Complete blood count |
| | Multiple myeloma | Serum protein electrophoresis |
| Immune system disorders | AIDS | HIV serology |
| | Amyloidosis | Mucosal biopsy |
| | Common variable immunodeficiency, IgA deficiency | Immunoglobin levels |
| Heavy metal poisoning | | Heavy metal screen |

$T_4$, thyroxine; ACTH, adrenocorticotropic hormone; TSH, thyroid-stimulating hormone; MEN, multiple endocrine neoplasia; VIP, vasoactive intestinal polypeptide; AIDS, acquired immunodeficiency syndrome; HIV, human immunodeficiency virus.

- Fecal impaction with overflow diarrhea
- Tube feeding
- Drug side effect

**7. What are the likely causes of osmotic watery diarrhea?**
Osmotic laxatives (e.g., $Mg^{2+}$, $PO^{3-}_4$, $SO^{2-}_4$) and carbohydrate malabsorption.

**8. List the likely causes of secretory watery diarrhea.**
- Congenital syndromes (e.g., congenital chloridorrhea)
- Bacterial toxins
- Ileal bile acid malabsorption
- Inflammatory bowel disease (ulcerative colitis, Crohn's disease, microscopic colitis [lymphocytic and collagenous colitis], diverticulitis)
- Vasculitis
- Drugs and poisons
- Stimulant laxative abuse
- Disordered motility/regulation (postvagotomy diarrhea, postsympathectomy diarrhea, diabetic autonomic neuropathy, amyloidosis, irritable bowel syndrome)
- Endocrine diarrhea (hyperthyroidism, Addison disease, gastrinoma, vipoma, somatostatinoma, carcinoid syndrome, medullary carcinoma of the thyroid, mastocytosis)
- Other tumors (colon cancer, lymphoma, villous adenoma)
- Idiopathic secretory diarrhea (epidemic secretory [Brainerd] diarrhea, sporadic idiopathic secretory diarrhea)

**9. List the likely causes of inflammatory diarrhea.**
- Inflammatory bowel disease (ulcerative colitis, Crohn's disease, diverticulitis, ulcerative jejunoileitis)
- Infectious diseases (pseudomembranous colitis, invasive bacterial infections [tuberculosis, yersiniosis], ulcerating viral infections [cytomegalovirus, herpes simplex], invasive parasitic infections [amebiasis, strongyloides])
- Ischemic colitis
- Radiation colitis
- Neoplasia (colon cancer, lymphoma)

## 10. List the likely causes of fatty diarrhea.

### MALABSORPTION SYNDROMES

- Mucosal disease (celiac disease, Whipple disease)
- Small bowel bacterial overgrowth
- Chronic mesenteric ischemia
- Short bowel syndrome
- Postgastrectomy syndrome

### MALDIGESTION

- Pancreatic exocrine insufficiency
- Orlistat ingestion
- Inadequate luminal bile acid concentration

## 11. Summarize the initial diagnostic scheme for patients with chronic diarrhea?

The scheme in Figure 56-2 is based on obtaining a careful history, looking for specific physical findings, and obtaining simple laboratory data to help classify the diarrhea as watery, fatty, or inflammatory. The value of obtaining a quantitative (as opposed to a spot) stool collection is debated among experts. A quantitative collection over 48 or 72 hours permits a better estimation of fluid, electrolyte, and fat excretion but is not absolutely necessary for the appropriate classification of diarrhea.

## 12. How do you distinguish secretory and osmotic watery diarrhea?

The most useful way to differentiate secretory and osmotic types of watery diarrhea is to measure fecal electrolytes and calculate the fecal osmotic gap. In many diarrheal conditions, sodium and potassium along with their accompanying anions are the dominant electrolytes in stool water. In secretory diarrhea, there is a failure to completely absorb electrolytes or actual electrolyte secretion by the intestine; sodium, potassium, and their accompanying anions are responsible for the bulk of osmotic activity in stool water and the retention of water within

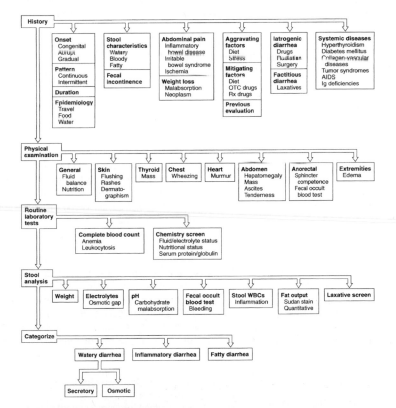

**Figure 56-2.** The initial evaluation plan for patients with chronic diarrhea is aimed at assessing the severity of the problem, looking for clues to etiology, and classifying the diarrhea as watery (with subtypes of osmotic and secretory diarrhea), inflammatory, or fatty. (From Fine KD, Schiller LR: AGA technical review on the evaluation and management of chronic diarrhea. Gastroenterology 116:1464–1486, 1999, with permission.)

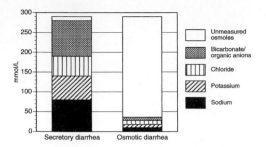

**Figure 56-3.** Electrolyte patterns differ between osmotic and secretory diarrhea. In secretory diarrhea, electrolytes account for the bulk of the osmotic activity of stool water. In contrast, in osmotic diarrhea electrolyte absorption is normal and therefore electrolyte concentrations are very low; most of the osmotic activity is due to unmeasured osmoles. (Bicarbonate concentrations are *virtual* and are not directly measurable in most circumstances due to reaction with organic acids generated by fermentation by colonic bacteria.)

the gut lumen. In contrast, in osmotic diarrhea, ingestion of poorly absorbed osmotically active substances is responsible for holding water within the gut lumen; electrolyte absorption is normal and thus sodium and potassium concentrations can become quite low (Figure 56-3). The fecal osmotic gap calculation takes advantage of these distinctions to differentiate the two conditions.

### 13. How is the fecal osmotic gap calculated?

Fecal osmotic gap represents the osmotic activity in stool water *not* due to electrolytes. The sum of the concentrations of sodium and potassium in stool water is multiplied by 2 to account for the anions that are also present and this product is subtracted from 290 mOsm/kg, the approximate osmolality of luminal contents within the intestine. (This number is a constant in this calculation because the relatively high permeability of the intestinal mucosa beyond the stomach means that osmotic equilibration with plasma will have taken place by the time that luminal contents reach the rectum.)

As an example, let us assume that a patient with watery diarrhea has a sodium concentration of 75 mmol/L and a potassium concentration of 65 mmol/L in stool water. Adding these together yields a concentration of 140 mmol/L. Doubling this to account for anions means that electrolytes account for 280 mOsm/kg of stool water osmolality. Subtracting this from 290 mOsm/kg yields an osmotic gap of 10 mOsm/kg. In contrast, if stool sodium was 10 mmol/L and potassium concentration was 20 mmol/L, the combined contribution of cations and anions in stool water would be only 60 mOsm/kg, yielding a fecal osmotic gap of 230 mOsm/kg. This represents the amount of some unmeasured substance that is contributing to fecal osmolality, presumably some poorly absorbed substance that is being ingested but not absorbed.

### 14. How is the fecal osmotic gap interpreted?

Fecal osmotic gaps less than 50 mOsm/kg correlate well with diarrheas caused by electrolyte secretion (or poor absorption). Fecal osmotic gaps greater than 50 mOsm/kg are associated with osmotic diarrheas.

### 15. What precautions are necessary when measuring fecal osmotic gaps?

Be certain that the stool has not been contaminated with either water or urine. Dilution by water or hypotonic urine will falsely lower fecal electrolyte concentrations and will elevate the calculated osmotic gap. This can be detected by actually measuring fecal osmolality; values that are substantially less than 290 mOsm/kg indicate dilution. Contamination with hypertonic urine may also affect fecal electrolyte concentrations but is harder to detect unless the sum of measured cations and assumed anions is much greater than 290 mmol/L.

### 16. How does one evaluate osmotic diarrhea?

Osmotic diarrheas are typically due to ingestion of poorly absorbed cations, such as magnesium, or anions, such as sulfate. In addition, carbohydrate malabsorption, such as that caused by ingestion of lactose in a patient with lactase deficiency, and ingestion of poorly absorbable sugar alcohols, such as sorbitol, can lead to an osmotic diarrhea.

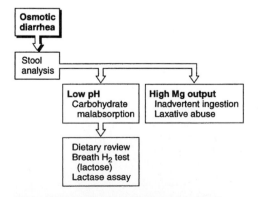

**Figure 56-4.** Once a diagnosis of osmotic diarrhea is made, evaluation is fairly straightforward; only a few etiologies are possible. (From Fine KD, Schiller LR: AGA technical review on the evaluation and management of chronic diarrhea. Gastroenterology 116:1464–1486, 1999, with permission.)

Measuring stool pH can help to distinguish between osmotic diarrheas due to poorly absorbed cations and anions and those due to ingestion of poorly absorbed carbohydrates and sugar alcohols. Carbohydrates and sugar alcohols are fermented by colonic bacteria, reducing fecal pH below 5 due to production of short-chain fatty acids. In contrast, ingestion of poorly absorbed cations and anions does not affect stool pH much and stool pH is typically 7 under these circumstances. Once acidic stools have been discovered, check the diet and inquire about food additives and osmotic laxative ingestion. Specific testing for magnesium and other ions in stool is readily available to confirm any suspicions (Figure 56-4).

### 17. Describe the evaluation of chronic secretory diarrhea.

Because there are many causes of chronic secretory diarrhea, an extensive evaluation is necessary (Figure 56-5). Rare cases of infection should be excluded by bacterial culture and examination of stool for parasites. Stimulant laxative abuse is best excluded by looking for laxatives in the urine or stool.

Structural disease and internal fistulas can be evaluated with small bowel radiography and computed tomography (CT) scanning of the abdomen and pelvis. Endoscopic examination of the upper gastrointestinal tract and colon is routine and should include biopsy of even normal-appearing mucosa, looking for microscopic evidence of disease. Systemic diseases such as hyperthyroidism, adrenal insufficiency, and defective immunity can be evaluated with appropriate tests (Table 56-2).

## 18. When should neuroendocrine tumors be suspected as a cause of chronic secretory diarrhea?

Neuroendocrine tumors are uncommon causes of chronic secretory diarrhea. For example, one VIPoma might be expected per 10 million people per year. Table 56-3 lists these tumors and their markers. Because of the rarity of these tumors as a cause for chronic diarrhea, other causes of secretory diarrhea should be considered first. If tumor is visualized by CT scan or if systemic symptoms (e.g., flushing) are present, evaluation for neuroendocrine tumors may have a better yield. Blanket testing for tumor-associated peptides is likely to yield many more false-positives than true-positives and therefore can be very misleading.

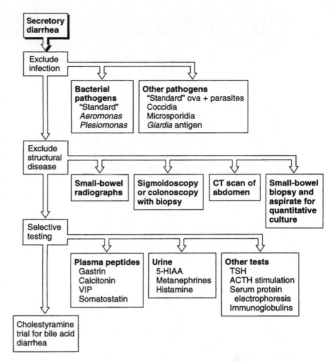

**Figure 56-5.** Evaluation of secretory diarrhea can be very complex. This *mind map* can be used to guide the evaluation, depending on the specifics of each case. Not every test needs to be done in every patient. (From Fine KD, Schiller LR: AGA technical review on the evaluation and management of chronic diarrhea. Gastroenterology 116:1464-1486, 1999, with permission.)

## 19. What is Bayes theorem? How does it relate to the diagnosis of peptide-secreting tumors?

Bayes theorem links the prevalence of the diagnosis to the positive predictive value of a diagnostic test. The positive predictive value of a test depends on the likelihood of the condition in the population to be tested, not only on the accuracy of the test. For example, peptide-secreting tumors are rare causes of chronic diarrhea with prevalences ranging from 1 per 5000 to 1 per 500,000 patients with chronic diarrhea, depending on tumor type. Bayes theorem can be expressed in the following simplified formula:

$$\text{Posttest odds of diagnosis} = \text{Pretest odds} \times \text{Likelihood ratio}$$

**TABLE 56-3.** Neuroendocrine Tumors Causing Chronic Diarrhea and Their Markers

| TUMOR | TYPICAL SYMPTOMS | MEDIATOR/TUMOR MARKER |
| --- | --- | --- |
| Gastrinoma | Zöllinger-Ellison syndrome: pancreatic or duodenal tumor, peptic ulcer, steatorrhea, diarrhea | Gastrin |
| VIPoma | Verner-Morrison syndrome: watery diarrhea, hypokalemia, achlorhydria, flushing | Vasoactive intestinal polypeptide |
| Medullary thyroid carcinoma | Thyroid mass, hypermotility | Calcitonin, prostaglandins |
| Pheochromocytoma | Adrenal mass, hypertension | Vasoactive intestinal polypeptide, norepinephrine, epinephrine |
| Carcinoid | Flushing, wheezing, right-sided cardiac valvular disease | Serotonin, kinins |
| Somatostatinoma | Nonketotic diabetes mellitus, steatorrhea, diabetes, gallstones | Somatostatin |
| Glucagonoma | Skin rash (migratory necrotizing erythema), mild diabetes | Glucagon |
| Mastocytosis | Flushing, dermatographism, nausea, vomiting, abdominal pain | Histamine |

where the likelihood ratio = true-positive/true-negative result. Because the pretest odds of a peptide-secreting tumor are so long and the false-positive rate of serum peptide assays for that diagnosis is so high (approximately 45%), the positive predictive value for serum peptide assays is substantially below 1%. An abnormal test result would be misleading more than 99% of the time.

**20. What is the likely outcome in patients with chronic secretory diarrhea in whom a diagnosis cannot be reached?**

Diagnostic testing may fail to reveal a cause for chronic diarrhea in up to 25% of patients with chronic diarrhea depending on referral bias and the extent of evaluation. Patients with continuous idiopathic secretory diarrhea have remarkably similar courses. In most cases diarrhea begins suddenly, is associated with some initial weight loss, and resolves in 1 to 2 years without recurrence. It is therefore preferable to treat patients with this form of diarrhea symptomatically rather than to endlessly repeat diagnostic testing once a thorough evaluation has been concluded.

**21. Describe the evaluation of chronic fatty diarrhea.**

Chronic fatty diarrhea is due to either maldigestion or malabsorption. Maldigestion can occur with pancreatic exocrine insufficiency and with ingestion of the lipase inhibitor Orlistat or if there is a bile acid deficiency, which reduces fat emulsification. Malabsorption typically is due to mucosal diseases such as celiac disease, bacterial overgrowth, or small bowel fistula or resection.

Pancreatic exocrine insufficiency can be evaluated with a secretin test or stool chymotrypsin or elastase measurement. Because these tests are not widely available or have poor specificity and sensitivity, clinicians often resort to a therapeutic trial of pancreatic enzymes. If this is done, the patient should be treated with a high dose of enzymes and the effect of this treatment on stool fat excretion as well as symptoms should be assessed.

Bile acid deficiency is a rare cause of maldigestion and is best assessed by direct measurement of duodenal bile acid concentration postprandially. Tests showing excess bile acid excretion in stool (radiolabeled bile acid excretion or total bile acid excretion tests) do not directly assess duodenal bile acid concentration, but if fecal bile acid excretion is high, reduced duodenal bile acid concentration can be inferred. Mucosal disease can be evaluated with small bowel biopsy and bacterial overgrowth can be assessed by breath hydrogen testing after an oral glucose load or by quantitative culture of intestinal contents (Figure 56-6).

**22. How does one make a diagnosis of celiac disease?**

Celiac disease is a common cause of chronic fatty diarrhea but may present without diarrhea. The population prevalence in the United States is estimated to be just less than 1%. Serologic testing for immunoglobulin A (IgA) antibodies against tissue transglutaminase (tTG) is the preferred noninvasive test, but small bowel mucosal biopsy is the definitive test. If serologic testing is done, IgA levels should be measured because 10% of patients with celiac disease may have IgA deficiency, which would produce a false-negative test result.

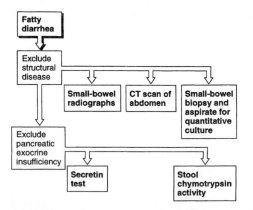

**Figure 56-6.** Evaluation of chronic fatty diarrhea is designed to determine whether malabsorption or maldigestion is the cause of the excess fecal fat excretion. (From Fine KD, Schiller LR: AGA technical review on the evaluation and management of chronic diarrhea. Gastroenterology 116:1464-1486, 1999, with permission.)

**23. Describe the further evaluation of chronic inflammatory diarrhea**

Inflammatory diarrheas can be due to idiopathic inflammatory bowel diseases, such as ulcerative colitis or Crohn's disease; invasive chronic infectious diseases, such as tuberculosis or yersiniosis; ischemic colitis; radiation colitis; and some tumors. To sort through these diagnoses, the most appropriate tests include colonoscopy to inspect the colonic mucosal visually, colonic biopsy to look for microscopic evidence of inflammation, small bowel radiography or CT scanning of the abdomen, and special cultures for chronic infections, such as tuberculosis or yersiniosis. In most cases, the diagnosis will be apparent after these tests are completed (Figure 56-7).

**24. How does one distinguish irritable bowel syndrome from chronic diarrhea?**

The diagnosis of irritable bowel syndrome should be based on the presence of abdominal pain that is associated with defecation and abnormal bowel habits. Chronic continuous diarrhea in the absence of pain is not irritable bowel syndrome, although it may be functional in nature. Symptom criteria (*Rome III criteria*) have been published for clinical and research purposes and include the presence of at least 3 days per month of abdominal pain or discomfort in the last 3 months that is associated with at least 2 of the following three features:

1. Relieved by defecation
2. Onset associated with a change in stool frequency
3. Onset associated with a change in stool form or appearance. Symptom onset must be at least 6 months prior to diagnosis.

## 25. What causes of chronic diarrhea may be difficult to diagnose?

- Fecal incontinence
- Iatrogenic diarrhea (drugs, surgery, radiation)
- Surreptitious laxative ingestion
- Microscopic colitis syndrome
- Bile acid–induced diarrhea
- Small bowel bacterial overgrowth
- Pancreatic exocrine insufficiency
- Carbohydrate malabsorption
- Peptide-secreting tumors
- Chronic idiopathic secretory diarrhea

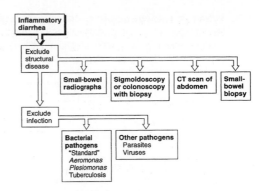

**Figure 56-7.** Chronic inflammatory diarrhea has a diverse differential diagnosis. Structural evaluation with endoscopic or radiographic techniques often yields a diagnosis. Mucosal biopsy may be needed to confirm the diagnosis. (From Fine KD, Schiller LR: AGA technical review on the evaluation and management of chronic diarrhea. Gastroenterology 116:1464-1486, 1999, with permission.)

These conditions are seen in referral centers after routine evaluation has failed to disclose a diagnosis. In general, the tests necessary to make these diagnoses are not difficult but have not been done because physicians have not considered these diagnoses in the differential diagnosis of chronic diarrhea.

## 26. What are common causes of iatrogenic diarrhea?

Most iatrogenic diarrheas are due to ingestion of drugs, some of which may not commonly cause diarrhea. About two-thirds of the drugs listed in the *Physician's Desk Reference* mention diarrhea as a possible side effect. Therefore, the physician should obtain a history of all ingested drugs, including prescription medications, over-the-counter drugs, and herbal remedies (Box 56-1). Other causes of iatrogenic diarrhea include operations, such as vagotomy, gastrectomy, and cholecystectomy, and radiation therapy during which the intestine is exposed to high doses of ionizing radiation.

## 27. What features should suggest surreptitious laxative ingestion?

Some patients who present with chronic diarrhea have diarrhea due to laxative abuse. In general, four groups of patients have this diagnosis:

- Bulimic patients: usually adolescent or young adult women concerned about body weight or with overt eating disorders
- Patients seeking a secondary gain: disability payments, concern or caring behavior by others
- Munchausen's syndrome: peripatetic patients who relish being diagnostic challenges; may undergo extensive testing repeatedly
- Polle syndrome (Munchausen syndrome by proxy): dependent child or adult given laxatives by caregiver to show effectiveness as a caregiver or to gain sympathy from others; may have a history of a sibling who died with chronic diarrhea

Laxatives can be detected by chemical testing of stool or urine. The diagnosis should be confirmed before confronting the patient, and psychiatric consultation should be available to help with further management.

**Box 56-1.** Drugs Associated With Diarrhea

- Antibiotics (most)
- Antineoplastic agents (many)
- Anti-inflammatory agents (e.g., NSAIDs, gold, 5-aminosalicylates)
- Antiarrhythmics (e.g., quinidine)
- Antihypertensives (e.g., β-receptor–blocking drugs)
- Antacids (e.g., those containing magnesium)
- Acid-reducing agents (e.g., $H_2$-receptor antagonists, proton pump inhibitors)
- Prostaglandin (e.g., misoprostol)
- Vitamin/mineral supplements
- Herbal products

## 28. What is microscopic colitis syndrome?

Microscopic colitis is a syndrome characterized by chronic secretory diarrhea, a normal gross appearance of the colonic mucosa, and a typical pattern of inflammation in colon biopsy specimens. This pattern includes changes of the surface epithelium (flattening and irregularity), intraepithelial lymphocytosis, and an increased density of inflammatory cells in the lamina propria. There are two varieties. The first type is collagenous colitis in which the subepithelial collagen layer is thickened, and the second type is lymphocytic colitis in which the subepithelial collagen layer is of normal thickness. Microscopic colitis is as common as Crohn's disease in the general population. It occurs frequently in older patients and may be associated with fecal incontinence. In many cases, a rheumatologic or autoimmune disorder may be present. Treatment is variably effective: budesonide has the most evidence for efficacy; bile acid–binding drugs and bismuth subsalicylate have some efficacy.

## 29. Define bile acid diarrhea.

In patients with ileal resection or disease, the part of the small intestine with high-affinity bile acid transporters has been removed or is dysfunctional. Thus, excessive bile acid finds its way into the colon. If the bile acid concentration in colonic contents reaches a critical level of approximately 3 to 5 mmol/L, salt and water absorption by the colonic mucosa is inhibited and diarrhea results. Patients who have had extensive small bowel resections (more than 100 cm) often have so much fluid entering the colon that this critical bile acid level is not reached (Figure 56-8).

In addition to this classic form of diarrhea caused by bile acid malabsorption, some investigators have speculated that bile acid malabsorption causes chronic diarrhea in some patients with an intact ileum. Although tests of bile acid absorption frequently are abnormal in patients with idiopathic diarrhea, treatment with bile acid–sequestering resins, such as cholestyramine, is not often as effective in this group of patients as in those who have had surgical resection of the ileum.

## 30. What is the likely outcome in chronic idiopathic secretory diarrhea?

Patients with chronic secretory diarrhea that evades a serious diagnostic evaluation often have a similar history of previous good health with the sudden onset of diarrhea, often accompanied by acute, but not progressive, weight loss. Although the acute onset suggests an acute infectious process, patients have negative microbiological studies and do not respond to empiric antibiotics. Diarrhea usually persists for 12 to 30 months and then gradually subsides. This condition can be sporadic or can occur in epidemics. The epidemic form (*Brainerd diarrhea*) seems to be associated with ingestion of potentially contaminated food or drink, but no organism has been implicated. Management consists of the effective use of nonspecific antidiarrheals until the process subsides.

## 31. What is the best nonspecific therapy for chronic diarrhea?

Because the evaluation of chronic diarrhea may extend over several weeks and since the diagnosis is not always forthcoming, patients may need symptomatic therapy. The most effective agents are opiates. Traditional antidiarrheal

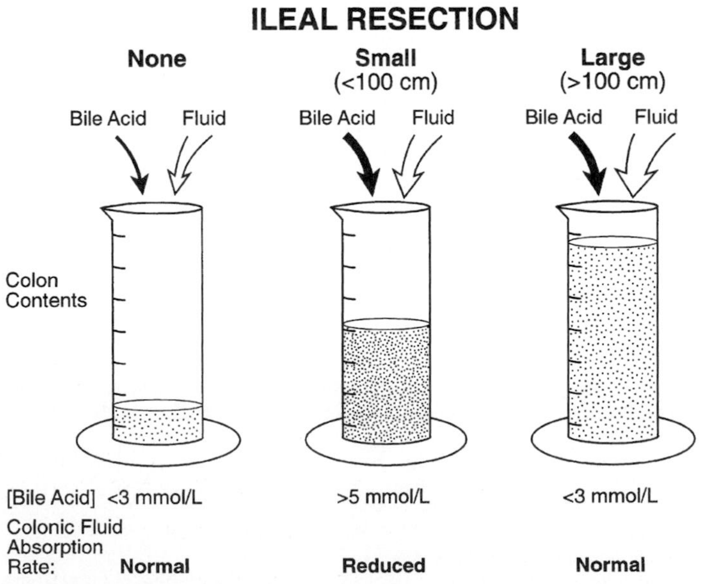

**ILEAL RESECTION**

**Figure 56-8.** Bile acid diarrhea occurs when bile acid malabsorption in the ileum is linked with relatively low fluid flows into the colon. As a result, the concentration of bile acid in colon contents is greater than the cathartic threshold of 3 to –5 mmol/L. If fluid flows are high (as with substantial small bowel resection), bile acid malabsorption may be just as severe, but bile acid concentrations are not high enough to impair absorption by the colon.

## TABLE 56-4. Nonspecific Therapy for Chronic Diarrhea

| DRUG CLASS | AGENT | DOSAGE |
|---|---|---|
| Opiates | **μ-Opiate receptor selective** | |
| | Diphenoxylate | 2.5 to 5 mg QID |
| | Loperamide | 2 to 4 mg QID |
| | Codeine | 15 to 60 mg QID |
| | Morphine | 2 to 20 mg QID |
| | Opium tincture | 2 to 20 drops QID |
| | **δ-Opiate receptor selective** | |
| | Racecadotril (acetorphan) | 1.5 mg/kg TID* |
| | Adrenergic agonist | |
| | Clonidine | 0.1 to 0.3 mg TID |
| | Somatostatin analogue | |
| | Octreotide | 50 to 250 µg TID (subcutaneously) |
| | Bile acid-binding resin | |
| | Cholestyramine | 4 g daily to QID |

*Not yet approved in the United States.

agents, such as diphenoxylate and loperamide, work well in many patients but should be given on a routine schedule in patients with chronic diarrhea rather than on an as-needed basis. Typical doses of 1 or 2 tablets or capsules of these agents before meals and at bedtime will improve symptoms in most people. When this therapy is ineffective, more potent opiates, such as codeine, opium, or morphine, can be used. With the stronger agents, doses should be low at first and increased gradually, so that tolerance to the central nervous system effects can develop. Fortunately, the gut does not become tolerant to these agents; thus, one can usually find a dose that will control symptoms without producing severe side effects. Other agents that are sometimes used to manage chronic diarrhea include clonidine, octreotide, and cholestyramine, but they tend to be less effective than opiates and are often less well tolerated by patients, making them second-line agents in most circumstances (Table 56-4).

## WEBSITES

http://content.nejm.org/cgi/content/extract/355/3/236

http://digestive.niddk.nih.gov/ddiseases/pubs/diarrhea/

http://www.gastro.org/userassets/Documents/02_Clinical_Practice/medical_position_stat ments/chronic_diarrhea_tr.pdf

http://www.uptodate.com/patients/content/topic.do?topicKey=digestiv/4974

www.cdc.gov/ncidod/dpd/parasites/diarrhea/factsht_chronic_diarrhea.htm

www.cdc.gov/ncidod/dpd/parasiticpathways/diarrhea.htm

## BIBLIOGRAPHY

1. Abraham B, Sellin JH. Drug-induced diarrhea. Curr Gastroenterol Rep 2007;9:365–72.
2. Fernandez-Banares F, Esteve M, Salas A, et al. Systematic evaluation of the causes of chronic watery diarrhea with functional characteristics. Am J Gastroenterol 2007;102:2520–8.
3. Hanauer SB. The role of loperamide in gastrointestinal disorders. Rev Gastroenterol Disord 2008;8:15–20.
4. Longstreth GF, Thompson WG, Chey WD, et al. Functional bowel disorders. Gastroenterology 2006;130:1480–91.
5. Schiller LR. Chronic diarrhea. Curr Treat Opt Gastroenterol 2005;8:259–66.
6. Schiller LR. Evaluation of small bowel bacterial overgrowth. Curr Gastroenterol Rep 2007;9:373–7.
7. Schiller LR. Malabsorption. In: Rakel RE, Bope ET, editors. Conn's Current Therapy 2008. Philadelphia: WB Saunders; 2008. pp. 534–40.
8. Schiller LR. Management of diarrhea in clinical practice: Strategies for primary care physicians. Rev Gastroenterol Disord 2007;7(Suppl. 3):S27–38.
9. Schiller LR, Sellin JH. Diarrhea. In: Feldman M, Friedman L, Brandt LJ, editors. Sleisenger & Fordtran's Gastrointestinal and Liver Disease. 8th ed. Philadelphia: WB Saunders; 2006. pp. 159–86.
10. Scott IA, Greenberg PB, Poole PJ. Cautionary tales in the clinical interpretation of studies of diagnostic tests. Intern Med J 2008;38:120–9.
11. Sellin JH. A practical approach to treating patients with chronic diarrhea. Rev Gastroenterol Disord 2007;7(Suppl. 3):S19–26.
12. Shelton JH, Santa Ana CA, Thompson DR, et al. Factitious diarrhea induced by stimulant laxatives: Accuracy of diagnosis by a clinical reference laboratory using thin layer chromatography. Clin Chem 2007;53:85–90.
13. Trinh C, Prabhakar K. Diarrheal diseases in the elderly. Clin Geriatr Med 2007;23:833–56.
14. Wall GC, Schirmer LL, Page MJ. Pharmacotherapy for microscopic colitis. Pharmacotherapy 2007;27:425–33.

# AIDS AND THE GASTROINTESTINAL TRACT

*George B. Smallfield, MD, and*
*C. Mel Wilcox, MD*

1. **What is the role of barium esophagram for patients with AIDS (acquired immunodeficiency syndrome) and esophageal symptoms?**

   Barium esophagram has a limited role in patients with AIDS. Infections are the most common cause of esophageal disease in patients with AIDS. Although many of these infections have a characteristic appearance on barium radiography, overlap is frequent, thus mandating a definitive diagnosis by other means before prescribing antimicrobial therapy. In addition, some therapies for these disorders (e.g., corticosteroids) may be associated with significant toxicity, further emphasizing the importance of a histologic diagnosis. Last, in patients with severe odynophagia, the barium study may be inadequate because severe pain on swallowing will limit the amount of barium that can be swallowed, thus limiting the quality of the study. For these reasons, endoscopy with biopsy is the preferred diagnostic modality in this group of patients as this will yield a definitive diagnosis in 75% of cases.

2. **What is the role of empiric therapy for new-onset esophageal symptoms in patients with AIDS?**

   Candida esophagitis is the most common cause of esophageal disease in patients with AIDS presenting with dysphagia or odynophagia (Fig. 57-1). Because of this high prevalence, an empiric approach to new-onset esophageal symptoms with potent antifungal therapy is commonly undertaken. A randomized study using a loading dose of 200 mg of fluconazole followed by 100 mg/day for 10-14 days showed both efficacy and cost-effectiveness, Because Candida esophagitis responds very rapidly to fluconazole, in the patient who does not symptomatically improve within the first few days of treatment, endoscopic evaluation to exclude other causes of disease (viral esophagitis) should be performed.

   With improving HIV/AIDS therapies, patient commonly have CD4 counts higher than 200 cells/mL. In these patients, an empiric trial of a proton pump inhibitor is reasonable for symptoms consistent with gastroesophageal reflux disease (GERD). If symptoms do not improve, endoscopic evaluation to exclude other causes of disease is indicated.

3. **What are the most common causes of esophageal ulceration in AIDS?**

   The most common causes are cytomegalovirus (CMV) and idiopathic esophageal ulcer (IEU). On endoscopy, CMV and IEU appear most often as large, well-circumscribed solitary ulcerations, with normal-appearing surrounding mucosa. Multiple ulcers may also be observed. Antiretroviral medications such as didanosine (ddI) and zidovudine (AZT) have also been associated with pill-induced esophagitis. Herpes simplex virus (HSV) is usually associated with multiple small, shallow esophageal ulcerations, often raised with a volcano crater appearance. GERD can also present with ulcerations of the distal esophagus generally involving the gastroesophageal junction; these lesions are generally linear and superficial. Neoplasms (e.g., lymphoma), parasites (e.g., leishmania), and fungal infections (e.g., histoplasmosis and *Candida* spp.) are rare causes of esophageal ulcers (Table 57-1).

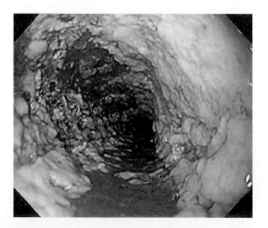

**Figure 57-1.** Candidal esophagitis. Yellow plaques coating the esophageal wall are typical for *Candida.* Note that on one portion of the wall, the material has been removed and the underlying mucosa is normal.

4. **What biopsy technique should be used to sample an esophageal ulcer?**

   The exact number of biopsies required for maximal sensitivity is not clearly established, but several studies suggest the range of 8 to 10. It is important to obtain biopsy samples from the ulcer margin and from the ulcer base. This is because biopsy of the ulcer edge reveals a cytopathic effect that is present in squamous epithelium associated with HSV; conversely, CMV resides in granulation tissue in the ulcer base. The role of culture and cytology for esophageal ulcers is not settled. If all biopsies are negative for viral, bacterial, fungal, and parasitic infections, a diagnosis of IEU can be made.

**Table 57-1.** Reported Causes of Esophageal Ulcers in AIDS

| | |
|---|---|
| Viruses | Cytomegalovirus, herpes simplex virus type II, Epstein-Barr virus, papovavirus, human herpes virus-6 |
| Fungi | *Candida* spp., *Histoplasma capsulatum, Cryptococcus neoformans,* mucormycosis, aspergillosis, *Penicillium chrysogenum, Exophiala jeanselmei* |
| Bacteria | *Mycobacterium avium*-complex, *Mycobacterium tuberculosis, Bartonella henselae, Nocardia asteroides, Actinomyces israelii* |
| Protozoa | Cryptosporidia, *Leishmania donovani, Pneumocystis carinii* |
| Tumors | Non-Hodgkin lymphoma, Kaposi sarcoma, cancer (squamous cell and adenocarcinoma), lymphoma |
| Pill-induced | Zalcitabine, zidovudine, other |
| Gastroesophageal disease, idiopathic | Idiopathic esophageal ulcer |

## 5. What is AIDS-cholangiopathy? How do patients present?

AIDS-cholangiopathy is a spectrum of biliary tract abnormalities resembling sclerosing cholangitis that can be caused by a wide array of microorganisms and neoplasms, usually in patients with advanced immunodeficiency. Almost all patients have a CD4 count less than 200 cells/mL and most have a CD4 count less than 50 cells/mL. Patients generally present with epigastric or right upper quadrant pain, fever, and malaise. Although AIDS-cholangiopathy is a cholestatic disease, jaundice and pruritus are uncommon. The most common laboratory finding in this syndrome is a markedly elevated alkaline phosphatase, usually more than three times the upper limits of normal. Typically bilirubin is not elevated and rarely exceeds 3 mg/dL, and transaminases are only mildly elevated. Generally, these patients have a dilated bile duct that is identifiable on abdominal ultrasonography. The diagnosis is best established by endoscopic retrograde cholangiopancreatography (ERCP). Several cholangiographic patterns have been described, including papillary stenosis, sclerosing cholangitis, combined papillary stenosis and sclerosing cholangitis, isolated intrahepatic disease, and long extrahepatic bile duct strictures. The most common pattern is papillary stenosis with intrahepatic sclerosing cholangitis. Endoscopic sphincterotomy is appropriate only for the relief of pain in patients with papillary stenosis. Unfortunately, the disease is progressive and antimicrobial therapy has no influence on its outcome. Treatment with highly active antiretroviral therapy (HAART) is associated with decreased mortality.

## 6. What are the most common causes of AIDS-cholangiopathy? How are they diagnosed?

1. *Cryptosporidium parvum*
2. Microsporidia
   *Enterocytozoon bieneusi*
   *Encephalitozoon intestinalis*
   *Encephalocytozoon cuniculi*
3. CMV
4. *Mycobacterium avium*-complex (MAC)
5. *Cyclospora cayetanensis*
6. Non-Hodgkin lymphoma
7. Kaposi sarcoma

The diagnosis is usually established by obtaining biopsy specimens of the ampulla or duodenal mucosa, bile duct biopsy, aspirated bile specimens, or biliary epithelial brush cytology. Despite its infectious origin, medical therapies aiming at the eradication of these organisms have not produced marked improvement in AIDS-cholangiopathy. Treatment with HAART is associated with decreased mortality.

## 7. What are the most common causes of pancreatitis in HIV-infected patients?

Several studies have documented chronic and/or recurrent elevations of serum amylase and lipase in up to 50% of patients with AIDS. Pancreatograms at the time of ERCP have shown abnormalities of the pancreatic ducts consistent with chronic pancreatitis. These findings have led many investigators to hypothesize that pancreatic insufficiency from chronic pancreatitis is an important cause of chronic diarrhea in AIDS; however, most cases of chronic pancreatitis are attributable to conditions, such as alcohol abuse. The most common medications associated with pancreatitis in AIDS are pentamidine, ddI, and zalcitabine (ddC). Protease inhibitors frequently cause hyperlipidemia. Ritonavir is associated with the most dramatic increases in triglycerides with 10% of patients developing severe hypertriglyceridemia. Pancreatitis is well described in patients with elevations in triglycerides from protease inhibitors. Reported infectious causes of pancreatitis include CMV, HSV, MAC, and tuberculosis. An infectious cause of pancreatitis is difficult to establish and would require pancreatic biopsy.

## 8. How has HAART affected the incidence of opportunistic gastrointestinal (GI) disorders?

Since the introduction of protease inhibitors and HAART in 1995, there has been a constant and dramatic decline of GI opportunistic disorders in AIDS patients. It is postulated that improvement in the immune status, as reflected by an increase in CD4 cells, prevents the development of opportunistic disorders. In several reports, symptoms resolved even before any changes in the total CD4 cell count were apparent, suggesting that the antiretroviral medications promote elimination of the offending GI infection, probably secondary to immune-boosting mechanisms independent of the CD4 cell count and intrinsic antimicrobial activity.

## 9. What is the recommended workup for diarrhea in AIDS?

When evaluating an AIDS patient with diarrhea, careful attention should be directed to the history and physical examination. Enteritis (small bowel diarrhea) is associated with voluminous, watery bowel movements, abdominal bloating, cramping, borborygmi, and nausea. Abdominal pain, if present, tends to be periumbilical or diffuse. Abdominal examination reveals an increase in number and frequency of bowel sounds, which may be high-pitched. Conversely, colitis (large bowel diarrhea) is characterized by frequent, small bowel movements, with the presence of mucus, pus, and/or blood (dysentery). Patients with prominent involvement of the distal colon also have proctitis symptoms, such as tenesmus, dyschezia (pain on defecation), and proctalgia (rectal pain) (Fig. 57-2).

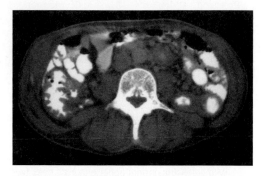

**Figure 57-2.** Cytomegalovirus colitis. Abdominal computed tomography scan shows colonic wall thickening most pronounced in the right colon.

It is also important to consider patient exposures. A history of new medications or an alteration in a current regimen, such as antiretrovirals or antibacterials, is important because many protease inhibitors are associated with diarrhea and antibacterials are associated with *Clostridium difficile* colitis. In febrile patients, blood cultures should be obtained for common bacteria. If the CD4 count is below 50 cells/mL, blood cultures for MAC should be obtained. If stool and blood culture studies are negative, the next step is endoscopic evaluation with biopsy. In the presence of colitis symptoms, flexible sigmoidoscopy or colonoscopy is recommended. Table 57-2 summarizes the studies and laboratory tests used in the evaluation of diarrhea in AIDS. Table 57-3 lists the most common infectious causes of diarrhea in AIDS. Table 57-4 lists common associations between exposures and infections.

## 10. Describe the clinical features of HSV proctitis in AIDS.

HSV proctitis is the most common cause of nongonococcal proctitis in sexually active homosexual men. HSV proctitis classically presents with tenesmus, purulent rectal discharge, severe proctalgia, fever, constipation, and anorectal bleeding. Painful inguinal lymphadenopathy is an almost universal finding. The pain tends to distribute in the region of the sacral roots (i.e., buttocks, perineal region, and posterior thigh). Because of the neural involvement by HSV and the presence of severe pain, patients may complain of impotence and difficulty in initiating micturition.

| **Table 57-2.** Studies and Laboratory Tests Used in the Evaluation of Diarrhea in AIDS | |
|---|---|
| Stool | Cultures (*Salmonella, Shigella, Campylobacter* spp.) |
| | Toxin (*Clostridium difficile*) |
| | Ova and parasites (*Giardia lamblia, Entamoeba histolytica, Cryptosporidium* spp.) |
| | Modified Kinyoun acid-fast (*Cryptosporidium* spp., *Isospora* belli) |
| | Concentrated stool (zinc sulfate, Sheather sucrose flotation) (microsporidia) |
| Blood | Cultures (*Mycobacterium avium*-complex, *Salmonella, Campylobacter* spp.) |
| | Antibodies (*Entamoeba histolytica*, cytomegalovirus [CMV]) |
| Gastrointestinal fluids | Duodenal aspirate (*Giardia lamblia*, microsporidia) |
| | Electron microscopy (*Cryptosporidium* spp., adenovirus) |
| Biopsy stains | Hematoxylin-eosin |
| | Giemsa or methenamine silver (fungi) |
| | Methylene blue–azure II–basic fuchsin (microsporidia) |
| | Fite (mycobacteria) |
| Immunohistochemical stains (CMV), immunologic methods | In situ hybridization (CMV) |
| | DNA amplification (CMV) |
| | Culture of tissue |
| | CMV |
| | Herpes simplex virus |
| | Mycobacteria |

**Table 57-3.** Infectious Causes of Diarrhea in AIDS

| VIRUSES | BACTERIA | PARASITES | FUNGI |
|---|---|---|---|
| Cytomegalovirus | *Salmonella* spp. | *Giardia lamblia* | *Histoplasma* |
| Astrovirus | *Shigella* spp. | *Entamoeba histolytica* | *capsulatum* |
| Picornavirus | *Campylobacter jejuni* | Microsporidia | *Candida albicans* |
| Coronavirus | *Clostridium difficile* | *Enterocytozoon bieneusi* | |
| Rotavirus | *Mycobacterium avium*-complex | *Encephalitozoon* | |
| Herpesvirus | *Treponema pallidum* | *intestinalis (formerly* | |
| Adenovirus | Spirochetes | *Septata)* | |
| Small round virus | *Neisseria gonorrhoeae* | *Cyclospora cayetanensis* | |
| HIV | *Vibrio cholerae* | *Cryptosporidium* spp. | |
| | *Aeromonas* spp. | *Isospora belli* | |
| | *Pseudomonas* spp. (?) | *Blastocystis hominis* (?) | |
| | *Staphylococcus aureus* | | |

**Table 57-4.** Sources of Infectious Diarrhea

| INFECTIOUS AGENT | ASSOCIATION |
|---|---|
| *C. difficile* | Recent antibiotics, nursing home or hospital exposures |
| Cryptosporidiosis Microsporidiosis | Recent visit to a farm, contact with farm animals, use of a public swimming pool |
| *Giardia* | Camping, stream water |
| *Mycobacterium avium* | CD4 count less than 50 |
| *Cyclospora cayetanesis* | Common cause of diarrhea in South America |
| Microsporidiosis | Uncommon in the southern United States |
| Rotavirus | Common cause of diarrhea in Australia |

Visual inspection and anoscopy commonly reveal the following lesions: vesicles, pustular rectal lesions, or diffuse ulcerations. HSV is a pathogen of the squamous mucosa; therefore, diffuse proctitis involving the entire rectum is rare. In severe cases, the columnar rectal and sigmoid mucosa has been involved. The differential diagnoses of HSV proctitis include lymphogranuloma venereum (*Chlamydia trachomatis*), *Entamoeba histolytica, Salmonella* spp., and *Campylobacter jejuni.*

11. **What is the preferred endoscopic procedure for the evaluation of diarrhea in AIDS?**
    The advantage of endoscopy is that it permits direct visualization of the mucosa and retrieval of tissue for histologic examination. The diagnostic yield of colonoscopy in HIV-infected patients with chronic diarrhea and negative stool studies ranges from 27% to 37%; CMV is the most common etiology identified. Because CMV colitis is usually present in the distal colon, sigmoidoscopy with biopsy may be a sufficient workup, but in 13% to 39% of cases of CMV enterocolitis, the virus can be detected in the right colon only. Therefore, if CMV is suspected as the cause of diarrhea, a full colonoscopy is warranted, especially if sigmoidoscopy is negative. However, it is still not clear whether colonoscopy has a higher yield than flexible sigmoidoscopy for the detection of organisms other than CMV. Evaluation with colonoscopy would be prudent if sigmoidoscopy is negative and right-sided abdominal complaints are reported. The value of upper endoscopy and small bowel biopsy in the evaluation of chronic diarrhea has also been demonstrated, although specific treatment options for most small bowel pathogens are limited. Some would obtain ileal biopsy at the time of colonoscopy rather than proceed with upper endoscopy and biopsy. The most commonly detected organisms involving the small bowel are cryptosporidia and microsporidia.

12. **What is the most common cause of viral diarrhea in AIDS?**
    CMV is one of the most common opportunistic infections in patients with AIDS, occurring late in the course of HIV infection when immunodeficiency is severe (CD4 lymphocyte count less than $100/mm^3$). CMV has been identified in mucosal biopsy samples in as many as 45% of patients with AIDS and diarrhea, especially in those patients with negative stool studies. CMV causes both enteritis and colitis. A number of other viral pathogens have been reported to involve the GI tract in patients with AIDS, but their clinical importance remains to be determined. Examples include adenovirus, rotavirus, astrovirus, picobirnavirus, and coronavirus. There are also reports that HIV itself can be isolated from enterocytes and colonic cells, but its role in causing disease is uncertain. HSV can cause proctitis that mimics diarrhea because of the rectal mucous discharge. However, HSV does not cause enterocolitis because it invades the squamous mucosa, not the columnar epithelium, such as the one lining the colonic and small bowel mucosa.

### 13. What are the treatment options for CMV enterocolitis?

The natural history of CMV colitis is variable. In untreated patients, it usually has a chronic course characterized by progressive diarrhea and weight loss, although occasionally symptoms and histologic abnormalities remit spontaneously. Unlike CMV retinitis, for which strong evidence supports induction therapy followed by lifelong maintenance therapy, the optimal duration of therapy and the need for maintenance therapy in CMV colitis are undefined. Consensus guidelines recommend 3 to 6 weeks of induction therapy followed by maintenance therapy if there is a history of relapses. Two antivirals (foscarnet and ganciclovir) have been studied extensively in the therapy of CMV colitis and/or enteritis. Cidofovir, the newest intravenous agent, has been used primarily in patients with retinal disease, but in our experience it is effective for GI disease as well. The newest agent is valganciclovir. This drug can be given orally and achieves serum levels similar to intravenous ganciclovir. Studies for GI disease are limited. Funduscopic examination at the time of diagnosis of CMV enterocolitis is mandatory, because duration of therapy is considerably longer for disseminated diseases than for disease limited to the GI tract.

A number of open-label trials of ganciclovir for HIV-infected patients with CMV GI disease have demonstrated clinical improvement in approximately 75% of patients. Open-label trials of foscarnet have yielded comparable results. The only placebo-controlled trial of ganciclovir in AIDS-associated CMV colitis found no clinically significant differences, probably because the treatment period was only 2 weeks. A randomized trial comparing ganciclovir with foscarnet in 48 AIDS patients with CMV GI disease found similar clinical efficacy (73%), regardless of the location of disease (esophagus vs. colon). Endoscopic improvement was documented in over 80% of patients. For all patients, institution of HAART is important and, if there is an immunologic response, long-term maintenance therapy can be discontinued.

### 14. Name the parasites that cause diarrhea in AIDS.

Among the protozoa, *C. parvum* is the most common parasite causing diarrhea in AIDS and has been identified in up to 11% of symptomatic patients. Although a cause of acute diarrhea, cryptosporidiosis is found most commonly in HIV-infected patients with chronic diarrhea. In some studies of HIV-infected patients with chronic diarrhea, microsporidia (*E. bieneusi* and *E. intestinalis*) are the most commonly identified pathogens. Giardia is also a consideration in patients with diarrhea, especially when chronic and associated with the upper gastrointestinal symptoms of nausea and bloating. *Isospora belli* is a rare GI pathogen in HIV-infected patients in North America, whereas it is endemic in many developing countries, such as Haiti.

### 15. Compare the clinical features and therapies for cryptosporidiosis and microsporidiosis.

Gastrointestinal microsporidial infection is generally attributed to two species: *E. bieneusi* and *E. intestinalis*. In general, intestinal disease is relatively mild in contrast to the severe diarrhea typical for cryptosporidiosis. Loose stools and mild weight loss are common with colonic symptoms typically absent. Gastrointestinal bleeding suggests another diagnosis as this infection does not cause mucosal ulceration. Although stool studies can establish the diagnosis, small bowel biopsies, of either the duodenum or ileum, with special stains are more sensitive. Although there is no effective antimicrobial therapy for *E. bieneusi*, albendazole is highly effective for *E. intestinalis*. As with all opportunistic infections in AIDS, HAART may result in clinical remission.

Cryptosporidia are a common cause of chronic diarrhea in HIV-infected patients with severe immunodeficiency. There are at least 40 species of Cryptosporidia, but the most common cause of human disease is *Cryptosporidium muri*. Cryptosporidia infect and then reproduce within the columnar small intestinal cells. Infection can occur from person-to-person or animal-to-person or from waterborne transmission (e.g., swimming pools, lakes). Therefore, a severely immunodeficient patient with AIDS not taking HAART should be advised to avoid contact with farm animals, public pools, and lakes. The life cycle is completed in a single host. Autoinfectious cycles follow ingestion of a few oocysts, leading to severe disease and persistent infection in severely immunodeficient hosts. The diarrhea is generally voluminous and watery. Dehydration and weight loss are common in patients with advanced immunodeficiency. Disease severity correlates with immune function. The stool may contain mucus but rarely contains blood or leukocytes. The disease may wax and wane, but persistent and/or progressive disease may be manifested by dehydration and electrolyte imbalances. Constitutional symptoms are prominent, including low-grade fever, malaise, anorexia, nausea, and vomiting. Both of these infections improve with reconstitution of the immune system following successful HAART.

### 16. Which bacteria most commonly cause diarrhea in AIDS?

*Campylobacter, Salmonella*, and *Shigella* spp. and *C. difficile. Yersinia enterocolitica, Staphylococcus aureus*, and *Aeromonas hydrophila* have also been associated with severe enterocolitis in HIV-infected patients. *C. difficile* colitis has become the most frequent bacterial cause of diarrhea in HIV-infected patients, perhaps because of frequent exposure to antimicrobials and requirement for hospitalization. MAC is a common pathogen in patients with advanced immunosuppression (i.e., CD4 count less than 50 cells/mm$^3$). An incidence of 39% has been described when the CD4 count remains less than 10/mm$^3$. Tuberculosis is most frequent in developing countries and is less likely to present with diarrhea alone.

## 17. What is bacillary peliosis hepatis (BPH)?

BPH produces multiple cystic blood-filled spaces in the liver. BPH is caused by an infection with the bacteria *Bartonella henselae* (formerly *Rochalimae*) and occurs in patients with advanced AIDS. Patients present with generalized and nonspecific symptoms, such as fever, weight loss, and malaise. Abdominal pain, nausea, vomiting, and diarrhea may be prominent. Skin manifestations include reddish vascular papules that can be confused with Kaposi sarcoma. On abdominal examination, hepatosplenomegaly and lymphadenopathy are the most prominent features. Histopathology of the liver lesions shows multiple cystic blood-filled spaces within fibromyxoid areas. The treatment of choice is erythromycin for at least 4 to 6 weeks, but doxycycline is a safe alternative.

## 18. Describe the management of HIV wasting syndrome.

AIDS wasting is defined as an involuntary weight loss of 10% from baseline over 12 months or 5% over 6 months. Approximately 20% of patients with HIV will develop wasting. With the advent of HAART, the incidence of AIDS wasting has decreased. However, the prevalence of wasting at the time of AIDS diagnosis has increased. The weight loss is typically lean muscle mass, which has a dramatic impact on quality of life. This loss of muscle mass is associated with increased mortality, accelerated disease progression, and impaired functioning. Many strategies have been developed to treat HIV wasting. Nutritional counseling and dietary supplements are effective in increasing fat free mass. Additionally, specific supplementation of L-glutamine, beta-hydroxy-beta-methylbutyrate, and L-arginine have been shown to increase lean muscle mass. Growth hormone and testosterone increase lean body mass, but these treatments have significant side effects. Some evidence shows anti–tumor necrosis factor therapies increase weight, but these agents present safety concerns in immunocompromised individuals. Resistance exercise provides significant increases in lean body mass as well as strength. Regimens vary, but typically they consist of a three-times-a-week regimen with a clearly defined number of repetitions and percent of maximal output for each repetition. Exercise is inexpensive and without reported side effects and thus is an ideal first-line therapy.

## 19. When do you initiate hepatitis B virus (HBV) therapy in the setting of HIV?

HBV/HIV coinfection represents a significant problem in HIV care. As HAART has improved the prognosis in HIV/AIDS, significant increases in morbidity and mortality due to liver disease have been observed. HBV and HIV are acquired by similar mechanisms and thus coinfection is common. Patients with coinfection of HIV and HBV have higher HBV DNA levels and are less likely to convert from HBeAg+ to HBeAb+, indicating a poorer response to HBV therapy. Patients with a HBV DNA greater than 2000 and F2 or greater fibrosis on biopsy should have HBV treatment. If a patient has cirrhosis, he or she should be treated if HBV DNA is greater than 200. For patients with a high CD4 count, HBV monotherapy that is not active against HIV should be first-line therapy. When initiating HAART, HBV also should be treated with two antiviral agents active against HBV. If CD4 counts are between 350 and 500 cells/mL, one can elect to treat both HIV and HBV. HAART with two agents active against HBV should be used instead of HBV monotherapy in these individuals.

## 20. Why is it important to know the HBV treatments that are also active in treating HIV?

Initiating HBV monotherapy that is also active in treating HIV can result in HIV resistance, potentially limiting HAART options. Furthermore, if HAART is initiated without concurrent HBV treatment, immune reconstitution can result in a potentially life-threatening flare of untreated HBV. Table 57-5 shows treatments active against HBV and HIV or HBV alone.

**Table 57-5.** Hepatitis B Treatments and HIV Activity

| TREATS HIV AND HBV | TREATS HBV WITHOUT HIV RESISTANCE |
|---|---|
| Lamivudine | Interferon/PEG-IFN |
| Tenofovir | Adefovir (at 10 mg dosing) |
| Emtricitabine | Telbivudine (in vitro) |
| Entecavir (in vivo) | |

## BIBLIOGRAPHY

1. Blanshard C, Francis N, Gazzard BG. Investigation of chronic diarrhoea in acquired immunodeficiency syndrome: A prospective study in 155 patients. Gut 1996;39:824–32.
2. Bonacini M, Young T, Laine L. The causes of esophageal symptoms in human immunodeficiency virus infection: A prospective study of 110 patients. Arch Intern Med 1991;151:1567–72.
3. Bush ZM, Kosmiski LA. Acute pancreatitis in HIV-infected patients: Are etiologies changing since the introduction of protease inhibitor therapy? Pancreas 2003;27:E1–5.
4. Call SA, Heudebert G, Saag M, et al. The changing etiology of chronic diarrhea in HIV-infected patients with CD4 cell counts less than 200 cells/mm³. Am J Gastroenterol 2000;95:3142–6.
5. Carr A, Marriott D, Field A, et al. Treatment of HIV-1-associated microsporidiosis and cryptosporidiosis with combination antiretroviral therapy. Lancet 1998;351:256–61.

6. Cello JP. Acquired immunodeficiency syndrome cholangiopathy: Spectrum of disease. Am J Med 1989;86:539.
7. Chen XM, LaRusso NF. Cryptosporidiosis and the pathogenesis of AIDS-cholangiopathy. Semin Liver Dis 2002;22:277–89.
8. Dieterich DT, Wilcox CM. Diagnosis and treatment of esophageal diseases associated with HIV-infection. Am J Gastroenterol 1996;91:2265–8.
9. Dore GJ, Marriott DJ, Hing MC, et al. Disseminated microsporidiosis due to Septata intestinalis in nine patients infected with the human immunodeficiency virus: Response to therapy with albendazole. Clin Infect Dis 1995;21:70–6.
10. Dungeon WD, Phillips Carson JA, et al. Counteracting muscle wasting in HIV-infected individuals. HIV Med 2006;7:299–310.
11. Dworkin MS, Williamson JM. AIDS wasting syndrome: Trends, influence on opportunistic infections, and survival. JAIDS 2003;33:267–73.
12. Goodgame RW. Understanding intestinal spore-forming protozoa: Cryptosporidia, microsporidia, isospora, and cyclospora. Ann Intern Med 1996;124:429–41.
13. Iser DM, Sasadeusz JJ. Current treatment of HIV/hepatitis B virus coinfection. J Gastroenterol Hepatol 2008;23:699–706.
14. Kearney DJ, Steuerwald M, Koch J, et al. A prospective study of endoscopy in HIV-associated diarrhea. Am J Gastroenterol 1999;94:556–9.
15. Mirete G, Masia M, Gutierrez A, et al. Acute pancreatitis as a complication of ritonavir therapy in a patient with AIDS. Eur J Clin Microbiol Infect Dis 1998;17:810–1.
16. Mohle-Boetani JC, Koehler JE, Berger TG, et al. Bacillary angiomatosis and bacillary peliosis in patients infected with human immunodeficiency virus: Clinical characteristics in a case-control study. Clin Infect Dis 1996;22:794–800.
17. Mönkemüller KE, Call SA, Lazenby AJ, et al. Decline in the prevalence of opportunistic gastrointestinal disorders in the era of HAART. Am J Gastroenterol 2000;95:457–62.
18. Mönkemüller KE, Wilcox CM. Diagnosis and treatment of colonic disease in AIDS. Gastrointest Endosc Clin North Am 1998;8:889.
19. Mönkemüller KE, Wilcox CM. Diagnosis and treatment of esophageal ulcers in AIDS. Semin Gastroenterol 1999;10:1.
20. Mönkemüller KE, Wilcox CM. Therapy of gastrointestinal infections in AIDS. Aliment Pharmacol Ther 1997;11:425–43.
21. Roubenoff R, McDermott A, Weiss L, et al. Short-term progressive resistance training increases strength and lean body mass in adults infected with human immunodeficiency virus. AIDS 1999;13:231–9.
22. Schwartz DA, Straub RA, Wilcox CM. Prospective endoscopic characterization of cytomegalovirus esophagitis in patients with AIDS. Gastrointest Endosc 1994;40:481–4.
23. Sullivan AK, Feher MD, Nelson MR, et al. Marked hypertriglyceridaemia associated with ritonavir therapy. AIDS 1998;12:1392–4.
24. Weber R, Bryan RT, Schwartz DA, et al. Human microsporidial infections. Clin Microbiol Rev 1994;7:426–61.
25. Wei-Fang K, Cello JP, Rogers SJ, et al. Prognostic factors for survival of patients with AIDS cholangiopathy. Am J Gastroenterol 2003;98:2176–81.
26. Wilcox CM. Etiology and evaluation of diarrhea in AIDS: A global perspective at the millennium. World J Gastroenterol 2000;6:177–86.
27. Wilcox CM, Clark WS, Thompson SE. Fluconazole compared with endoscopy for human immunodeficiency virus-infected patients with esophageal symptoms. Gastroenterology 1996;110:1803–8.
28. Wilcox CM, Schwartz DA, Clark WS. Causes, response to therapy, and long-term outcome of esophageal ulcer in patients with human immunodeficiency virus infection. Ann Intern Med 1995;122:143–9.

# ISCHEMIC BOWEL DISEASE

Arvey I. Rogers, MD, FACP, and
Amar R. Deshpande, MD

# CHAPTER 58

## 1. What is ischemic bowel disease?

It is a disorder that results from a sustained reduction in mesenteric blood flow, reduced oxygen content of red blood cells distributed via the mesenteric arterial circulation, or mesenteric venous stasis, any of which can lead to tissue hypoxia and ischemic injury. This injury principally affects the small and/or large intestine and is manifested clinically as acute or chronic mid-abdominal pain (meal-induced), vomiting, sitophobia (fear of eating), weight loss, diarrhea, ileus, gastrointestinal bleeding, intestinal infarction, peritonitis, or fibrotic strictures.

## 2. Describe the gross anatomy of the mesenteric vascular system.

The mesenteric circulation consists of three major arteries (celiac axis, superior mesenteric artery [SMA], and inferior mesenteric artery [IMA]) and two major veins (superior [SMV] and inferior mesenteric [IMV] veins), connected by arterioles, capillaries, and venules. This cascade, referred to as the *splanchnic circulation*, courses through the mesentery, providing blood to and draining it from the digestive organs.

The celiac axis provides blood to the stomach, proximal duodenum, part of the pancreas, spleen, liver, gallbladder, and biliary tree. The rest of the duodenum and pancreas, the entire small intestine, and the large intestine up to the splenic flexure receive arterial blood via the SMA. The IMA provides blood to the remainder of the colon and rectum, the latter dually perfused by branches of the internal iliac arteries (Fig. 58-1).

The IMV joins the splenic vein, and the SMV and splenic vein anastomose to form the portal vein. As with the arterial supply, there is a dual venous drainage from the rectum into the systemic circulation through the inferior vena cava (IVC) via the internal iliac veins as well as into the portal circulation via the IMV.

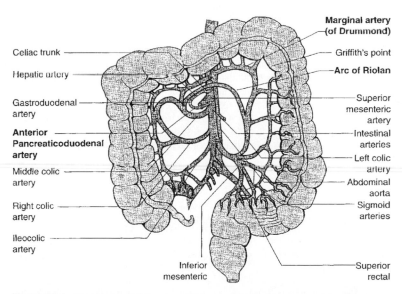

**Figure 58-1.** Mesenteric arterial anatomy. Three unpaired arterial branches of the aorta (celiac, superior mesenteric, and inferior mesenteric arteries) provide oxygenated blood to the small and large intestines. In most instances, veins parallel arteries. The superior mesenteric vein joins the splenic vein to form the portal vein, which enters the liver at its hilum. The inferior mesenteric vein joins the splenic vein near the juncture of the superior mesenteric and splenic veins. (Adapted from Rogers AI, Rosen CM: Mesenteric vascular insufficiency. In Schiller LR, ed.: Small Intestine, Current Medicine. Philadelphia, Lange, 1997, with permission.)

### 3. An extensive collateral circulatory system exists between the systemic and splanchnic vascular networks. Describe this system.

The several systemic-splanchnic and intersplanchnic collateral channels that anastomose the three major mesenteric arteries and their branches become apparent in the event of occlusion of one of the major branches (Fig. 58-2):

- *Pancreaticoduodenal arcade* provides collateral channels between the celiac axis and SMA (the superior pancreaticoduodenal arteries of the celiac axis collateralize with the inferior pancreaticoduodenal arteries of the SMA).
- *Marginal artery of Drummond*, composed of branches of the SMA and IMA, is a continuous arterial pathway that runs parallel to the entire colon.
- The middle colic branch of the SMA and the left colic branch of the IMA are anastomosed by the *arc of Riolan*.

Slowly developing occlusion of the mesenteric arteries, as in atherosclerotic disease, promotes the opening of these collateral channels to ensure the maintenance of arterial flow to and oxygenation of the small and large intestines. As a result, chronic mesenteric arterial insufficiency (i.e., abdominal angina) is distinctly unusual unless there is virtually complete occlusion of two of the three major mesenteric arteries, including the SMA.

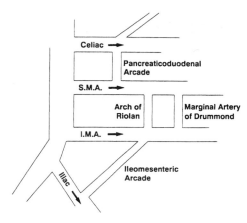

**Figure 58-2.** Schematic representation of collateral channels between the three major mesenteric arteries. The development of alternative anastomoses and collateral flow makes it theoretically possible that any single artery could supply all of the abdominal viscera with arterial blood given sufficient time and opportunity, that is, gradual occlusion of one or two of the other major arterial vessels. One major anastomosis exists between the left branch of the middle colic artery (from the superior mesenteric artery [SMA]) and the left colic artery from the inferior mesenteric artery (IMA), forming the meandering mesenteric artery or the arc of Riolan. Its demonstration by angiography indicates occlusion of the SMA or IMA. The marginal artery of Drummond is an arterial connection that provides a continuous channel of collateral flow via the vasa recta to the small and large intestines. The ileomesenteric arcade establishes an important anastomosis between the mesenteric and systemic circulation between the superior hemorrhoidal artery, a branch of the IMA, and the hypogastric artery, a branch of the iliac artery. (Adapted from Rogers AI, Rosen CM: Mesenteric vascular insufficiency. In Shiller LR, ed.: Small intestine, Current Medicine. Philadelphia, Lange, 1997, with permission.)

### 4. What is meant by *autoregulation*?

A unique intramucosal microcirculation functions to maintain oxygen delivery to the intestines under circumstances that compromise blood flow; it consists of arterioles, capillaries, and venules. Arterioles resist and therefore regulate the flow of blood through the tissues. A steep gradient of pressure exists between the artery and proximal portion of the arteriole. When arterial perfusion pressure is reduced, or if demand increases (as in the postprandial state), the arterioles dilate and underperfused capillaries are recruited, thereby compensating for the steep gradient in tissue oxygen levels and preventing tissue hypoxia. The venules store blood for short periods before it is returned to the heart; in the face of systemic hypotension, the tone of the venous system is increased, enhancing venous return to the heart to ensure maintenance of cardiac output. In this manner, blood flow can remain relatively constant, a concept known as *autoregulation* (Fig. 58-3).

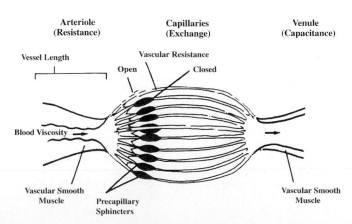

**Figure 58-3.** Intramural vascular anatomy. The assured delivery of oxygen-rich arterial blood to the various layers of the small and large intestinal wall during basal, meal-stimulated, and stress states depends on the interplay between various anatomic and physiologic factors, including blood viscosity, red blood cell oxygen saturation, arteriole length and resistance to flow, tone of precapillary sphincters, tone of vascular smooth muscle, and venous capacitance. (Adapted from Rogers AI, Rosen CM: Mesenteric vascular insufficiency. In Schiller, LR, ed.: Small intestine, Current Medicine. Philadelphia, Lange, 1997, with permission. The publisher is Lange [a book].)

## 5. What are the different varieties of ischemic bowel disease?

The different varieties are defined by the vascular component affected (i.e., arterial or venous), the duration of the reduction in flow through the affected vessel (i.e., acute or chronic), and the pathophysiology underlying the reduction in flow (i.e., occlusive or nonocclusive). Ischemic bowel disease can also be divided into clinical entities: acute mesenteric ischemia (AMI), the result of emboli, thrombi, or vasoconstriction; chronic mesenteric ischemia (CMI), usually from atherosclerotic disease; and colonic ischemia (CI), typically due to transient hypoperfusion (Fig. 58-4).

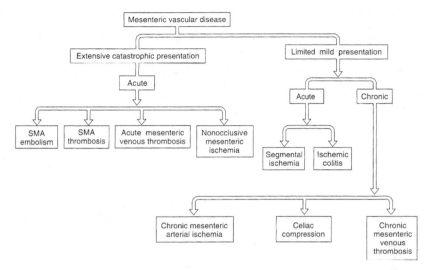

**Figure 58-4.** Classification of mesenteric vascular disease based on the extent of resulting ischemia. This particular classification, proposed by Williams may facilitate more effective evaluation and management by focusing on extent of gut involvement (From Williams LF. Mesenteric ischemia. Surg Clin North Am 1988;68:331–53.)

## 6. What clinical circumstances predispose to ischemic bowel disease?

### ARTERIAL

#### OCCLUSIVE MESENTERIC ISCHEMIA

- Embolus: cardiac dysrhythmias, valvular heart disease, myocardial infarction, mural thrombus, atrial myxoma, angiography
- Thrombosis: atherosclerosis, hypercoagulable states (e.g., pregnancy, hyperhomocysteinemia, antiphospholipid syndrome, birth control pills, neoplasms, polycythemia vera, essential thrombocytosis, and paroxysmal nocturnal hemoglobinuria), vascular aneurysms or dissections, vasculitides

#### NONOCCLUSIVE MESENTERIC ISCHEMIA

- Cardiac dysrhythmias, hypoperfusion (cardiogenic shock, hypovolemia, sepsis), and vasoconstricting drugs (digoxin, cocaine)

### VENOUS

- Hypercoagulable states (see Arterial entries, plus deficiencies of factor V Leiden, protein C or S, or antithrombin III), congestive heart failure, shock, portal hypertension, Budd-Chiari syndrome, malignancy, trauma, sclerotherapy, peritonitis, diverticulitis, pancreatitis, inflammatory bowel disease, intestinal obstruction, postoperative states, trauma

## 7. Describe the pathophysiology of occlusive AMI.

Intestinal ischemia results from tissue hypoxia, which occurs when blood volume, red blood cell (RBC) mass, flow rate, or RBC oxygen content is altered in the mesenteric arterial or venous circulation. As the radius of an artery decreases, regardless of etiology, the resistance to flow increases by a power of 4. Autoregulation (see Question 4) results in vasodilation to maintain flow up to a critical point; beyond this level, flow decreases. Decreased flow affecting the arterial vasculature can result from an obstruction caused by a thrombus (acute or chronic), embolus (acute), or transient vasoconstriction.

**8. What is abdominal angina? What is its clinical significance?**

Abdominal angina refers to chronic, recurring abdominal pain due to diminished arterial flow through mesenteric arteries narrowed by thrombosis. Pain radiating to the mid-back may be experienced as well. Affected patients are often dyslipidemic, diabetic, or chronic tobacco users and have associated peripheral vascular (arterial) disease. It can be viewed as intermittent claudication of the gut. The equivalent of an exercise stimulus is a meal; the pain is experienced 30 to 90 minutes postprandially and can last up to 4 hours. As food enters the stomach and the demand for oxygen increases, the flow of blood to the small intestine diminishes (*steal phenomenon*). Although minimal at first, postprandial abdominal pain increases progressively in severity over weeks to months. Profound and prolonged hypoxia of small intestinal mucosa may result in villous atrophy, leading to diarrhea, protein-losing enteropathy, steatorrhea, weight loss, and malnutrition.

**9. Describe the pathophysiology of nonocclusive mesenteric ischemia.**

Shock, profound hypovolemia, impaired cardiac output, and major thoracic or abdominal surgery are risk factors for intestinal hypoperfusion due to vasoconstriction of the mesenteric vasculature. This condition is known as nonocclusive mesenteric ischemia (NOMI), as no occluding thrombus or embolus is present. NOMI is encountered most commonly in patients who have undergone major abdominal or thoracic surgery complicated by pulmonary edema, cardiac dysrhythmia, or shock. Digoxin can aggravate mesenteric vasoconstriction; affected patients manifest the same symptoms and signs as those with occlusive disease.

**10. What should I know about mesenteric *venous* occlusion as a cause of ischemic bowel disease?**

Mesenteric venous occlusion is an infrequent cause of ischemic bowel disease. Just as in AMI, most patients present with severe mid-abdominal pain that is disproportionate to the minimal findings on physical examination of the abdomen. The abdominal pain may present acutely or subacutely (weeks to months). An accurate diagnosis requires a high index of suspicion triggered by the recognition of predisposing factors (see Question 6). Abdominopelvic computed tomography (CT) with contrast enhancement is the diagnostic test of choice, revealing findings consistent with venous occlusion in more than 90% of patients. These findings include thickening and contrast enhancement of the bowel wall (the result of delayed venous flow), enlarged SMV, thrombosis in the lumen of the SMV, and prominent collateral vessels. If there are no signs of intestinal infarction, patients should be treated with anticoagulation and possibly thrombolytics. If infarction is strongly suspected, patients should be operated on immediately to avert extensive irreversible ischemic injury and large volume resection.

**11. What is focal segmental (short segment) ischemia?**

The same pathophysiologic processes (embolus, thrombosis, venous occlusion, NOMI) capable of causing extensive bowel ischemia can also lead to a form of ischemia limited to a short segment of bowel. It is the result of the involvement of a few small arteries or veins and is known as focal segmental ischemia.

**12. What are the common symptoms of occlusive mesenteric ischemia?**

Presenting complaints vary with the etiology of the ischemia. Most patients with intestinal ischemia complicating acute embolic or thrombotic occlusion of the SMA present with the abrupt onset of severe abdominal pain, usually mid-abdominal in location and colicky in character. Simultaneously, involuntary evacuation of bowel contents may occur because of the intense tonic contractions of gut smooth muscle provoked by ischemia. Abdominal pain resulting from smooth muscle spasm presents with few abdominal physical findings. Abdominal distention and guaiac-positive stool *(late findings)* may be the only presenting signs in the demented or altered patient or the patient in the intensive care unit who is incapable of complaining of abdominal pain.

Patients with AMI secondary to thrombotic occlusion may have a history consistent with mesenteric angina, characterized by recurrent postprandial mid or diffuse abdominal pain, sometimes with a back-radiation component. Weight loss usually ensues because of sitophobia. Diarrhea, steatorrhea, and/or protein-losing enteropathy may complicate chronic ischemia-induced atrophy of the small intestinal mucosa.

Venous occlusive disease may have a more insidious onset, characterized by vague abdominal pain, diarrhea, and vomiting. It should be suspected in the appropriate clinical setting (e.g., abdominal sepsis, hypercoagulability, birth control pills). Venous disease results in ischemia due to massive influx of fluid into the bowel wall and lumen, thereby resulting in systemic hypotension and eventually reduced arterial inflow.

**13. What are the physical findings in a patient with mesenteric ischemia?**

These vary with the etiology and duration of the ischemia. In the appropriate clinical setting, acute occlusion of the SMA via embolism or thrombosis should be suspected when a striking disparity exists between the complaint of severe, diffuse abdominal pain and the minimal findings on abdominal examination. Early in the course of disease, only mild distention and normal or hyperactive bowel sounds are likely to be encountered; abdominal arterial bruits are too nonspecific to be of value. As the ischemic injury progresses, ileus develops, bowel sounds diminish, and abdominal distention worsens. Stools become guaiac positive, and even bloody diarrhea can occur. Hypotension and tachycardia signal volume sequestration, whereas fever and peritoneal signs indicate transmural injury and probable infarction.

Nonocclusive ischemia should be considered in the appropriate clinical setting (see Question 9). Early complaints are less dramatic than with acute arterial occlusion and physical findings vary with the duration of ischemia. Chronic, recurring abdominal pain on the basis of compromised flow through the SMA (abdominal angina) is not associated with specific physical findings. Most patients have evidence of peripheral vascular disease and may exhibit features of weight loss.

Physical findings in venous occlusive disease depend on its severity and etiology (e.g., congestive heart failure, stigmata of chronic liver disease and portal hypertension, hypercoagulability, abdominal mass). Tachycardia and hypotension are present if splanchnic volume has been sequestered.

### 14. Do laboratory findings help at all?

Laboratory findings in mesenteric ischemia are usually nonspecific and vary with the etiology, duration, severity, and extent of ischemic injury (i.e., which organs are involved and the potential for reversing precipitating and complicating events). In the early stages, there are no abnormalities other than those associated with the disorder that may have predisposed to mesenteric ischemia. Abnormal laboratory findings related to ischemia and/or infarction per se are the consequence of volume sequestration, tissue hypoxia, inflammation, and necrosis; they include hemoconcentration, leukocytosis, and lactic acidosis.

### 15. What are the differential diagnostic considerations in a patient with suspected AMI, and how do plain abdominal radiographs help elucidate the disorder?

Unless there is a clear diagnosis of ischemia in the absence of mimicking etiologies, abdominal plain films (flat and upright) should be obtained first. Helpful clues to diagnose the cause of abdominal pain that may be seen on plain radiographs of the abdomen are listed in Table 58-1.

Contrast-enhanced CT, Doppler ultrasound of mesenteric vessels, mesenteric angiography (magnetic resonance angiography or invasive arteriography), laparoscopy, and enteroscopy are among the diagnostic techniques most frequently used. The clinical circumstances dictate which tests to perform and in what sequence.

The administration of barium for a small bowel study should be avoided if a contrast CT or angiogram is being considered, as the oral contrast interferes with the ability to perform and/or interpret findings of these studies. As mentioned earlier (see Question 10), a dynamic, contrast-enhanced abdominal CT can be very valuable in diagnosing venous occlusive disease. Both plain abdominal radiographs and CT scans show only nonspecific abnormalities in 35% of patients with infarcted bowel. Angiography is superior to CT for the identification of mesenteric arterial occlusion or NOMI.

### 16. What is the role of magnetic resonance angiography (MRA) in patients with suspected abdominal angina?

Gadolinium-enhanced MRA may be useful in patients with chronic mesenteric ischemia who have severe iodine allergies. Three-dimensional reconstruction may also be feasible with MRA, allowing for visualization of the orifices of the splanchnic arteries. Correlation with conventional angiography is considered to be good. In patients with impaired kidney function, gadolinium may not cause the same contrast-induced nephropathy as iodine, but it can lead to an irreversible condition known as nephrogenic systemic fibrosis.

### Table 58-1. Radiographic Clues to Diagnosis

| DISORDER | FINDING ON PLAIN ABDOMINAL RADIOGRAPHS |
| --- | --- |
| Small bowel obstruction | Dilated loops of bowel with or without air-fluid levels<br>Stair-step overlapping of loops of small bowel<br>Termination of luminal small bowel air at transition point of obstruction |
| Pancreatitis | Sentinel loop of jejunum or colon cut-off sign |
| Volvulus | Characteristic jejunal, sigmoid, or cecal dilation (sigmoid volvulus—coffee bean sign) |
| Intra-abdominal sepsis (appendicitis, diverticulitis) | Air in the hepatic/portal venous system (portal venous gas) |
| Perforation | Free air under the diaphragm<br>Air dissecting between bowel loops or seen retroperitoneally |
| Bowel ischemia | Bowel wall thickening, loop separation, thumbprinting |
| Pneumatosis intestinalis and portal venous gas | Late signs and ominous for impending or frank infarction |
| Emphysematous cholecystitis | Air within the gallbladder wall, air-fluid level in the gallbladder (also caused by gas-forming organisms) |

### 17. Describe the role of Doppler ultrasound studies in diagnosis.

Duplex ultrasound (fasting and meal-stimulated) is a noninvasive test that can be used to assess the patency of and blood flow through the major mesenteric vessels. Its greatest use is in diagnosing multivessel stenosis in cases of suspected mesenteric angina; findings include narrowing or occlusion at a vessel origin and excessively turbulent flow. The value of transabdominal ultrasound is diminished in obese patients, as ultrasound waves must penetrate through body tissue to produce a quality diagnostic image.

### 18. What is the diagnostic role of endoscopy (sigmoidoscopy, colonoscopy, enteroscopy) and laparoscopy?

Conventional enteroscopy should not be undertaken for purposes of diagnosing small bowel ischemic disease. Despite the fact that scattered case reports describe diagnostic findings in selected clinical settings, enteroscopy can be dangerous, with a significant risk of perforation. Lower endoscopy (sigmoidoscopy or colonoscopy), however, is relatively safe and may be highly informative in patients with suspected ischemic colitis (see Questions 24–28).

Laparoscopy is another way to diagnose and assess the severity of ischemic injury to the gut. This invasive but relatively safe technique can diagnose full-thickness mesenteric injury, a late finding; its limitation is that it will miss earlier stages of potentially reversible ischemia. While the serosa can appear completely benign on laparoscopy, the mucosal surface may still be undergoing necrosis, as ischemic injury affects the mucosal surface first. Another concern of laparoscopy is that splanchnic blood flow decreases when intraperitoneal pressure exceeds 20 mm Hg, a level often reached after insufflation during laparoscopy.

### 19. When should you undertake invasive mesenteric angiographic studies?

Early diagnosis and definitive therapy are important in patients with suspected ischemic bowel disease. The mortality rate is quite high when diagnosis and therapy are delayed and when peritoneal signs and acidosis ensue. Angiography is the gold standard for the diagnosis of mesenteric arterial occlusion and sometimes differentiates an embolic from a thrombotic event. The angiographic demonstration of an abrupt cutoff of a major artery in the absence of collateral vessel enlargement suggests an acute embolic occlusion, whereas vessel narrowing by atherosclerosis in association with the development of prominent collaterals is more consistent with thrombosis. The venous phase of the angiogram may demonstrate veno-occlusive disease. The angiographic findings in NOMI include vessel narrowing or spasm and arterial beading.

On occasion, angiography also can be therapeutic, allowing for the selective infusion of vasodilating drugs (e.g., papaverine) or thrombolytic agents into the spastic or acutely occluded artery(ies), respectively, or the performance of therapeutic angioplasty, balloon embolectomy, or stent placement. The infusion of thrombolytic agents should probably be limited to tertiary care centers with technical expertise, to patients considered poor surgical candidates without peritoneal signs, and to those in whom the ischemic event is considered to be reversible and/or of short duration. Angiography is an invasive procedure associated with definite risks. In the patient population with atherosclerotic mesenteric arterial disease, atherosclerosis commonly involves the femoral artery (the usual site of entry for the angiographic catheter as well), which can make accessing the mesenteric system challenging and possibly cause the release of an arterial plaque resulting in distal embolic arterial occlusion. Also, infusion of iodinated contrast in the presence of hypovolemia, impaired cardiac output, or reduced renal blood flow increases the likelihood of developing renal insufficiency, especially if the patient is diabetic. Nonetheless, angiography is the only definitive technique short of exploratory surgery to establish the diagnosis of mesenteric occlusive or nonocclusive ischemia early in the disease and to provide potentially therapeutic interventions.

### 20. Is there any medical treatment for mesenteric ischemia?

Yes, there are conservative measures that can be undertaken in mesenteric ischemia:

- Management of underlying disease (e.g., aspirin and Plavix for vascular disease, correcting dyslipidemic states, optimizing heart failure therapy, controlling volume status, treating sepsis)
- Anticoagulation for arterial thromboembolic and venous occlusive disease
- Adequate pain control (being careful to minimize opiates, which inhibit peristalsis and aggravate ischemia)
- Theoretical: eat small meals, suppress gastric acid secretion to reduce mucosal oxygen demand during meals, vasodilators, refrain from smoking

### 21. What is the role of angioplasty and stenting in the management of ischemic bowel disease?

Percutaneous transluminal angioplasty with or without stent placement may have a role in some selected patients with intestinal angina. Lesions located at the aortic orifices of the mesenteric arteries may not be as amenable to dilation and angioplasty because of their fixed diameter, but more distal lesions can be dilated without the morbidity and mortality of surgical intervention.

### 22. When should a patient with ischemic bowel disease be sent to the operating room?

A clinical picture compatible with acute ischemic bowel disease when other diagnoses have been excluded should prompt angiography. If the findings are amenable to nonoperative management (e.g., NOMI treated with papaverine infusion or acute embolism treated with embolectomy or thrombolysis) and there is no sign of bowel necrosis, patients can be treated nonsurgically. Otherwise, patients should be taken to the operating room to:

- Assess the degree and extent of gut injury (bowel viability may be assessed by the injection of fluorescein dye)
- Identify the site of and relieve arterial occlusion
- Resect irreversibly damaged bowel and preserve presumably viable bowel
- Undergo revascularization

Surgical revascularization probably should be limited to a select group of patients. Indications include typical, disabling symptoms of abdominal angina (chronic postprandial abdominal pain, sitophobia, weight loss), angiographic evidence of occlusion of at least two of the three major mesenteric arteries (inclusive of the SMA), and an acceptable risk of surgery. Whether multiple vessels or only the SMA should be revascularized is controversial. Keep in mind that resection of long segments of bowel (ileum more so than jejunum) can result in short bowel syndrome and its myriad consequences.

### 23. What is meant by a *second-look* operation?
At the time of initial surgery there may have been some doubt about the viability of a segment of bowel left intact, whether or not revascularization had been attempted. Under such circumstances, the patient may undergo a second operation 24 to 48 hours later to assess bowel viability. This is an area of ongoing, active controversy.

### 24. Can ischemia be isolated to the colon?
Yes. In fact, ischemic colitis is the most common form of intestinal ischemia. Most affected patients are elderly with impaired cardiac output, and the underlying pathophysiology is usually nonocclusive in nature. However, in the younger population, the etiology can be occlusive (e.g., sickle cell disease, estrogen use, pregnancy, hypercoagulable states) or nonocclusive (e.g., cocaine use, long-distance running, vasculitis).

### 25. How does ischemic colitis present clinically?
The most common presenting symptoms are the sudden onset of cramping, mild, left lower quadrant abdominal pain and the urge to defecate. Bright red blood per rectum or hematochezia may be seen. Abdominal tenderness can be elicited over the involved segment of bowel. In the postoperative state, mild symptoms are often dismissed. The differential diagnosis includes infectious colitis, diverticulitis, and inflammatory bowel disease.

### 26. How do you confirm a suspected diagnosis of ischemic colitis?
Abdominal plain films may demonstrate "thumbprinting" along the wall of an affected colonic segment (often the splenic flexure), the result of subepithelial edema and hemorrhage. If ischemic colitis is suspected and there are no clinical features to suggest peritoneal irritation, a colonoscopy should be undertaken to confirm the diagnosis. Any region of the colon may be affected, but the key endoscopic feature of ischemic colitis is the tendency for *segmental* distribution, classically at the watershed areas between the arterial distributions of the SMA and IMA. The rectosigmoid (20%), descending colon (20%), splenic flexure (11%), and all three in combination (14%) are affected most commonly. Changes may be isolated to the rectum (6%) or right colon (8%). Flexible sigmoidoscopy may be nondiagnostic in those with more proximal disease (e.g., isolated to the splenic flexure). When the rectosigmoid region is involved with sparing of the rectum, the diagnosis is strongly suspected (the rectum is infrequently involved because of its dual blood supply derived from the inferior mesenteric and internal iliac arterial branches). Barium enema is less sensitive than colonoscopy for detecting mucosal changes but may reveal thumbprinting abnormalities. Angiography is not indicated in ischemic colitis because the predisposing nonocclusive vascular factors are often not demonstrable by angiography once ischemic injury has occurred (Fig. 58-5).

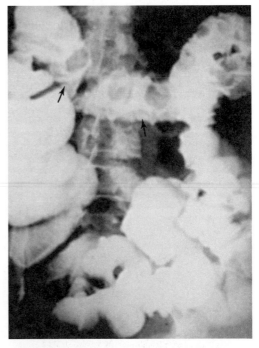

**Figure 58-5.** Fluoroscopic view of thumbprinting in ischemic colitis. Note the appearance of thumbprints in the transverse colon (*arrows*) seen on barium enema. (From Brandt LJ: Intestinal ischemia. In Feldman M, Friedman LS, Brandt LJ [eds]: Sleisenger & Fordtran's Gastrointestinal and Liver Disease. Philadelphia, Elsevier, 2006, pp. 2575–2576.)

**27. What are the sequelae of ischemic colitis? Can anything be done to modify the course of the disease?**

Optimizing cardiac function is imperative; impaired cardiac output and cardiac dysrhythmias should be corrected. Factors predisposing to vasoconstriction, digoxin therapy, vasopressor agents, and hypovolemia should be avoided when possible. Vasodilating agents are ineffective because low colonic blood flow has often already returned to normal by the time the ischemia has occurred. The bowel should be placed at rest, broad-spectrum antibiotics and intravenous fluids should be administered, and a distended colon should be decompressed colonoscopically, by placement of a rectal tube, or by rolling the patient from a supine position to right and left lateral decubitus positions. If the precipitating event is occlusive in nature, the underlying etiology should be corrected, possibly including prolonged anticoagulation.

Ischemic colitis is reversible in more than 50% (and maybe up to 70% to 80%) of patients whose symptoms abate within 24 to 48 hours; in these patients, healing occurs without stricture in 1 to 2 weeks. The severely injured colon may require 1 to 6 months to heal completely. Irreversible damage occurs in less than 50% and can lead to toxic megacolon, gangrene and perforation, fulminant colitis (all ominous signs), and ischemic stricture; the course cannot be predicted at the time of initial presentation. Isolated right-sided ischemic colitis has a higher mortality and need for surgery, possibly because its pathophysiology may be more closely related to acute mesenteric ischemia.

**28. When is surgery indicated in patients with ischemic colitis?**

Surgery is indicated in patients who present with or develop peritoneal signs, massive bleeding, gangrene or perforation, evidence of toxic megacolon, or fulminant colitis. It should be considered even with apparent healing in patients who have recurrent bouts of sepsis and in patients who fail to respond to conservative measures over 2 to 3 weeks. Symptomatic colon strictures may also warrant surgical or endoscopic correction (e.g., balloon dilation or stent placement).

## BIBLIOGRAPHY

1. Brandt LJ, Boley SJ. AGA technical review on intestinal ischemia. Gastroenterology 2000;118:954–68.
2. Brandt LJ, Boley SJ. Sleisenger & Fordtran's Gastrointestinal and Liver Disease. 7th ed. Philadelphia: Saunders; 2002.
3. Burns BJ, Brandt LJ. Intestinal ischemia. Gastroenterol Clin North Am 2003;32:1127–43.
4. Chang RW, Chang JB, Longo WE. Update in management of mesenteric ischemia. World J Gastroenterol 2006;2:3243–7.
5. Chang JB, Stein TA. Mesenteric ischemia: Acute and chronic. Ann Vasc Surg 2003;17:323–8.
6. Herbert GS, Steele SR. Acute and chronic mesenteric ischemia. Surg Clin North Am 2007;87:1115–34.
7. Jakribettuu VS, Levine JS. Ischemia and ischemic colitis. Clinical Gastroenterology and Hepatology. Weinstein WM, Hawkey CJ, Bosch J, eds. Spain: Mosby; 2005.
8. Kim AY, Ha HK. Evaluation of suspected mesenteric ischemia: Efficacy of radiologic studies. Radiol Clin North Am 2003;41:327–42.
9. Kougias P, El Sayed HF, Zhou W, et al. Management of chronic mesenteric ischemia: The role of endovascular therapy. J Endovasc Ther 2007;14:395–405.
10. Lefkovitz Z, Cappell MS, Lookstein R, et al. Radiologic diagnosis and treatment of gastrointestinal hemorrhage and ischemia. Med Clin North Am 2002;86:1357–99.
11. Mallick IH, Yang W, Winslet MC, et al. Ischemia-reperfusion injury of the intestine and protective strategies against injury. Dig Dis Sci 2004;49:1359–77.
12. Oldenburg WA, Lau LL, Rodenberg TJ, et al. Acute mesenteric ischemia: A clinical review. Arch Intern Med 2004;164:1054–62.
13. Sotiriadis J, Brandt LJ, Behin DS, et al. Ischemic colitis has a worse prognosis when isolated to the right side of the colon. Am J Gastro 2007;102:2247–52.
14. Sreenarasimhaiah J. Chronic mesenteric ischemia. Best Pract Res Clin Gastroenterol 2005;19:283–95.
15. Sreenarasimhaiah J. Diagnosis and management of intestinal ischemic disorders. BMJ 2003;326:1372–6.
16. vanBockel JH, Geelkerken RH, Kolkman JJ. Splanchnic vascular disorders. In: Clinical Gastroenterology and Hepatology. Weinstein WM, Hawkey CJ, Bosch J, eds. Spain: Mosby; 2005. pp. 479–84.
17. Williams LF. Mesenteric ischemia. Surg Clin North Am 1988;68:331–53.

# NUTRITION, MALNUTRITION, AND PROBIOTICS

## CHAPTER 59

*Peter R. McNally, DO, FACP, FACG*

### 1. What is meant by *nutritional status*?

Nutritional status reflects how well nutrient intake contributes to body composition and function in the face of the existing metabolic needs. The four major body compartments are water, protein, mineral, and fat. The first three compose the lean body mass (LBM); functional capacity resides in a portion of the LBM called the body-cell mass. Nutritionists concentrate their efforts on preservation or restoration of this vital component.

### 2. Define *malnutrition.*

Malnutrition refers to states of overnutrition (obesity) or undernutrition relative to body requirements, resulting in dysfunction.

### 3. How do different types of malnutrition affect function and outcome?

- *Marasmus* is protein–calorie undernutrition associated with significant physical wasting of energy stores (adipose tissue and somatic muscle protein) but preservation of visceral and serum proteins. Patients are not edematous and may have mild immune dysfunction.
- *Hypoalbuminemic malnutrition* occurs with stressed metabolism and is common in hospitalized patients. They may have adequate energy stores and body weight but have expanded extracellular space, depleted intracellular mass, edema, altered serum protein levels, and immune dysfunction.
- A similar state of relative protein deficiency occurs in classic *kwashiorkor*, in which caloric provision is adequate but quantity and quality of protein are not.

### 4. How do you perform a simple nutritional assessment?

Simple bedside assessment may be as valuable for predicting nutrition-associated outcomes as sophisticated composition and function tests. Two popular methods, the Subjective Global Assessment (SGA) and the Mini Nutritional Assessment (MNA) are simple-to-use validated nutritional assessment tools. Each incorporates basic questions about weight history, intake, gastrointestinal (GI) symptoms, disease state, functional level, and a physical examination to classify patients as well-nourished, mildly to moderately malnourished, or severely malnourished. See Figure 59-1.

A weight history, estimate of recent intake, brief physical exam, consideration of disease stress/medications, and assessments of functional status and wound healing allow a good estimate of nutritional status. They predict the risk for malnutrition-associated complications as well as or better than laboratory data. Poor intake for longer than 1 to 2 weeks, a weight loss of more than 10%, or a weight less than 80% of desirable warrants closer nutritional assessment and follow-up.

### 5. Serum proteins are a marker of overall nutritional health. Which plasma proteins will have the most sensitive turnover rate?

| | |
|---|---|
| Ferritin | 30 hours |
| Retinol binding protein | 2 days |
| Prealbumin | 2 to 3 days |
| Transferrin | 8 days |
| Albumin | 18 days |

### 6. What simple blood tests offer an *instant* nutritional assessment?

Serum albumin → abnormal if <3.5 g%

Total lymphocyte count → abnormal if <1500/mm³

NESTLÉ NUTRITION SERVICES

**Nestlé**

# Mini Nutritional Assessment
## MNA®

| Last name: | First name: | Sex: | Date: |

| Age: | Weight, kg: | Height, cm: | I.D. Number: |

*Complete the screen by filling in the boxes with the appropriate numbers.*
*Add the numbers for the screen. If score is 11 or less, continue with the assessment to gain a Malnutrition Indicator Score.*

### Screening

A  Has food intake declined over the past 3 months due to loss of appetite, digestive problems, chewing or swallowing difficulties?
0 = severe loss of appetite
1 = moderate loss of appetite
2 = no loss of appetite □

B  Weight loss during the last 3 months
0 = weight loss greater than 3 kg (6.6 lbs)
1 = does not know
2 = weight loss between 1 and 3 kg (2.2 and 6.6 lbs)
3 = no weight loss □

C  Mobility
0 = bed or chair bound
1 = able to get out of bed/chair but does not go out
2 = goes out □

D  Has suffered psychological stress or acute disease in the past 3 months
0 = yes        2 = no □

E  Neuropsychological problems
0 = severe dementia or depression
1 = mild dementia
2 = no psychological problems □

F  Body Mass Index (BMI) (weight in kg) / (height in m)²
0 = BMI less than 19
1 = BMI 19 to less than 21
2 = BMI 21 to less than 23
3 = BMI 23 or greater □

**Screening score** (subtotal max. 14 points) □ □
12 points or greater   Normal – not at risk – no need to complete assessment
11 points or below   Possible malnutrition – continue assessment

### Assessment

G  Lives independently (not in a nursing home or hospital)
0 = no        1 = yes □

H  Takes more than 3 prescription drugs per day
0 = yes        1 = no □

I  Pressure sores or skin ulcers
0 = yes        1 = no □

Ref.: Guigoz Y, Vellas B and Garry PJ. 1994. Mini Nutritional Assessment: A practical assessment tool for grading the nutritional state of elderly patients. *Facts and Research in Gerontology*. Supplement #2:15-59.
Rubenstein LZ, Harker J, Guigoz Y and Vellas B. Comprehensive Geriatric Assessment (CGA) and the MNA: An Overview of CGA, Nutritional Assessment, and Development of a Shortened Version of the MNA. In: "Mini Nutritional Assessment (MNA): Research and Practice in the Elderly". Vellas B, Garry PJ and Guigoz Y, editors. Nestlé Nutrition Workshop Series. Clinical & Performance Programme, vol. 1. Karger, Bâle, in press.

© Nestlé, 1994, Revision 1998. N67200 12/99 10M

J  How many full meals does the patient eat daily?
0 = 1 meal
1 = 2 meals
2 = 3 meals □

K  Selected consumption markers for protein intake
• At least one serving of dairy products (milk, cheese, yogurt) per day?   yes □ no □
• Two or more servings of legumes or eggs per week?   yes □ no □
• Meat, fish or poultry every day   yes □ no □
0.0 = if 0 or 1 yes
0.5 = if 2 yes
1.0 = if 2 yes □ . □

L  Consumes two or more servings of fruits or vegetables per day?
0 = no        1 = yes □

M  How much fluid (water, juice, coffee, tea, milk…) is consumed per day?
0.0 = less than 3 cups
0.5 = 3 to 5 cups
1.0 = more than 5 cups □ . □

N  Mode of feeding
0 = unable to eat without assistance
1 = self-fed with some difficulty
2 = self-fed without any problem □

O  Self view of nutritional status
0 = views self as being malnourished
1 = is uncertain of nutritional state
2 = views self as having no nutritional problem □

P  In comparison with other people of the same age, how does the patient consider his/her health status?
0.0 = not as good
0.5 = does not know
1.0 = as good
2.0 = better □ . □

Q  Mid-arm circumference (MAC) in cm
0.0 = MAC less than 21
0.5 = MAC 21 to 22
1.0 = MAC 22 or greater □ . □

R  Calf circumference (CC) in cm
0 = CC less than 31        1 = CC 31 or greater □

**Assessment** (max. 16 points) □ □ . □

**Screening score** □ □

**Total Assessment** (max. 30 points) □ □ . □

**Malnutrition Indicator Score**
17 to 23.5 points        at risk of malnutrition □
Less than 17 points      malnourished □

**Figure 59-1.** Mini Nutritional Assessment.

**7. List desirable weights for men and women (according to the 1983 Metropolitan Height and Weight Tables).**
• Men: 135 lb for the first 5 feet 3 inches of height plus 3 lb per additional inch (±10%)
• Women: 119 lb for the first 5 feet 0 inches of height plus 3 lb per additional inch (±10%)

Basal energy expenditure (BEE) in calories can be derived from the Harris Benedict equation:

$$\text{BEE for } \male : 66 + [13.7 \times \text{weight (kg)}] + [5.0 \times \text{height (cm)}] - [(6.8 \times \text{age})] = \text{kcal/day}$$

$$\text{BEE for } \female : 655 + [9.6 \times \text{weight (kg)}] + [1.8 \times \text{height (cm)}] - [(4.7 \times \text{age})] = \text{kcal/day}$$

$$\text{BEE} \times \text{Stress factor} = \text{daily caloric need}$$

| STRESS | FACTOR |
|---|---|
| Mild stress | (× 1 to 1.3) |
| Moderate stress | (× 1.3 to 1.4) |
| Severe stress | (× 1.5) |

See Table 59-1.

**Table 59-1.** Quick Formulas for Calculation of Protein and Caloric Requirements

| ILLNESS SEVERITY | PROTEIN, G/KG/DAY | CALORIES, KCAL/KG/DAY |
|---|---|---|
| Minimal | 0.8 | 20 to 25 |
| Moderate | 1 to 1.5 | 25 to 30 |
| Severe | 1.5 to 2.5 | 30 to 35 |

## 8. Describe the types of commonly prescribed oral diets.

The clear liquid diet supplies fluid and calories in a form that requires minimal digestion, stimulation, and elimination by the GI tract. It provides about 600 cal and 150 g carbohydrate but inadequate protein, vitamins, and minerals. Clear liquids are hyperosmolar; diluting the beverages and eating slower may minimize GI symptoms. If clear liquids are needed for longer than 3 days, a dietitian can assist with supplementation.

The full liquid diet is used often in progressing from clear liquids to solid foods. It also may be used in patients with chewing problems, gastric stasis, or partial ileus. Typically, the diet provides more than 2000 cal and 70 g protein. It may be adequate in all nutrients (except fiber), especially if a high-protein supplement is added. Patients with lactose intolerance need special substitutions. Progression to solid foods should be accomplished with modifications or supplementation, as needed.

## 9. What is a *hidden* source of calories in the intensive care unit?

Watch out for significant amounts of lipid calories from propofol, a sedative in 10% lipid emulsion (1.1 kcal/mL).

## 10. Summarize the typical findings in deficiency or excess of various micronutrients

See Table 59-2.

## 11. What are the nutritional concerns in patients with short bowel syndrome?

Loss of bowel surface puts the patient at great risk for dehydration and malnutrition. The small bowel averages 600 cm in length and absorbs about 10 L/day of ingested and secreted fluids. A patient may tolerate substantial loss of small bowel, although preservation of less than 2 feet with an intact colon and ileocecal valve or less than 5 feet in the absence of the colon and ileocecal valve may make survival impossible when just the enteral route of nutrition is used. In addition, the loss of the distal ileum precludes absorption of bile acids and vitamin $B_{12}$. Remaining bowel, especially ileum, may adapt its absorptive ability over several years, but underlying disease may hamper this process.

## 12. Describe the management of nutritional problems in patients with short bowel syndrome.

Therapy in the acute postsurgical phase is aimed at intravenous fluid and electrolyte restoration. Parenteral nutrition may be required while the remaining gut function is assessed and adaptation takes place. Attempts at oral feeding should include frequent, small meals with initial limitations in fluid and fat consumption. Osmolar sugars (e.g., sorbitol), lactose, and high-oxalate foods are best avoided. In patients with small bowel–colon continuity, increased use of complex carbohydrates may allow the salvage of a few hundred calories from colonic production and absorption of short-chain fatty acids. Antimotility drugs and gastric acid suppression should be used if stool output remains high. Oral rehydration with glucose- and sodium-containing fluids (e.g., sports drinks) may help to prevent dehydration. Pancreatic enzymes, bile acid–binding resins (if bile acids are irritating the colon), and octreotide injections may play a role in selected cases. If oral diets fail, the use of elemental feedings may enhance absorption and nutritional state. Studies of gut rehabilitation with growth hormone and glutamine, as well as intestinal or combined intestinal-liver transplantation, are available at selected centers.

## 13. Describe the approach to nutritional support in patients with acute pancreatitis.

Pancreatitis can resemble other cases of stressed metabolism. If severe pancreatitis precludes the resumption of food intake beyond 4 to 5 days, consideration should be given to nutrition support. The route of feeding remains controversial; neither bowel/pancreatic rest nor nutritional support has been shown conclusively to alter the clinical course beyond improvement of the nutritional state. Several recent randomized trials suggest that distal (jejunal) enteral feeding may be tolerated as well as bowel rest/total parenteral nutrition (TPN), with fewer complications. See Figure 59-2. The enteral route may be tried in the absence of GI dysfunction (e.g., ileus). Energy expenditure is variable, but most likely only 20%

**Table 59-2.** Vitamin and Mineral Deficiencies and Toxicities

| MICRONUTRIENT | DEFICIENCY | TOXICITY |
|---|---|---|
| Vitamin A | Follicular hyperkeratosis, night blindness, corneal drying, keratomalacia | Dermatitis, xerosis, hair loss, joint pain, hyperostosis, edema, hypercalcemia, hepatomegaly, pseudotumor |
| Vitamin D | Rickets, osteomalacia, hypophosphatemia, muscle weakness | Fatigue, headache, hypercalcemia, bone decalcification |
| Vitamin E | Hemolytic anemia, myopathy, ataxia, ophthalmoplegia, retinopathy, areflexia | Rare: possible interference with vitamin K, arachidonic acid metabolism; headache, myopathy |
| Vitamin K | Bruisability, prolonged prothrombin time | Rapid intravenous infusion: possible flushing, cardiovascular collapse |
| Vitamin C | Scurvy: poor wound healing, perifollicular hemorrhage, gingivitis, dental defects, anemia, joint pain | Diarrhea; possible hyperoxaluria, uricosuria; interference with glucose, occult blood tests; dry mouth, dental erosion |
| Vitamin B$_1$ (thiamine) | Dry beriberi (polyneuropathy): anorexia, low temperature<br>Wet beriberi (high-output congestive heart failure): lactic acidosis<br>Wernicke-Korsakoff syndrome: ataxia, nystagmus, memory loss, confabulation, ophthalmoplegia | Large-dose intravenous: anorexia, ataxia, ileus, headache, irritability |
| Vitamin B$_2$ (riboflavin) | Seborrheic dermatitis, stomatitis, cheilosis, geographic tongue, burning eyes, anemia | None |
| Vitamin B$_3$ (niacin) | Anorexia, lethargy, burning sensations, glossitis, headache, stupor, seizures<br>Pellagra: diarrhea, pigmented dermatitis, dementia | Hyperglycemia, hyperuricemia, GI symptoms, peptic ulcer, flushing, liver dysfunction |
| Vitamin B$_6$ (pyridoxine) | Peripheral neuritis, seborrhea, glossitis, stomatitis, anemia, CNS/EEG changes, seizures | Metabolic dependency, sensory neuropathy |
| Vitamin B$_{12}$ | Glossitis, paresthesias, CNS changes, megaloblastic anemia, depression, diarrhea | None |
| Folic acid | Glossitis, intestinal mucosal dysfunction, megaloblastic anemia | Antagonizes antiepileptic drugs, decreases zinc absorption |
| Biotin | Scaly dermatitis, hair loss, papillae atrophy, myalgia, paresthesias, hypercholesterolemia | None |
| Pantothenic acid | Malaise, GI symptoms, cramps, paresthesias | Diarrhea |
| Calcium | Paresthesias, tetany, seizures, osteopenia, arrhythmia | Hypercalciuria, GI symptoms, lethargy |
| Phosphorus | Hemolysis, muscle weakness, ophthalmoplegia, osteomalacia | Diarrhea |
| Magnesium | Paresthesias, tetany, seizures, arrhythmia | Diarrhea, muscle weakness, arrhythmia |
| Iron | Fatigue, dyspnea, glossitis, anemia, koilonychia | Iron overload (hepatic, cardiac), possible oxidation damage |
| Iodine | Goiter, hypothyroidism | Goiter, hypo/hyperthyroidism |
| Zinc | Lethargy, anorexia, loss of taste/smell, rash, hypogonadism, poor wound healing, immunosuppression | Impaired copper, iron metabolism, reduced HDL, immunosuppression |
| Copper | Anemia, neutropenia, lethargy, depigmentation, connective tissue weakness | GI symptoms, hepatic damage |
| Chromium | Glucose intolerance, neuropathy, hyperlipidemia | None |
| Selenium | Keshan's cardiomyopathy, muscle weakness | GI symptoms |
| Manganese | Possible weight loss, dermatitis, hair disturbances | Inhalation injury only |
| Molybdenum | Possible headache, vomiting, CNS changes | Interferes with copper metabolism, possible gout |
| Fluorine | Increased dental caries | Teeth mottling, possible bone integrity/fluorosis |

CNS, central nervous system; EEG, electroencephalography; GI, gastrointestinal; HDL, high-density lipoproteins.

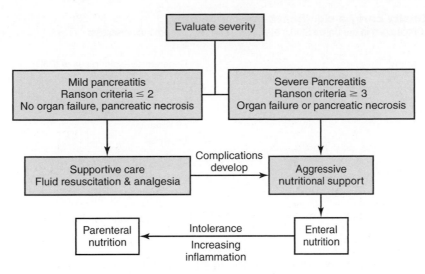

**Figure 59-2.** Nutrition for pancreatitis.

to 30% above basal. Use partial parenteral nutrition (PPN) or TPN if the enteral approach fails. Experiments suggest that parenteral nutrition, including intravenous fat, elicits little significant pancreatic secretion; however, all patients with pancreatitis should be monitored to exclude severe hypertriglyceridemia.

14. **What adverse GI effects may be encountered in a patient using herbal supplements?**
It is estimated that one third to one half of the U.S. population uses herbal products in supplementary form and that 60% to 75% do not inform health care providers. Because herbal products are not regulated and their composition is not standardized, toxicity data are less clear than with regulated pharmaceuticals. However, popular products that may cause adverse GI effects include saw palmetto, *Ginkgo biloba* (nonspecific GI upset), garlic (nausea, diarrhea), ginseng (nausea, diarrhea), aloe (diarrhea, abdominal pain), and guar gum (obstruction). In addition, hepatotoxicity (ranging from asymptomatic enzyme elevation to fulminant necrosis) has been documented with germander, chaparral, senna, atractylis, and *Callilepis*. Hepatotoxicity associated with the use of valerian, mistletoe, skullcap, and various Chinese herbal mixtures has been noted but awaits a cause-and-effect confirmation. The pyrrolizidine alkaloids in *Crotalaria, Senecio, Heliotropium*, and comfrey have long been implicated in cases of veno-occlusive liver disease.

15. **How is *obesity* defined, and how common is it among U.S. residents?**
Body mass index (BMI) has become the standard of measurement for obesity.

$$BMI = Weight (kg) \times body surface area (m^2)$$

- A BMI higher than $30 \, kg/m^2$ is defined as obese.

| BODY MASS INDEX CATEGORY | BMI, KG/M² | | | | |
|---|---|---|---|---|---|
| Normal | 18.5 to 24.9 | | | | |
| Overweight | 25 to 29.9 | | | | |
| Obesity | 30 to 39.9 | | | | |
| Morbid/extreme | 40 to 49.9 | | | | |
| Superobesity | >50 | | | | |
| ADULTS | 1988–1994 | 1995 | 1999–2000 | 2000 | 2008 |
| Obese | 22.9% | 15.9% | 30.5% | 20% | 26.6% |
| Overweight | 55.9% | 35.5% | 64.5% | 36.7% | 36.6% |
| Extremely obese | 2.9% | | 4.7% | | |

While the number of adults has doubled since 1980, the number of obese adults has quadrupled; approximately 72 million adults in the United States are obese: http: //apps. need. cdc. gov/brfss/

16. **In 2007, what U.S. state had an obesity rate of less than 20%?**
Colorado. Open the link showing the percentage of each state's population that is obese: http://www.cdc.gov/nccdphp/dnpa/obesity/trend/maps/

### 17. Does obesity carry a significant risk for death?

Yes, 300,000 persons in the United States die annually from obesity-related diseases:

| | |
|---|---|
| Cardiomyopathy | Degenerative joint disease (DJD) |
| Coronary artery disease | Immobility |
| Dyslipidemia | Depression |
| Hypertension | Low self-esteem |
| Diabetes | Malignancy |
| Infertility | Dyspnea |
| Fatty liver | Obstructive sleep apnea |
| Deep vein thrombosis (DVT) | Obesity hypoventilation |
| Gallstones | Chronic fatigue |
| Pulmonary embolus | Venous stasis |
| Urinary stress incontinence | Gastroesophageal reflux disease (GERD) |

### 18. What are the medical therapies for obesity?

Dietary restriction of calories, while maintaining adequate protein, fluid electrolyte, mineral, and vitamin intake, is the key. A sensible weight reduction program targets gradual weight reduction by behavior modification, including dietary and activity changes. Numerous fad diets claim success, but key to the weight loss is patient commitment and total lifestyle modification.

### 19. What are the surgical options for obesity?

Bariatric surgery dates to the 1950s when intestinal bypass was first performed. The total weight lost correlates with the total length of bowel bypassed. Gastric bypass (GBP) is the most common weight loss surgery performed in the United States. See Chapter 79.

### 20. What are the National Institutes of Health consensus criteria thought to be viable indications for bariatric surgery?

Failure of a major weight-loss program plus morbid obesity BMI >40 kg/m²

**or**

Failure of a major weight-loss program plus BMI >35 kg/m²

**and**

Obesity-related comorbidities*

### 21. What is the operative mortality of GBP surgery?

Operative mortality ranges from 0.3% to 1.6%, and perioperative complications occur in 10% of patients:

#### PERIOPERATIVE COMPLICATIONS

- Splenic injury
- Pneumonia
- Wound infection
- Thrombotic events
- Anastomotic leaks
- Hemorrhage
- Pulmonary failure
- Cardiac events
- Wound dehiscence
- Thrombocytopenia
- Intra-abdominal sepsis
- Death

---

*Hypertension, type 2 diabetes mellitus, DJD and disc disease, GERD, sleep apnea, obesity hypoventilation, severe venous stasis, abdominal wall hernias, and pseudotumor cerebri.

## 22. What are medical benefits of bariatric surgery?

- *Diabetes*: 83% of patients with non–insulin-dependent diabetes mellitus (NIDDM) and 99% of those with glucose intolerance maintained normal levels of plasma glucose, glycosylated hemoglobin, and insulin—88% of diabetics no longer required medication.
- *Cardiovascular*: 15% decrease in cholesterol, 50% decrease in triglycerides, hypertension 58% rx treated to 14%
- *Pulmonary*: 14% preoperative have obstructive or hypoventilation syndrome, with most improved

## 23. What nutritional deficiencies are seen with bariatric surgery?

- Fat malabsorption
- $B_{12}$ deficiency: 37% develop $B_{12}$ deficiency
- Folate deficiency
- Fat-soluble vitamin deficiency
- Iron deficiency and anemia seen in 33% and 30%, respectively

### RECOMMENDED SUPPLEMENTS

- Iron 325 mg twice daily
- $B_{12}$ as part of a multivitamin
- Folate as part of a multivitamin
- 1200 to 1500 mg calcium in divided doses over the day. Calcium citrate is better absorbed in low acid environment.

## 24. Is the number of bacteria populating the human intestine greater than the total number of cells in the human body?

Yes. The average human body consists of about 10 trillion cells, while there are about 10 times that number of microorganisms in the gut.

## 25. What value is gut microbiotica to human existence?

There are estimated to be 200 to 300 colonic species of bacteria in the gut, each with a unique function. See Table 59-3.

## 26. Is there a link between gut microbiotica and obesity?

Yes. Intestinal microbiotica of obese *(ob/ob)* mice were examined and compared to wild-type *(WT/WT)* mice and it was found that *ob/ob* animals have a 50% reduction in the abundance of Bacteroidetes and a proportional increase in Firmicutes species that are more efficient in extracting calories from otherwise nondigestible polysaccharides in our diet and ultimately generating short-chain fatty acids (SCFAs).

## 27. What is the definition of a *probiotic*?

Live microbial food supplements that beneficially affect the host by improving intestinal microbial balance but must fulfill the following criteria:

- When ingested, survive and colonize gut, but rapidly disappear when discontinued
- Human origin
- Do not produce plasmids

## 28. What are some of the common probiotics?

Probiotics are generally derived from four bacterial species: *Lactobacillus, Bifidobacter, Streptococcus,* and *Escherichia coli.* See Table 59-4.

| Table 59-3. Commensal Effects of Gut Microbiotica on Humans | |
| --- | --- |
| ACTION | EFFECT |
| Carbohydrate fermentation | Reduction of intraluminal colonic pH |
| Protein fermentation | Production of $NH_4$ and sympathetic amines |
| Synthesis of short-chain free fatty acids (SCFAs) | Main source of energy and nutrition for colon |
| Synthesis of vitamins K, $B_1$, B6$_1$, and $B_{12}$, folic acid, and pantothenic acid | Essential components for biologic processes |
| Deconjugation of bile salts, bilirubin, drugs, and steroid hormones | Biotransformation and absorption |
| Fat malabsorption | Regulation of plasma levels of cholesterol and triglycerides |

## Table 59-4. Common Probiotics

| LACTOBACILLUS (LAB) | BIFIDOBACTERIA | STREPTOCOCCUS | ESCHERICHIA COLI |
|---|---|---|---|
| L. acidophilus | B. bifidum | S. thermophilus | Nissle 1917 |
| L. casei GG | B. infantis | S. lactis | Serotype |
| L. rhamnosom | B. longum | S. salivarius | 06:K5:H1 |
| L. salavarius | B. thermophilum | | |
| L. delbruecki | B. adolescents | | |
| L. reuteri | | | |
| L. brevis | | | |
| L. plantarium | | | |

**29. Have probiotics been shown to benefit the treatment of gastrointestinal disorders?**
Yes.

| DISEASE STATE | PROBIOTIC |
|---|---|
| Irritable bowel disease | *Bifidobacter,* VSL#3* |
| Ulcerative colitis | VSL#3* |
| Traveler's diarrhea | *Lactobacillus,* VSL#3* |
| Antibiotic-related diarrhea | Nonpathologic *E. coli* sero O6:K5:H1 Nissle 1917 |
| Relapsing *Clostridium difficile* diarrhea | *Saccharomyces boulardii* |
| Recurrent pouchitis | VSL#3* |

*VSL#3 is a concentration of eight strains of bacteria.

**30. How are probiotics believed to exert beneficial effect on the gut?**
- Immune actions
  - Decrease tumor necrosis factor (TNF) and interferon (IFN)
  - Induce T reg cells
  - Induce T-cell apoptosis
  - Dendritic cell modulation
- Antimicrobial activity
  - Limited adhesion
  - Stimulate↑ IgA
  - Reduced chloride secretion
- Enhanced barrier integrity
  - Increase mucus secretion (increase in interleukins 10 and 12)
  - Enhance tight junctions

# WEBSITES

http://www.cdc.gov/nccdphp/dnpa/nutrition/index.htm

http://www.cdc.gov/nccdphp/dnpa/obesity/trend/maps/

http://www.halls.md/ideal-weight/body.htm

http://www.mypyramid.gov/

http://www.nestle-nutrition.com/Clinical_Resources/Mini_Nutritional_Assessment.aspx

http://www.nutrition.gov/

## BIBLIOGRAPHY

1. Buddeberg-Fischer B, Klaghofer R, Sigrist S, et al. Impact of psychosocial stress and symptoms on indication for bariatric surgery and outcome in morbidly obese patients. Obes Surg 2004;14:361–99.
2. Byrne TK. Complications of surgery for obesity. Surg Clin North Am 2001;81:1181–93.
3. Caba D, Ochoa JB. How many calories are necessary during critical illness? Gastrointest Endoscopy Clin N Am 2007;17:703–10.

4. DeLegge MH, Drake LM. Nutritional assessment. Gastroenterol Clin N Am 2007;36:1–22.
5. Floch MH, Montrose DC. Use of probiotics in humans: An analysis of the literature. Gastroenterol Clin N Am 2005;34:547–70.
6. Francesco FW, Regano N, Mazzuoli S, et al. Cholestasis induced by total parenteral nutrition. Clin Liver Dis 2008;12:97–110.
7. Fuller R. Probiotics in man and animals. J Appl Bacteriol 1989;66:365–78.
8. Harrison GG. Height-weight tables. Ann Intern Med 1985;103:489–94.
9. Lee WJ, Wang W, Chen TC, et al. Clinical significance of central obesity in laparoscopic bariatric surgery. Obes Surg 2003;13:921–5.
10. Ley RE, Turnbaugh PJ, Klein S, et al. Microbial ecology: Human gut microbes associated with obesity. Nature 2006;444:1022–3.
11. Maroo S, Lamont JT. Recurrent *Clostridium difficile* related antibiotic diarrhea. Gastroenterology 2006;130:1311–6.
12. Nisha R, Punjabi NM. Sleep apnea and metabolic dysfunction: Cause or co-relation? Sleep Med Clin 2007;2:237–50.
13. Ochoa JB, Caba D. Advances in surgical nutrition. Surg Clin N Am 2006;86:1483–93.
14. Pai MP, Paloucek FP. The origin of the "ideal" body weight equations. Ann Pharmacol 2000;34:1066–9.
15. Pinkney J, Kerrigan D. Current status of bariatric surgery in the treatment of type 2 diabetes. J Obes Rev 2004;5:69–78.
16. Quigley EM. Bacteria: a new player in gastrointestinal motility disorders—Infections, bacterial overgrowth and probiotics. Gastroenterol Clin N Am 2007;36:735–48.
17. Shen B. Managing pouchitis. Am J Gastroenterol 2007;102:S60–4.
18. Skelton JA, DeMattia L, Miller L, et al. Obesity and its therapy: from genes to community action. Pediatr Clin N Am 2006;53:777–94.
19. Tenenhaus M, Rennekampff HO. Burn surgery. Clin Plast Surg 2007;34:697–715.
20. Tucker ON, Szomstein S, Rosenthal RJ, et al. Nutritional consequences of weight-loss surgery. Med Clin N Am 2007;91:499–514.

## SMALL INTESTINE

### 1. What are the morphologic features of celiac disease?

The normal duodenal mucosa has numerous *fingerlike* projections or villi as shown in Figure 60-1*A*, while in celiac disease the normal villous architecture is lost (blunted villi and crypt hyperplasia) and intraepithelial lymphocytes (IELs) are increased, as shown in Figure 60-1*B*. The Marsh Criteria represent a morphologic classification that defines the many histologic features of this entity. See Table 60-1.

The modified classification subdivides Marsh III into A, B, and C as partial, subtotal, or total villous atrophy, respectively. Increased intraepithelial lymphocytes are seen more toward the tips of the villi. These are T lymphocytes that can be highlighted by CD3 immunohistochemical stain.

Treated celiac disease may show normal villous architecture but the intraepithelial lymphocytes are still increased.

### 2. What is the differential diagnosis of the biopsy showing villous blunting?

- Allergy to other proteins, i.e., cow's milk (in pediatric population)
- Dermatitis herpetiformis
- Nonsteroidal anti-inflammatory drugs (NSAIDs)
- Peptic duodenitis
- Giardiasis
- Tropical sprue
- Crohn's disease
- Severe malnutrition
- Bacterial overgrowth
- Common variable immunodeficiency
- Autoimmune enteropathy
- Graft-versus-host disease
- Zöllinger-Ellison syndrome
- Chemotherapy effect

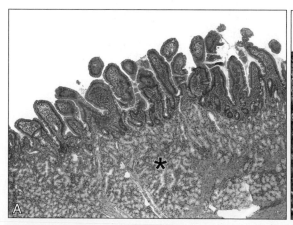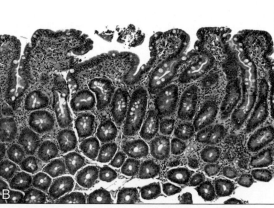

**Figure 60-1.** Photomicrographs of *A*, Duodenum (normal) with underlying Brunner glands (*asterisk*). *B*, Celiac disease. Villous blunting with crypt hyperplasia and increased intraepithelial lymphocytes (tip heavy pattern). Hematoxylin and eosin stain.

**Table 60-1.** Marsh Criteria

| MARSH CLASSIFICATION | DUODENAL VILLI | INTRAEPITHELIAL LYMPHOCYTES (IELS) | CRYPTS |
|---|---|---|---|
| 0 | Normal | Normal number of IELs | Normal |
| I (infiltrative) | Normal | ↑↑ IELs | Normal |
| II (hyperplastic) | Normal | ↑↑ IELs | Crypt hyperplasia |
| III (destructive) | Blunting | ↑↑ IELs | Crypt hyperplasia |
| IV (hypoplastic) | Total villous atrophy | ↑↑ IELs | Atrophic crypts |

### 3. What are the complications of celiac sprue?

- *Collagenous sprue:* Some cases of longstanding sprue, unresponsive to gluten-free diet, exhibit a thickened subepithelial collagen table greater than 10 microns along with marked villous blunting.
- *Ulcerative jejunoileitis:* Characterized by multiple transverse ulcers in the small intestine predominantly in jejunum.
- *Enteropathy-associated T-cell lymphoma:* Mostly seen in elderly patients with celiac disease.
- *Small bowel adenocarcinoma*

### 4. Histologically, what findings suggest peptic duodentitis versus Crohn's disease?

- *Peptic duodenitis:* Gastric foveolar metaplasia is seen in the villi, which may be focal, along with cryptitis. Rarely, *Helicobacter* organisms may be identified in cases with extensive foveolar metaplasia.
- *Crohn's disease:* Like biopsies from terminal ileum mucosa (Fig. 60-2), duodenal biopsies show superficial ulcers/erosions (aphthous ulcers), blunting of villi, foci of cryptitis, crypt abscesses, increased chronic inflammation in the lamina propria, pyloric metaplasia, and prominent Peyer patches. Foci uninvolved by inflammation are generally present. Occasionally, granulomas can be seen. The differential diagnosis of focal cryptitis (and lack of features of chronicity) also includes NSAID mucosal injury and infections.

### 5. Discuss a few causes of infectious enteritis.

- *Giardiasis: Giardia lamblia* is seen as a pear-shaped organism, which resides in the upper small intestine (duodenum and jejunum) (Fig. 60-3) and exists in two forms—trophozoite and cyst. The trophozoite form (7 microns wide, 14 microns long) shows two symmetrical nuclei with nucleoli and four pairs of flagella. On longitudinal sections, it appears as a long, curved organism
- *Mycobacterium avium intracellulare infection:* This opportunistic infection affects both small and large bowel in immunocompromised hosts in a patchy distribution. Histology shows numerous histiocytes in the lamina propria (Fig. 60-4A) that contain numerous acid-fast bacilli highlighted by Kinyoun stain (Fig. 60-4B). Granulomas may not be identified.

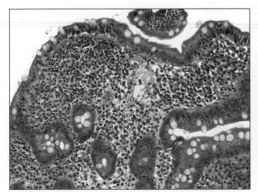

**Figure 60-2.** Photomicrograph of Crohn's disease involving ileum. Note the villous blunting and the increased inflammation in the lamina propria. Hematoxylin and eosin stain.

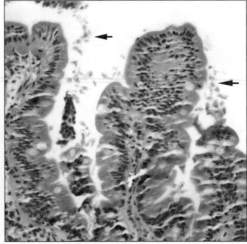

**Figure 60-3.** Photomicrograph of *Giardiasis*. Small bowel biopsy shows pear-shaped trophozoite forms (*arrows*) on the luminal surface. Hematoxylin and eosin stain. (Courtesy of Dr. Loretta Gaido, Denver Health Medical Center, Denver, CO.)

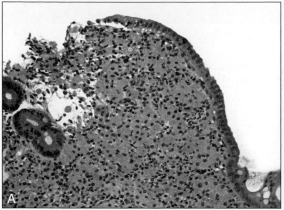
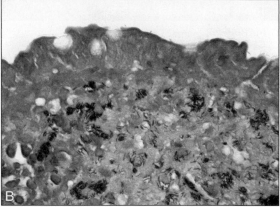

**Figure 60-4.** Photomicrographs of *A, Mycobacterium avium intracellulare.* There is marked expansion of the lamina propria by plump histiocytes (hematoxylin and eosin stain). *B, Mycobacterium avium intracellulare.* Acid-fast bacilli (magenta staining rods within histiocytes) highlighted by the Kinyoun stain. The *Tropheryma whippeli* organisms are not acid fast.

- *Whipple disease: Tropheryma whippeli* infects the small intestine, cardiac valves, nervous system, and lymph nodes. Histology shows expansion of lamina propria by PAS-positive Whipple bacilli that are negative with acid-fast bacilli stain. The other feature that points to Whipple infection is the dilated lymphatics in the lamina propria caused by obstruction of the lymphatic ducts by bacilli. The other tests that can be used include polymerase chain reaction (PCR) assay and electron microscopy.
- Other infections include *cryptosporidium*, disseminated *histoplasmosis, Isospora belli, Microsporidium* sp. *(Enterocytozoon bieneusi, Enterocytozoon intestinalis), strongyloides,* and *Yersinia* sp.

## MISCELLANEOUS CONDITIONS

- *Lymphangiectasia:* Primary lymphangiectasia presents in the pediatric age group generally before 3 years. The biopsy sample shows dilated lymphatics in the superficial lamina propria (Fig. 60-5). Secondary causes will show similar histology and include local inflammatory or a neoplastic process.
- *Ischemic enteritis:* This is often the result of mechanical obstruction and, histologically, shows hemorrhage in the lamina propria or transmural hemorrhage with mucosal sloughing.
- *Graft-versus-host disease (GVHD):* Histology is graded as follows:
  - Grade 1—Apoptosis (single cell necrosis) of the crypt epithelium
  - Grade 2—Apoptosis with crypt abscesses
  - Grade 3—Individual crypt necrosis/crypt drop-out
  - Grade 4—Total surface denudation of areas of bowel
- *Eosinophilic gastroenteritis:* The biopsy shows villous blunting with numerous eosinophils in the lamina propria forming clusters or sheets. The etiologies include food allergies, parasites, drugs, hypereosinophilic syndrome, and idiopathic.

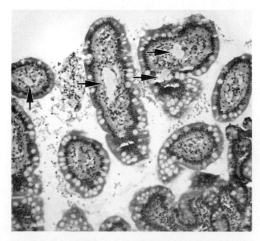

**Figure 60-5.** Photomicrograph of lymphangiectasia (secondary). Small bowel biopsy showing villi with dilated lacteals (*arrows*). Hematoxylin and eosin stain.

## SMALL INTESTINAL NEOPLASMS

- *Peutz-Jeghers polyps:* The small intestine is the most common site for polyps in Peutz-Jeghers syndrome. Histology shows arborizing smooth muscle bundles in the lamina propria without much expansion of lamina propria by inflammatory infiltrate (Fig. 60-6). The overlying epithelium is that of small intestinal type and may show hyperplasia. Dysplasia can occasionally be seen in these polyps.
- *Adenomas:* Duodenum is the most common upper gastrointestinal site for an adenoma. The morphology is similar to that in colon: tubular, tubulovillous, or villous patterns are seen. Ampullary adenomas arise in the ampulla or periampullary region and are indistinguishable from each other based on morphology.
- *Adenocarcinomas:* The primary adenocarcinoma of the small intestine is uncommon (2% of gastrointestinal [GI] tract tumors), and duodenum is the most common site. Usually, these arise from a sporadic adenoma.

Histology resembles colonic adenocarcinoma. Other predispositions include familial adenomatous polyposis (FAP), nonpolyposis colorectal cancer (HNPCC), or hamartomatous polyp syndromes. Chronic inflammatory conditions that are the risk factors include celiac disease, Crohn's disease, ileostomy, and protein-losing enteropathy.

### 6. Discuss the neuroendocrine tumors.

- *Carcinoid tumor* (Fig. 60-7): Duodenum is the most common site of these well-differentiated neuroendocrine tumors. These can be functional or nonfunctional in the production of hormones.
  - Serotonin production is common in ileal carcinoids.
  - Gastrin production is common in duodenal carcinoids.

Immunohistochemical stains cannot be used to predict the functional status of the tumor. All carcinoids are considered to have metastatic potential. Histologic architecture varies from nested, trabecular, cords, or glandular morphology and

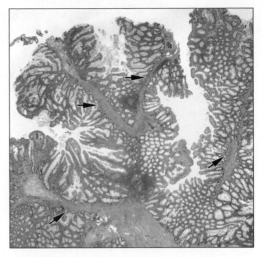

**Figure 60-6.** Photomicrograph of Peutz-Jeghers polyp. Note the arborizing smooth muscle bundles (*arrows*) traversing the lamina propria. Hematoxylin and eosin stain.

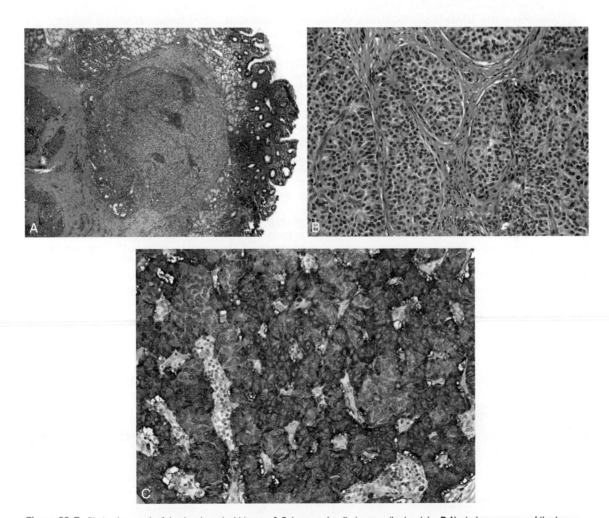

**Figure 60-7.** Photomicrograph of duodenal carcinoid tumor. *A,* Submucosal well-circumscribed nodule. *B,* Nested appearance of the tumor and cells with round-to-ovoid nuclei and salt-pepper chromatin. Hematoxylin and eosin stain. *C,* Same case of carcinoid tumor showing strong immunoreactivity with chromogranin stain.

consists of cells with scant amphophilic cytoplasm that show a salt-and-pepper chromatin pattern in the round/ovoid nuclei with inconspicuous nucleoli. Mitotic figures are rare. Gastrin-producing, somatostatin cell and serotonin-producing tumors have aggressive behavior and metastasize.

- *Gangliocytic paragangliomas* are usually benign infiltrative lesions and consist of ganglion cells, spindle cells (neural), and epithelial cells forming trabeculae, nests, and pseudoglandular architecture. Occasional large tumors (more than 2 cm) may spread to the lymph nodes.
- *Small cell carcinoma* is the other end of spectrum of neuroendocrine tumors. These are malignant tumors with small cell morphology, necrosis, and increased mitotic activity.

### SMALL INTESTINAL LYMPHOMAS

- Small intestinal lymphomas are less common than gastric lymphomas and include extranodal marginal zone lymphoma (low-grade mucosa-associated lymphoid tissue [MALT] MALToma or MALT lymphoma) (Fig. 60-8), mantle cell lymphoma, Burkitt lymphoma, immunoproliferative small intestinal disease (IPSID), and enteropathy-like T-cell lymphoma (rare).
- IPSID is seen exclusively in Mediterranean and Middle Eastern regions. This is a variant of MALT lymphoma that secretes defective alpha heavy chains. The infiltrate consists of plasma cells with small lymphocytes, and monoclonal alpha heavy chain can be demonstrated in the cytoplasm of neoplastic cells. Transformation to large B-cell lymphoma is frequent in late stages.

## LARGE INTESTINE

### 7. What are the histologic features of idiopathic inflammatory bowel disease (IBD)?

- *Chronic ulcerative colitis (UC)*: Grossly, there is diffuse involvement of rectosigmoid and left-sided colon, and proximal extent of the disease varies. Infections such as *cytomegalovirus, Salmonella, Shigella,* and *Clostridium difficile* can complicate UC. Toxic megacolon is a fulminant acute complication of the disease. Histologically, the features of acute disease include cryptitis (neutrophilic infiltration in the crypt epithelium), crypt abscesses (neutrophils in the crypt lumens), and mucosal erosions/ulcers. The features of chronicity include architectural distortion of crypts (crypt dropout, bifid crypts, crypt branching), mucin depletion (loss of goblet cells), Paneth cell metaplasia, basal plasmacytosis, increased eosinophils, and prominent lymphoid aggregates. These changes are diffuse except in resolving phase where these may be focal (should not be confused with Crohn's disease). Fibrosis is unusual in UC in contrast to Crohn's disease. The differential diagnosis, especially in the acute disease process, includes infection, NSAID-associated colitis, ischemic colitis, and Crohn's disease.
- *Quiescent colitis* shows mucosal atrophy (short crypts, loss of crypts, and crypt distortion), thickened muscularis mucosae, and normal inflammatory component in the lamina propria. Inflammatory pseudopolyps can be seen in longstanding cases.
- *Backwash ileitis* is seen in some patients with pancolitis, and the biopsy sample shows acute disease without features of chronicity.
- *Crohn's disease*: Colon biopsy samples show variable morphology. Some foci may appear normal and the others show aphthous ulcers, cryptitis, glandular distortion and loss, and occasionally, granulomas (Fig. 60-9). Transmural inflammation is characteristic of Crohn's disease and a distinguishing feature from UC. Rectum is usually spared. The resection (done in complicated cases) specimen shows segmental involvement with *skip areas*, linear ulcers, cobblestoning, strictures, fissures/fistulas, inflammatory pseudopolyps, serosa with *creeping fat,* and a firm pipelike bowel due to fibrosis. Involvement of terminal ileum shows villous blunting and increased inflammation in the lamina propria.

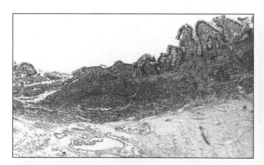

**Figure 60-8.** Photomicrograph of mucosa-associated lymphoid tissue [MALT] lymphoma in a resection specimen. Note the expansion of the lamina propria by the neoplastic lymphoid infiltrate extending into the adjacent submucosa. Hematoxylin and eosin stain.

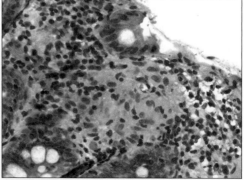

**Figure 60-9.** Photomicrograph of Crohn's disease. A microgranuloma is seen in the lamina propria in this biopsy from transverse colon. Note the epitheloid histiocytes with ample eosinophilic cytoplasm and ovoid nuclei. Hematoxylin and eosin stain.

## 8. Discuss colitis-associated dysplasia in IBD.

- Dysplasia can be flat or form a mass (dysplasia associated lesion/mass [DALM]). Dysplasia in UC is graded as negative, indefinite, low grade, high grade, or carcinoma.
- The differential diagnosis of DALM is sporadic adenoma. The distinction between the two is difficult and requires clear communication between the pathologist and the endoscopist. If the lesion is isolated from the areas affected by colitis, then the diagnosis is usually a sporadic adenoma. A DALM lesion shows foci of dysplastic epithelium associated with areas of colitis. The pattern of dysplasia may not be uniform. Positive staining with beta-catenin may help in these cases that are negative for p53. Both DALM of any grade and flat high-grade dysplasias are associated with the increased risk of invasive adenocarcinomas and total colectomy is usually recommended in UC cases.

## 9. What is the differential diagnosis of focal active colitis?

- Infectious colitis
- Crohn's disease
- UC early or resolving
- Bowel preparation artifact

## 10. What is the differential diagnosis of pseudomembranes?

- *Pseudomembranous colitis* is a complication of antibiotic-associated colitis caused by C. *difficile*. Not all *C. difficile* infections produce pseudomembranous colitis. Grossly, discrete gray-white patches of pseudomembranes are identified. The histologic features include loosely adherent fibrinopurulent exudate on the luminal surface (pseudomembrane) with associated superficial mucosal necrosis (Fig. 60-10).
- *Ischemic colitis*: Features of ischemic damage include mucosal necrosis, hemorrhage with congestion in the lamina propria, hyalinization of lamina propria, occasional fibrin thrombi, and pseudomembrane (neutrophilic-fibrinous exudate) formation. In longstanding ischemic bowel, mucin depletion, regenerative change, lymphoplasmacytic infiltrate, hemosiderin pigment, and fibrosis of lamina propria are seen. Systemic vasculitis should be considered in the differential diagnosis in these cases.

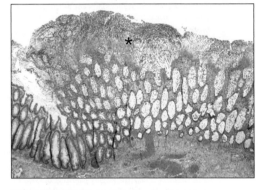

**Figure 60-10.** Microscopically, pseudomembrane (*asterisk*) is seen as necroinflammatory exudate on the luminal surface. Hematoxylin and eosin stain.

## 11. Histologically, which findings help differentiate infectious colitis and NSAID-associated colitis?

- *Infectious colitis*: Histology shows acute inflammation in the lamina propria with cryptitis, crypt abscesses, and lack of prominent chronic inflammatory infiltrate, basal plasmacytosis (as seen in IBD). Chronic architectural changes may not be pronounced. Causative organisms include *Escherichia coli* 0157:H7, *Salmonella*, *Shigella*, *Clostridium*, *Campylobacter*, *Yersinia*, cytomegalovirus colitis (Fig. 60-11), amebic colitis, and histoplasmosis. Granulomas can be seen in tuberculosis, *Yersinia pseudotuberculosis,* and *Chlamydia* infections.

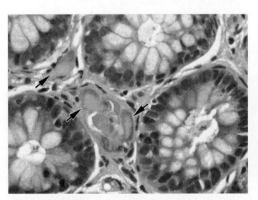

**Figure 60-11.** Photomicrograph of cytomegalovirus colitis. Note the large eosinophilic intranuclear viral inclusions (*arrows*). Hematoxylin and eosin stain.

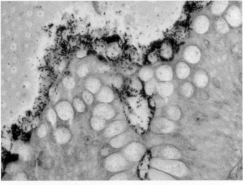

**Figure 60-12.** Photomicrograph of intestinal spirochetosis. Steiner stain highlights the spirochetes obscuring the luminal border. No significant inflammation was seen within crypts or lamina propria.

- *Intestinal spirochetosis* (Fig. 60-12, Steiner stain) shows organisms on the luminal surface that may not cause an active inflammatory response or injury in the mucosa. These anaerobic organisms belong to *Brachyspira* sp.
- *NSAID-associated colitis*: Changes are patchy, may involve any part of the colon, and histologically include focal active colitis, erosions/ulcers, increased apoptosis in crypts, and diaphragm strictures. *Diaphragm-like* strictures are formed as a result of repeated injury and repair and are seen microscopically as mucosal and submucosal fibrosis. These may cause luminal narrowing and occasionally serosal strictures. Thickened subepithelial collagen layer in longstanding cases has been associated with NSAIDs that can be confused with collagenous colitis and requires correlation with clinical history and endoscopic findings.

## 12. What are the histologic features of microscopic colitis?

- This term encompasses *collagenous* and *lymphocytic* colitis. Both of these conditions present as chronic watery diarrhea, are associated with autoimmune diseases, and show a near normal endoscopic examination. Histologically, collagenous colitis (Fig. 60-13*A*) shows thickened subepithelial collagen layer that has irregular edges, is infiltrated by a few lymphocytes and eosinophils, and has dilated vessels. A few intraepithelial lymphocytes may be seen. The collagen band can be highlighted by trichrome stain (Fig. 60-13*B*). The differential diagnosis also includes ischemic colitis, NSAID-associated injury, IBD, diverticular disease, radiation injury, mucosal prolapse, and amyloidosis.
- Lymphocytic colitis shows increased intraepithelial lymphocytes more on the surface epithelium. Both of the conditions show increased chronic inflammation in the lamina propria with increased eosinophils seen in collagenous colitis. An association between lymphocytic colitis and celiac disease is well known.

### MISCELLANEOUS CONDITIONS

- *Irritable bowel syndrome*—Histologically, the biopsy samples do not show significant abnormality in these cases and appear normal.
- *Radiation colitis*—The histology mimics ischemic colitis and shows enlarged nuclei and cells with hyalinization of lamina propria and vessel walls with scattered atypical stromal cells.
- *Eosinophilic colitis*—Microscopically, abundant eosinophils in the mucosa extending into submucosa are seen with minimal architectural distortion, if any.
- *Diversion colitis*—Mild colitis is seen on microscopic examination. Follicular lymphoid hyperplasia may be seen. The condition reverses on treatment with short-chain fatty acids [SCFAs].
- *Pouchitis*—This is a complication following ileal-pouch anal anastomosis for refractory UC. The pattern of inflammation mimics UC and there are no specific histologic criteria to distinguish recurrent UC from nonspecific inflammation of the pouch. Comparison with the biopsy samples from the nonpouch portion of the ileum may help.
- *Diverticular disease–associated colitis*—It is seen in the areas around diverticular orifices. Histologically, the findings are similar to those seen in IBD. Correlation with endoscopic findings and clinical history is essential.
- *Melanosis coli*—The biopsy sample shows numerous brown pigment–laden macrophages (lipofuscin) in the lamina propria (Fig. 60-14). These are negative for staining on iron stains. There are no significant acute or chronic changes in the biopsy sample.
- *Endometriosis*—The common site in GI tract is the sigmoid colon. The biopsy sample shows endometrial glands and stroma with hemorrhage or hemosiderin pigment (Fig. 60-15). Any or all the components may be present.

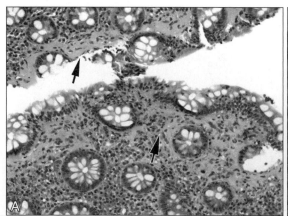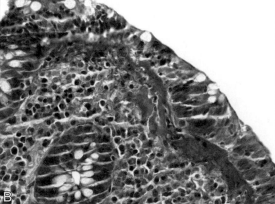

**Figure 60-13.** Photomicrographs of *A,* Collagenous colitis. Note the thickened subepithelial collagen table (*arrows*) with entrapped capillaries and inflammatory infiltrate. Hematoxylin and eosin stain. *B,* Collagenous colitis (trichrome stain). The stain highlights the thickened band that shows irregular edges.

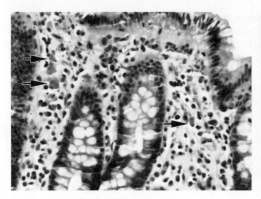

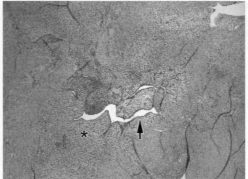

**Figure 60-14.** Photomicrograph of melanosis coli. Pigment laden macrophages in the lamina propria (*arrows*). Hematoxylin and eosin stain.

**Figure 60-15.** Photomicrograph of rectal endometriosis. Note the endometrial glands (*arrow*) surrounded by hemorrhage and stroma (*asterisk*). Hematoxylin and eosin stain.

**13. What is the differential diagnosis of polypoid lesions that can mimic adenoma?**
- Mucosal prolapse/solitary rectal ulcer syndrome/colitis cystica profunda/eroded polypoid hyperplasia—These are seen in rectosigmoid colon as an ulcerated or a polypoid lesion in patients with history of constipation or straining during defecation. The histology shows surface erosion, epithelial hyperplasia with distorted and dilated crypts, vertical stranding of muscle fibers in the lamina propria, fibrosis, and lymphoplasmacytic infiltrate. Inflammatory cloacogenic polyps are present at the anorectal junction and show similar histology with both squamous and colonic epithelia.
- *Lymphoid polyps:* These are benign reactive lymphoid aggregates in the mucosa.
- *Inflammatory polyps*: Generally associated with IBD or diverticulitis and consist of marked inflammation in the lamina propria with granulation tissue and fibrosis. The mucosal lining may show regenerative change and/or erosions.

## POLYPS AND NEOPLASMS

**14. What are the histologic features of conventional adenomas?**
*Tubular adenoma, tubulovillous adenoma, villous adenoma*: Tubular adenomas (Fig. 60-16) have a tubular architecture with the surface epithelium showing low-grade dysplasia that extends downward in the base. These can show focal areas of high-grade dysplasia with architectural complexity and marked cytologic atypia. Focal high-grade dysplasia does not have a metastatic potential. The tubulovillous adenomas (Fig. 60-17) show a combination of tubular and villous architecture (villous component greater than 25%). Villous adenoma displays a predominant villous architecture (greater than 75%) and has a greater propensity for malignant transformation. All of these can have focal areas of pseudoinvasion that should not be interpreted as intramucosal carcinoma. The conventional adenomas show *KRAS* mutations (*BRAF* negative).

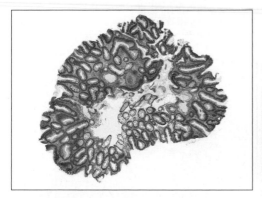

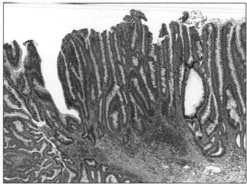

**Figure 60-16.** Photomicrograph of tubular adenoma. Polyp showing tubular architecture lined by cells with nuclear stratification and hyperchromasia. Hematoxylin and eosin stain.

**Figure 60-17.** Photomicrograph of tubulovillous adenoma. Polyp showing villous architecture in addition to typical tubular areas. Hematoxylin and eosin stain.

**15. What is meant by intramucosal carcinoma in an adenoma?**

Invasion of dysplastic glands into the lamina propria is intramucosal carcinoma. In the colon, it is equivalent to high-grade dysplasia, since it is not associated with metastatic potential and a polypectomy with negative margins should suffice.

**16. What is meant by the term *depressed* or *flat* adenoma?**

Endoscopically (Fig. 60-18*A*), it shows subtle depression in the mucosa or may be flat. Histologically (Fig. 60-18*B*), the adenomatous glands show long tubular architecture with a narrow opening at the surface and are lined by dysplastic epithelium. These tend to have high-grade dysplasia more often than the tubular adenomas and are more aggressive.

**17. What is the difference between hyperplastic polyp (HP), traditional serrated adenoma (TSA), and sessile serrated adenoma (SSA)?**

- *Hyperplastic polyp*: Polyps characterized by serrated crypt lumens that are lined by normal epithelial cells that lack dysplasia (Fig. 60-19).
- *Traditional serrated adenoma*: These polyps show serrated crypt lumens with stratified *pencil-like* nuclei at the base of crypts (Fig. 60-20) that resemble the ones seen in tubular adenoma. Some authors have described ectopic crypt formation (ECF) in TSA. These are short crypts away from muscularis mucosae and are considered precursors to colorectal cancer (CRC).
- *Sessile serrated adenoma*: These are seen more on the right side of colon in elderly women and are always sessile. A few (10%) may occur in the left colon. In various studies, these account for 4% to 15% of serrated polyps. Architecturally, it differs and shows serrated mucosal glands with a broad or boat-shaped base. The lining epithelium has pink cytoplasm and lacks conventional dysplasia. Mild nuclear atypia is seen. A subset of these polyps may show focal conventional dysplasia; however, architecture is the key finding. This adenoma has been associated with MSI-H (microsatellite instability-high)–related sporadic CRCs (hypermethylation of promoter gene). The majority of these show *BRAF* mutation, and approximately 1 in 25 (4%) of these will progress to cancer.
- *Mixed polyps:* These are hyperplastic polyps with typical adenoma foci.

**18. What are the genetic abnormalities in conventional CRCs?**

- Colorectal adenocarcinoma usually arise from adenomas and can be sporadic (85%) or syndromic. These are graded as well, moderately, or poorly differentiated based on the glandular differentiation (Fig. 60-21). The variants include

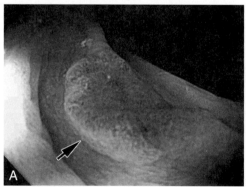

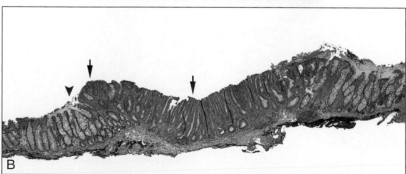

**Figure 60-18.** ***A,*** Depressed adenoma (*arrow*), endoscopic view. ***B,*** Photomicrograph of depressed adenoma, morphology. Note the abrupt junction between normal (*arrowhead*) and abnormal (*arrow*) and the depression with tubular glands showing narrow openings at the surface (*central arrow*). Hematoxylin and eosin stain. (**A,** Courtesy of Dr. Norio Fukami, University of Colorado Denver Health Sciences Center.)

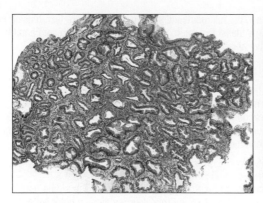

**Figure 60-19.** Photomicrograph of hyperplastic polyp. Polyp with hyperplastic glands showing serrated lumens lined by epithelial cells without dysplasia. Hematoxylin and eosin stain.

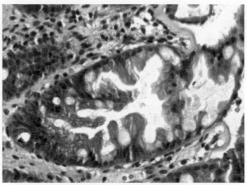

**Figure 60-20.** Photomicrograph of traditional serrated adenoma (TSA). Note the serrated lumens (as seen in hyperplastic polyps) lined by cells that show pencillate nuclei and stratification (as seen in tubular adenomas). Hematoxylin and eosin stain.

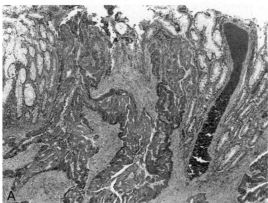

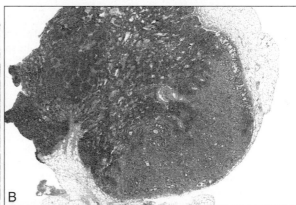

**Figure 60-21.** Photomicrographs of **A,** Colon adenocarcinoma, moderately differentiated. Note the infiltrating neoplastic glands with surface involvement in the center of the image and the non-neoplastic epithelium adjacent to it (for comparison). **B,** Lymph node with metastasis from colon adenocarcinoma (*right*). Hematoxylin and eosin stain.

mucinous (greater than 50% mucinous morphology) (Fig. 60-22) and signet ring cell carcinomas (greater than 50% signet ring cell morphology). Histologically, neoplastic glands with necrotic debris show invasion through the muscularis mucosa into the submucosa. On immunohistochemistry, these usually show staining with cytokeratin 20 and CDX2 and are negative for staining with cytokeratin 7. The most common genetic alteration (somatic) in sporadic CRCs is inactivation of APC/beta-catenin pathway that can have multiple consequences. Clonal accumulation of additional genetic alterations then occurs, including activation of proto-oncogenes such as *c-myc* and *ras* and inactivation of additional tumor suppressor genes (*TP53* on chromosome 17). These tumors are microsatellite stable (MSS). *BRAF* mutation is not common and seen in a few (less than 10%) conventional CRCs.

- *Small cell carcinoma*: This is a rare variant of CRC with poor prognosis, which shows small cell morphology and positive immunostaining with neuroendocrine markers such as chromogranin, synaptophysin, and NCAM (CD56). These are not associated with carcinoid tumors (well-differentiated neuroendocrine tumors) and may be seen with conventional CRC.

## 19. What genetic abnormalities point to HNPCC?

HNPCC presents in a younger age group and has an autosomal dominant pattern of inheritance. Revised Bethesda Criteria are set to screen the patients for microsatellite instability (MSI). DNA mismatch repair *(MMR)* gene defect is tested for *hMLH1* (50%), *hMSH2* (39%), *hMSH6* (8%), and *hPMS2* (1%) genes.

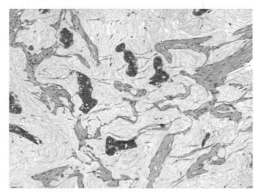

**Figure 60-22.** Photomicrograph of mucinous adenocarcinoma. Note the mucin pools with floating neoplastic cell clusters. Hematoxylin and eosin stain.

These defects result in insertion or deletion of nucleotides in the microsatellite sequences, which are tested using PCR and reported as high (MSI-H), low (MSI-L), or stable (MSS). At least five microsatellite sequences are tested and MSI-H is defined as instability in 30% to 40% of markers (two of five at least).

- Loss of *hMSH2*—indicates HNPCC
- Loss of *hMLH1*—HNPCC or sporadic CRC (loss due to hypermethylation of *hMLH1* promoter in sporadic CRC)
- The immunohistochemistry (IHC) on paraffin sections (of normal and tumor) to test for mismatch repair is also done, which shows loss of staining in the tumor (due to mutated gene) compared with the normal. Loss of *hMSH2* and/or *hMSH6* is highly associated with Lynch syndrome. Direct gene sequencing can be done in highly susceptible cases and to confirm the results of MSI and IHC. A negative test in an at-risk patient does not rule out other hereditary causes of CRC.

### 20. What histologic features seen in CRCs can predict MSI-H?

These tumors are usually right sided, show a medullary/syncytial growth pattern, have mucinous or signet ring cell features, are poorly differentiated, and show lymphocytic infiltration. Also, a Crohn-like reaction (nodular lymphoid aggregates) is seen beyond the advancing edge of the tumor. These features along with the age at diagnosis are used to determine MsPath score (Microsatellite instability by pathology). This scoring system can be used as a triage procedure for prioritizing CRCs for MSI testing. This scoring does not exclude other forms of hereditary CRC.

### 21. What is the abnormality in MSI unstable sporadic CRCs?

These constitute about 12% to 15% of CRCs. The MSI-H is caused by somatic inactivation of *hMLH1* mismatch repair gene due to hypermethylation of the promoter region preceding the gene sequence, whereas in HNPCC, the instability is due to germline mutation in the *MMR* genes. Most of the sporadic ones show *BRAF* mutations (*V600E* mutation of *BRAF* oncogene). The histology is similar to that seen in HNPCC.

## POLYPOSIS SYNDROMES

### 22. Name the hamartomatous polyp syndromes.

- *Hamartomatous polyps:* Includes juvenile hamartomatous polyp and the hamartomatous polyp of Peutz-Jeghers type.
- *Peutz-Jeghers syndrome:* Involves entire GI tract (small intestine most common); 93% lifetime risk of cancer. Sporadic Peutz-Jeghers polyps can occur but are extremely rare. Follow-up of these patients is warranted. Histologically, these typically show arborizing smooth muscle bundles in the lamina propria lined by normal or hyperplastic epithelium, occasionally with dysplastic foci.
- *Juvenile polyposis syndrome:* Involves colon or entire GI tract (pedunculated polyps); risk of colorectal cancer is about 30% to 40% and is less (10% to 15%) for upper GI cancer. This is the most common polyp in juvenile population. Germline mutation in *SMAD4/DPC4* tumor suppressor gene accounts for half the cases. Histologically, these are lobulated polyps with cystically dilated crypt (mucus retention cysts) with inflamed edematous lamina propria and occasionally with superficial erosions. Other than juvenile polyp syndromes, juvenile polyps are seen in Cowden syndrome and Bannayan-Riley-Ruvalcaba syndrome.
- *Cowden syndrome:* Involves entire GI tract from esophagus to rectum; risk of developing CRC is generally not increased. Most commonly recognized cancer is breast, followed by thyroid. Arises from *PTEN* germline mutation. Histologically, juvenile polyps are common; also seen are hyperplastic polyps, adenomas, lipomas, and, rarely, ganglioneuromas.
- *Bannayan-Riley-Ruvalcaba syndrome:* Variant of Cowden syndrome with similar histologic features.
- *Cronkhite-Canada syndrome:* Any portion of GI tract (sessile polyps); risk of developing cancer is not well described; Histologically, the polyps seen are similar to juvenile-type (retention) polyps with marked edema in the lamina propria; the intervening mucosa shows similar changes in the lamina propria. Differential diagnosis includes Ménétrier disease and juvenile polyposis syndrome.
- *Hyperplastic polyposis:* A rare syndrome with an increased risk for colorectal cancer. It is characterized by the presence of hyperplastic polyps predominantly (adenomas - tubular or serrated also can be seen) in the colon proximal to sigmoid colon. The number of polyps ranges from 5 to 100. Most of these are nonfamilial and the genetic abnormalities include *BRAF* and *KRAS* mutations.

All are hereditary except Cronkhite-Canada syndrome and hyperplastic polyposis.

### 23. Name the adenomatous polyp syndromes.

- FAP; entire colon and rectum; 100% risk of cancer. Histologically, tubular adenomas and occasionally tubulovillous and villous adenomas are identified.
- The variants include attenuated FAP, Gardner syndrome, Turcot syndrome, hereditary flat adenoma syndrome, and Muir-Torre syndrome.

All are hereditary syndromes.

## 24. How are neuroendocrine tumors classified?

The spectrum ranges from well-differentiated neuroendocrine tumors (carcinoid tumors) to poorly differentiated (small cell carcinomas) and large cell neuroendocrine carcinomas. The common site of involvement is rectum, followed by cecum and sigmoid colon. The histologic characteristics are similar to those described in the small intestine section. These are sporadic tumors. The malignancy rate of 11% to 14% has been calculated for rectal carcinoids. The malignancy criteria include size greater than 2 cm, invasion into muscularis propria, and increased mitoses.

## 25. What are the most common primary tumor sites that can show colon metastases?

These include lung, stomach, breast, ovary, endometrium, and melanoma. These tumor cells creep under the surface epithelium or form submucosal nodules of varying sizes. More than one focus is generally seen. The surface epithelium lacks dysplasia (expected with primary colon adenocarcinomas). Immunohistochemistry may be helpful in poorly differentiated neoplasms. Usually primary colonic adenocarcinomas show immunoreactivity with cytokeratin 20 (95%) and CDX2 (intestinal epithelium marker). Difficulty arises in some poorly differentiated tumors that have lost antigenicity or show lineage infidelity.

## 26. What is the differential diagnosis of stromal tumors in colon?

- *Gastrointestinal stromal tumors* (GISTs) (Fig. 60-23): The most common site in GI tract is stomach (50%), followed by small bowel (25%), colon and rectum (10%), and, least common, esophagus (5%). Histologically, these can be spindled or epitheloid and show strong reactivity with CD117 (95%), and 60% to 70% show positive staining with CD34. Around one third can also show reactivity with smooth muscle markers (smooth muscle actin). These arise from interstitial cells of Cajal, and *KIT* mutations are seen in 85% to 90% of GISTs. Approximately 5% show mutation within *PDGFRA* gene and these are seen in gastric GISTs. These have epithelioid morphology and a less aggressive clinical course. All the GISTs are potentially aggressive. The clinical behavior can be predicted on the basis of size, mitotic figures, and site. Gastric GISTs have a better prognosis than the small bowel GISTs. The GISTs with *exon 11* mutation have a low risk for progressive disease (as opposed to *exon 9* mutation) and respond better to imatinib mesylate in the metastatic disease setting.
- *Schwannoma*: These are well-circumscribed, nonencapsulated spindle cell tumors with strong immunoreactivity with S100 protein. Dense lymphoid cuffing is seen around schwannomas.
- *Leiomyoma* (Fig. 60-24): Another spindle cell tumor arising from the smooth muscle in muscularis mucosae that shows strong positive immunostaining with smooth muscle actin.
- *Lipoma*: Sporadic benign well-circumscribed submucosal lesion of adipose tissue.

### VASCULAR LESIONS

- *Kaposi sarcoma*—This lesion shows proliferation of slit-like vascular channels, spindle cells, and inflammatory infiltrate (Fig. 60-25). It is seen in some patients with human immunodeficiency virus (HIV) infection and is associated with HHV-8 virus.
- Other lesions include hemangiomas, lymphangiomas, vascular malformations, and, rarely, angiosarcomas.

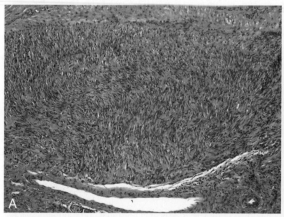
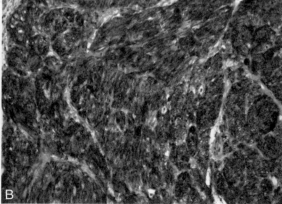

**Figure 60-23.** Photomicrographs of *A,* Gastrointestinal stromal tumor (GIST). Spindle cell tumor in the submucosa (hematoxylin and eosin stain). *B,* GIST. CD117 immunostain showing strong staining in the spindle cells.

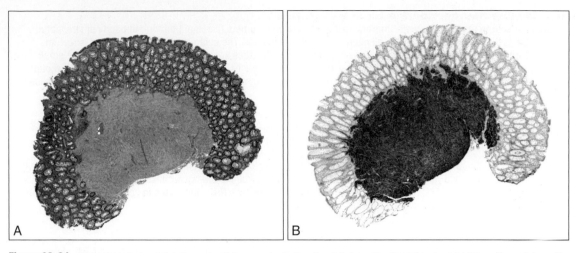

**Figure 60-24.** Photomicrographs of **A,** Leiomyoma. Submucosal spindle cell nodule (hematoxylin and eosin stain) (**B**) positive staining with smooth muscle actin immunostain.

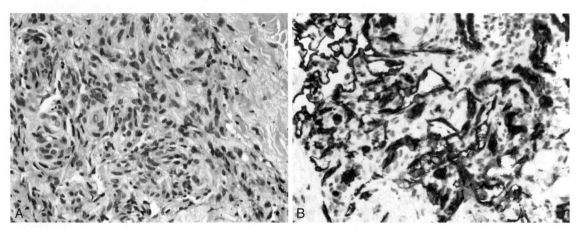

**Figure 60-25.** Photomicrographs of Kaposi sarcoma. **A,** Proliferation of irregular slit-like vessels (hematoxylin and eosin stain) highlighted by (**B**) the endothelial cell marker CD31.

## DISEASES OF THE APPENDIX

### 27. What is the effect of IBD on the appendix?
The appendix is involved in 50% of cases with ileal Crohn's disease and UC with cecal involvement. Isolated involvement is rare.

### 28. Describe the mucinous lesions of appendix.
- *Mucocele*: This is a cystically dilated appendiceal lumen containing mucus. They can be non-neoplastic or neoplastic. Any obstruction of the lumen can give rise to mucocele.
- *Low-grade mucinous adenocarcinomas, with pseudomyxoma peritonei (PMP):* The mucin dissects through the wall of the appendix into the peritoneum. Most cases of synchronous tumors in the ovary and appendix are now considered metastases from the appendiceal tumor. Acellular pools of mucin pose a diagnostic problem. A diagnosis of adenoma (or cystadenoma) should be rendered only if the entire muscularis mucosae is intact. A diagnosis of "uncertain malignant potential" is favored in the cases where an intact muscularis mucosae cannot be seen.
- *Mucinous adenocarcinomas with mucinous carcinomatosis*: Includes signet ring cell carcinomas, invasive well-differentiated carcinomas, and cystadenocarcinoma.

### 29. What is the incidence of carcinoid tumors in appendectomy specimens (performed for appendicitis)?
Appendiceal carcinoid has been reported in 0.3% to 0.9% of appendectomy specimens. It is the most common appendiceal neoplasm. The functioning tumors are commonly serotonin-producing neoplasms. The risk factors for malignancy include size greater than 2 cm and invasion of mesoappendix.

**30. What are the histologic types of mixed endocrine-exocrine neoplasms?**

These include goblet cell carcinoid, tubular carcinoid, and mixed carcinoid-adenocarcinoma. Mixed carcinoid-adenocarcinoma carries the worst prognosis.

## DISEASES OF THE ANAL CANAL

**31. The typical findings of Hirschsprung disease include absence of ganglion cells. What other stain can help support the diagnosis, and what is the ideal site of biopsy?**

Acetylcholinesterase stain highlights the proliferation of thickened nerve fibers in the lamina propria and muscularis mucosae. This stain is done on the frozen tissue. So, ideally, two biopsy samples are sent—one in formalin and another fresh for freezing. The site of biopsy is at least 2 cm above the dentate line. The lower rectum (adjacent to dentate line) is physiologically hypoganglionic. Also, submucosa should be included in the biopsy samples to assess nerves in both the lamina propria and muscularis mucosae.

**32. How is anal intraepithelial neoplasia (AIN) graded and what is the risk of progression to squamous cell carcinoma (SCC)?**

AIN is graded as low grade (AIN I or mild dysplasia) and  high grade (encompasses AIN II and AIN III or moderate and severe dysplasia/carcinoma in-situ respectively). The term 'Bowen disease' (Fig. 60-26A) is used for lesions with severe dysplasia (carcinoma in-situ)  seen at anal verge/perianal skin. The high grade lesions are associated with high risk human papillomavirus (HPV) 16 and 18, among others. These lesions are known to recur after local treatment. The risk of progression to squamous cell carcinoma (Fig. 60-26B) is low (approximately 5%).

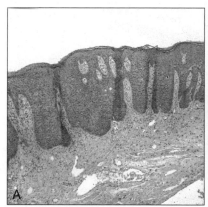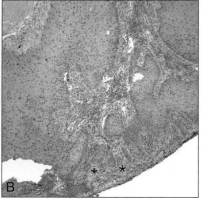

**Figure 60-26.** Photomicrographs of **A,** Bowen disease. Note the thickened squamous epithelium showing severe full-thickness dysplasia. **B,** Squamous cell carcinoma (asterisks) at another focus within the same specimen. Hematoxylin and eosin stain.

**33. What are the cells of origin and the immunohistochemical profile of Paget disease?**

The Paget cells (intraepithelial large cells with pale pink cytoplasm and large nuclei) are believed to be of apocrine lineage and show immunoreactivity with low-molecular-weight keratins Cam 5.2, CK7, and carcinoembryonic antigen (CEA). Mucin stain may be positive. The differential diagnosis includes pagetoid spread from adjacent CRC and melanoma in situ. The immunoprofile helps.

## BIBLIOGRAPHY

1. Al-Daraji WI, Montgomery E. Serrated polyps of the large intestine: A practical approach. Pathol Case Rev 2007;12:129–35.
2. Carvajal-Carmona LG, Howarth KM, Lockett M, et al. Molecular classification and genetic pathways in hyperplastic polyposis syndrome. J Pathol 2007;212:378–85.
3. Check W. Lynch syndrome testing—When and how? CAP Today 2007. December, 2007. http://www.cap.org.
4. Demetri GD, Benjamin RS, Blanke CD, et al. NCCN Task Force Report: Management of patients with gastrointestinal stomal tumor (GIST)—Update of the NCCN clinical practice guidelines. JNCCN 2007;5(Suppl. 2):S1–29.
5. Hamilton SR, Aaltonen LA, editors. WHO Classification of Tumors: Pathology and Genetics of the Digestive System. Lyon: IARC Press; 2000. pp. 96–8 105–136.
6. Issacson PG, Muller-Hermelink HK, Piris MA, et al. WHO Classification of Tumors: Tumors of Hematopoietic and Lymphoid Tissues. Lyon: IARC Press; 2001. pp. 157–60.
7. Jenkins MA, Hayashi S, O'Shea A, et al. Pathology features in Bethesda guidelines predict colorectal cancer microsatellite instability: A population-based study. Gastroenterology 2007;133:48–56.
8. Marsh MN. Gluten, major histocompatibility complex, and the small intestine. A molecular and immunobiologic approach to the spectrum of gluten sensitivity ("celiac sprue"). Gastroenterology 1992;102:330–54.
9. Miettinen M, Lasota J. Gastrointestinal stromal tumors: Pathology and prognosis at different sites. Semin Diagn Pathol 2006;23:111–9.
10. Montgomery EA. Biopsy Interpretation of the Gastrointestinal Tract Mucosa. Philadelphia: Lippincott Williams & Wilkins; 2006.
11. Noffsinger A, Fenoglio-Presiser C, Maru D, et al. Gastrointestinal Diseases: Atlas of Nontumor Pathology, first series. Washington, DC: American Registry of Pathology in collaboration with Armed Forces Institute of Pathology; 2007. pp. 635–6.
12. Odze R. Diagnostic problems and advances in inflammatory bowel disease. Mod pathol 2003;347–58.
13. Snover DC, Jass JR, Fenoglio-Preiser C, et al. Serrated polyps of the large intestine: A morphologic and molecular review of an evolving concept. Am J Clin Pathol 2005;124:380–91.
14. Snover DC, Weisdorf SA, Vercellotti GM, et al. A histopathologic study of gastric and small intestinal graft-versus-host disease following allogenic bone marrow transplantation. Hum Pathol 1985;16:387–92.
15. Tchana-Sato V, Detry O, Polus M, et al. Carcinoid tumor of appendix: a consecutive series from 1237 appendectomies. World J Gastroenterol 2006;12:6699–701.
16. Torlakovic EE, Gomez JD, Driman DK, et al. Sessile serrated adenoma (SSA) vs traditional serrated adenoma (TSA). Am J Surg Pathol 2008;32:21–9.

# FOREIGN BODIES AND THE GASTROINTESTINAL TRACT

*George Triadafilopoulos, MD*

# CHAPTER 61

**1. How common are foreign bodies in the gastrointestinal (GI) tract?**

Every year, millions of foreign bodies enter the GI tract through the mouth or anus, and about 1500 to 3000 people die every year from ingestion of foreign objects. However, only about 10% to 20% of foreign bodies require removal through some form of therapeutic intervention; the rest pass through the GI tract without incident.

**2. Which populations are at risk for foreign-body ingestion?**

Eighty percent of foreign-body ingestions occur in children, whereas almost all foreign bodies inserted into the rectum are described in adults. Other groups at increased risk for foreign-body ingestion include psychiatric patients, inmates, and people who frequently use alcohol or sedative-hypnotic medications. Also at risk are elderly subjects, who may have poorly fitting dentures, impaired cognitive function due to medications, or dementia and/or dysphagia after stroke. Intentional ingestion of foreign objects is well described in smugglers of illicit drugs, jewels, or other valuable items.

**3. Which areas of the GI tract lead to problems in the passage of foreign bodies?**

Several areas of anatomic or physiologic narrowing exist along the GI lumen and may compromise the spontaneous passage of foreign bodies: cricopharyngeal muscle, extrinsic compression of the middle esophagus from the aortic arch, lower esophageal sphincter, pylorus, ileocecal valve, rectal valves of Houston, and anal sphincters. In addition, numerous pathologic abnormalities, such as strictures or tumors, may impair spontaneous passage of foreign bodies (see Question 12).

**4. What objects are commonly ingested?**

The object ingested most commonly by children is a coin. Meat boluses impacted above an esophageal stricture, Schatzki ring, or eosinophilic esophagitis account for most adult cases (Fig. 61-1). Accidental loss of sex stimulant devices account for over one half of foreign objects introduced through the anus.

**5. Describe the typical clinical presentation of foreign-body ingestion.**

Adults trace the onset of symptoms to the ingestion of a specific meal or foreign body. Most commonly, acute dysphagia, odynophagia, and chest pain reflect underlying esophageal obstruction. Respiratory distress, stridor, and inability to handle oral secretions suggest the need for urgent intervention. Persons with developmental disabilities, psychiatric patients, or children may remain asymptomatic for months after ingestion, or they may not volunteer the history. Patients with impacted anorectal foreign bodies may relate a wide variety of medical histories to account for their predicament, ranging from accidents or assault to medical remedies.

**6. What is suggested by respiratory symptoms related to foreign-body ingestion?**

Patients with wheezing, stridor, cough, or dyspnea after foreign-body ingestion may have foreign body entrapment in the hypopharynx, trachea, pyriform sinus, or Zenker diverticulum.

**7. Do ingested sharp objects perforate the intestine?**

On rare occasions, sharp objects, such as pins, needles, nails, and toothpicks, may perforate the intestine, but in 70% to 90% of cases they pass through the alimentary tract without complication. Two phenomena in the intestine allow safe passage: (1) foreign bodies pass with axial flow down the lumen, and (2) reflex relaxation and slowing of peristalsis cause sharp objects to turn around in the lumen so that the sharp end trails down the intestine. In the colon, the foreign object is centered in the fecal bolus, which further protects the bowel wall.

**8. Why is it important to identify the type of foreign body ingested?**

Although most foreign bodies traverse the GI tract without complication, specific exceptions require special attention. Button alkaline batteries may cause coagulation necrosis in the esophagus, but once they reach the stomach, gastric acid neutralizes their risk. Sharp objects can perforate any part of the alimentary tract. There is no known absolute size of a foreign body that dictates surgical intervention since the shape, composition, and sharpness of edges may play a

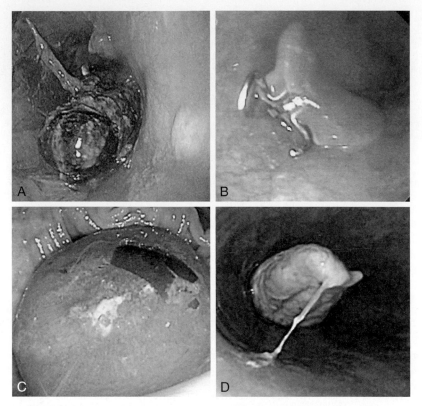

**Figure 61-1.** Several examples of foreign bodies in the gastrointestinal tract. **A,** Meat bolus ($3 \times 1$ cm) impacted in the mid esophagus of a patient with diffuse esophageal spasm. **B,** Inadvertenty swallowed partial denture ($3 \times 2$ cm), with exposed hooks, in the esophagus of a patient without underlying esophageal pathology. **C,** Dried apricot ($2 \times 2$ cm) in the colon of a patient with intermittent abdominal pain. **D,** Chicken bolus ($2 \times 2$ cm) impacted in distal esophagus of a patient with underlying eosinophilic esophagitis.

key role. In general, inert, blunt objects measuring $3 \times 3$ cm pass through the intestine, while objects longer than 6 cm may become lodged in the C-loop of the duodenum. Ingested magnets from magnetic toy sets may be attracted to one another across multiple loops of bowel and lead to intestinal perforation caused by bowel wall erosion and necrosis between the magnets.

### 9. How urgent is removal of a foreign body after ingestion?

Button batteries or magnets, ingested typically by small children, need to be removed urgently because of the severe trauma that they may cause in the esophagus. Any sharp object that carries a high risk for perforation should be removed as soon as possible before it passes to a level that is beyond the reach of an endoscope. For the same reasons, long objects (larger than 6 cm) should be removed when identified. Finally, objects lodged in the esophagus that compromise ability to handle oral secretions should be removed urgently to reduce the risk of aspiration.

### 10. Describe the signs and symptoms of a complication related to foreign-body ingestion.

Respiratory symptoms suggest entrapment of the foreign body in the hypopharynx, trachea, pyriform sinus, or Zenker diverticulum (see Question 6). Sharp objects may penetrate, obstruct, or perforate the esophagus or intestine, presenting with chest, neck, or abdominal pain that varies from mild discomfort to symptoms and signs of acute abdomen. Injury to the esophagus can lead to hematemesis, fever, tachycardia, neck swelling, and crepitus. Excessive drooling and inability to swallow saliva suggest complete esophageal obstruction. Abdominal distention, vomiting, and hyperactive bowel sounds suggest intestinal obstruction. Hypoactive or absent bowel sounds, guarding, rebound, and abdominal pain are seen with wall penetration or free perforation. Aortoenteric fistula due to ingestion of a sharp foreign body may cause massive hematemesis.

### 11. How should foreign bodies be removed?

Once identified, nearly all objects can be removed endoscopically. Other modalities have been used with variable success, although major complications have been reported. Prior to endoscopy, a rehearsal of what will be done using retrieval devices that would capture similar-shaped foreign objects is useful. Several endoscopic retrieval tools, such as rat tooth, grasping forceps, baskets, snares, Roth retrieval net, and overtube, are available (Fig. 61-2). Protection of the airway, especially in children or combative or elderly patients with poor reflexes and cardiopulmonary reserve, is essential. Consultation with a surgeon is appropriate for cases in which perforation or other major complications are probable. Minimally invasive surgery alone or combined with endoscopy is used increasingly.

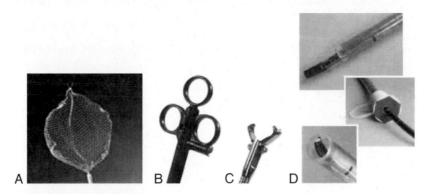

**Figure 61-2.**  Several examples of foreign body removal tools: **A,** Roth net. **B,** Standard polypectomy snare. **C,** Rat-tooth grasper. **D,** Overtube for extraction of sharp foreign bodies.

## 12. Which anatomic/functional defects of the GI tract contribute to foreign-body obstruction?
See Table 62-1.

**Table 61-1.** Anatomic/Functional Defects of the Gastrointestinal Tract That Contribute to Foreign-Body Obstruction

| INTESTINAL SITE | ANATOMIC DEFECT | FUNCTIONAL DEFECT |
|---|---|---|
| Esophagus | Stenosis, atresia, rings, webs, benign/malignant stricture, eosinophilic esophagitis, diverticula, vascular anomalies | Scleroderma, achalasia, Chagas disease |
| Stomach | Pyloric stenosis (congenital, malignancy, postoperative, gastroduodenal ulcer disease) | Gastroparesis (uremia, diabetes, hypothyroidism) |
| Intestine | Postoperative adhesion, Meckel diverticulum, strictures (ischemic, anastomotic, Crohn's disease), malignancy | Idiopathic intestinal pseudo-obstruction, scleroderma |
| Colon | Strictures (ischemic, anastomotic, ulcerative colitis, Crohn's disease, radiation, trauma, infection, surgery), diverticular disease, malignancy | Cathartic colon, idiopathic constipation, familial megacolon, Idiopathic intestinal pseudo obstruction |
| Anus | Stenosis (Crohn's disease, trauma, radiation, infection, surgery) | Hirschsprung disease |

### BIBLIOGRAPHY

1. Arana A, Hauser B, Hachimi-Idrissi S, et al. Management of ingested foreign bodies in childhood and review of the literature. Eur J Pediatr 2001;160:468–72.
2. Barone JE, Yee J, Nealon Jr TF. Management of foreign bodies and trauma of the rectum. Surg Gynecol Obstet 1983;156:453–7.
3. Bounds BC. Endoscopic retrieval devices. Tech Gastrointest Endosc 2006;8:16–21.
4. Busch DB, Starling JR. Rectal foreign bodies: Case reports and a comprehensive review of the world's literature. Surgery 1986;100:512–9.
5. Caratozzolo E, Massani M, Antoniutti M, et al. Combined endoscopic and laparoscopic removal of ingested large foreign bodies: Case report and decisional algorithm. Surg Endosc 2001;15:1226.
6. Cheng W, Tam PK. Foreign-body ingestion in children: Experience with 1,265 cases. J Pediatr Surg 1999;34:1472–6.

7. Katsinelos P, Kountouras J, Paroutoglou G, et al. Endoscopic techniques and management of foreign body ingestion and food bolus impaction in the upper gastrointestinal tract: A retrospective analysis of 139 cases. J Clin Gastroenterol 2006;40:784–9.

8. Li ZS, Sun ZX, Zou DW, et al. Endoscopic management of foreign bodies in the upper-GI tract: Experience with 1088 cases in China. Gastrointest Endosc 2006;64:485–92.

9. Mehta D, Attia M, Quintana E, et al. Glucagon use for esophageal coin dislodgment in children: A prospective, double-blind, placebo-controlled trial. Acad Emerg Med 2001;8:200–3.

10. Mosca S, Manes G, Martino R, et al. Endoscopic management of foreign bodies in the upper gastrointestinal tract: Report on a series of 414 adult patients. Endoscopy 2001;33:692–6.

11. Pavlidis TE, Marakis GN, Triantafyllou A, et al. Management of ingested foreign bodies. How justifiable is a waiting policy? Surg Laparosc Endosc Percutan Tech 2008;18:286–7.

12. Rodríguez-Hermosa JI, Codina-Cazador A, Ruiz B, et al. Management of foreign bodies in the rectum. Colorectal Dis 2007;9:543–8.

# FUNCTIONAL GASTROINTESTINAL DISORDERS AND IRRITABLE BOWEL SYNDROME

*Erica N. Roberson, MD, and Arnold Wald, MD*

CHAPTER 62

**1. What are functional gastrointestinal (GI) disorders?**

Functional GI disorders cause diverse symptoms such as pain, bloating, nausea, and altered bowel habits in the absence of an organic etiology identifiable by current laboratory, imaging, or endoscopy methods. These common disorders often have a significant negative effect on quality of life. The pathogenesis of these disorders is incompletely understood but likely involves a complex interaction between the central and peripheral nervous systems, gut mucosa, motility, and immune system. The Rome III symptom–based classification, published in 2006, provides a framework for research and treatment of these disorders.

**2. Define *irritable bowel syndrome* (IBS).**

IBS is a functional GI disorder characterized by chronic, recurrent abdominal pain or discomfort associated with disturbed bowel habits. As defined by Rome III (Box 62-1), symptoms must be present for at least 6 months and often occur intermittently with asymptomatic intervals. IBS has been further classified as diarrhea-predominant, constipation-predominant, or mixed habit depending on the predominant symptom patterns. These symptoms often change over time, resulting in redefinition of their subtype. Because IBS is a functional disorder, the symptom-based Rome III criteria may be useful in forming a positive diagnosis in clinical practice as well as assisting in research on IBS.

**3. Discuss the epidemiology of IBS.**

Although the prevalence of IBS has varied according to the definitions used, most population studies report a prevalence of up to 15% of adults in the United States and Europe. IBS is more common in women and peaks in the third and fourth decades of life but is seen in all age groups and races. Fortunately, only a minority of patients seek medical care for IBS; nevertheless, IBS is the most common outpatient disorder seen by gastroenterologists and accounts for at least 28% of referrals.

**4. What is the natural history of IBS?**

Studies have shown that most patients with IBS continue to have symptoms over many years. The overall prevalence of each subgroup (constipation-predominant, diarrhea-predominant, mixed) is stable over time, but individual patients often have a change in their subgroup. IBS is not a risk factor for organic gastroenterologic disease and, once the diagnosis is made, only a very small percentage are diagnosed with an alternative organic disorder to explain their symptoms. IBS is not linked to an increase in mortality, but it is associated with increased diagnostic testing and surgical interventions, especially in women.

**5. Discuss the current pathophysiology of IBS.**

The pathophysiology of IBS is incompletely understood; it is likely multifactorial and involves visceral hypersensitivity and altered motility, immune activation, and stress response. Because IBS clusters in families, there may be a genetic component and some proposed genes include those encoding the serotonin transport protein or inflammatory marker

---

**Box 62-1.** Rome III Symptoms Based Criteria* for Irritable Bowel Syndrome.

Recurrent abdominal pain or discomfort at least 3 days per month in the last 3 months,† associated with two or more of the following:
1. Improvement with defecation
2. Onset associated with a change in frequency of stool
3. Onset associated with a change in form (appearance) of stool

*Criteria must be fulfilled for the last 3 months with symptom onset at least 6 mo prior to diagnosis.
†Discomfort means an uncomfortable sensation not described as pain. Pain or discomfort frequency of least 2 days a week during screening should be present for clinical trial eligibility.

production. However, studies have noted that concordance between parents and children is greater than that between twins, suggesting a more significant role for environment than for genetics.

Disturbances in colonic motility patterns have been observed in IBS. In general, diarrhea-predominant IBS has accelerated transit and more high-amplitude propagating contractions (HAPCs), whereas constipation-predominant IBS has slower transit and fewer HAPCs. This may, in part, be related to serotonin, a stimulant of GI motility, as patients with diarrhea-predominant IBS have high levels of serotonin and patients with constipation-predominant IBS have low plasma serotonin levels. Small bowel motility is also altered in IBS, especially in patients with diarrhea-predominant IBS, as increased frequency of migrating motor complex (MMC) and discrete cluster contractions have been reported. Both the small and large bowels have exaggerated responses to meal ingestion and corticotrophin-releasing hormone (CRH) (see later).

Visceral hypersensitivity has been observed in about 60% of patients with IBS and perhaps involves alterations in interactions of the central and peripheral nervous systems with the GI tract. This results in the perception or exaggerated sensation of abdominal pain and disordered bowel movements. Peripheral nerve endings are stimulated by inflammation to increase their excitability, resulting in lower thresholds for perceived pain and modified responses to external stressors. Peripheral nerve stimulation causes recruitment of other nerves, a process called *central sensitization,* and therefore amplification of the perception of pain. Functional neuroimaging studies have shown that patients with IBS may have altered somatosensory processing in the thalamus and cortex and altered cognitive/affective processing in the cingulate gyrus and insula. A recent study suggests that altered motility and visceral hypersensitivity work independently to contribute to the symptoms of IBS.

Altered immune activation may also play a role in the development of IBS. Recent studies have shown that some patients with IBS have elevated inflammatory markers compared with healthy controls. Also, a genetic polymorphism that increases production of tumor necrosis factor-alpha is more common in patients with IBS.

Finally, recent studies have focused on *altered stress circuits* in patients with IBS. The hypothalamus-pituitary-adrenal (HPA) axis starts in the hypothalamus, which produces CRH. CRH then stimulates the pituitary to release adrenocorticotropic hormone (ACTH), which stimulates the adrenal medulla to produce cortisol. As altered response to stress is well described in IBS patients, physical and psychological stress may result in exaggerated responses to stress, as exemplified by elevated secretion of ACTH and cortisol in response to infusion of CRH.

## 6. Discuss the interplay of IBS and psychiatric disorders.

The relationship between IBS and psychiatric disorders is complex. Although psychiatric disorders do not cause IBS, they may contribute to exacerbations of symptoms, increased health care utilization, and reduced success of treatment. Patients with IBS who present for medical care have a higher prevalence of psychiatric comorbidities, including depression, anxiety, and somatization, compared with the general population. Screening for psychiatric disorders is important as patients with IBS and untreated depression and anxiety are often resistant to treatment.

## 7. Discuss important aspects in the patient's history to diagnosing IBS.

The history should include assessment of abdominal pain, bowel function, and chronicity of symptoms. Although variable, abdominal pain is often diffuse, crampy, and intermittent. Altered bowel habits include diarrhea, constipation, or both, often alternating with normal bowel activity. Diarrhea is described as frequent, loose stools that may be associated with urgency; stool volume is normal. Constipation is characterized by pellet-like stools associated with straining, sense of incomplete evacuation, and passage of mucus. Again, the predominant symptom patterns often change over time and are interspersed with asymptomatic periods. Symptoms may be exacerbated by psychosocial stressors and in some patients are preceded by a discrete diarrheal illness (see Question 11). The presence of so-called *alarm symptoms* should be evaluated (see Question 14).

## 8. Discuss clinical assessment of psychological disorders.

Simple questions or short questionnaires may be used to screen patients for psychological disorders such as depression and anxiety. Examples of such questions include the following:

- Do you feel down or have you lost interest in things you normally enjoy?
- Have you had sudden unprovoked attacks of fear or anxiety?
- Do you worry or feel anxious most of the time?
- Do you have a fear of embarrassment or criticism when in public situations?

Two examples of short-form questionnaires are the Patient Health Questionnaire (PHQ 15), which helps to identify somatization, and the Hospital Anxiety and Depression Scale (HADS), which assesses anxiety and depression. (See Websites.)

9. **List the differential diagnosis for IBS.**

The differential diagnosis of diarrhea-predominant IBS may include, among others, celiac disease, microscopic colitis, inflammatory bowel disease, giardiasis, lactose intolerance, small bowel bacterial overgrowth, and bile salt malabsorption. The differential diagnosis for constipation-predominant IBS includes chronic functional constipation, medications, and diverticular disease. Colon cancer should be considered in any person with new GI complaints, especially if the patient is older than 50 years, has blood in stools, or has a family history of colon cancer.

10. **Discuss postinfectious IBS and related pathology.**

Approximately 7% to 30% of persons who experience an episode of infectious diarrhea associated with bacteria or a virus develop IBS symptoms. Risk factors for the development of postinfectious IBS include severity and length of illness, use of antibiotics, female gender, and presence of psychosocial factors such as anxiety and depression. The development of postinfectious IBS is independent of the cause of infectious diarrhea and symptoms are classically diarrhea-predominant. Rectal biopsy samples obtained from affected patients have shown hyperplasia of enterochromaffin cells; these store and release serotonin, which is known to increase peristalsis and intestinal secretions. Studies have also shown increased lymphocytes in the lamina propria, which may promote secretion of cytokines and other inflammatory markers. Increase in mast cell activation and release of histamine also contribute to an increase in gut permeability in some patients.

11. **Discuss the physical exam pertinent for IBS.**

The physical exam should include an abdominal and rectal exam. Abdominal exam may be normal or may elicit abdominal tenderness, which is characteristically nonfocal, reflecting its visceral origin. Rectal exam is performed to assess for perianal disease, rectal masses, and sphincter tone. Perianal disease should raise suspicion for Crohn's disease. Stool examination should be performed to assess for occult blood. The presence of a rectal mass or positive stool guaiac should prompt evaluation with colonoscopy to evaluate for colon cancer.

12. **What is Carnett test?**

Carnett test is a physical finding that helps to distinguish abdominal wall pain from intraperitoneal pain. Patients should fold their arms across their chest and raise their head off the pillow while the physician palpates the abdomen. If focal tenderness improves or disappears, the etiology is likely visceral in origin. However, if the tenderness is worse with this motion, the origin is the abdominal wall. Abdominal wall tenderness can be due to a muscle injury, trapped nerve, or hernia. Resolution of the pain after a trigger point injection with 1% Xylocaine with or without 20 to 40 mg triamcinolone confirms that the origin was in the abdominal wall.

13. **What laboratory studies should be performed in all patients with IBS?**

Guidelines may vary, but laboratory evaluations should be limited: complete blood count (CBC), sedimentation rate, celiac antibody tests, thyroid function, and stool for parasite and guaiac.

14. **What are alarm symptoms that should alert the clinician to investigate further?**

So-called *alarm symptoms* in the history include fever, weight loss, passage of blood per rectum, age greater than 50 years, a major change in symptoms, short history of symptoms, nocturnal symptoms, recent antibiotics, and a family history of colon or ovarian cancer or inflammatory bowel disorder. The presence of an abdominal mass or rectal mass on examination should alert the physician to investigate further. Laboratory results revealing anemia, elevated inflammatory markers, and positive celiac antibodies should also prompt investigation. If alarm symptoms are present, exclusion of organic pathology by appropriate testing is necessary before a diagnosis of IBS is made.

15. **Should a colonoscopy be performed on all patients with IBS?**

A colonoscopy is not routinely recommended for the diagnosis of IBS by any guideline. IBS is not a risk factor for developing colon cancer as the incidence of colon cancer is the same in IBS patients as among the general population. If a patient is older than 50 years, he or she should undergo a screening colonoscopy as a part of preventative health care. If alarm symptoms are present or if the clinical picture is suggestive, a colonoscopy may be an appropriate test.

16. **How is IBS diagnosed?**

Although experts state that IBS should be a positive diagnosis based on history, physical exam, and judiciously used investigations, in clinical practice IBS is often a diagnosis of exclusion. Abdominal pain or discomfort should be present intermittently for longer than 6 months. This discomfort is associated with a change in bowel habits and symptoms may be worse with psychosocial stress. IBS can be subclassified as diarrhea-predominant, constipation-predominant, or mixed based on stool consistency. Physical exam and laboratory tests may be normal. If alarm symptoms are present, further investigation should be performed to exclude an organic cause. A clinical diagnosis of IBS can then be made with confidence.

## 17. Discuss the general approach to patients with IBS.

As is true for all medical disorders, the key to successful management of IBS is to establish a good physician-patient relationship. Patients with chronic disorders like IBS benefit from continuity of care and a therapeutic liaison with their health care provider. Components of a good relationship include good eye contact, appropriate body language, open-ended questions, and empathy. It is important that the patient does not feel symptoms are being trivialized or that it is *all in the head*. The clinician should establish why the patient is seeking care:

- What does the patient believe is causing the symptoms?
- Is there a fear of cancer or secondary gain?
- Are any psychosocial factors present?

The patient should be reassured that IBS has no effect on mortality and is not a risk factor for other GI diseases.

## 18. Describe the initial and general treatment of IBS.

Crucial to the initial treatment of IBS are education and healthy lifestyle modifications. As with all chronic disorders, education improves clinical outcome by giving patients the knowledge and coping skills to manage their IBS. Studies have also shown that most patients with IBS desire more education about what causes IBS, what foods to avoid, and coping strategies to reduce symptoms. They also want to know about medications to prevent attacks, psychological factors in IBS, and availability of research studies.

Lifestyle modifications should focus on diet, stress management, and exercise. Patients may benefit from keeping a daily diary to help identify factors that trigger symptoms such as food, stressors, or moods. Certain foods such as cabbage, beans, broccoli, and cauliflower may trigger symptoms. If bloating is problematic, carbonated beverages, gum, and artificial sweeteners containing sucralose should be avoided. Stress reduction techniques include relaxation through meditation, as well as coping skills. The benefits of exercise include reduced stress and improved well-being and functional status. Patients should be encouraged to obtain adequate sleep as many patients with IBS have impaired sleep quality and sleep fragmentation.

Medical management should be tailored to the predominant symptoms of each individual and multiple medications are often required. As symptoms frequently change over time, medications may need parallel adjustments. For instance, a patient with abdominal pain could be prescribed a tricyclic antidepressant (TCA) such as amitriptyline (see Question 21), which is a good choice for patients with diarrhea-predominant symptoms. Low-dose selective serotonin reuptake inhibitors (SSRIs) are also reasonable to use with pain-predominant symptoms and may be a better choice than tricyclic antidepressants in a patient with constipation-predominant symptoms (see Question 26). For a patient with unpredictable episodic abdominal cramps, hyoscyamine sublingual (0.125 mg) is a reasonable choice.

For patients with mild constipation, non–gas-producing osmotic laxatives, such as polyethylene glycol or stimulant laxatives, may be tried. As noted earlier, only in unresponsive patients should more expensive medications like lubiprostone and tegaserod be considered. Patients with mild diarrhea can be treated with loperamide (2 mg daily or twice a day). TCAs are also good options for patients with more persistent diarrhea. Alosetron is a restricted medication that should be used only in refractory cases (see Question 20).

For selected patients with refractory IBS, cognitive-behavioral therapy (CBT) and hypnotherapy may be very effective. In contrast, acupuncture has not shown to be effective.

## 19. What medical therapies are helpful for diarrhea-predominant IBS?

Loperamide can be titrated to control diarrhea in patients with IBS (see earlier). Several older small studies found that loperamide improved bowel frequency and urgency but not pain. TCAs are a good choice for some patients with pain as a predominant symptom and improve overall well-being (see Question 21). Despite the paucity of evidence in the literature due to lack of large randomized controlled trials, antispasmodic medications such as hyoscyamine (0.125 mg, sublingual) are often effective options for patients with episodic pain and may be used on an as-needed basis.

## 20. What is the current role for alosetron in IBS?

Alosetron is a (5-hydroxytryptamine$_3$) (5-HT$_3$) receptor antagonist that has been shown to improve urgency, bowel frequency, abdominal pain, and global symptoms in women with diarrhea predominant IBS. One meta-analysis of multicenter randomized placebo-controlled studies confirmed that both men and women taking alosetron also have significant global improvement of overall symptoms and pain.

Alosetron was originally approved in 2000 by the U.S. Food and Drug Administration (FDA) for diarrhea-predominant IBS. Later that year, the drug was withdrawn because of concerns about ischemic colitis (0.15% compared to

0.0% in placebo). In 2002, alosetron (1 mg daily to twice daily) was reintroduced with restriction to women with longstanding diarrhea-predominant IBS is refractory to other therapies. Physicians prescribing this drug must be part of a physician-prescribing program (http://www.lotronex.com). Patients taking alosetron must sign a patient-physician agreement indicating they have been informed of and understand the associated risks.

## 21. What role do TCAs play in the treatment of IBS?
TCAs are thought to work in IBS by improving visceral pain, and they may also modulate gut function, particularly in patients with diarrhea-predominant symptoms. Because TCAs have anticholinergic properties, side effects include constipation, urinary retention, and dry mouth. Doses much lower than those used for depression are often effective for pain associated with IBS. Effects are independent of improvement in anxiety or depression.

Although these medications are used frequently in IBS, supportive data are limited. Desipramine 150 mg daily did not show statistically significant improvement compared with placebo in a 12-week multicenter trial of women with functional abdominal pain. However, when only patients who remained on the drug were analyzed, desipramine had a significantly higher response with a number needed to treat (NNT) of 4.3. A recent double-blind study of amitriptyline in adolescents with IBS showed significant improvement in quality of life, abdominal pain, and diarrhea compared with placebo that persisted after discontinuation of the drug. Another small randomized double-blind study of adults with diarrhea-predominant IBS showed significantly improved abdominal pain and bowel habits with amitriptyline 10 mg daily compared with placebo.

Our approach is to start with low doses (10 to 25 mg daily) of one of four drugs: amitriptyline or its tertiary amine, nortriptyline, or imipramine or its tertiary amine, desipramine. The dose may be increased by 10 mg daily every 2 to 3 weeks as tolerated and according to symptomatic response. If unacceptable side effects occur, the drug is stopped and another TCA is substituted. There is no fixed or standard dose and it may take 2 to 3 weeks to see a beneficial effect. An overall response rate of approximately 80% has been reported and is consistent with our experience.

## 22. Discuss therapeutic options for constipation-predominant IBS.
Although fiber has been traditionally used as a first-line agent for constipation-predominant IBS, no clinical trial has shown a benefit. Fiber intake should be minimized to avoid side effects, such as bloating, which often limit use. Osmotic laxatives, such as polyethylene glycol, can be effective but gas-producing laxatives, such as lactulose, should be avoided as they may exacerbate bloating. Although good randomized controlled trials are lacking, SSRIs may be beneficial in patients with constipation-predominant symptoms. Therapeutic agents such as tegaserod and lubiprostone should be limited to severe, refractory cases.

## 23. Discuss the controversy behind fiber and IBS.
A recent Cochrane Review did not find significant benefit of bulking agents on abdominal pain, global assessment of pain, or symptom score. However, the heterogeneity of IBS symptoms in the studies limits the conclusion that bulking agents are not useful for some patients. Another meta-analysis evaluated 13 placebo-controlled trials and found that bulking agents, such as fiber, improve global IBS symptoms in IBS. However, when poor-quality studies were removed from the analysis, there was no significant difference in symptoms compared with placebo. An additional systematic review of 17 studies found that patients with constipation-predominant IBS had improvement in global symptoms and constipation from soluble fiber, in contrast to insoluble fiber, which improved constipation but not global well-being. Also, neither type of fiber improved abdominal pain. Several studies have noted that insoluble fiber, specifically bran, may worsen bloating and abdominal pain. We start with small amounts of soluble fiber and limit insoluble fiber (bran). Fiber should be slowly increased if no intensification of bloating or abdominal pain is noted.

## 24. What is the current role for tegaserod in IBS?
Tegaserod is a partial 5-HT$_4$ agonist approved by the FDA in 2002 for constipation-predominant IBS. Studies have reported a modest increase in global response rate above placebo and the number needed to treat (NNT) was 17 (i.e., 17 patients had to be treated to obtain a benefit for 1 patient compared with placebo).

However, the FDA removed tegaserod from the market in March 2007 because of a small increase in cardiovascular events during post-marketing studies. All patients who developed cardiovascular events were known to have coronary risk factors or cardiovascular disease. In July 2007, the FDA approved tegaserod as an investigational drug to be used only in women younger than age 55 who did not have cardiovascular risk factors and had chronic constipation or constipation-predominant IBS that does not respond to other treatments.

## 25. What is the current role for lubiprostone in IBS?
Lubiprostone is a prostaglandin E$_1$ analog and activates intestinal chloride-2 channels to increase chloride and fluid secretion into the lumen. This should increase bowel movement frequency and soften stools. Originally approved in

January 2008 for chronic constipation, it was approved by the FDA in April 2008 for women with constipation-predominant IBS. The package insert states that in the two pivotal studies, response rates were 14% and 12%, higher than placebo response rates of 8% and 6%, respectively. The recommended dose of 8 mcg twice daily is lower than that used for chronic constipation (24 mcg twice daily). The most common side effects are nausea and diarrhea. We consider this medication only after other available treatments have failed.

### 26. What role do SSRIs and serotonin-norepinephrine reuptake inhibitors (SNRIs) have in the treatment of IBS?

SSRIs may be useful to manage abdominal pain in some patients with IBS independent of their antidepressant effects. They are often used at doses lower than those used for mood disorders. The exact mechanisms by which SSRIs benefit IBS patients are unclear, although serotonin is a key neurotransmitter in the central processing of visceral afferent information and has effects on GI motility. In contrast to the paucity of published data on SNRIs (duloxetine, venlafaxine) in IBS, there have been published studies of paroxetine, fluoxetine, and citalopram in the treatment of IBS. In a randomized double-blind study, paroxetine (20 mg daily for 3 weeks, then 40 mg daily for 3 weeks) improved well-being in 63% of patients with IBS compared to 26% with placebo. Benefit occurred in both depressed and nondepressed patients but there were no differences in abdominal pain or bloating. In another study of severe IBS, paroxetine (20 mg daily) reduced frequency of abdominal pain at 3 months and improved health-related quality of life at 3 and 12 months. In a randomized, double-blinded study, fluoxetine (20 mg daily) improved bowel movements and decreased abdominal discomfort in patients with constipation predominant IBS compared with placebo. Improvement persisted 4 weeks after discontinuation of the medication. Citalopram (20 mg daily for 3 weeks, then 40 mg daily for 3 weeks) significantly improved overall well-being, abdominal pain, bloating, and bowel movements in a 6-week double-blind cross-over study, and improvement was also independent of the presence of depression and anxiety. In our practice, we prefer these agents in patients with constipation-predominant IBS and in patients with IBS who do not tolerate or respond to TCAs.

### 27. Discuss the role of CBT and hypnotherapy in treating IBS.

CBT is based on the theory that the symptoms of IBS are due to maladaptive responses. Specifically, CBT is a structured, problem-based therapy that consists of education on the influence of stress on symptoms, coping skills to deal with stress including relaxation techniques and strategies to deal with stress, and modification of emotional and physiologic reactions to stress (behavioral self-care skills). A recent meta-analysis showed that the NNT for more than 50% relief of symptoms was only two compared to controls. A pilot study found that patient-administered CBT (also called minimal contact CBT [MC-CBT]) may be as effective as therapist-administered CBT. Such patient-administered CBT overcomes some of the limitations of CBT including the number of sessions, therapist time, and cost.

The aim of hypnotherapy (also called gut-directed hypnotherapy [GDH]) is to control gut function by using therapist and self-induced hypnosis to induce progressive relaxation. Hypnotherapy has been found to be superior to wait-listed controls for symptoms of IBS. GDH is appropriate for selected (hypnotizable) patients for whom conservative and medical therapy has failed. Current studies show that GDH decreases health care utilization and improves quality of life; it is hoped that future studies will define its precise role in the management of IBS.

### 28. Do probiotics and antibiotics have a role in the management of IBS?

Recent studies have suggested that nonabsorbable antibiotics, such as rifaximin, may be beneficial in IBS by decreasing bloating. We are skeptical of this practice because of the potential harmful effects of using antibiotics on colonic bacterial flora and because similar effects can be achieved at less cost and less risk with carbohydrate-restricted diets (so-called Atkins diet).

Probiotics in diet and in pill form have gained popularity for IBS in recent years, particularly for bloating and flatulence. There is little supporting evidence for their use in IBS and they are not a part of our routine practice. However, many patients do use them and we do not actively discourage their use.

## WEBSITES

http://www.cignabehavioral.com/web/basicsite/provider/newsAndLearning/clinicalScreeningTools/phq15.pdf

http://www.eardoctor.org/pdf/Hospital%20Anxiety%20and%20Depression%20Scale.pdf

http://www.aboutibs.org

http://www.digestive.niddk.nih.gov/

# BIBLIOGRAPHY

1. Andresen V, Montori VM, Keller J, et al. Effects of 5-hydroxytryptamine (serotonin) type 3 antagonists on symptom relief and constipation in nonconstipated irritable bowel syndrome: A systematic review and meta-analysis of randomized controlled trials. Clin Gastroenterol Hepatol 2008;6:545–55.
2. Azpiroz F, Bouin M, Camilleri M, et al. Mechanisms of hypersensitivity in IBS and functional disorders. Neurogastroenterol Motil 2007;19:62–88.
3. Bahar RJ, Collins BS, Steinmetz B, et al. Double-blind placebo-controlled trial of amitriptyline for the treatment of irritable bowel syndrome in adolescents. J Pediatr 2008;152:685–9.
4. Cash BD, Schoenfeld P, Chey WD. The utility of diagnostic tests in irritable bowel syndrome patients: A systematic review. Am J Gastroenterol 2002;97:2812–9.
5. Dalrymple J, Bullock I. Diagnosis and management of irritable bowel syndrome in adults in primary care: Summary of NICE guidance. BMJ 2008;336:556–8.
6. Dinan TG, Quigley E, Ahmed S, et al. Hypothalamic-pituitary-gut axis dysregulation in irritable bowel syndrome: Plasma cytokines as a potential biomarker? Gastroenterology 2006;130:304–11.
7. Halpert A, Dalton CB, Palsson O, et al. What patients know about irritable bowel syndrome (IBS) and what they would like to know. National Survey on Patient Educational Needs in IBS and development and validation of the Patient Educational Needs Questionnaire (PEQ). Am J Gastroenterol 2007;102:1972–82.
8. Johanson JF, Drossman DA, Panas R, et al. Clinical trial: Phase 2 study of lubiprostone for irritable bowel syndrome with constipation. Aliment Pharmacol Ther 2008;27:685–96.
9. Kanazawa M, Palsson O, Thiwan S, et al. Contributions of pain sensitivity and colonic motility to IBS symptom severity and predominant bowel habits. Am J Gastroenterol 2008;103:2550–61.
10. Lackner JM, Jaccard J, Krasner S, et al. Self-administered cognitive behavior therapy for moderate to severe irritable bowel syndrome: Clinical efficacy, tolerability, feasibility. Clin Gastroenterol Hepatol 2008;6:899–906.
11. Longstreth GF, Thompson WG, Chey WD, et al. Functional bowel disorders. Gastroenterology 2006;130:1480–91.
12. Lubiprostone (Amitiza) for irritable bowel syndrome with constipation. Med Lett Drugs Ther 2008;50:53–4.
13. Mayer EA. Clinical practice. Irritable bowel syndrome. N Engl J Med 2008;358:1692–9.
14. Quartero AO, Meineche-Schmidt V, Muris J, et al. Bulking agents, antispasmodic and antidepressant medication for the treatment of irritable bowel syndrome. Cochrane Database Syst Rev 2005; CD003460.
15. Rahimi R, Nikfar S, Abdollahi M. Efficacy and tolerability of alosetron for the treatment of irritable bowel syndrome in women and men: A meta-analysis of eight randomized, placebo-controlled, 12-week trials. Clin Ther 2008;30:884–901.
16. Rhodes DY, Wallace M. Post-infectious irritable bowel syndrome. Curr Gastroenterol Rep 2006;8:327–32.
17. Spiller R. Review article: Probiotics and prebiotics in irritable bowel syndrome. Aliment Pharmacol Ther 2008;28:385–96.
18. Spiller R, Aziz Q, Creed F, et al. Guidelines on the irritable bowel syndrome: Mechanisms and practical management. Gut 2007;56:1770–98.
19. Tack J, Broehaert D, Fischler B, et al. A controlled crossover study of the selective serotonin reuptake inhibitor citalopram in irritable bowel syndrome. Gut 2006;55:1095–103.
20. Vahedi H, Merat S, Momtahen S, et al. Clinical trial: The effect of amitriptyline in patients with diarrhoea-predominant irritable bowel syndrome. Aliment Pharmacol Ther 2008;27:678–84.
21. Vahedi H, Merat S, Rashidioon A, et al. The effect of fluoxetine in patients with pain and constipation-predominant irritable bowel syndrome: A double-blind randomized-controlled study. Aliment Pharmacol Ther 2005;22:381–5.
22. Wald A, Rakel D. Behavioral and complementary approaches for the treatment of irritable bowel syndrome. Nutr Clin Pract 2008;23:284–92.
23. Wilson S, Maddison T, Roberts L, et al. Systematic review: The effectiveness of hypnotherapy in the management of irritable bowel syndrome. Aliment Pharmacol Ther 2006;24:769–80.

# ENDOSCOPIC CANCER SCREENING AND SURVEILLANCE

*Joel Z. Stengel, MD, and*
*David P. Jones, DO*

**1. What is endoscopic cancer screening and surveillance?**

*Endoscopic screening* for premalignant or malignant conditions is the one-time application of a test to search for lesions in asymptomatic persons in the hope that an early diagnosis will have an impact on disease outcomes. *Endoscopic surveillance* in patients with known premalignant or malignant conditions is the repeated application of a test over time to search for lesions in patients at increased risk.

**2. Why is endoscopic cancer screening and surveillance performed for gastrointestinal (GI) cancers?**

GI cancers are annually reported as one of the most common causes of cancer death. Many GI cancers have well-defined premalignant lesions that are easily indentified on endoscopy; examples include Barrett's esophagus and colorectal adenomas.

## ESOPHAGUS

**3. Endoscopic cancer screening of the esophagus is primarily undertaken for what two types of esophageal cancer? What risk factors are associated with these two types of cancer?**

- *Adenocarcinoma* is the most common type of esophageal cancer in the United States and is associated with Barrett's esophagus and obesity.
- *Squamous cell carcinoma* (SCC) is a less frequent cause of esophageal cancer in the United States. The risk factors for esophageal SCC include alcohol, tobacco smoking, achalasia, caustic injury, tylosis, prior or concurrent head and neck SCC, and Plummer-Vinson syndrome.

**4. What is Barrett (metaplasia) esophagus? Why is endoscopic screening and surveillance for Barrett's esophagus necessary?**

Barrett's esophagus is specialized intestinal metaplasia of the distal tubular esophagus, which has been identified as a premalignant precursor to adenocarcinoma. The incidence of esophageal adenocarcinoma is currently increasing at a rate greater than that of any other cancer in the Western world. The 5-year survival rate for late-stage esophageal adenocarcinoma is poor and the only hope for improved survival is early detection of the cancer.

**5. Which patients should undergo endoscopic screening for Barrett's esophagus?**

Screening for Barrett's esophagus in the general population is not recommended at this time, but should be considered in selected patients with frequent heartburn (several times per week), longstanding (more than 5 years) gastroesophageal reflux disease. Patients at increased risk for Barrett are typically white men older than 50 years and those with nocturnal reflux. After a negative screening examination, surveillance endoscopy is not indicated.

**6. What techniques are used to perform endoscopic screening in Barrett's esophagus?**

A complete direct visual examination of the esophagus with a white light high-resolution and high-definition endoscope is the standard for endoscopic screening of Barrett's esophagus. Esophageal capsule endoscopy is a new technique that can provide a noninvasive assessment of suspected Barrett's esophagus, but the capsule is expensive and early studies have demonstrated varying sensitivity with the device.

**7. What is the rationale for endoscopic surveillance in Barrett's esophagus?**

Barrett's esophagus surveillance programs attempt to detect adenocarcinoma or high-grade dysplasia (HGD) at an earlier, potentially curable stage and have been shown to significantly improve 5-year survival compared with similar patients not undergoing routine endoscopic surveillance.

**8. What techniques are used to perform endoscopic surveillance in Barrett's esophagus?**

Surveillance endoscopy should only be performed after patients have their reflux aggressively controlled with a proton pump inhibitor because any inflammation may interfere with the endoscopic and microscopic identification of dysplasia. Endoscopic surveillance involves systematic four-quadrant biopsies at 1- to 2-cm intervals along the entire length of the Barrett segment. Biopsies should also specifically target any luminal irregularity in the Barrett segment (e.g., ulceration, erosion, nodule, or stricture) because there is an association of such lesions with underlying cancer. The use of *jumbo* biopsy forceps may improve the yield of the biopsies and should be considered, especially in patients with previous dysplasia.

**9. How often should patients with Barrett's esophagus undergo endoscopic surveillance?**

Endoscopic surveillance intervals are determined by the presence and grade of dysplasia found in patients with Barrett's esophagus. In general, Barrett's esophagus patients without dysplasia are recommended to undergo two negative upper endoscopies (within 1 year) with systematic four-quadrant biopsies prior to initiating surveillance endoscopies every 3 years (Table 63-1).

**10. How do you manage low-grade dysplasia (LGD) in patients with Barrett's esophagus?**

LGD must be confirmed on a repeat esophagogastroduodenoscopy (EGD) within 6 months and an expert GI pathologist is also required to review the biopsy samples before the initiation of annual endoscopic surveillance. Surveillance endoscopy continues until the lesion disappears on two consecutive endoscopic exams. Patients can be reassured that 60% of patients with LGD will regress to no dysplasia after a mean follow-up of 4 years.

**11. How do you manage HGD in patients with Barrett's esophagus?**

HGD is associated with 30% risk of developing esophageal adenocarcinoma. If HGD is confirmed by an expert GI pathologist, there is currently no agreement on the most appropriate management of these patients. Treatment options available to patients include intensive endoscopic surveillance with four-quadrant biopsies every 1 cm performed every 3 months, endoscopic ablation therapy, or surgical resection. All of these treatment options have produced similar outcomes for patients in retrospective cohort studies performed at expert centers. Optimal treatment is therefore determined on a case-by-case basis taking into account the patient's age, comorbidities, and ability to comply with an aggressive surveillance program and local surgical expertise.

**12. What is the principal role of endoscopic ultrasound (EUS) in evaluating patients with HGD?**

EUS can be used to exclude the presence of occult cancer, submucosal invasion, and malignant lymphadenopathy in patients with Barrett's esophagus of HGD. This information is particularly important when determining the appropriate selection of patients if endoscopic management is considered. Routine application of EUS in Barrett's esophagus with LGD or without dysplasia is not recommended because the risk of malignancy is so low.

**13. What is the next step if adenocarcinoma is identified while performing endoscopic surveillance for Barrett's esophagus?**

Once esophageal adenocarcinoma is confirmed by an expert GI pathologist, staging of the cancer is performed with a computed tomography (CT) scan, preferably integrated positron emission tomography/CT, to evaluate for the presence of metastatic disease. Next, patients without evidence of metastatic disease by CT would undergo EUS for regional staging to provide detailed images of the esophageal masses and their relationship within the structure of the esophageal wall. EUS with fine-needle aspiration (FNA) can also be used for lymph node staging. Finally, depending on the stage of the cancer, the patient should be referred to oncology, radiation oncology, and/or surgery for treatment.

**Table 63-1.** 2008 American College of Gastroenterology Practice Guidelines for Endoscopic Surveillance of Barrett's Esophagus

| DYSPLASIA | DOCUMENTATION | FOLLOW-UP INTERVAL |
|---|---|---|
| None | Two negative EGDs (within 1 year) with four quadrant biopsies every 2 cm in the Barrett segment | Surveillance EGD every 3 years |
| Low grade | Expert GI pathologist confirmation | Confirmed on repeat EGD within 6 months, 1 year interval (EGD) until no dysplasia × 2 |
| High grade | Expert GI pathologist confirmation Endoscopic mucosal resection (EMR) of any mucosal irregularities, Intensive biopsy protocol with biopsies every 1 cm | Repeat EGD within 3 months Expert pathologist confirmation Management dependent on local expertise (surgery vs. endoscopic therapy) |

EGD, esophagogastroduodenoscopy; GI, gastrointestinal; EMR, endoscopic mucosal resection.

## 14. What new imaging modalities are available for Barrett's esophagus endoscopic screening and surveillance?

Narrow band imaging (NBI) is a new technique that filters the illuminating white light on the endoscope into two colors (blue and green), which are avidly absorbed by blood vessels to allow for better visualization of the mucosa. In one study of patients with Barrett's esophagus, the sensitivity of NBI detection for an irregular mucosal pattern was 100% with a specificity of 98.7%. Chromoendoscopy may also be used to stain the esophagus with agents like methylene blue, crystal violet, indigo carmine, and acetic acid that are applied to the mucosa to enhance the detection of abnormal mucosal patterns in Barrett's esophagus.

## 15. Do patients with achalasia have an increased risk of esophageal cancer?

Individuals with achalasia have as much as a 33-fold greater risk of developing SCC of the esophagus compared with the general population. On average, patients with achalasia will have had at least 15 years of symptoms prior to the diagnosis of esophageal cancer. Patients with achalasia have a generally poor prognosis once esophageal cancer is diagnosed.

## 16. What is the role of endoscopic cancer surveillance in patients with achalasia?

Currently, there are insufficient data to support routine endoscopic surveillance in patients with achalasia. Endoscopic surveillance in patients with achalasia has not been found to be cost effective, but it may be considered 15 years after the onset of symptoms. All surface abnormalities of esophagus identified during the exam should undergo biopsy, and the recommended timing of any surveillance endoscopy has not been defined.

## 17. Is there a link between caustic ingestion and the development of esophageal cancer?

Yes. A caustic injury to the esophagus, most commonly after lye ingestion, appears to be associated with an increased risk of developing SCC of the esophagus. A history of caustic ingestion is present in 1% to 4% of patients with esophageal cancer. A single Finnish study found the magnitude of risk was approximately 1000-fold increased compared with the general population.

## 18. What are the clinical characteristics of patients who develop esophageal cancer after a caustic injury?

- Mean age of onset 35 to 51 years
- Average interval between caustic injury and development of esophageal cancer approximately 40 years
- Cancers located in the mid-esophagus

## 19. How is endoscopic surveillance used in patients with a history of caustic ingestion?

Endoscopic surveillance should begin 15 to 20 years after the caustic ingestion and the interval between exams should not be more frequent than every 1 to 3 years. Any reported swallowing problems should be investigated immediately with endoscopy in this patient population.

## 20. What rare genetic disorder is associated with a high incidence of SCC of the esophagus?

*Tylosis* is an uncommon autosomal dominant disorder that is distinguished by thickening of the skin (hyperkeratosis) on the palms and soles. The syndrome is associated with a 27% incidence of SCC of the esophagus. The average age at onset of esophageal cancer is 45 years and death from esophageal cancer can occur in patients as young as 30 years.

## 21. What type of endoscopic surveillance is recommended in patients with tylosis?

Patients with tylosis should begin endoscopic surveillance at the age of 30. Most cases of esophageal cancer in these patients have been noted in the distal esophagus so attention should be focused in this area during the exam. Repeat endoscopy should not be conducted more frequently than every 1 to 3 years in these patients.

## 22. Are patients with a history of head and neck, lung, or esophageal SCC at risk for synchronous or metachronous cancer of the esophagus?

Yes. The incidence of multiple SCCs of the upper aerodigestive tract has been reported to range from 3.7% to 30% and the risk does not appear to diminish over time.

## 23. Are endoscopic screening and surveillance warranted in patients with aerodigestive SCC?

Currently, insufficient data (survival benefit or cost-effectiveness) are available to support routine endoscopic surveillance for patients with previous aerodigestive squamous cell cancer. A single endoscopy may be indicated to identify synchronous esophageal cancer. Lugol dye staining has been effectively used during endoscopic surveillance in these patients to improve the detection of early esophageal cancer and dysplasia.

## STOMACH AND SMALL BOWEL

**24. What is the malignant potential of gastric polyps?**

Gastric polyps are often found incidentally during endoscopy and are classified as hyperplastic, fundic gland, or adenomatous polyps histologically.

- *Hyperplastic polyps* are the most commonly encountered type of gastric polyp (70% to 90%) and may have malignant potential. Recent clinical studies have demonstrated dysplasia in up to 19% of hyperplastic polyps and there have been several reports of focal cancer.
- *Fundic gland polyps* have not been associated with an increased risk of gastric cancer but may develop in association with long-term use of proton pump inhibitors or may occur in association with familial adenomatous colorectal polyps.
- *Gastric adenomatous polyps* do have malignant potential, which correlates with the size of the polyp and the age of patient.

**25. How are gastric polyps managed when encountered radiographically or endoscopically?**

Endoscopic evaluation is warranted for polyps of any size that are detected radiographically. During endoscopy, gastric polyps should be removed whenever possible because the gross appearance of polyps cannot be used to differentiate the histologic subtypes. A representative biopsy should be performed on the largest polyp if multiple polyps are encountered or if a polypectomy is not possible. Surgical resection may be considered for any large adenomatous polyps or polyps containing dysplastic tissue.

**26. Is endoscopic surveillance required after the removal of a gastric polyp?**

Surveillance endoscopy is not necessary after the adequate sampling or the excision of a nondysplastic polyp. Gastric polyps with HGD or early gastric cancer necessitate individualized surveillance programs. Surveillance endoscopy should begin 1 year after removal of all adenomatous gastric polyps to assess for any recurrence and/or new or previously missed polyps. If the initial surveillance exam is negative, then repeat endoscopy should be repeated no earlier than every 3 to 5 years.

**27. What is gastric intestinal metaplasia (GIM)?**

GIM has been identified as a premalignant condition that may be the result of an adaptive response to a variety of environmental insults, such as *Helicobacter pylori* infection, smoking, or high salt intake. GIM is histologically identically to esophageal intestinal metaplasia.

**28. How common is GIM? What is its malignant potential?**

GIM is extremely common in Western countries; up to 25% to 30% of the population can be affected. Individuals with GIM, especially in certain geographical regions (e.g., Japan) and in those infected with *H. pylori*, have greater than a 10-fold increased risk of developing gastric cancer. Patients found to have GIM with HGD are at a significant risk for developing gastric cancer and should proceed immediately to gastrectomy or endoscopic mucosal resection.

**29. What role does endoscopic surveillance have in GIM?**

Endoscopic surveillance is not uniformly recommended for gastric intestinal metaplasia. GIM has not been extensively studied in the United States, and recent reports suggest that the risk of progression to cancer is low for most patients. Patients at increased risk for gastric cancer, based on ethnicity or family history, may benefit from surveillance. Topographic mapping of the entire stomach should be performed if endoscopic surveillance is to be undertaken.

**30. Are patients with pernicious anemia at an increased risk for gastric cancer? Is endoscopic screening or surveillance required?**

Yes. Individuals with pernicious anemia have an estimated 2- to 3-fold increased risk of developing gastric cancer. The risk for developing gastric cancer in patients with pernicious anemia is highest within the first year of diagnosis so a single endoscopy should be considered to identify prevalent neoplasia. There are insufficient data to support subsequent endoscopic surveillance.

**31. What is the frequency of gastric cancer in patients who have undergone a partial gastrectomy?**

Patients with a history of benign gastric or duodenal ulcers requiring treatment with gastric surgery may be at an increased risk for neoplasia in the gastric remnant. Endoscopic surveillance studies have detected gastric cancer in 4% to 6% of these patients, but population-based studies have failed to confirm an increased risk.

**32. What are the endoscopic surveillance recommendations for postgastrectomy surgery patients?**

All postgastrectomy patients with a history of peptic ulcer disease should have an index endoscopy to asses for *H. pylori*, chronic gastritis, and/or intestinal metaplasia. Routine endoscopic surveillance is not recommended for these patients but may be considered after an interval of 15 to 20 years. During the endoscopic exam, multiple biopsy samples should be taken from the anastomosis and gastric remnant. In general, however, there should be a low threshold for endoscopy in postgastrectomy patients with upper GI symptoms.

### 33. Who is at risk for ampullary and nonampullary duodenal adenomas?

Ampullary and nonampullary duodenal adenomas can occur sporadically or in association with genetic syndromes, such as familial adenomatous polyposis (FAP) or Peutz-Jeghers syndrome (PJS). Ampullary adenomas are considered premalignant lesions that can be treated surgically or endoscopically. Nonampullary duodenal adenomas have the potential for malignant transformation and are usually removed endoscopically.

### 34. What is the upper GI tract endoscopic surveillance strategy for patients with FAP?

Individuals with FAP should undergo endoscopic surveillance for duodenal adenomas with exams beginning around the time the patient is being considered for colectomy or early in the third decade of life. The upper endoscopy needs to be performed with both end-viewing and side-viewing endoscopes. If no adenomas are found, then the exam should be repeated in 5 years.

### 35. How often is surveillance endoscopy performed on patients who have undergone endoscopic resection of ampullary adenomas?

Patients who have undergone endoscopic management of ampullary adenomas should have regular endoscopic surveillance for the detection of recurrent dysplasia with both a forward and a side-viewing endoscope. Follow-up endoscopy and multiple biopsies should be performed every 6 months for a minimum of 2 years with repeated endoscopic exams at 3-year intervals.

### 36. When should surveillance endoscopy begin for patients with PJS?

PJS places patients at 5% to 10% increased risk of gastric malignancy. The lifetime risk of developing small bowel cancer in PJS is 13%. Endoscopic surveillance of the stomach and duodenum with upper endoscopy should be performed every 2 years beginning at age 10. All visible polyps should be removed during the endoscopic exams.

### 37. What is the role of capsule endoscopy in small bowel surveillance for PJS?

Patients with PJS have a significantly increased risk of developing dysplastic polyps and malignancies along the entire length of the small bowel. Capsule endoscopy is the method of choice for small bowel surveillance in PJS and should be performed every 2 years beginning at age 10.

### 38. What are the endoscopic surveillance guidelines for sporadic duodenal adenomas?

Sporadic duodenal adenomas are usually removed completely with endoscopic techniques and surveillance endoscopy is usually performed to ensure complete tissue removal and to assess for recurrence. Currently, the surveillance interval for patients with sporadic duodenal adenomas is unavailable because of lack of data. Patients discovered to have advanced (stage IV) duodenal polyposis require surgical consultation for possible resection. All patients found to have duodenal adenomas should be offered colonoscopy because they are at increased risk for colorectal polyps.

## PANCREAS

### 39. Who should undergo endoscopic screening and surveillance for pancreatic cancer?

Endoscopic screening and surveillance for pancreatic cancer is not recommended for the general population due to the low prevalence of the disease, the inaccuracy of available testing modalities, and the high expense. Some medical centers advocate that first-degree relatives of patients with familial pancreatic cancer and individuals with genetic syndromes associated with pancreatic cancer (such as hereditary nonpolyposis colorectal cancer [CRC], familial atypical mole melanoma, or PJS) undergo endoscopic screening and surveillance. CT scan, combined with EUS, is considered to be the best available method for pancreatic cancer screening because of their high sensitivity/specificity and high negative predictive value for pancreatic malignancy.

### 40. When should endoscopic screening begin for patients at increased risk for pancreatic neoplasia?

At this time, no standardized recommendations are available for the endoscopic screening of individuals at high risk for pancreatic cancer. Small clinical studies have suggested some benefit with endoscopic screening with EUS for individuals with genetic syndromes associated with pancreatic cancer beginning at the age of 30. First-degree relatives of patients diagnosed with pancreatic cancer should begin endoscopic screening with EUS around the age of 40, or 10 years younger than the earliest age of pancreatic cancer development. Smokers should be screened at an earlier age because smoking decreases the age of onset for familial pancreatic cancer by 10 to 20 years.

**41. What is the recommended endoscopic surveillance interval for patients at high risk for pancreatic cancer?**

There is currently no consensus for the optimum endoscopic surveillance interval in individuals determined to be at increased risk for pancreatic neoplasia. Some medical centers advocate surveillance EUS in high-risk patients every 2 to 3 years with the interval decreasing to every 12 months as the patient approaches the age when pancreatic cancer developed in the youngest affected relative.

## COLON

**42. At what age is CRC screening recommended for average-risk patients? What are the preferred testing modalities for CRC screening?**

CRC screening should be offered to average-risk (asymptomatic) individuals beginning at the age of 50. It is also now recommended that African Americans should start CRC screening at the age of 45. The risks and benefits of each CRC screening method must be discussed between the physician and the individual patient (Table 63-2).

**43. When should endoscopic screening begin for individuals with a family history of CRC? How often should endoscopic surveillance be performed in these individuals?**

Endoscopic screening for CRC should begin at age 40 or 10 years younger than the affected relative in individuals with a first-degree relative with CRC. Surveillance endoscopy should be scheduled every 3 to 5 years if the relative was younger than age of 60 at diagnosis. Individuals with a first-degree relative with CRC or advanced adenomas diagnosed at age ≥60 years can be screened like average-risk persons. Patients with a second- or third-degree relative with CRC should adhere to average-risk screening recommendations.

**44. What are the endoscopic surveillance guidelines for individuals with a personal history of colon cancer?**

If a complete endoscopic examination was not performed at the time of colon cancer diagnosis, a colonoscopy should be performed within 6 months after surgical resection. Endoscopic surveillance should begin 1 year after surgery and continue in 3- to 5-year intervals if the colonoscopy results are normal.

**45. Outline the endoscopic surveillance guidelines for individuals with a personal history of *rectal* cancer**

- Colonoscopy at time of surgical resection
- Colonoscopy at 1 year and 4 years after resection, then at 5-year intervals
- Flexible sigmoidoscopy every 6 months for the first 2 years postoperatively for patients who did not receive pelvic radiation or those who underwent nonmesorectal resection

**46. What is the role of EUS in the endoscopic surveillance of individuals with a personal history of rectal cancer?**

After surgical resection, the local recurrence rate for advanced rectal cancer is approximately 25% and the risk of recurrence is greatest in the first 2 years after surgery. EUS may be used to accurately detect recurrent rectal cancer and provide pathologic confirmation via FNA. The optimal interval for performing EUS following surgical resection has not been established. Currently, rectal EUS is recommended every 6 months for the first 2 years after low anterior resection or transanal excision to screen for recurrent rectal cancer.

**47. Do individuals with a first-degree relative diagnosed with adenomatous polyps require earlier screening for CRC? Do they have an increased risk for CRC?**

Yes. Persons with a first-degree relative diagnosed with an advanced adenomas (an adenoma ≥ 1 cm in size, or with high-grade dysplasia, or with villous elements) before the age of 50 should begin CRC screening at the age of 40 or 10 years younger than the affected relative. A first-degree relative with adenomatous polyps increases an individual's risk for CRC by 2- to 4-fold.

**48. What are the surveillance recommendations for a patient with a previous history of adenomatous colon polyps?**

After the removal of an adenomatous polyp, colonoscopy is the recommended method of surveillance because it has been shown to significantly reduce subsequent CRC incidence (Table 63-3).

**Table 63-2.** CRC Screening Recommendations

| | |
| --- | --- |
| Preferred method | Colonoscopy every 10 years |
| Alternative methods | Annual fecal immunochemical test (FIT) |
| | Flexible sigmoidoscopy every 5 years |
| | CT colonography every 5 years |
| | Double-contrast barium enema every 5 to 10 years |

**Table 63-3.** Colonoscopy Surveillance Recommendations

| PERSONAL HISTORY | SURVEILLANCE RECOMMENDATION |
|---|---|
| ≤2 small tubular adenomas (<1 cm) and only low-grade dysplasia | No earlier than 5 years |
| Advanced neoplasia or 3 to 10 adenomas | 3 years |
| More than 10 adenomas | Within 3 years |
| Large, sessile polyp with incomplete excision | 2 to 6 months |
| Negative surveillance colonoscopy | No earlier than 5 years |

### 49. Define *familial adenomatous polyposis syndrome*. What is the risk of developing CRC in patients with FAP syndrome?

FAP syndrome presents as more than 100 adenomas throughout the colon and is caused by mutations in the adenomatous polyposis coli *(APC)* gene. The risk of developing CRC in patients with FAP is almost 100% by age 40 to 50 years. Total colectomy is indicated in patients with FAP who develop multiple, diffuse adenomas in the colon.

### 50. When should endoscopic screening begin in patients with FAP?

Prior to endoscopic screening, genetic testing should be offered to all patients at risk for FAP and to family members. Beginning at age 10 to 12, individuals at risk for FAP should undergo annual flexible sigmoidoscopy until 40 years of age and then every 3 to 5 years thereafter. Family members are assumed not to be affected if their genetic test is negative and the index case is positive but can be offered sigmoidoscopy every 7 to 10 years to account for any potential errors in the test.

### 51. Do patients with PJS require endoscopic screening and surveillance for CRC?

CRC surveillance endoscopy is offered to patients with PJS syndrome because the lifetime risk of CRC for these individuals ranges from 10% to 20%. Several surveillance protocols have been published, but the true efficacy of aggressive CRC surveillance for these patients has yet to be established. Most endoscopic surveillance protocols suggest colonoscopic exams begin around the age of 18 with 3-year surveillance intervals.

### 52. What is hereditary nonpolyposis colorectal cancer syndrome (HNPCC)?

HNPCC syndrome is an autosomal dominant disorder distinguished by the early development of CRC (average age is 44). The diagnostic clinical criteria used to help establish the diagnosis of HNPCC include the Amsterdam (modified) and Bethesda classification systems.

### 53. What are the endoscopic screening and surveillance guidelines for HNPCC?

Colonoscopy should be performed every 1 to 2 years in patients at risk for HNPCC beginning at age 20 to 25 years or 10 years younger than the age of the earliest diagnosis of cancer in the family. The screening interval for endoscopic surveillance changes to yearly beginning at age 40.

### 54. Do patients with ulcerative colitis (US) and Crohn's disease require endoscopic surveillance?

Yes. Longstanding UC and extensive Crohn's disease increase an individual's risk for the development of dysplasia and/or CRC.

### 55. Which clinical characteristics increase the risk of CRC in patients with UC and Crohn's disease?

In patients with UC and Crohn's disease, the risk of CRC increases with longer duration and extensive (more than one-third colonic involvement) severe colitis, a family history of CRC, young age at onset of disease, presence of backwash ileitis, and personal history of primary sclerosing cholangitis. The presence of proctitis alone does not increase the risk for CRC.

### 56. How should endoscopic surveillance be performed in patients with UC and Crohn's disease?

Surveillance colonoscopy should be performed in patients with UC or extensive Crohn's disease every 1 to 2 years beginning 8 to 10 years after the clear onset of disease symptoms. During the colonoscopy, four-quadrant biopsy samples should be obtained every 10 cm from the cecum to the rectum (minimum of 32 biopsy samples) in these patients. Biopsies targeted at macroscopically involved segments may be adequate for endoscopic surveillance in patients with less extensive colitis.

### 57. What is the treatment strategy for dysplasia in patients with UC or Crohn's disease?

If dysplasia is identified during endoscopic screening, it should be confirmed by a second GI pathologist. HGD or multifocal LGD detected during endoscopy in an area of flat mucosa is an indication for colectomy. The management of unifocal LGD is controversial, as some experts recommend colectomy.

**58. How are adenomatous-appearing polyps managed in patients with UC and Crohn's disease?**

Adenomatous-appearing polyps should be completely removed by polypectomy and biopsy specimens should be obtained from the adjacent flat mucosa to determine the presence of dysplasia. If no dysplasia or inflammation is found in the surrounding mucosa, then this can be managed as a sporadic adenomatous polyp. Colectomy is indicated if dysplasia is identified in an area of active inflammation, also known as dysplasia-associated lesion or mass (DALM), and there is evidence of dysplasia in the adjacent mucosa. Repeat colonoscopy in 3 to 6 months and close follow-up are warranted when indefinite dysplasia is detected. Mucosal tattooing often assists in identifying the area in question on subsequent endoscopies.

## WEBSITES

### GENERAL SCREENING/SURVEILLANCE

http://www.acg.gi.org

http://www.asge.org/PublicationsProductsindex.aspx?id=352

http://www.gastro.org/wmspage.cfm?parm1=4453

### UPPER GASTROINTESTINAL (ESOPHAGUS, STOMACH, AND SMALL BOWEL)

http://www.emedicine.com/med/topic2642.htm

http://www.entusa.com/esophagoscopy_5.htm

http://www.mayoclinic.org/barretts-esophagus/

### PANCREATIC ENDOSCOPIC ULTRASOUND

http://daveproject.org/viewFilms.cfm?film_id=57

http://www.vhjoe.org/Volume1Issue4/1-4-3.htm

### COLON

http://daveproject.org/ViewFilms.cfm?Film_id=619

## BIBLIOGRAPHY

1. Adler DG, Qureshi W, Davila R, et al. The role of endoscopy in ampullary and duodenal adenomas. Gastrointest Endosc 2006;64:849–54.
2. Ahsan H, Neugut AI, Waye JD, et al. Family history of colorectal adenomatous polyps and increased risk for colorectal cancer. Ann Intern Med 1998;128:900–5.
3. ASGE guideline: colorectal cancer screening and surveillance. Gastrointest Endosc 2006;63:546–57.
4. Brucher B.L., Stein HJ, Bartels H, et al. Achalasia and esophageal cancer: Incidence, prevalence, and prognosis. World J Surg 2001;25:745–9.
5. Burke CA, Santisi J, Church J, et al. The utility of capsule endoscopy small bowel surveillance in patients with polyposis. Am J Gastroenterol 2005;100:1498–1502.
6. Buttar NS, Wang KK, Sebo TJ, et al. Extent of high grade dysplasia in Barrett's esophagus correlates with risk of adenocarcinoma. Gastroenterology 2001;120:1630–9.
7. Canto MI, Goggins M, Hruban RH, et al. Screening for early pancreatic neoplasia in high-risk individuals: A prospective controlled study. Clin Gastroenterol Hepatol 2006;4:766–81.
8. Corley DA, Levin TR, Habel LA, et al. Surveillance and survival in Barrett's adenocarcinomas: A population-based study. Gastroenterology 2002;122:633–40.
9. Davila RE, Rajan E, Adler D, et al. ASGE guideline: The role of endoscopy in the diagnosis, staging, and management of colorectal cancer. Gastrointest Endosc 2005;61:1–7.
10. Erkal HS, Mendenhall WM, Amdur RJ, et al. Synchronous and metasynchronous squamous cell carcinomas of the head and neck mucosal sites. J Clin Oncol 2001;19:1358–62.
11. Giardiello FM, Brensinger JD, Tersmette AC, et al. Very high risk of cancer in familial Peutz-Jeghers syndrome. Gastroenterology 2000;119:1447–53.
12. Ginsberg GG, Al-Kawas FH, Fleishcher DE, et al. Gastric polyps: Relationship of size and histology to cancer risk. Am J Gastroenterol 1996;91:714–7.
13. Hirota WK, Zuckerman MJ, Adler DG, et al. The role of endoscopy in the surveillance of premalignant conditions of the upper GI tract. Gastrointest Endosc 2006;63:570–80.

14. Kimmey MB, Bronner MP, Byrd DR, et al. Screening and surveillance for hereditary pancreatic cancer. Gastrointest Endosc 2002;56:S82–6.
15. Leighton JA, Shen B, Baron TH, et al. ASGE Guideline: Endoscopy in the diagnosis and treatment of inflammatory bowel disease. Gastrointest Endosc 2006;63:558–65.
16. Leung WK, Sung JJY. Review article: Intestinal metaplasia and gastric carcinogenesis. Aliment Pharmacol Ther 2002;16:1209–16.
17. Maillefer RH, Greydanus MP. To B or not B: Is tylosis B truly benign? Two North American genealogies. Am J Gastroenterol 1999;94:829–34.
18. Pohl H, Welch HG. The role of overdiagnosis and reclassification in the marked increase of esophageal adenocarcinoma incidence. J Natl Cancer Inst 2005;97:142–6.
19. Sharma P, Bansal A, Mathur S, et al. The utility of a novel narrow band imaging endoscopy system in patients with Barrett's esophagus. Gastrointest Endosc 2006;64:167–75.
20. Skacel M, Petras RE, Gramlich TL, et al. The diagnosis of low-grade dysplasia in Barrett's esophagus and its implications for disease progression. Am J Gastroenterol 2000;95:3383–7.
21. Toh BH, van Driel IR, Gleeson PA. Pernicious anemia. N Engl J Med 1997;337:1441–8.
22. Wang KK, Sampliner RE. Updated guidelines 2008 for the diagnosis, surveillance and therapy of Barrett's esophagus. Am J Gastroenterol 2008;103:788–97.
23. Kiviranta UK. Corrosion carcinoma of the esophagus. Acta Otolaryngol 1952;42:89–95.
24. Lundergardh G, Adami HO, Helmick C. Stomach cancer after partial gastrectomy for benign ulcer disease. N Engl J Med 1988;319:195–200.
25. McGarrity TJ, Kulin HE, Zaino RJ. Peutz-Jeghers syndrome. Am J Gastroenterol 2000;95:596–604.
26. Rex DK, Johnson DA, Anderson JC, Schoenfeld PS, Burke CA, Inadomi JM. American college of gastroenterology guidelines for colorectal cancer screening 2008. Am J Gastroenterol 2009 Mar;104(3): 739–50.

# RHEUMATOLOGIC MANIFESTATIONS OF GASTROINTESTINAL DISEASES

*Sterling G. West, MD*

**CHAPTER 64**

## ENTEROPATHIC ARTHRITIS

**1. How often does an inflammatory peripheral or spinal arthritis occur in patients with idiopathic inflammatory bowel disease (IBD)?**

Arthritis of either type is the most common extraintestinal manifestation (EIM) of either type of IBD affecting up to 20% of patients (Table 64-1).

**Table 64-1.** Frequency of Peripheral or Spinal Arthritis in Inflammatory Bowel Disease

|  | ULCERATIVE COLITIS | CROHN'S DISEASE |
| --- | --- | --- |
| Peripheral arthritis | 10% | 20% |
| Sacroiliitis | 15% | 15% |
| Sacroiliitis/spondylitis* | 5% | 5% |

*Some studies report that ankylosing spondylitis occurs more commonly in Crohn's disease than in ulcerative colitis.

**2. What are the most common joints involved in ulcerative colitis and Crohn's disease patients with an inflammatory peripheral arthritis?**

Upper extremity and small joint involvement is more common in ulcerative colitis than in Crohn's disease. Both ulcerative colitis– and Crohn's disease–related arthritis affect the knee and ankle predominantly (Fig. 64-1).

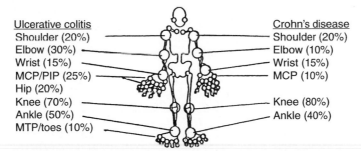

Ulcerative colitis
Shoulder (20%)
Elbow (30%)
Wrist (15%)
MCP/PIP (25%)
Hip (20%)
Knee (70%)
Ankle (50%)
MTP/toes (10%)

Crohn's disease
Shoulder (20%)
Elbow (10%)
Wrist (15%)
MCP (10%)
Knee (80%)
Ankle (40%)

**Figure 64-1.** Joints commonly involved as an extraintestinal manifestation of ulcerative colitis and Crohn's disease.

**3. Describe the clinical characteristics of the inflammatory peripheral arthritis associated with idiopathic IBD.**

The most common type of arthritis (type 1) occurs equally in males and females, and children are affected as often as adults. The arthritis is typically acute in onset and asymmetric and usually involves fewer than five joints (i.e., pauciarticular). It occurs early in the course of the bowel disease and is strongly associated with flares of IBD and other extra-articular manifestations. Synovial fluid analysis reveals an inflammatory fluid with up to 50,000 WBC/mm$^3$ (predominantly neutrophils) and negative findings on crystal examination and cultures. There is an increased prevalence of *HLA-B35* and *HLA-DRB1*0103* in this type of arthritis. Most arthritic episodes are self-limited (90% within 6 months) and do not result in radiographic changes or deformities.

A second type of arthritis (type 2) is less common (less than 5%) but tends to be polyarticular (metacarpophalangeal joints more than other joints), runs a course independent of the activity of IBD, and does not coincide with extra-articular manifestations. Active synovitis persists for months and episodes of exacerbations and remissions may continue for years. Due to its chronicity, this type of arthritis can cause erosions and deformities. There is an association of this arthritis with *HLA-B44* but not with *HLA-B27*.

**4. What other extraintestinal manifestations commonly occur in patients with idiopathic IBD and inflammatory peripheral arthritis?**
Approximately 25% of patients with IBD have a combination of EIMs. The development of one manifestation increases the risk of developing others. In IBD patients with arthritis, the following EIM may be seen:

**P** = Pyoderma gangrenosum (less than 5%)
**A** = Aphthous stomatitis (less than 10%)
**I** = Inflammatory eye disease (acute anterior uveitis) (5% to 15%)
**N** = Nodosum (erythema) (less than 10%)

**5. Do the extent and activity of IBD correlate with the activity of the peripheral inflammatory arthritis?**
Patients with ulcerative colitis and Crohn's disease are more likely to develop a peripheral arthritis if the colon is extensively involved. In patients with type1 arthritis, most arthritic attacks occur during the first few years following onset of the bowel disease but late occurrences also occur. The episodes coincide with flares of bowel disease in 60% to 70% of patients. Occasionally, the arthritis may precede symptoms of IBD, especially in children with Crohn's disease. Consequently, lack of gastrointestinal (GI) symptoms and even a negative stool guaiac test do not exclude the possibility of occult Crohn's disease in a patient who presents with a characteristic arthritis.

**6. Which points in the history and physical examination are helpful in separating inflammatory spinal arthritis from mechanical low back pain in an IBD patient?**
On the basis of history and physical examination, 90% of patients with inflammatory spinal arthritis can be differentiated from patients with mechanical low back pain (Table 64-2).

**Table 64-2.** Clinical Differentiation of Inflammatory Spinal Arthritis (SA) and Mechanical Low Back Pain (LBP)

|  | INFLAMMATORY SA | MECHANICAL LBP |
|---|---|---|
| Onset of pain | Insidious | Acute |
| Duration of morning stiffness | >60 min | <30 min |
| Nighttime pain | Yes | Infrequent |
| Exercise effect on pain | Improvement | Worsen |
| Sacroiliac joint tenderness | Usually | No |
| Range of back motion | Global loss of motion | Abnormal flexion |
| Reduced chest expansion | Sometimes | No |
| Neurologic deficits | No | Possible |
| Duration of symptoms | >3 mo | <4 wk |

**7. Does the activity of inflammatory spinal arthritis correlate with the activity of the IBD?**
No. The onset of sacroiliitis or spondylitis can precede by years, occur concurrently, or follow by years the onset of IBD. Furthermore, the course of the spinal arthritis is completely independent of the course of IBD.

**8. What human leukocyte antigen (HLA) occurs more commonly than expected in patients with inflammatory spinal arthritis associated with IBD?**
*HLA-B27* is found in 55% of Crohn's disease patients and 70% of ulcerative colitis patients with inflammatory sacroiliitis/spondylitis. This contrasts with an 8% frequency of *HLA-B27* in a normal healthy, white population. Thus, a patient with IBD who possesses the *HLA-B27* gene has 7 to 10 times increased risk of developing inflammatory sacroiliitis/spondylitis compared with IBD patients who are *HLA-B27* negative.

**9. What serologic abnormalities are seen in patients with IBD?**
- Erythrocyte sedimentation rate (ESR) and C-reactive protein (CRP) are elevated, while rheumatoid factor and anti–nuclear antibody (ANA) are negative.
- Anti–neutrophil cytoplasmic antibody (ANCA)—up to 50% to 60% of ulcerative colitis patients can have pANCA, which is directed against bactericidal permeability increasing protein (BPI), cathepsin G, lactoferrin, lysozyme, or elastase but not myeloperoxidase (MPO).
- Up to 50% of Crohn's disease patients can have antibodies against *Saccharomyces cerevisiae*.

## 10. Describe the typical radiographic features of inflammatory sacroiliitis and spondylitis in IBD patients.

The radiographic abnormalities in IBD patients with inflammatory spinal arthritis are similar to those seen in ankylosing spondylitis. Patients with early inflammatory sacroiliitis frequently have normal plain radiographs. In these patients, magnetic resonance (MR) imaging of the sacroiliac joints demonstrates inflammation and edema (Fig. 64-2, *A*). Over several months to years, patients develop sclerosis and erosions in the lower two-thirds of the sacroiliac joint (Fig. 64-2 *B*). In some patients, these joints may completely fuse.

Patients with early spondylitis may also have normal radiographs. Later, radiographs may show shiny corners at the insertion of the annulus fibrosis, anterior squaring of the vertebrae, and syndesmophyte formation (Fig. 64-3, *A*). Syndesmophytes (calcification of annulus fibrosis) are thin, marginal, and bilateral. A "bamboo spine" (bilateral syndesmophytes traversing the entire spine from lumbar to cervical) (Fig. 64-3, *B*) occurs in 10% of patients. Patients who develop inflammatory hip disease may be at increased risk for subsequently developing a bamboo spine.

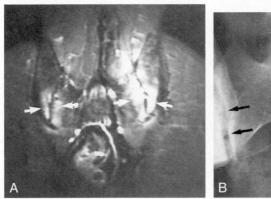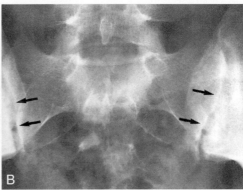

**Figure 64-2.** *A,* MR image of the sacroiliac joints showing inflammation (*arrows*) (T2-weighted image, TE50, TR2500). *B,* Radiograph showing early bilateral sacroiliitis (*arrows*).

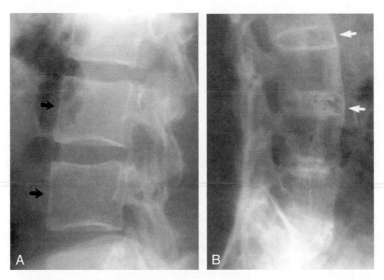

**Figure 64-3.** *A,* Radiographs showing anterior squaring of the vertebrae in a patient with early inflammatory spondylitis. *B,* Radiograph showing thin, marginal syndesmophytes (*arrows*) causing bamboo spine in a patient with Crohn's disease with advanced inflammatory spondylitis.

## 11. What other rheumatic problems occur with increased frequency in IBD patients?

- Achilles tendon/plantar fascia enthesitis
- Clubbing of fingernails (5%)
- Hypertrophic osteoarthropathy (periostitis)
- Psoas abscess or septic hip from fistula formation (Crohn's disease)
- Osteoporosis secondary to medications (i.e., prednisone)

- Granulomatous lesions of bone and joints
- Vasculitis
- Amyloidosis

## 12. Can treatment alleviate the symptoms of inflammatory peripheral arthritis and/or spinal arthritis in IBD patients?

See Table 64-3.

**Table 64-3.** Alleviation of Arthritic Symptoms in Inflammatory Bowel Disease (IBD)

|  | PERIPHERAL ARTHRITIS | SACROILIITIS/SPONDYLITIS |
|---|---|---|
| NSAIDs* | Yes | Yes |
| Intra-articular corticosteroids | Yes | Yes (sacroiliitis) |
| Sulfasalazine | Yes | No |
| Immunosuppressives | Yes | No |
| Anti–tumor necrosis factor (TNF)α | Yes | Yes |
| Bowel resection |  |  |
| Ulcerative colitis (UC) | Yes | No |
| Crohn's disease (CD) | No | No |

*Nonsteroidal anti-inflammatory drugs (NSAIDs) may exacerbate IBD. Sulfasalazine helps the peripheral arthritis in UC patients more than CD patients. Anti–TNFα agents that are effective include infliximab and adalimumab.

## 13. What rheumatic disorders are associated with pouchitis, lymphocytic colitis (LC), and/or collagenous colitis (CC)?

See Table 64-4.

**Table 64-4.** Rheumatic Disorders Associated With Pouchitis, Microscopic (Lymphocytic) Colitis (MC), and/or Collagenous Colitis (CC)

|  | POUCHITIS | MC | CC |
|---|---|---|---|
| IBD-like peripheral inflammatory arthritis | Yes | Yes | Yes (10%) |
| Rheumatoid arthritis | No | Yes | Yes |
| Ankylosing spondylitis* | No | No | No |
| Thyroiditis/other autoimmune disease | No | Yes | Yes |

*Up to 60% of patients with ankylosing spondylitis have asymptomatic Crohn-like lesions on right-sided colon biopsies. However, only 4% to 5% will evolve into overt inflammatory bowel disease (IBD).

## 14. Why are patients with IBD more prone to develop an inflammatory arthritis?

Environmental antigens capable of inciting rheumatic disorders enter the body's circulation by traversing the respiratory mucosa, skin, or GI mucosa. The human GI tract has an estimated surface area of $1000\,m^2$ and functions not only to absorb nutrients but also to exclude potentially harmful antigens. The gut-associated lymphoid tissue (GALT), which includes Peyer patches, the lamina propria, and intraepithelial T cells, constitutes 25% of the GI mucosa and helps to exclude entry of bacteria and other foreign antigens. Although the upper GI tract is normally not exposed to microbes, the lower GI tract is constantly in contact with millions of bacteria (up to $10^{12}/g$ of feces).

Inflammation, whether from idiopathic IBD or from infection with pathogenic microorganisms, can disrupt the normal integrity and function of the bowel, leading to increased gut permeability. This increased permeability may allow nonviable bacterial antigens in the gut lumen to enter the circulation more easily. These microbial antigens could either deposit directly in the joint synovia, leading to a local inflammatory reaction, or cause a systemic immune response, resulting in immune complexes that then deposit in joints and other tissues.

## REACTIVE ARTHRITIS

## 15. What is reactive arthritis, and what are the most common GI pathogens that cause it?

A reactive arthritis is a sterile inflammatory arthritis that occurs within 1 to 3 weeks following an infection by an organism that infects mucosal surfaces, especially the urethra or large bowel. The most common GI pathogens causing reactive arthritis are:

- *Yersinia enterocolitica* (0:3 and 0:9) or *Y. pseudotuberculosis*
- *Salmonella enteritidis* or *S. typhimurium*
- *Shigella flexneri* > *S. dysenteriae* > *S. sonnei*

- *Campylobacter jejuni*
- *Clostridium difficile*

Approximately 1% to 3% of patients who have an infectious gastroenteritis during an epidemic subsequently develop a reactive arthritis. It may be as high as 20% in *Yersinia*-infected individuals. Recently, joint pain following a diarrheal illness due to pathogenic *Escherichia coli* has been reported.

**16. Which joints are most commonly involved in a reactive arthritis following a bowel infection (i.e., postenteritic reactive arthritis)?**
See Figure 64-4.

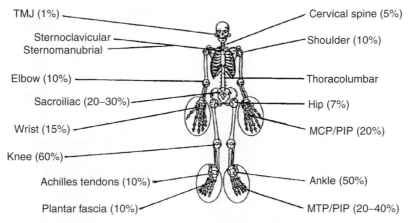

TMJ (1%)

Sternoclavicular
Sternomanubrial

Elbow (10%)

Sacroiliac (20–30%)

Wrist (15%)

Knee (60%)

Achilles tendons (10%)

Plantar fascia (10%)

Cervical spine (5%)

Shoulder (10%)

Thoracolumbar

Hip (7%)

MCP/PIP (20%)

Ankle (50%)

MTP/PIP (20–40%)

**Figure 64-4.** Joints commonly involved in reactive arthritis after bowel infection.

**17. Describe the clinical characteristics of postenteritic reactive arthritis.**
- Demographics—males > females; average age is 30 years old
- Onset of arthritis—abrupt, acute
- Distribution of joints—asymmetric, pauciarticular; lower extremity involved in 80% to 90%; sacroiliitis in 20% to 30%; enthesitis (Achilles tendon, plantar fascia attachments); toe dactylitis
- Synovial fluid analysis—inflammatory fluid (usually 10,000-50,000 WBC/mm³), no crystals, negative cultures
- Course and prognosis—80% resolve in 1 to 6 months; 20% have chronic arthritis with radiographic changes of peripheral and/or sacroiliac joints

**18. What extra-articular manifestations can occur in patients with postenteritic reactive arthritis?**
- Sterile urethritis (15% to 70%)
- Conjunctivitis
- Acute anterior uveitis (iritis)
- Oral ulcers (painless or painful)
- Erythema nodosum (5% of *Yersinia* infections)
- Circinate balanitis
- Keratoderma blennorrhagicum

**19. How commonly do patients with postenteritic reactive arthritis have the clinical features of Reiter syndrome?**
The triad of inflammatory arthritis, urethritis, and conjunctivitis/uveitis with or without mucocutaneous lesions that characterize Reiter syndrome may develop 2 to 4 weeks after an acute urethritis or diarrheal illness. The frequency varies with the causative enteric organism:

- *Shigella*, 85%
- *Yersinia*, 10%
- *Salmonella*, 10% to 15%
- *Campylobacter*, 10%

**20. How do the radiographic features of inflammatory sacroiliitis and spondylitis due to postenteritic reactive arthritis differ from those in IBD patients?**
See Table 64-5 and Figure 64-5.

**Table 64-5.** Radiologic Comparison of Spinal Arthritis in Postenteritic Reactive Arthritis Versus Inflammatory Bowel Disease (IBD)

| | REACTIVE ARTHRITIS | IBD |
|---|---|---|
| Sacroiliitis | Unilateral, asymmetric | Bilateral, sacroiliac involvement |
| Spondylitis | Asymmetric, nonmarginal, jug-handle syndesmophytes | Bilateral, thin, marginal syndesmophytes |

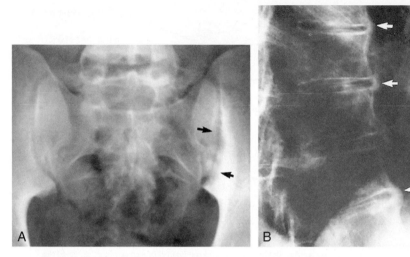

**Figure 64-5.** *A,* Radiograph showing unilateral sacroiliitis (*arrows*) in a patient with reactive arthritis. *B,* Radiograph showing large, nonmarginal syndesmophytes (*arrows*) of the spine in a patient with reactive arthritis.

21. **Discuss the relationship of *HLA-B27* positivity in patients with postenteritic reactive arthritis compared with a normal healthy population.**
    - Reactive arthritis patients, 60% to 80% *HLA-B27* positive; normal healthy controls, 4% to 8% *HLA-B27* positive.
    - Caucasians and patients with radiographic sacroiliitis and/or uveitis are more likely to be *HLA-B27* positive.
    - A person who is *HLA-B27* positive has a 30 to 50 times increased risk of developing reactive arthritis following an episode of infectious gastroenteritis compared to a person who does not have the *HLA-B27* gene.
    - Only 20% to 25% of all *HLA-B27*–positive individuals who get an infectious gastroenteritis from *Shigella, Salmonella,* or *Yersinia* go on to develop a postenteritic reactive arthritis.

22. **Explain the current theory for the pathogenesis of a postenteritic reactive arthritis.**
    Bacterial lipopolysaccharide antigens (but not viable organisms or nucleotides) from the pathogens (*Yersinia, Shigella, Salmonella*) causing the infectious gastroenteritis have been shown to be deposited in the joints of patients who develop a postenteritic reactive arthritis. These bacterial cell wall components are thought to incite inflammation in the joint. The role that *HLA-B27* plays in the pathogenesis is debated. One possibility is that recirculating *HLA-B27*–restricted T cells present bacteria-derived peptides with arthritogenic properties to the immune system in a unique way, leading to inflammation. Another postulate is that there is molecular mimicry between the *HLA-B27* molecule and the bacterial antigens, causing an aberrant immune response leading to altered or defective intracellular killing by *HLA-B27*–positive cells, resulting in persistence of arthritogenic pathogens. A third hypothesis relates to the tendency for the *HLA-B27* heavy chain to misfold when the cell is under stress. This results in heavy chains accumulating in the endoplasmic reticulum leading to an "unfolded protein response," causing the release of inflammatory cytokines. The chronic persistence of bacterial antigens may stress the *HLA-B27*–positive cells, leading to *B27* heavy chain misfolding and the unfolded protein response. However, because *HLA-B27* positivity is neither necessary nor sufficient to cause reactive arthritis, additional genetic and environmental factors likely play a role in the pathogenesis of postenteritic reactive arthritis.

23. **Is any therapy beneficial for postenteritic reactive arthritis?**
    See Table 64-6.

**Table 64-6.** Treatment of Postenteritic Reactive Arthritis

| TREATMENT | PERIPHERAL ARTHRITIS | | SACROILIITIS |
| --- | --- | --- | --- |
| | ACUTE | CHRONIC | |
| NSAIDs | Yes | Yes | Yes |
| Corticosteroids | | | |
|   Intra-articular | Yes | Yes | Yes |
|   Oral only if used in high doses | No | No | |
| Antibiotics | | | |
|   2-wk course | No | No | No |
|   3-mo course | NA | No | No |
| Sulfasalazine | NA | Yes | No |
| Methotrexate | NA | Yes | No |
| Anti–tumor necrosis factor (TNF)α | NA | Yes | Yes |

NA, not applicable.
*Anti–TNF α agents include etanercept, infliximab, and adalimumab.

# WHIPPLE DISEASE

## 24. Who was Whipple?

George Hoyt Whipple, MD, in 1907 reported the case of a 36-year-old medical missionary with diarrhea, malabsorption with weight loss, mesenteric lymphadenopathy, and migratory polyarthritis. He named this disease "intestinal lipodystrophy," but it is now known as Whipple disease. Dr. Whipple also became a Nobel laureate in physiology in 1934 and was the founder of the University of Rochester Medical School.

## 25. What are the multisystem manifestations of Whipple disease?

**W** = Wasting/weight loss   **D** = Diarrhea
**H** = Hyperpigmentation (skin)  **I** = Interstitial nephritis
**I** = Intestinal pain     **S** = Skin rashes
**P** = Pleurisy       **E** = Eye inflammation
**P** = Pneumonitis      **A** = Arthritis
**L** = Lymphadenopathy    **S** = Subcutaneous nodules
**E** = Encephalopathy     **E** = Endocarditis
**S** = Steatorrhea

## 26. Describe the clinical characteristics of the arthritis associated with Whipple disease.

Whipple disease occurs most commonly in middle-aged white men (male/female ratio, 9:1). Seronegative oligoarthritis or polyarthritis (knees, ankles, wrists) is the presenting symptom in 60% of patients and may precede the intestinal symptoms by up to 5 years. More than 70% of patients will develop arthritis at some time during their disease course. The arthritis is inflammatory, is often migratory, and does not correlate with intestinal symptoms. Sacroiliitis or spondylitis occurs in 5% to 10% of patients, especially in those who are *HLA-B27* positive (33% of patients). Synovial fluid analysis shows an inflammatory fluid with 5000 to 100,000 cells/mm$^3$ (predominantly neutrophils). Radiographs usually remain unremarkable.

## 27. What is the etiology of Whipple disease?

Multiple tissues show deposits in macrophages that stain with periodic acid–Schiff (PAS). These deposits contain rod-shaped free bacilli seen on electron microscopy. Recently, these bacilli have been shown to be a new organism, a gram-positive actinomycete called *Tropheryma whippelii*. The diagnosis is usually made by demonstrating PAS-positive inclusions in macrophages in small bowel or lymph node biopsy samples. Recently, a more accurate diagnosis can be made by polymerase chain reaction of the DNA sequence of the 16S-ribosomal RNA gene sequence of *T. whippelii* in synovial fluid, cerebrospinal fluid, or small bowel biopsy samples.

## 28. How is Whipple disease best treated?

Tetracycline, penicillin, erythromycin, or trimethoprim–sulfamethoxazole (TMP/SMX) for more than 1 year. Relapses can occur (particularly in patients with central nervous system involvement [30%]). Chloramphenicol or TMP/SMX is recommended if the central nervous system is involved.

## OTHER GASTROINTESTINAL DISEASES

### 29. What rheumatic manifestations have been described in patients with celiac disease (gluten-sensitive enteropathy)?

Celiac disease is an enteropathy resulting from an autoimmune reaction to wheat gliadins. It is primarily seen in whites and is associated with *HLA-DQ2* and/or *-DQ8*, usually in linkage with *HLA-DR3*. The most frequent rheumatic manifestations include:

- Arthritis (4% to 26%)—symmetric polyarthritis involving predominantly large joints (knees and ankles > hips and shoulders); may precede enteropathic symptoms in 50% of cases. Oligoarthritis and sacroiliitis can also occur.
- Osteomalacia—due to steatorrhea from severe enteropathy causing vitamin D deficiency
- Dermatitis herpetiformis

These rheumatic manifestations can respond dramatically to a gluten-free diet but not always.

### 30. Describe the intestinal bypass arthritis-dermatitis syndrome.

This syndrome occurs in 20% to 80% of patients who have undergone intestinal bypass (jejunoileal or jejunocolic) surgery for morbid obesity. The arthritis is inflammatory, polyarticular, symmetric, and frequently migratory and affects both upper and lower extremity small and large joints. Radiographic findings usually remain normal, despite 25% of patients having chronic recurring episodes of arthritis. Up to 80% develop dermatologic abnormalities, the most characteristic of which is a maculopapular or vesiculopustular rash.

The pathogenesis involves bacterial overgrowth in the blind loop, resulting in antigenic stimulation that purportedly causes immune complex formation (frequently cryoprecipitates containing secretory IgA and bacterial antigens) in the serum that deposits in the joints and skin. Treatment includes NSAIDs and oral antibiotics, which usually improve symptoms. Only surgical reanastomosis of the blind loop can result in complete elimination of symptoms. Fortunately, this surgery is no longer done for morbid obesity. However, this syndrome can also occur in patients who have intestinal derangements causing bacterial overgrowth from postoperative, inflammatory, or diverticular conditions.

### 31. What types of arthritis can be associated with carcinomas of the esophagus and colon?

Carcinomatous polyarthritis can be the presenting feature of an occult malignancy of the gastrointestinal tract. The arthritis is typically acute in onset and asymmetric and predominantly involves lower extremity joints while sparing the small joints of the hands and wrists. Patients have an elevated ESR and a negative rheumatoid factor. Another type of arthritis associated with colorectal malignancy is septic arthritis caused by *Streptococcus bovis*.

### 32. What are the clinical features of the pancreatic panniculitis syndrome?

Pancreatic panniculitis is a systemic syndrome occurring in some patients with pancreatitis or pancreatic acinar cell carcinoma. Its clinical manifestations can be remembered by the following mnemonic:

**P** = Pancreatitis

**A** = Arthritis (60%) and arthralgias, usually of the ankles and knees. Synovial fluid is typically noninflammatory and creamy in color due to lipid droplets that stain with Sudan black or oil red O.

**N** = Nodules that are tender, red, and usually on extremities. These are frequently misdiagnosed as erythema nodosum but really are areas of lobular panniculitis with fat necrosis.

**C** = Cancer of the pancreas more commonly causes this syndrome than does pancreatitis.

**R** = Radiologic abnormalities due to osteolytic bone lesions from bone marrow necrosis (10%).

**E** = Eosinophilia.

**A** = Amylase, lipase, and trypsin released by the diseased pancreas causes fat necrosis in skin, synovium, and bone marrow.

**S** = Serositis including pleuropericarditis frequently with fever.

### 33. What musculoskeletal problem can occur with pancreatic insufficiency?

Osteomalacia due to fat-soluble vitamin D malabsorption.

**BIBLIOGRAPHY**

1. Andras C, Csiki Z, Ponyi A, et al. Paraneoplastic rheumatic syndromes. Rheumatol Int 2006;26:376–82.
2. Dahl PR, Su WP, Cullimore KC, et al. Pancreatic panniculitis. J Am Acad Dermatol 1995;33:413–7.
3. Fenollar F, Puechal X, Raoult D. Whipple's disease. N Engl J Med 2007;356:55–66.
4. Green PHR, Cellier C. Celiac sprue. N Engl J Med 2007;357:1731–43.
5. Holden W, Orchard T, Wordsworth P. Enteropathic arthritis. Rheum Dis Clin N Am 2003;29:513–30.

6. Kethu SR. Extraintestinal manifestations of inflammatory bowel diseases. J Clin Gastroenterol 2006;40:467–75.
7. Lichtenstein GR, Sands BE, Pazianas M. Prevention and treatment of osteoporosis in inflammatory bowel disease. Inflamm Bowel Dis 2006;12:797–813.
8. Lubrano E, Cicacci C, Amers PR, et al. The arthritis of coeliac disease: Prevalence and pattern in 200 adult patients. Br J Rheumatol 1996;35:1314–8.
9. Reveille JD. Major histocompatibility genes and ankylosing spondylitis. Best Pract Res Clin Rheumatol 2006;20:601–9.
10. Roubenoff R, Ratain J, Giardiello I, et al. Collagenous colitis, enteropathic arthritis, and autoimmune diseases: Results of a patient survey. J Rheumatol 1989;16:1229–32.
11. Schiellerup P, Krogfelt KA, Locht H. A comparison of self-reported joint symptoms following infection with different enteric pathogens: Effect of HLA-B27. J Rheumatol 2008;35:480–7.
12. Yu D, Kuipers JG. Role of bacteria and HLA-B27 in the pathogenesis of reactive arthritis. Rheum Dis Clin N Am 2003;29:21–36.

# 65

# DERMATOLOGIC MANIFESTATIONS OF GASTROINTESTINAL DISEASE

*James E. Fitzpatrick, MD, and*
*Lori Prok, MD*

### 1. At what serum level of bilirubin do adults and infants develop clinically noticeable jaundice?

Adults develop clinically detectable jaundice when serum levels of bilirubin reach 2.5 to 3.0 mg/dL, whereas infants may not demonstrate visually detectable jaundice until serum levels reach 6.0 to 8.0 mg/dL. Hyperbilirubinemia precedes jaundice by several days because the bilirubin has not yet bound to tissue. After serum levels of bilirubin normalize, patients may remain visually jaundiced, as it takes several days for tissue-bound bilirubin to be released.

### 2. Where is clinical jaundice first visible?

The mucosae of the soft palate and sublingual region are often the first cutaneous surfaces to appear yellow in response to hyperbilirubinemia. This is likely because of the thin mucosal surface in these anatomic locations. Bilirubin also has a strong affinity for elastin, which accounts for its early appearance in the sclera of the eye.

### 3. What other conditions produce yellowish discoloration of the skin?

Carotenoderma due to excessive ingestion of carotene (e.g., yellow and orange vegetables such as carrots and squash), lycopenodermia due to excessive ingestion of lycopenes (e.g., red vegetables such as tomatoes and rose hips), and systemic administration of quinacrine can all cause yellowish skin discoloration unrelated to hyperbilirubinemia. The skin may also demonstrate a sallow, subtle yellowish hue in patients with profound hypothyroidism.

### 4. What are Terry nails and Muehrcke nails?

Terry nails are characterized by uniform white discoloration of the nail, with the distal 1 to 2 mm remaining pink. The white color results from abnormalities in the nail bed vasculature and is most commonly seen in patients with liver cirrhosis, heart disease, and diabetes. Muehrcke nails are characterized by double white transverse lines across the nails that disappear when pressure is applied. These lines are also caused by abnormal vasculature of the nail bed. They are most commonly seen in liver disease associated with hypoalbuminemia.

### 5. What gastrointestinal disease is associated with blue lunulae?

The lunula is the moon-shaped white area present at the proximal nail plate. Blue lunulae are seen in Wilson disease (hepatolenticular degeneration), which is caused by an autosomal recessive defect in ATP7B and copper transport. Copper accumulates in the liver, brain, cornea, skin, nails, and other tissues. Patients may also demonstrate pretibial hyperpigmentation. Kayser-Fleischer rings (brown to green circle of pigment in Descement membrane of the eye) are pathognomonic of Wilson disease.

### 6. What are spider angiomas? Why are they associated with liver disease?

Spider angiomas (nevus araneus) are vascular lesions characterized by a central arteriole and horizontal radiating thin-walled vessels that produce the *legs* of the vascular spider (Figure 65-1). The pulsation of the central vertically oriented arteriole in larger lesions can be visualized with diascopy (observing the lesion through a glass slide firmly pressed on the lesion). The pathophysiologic mechanism is not proved, but the high incidence of spider angiomas in alcohol-associated hepatitis and pregnancy suggests that elevated levels of estrogens, due to higher production or decreased metabolism, is responsible. Patients with liver cirrhosis and spider angiomas have elevated plasma levels of vascular endothelial growth factor, which may play a role in the development of spider angiomas.

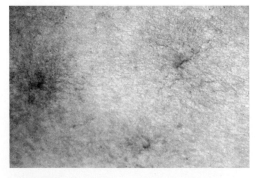

**Figure 65-1.** Three spider angiomas demonstrating central arteriole and radiating dilated blood vessels.

### 7. Do the number of spider angiomas correlate with the severity of alcohol-induced liver disease?

Yes, although there is some degree of individual susceptibility to spider angiomas. However, the correlation is high enough that one report suggests that barmaids in New York used to guess the degree of severity of liver cirrhosis of their customers based on the number of visible spider angiomas! The number of spider angiomas also correlates with the presence of esophageal varices. One study demonstrated that the presence of more than 20 spider angiomas correlated with a 50% chance of esophageal bleeding.

### 8. Why do many patients with hepatobiliary disease itch?

Approximately 40% of patients with hepatic cirrhosis demonstrate moderate to severe pruritus. The mechanism of pruritus associated with hepatobiliary disease has not been firmly established but is likely due to elevated levels of bile acids secondary to cholestasis. Serum bile acids are frequently elevated in patients with hepatobiliary disease and pruritus, and bile acid–binding resins relieve the pruritus. Studies on purified bile salts placed on blister bases have shown that all bile salts produced pruritus, but unconjugated chenodeoxycholate is the most potent.

### 9. A 64-year-old alcoholic man presents with blisters on the dorsal hands and sclerotic changes of the facial skin. For what chronic liver disease should he be screened?

This patient most likely has porphyria cutanea tarda, and he should be evaluated for hepatitis C virus infection. Patients with hepatitis C can present with a variety of cutaneous eruptions, including pruritus, vasculitis, lichen planus, cryoglobulinemic purpura, and porphyria cutanea tarda (PCT). PCT is characterized by photosensitivity, skin fragility resulting in vesicles and bullae of sun-exposed skin, dyspigmentation, alopecia, hirsutism, and skin thickening. It is caused by reduced hepatic uroporphyrinogen decarboxylase activity, which results in overproduction of blood and urine porphyrins. Hepatitis C virus (HCV) may cause hepatic iron overload in genetically susceptible individuals, leading to the clinical manifestations of PCT. Concomitant alcohol abuse, or other diseases or medications resulting in excess estrogens, increases the risk of developing PCT in these patients.

### 10. A 25-year-old woman presents with painful, tender, red-to-violaceous subcutaneous nodules of the pretibial skin associated with diarrhea. What is the skin lesion?

The patient most likely has erythema nodosum. The differential diagnosis also includes other types of panniculitis (e.g., erythema induratum, pancreatitis-associated panniculitis), infection, and deep vasculitis (e.g., periarteritis nodosum). Erythema nodosum is a form of hypersensitivity panniculitis that preferentially affect the fibrous septae between the fat lobules. Clinically, erythema nodosum most commonly presents on the anterior surface of the legs as painful red to violaceous subcutaneous nodules without overlying scale (Figure 65-2). Lesions are typically bilateral but unilateral and even annular variants exist. Typical lesions resolve over a period of 3 to 6 weeks but atypical lesions may persist for months. The diagnosis is usually made clinically but occasional cases require biopsy. The pathogenesis is not understood. Ulcerative colitis,

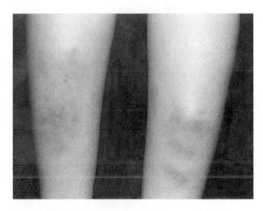

**Figure 65-2.** Typical lesions of erythema nodosum demonstrating bilateral, red, tender subcutaneous nodules on the anterior lower legs.

Crohn's disease, and infectious colitis (e.g., *Salmonella* and *Yersinia enterocolitis*) are the most common gastrointestinal (GI) diseases associated with erythema nodosum. In patients with inflammatory bowel disease, erythema nodosum is most commonly associated with ulcerative colitis (up to 7% of patients) and less commonly with Crohn's disease. The disease activity of erythema nodosum often parallels the activity of the bowel disease.

### 11. A 22-year-old woman presents with low-grade fever and an expanding oozing ulcer of the hand that is rapidly increasing in size despite aggressive surgical debridement and intravenous antibiotics. What does this patient have?

The patient most likely has pyoderma gangrenosum. Pyoderma gangrenosum usually affects the lower legs but can involve any cutaneous surface and the mucosal surfaces of the eye and oral cavity. The lesion begins as a tender red papule or pustule that rapidly increases in size to form an ulcer with an undermined border (Figure 65-3). Lesions of pyoderma gangrenosum may remain fixed or may rapidly expand at a rate of more than 1 cm per day. Pyoderma gangrenosum often demonstrates *pathergy*, which is the development of skin lesions at the site of trauma. Pyoderma gangrenosum mistaken for bacterial pyodermas may be treated with surgical debridement, which often makes the lesion worse. The pathogenesis of pyoderma gangrenosum is controversial. Histologically, the predominant effector cells are neutrophils and some authorities have even considered it to be a form of vasculitis. More recent evidence suggests that it is probably lymphocyte mediated, which accounts for its marked response to cyclosporine.

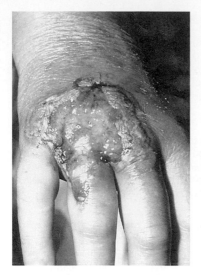

**Figure 65-3.** Typical lesion of pyoderma gangrenosum demonstrating tender, rapidly expanding ulcer with undermined edge.

### 12. List the GI diseases most commonly associated with pyoderma gangrenosum.

Like erythema nodosum, pyoderma gangrenosum is associated with ulcerative colitis (most common), Crohn's disease, and chronic infectious hepatitis. One study reported that 50% all cases of pyoderma gangrenosum are associated with ulcerative colitis but less than 10% of all patients with ulcerative colitis will develop pyoderma gangrenosum. A separate study reported that one-third of patients with pyoderma gangrenosum had inflammatory bowel disease; ulcerative colitis and Crohn's disease were equally represented.

### 13. What are the cutaneous manifestations of pancreatitis?

Cutaneous manifestations of pancreatitis include Cullen sign, Grey Turner sign, and pancreatic fat necrosis. Cullen sign is a hemorrhagic discoloration of the umbilical area due to intraperitoneal hemorrhage from any cause; one of the more frequent causes is acute hemorrhagic panniculitis. Grey Turner sign is a discoloration of the left flank associated with acute hemorrhagic pancreatitis. Acute and chronic pancreatitis and pancreatic carcinoma may also produce pancreatic fat necrosis, which presents as very tender, erythematous nodules of the subcutaneous fat that may spontaneously drain necrotic material (Figure 65-4). Patients also often have associated acute arthritis that may be crippling. Histologically pancreatic fat necrosis demonstrates diagnostic changes manifesting as necrosis and saponification of the fat associated with acute inflammation. The fat necrosis is thought to be due to release of lipase and amylase, which have been demonstrated to be elevated within lesions.

### 14. A 32-year-old man presents with a 2-year history of recurrent blisters that are intensely pruritic and have been recalcitrant to antihistamines and topical corticosteroids. They are primarily located on the elbows, knees, and buttocks. What does this patient most likely have?

This patient most likely has dermatitis herpetiformis, an autoimmune vesiculobullous disease characterized by intensely pruritic blisters that are often grouped (herpetiform) or less commonly plaques studded with vesicles or bullae (Figure 65-5). Dermatitis herpetiformis has a classic symmetric distribution; the characteristic sites are the elbows, knees, buttocks, and scalp. Because of the intense pruritus, patients often present with excoriations only. The diagnosis is usually established by demonstrating the presence of IgA autoantibodies along the dermoepidermal junction by direct immunofluorescence.

### 15. What GI disease is most commonly associated with dermatitis herpetiformis?

Celiac disease (gluten-sensitive enteropathy). Although almost all patients demonstrate histologic findings of celiac disease in the gastrointestinal tract, only one-third demonstrate clinical symptoms of celiac disease. Both celiac disease and dermatitis herpetiformis respond to a gluten-free diet. Oral dapsone results in rapid improvement of the characteristic skin lesions and associated pruritus of dermatitis herpetiformis.

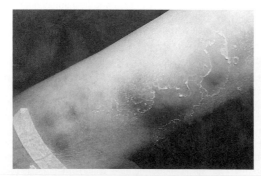

**Figure 65-4.** Pancreatic fat necrosis in a patient with alcohol-associated pancreatitis. Unlike erythema nodosum, epidermal changes (note scale) and ulceration are common.

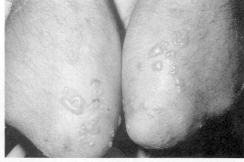

**Figure 65-5.** Grouped vesicles and bullae on the elbows of a patient with dermatitis herpetiformis.

**16. A 30-year-old man presents with acute GI bleeding. He has yellowish pebbly papules that coalesce into plaques of the neck, antecubital fossae, and axillae. Similar lesions are also present on his lower lip. What does he have?**

The patient has pseudoxanthoma elasticum (PXE), a disorder characterized by progressive calcification of elastic fibers. It is most commonly inherited in an autosomal dominant fashion but autosomal recessive variants have also been described. Mutations in the *ABCC6* gene have been demonstrated to be the genetic defect but how this defect produces PXE is not understood. The mucocutaneous manifestations are described as looking like *plucked chicken skin* (Fig. 65-6). The histologic findings are diagnostic and demonstrate fragmentation of abnormal elastic fibers in the dermis associated with calcification. Identical yellowish papules are seen in the GI mucosa including the mouth, esophagus, and stomach. Involvement of the elastic fibers in gastric arteries may result in acute and sometimes massive hemorrhage. Additional findings associated with PXE include angioid streaks of the retina, claudication, premature angina, and hypertension.

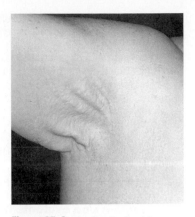

**Figure 65-6.** Confluent yellowish papules with appearance of "plucked chicken skin" in a patient with pseudoxanthoma elasticum.

**17. A 24-year-old man presents with a history of unexplained melena, nose bleeds, and red macular lesions of his lips and fingers. What does he have?**

This patient most likely has hereditary hemorrhagic telangiectasia (HHT), also known as Osler-Weber-Rendu disease. This uncommon genetic disorder is inherited in an autosomal dominant fashion and is the result of mutations of two genes: *ENG* (HHT1) and *ALK1* (HHT2). The cutaneous lesions typically present at the time of puberty or later and manifest as linear, punctate, or macular lesions that most commonly affect the skin surfaces of the face, finger, and toes. Similar lesions are also found in many types of mucosal surfaces including the nasal mucosa, lips, entire gastrointestinal tract, and urinary tract. Arteriovenous malformations also may develop in the central nervous system, eye, lungs, and liver. Patients continue to develop new lesions during their lifetime and may experience chronic iron-deficiency anemia due to chronic low-grade blood loss from the GI tract.

**18. During evaluation for GI bleeding, a 25-year-old man is noted to have 2- to 4-mm pigmented macules of the lips and buccal mucosa. What does he most likely have?**

This patient most likely has Peutz-Jeghers syndrome, an autosomal dominant disorder associated with germline mutations of the *STKII/LKB1* tumor suppressor gene. It is characterized by round to oval pigmented macules that vary from brown to blue-brown in color and small intestine hamartomatous polyps. The pigmented macules are usually present at birth or develop during infancy. The most commonly affected areas are the lips, buccal mucosa, hard palate, gingival, anus, palms, and soles. Since pigmented macular lesions may be seen in these areas in normal individuals and in association with other syndromes, clinical and historical correlation is necessary to make establish a diagnosis of Peutz-Jeghers syndrome. The lifetime risk of developing adenocarcinoma in the GI polyps seen in Peutz-Jeghers is calculated to be between 2% to 13%. Patients also demonstrate an increased incidence of other types of neoplasia, including breast carcinoma, cervical adenocarcinoma, and both benign and malignant tumors of the ovary and testes.

**19. During evaluation for numerous polyps of the colon, a 19-year-old man is noted to have multiple cysts of the skin and an osteoma. What does he most likely have?**

Gardner syndrome, which is inherited in an autosomal dominant fashion, is due to a mutation in the *APC* gene located at 5q21. This rare disorder occurs in 1 of every 14,000 births. The polyps resemble the polyps of familial adenomatous polyposis. Patients have colonic polyps and 10% have small intestine polyps. The cutaneous manifestations consist of epidermoid cysts (epidermal inclusion cysts), lipomas, fibromas, desmoid tumors, and rarely pilomatricomas (uncommon hair follicle tumors). Patients often have bone tumors, most of which are osteomas; supernumerary teeth; and congenital hypertrophy of the retinal pigmented epithelium. The lifetime risk of colon cancer in Gardner syndrome approaches 100%. Proctocolectomy is recommended for all patients, followed by periodic monitoring of the rectal mucosal remnant and the upper GI tract. Patients with Gardner syndrome also have a higher incidence of extracolonic malignancies, including papillary thyroid carcinoma, adrenal carcinoma, hepatoblastoma, periampullary carcinoma, and duodenal carcinoma.

**20. A 44-year-old man presents with multiple hamartomatous polyps of the small and large bowel. Cutaneous examination reveals *cobblestoning* of the oral mucosa and multiple small papules and verrucous papules of this face. What does this patient most likely have?**

Cowden disease, which is also known as multiple hamartoma syndrome. This rare syndrome is inherited in an autosomal fashion and is due to mutations in *PTEN,* a tumor suppressor gene located on chromosome 10q23.

The mucocutaneous manifestations include small papules of the oral mucosa that are usually most prominent on the gingival, are often numerous, and have been described as resembling cobblestones; papules and verrucous papules, usually located on the face that are trichilemmomas (benign follicular tumors), hyperkeratotic papules of the extremities, and firm nodules called sclerotic fibromas. Sclerotic fibromas are uncommon benign fibrous tumors that are typically solitary. Multiple sclerotic fibromas are considered to be a specific marker for Cowden disease; the incidence approaches 100% if two or more are present. Polyps are present in the GI tract in approximately 30% of patients and may be present at any site. The polyps associated with Cowden syndrome do not demonstrate an increased risk of malignancy. However, patients with Cowden syndrome demonstrate an increased incidence of thyroid disease; up to two-thirds have goiter and 10% develop thyroid carcinoma. Seventy-five percent of women with Cowden demonstrate breast neoplasia manifesting as fibrocystic breast disease, fibroadenomas, and breast carcinoma.

### 21. A 60-year-old man has had multiple keratoacanthomas removed from his skin and recently had a biopsy of a sebaceous adenoma of the cheek. For what syndrome should he be evaluated?

This patient should be evaluated for Muir-Torre syndrome, which is characterized by multiple benign and/or malignant cutaneous sebaceous neoplasms, and an increased risk of gastrointestinal malignancies (colon adenocarcinoma, genitourinary tract carcinoma, and lymphoma). Patients may also demonstrate multiple keratoacanthomas (well-differentiated squamous cell carcinomas of the skin). Muir-Torre syndrome is inherited in an autosomal dominant manner and is caused by a defect in the DNA mismatch repair genes *MSH1* and *MSH2*. Most recently, defects in *MSH6* have also been identified in several patients. Because the cutaneous neoplasms occur prior to the development of internal malignancy in these patients, appropriate workup and genetic counseling can be lifesaving.

### 22. What is Trousseau sign?

Trousseau sign consists of superficial migratory thrombophlebitis associated with an underlying malignancy. Clinically it presents as erythematous linear cords that affect the superficial veins of the extremities and trunk. Patients typically continue to develop new lesions at multiple sites that may appear to *migrate*. Trousseau sign may be seen in association with many types of GI malignancies (e.g., gastric carcinoma, pancreatic adenocarcinoma) in addition to lung carcinoma, multiple myeloma, and Hodgkin disease. The pathogenesis is not understood and the thrombophlebitis is notoriously resistant to anticoagulant therapy. It was a cruel coincidence that the physician who described this sign, Dr. Trousseau was himself to develop Trousseau sign secondary to his underlying gastric carcinoma, which was ultimately fatal.

### 23. A 50-year-old woman presents with alopecia, unexplained 20-pound weight loss, and very superficial flaccid vesicles and erosions on an erythematous base that preferentially involves the perioral and perianal areas. What does she most likely have?

The cutaneous lesions are consistent with necrolytic migratory erythema, a paraneoplastic cutaneous finding associated with alpha-2-glucagon–producing islet cell tumors of the pancreas. The cutaneous lesions characteristically start as broad areas of erythema that preferentially affect the face, intertriginous areas, ankles, and feet. The skin often appears to peel or demonstrate superficial vesicles. Patients also may demonstrate stomatitis, glossitis, alopecia, nail dystrophy, weight loss, diabetes mellitus, and anemia. Resection of the glucagon-producing tumor produces prompt resolution of the skin lesions.

### 24. Who was Sister Mary Joseph and what is a Sister Mary Joseph nodule?

Sister Mary Joseph was the first surgical assistant to Dr. W.J. Mayo, who eventually became the superintendent of St. Mary's Hospital in Rochester, Minnesota. A Sister Mary Joseph nodule is an umbilical metastasis of an internal malignancy. In the largest series reported, the most common primary malignancies were stomach (20%), large bowel (14%), ovary (14%), and pancreas (11%). In 20% of cases, the primary could not be established. In 14% of cases, a Sister Mary Joseph nodule was the initial presentation of the internal malignancy. Umbilical metastases usually indicate advanced disease; the average survival is 10 months. Although it was Dr. Mayo who described the clinical features of nodular umbilical metastases, Sister Mary Joseph is credited with being the first to appreciate that patients with this finding had a poor prognosis.

## WEBSITE

http://www.derm.ubc.ca

## BIBLIOGRAPHY

1. Callen JP, Jackson JM. Pyoderma gangrenosum: An update. Rheumatol Dis Clin N Am 2007;33:787–802 vi.
2. Chhibber V, Dresser K, Mahalingam M. MSH-6: Extending the reliability of immunohistochemistry as a screening tool in Muir-Torre syndrome. Mod Pathol 2008;21:159–64.
3. Galossi A, Guarisco R, Bellis L, et al. Extrahepatic manifestations of chronic HCV infection. J Gastrointest Liver Dis 2007;16:65–73.
4. Ghosn SH, Kibbi AG. Cutaneous manifestations of liver diseases. Clin Dermatol 2008;26:274–82.
5. Li CP, Lee FY, Hwang SJ, et al. Spider angiomas in patients with liver cirrhosis: Role of vascular endothelial growth factor and basic fibroblast growth factor. World J Gasteroenterol 2003;9:2832–3.
6. Marsh R, de W, Hagler KT, Carag HR, et al. Pancreatic panniculitis. Eur J Surg Oncol 2005;31:1213–5.
7. Masmoudi A, Boudaya S, Charfeddine A, et al. Sister Mary Joseph's nodule: Report of five cases. Int J Dermatol 2008;47:134–6.
8. McDonald J, Bayrak-Toydemir P. Hereditary hemorrhagic telangiectasia. Haematologica 2005;90:728–32.
9. Wahie S, Lawrence CM. Cutaneous signs as a presenting manifestation of alcohol excess. Br J Dermatol 2006;155:195–7.

# ENDOCRINE ASPECTS OF GASTROENTEROLOGY

*Tom J. Sauerwein, MD, FACE, and*
*Kevin J. Franklin, MD, FACP*

**1. What are the etiologies of diabetic gastroparesis? How should it be treated?**

Diabetic gastroparesis can occur with both type 1 and type 2 diabetes, usually of at least 10 years' duration. Patients often have associated end organ damage such as peripheral neuropathy, nephropathy, or retinopathy. Gastric emptying mechanisms are deranged to include vagal nerve neuropathy, reduction in intrinsic inhibitory neurons critical for motor conduction, a reduction in gastric pacemaker cells (interstitial cells of Cajal), and increased glucagon levels. Gastric emptying can also be retarded in acute hyperglycemia with blood glucose levels greater than 180 mg/dL. Neurohormonal dysfunction and hyperglycemia also reduce the frequency of antral contractions. Behavioral, medical, and surgical treatment strategies of gastroparesis are outlined in Table 66-1.

**2. Describe the mechanisms of chronic diarrhea in diabetes mellitus and their treatments.**

Chronic diarrhea in patients with diabetes mellitus usually is related to either chronic autonomic dysfunction, steatorrhea, or associated diseases that are more prevalent in the diabetic population. The most common cause of nondiabetic diarrhea in diabetics is a side effect of drug therapy associated with metformin. Treatment strategies based on the primary cause of the diabetic diarrhea are depicted in Table 66-2.

**3. Patients with primary biliary cirrhosis (PBC) are at increased risk for what endocrine disorders?**

Patients with PBC have an approximately 22% prevalence rate for hypothyroidism overall with a 12% prevalence rate of newly diagnosed primary hypothyroidism after PBC has been diagnosed. Antimicrosomal antibodies are positive in 34% and antithyroglobulin antibodies are positive in 20% of patients with PBC, but not all patients with antibodies have hypothyroidism.

**Table 66-1.** Management of Diabetic Gastroparesis Based on Severity of Disease

| TREATMENT | SEVERITY OF DISEASE (TYPICAL GASTRIC RETENTION OF SOLID FOOD AT 4 HOURS) | | |
|---|---|---|---|
| | **MILD (10% TO 15%)** | **MODERATE (16% TO 35%)** | **SEVERE (>35%)** |
| Homogenized food consumption | When symptomatic | When symptomatic | Routinely |
| Nutritional supplementation | Rare | Caloric liquids orally, rare PEJ | PEJ tube may be needed |
| Pharmacologic treatment | Reglan 10 mg PRN Dramamine 50 mg PRN | Reglan 10 mg QAC Domperidone 10 to 20 mg QAC Erythromycin 40 to 250 mg QAC Dimenhydrinate 50 mg PRN Compazine 25 mg PRN | Reglan 10 mg QAC Domperidone 10 to 20 mg QAC Erythromycin 40 to 250 mg QAC Dimenhydrinate 50 mg PRN Compazine 25 mg PRN Zofran 4 to 8 mg PRN |
| Nonpharmacologic treatment | None | None | PEG decompression PEJ feeding TPN Gastric electrical stimulation |

PEG, percutaneous endoscopic gastrostomy; PEJ, percutaneous endoscopic jejunostomy; PRN, pro re nata (as needed); QAC, before meals; TPN, total parenteral nutrition.
Modified from Camilleri M: Diabetic gastroparesis. N Engl J Med 356:823, 2007.

**Table 66-2.** Causes and Treatment of Diabetic Diarrhea

| CAUSE OF DIABETIC DIARRHEA | TREATMENT |
|---|---|
| Metformin induced | Prescribe metformin 250 to 500 mg with evening meal and instruct to slowly increase as tolerated to effective dose. |
| Intestinal bacterial overgrowth | Tetracycline, metronidazole, cephalosporins, quinolones, amoxicillin-clavulanic acid, trimethoprim–sulfamethoxazole, norfloxacin, gentamicin, rifaximin (7 to 10 days)—monotherapy or combination or rotating therapy |
| Celiac disease | Gluten-free diet |
| Use of dietetic foods | Avoid sorbitol products |
| Pancreatic exocrine deficiency | Pancreatic enzymes |
| Bile acid malabsorption | Cholestyramine (4 to 16 g/day), Colestipol (2 g 1 to 2 times daily) |
| Abnormal colonic motility | Loperamide (2 to 4 mg/day), diphenoxylate (5 mg four times daily), codeine (30 mg four times daily) |
| Altered intestinal secretion | Octreotide (50 to 75 mcg subcutaneously before meals), clonidine |
| Anorectal dysfunction | Biofeedback |

Freiling T: Diabetic autonomic neuropathy of the gastrointestinal tract. In Rose BD (ed): Waltham, MA, updateonline.com, 2008. Modified from Liver Secrets, 3rd edition, page 569.

Osteoporosis, but not osteomalacia, occurs at an increased rate (RR: 3.83) in female patients with PBC compared with age-matched controls. The 32.4% prevalence was associated with age, longer PBC duration, and higher Mayo risk score. There is a modest 2-fold relative increased risk of fracture also seen in patients with PBC.

Hyperlipidemia is seen in 10% of patients and its appearance is similar to dysbetalipoproteinemia-tuberous xanthomas and palmar xanthomas. Xanthomas develop in patients with extremely high cholesterol levels.

4. **What are the most prominent GI manifestations seen in hyperthyroidism and in hypothyroidism?**
   - *Hyperthyroidism:* Gastritis occurs in 80% of patients and is associated with decreased acid secretion. Hyperdefecation, malabsorption, and rarely steatorrhea are seen secondary to altered intestinal motility. Hyperphagia is seen in most patients, while anorexia may be prominent in elderly patients. The liver is the primary organ of thyroid hormone metabolism and elevated liver function tests can be seen in up to 90% of patients. Hypoxia secondary to increased oxygen utilization may not be totally compensated by hepatic blood flow, which results in pericentral hepatic acini damage.
   - *Hypothyroidism:* Constipation, obstipation, and colonic gas retention are seen secondary to prolonged gastrointestinal (GI) transit times. Hepatomegaly and mild elevations in liver function tests are seen frequently and pathologic examination reveals central *congestive* fibrosis. Infiltration of the submucosa by lymphocytes and plasma cells as well as a myxedematous infiltration of the stroma are found.

5. **Name the two metabolic causes of acute pancreatitis. Which diabetic medication may cause acute pancreatitis?**
   Hypertriglyceridemia and hypercalcemia are the two metabolic disturbances that can precipitate acute pancreatitis. Triglyceride concentrations above 1000 mg/dL (11 mmol/L) may account for 1.3% to 3.8% of acute pancreatitis cases. The pathogenesis in this setting is unclear. Hypertriglyceridemia may be overlooked as a cause due to low serum amylase levels and normalization of triglyceride levels with fasting. Hypercalcemia of any etiology can cause acute pancreatitis, but it is rare. Proposed mechanisms include calcium activation of trypsinogen in the pancreatic parenchyma and the deposition of calcium in the pancreatic duct.

   Acute pancreatitis has been reported in patients taking exenatide (Byetta) and is suspected as being causative. While 90% of patients had other risk factors for acute pancreatitis, 73% improved following discontinuation of exenatide. When rechallenged, 10% of patients had recurrent symptoms.

6. **Define *hypoglycemia* and list the counter-regulatory response to hypoglycemia.**
   A clinical condition in which the plasma glucose levels fall below 50 mg/dL (2.8 mmol/L) resulting in adrenergic symptoms or neuroglycopenia (Table 66-3).

**Table 66-3.** Physiologic Response to Hypoglycemia

| RESPONSE | GLYCEMIC THRESHOLD, mg/dL (mmol/L) | ROLE IN THE PREVENTION OR CORRECTION OF HYPOGLYCEMIA (GLUCOSE COUNTERREGULATION) |
| --- | --- | --- |
| ↓Insulin | 80 to 85 (4.4 to 4.7) | *Primary* glucose regulatory factor/first defense against hypoglycemia |
| ↑ Glucagon | 65 to 70 (3.6 to 3.9) | *Primary* glucose counter-regulatory factor/second defense against hypoglycemia |
| ↑ Epinephrine | 65 to 70 (3.6 to 3.9) | Third defense against hypoglycemia, critical when glucagon is deficient |
| ↑ Cortisol and growth hormone | 65 to 70 (3.6 to 3.9) | Involved in defense against *prolonged* hypoglycemia, not critical |
| Adrenergic symptoms | 50 to 55 (2.8 to 3.1) | Prompt behavioral defense against hypoglycemia (food ingestion) |
| ↓ Cognition (neuroglycopenia) | <50 (2.8) | Compromises behavioral defense against hypoglycemia |

Modified from Harrison's Principles of Internal Medicine, 17th ed (2008), New York, McGraw-Hill, Table 339-2.

### 7. What is Whipple triad? Why is it important?

Whipple described the following triad of findings that should exist before insulin levels are measured and other elaborate testing performed in the pursuit of a rare insulinoma (Fig. 66-1):

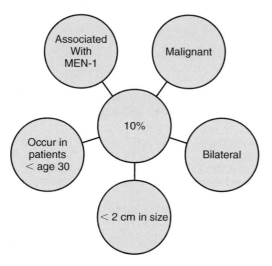

**Figure 66-1.** Rule of 10s for insulinoma

- Presence of neuroglycopenic* symptoms consistent with hypoglycemia
- Documentation of low plasma glucose with a reliable assay
- Relief of symptoms after the plasma glucose is normalized

### 8. Which GI and hepatic disturbances are associated with hypoglycemia?

Hypoglycemia (less than 50 mg/dL) may occur in either the fasting state or the postprandial state (reactive). Etiologies that cause fasting hypoglycemia are predominantly organic and result in neuroglycopenia. There is either underproduction or overutilization of glucose. Overutilization may be further classified as insulin dependent or insulin independent. Etiologies that cause reactive hypoglycemia are functionxal and typically result in adrenergic symptoms. Fasting hypoglycemia is diagnosed with a supervised 72-hour fast, while postprandial hypoglycemia is diagnosed with a mixed meal test (Fig. 66-2).

### 9. How does ethanol cause hypoglycemia?

- Associated with poor food intake and occurs only after hepatic glycogen stores have been depleted
- Ethanol impairs gluconeogenesis through depletion of $NADH_2$ to NAD and decreases uptake of lactate, alanine, and glycerol (gluconeogenesis substrates)
- Alcohol dampens the normal growth hormone, corticotropin, cortisol, and glucagon responses to induced hypoglycemia
- Ethanol does not impair glycogenolysis

### 10. Should routine screening for polyps and colorectal cancer be performed in patients with acromegaly?

Acromegaly appears to be associated with an increased risk of colonic adenomatous polyps and colorectal cancer. Studies have reported conflicting results. Several mechanisms are thought to be causative to include an IGF-1 trophic effect on epithelial cell proliferation and a reduced expression of the peroxisome proliferator-activated receptor *(PPAR)*

---

* *Neuroglycopenic* symptoms due to cerebral glucose deprivation include confusion, difficulty thinking, a sense of increased warmth, weakness, fatigue, bizarre behavior, seizures, and coma as opposed to reactive *adrenergic* symptoms like tremulousness, anxiety, and palpitations, sweating, and paresthesia.

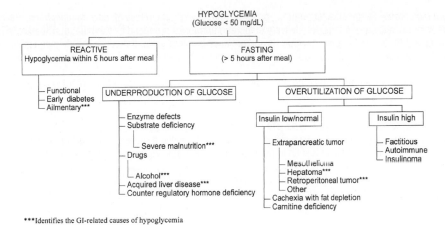

**Figure 66-2.** Contributions of gastrointestinal and hepatic disturbances to the development of hypoglycemia.

gene. Colonoscopy is currently recommended in patients with acromegaly over 50 years old at 3- to 5-year intervals. The shorter interval should be offered to patients with adenomas at index colonoscopy or those with IGF-1 levels above the maximum age-corrected normal range.

## 11. What GI symptoms may be seen with hypercalcemia?

The most common gastrointestinal symptoms associated with hypercalcemia are constipation (33%), abdominal pain (29%), nausea (28%), vomiting (19%), and duodenal ulcer (12%). The exact mechanism of these symptoms in hypercalcemia is not known. Anorexia, nausea, and vomiting appear early in hypercalcemic crisis. Poor oral intake and accelerated water loss from hypercalcemia-induced nephrogenic diabetes insipidus result in polyuria, dehydration, decreased renal blood flow, and a fall in glomerular filtration rate; this leads to increased proximal tubular sodium reabsorption. Enhanced calcium reabsorption, linked to the latter, increases sodium uptake, further exacerbating the hypercalcemia and can result in stupor, coma, and even death. Duodenal ulcers appear to occur with greater frequency in association with hyperparathyroidism. The incidence is reported as high as 20% to 30%. Hypercalcemia is thought to increase gastric secretion by stimulating antral gastrin release.

## 12. What are the National Institutes of Health (NIH) criteria for bariatric surgery?

- Body mass index = 40 kg/m²
- Body mass index = 35 kg/m² plus an obesity-related condition
- Documented failure to control weight with pharmacologic lifestyle means
- Absence of medical or psychological contraindications
- Good understanding of the procedure's risks and expected outcomes
- Awareness of and motivation to comply with the postoperative regimen
- Supportive social environment

## 13. How effective are bariatric surgical procedures for long-term control of morbid obesity?

See Table 66-4.

**Table 66-4.** Pooled Weight Loss Results Following Bariatric Surgery

| PROCEDURE | 12-MONTH WEIGHT LOSS, kg (95% CI) | >36-MONTH WEIGHT LOSS, kg (95% CI) |
|---|---|---|
| Roux-en-Y gastric bypass | 43.46 (41.24 to 43.46) | 41.46 (37.36 to 45.56) |
| Vertical banded gastroplasty | 32.16 (29.92 to 34.41) | 32.03 (27.67 to 36.38) |
| Adjustable gastric banding | 30.19 (27.95 to 32.42) | 34.77 (29.47 to 40.07) |

Modified from Maggard MA, Shugarman LA, Suttopr M, et al: Meta to analysis: Surgical treatment of obesity. Ann Intern Med 142:547–559, 2005.

## 14. Describe gut hormone changes following Roux-en-Y gastric bypass (RYGB) that theoretically may explain the development of nesidioblastosis.

Ghrelin, which is produced by the stomach and duodenum, is an orexigenic hormone that antagonizes insulin secretion. Following RYGB, ghrelin levels decline and lose its prandial pattern. Since ghrelin antagonizes insulin secretion and action, lower levels enhance insulin secretion and action.

- *Foregut hypothesis:* Surgical isolation of the proximal intestine results in loss of, as yet unidentified, anti-incretin factors, thereby allowing unimpeded delivery of incretin hormones produced by the hindgut. The excess incretin hormones are theorized to prevent apoptosis and enhance proliferation of beta cells resulting in nesidioblastosis.
- *Hindgut hypothesis:* Rapid nutrient transport to the ileum enhances L-cell production of glucagon-like peptide 1 (GLP-1).
- It appears that RYGB produces maximum incretin action by surgically excluding the foregut and effectively advancing the hindgut in nutrient transit.

### 15. What is multiple endocrine neoplasia type 1 (MEN1)?

Also known as Wermer syndrome, it is an autosomal dominant inheritable disorder with an estimated prevalence of 2 to 20 per 100,000 patients. The syndrome results from mutations in the tumor suppression gene *menin* that is located on the long arm of chromosome 11. Almost 300 independent mutations have been described, which result in hyperparathyroidism (95% to 100%) from parathyroid hyperplasia, followed by pancreatic islet tumors (30 % to 80%), and finally multicentric pituitary tumors (20% to 25%). Carcinoid tumors, almost exclusively foregut carcinoids (thymic, bronchial, gastric), are seen with increased frequency in MEN1. Thymic carcinoids occur more frequently in men and bronchial carcinoids in women.

### 16. List the order of pancreatic islet cell tumor prevalence in MEN1 and their clinical manifestations.

See Table 66-5.

**Table 66-5.** Pancreatic Islet Cell Tumor Prevalence

| TUMOR TYPE | PREVALENCE | CLINICAL MANIFESTATION |
| --- | --- | --- |
| Gastrinoma | 60% | Recurrent refractory peptic ulcers |
| Insulinoma | 30% | Hypoglycemia, weight gain, neuroglycopenia, esophagitis, diarrhea |
| Glucagonoma | 5% | Hyperglycemia, anorexia, glossitis, anemia, migratory necrolytic erythema |
| VIPoma | 3% | Watery diarrhea, hypokalemia, hypercalcemia, hypochloremic metabolic alkalosis |
| Somatostatinoma | 1% | Diabetes mellitus, diarrhea, steatorrhea, cholelithiasis |
| Other | 1% | |

### 17. Are patients with MEN1 and gastrinomas at greater risk for esophageal complications compared with gastrinoma patients without MEN1?

When patients with MEN1/Zöllinger-Ellison syndrome (ZES) are compared with patients with just ZES, those with MEN1 have a 3-fold higher incidence of esophageal strictures, a 5-fold higher incidence of Barrett esophagus, and an 8-fold higher incidence of dysplasia. In a recent study, one of 80 patients with MEN1/ZES died of esophageal adenocarcinoma, whereas none of the 215 patients with ZES alone died.

### 18. Define *carcinoid syndrome*

*Carcinoid syndrome* is the term given to a constellation of symptoms mediated by a variety of humoral factors elicited by some carcinoid tumors including polypeptides, prostaglandins, and biogenic amines. The syndrome is found in 5% to 20% of patients. Typical symptoms include cutaneous flushing, diarrhea, and bronchospasm. Other features include hypotension, the development of venous telangiectasias, and right-sided cardiac valvular lesions.

### 19. How are carcinoid tumors classified?

Traditionally, carcinoid tumors are classified according to their embryologic site of origin into foregut (lungs, bronchi, stomach, duodenum, pancreas), midgut (small intestine, appendix, proximal colon) and hindgut (distal colon, rectum, genitourinary tract). Midgut tumors are derived from serotonin-containing enterochromaffin cell (EC) cells and may secrete serotonin while foregut tumors are derived from histamine-containing enterochromaffin like cell (ECL) cells. Gastric carcinoids have been categorized according to their pathobiological behaviors into types I, II, and III (Table 66-6).

### 20. Where do carcinoid tumors occur, and what are the characteristic features of carcinoid tumors by site of origin?

- *Gastric* (7%): Most gastric carcinoids are asymptomatic and discovered incidentally during endoscopy. One-half of gastric carcinoids are multifocal, but less than 10% metastasize.
- *Small intestinal* (45%): Frequently located in the distal ileum in patients older than 60 years with chronic abdominal pain or small bowel obstruction. Lymph node or hepatic metastases are common (20%). Only 5% to 7% manifest carcinoid syndrome. May be multicentric with dozens of lesions lining the small bowel.

**Table 66-6.** Classification of Gastric Carcinoid Tumors

|  | TYPE I | TYPE II | TYPE III |
|---|---|---|---|
| Percent | 70 to 80 | 5 to 10 | 15 to 20 |
| Association | CAG/PA | MEN-1 ZES | Sporadic |
| Mucosa | Atrophy | Hypertrophy | Normal |
| Metastasis (%) | <5 | 7 to 10 | >50 |

CAG, chronic atrophic gastritis MEN, multiple endocrine neoplasia; PA, pernicious anemia; ZES, Zollinger Ellison syndrome
Modified from Hou W, Shubert ML: Treatment of gastric carcinoids. Curr Treat Opt Gastroenterol 10:125, 2007.

- *Appendicle* (16%): Most common tumor of the appendix. Presents in patients 40 to 50 years of age. More common in women. Less than 10% cause symptoms and metastases are rare.
- *Colonic* (11%): Presents in the seventh decade of life. Less than 5% manifest carcinoid syndrome. Two-thirds are found in the right colon.
- *Rectal* (20%): Most present in the sixth decade of life. Usually contain glucagon- and glicentin-related peptides rather than serotonin. One-half are asymptomatic. The remainder present with rectal bleeding, pain, or constipation.

### 21. How is carcinoid syndrome treated?

General treatment measures and agents to ameliorate symptoms associated with carcinoid syndrome are depicted in Table 66-7.

**Table 66-7.** Treatment of Carcinoid Syndrome

| CARCINOID SYMPTOM/PROBLEM | INTERVENTION |
|---|---|
| General | Niacin supplementation to compensate for accelerated conversion of tryptophan to serotonin<br>High-protein diet<br>Avoidance of precipitants for spells, such as sympathomimetics, alcohol, and stress |
| Flushing | Somatostatin analogs<br>H1 and H2 blockers (especially for gastric carcinoid)<br>Interferon<br>Phenoxybenzamine |
| Diarrhea | Loperamide and diphenoxylate<br>Antiserotonin agents (methysergide, cryproheptadine)<br>Somatostatin analogs<br>Cholestyramine |
| Asthma and bronchospasm | Methylxanthines and glucocorticoids are the most commonly used agents. Beta-agonists and epinephrine should be avoided because they may precipitate attacks. |
| Excessive tumor burden | Surgery<br>Hepatic artery embolization or ligation<br>Chemotherapy (streptoxocin and fluorouracil; methotrexate and cyclophosphamide; interferon; doxorubicin; cisplatinum; etoposide)<br>Radiolabeled somatostatin analogs |

### 22. What hepatic effects are seen in patients with adrenal disorders?

Patients with adrenal insufficiency have been reported to have elevated serum aminotransferase concentrations. These levels tend to normalize with appropriate hormone replacement. Hypercortisolism (Cushing syndrome) has been associated with fatty infiltration of the liver in 50% of patients, which may progress to nonalcoholic steatohepatitis (NASH). NASH has an estimated prevalence of 20% to 50% in patients with Cushing syndrome.

**BIBLIOGRAPHY**

1. Ahmad SR, Swann J. Exenatide and rare adverse events. N Engl J Med 2008;358:1969–72.
2. Arky RA. Hypoglycemia associated with liver disease and ethanol. Endocrinol Metab Clin North Am 1989;18:75.
3. Elta GH, Sepersky RA, Goldbery MJ, et al. Increased incidence of hypothyroidism in primary biliary cirrhosis. Dig Dis Sci 1983;28:971–5.

4. Folaron I, Sauerwein T. Hyperinsulinemic hypoglycemia after gastric bypass. Pract Diabetol 2008.

5. Gardener DG, Shoback D. Greenspan's basic & clinical endocrinology. 8th ed. New York: McGraw-Hill; 2007. pp. 831–4.

6. Gardner EC, Hersh T. Primary hyperparathyroidism and the gastrointestinal tract. South Med J 1981;74:197–9.

7. Gastrointestinal Surgery for Severe Obesity. National Institutes of Health consensus development conference statement. Am J Clin Nutr 1992;55(Suppl. 2):61S–9.

8. Guanabens N, Pares A, Ros I, et al. Severity of cholestatis and advanced histological stage but not menopausal status are the major risk factors for osteoporosis in primary biliary cirrhosis. South J Hepatol 2005;42:573–7.

9. Hoffmann KM, Gibril F, Entsuah LK, et al. Patients with multiple endocrine neoplasia type 1 with gastrinomas have an increased risk of severe esophageal disease including stricture and the premalignant condition, Barrett's esophagus. J Clin Endocinol Metab 2006;91:204–12.

10. Hou W, Shubert ML. Treatment of gastric carcinoids. Curr Treat Opt Gastroenterol 2007;10:123–33.

11. Jenkins PJ, Fairclough PD. Screening guidelines for colorectal cancer and polyps in patients with acromegaly. Gut 2002;51(Suppl. V):13v–14.

12. Kulke MH, Mayer RJ. Carcinoid tumors. N Engl J Med 1999;18:858.

13. Larson AM, Kowdley KV. Clinical Practice of Gastroenterology. Philadelphia, Churchill Livingstone, 1999, p.1509.

14. Marx SJ. Hyperparathyroid and hypoparathyroid disorders. N Engl J Med 2000;343:1863–75.

15. Melmed S. Clinical manifestations of acromegaly. In: Rose BD, editor. Waltham, MA: UpToDateOnline.com, 2008.

16. Santhi SV, Chari ST. Etiology of acute pancreatitis. In: Rose BD, editor. Waltham, MA: UpToDateOnline.com, 2008.

17. Shimizu Y. Liver in systemic disease. World J Gastroenterol 2008;14:4115.

18. Solaymani-Dodaran M, Card TR, Aithal GP, et al. Fracture risk in people with primary biliary cirrhosis: A population-based cohort study. Gastroenterology 2006;131:1752–7.

19. Soylu A, Taskale MG, Ciltas A, et al. Intrahepatic cholestasis in subclinical and overt hyperthyroidism: Two case reports. J Med Case Rep 2008;2.116.

20. Vassilopoulou-Sellin R, Ajani J. Neuroendocrine tumors of the pancreas. Endocrinol Metab Clin North Am 1994;23:53.

# RADIOGRAPHY AND RADIOGRAPHIC-FLUOROSCOPIC CONTRAST EXAMINATIONS

*Bernard E. Zeligman, MD*

**CHAPTER 67**

## 1. When requesting an imaging examination, what information should a clinician provide for a radiologist?

By communicating the following information, a clinician helps ensure that an imaging examination will be conducted and interpreted optimally for each patient.

- Known major diagnoses
- Clinical information pertinent to the examination: (a) key findings from history, physical examination, and/or laboratory tests that suggest the diagnoses in question and (b) any surgical alteration of the anatomy to be examined with imaging
- The purpose of the examination: possible diagnoses, possible complications of a procedure, or an established diagnosis or finding to follow for change
- The precise name of the requested examination. Using the following expressions precisely should minimize the possibility that the wrong procedure will be done:
  - *Barium swallow:* an examination for anatomic and functional abnormalities of *swallowing* (oral-pharyngeal and/or esophageal). Examining the esophagus should include checking for a hiatus hernia and for gastric outlet obstruction, two predispositions to gastroesophageal reflux.
  - *Upper GI series:* an examination of the esophagus, stomach, and duodenum. The esophagus is examined less thoroughly than during a barium swallow.
  - *Small bowel follow-through:* an examination, with barium taken orally (or introduced via a tube into the stomach), of the jejunum and ileum.

## ABDOMINAL RADIOGRAPHY

## 2. Which radiographs should constitute an acute abdominal series?

The optimal series, sometimes called a *three-way abdomen*, includes:

1. Posteroanterior (PA) upright chest
2. Supine abdomen
3. Upright abdomen

If limited patient mobility precludes upright positioning, the series should include:

1. Anteroposterior (AP) supine (or semiupright) chest
2. Supine abdomen
3. Left lateral decubitus abdomen

If clinical suspicion of one particular diagnosis, such as acute appendicitis or acute cholecystitis, is strong, the first imaging procedure should be the best one for that condition. Otherwise, the first imaging test for an acute abdomen should be the radiographic acute abdominal series—the *entire* series. An upright abdomen radiograph—which is (on average) less sensitive than either an upright chest or left lateral decubitus abdomen for pneumoperitoneum and is also (on average) less diagnostic than a supine abdomen for bowel obstruction—should *never* be the *only* radiograph for possible perforation or obstruction of the gut. An upright chest radiograph, although the *single* most sensitive for pneumoperitoneum, should *never* be the *only* image for suspected perforation of the gut. If the patient cannot stand, a radiograph of the entire chest should still be part of the series because pneumonia and pulmonary embolism, even if *high* in the chest (and above the field of view of a computed tomography [CT] scan of the abdomen), may present clinically as an acute abdomen (Fig. 67-1).

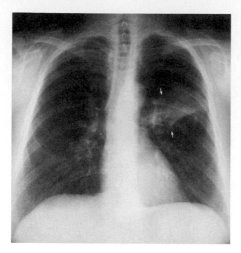

**Figure 67-1.** Pneumonia presenting as an acute abdomen. The abdomen radiographs were normal, but this posteroanterior chest radiograph shows fluffy opacification *(arrows)* in the left *upper* lobe.

### 3. What is the key radiographic finding of bowel obstruction?

The hallmark of obstruction, whether mechanical or functional, is *dilatation* of bowel. If bowel is dilated all the way down to the anorectal junction, the obstruction is functional (unless from anorectal malformation in a newborn). Alternatively, if bowel is dilated not down to the anorectal junction but to a point of transition to normal or smaller than normal caliber, mechanical obstruction (Figs. 67-2 and 67-3) is most likely, but functional obstruction (Fig. 67-4) and bowel ischemia are two alternative possible causes.

Two old axioms—(a) that gas in the lumen of duodenal loop, jejunum, or ileum is abnormal and (b) that gas-fluid levels in any of those locations or in the colon are abnormal—are excessively strict. Gas, with or without fluid levels, can be normal in any part of the intestine.

Abdomen radiographs can be falsely negative for obstruction, even if of high grade.

### 4. What are causes of pneumatosis intestinalis?

The reported causes of pneumotosis (Figs. 67-5 and 67-6*B*, Table 67-1) are numerous, but a logical approach based on pathophysiology will bring the common causes to mind.

1. The gas in the bowel wall came from one of two sites: the lungs or the gut lumen.
2. Gas (or gas-producing bacteria) that entered the wall from the lumen did so by one of two mechanisms: loss of mucosal integrity or increased intraluminal pressure. (Increased pressure probably must tear the mucosa to cause pneumatosis but is a mechanism fundamentally different from loss of mucosal integrity, alone.)
3. For each possible mechanism, think of common etiologies. Because of its urgency, think first of one cause of loss of mucosal integrity: bowel ischemia.

### 5. What distinguishes portal venous gas from pneumobilia?

Although in both conditions gas is in a branching, tapering pattern, the location within the liver of the gas is usually distinctive. Because portal venous blood normally flows toward the periphery, gas in portal veins tends to accumulate in the periphery of the liver (Fig. 67-5). Because bile normally flows toward the hilum, biliary gas tends to be near the

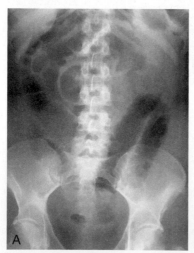

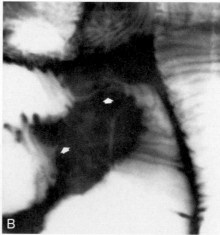

**Figure 67-2.** Mechanical small bowel obstruction. *A*, Supine abdomen radiograph. Because small bowel dilatation does not reach the right lower quadrant, high-grade mechanical obstruction of upper small bowel (above the lower ileum) is likely. *B*, The appropriate fluoroscopic-radiographic examination, a small bowel follow-through, shows partial obstruction of two nearby foci of jejunum *(arrows)* and strongly suggests the cause: an adhesion.

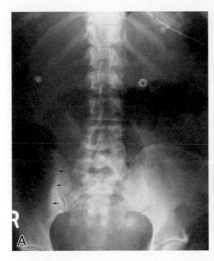
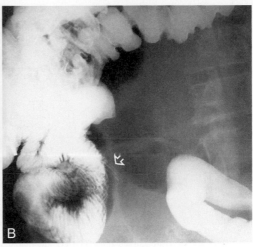

**Figure 67-3.** Mechanical small bowel obstruction. *A*, Supine abdominal radiograph. Because small bowel is dilated in the right lower quadrant *(arrows)* but colon is not dilated, high-grade mechanical obstruction low in the ileum is likely. *B*, The appropriate fluoroscopic-radiographic examination, a single-contrast barium enema, excluded obstruction of the colon, shows complete obstruction to retrograde flow of barium at a tapered narrowing *(arrow)* of ileum, and strongly suggests the cause: an adhesion.

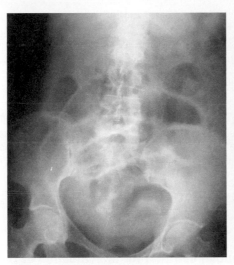
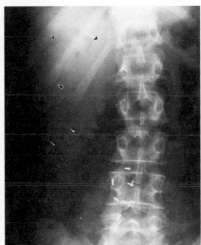

**Figure 67-4.** Portable supine abdomen radiograph. Because dilatation of small bowel does not reach the right lower quadrant, mechanical obstruction of small bowel substantially upstream of the terminal ileum is probable. This obstruction, however, was functional, a result of acute pancreatitis

**Figure 67-5.** Supine abdomen radiograph. These two patterns of pneumatosis intestinalis—linear and bubbly *(arrows)*—are consistent with, but not diagnostic of, bowel ischemia. (A third pattern of pneumotosis, not shown here—cystic in the colon—indicates pneumatosis cystoides coli and is rarely if ever from ischemia.) Other gas in an abnormal location—branching and tapering in the liver *(arrowheads)*—as its predominantly peripheral location favors, is not in bile ducts but in portal veins.

hilum (Fig. 67-6*A*). These rules fail occasionally, however, because at the instant a radiograph is exposed the location of the constantly moving gas may transiently be atypical (Fig. 67-6*B*).

## CONTRAST MEDIA

6. **When is barium preferable to iodinated contrast media to opacify the lumen of the gastrointestinal (GI) tract?**

Barium contrast media, which consist of barium sulfate particles suspended in water, are usually far superior to iodinated contrast because they produce better images, are less costly, and rarely do harm. For examinations for bowel obstruction, barium is the better choice except for two situations in which barium may do harm:

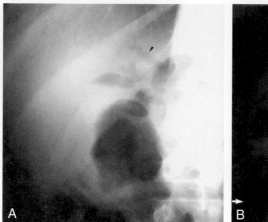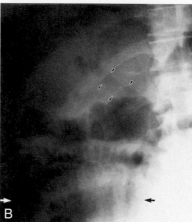

**Figure 67-6.**  A branching and tapering gas pattern in the liver, if predominantly near the hilum *(arrowheads)*, usually is biliary (*A*) but occasionally is in portal veins. *B*, Bubbly and linear pneumatosis *(arrows)* below the liver is consistent with bowel ischemia.

---

**Table 67-1.**  Common Causes of Pneumatosis Intestinalis

| SOURCE OF GAS: LUNGS | | SOURCE OF GAS: GUT LUMEN |
|---|---|---|
| • Barotrauma<br>• COPD<br>• Idiopathic | ***Mechanism:*** Increased intraluminal pressure<br>• Air insufflation (endoscopy)<br>• Bowel obstruction (mechanical or functional) | ***Mechanism:*** Loss of mucosal integrity<br>• Ischemia<br>• Inflammation (infectious or noninfectious)<br>• Drugs (e.g., glucocorticoids) |

---

- Because barium (at least theoretically) upstream of a partial obstruction of the *colon* may become inspissated and then worsen the obstruction, a large volume of barium should be avoided upstream of a mechanical colon obstruction.
- If mechanical small bowel obstruction is both severe and inoperable (a situation usually caused by peritoneal carcinomatosis) or if functional small bowel obstruction is both chronic and severe, barium may remain in small bowel long enough to become inspissated.

Adequate assessment of oral and pharyngeal swallowing dysfunction requires barium. The small volumes of barium that enter the larynx during many of such examinations, and that enter the lungs during a small percentage of them do no harm (even in the occasional cases in which barium is conspicuous on chest radiographs for months afterward).

### 7. What is the role of iodinated (water-soluble) contrast for opacification of the lumen of the GI tract?

The major reason to use iodinated contrast instead of barium is possible intraperitoneal or retroperitoneal perforation of the gut. If extravasated into these spaces, iodinated contrast is safer than barium. Because of its lower contrast resolution, however, iodinated contrast is less likely than barium to show a small or walled-off perforation. If no extravasation of iodinated contrast is evident, examination with barium should follow because the benefit of detecting an otherwise inconspicuous perforation exceeds the possible harm from extravasation of a small volume of barium.

To examine the esophagus for perforation, some physicians begin with barium because extravasation of barium into the mediastinum and pleural cavity has not been proved harmful. Beginning with iodinated contrast and following with barium if no extravasation of iodinated contrast is apparent is preferable, however, because extravasation of a large volume of barium may result in permanent residual barium that could interfere with imaging of the chest thereafter.

### 8. Are some iodinated contrast media better than others?

Iodinated contrast media are either *high osmolality* or *low osmolality*. Because high osmolality contrast, if a substantial volume enters the lungs, may cause potentially fatal pulmonary edema, contrast that will be swallowed or instilled through a tube into the esophagus or stomach should be low osmolality. Contrast introduced through a tube directly into the intestinal lumen, however, can be either low osmolality or a less costly high osmolality medium on the market for intravascular use. For the *distal intestinal obstruction syndrome* of cystic fibrosis, in which copious viscid intraluminal material accumulates in the colon and/or lower ileum, an enema (during fluoroscopic monitoring) of high-osmolality contrast may stimulate evacuation when other methods have failed.

## SWALLOWING STUDIES

**9. What is a barium swallow?**

*Barium swallow* is the general term for a fluoroscopic-radiographic examination of oral, pharyngeal, and/or esophageal swallowing. Each examination should be tailored to the patient.

For symptoms, such as retrosternal dysphagia, that may be of esophageal but not of oral or pharyngeal cause, the examination should be directed to the esophagus.

Other symptoms, such as coughing and choking with swallowing and a sensation that swallowed boluses stick in the throat, suggest abnormalities of oral-pharyngeal swallowing. Possible etiologies include diseases of the central nervous system, cranial nerves, neuromuscular junction (myasthenia gravis), and muscle (dermatomyositis, polymyositis, muscular dystrophy) (see Chapter 1). An examination for such symptoms, however, should include not only oral and pharyngeal swallowing but also the *esophagus* because:

- A sensation that swallowed boluses stick in the throat is often of esophageal cause and referred upward.
- Chronic esophageal disease—achalasia and probably also gastroesophageal reflux disease (GERD)—can cause pharyngeal abnormalities.
- Esophageal abnormalities coexisting with but unrelated to oral-pharyngeal swallowing dysfunction may contribute to the dysphagia and tend to be more amenable to treatment than neurogenic oral-pharyngeal dysfunction.
- Several diseases—Parkinson disease, myotonic dystrophy, and collagen-vascular diseases—can simultaneously impair both oral-pharyngeal and esophageal swallowing.
- Examinations *limited to* oral and pharyngeal swallowing are appropriate to follow known abnormalities and to assess for oral-pharyngeal dysfunction of patients too ill for a complete barium swallow.

**10. What can a barium swallow contribute to an evaluation for dysphagia?**

The many possible causes of dysphagia can be difficult to distinguish by history. In addition, several abnormalities—functional and/or structural—and oral, pharyngeal, and/or esophageal—often coexist. A barium swallow is the only single procedure than can demonstrate both functional and structural abnormalities and that can examine all three phases of swallowing (Fig. 67-7). The first procedure to investigate the cause of dysphagia should be a barium swallow.

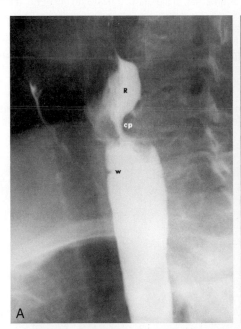
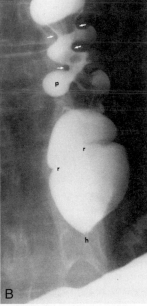

**Figure 67-7.** This man complained that swallowed boluses stuck in his throat, but abnormalities shown by barium swallow were numerous and widespread. **A,** Occasionally, before initiation of oral swallowing, portions of some boluses leaked from mouth to pharynx and were then aspirated. Less than normal pharyngeal muscle contraction (and maybe also partial luminal obstruction from incomplete opening of the cricopharyngeus [cp] contributed to pharyngeal barium residual [R]), which became more apparent as this procedure progressed. A cervical esophageal web (w) is small. **B,** Other abnormalities were spasm *(arrows)* and a pulsion diverticulum (p) low in the esophagus; a sliding hiatus hernia (not completely reducible) between a Schatzki ring (r) and the esophageal hiatus (h); and esophageal barium residual, a result of the spasm and maybe also of weakness and breakup of peristalsis.

## 11. Which esophageal motility disorders are diagnosable by barium swallow?

Of the five primary esophageal motility disorders, three may be diagnosed by barium swallow: achalasia, esophageal spasm, and ineffective esophageal motility. In achalasia, peristalsis in the pure smooth muscle part (the most inferior 60%) of the esophagus is absent, and there is a lower esophageal *beak*. Although a barium swallow, like manometry, may be falsely negative for spasm because spasm may be intermittent and therefore absent during the procedure, nonperistaltic contractions obliterating or nearly obliterating the lumen during at least 20% of swallows indicate spasm. Nonperistaltic contractions that do not obliterate or nearly obliterate the lumen, however, are insignificant. Esophageal residuals resulting from breakup or weakness of peristalsis in the pure smooth muscle part of the esophagus during at least 50% of swallows indicate ineffective esophageal motility if no other possible condition, such as diabetic autonomic neuropathy or scleroderma, may be present.

The two primary motility disorders that cannot be diagnosed by barium swallows are "nutcracker esophagus" and hypertensive lower esophageal sphincter (LES). In those cases of hypertensive LES in which spasm above the LES accompanies the high resting LES pressure, a radiologic diagnosis of spasm would be made instead of hypertensive LES with accompanying spasm.

## 12. What may a barium swallow contribute to diagnosis and management of GERD?

A barium swallow is the best examination for the common predisposing condition (hiatus hernia) and for a less common predisposing condition (mechanical gastric outlet obstruction) and may suggest another uncommon predisposing condition (gastric hypomotility). Free gastroesophageal reflux of barium is diagnostic of, but uncommon in, GERD. Minimal reflux of barium is not definitely abnormal, and absence of reflux during the short period of observation provided by a barium swallow is meaningless. A barium swallow may demonstrate esophagitis or Barrett's esophagus but can exclude neither.

A barium swallow, therefore, should not be requested to establish or exclude the diagnosis of GERD but may contribute useful information in the setting of GERD:

1. *Dysphagia.* The cause of the dysphagia may be unrelated to the GERD. If related to the GERD, the cause may be morphologic and/or functional—and, for dysphagia perceived in the throat, the cause may be esophageal and/or pharyngeal. As is true for dysphagia in general, the best first test is a barium swallow.
2. *Assessment for surgery.* (a) Assessment of barium transport by the esophagus is one way to assess for ineffective esophageal motility, which is common in GERD and may predispose, especially if severe, to dysphagia after a fundoplication. (b) The presence or absence of a hiatus hernia and its size when maximally reduced can help a surgeon choose the appropriate operation and estimate the complexity of, and time needed for, the operation.
3. *Postoperative symptoms.* A barium swallow can show such causes of symptoms as excessive esophageal narrowing by a fundoplication, disruption of or *slip* of a fundoplication, and a hiatus hernia (sliding and/or paraesophageal).

## 13. How can a barium swallow distinguish achalasia from scleroderma?

If the condition results in dysmotility that is at least moderately severe, barium swallow abnormalities are usually different in these two conditions (Fig. 67-8, Table 67-2).

## 14. What findings help distinguish achalasia secondary to cancer from primary achalasia?

If achalasia is secondary to cancer, the beak, the narrowing at the LES, may be irregular, eccentric, and/or abruptly marginated. Two other characteristics, however, are more sensitive for secondary achalasia:

- A relatively long length, longer than 3.5 cm, of the beak
- Relatively minimal dilatation, to a caliber less than 4.0 cm, above the beak.

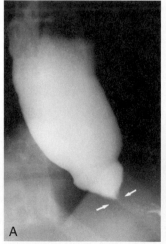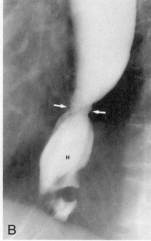

**Figure 67-8.** Lower esophagus. *A,* Achalasia. Dilatation is marked above a "beak" *(arrows)* formed by the closed lower sphincter. *B,* Scleroderma. Dilatation is moderate above a cylindrical reflux esophagitis stricture *(arrows),* below which is a sliding hiatus hernia (H).

**Table 67-2.** Achalasia Versus Scleroderma

| | ESOPHAGEAL DILATATION | PERISTALSIS IN PURE SMOOTH MUSCLE PART OF ESOPHAGUS | ESOPHAGOGASTRIC JUNCTION |
|---|---|---|---|
| Achalasia | May be marked | Absent | Beak: smooth, concentric, tapered, flexible<br>No hiatus hernia |
| Scleroderma | Minimal or moderate | Weak, incomplete, or absent | Stricture from esophagitis: cylindrical, rigid, sometimes irregular and/or ulcerated<br>Often a sliding hiatus hernia |

## UPPER GASTROINTESTINAL SERIES

### 15. Can benign and malignant gastric ulcers be distinguished?

Imaging features—shown best with biphasic technique, which consists of both a double-contrast and a single-contrast phase—allow an estimate of the likelihood of malignancy. A malignant or possibly malignant appearance warrants endoscopy and biopsy. For unequivocally benign radiographic features, radiologic follow-up is a less costly and adequate alternative. If, on follow-up, healing is complete and features of any scar that has developed are unequivocally benign, further assessment for malignancy is unnecessary. If healing is only partial but the appearance remains benign, a second follow-up upper GI series is sufficient. If features of or equivocal for malignancy develop during follow-up or if healing fails despite adequate medical therapy, endoscopy and biopsy are indicated (Table 67-3).

**Table 67-3.** Gastric Ulcers on Upper Gastrointestinal Series: Benign and Malignant Features

| FINDINGS | BENIGN | MALIGNANT |
|---|---|---|
| Location in stomach | Other than upstream half of stomach along greater curvature | Upstream half of stomach along greater curvature |
| Profile view: Relationship of ulcer to lumen | Beyond expected lumen | Within expected lumen |
| Radiating folds | Regular<br>To margin of ulcer or to ulcer mound (of edema) | Nodular, irregular, fused, clubbed, amputated, or nodular<br>May not reach ulcer margin |
| *If* ulcer is within a mass | Ulcer location in mass: central<br>Mass: smooth<br>Junction with wall: obtuse angle | Ulcer location in mass: eccentric<br>Mass: Irregular<br>Junction with wall: acute angle |
| Surrounding mucosa | Intact | Distorted or obliterated |
| Ulcer shape | Round, oval, or linear | Angular |
| Other | Hampton line | |
| Healing | Complete | Usually incomplete<br>Occasionally complete, but scar:<br>Is nodular<br>Radiating folds with malignant characteristics |

## SMALL BOWEL

### 16. What are advantages and disadvantages of, and indications for, enteroclysis (small bowel enema)?

#### ADVANTAGES

Enteroclysis, for two reasons, provides more anatomic detail than does a follow-through:

- Barium can be introduced into the bowel lumen at whatever rate distends the bowel optimally.
- Double-contrast examination of the jejunum and the upper ileum is possible by instilling air or methylcellulose through the tube immediately after barium instillation. (Double-contrast examination of the lower ileum—a technique called *peroral pneumocolon* because air is introduced per rectum—may accompany either a follow-through or enteroclysis.)

### DISADVANTAGES

- Greater cost
- More patient discomfort
- Greater radiation exposure
- Nonphysiologic examination

### INDICATIONS

Opinions vary, but the following guidelines are commonly followed. A follow-through is the routine examination. Enteroclysis is reserved for situations in which the superior demonstration of anatomy is especially advantageous:

- Suspected mechanical obstruction of *low* grade
- Gastrointestinal bleeding unexplained by examination of the upper GI tract and colon

To investigate bleeding, three techniques—enteroclysis, push enteroscopy, and capsule endoscopy—are complementary. Enteroclysis, unlike enteroscopy and capsule endoscopy, cannot show flat vascular lesions. Capsule endoscopy may miss a small lesion that push enteroscopy and enteroclysis may show.

**17. When information from imaging, beyond that provided by radiographs, is indicated for suspected small bowel obstruction, which fluoroscopic-radiographic contrast examination is best?**

For low-grade obstruction, enteroclysis is more likely than a follow-through to distend the bowel adequately to show a minimal narrowing. For high-grade (see Fig. 67-2), however, a follow-through is more likely than enteroclysis to be diagnostic (unless luminal decompression by a long tube precedes enteroclysis) (Table 67-4).

**Table 67-4.** Choice of Fluoroscopic-Radiographic Examination for Suspected Small Bowel Obstruction

| SETTING | SUSPECTED OBSTRUCTION | BEST EXAMINATION |
|---|---|---|
| Illness too mild for hospitalization *and* any abdomen radiographs taken do not show dilated small bowel | Low-grade | Enteroclysis |
| Radiographs show dilated small bowel, but not as far down as right lower quadrant | High-grade<br>Above lower ileum | Small bowel follow-through |
| Radiographs show dilated small bowel, including in right lower quadrant | High-grade<br>Near terminal ileum | Barium enema: single contrast, no preparation |
| Illness characteristic of high-grade obstruction, but radiographs show no small bowel dilatation | High-grade<br>Anywhere | Small bowel follow-through |

For suspected obstruction of or near the terminal ileum, a single-contrast barium enema is best for two reasons:

- The radiographic bowel gas pattern characteristic of obstruction low in the ileum is sometimes caused by obstruction of the colon—a diagnosis obvious on barium enema.
- Barium introduced per rectum often will flow across the ileocolic junction and show an obstruction low in the ileum (see Fig. 67-3) and, if so, will establish the diagnosis much faster than will barium taken orally.

**18. When is CT preferable to a fluoroscopic-radiographic contrast study for small bowel obstruction?**

The most important question the examination is to answer should determine the choice. CT is better for hernias, can show more abdominal abnormalities outside the gut, and, unlike fluoroscopic-radiographic studies, can show if the obstruction may be strangulated. Fluoroscopic-radiographic examinations show more conclusively the presence or absence of, and severity of, mechanical obstruction. If which type of procedure to choose is unclear, CT is the better choice because a CT scan will delay a subsequent fluoroscopic examination less than a fluoroscopic procedure will delay a subsequent CT scan.

**19. When is a retrograde examination of small bowel indicated?**

Although a single-contrast barium enema for suspected obstruction low in the ileum may be considered a limited retrograde small bowel study, this question refers to an examination of the entire small bowel by retrograde instillation of barium, a procedure that is feasible if barium is introduced through an ileostomy. This examination is faster than either enteroclysis or a follow-through and shows anatomy as well as single-contrast enteroclysis—with less cost, less radiation exposure, and less discomfort. If an ileostomy is present, a small bowel examination should be done retrograde unless the suspected abnormality is in the duodenum or upper jejunum.

## COLON AND RECTUM

**20. What are indications for single-contrast and double-contrast techniques of barium enema examination?**

- *Single contrast:* for obstruction or for fistula or sinus track
- *Double contrast:* for polyps, cancer, or colitis

Single-contrast technique, which requires less patient mobility than does double contrast, is necessary regardless of the purpose of the examination if mobility is inadequate for double contrast.

Detection of incidental adenomas and carcinomas during barium enemas undertaken for other purposes presumably prevents some deaths from colon cancer. Because, in the general population, adenomas are prevalent among those 40 years of age and older, double contrast is preferable in that age group unless there is a special indication for single contrast.

**21. What are advantages and disadvantages of screening for colon cancer with a barium enema instead of colonoscopy?**

### ADVANTAGES

- Lower cost
- Greater safety
- Greater likelihood the entire colon will be examined

### DISADVANTAGES

- Lower sensitivity for polyps (especially diminutive ones)
- Some false positive interpretations (because of adherent stool) for polyps
- A positive (true or false) result requires a second procedure: endoscopy for polypectomy or biopsy.

**22. What is the role of defecography (evacuation proctography)?**

Symptoms of are of limited value in distinguishing constipation caused by slow colonic transit from that caused by anorectal dysfunction or both. Defecography may clarify the cause and help direct therapy if there is anorectal dysfunction (Fig. 67-9). For this procedure, barium contrast of paste consistency is introduced through the anal canal into the rectum. Barium is also usually given orally and introduced vaginally (most patients are female) so that the location of the ileum and vagina will be apparent. Rectal evacuation that is slower or less complete than normal, without some other evident cause, indicates probable dyssynergic defecation, which may respond to biofeedback. Defecography may also show one or more of the following—rectocele, rectal intussusception (rectorectal or intra-anal), external rectal prolapse, enterocele, sigmoidocele, peritoneocele, and excessive descent of the posterior part of the pelvic floor or of the perineum—which are often complications of dyssynergic defecation, some of which may be inapparent on physical examination, and which may warrant surgical correction. Optimal diagnosis and management require correlation of defecography findings with history, physical examination, nonimaging tests of anorectal function, and often endoanal ultrasound.

## CHOLANGIOPANCREATOGRAPHY

**23. What cholangiopancreatographic features distinguish pancreatitis from ductal adenocarcinoma of the pancreatic head?**

The details of the abnormalities of both ductal systems (Figs. 67-10 and 67-11) are clues to this distinction (Table 67-5).

**24. What is the double duct sign of cholangiopancreatography?**

A stricture or complete obstruction of the intrapancreatic common bile duct and another stricture or complete obstruction of the main pancreatic duct nearby (Fig. 67-12) constitute the double duct sign. The most common malignant cause is ductal adenocarcinoma of the pancreatic head; cholangiocarcinoma, lymphoma, and metastasis are occasional causes. The benign cause is chronic pancreatitis.

A different double duct sign—dilatation of the biliary tract and of the pancreatic duct—is sometimes used during interpretation of CT scans but is less predictive of a lesion in the pancreatic head, or of any particular diagnoses, than is the double duct sign of cholangiopancreatography.

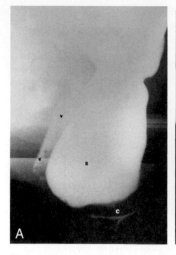
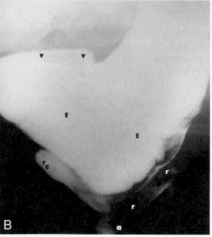
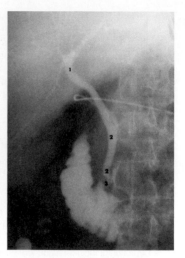

**Figure 67-9.** Lateral views from a defecogram of a woman who complained of difficult and incomplete rectal evacuation. *A,* The appearance before evacuation was normal. Barium paste opacifies the rectum (R) and anal canal (C). A contrast-impregnated tampon (we now use thick liquid barium instead of a tampon) indicates the location of the vagina (v). *B,* Evacuation was slow and incomplete. Intussuscepting rectal tissue (radiolucency demarcated anteriorly and posteriorly by linear barium) has descended into and now obstructs the lower rectum (r) and anal canal (a). A rectocele (rc) retains rectal contents. An enterocele (E) is very large: numerous loops of ileum, opacified by barium taken orally earlier, have descended into the pelvis between the rectum and vagina (v) and widely separate them.

**Figure 67-10.** Common sites of extrahepatic biliary obstruction are indicated on this operative cholangiogram. (1) Hepatic duct confluence. (2) Intrapancreatic portion of common bile duct. (3) Intraduodenal portion of common bile duct (and/or common channel of individuals whose common bile and pancreatic ducts fuse before reaching the duodenal lumen).

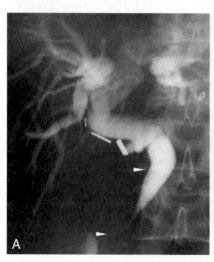
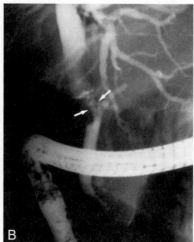

**Figure 67-11.** Strictures of intrapancreatic common bile duct. *A,* Percutaneous transhepatic cholangiogram. This stricture *(arrowheads),* with all the characteristics of benignity, is caused by pancreatitis. *B,* Endoscopic retrograde cholangiogram (ERC). This stricture *(arrows),* with all the characteristics of malignancy, is from ductal adenocarcinoma of the pancreatic head.

**Table 67-5.** Pancreatitis Versus Cancer of the Pancreatic Head: Cholangiopancreatographic Features

|  | **PANCREATITIS** | **CARCINOMA** |
| --- | --- | --- |
| Pancreatogram | If chronic: widespread ductal abnormalities: dilatations, strictures, and/or calcifications | Focal abnormality of main duct in pancreatic head (obstruction, stricture, or disruption) |
| Cholangiogram (stricture of intrapancreatic common bile duct) | Smooth<br>Tapered<br>Concentric<br>Of entire intrapancreatic portion | Irregular<br>Abrupt margins<br>Eccentric<br>Only of part of the intrapancreatic portion (usually) |

## 25. What pancreatographic features distinguish pancreas divisum from complete obstruction of the main pancreatic duct?

Although the main duct opacified via the major papilla is shorter than normal in both conditions, their pancreatographic appearances are usually distinctive.

- With obstruction (Fig. 67-12), the main duct appears *truncated*. Caliber of the opacified part of main duct and its branches is normal, and upstream termination of the main duct is abrupt. (Two other conditions—traumatic disruption of the main duct and excision of the pancreatic tail and body—can have this same appearance.)
- In divisum (Fig. 67-13), the ductal system appears *minified*. Caliber of the main duct and its branches is small, and the main duct terminates upstream not abruptly but by branching and tapering.

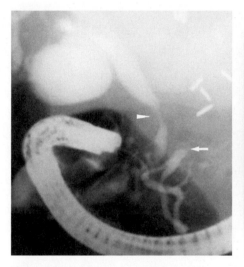
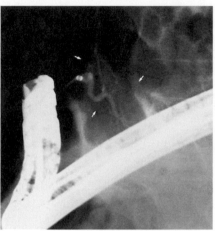

**Figure 67-12.**  Double duct sign. The stricture (*arrowhead*) of the intrapancreatic common bile duct, though smooth and predominantly tapered, is probably malignant because it is short and eccentric. Nearby is a complete obstruction (*arrow*) of the pancreatic duct. No abnormalities of chronic pancreatitis involve the *truncated* opacified part of the pancreatic duct. Diagnosis: ductal adenocarcinoma of the pancreatic head.

**Figure 67-13.**  Pancreas divisum. This short pancreatic ductal system (*arrows*), opacified via the major papilla, is *minified*.

## OTHER

## 26. What are advantages of fistulography?

For a suspected fistula between skin and gut lumen, a fistulagram is usually the most informative imaging examination. A fistulagram not only usually provides adequate assessment for obstruction of the gut downstream of a fistula but, compared to barium studies of the gut:

- Is more likely to show a fistula
- Demonstrates anatomy of a track more completely, and the site of the gut in continuity with the track more precisely
- Does not delay percutaneous therapy. Immediately after diagnostic fistulography, a catheter may be introduced for drainage or injection of fibrin sealant

## WEBSITES

http://radiology.duke.edu/modules/dept_rad_msedu/index.php?id=6

http://www.radrounds.com/

http://www.vhjoe.com

## BIBLIOGRAPHY

1. Levine MS, Creteur V, Kresel HY. Benign gastric ulcers: Diagnosis and follow-up with double-contrast radiography. Radiology 1987;164:9.
2. Levine MS, Glick SN, Rubesin SE, et al. Double-contrast barium enema examination and colorectal cancer: A plea for radiologic screening. Radiology 2002;222:313–5.
3. McMahon PM, Bosch JL, Gleason S, et al. Cost-effectiveness of colorectal cancer screening. Radiology 2001;219:44–50.
4. Woodfield CA, Levine MS, Rubesin SE, et al. Diagnosis of primary versus secondary achalasia: Reassessment of clinical and radiographic criteria. Am J Roentgenol AJR 2000;175:727–31.

# INTERVENTIONAL RADIOLOGY: CROSS-SECTIONAL IMAGING PROCEDURES

Kimi L. Kondo, DO, Paul D. Russ, MD, and
Stephen W. Subber, MD

### 1. What common percutaneous procedures are performed using cross-sectional imaging guidance?

The two basic procedures performed in abdominal imaging are biopsies of masses and drainage of fluid collections. Masses and fluid collections of the solid organs, peritoneum, retroperitoneum, vertebrae, psoas, and paraspinous muscles are usually accessible.

*Biopsies* can be categorized as fine-needle aspiration (FNA), which yields clusters of cells and occasionally small tissue fragments for cytopathology, or core biopsy, which yields cylinders of tissue, 1 to 2 cm long, with preserved architecture for histopathologic analysis.

*Fluid collections* can be needled for Gram stain and culture and aspirated for diagnosis and/or therapeutic decompression. They can be drained with percutaneous catheters for cure or for temporization and medical stabilization before surgery. Some cystic lesions and collections are catheterized for purposes of drainage and subsequent treatment (e.g., sclerotherapy)

### 2. What materials and equipment are used for FNAs, core biopsies, and percutaneous catheter drainages?

- Most *FNAs* are performed using 21- to 23-gauge *skinny* needles; 20-gauge needles are of intermediate size and should be avoided in cases involving the bowel, bile ducts or large vessels.
- *Core biopsies* usually are obtained with 18-gauge disposable, spring-loaded, automated guns. For most focal pathology, 18-gauge specimens are as diagnostic as those obtained with 14- to 16-gauge devices and there is a decreased risk of bleeding complications. In most cases, better samples are obtained with 18-gauge than 20-gauge guns. Needle size and number of specimens needed for pathologic diagnosis often vary by institution and are dependent on the experience and expertise of the pathology department. Evaluation for adequacy of the FNA or *touch prep* of the core biopsy by the cytopathologist during the procedure significantly reduces the need for repeat biopsies due to *inadequate sample*.
- The vast majority of *fluid collections* can be drained and treated with 8- to 14-Fr self-retaining, pigtail catheters. Except for some percutaneous gallbladder and ascitic fluid drainages, catheters smaller than 8-Fr offer no advantages, are often more difficult to place, and are dislodged more frequently. The size of the catheter used is often operator dependent. The viscosity of the fluid to be drained, the size of the collection, and location of the puncture site (e.g., intercostal, subphrenic, transgluteal) are factors to consider when choosing a catheter size. Smaller catheters tend to kink easier and are more prone to clogging of the side holes.

### 3. What are the indications for percutaneous image-guided biopsy?

1. Establish a malignant diagnosis (either primary or metastatic).
2. Establish a benign diagnosis.
3. Obtain material for culture or other laboratory studies.

### 4. What four conditions must be satisfied before a percutaneous procedure can be performed?

1. The patient or patient representative must provide written informed consent for both the procedure and anticipated intravenous conscious sedation.
2. The referring physician must order antibiotic coverage if there is any possibility that the lesion or fluid collection is infected.
3. The patient's coagulation profile must be determined.
4. The patient must be voluntarily cooperative during the procedure.

### 5. What coagulation parameters are assessed before a percutaneous procedure?

The patient history should be reviewed for bleeding risks, such as anticoagulant (warfarin [Coumadin], low-molecular-weight heparin) or platelet-inhibitor agents (aspirin, clopidogrel [Plavix]), uremia, or hepatocellular disease.

At a minimum, prothrombin time (PT), international normalized ratio (INR), partial thromboplastin time (PTT), and platelet count should be assessed in all patients, regardless of the procedure. An INR greater than 2.0, a PTT greater than 1.5 times normal, or a platelet count less than 50,000/μL are each a relative contraindication for most procedures. However, after the discontinuation or reversal of anticoagulants, administration of fresh frozen plasma, and/or platelet transfusion, many coagulopathies can be corrected temporarily to allow for intervention.

**6. Which imaging modalities are used to guide interventional procedures?**

Fluoroscopy, ultrasound (US), computed tomography (CT), and magnetic resonance imaging (MRI) can be used to guide interventions. US and CT are used most often (Fig. 68-1).

**7. Summarize the advantages and disadvantages of US.**

### ADVANTAGES

- Widely available and portable
- Allows relatively easy scanning in nonorthogonal planes
- Imaging and needle passage can be viewed in real time
- No ionizing radiation
- Low cost
- Vasculature can be readily identified using color and power Doppler

### DISADVANTAGES

- Inadequate visualization of the target lesion. This can be due to patient body habitus, obscuration of the target lesion by overlying bowel gas, air, or bone or deep lesion location.
- Inadequate visualization of the needle. Use of US guidance is operator dependent and visualization requires the needle to be in the scan plane of the transducer. Needle guides and needles with tips enhanced for US use are commercially available and may be helpful.

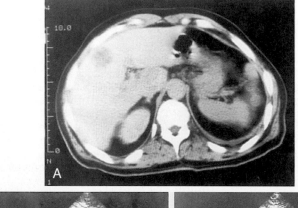

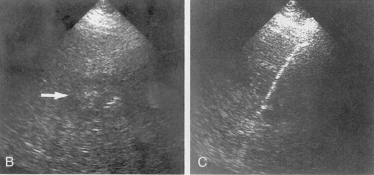

**Figure 68-1.** Metastatic colon cancer to the liver. **A,** Contrast-enhanced computed tomography scan of the liver demonstrates a 3-cm hypodense mass. **B,** Ultrasound of the liver reveals the mass to be primarily hypoechoic (*arrow*). **C,** The needle tract is conspicuously demonstrated during ultrasound-guided biopsy.

## 8. Summarize the advantages and disadvantages of CT (Fig. 68-2).

### ADVANTAGES

- Ability to image areas difficult to visualize with US (lung, bone, areas of the abdomen obscured by bowel gas)
- Ability to visualize deep targets

### DISADVANTAGES

- Not portable
- Needle passage cannot be viewed in real time unless CT fluoroscopy is available. Additionally, in units with CT fluoroscopy capability, several images must be acquired after each needle/wire manipulation for visualization, which can result in prolonged procedure times.
- Angled approaches not in the axial plane can be difficult.
- Ionizing radiation and potential for significant radiation exposure especially with CT fluoroscopy

## 9. Summarize the advantages and disadvantages of conventional fluoroscopy.

### ADVANTAGES

- Widely available
- Needle passage viewed in real time
- Low cost

### DISADVANTAGES

- Ionizing radiation
- Single-dimension imaging unless using a C-arm, which allows imaging in multiple projections without having to move the patient
- Unable to adequately visualize structures between the skin surface and the target

Fluoroscopy is often used in combination with US guidance for placement of drainage catheters. The needle is placed using US guidance and wire passage and catheter placement are performed using fluoroscopy for real-time visualization and precise positioning. Fluoroscopy is also used for sinograms and abscessograms. Fluoroscopy is recommended by many authors during hepatic and renal cyst sclerotherapy to check for communication with the biliary tree and urinary tract, respectively.

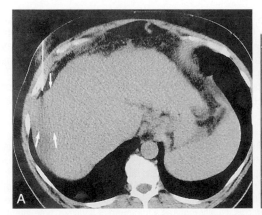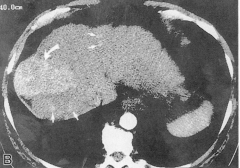

**Figure 68-2.** Biopsy of a hepatic mass in a 54-year-old man with end-stage alcoholic cirrhosis. *A,* Noncontrast computed tomography (CT) scan performed during percutaneous biopsy of a large, solid liver lesion shows an isodense lobulation (*arrows*) of the right lobe corresponding to a tumor better demonstrated by previous dynamic CT scan. Two 21-gauge FNAs and two 18-gauge core biopsies of the lesion confirmed hepatocellular carcinoma. CT guidance allowed a tract to be selected that avoided aerated lung; thus, a pneumothorax was avoided. *B,* After chemoembolization, the stained carcinoma is more conspicuously shown with CT (*curved arrow*). Small satellite foci are also depicted (*small, straight arrows*).

**10. Summarize the advantages and disadvantages of MRI.**

### ADVANTAGES

- Multidimensional imaging
- No ionizing radiation
- Better soft tissue contrast resolution than CT. MRI may be the only modality that depicts the lesion.
- Heat-sensitive pulse sequences provide unique information during thermal ablations.

### DISADVANTAGES

- Less widely available
- Requires use of MR-compatible monitoring equipment and devices, which are not widely available
- Contraindicated in patients with pacemakers, implanted cardiac defibrillators, and cochlear implants
- Longer imaging time
- Image artifacts

**11. What two techniques can be used to drain fluid collections?**
- With the *Seldinger technique*, a drainage catheter is placed over a guidewire after needle puncture and tract dilatation.
- With the trocar technique, the fluid collection is punctured directly with the catheter mounted on a removable sharp-tipped trocar.

**12. Which technique is used more often?**
The Seldinger technique is used more often, because it starts with a smaller needle, and because catheter insertion over a guidewire is more controlled. The trocar technique is a faster, one-step procedure, but some control and access may be lost during catheter insertion compared with the Seldinger method. The trocar technique usually is reserved for large, superficial fluid collections or for draining a large volume of ascites.

**13. What pharmacologic agents can be injected into septated or viscous abdominal fluid collections to improve drainage?**
Intracavitary fibrinolysis therapy with either urokinase or tissue plasminogen activator (tPA) can be performed through the drainage catheters to shorten treatment time and improve the clinical course of patients treated with percutaneous drainage catheters. tPA is probably more commonly used today than urokinase. Optimal dosing regimens have not been determined. Typical doses of tPA range from 2 to 10 mg of tPA diluted in 25 to 50 mL saline. The total volume of fluid depends on the size of the cavity. The dose is injected into the catheter, which is clamped for 1 hour after the dose is administered. After unclamping, the dose is allowed to drain spontaneously. The dose can be administered 1 or 2 times daily. Total number of doses varies depending on output response. Typical doses of urokinase range between 12,500 and 150,000 units. With both agents, caution should be used with hepatic abscesses or in patients who are coagulopathic.

**14. What should you suspect if the drainage catheter has persistently elevated outputs?**
If a catheter has persistently elevated outputs, a sudden increase in drainage, or a change in the composition of the effluent, a fistula should be suspected. Injection of contrast into the catheter under fluoroscopy often demonstrates the fistula, which can be to the gastrointestinal tract, pancreatic duct, biliary system, or to the genitourinary tract. Occasionally, an alternative study is necessary such as a small bowel follow-through (SBFT) if the fistula acts as a one-way valve and is not demonstrated by injection of the drainage catheter. Often the fistula will heal but prolonged drainage is required and can last as long as 2 to 4 weeks or more. The catheter should not be removed until the fistula has healed or has been repaired.

**15. When should you remove the drainage catheter?**
If the catheter output is less than 10 to 20 mL per 24 hours, there are no other reasons for the decreased outputs (e.g., catheter clogged, kinked, or malpositioned), and the patient has clinically improved, the catheter can be removed. Repeat imaging with US, CT, or contrast injection under fluoroscopy is not necessary unless the patient has a known fistula or is still clinically symptomatic or the overall output is less than expected. An exception to these criteria for catheter removal is percutaneous cholecystostomy catheters. Percutaneous cholecystostomy catheters require an epithelialized tract to form before removal to prevent bile leakage and bile peritonitis. This usually requires a minimum of 3 weeks' time, but if the patient is immunocompromised or in the intensive care unit, the process can take even longer.

**16. What are the major complications of percutaneous procedures?**
The major complications of percutaneous procedures are hemorrhage, infection, sepsis, solid organ injury, bowel perforation, and pneumothorax. The complication rate of skinny needle interventions is about 0.06% to 0.6%. The complication rate of catheter drainage is 3% to 4%. The increased risk of large needle procedures compared with

skinny needle procedures is the subject of some debate. However, it seems intuitive that the smallest adequate needle or catheter should be used for every procedure.

**17. How common is seeding of the needle tract during routine tumor biopsy?**

Seeding the needle tract is rare with skinny needle FNAs and 18-gauge core biopsies. A few cases of needle tract seeding have been reported for biopsy of solid, neoplastic masses of the abdomen and retroperitoneum. Although this potential complication should be discussed with the patient prior to the procedure, it should not be considered a contraindication to FNA or core biopsy.

However, cystic lesions like suspected cystadenomas or cystadenocarcinomas of the ovary or pancreas should not be sampled percutaneously, even with small, skinny needles. This is associated with a significant risk of postprocedure needle-tract seeding and subsequent pseudomyxoma peritonei or peritoneal carcinomatosis.

Of note, *percutaneous thermal ablation* (radiofrequency [RF], microwave, laser) of hepatocellular carcinoma (HCC) and hepatic colorectal cancer metastases, which uses probes as large as 14 gauge, is currently associated with tumor seeding of the tract in about 2% to 3% of patients.

## HEPATIC INTERVENTIONS

**18. What image-guided procedures are performed in the liver?**

Cross-sectional imaging is used to perform:

- FNAs and core biopsies of primary and metastatic tumors
- Catheter drainage of abscesses and other fluid collections
- Sclerotherapy of simple hepatic cysts
- Percutaneous thermal and chemical ablation of liver tumors

**19. How is hepatic metastatic disease diagnosed?**

FNA is a simple and quick way to diagnose hepatic metastatic disease. Because of the marked difference between metastatic neoplastic cells and background hepatocytes, cytology alone is frequently diagnostic and core biopsies unnecessary. In difficult cases, comparison with previously obtained specimens of the primary tumor can help to establish the diagnosis.

**20. How is malignant, primary hepatic neoplasm diagnosed?**

Primary hepatic neoplasm can be diagnosed with FNA alone, depending on the tumor cytomorphology and the experience of the cytopathologist. However, because many primary hepatic tumors require histologic evaluation, core biopsies are often needed (Fig. 68-2). With current biopsy gun technology, 18-gauge cores are recommended. Core biopsy of background liver is helpful to the pathologist in cases of well-differentiated neoplasm and assists the hepatologist to choose among treatment options by detecting the presence and severity of underlying hepatocellular disease.

**21. How are pyogenic hepatic or parahepatic abscesses treated?**

At least 90% of pyogenic hepatic or parahepatic abscesses can be successfully drained percutaneously. Almost all pyogenic abscesses can be drained with an 8- to 14-Fr, self-retaining, pigtail catheter. After needle puncture, caution should be exercised during wire placement, dilatation, and catheter insertion; frequent imaging is necessary to ensure that the drainage devices have not migrated beyond the soft margin of the abscess, which can result in significant complications. It should be noted that early (1 to 14 days), postprocedure CTs can result in the underestimation of the therapeutic effectiveness of percutaneous hepatic abscess drainage. Evidence for resolution of the hepatic abscess at early follow-up CT often lags behind the clinical improvement of the patient. The decision to alter patient management or to re-intervene should not be based on the imaging alone.

Although rare, the possibility of an abscess complicating an underlying hepatic neoplasm should always be considered. Material for cytology should always be sent at the initial aspiration of an hepatic abscess. Follow-up CT scans at 3, 6, and 12 months should always be obtained to document eventual complete resolution of the lesion. Consideration should be given for FNA or core biopsy of any persistent abnormality to exclude occult hepatic tumor.

**22. Describe the treatment of simple, benign, epithelialized hepatic cysts**

Epithelialized hepatic cysts can be drained successfully and obliterated with alcohol sclerotherapy. A self-retaining, pigtail catheter can be used. After catheter placement with US or CT guidance, and complete cyst aspiration, samples

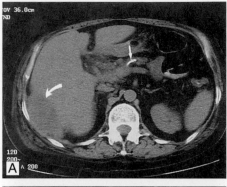

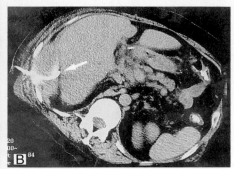

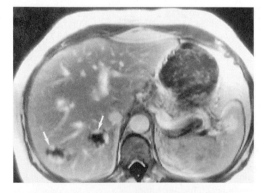

**Figure 68-3.** Parahepatic abscess in a 60-year-old woman, at first diagnosed with acute pancreatitis. **A,** After she failed to respond to initial management, including pancreatic duct stenting (*straight arrow*), computed tomography scan revealed a fluid collection (*curved arrow*) adjacent to the liver. **B,** An 8-Fr pigtail catheter successfully drained the *Streptococcus milleri* abscess (*straight arrow*). **C,** A hepatic flexure mass (*curved arrow*) was suspected to be the site of origin of the parahepatic abscess.

are sent for culture and cytology. Subsequently, water-soluble contrast is injected through the catheter under fluoroscopic guidance to ensure that there is no communication with the biliary tree. If no connection to the bile ducts is demonstrated, then 33% to 50% of the original cyst volume is replaced with sterile, absolute alcohol (not to exceed 100 mL). The patient is rotated into multiple positions until the entirety of the cyst wall has been in contact with the sclerosing agent for 20 to 30 minutes. The entire volume of alcohol and residual cyst contents are then completely aspirated through the catheter. Large cysts may require repeat treatments. After the final treatment and aspiration, the catheter is removed.

Solitary hepatic cysts are more often successfully sclerosed than cysts in patients with polycystic liver disease. In polycystic liver disease, cysts tend not to collapse, presumably because the surrounding liver is less pliable, making cyst wall apposition and subsequent scarring of the cavity less likely (Fig. 68-3). In cases of polycystic liver disease, laparoscopic unroofing or surgical removal of multiple, symptomatic cysts is replacing alcohol sclerotherapy.

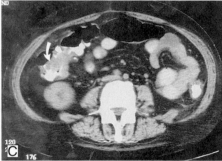

**Figure 68-4.** Dynamic, gadolinium-enhanced. T1-weighted magnetic resonance (MR) scan of the liver shows two lesions (*arrows*) with perfusion patterns characteristic of hemangiomas. Their distinctive MR features allow conservative management with surveillance imaging, obviating biopsy. Incidental note is made of a nonspecific hyperintensity in the spleen.

### 23. Is FNA or core biopsy safe for all hepatic lesions?

FNA or core biopsy of some hepatic lesions is contraindicated. Carcinoid crisis characterized by profound hypotension can be precipitated by FNA of hepatic carcinoid metastases. Hepatic hemangiomas should not be intentionally needled or biopsied. Because of the ability to characterize most hemangiomas noninvasively with cross-sectional imaging, obtaining specimens for cytology or histology is unnecessary in the management of most patients with typical hemangiomas (Fig. 68-4). Amebic abscesses respond well to medical treatment with metronidazole and usually do not require catheter drainage. However, indications for aspiration or drainage of amebic abscesses include imminent rupture, bacterial superinfection, or failure of medical treatment (Fig. 68-5). In the United States, percutaneous aspiration and drainage of a suspected echinococcal lesion should not be performed; other options should be considered.

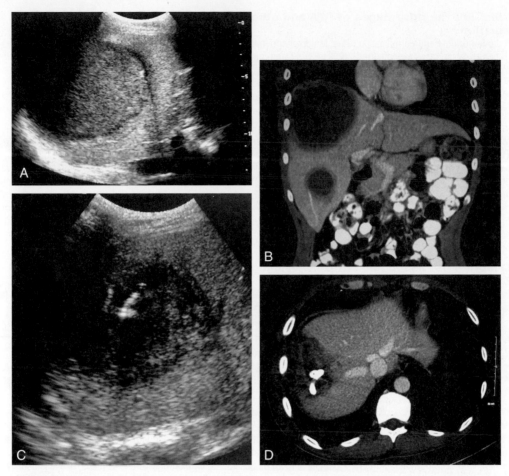

**Figure 68-5.** Percutaneous drainage of an amebic abscess in a 43-year-old Mexican immigrant who presented with abdominal pain, vomiting, night sweats, and fever. *A,* Ultrasound of the liver demonstrates a 9 × 10 cm well-defined, homogeneously echogenic abscess. *B,* Coronal image from a contrast-enhanced computed tomography (CT) scan of the abdomen obtained 9 hours later for worsening right upper quadrant pain and fever despite intravenous metronidazole. The large abscess in the right hepatic dome has increased to 9.6 × 13 cm, concerning for imminent rupture. A second smaller abscess is in the inferior right lobe. *C,* Ultrasound guided placement of 14-Fr pigtail catheter. The echogenic puncture needle is well-visualized in the center of the abscess at sonography, and 500 mL of thick, brownish material was evacuated with immediate pain relief. *D,* CT scan obtained 1 week later demonstrates significant decrease in the size of the abscess.

## 24. Describe the percutaneous thermal ablative treatments for HCC?

Four different technologies for image-guided percutaneous thermal tumor destruction have been developed and clinically tested: radiofrequency ablation (RFA), microwave ablation, laser ablation, and cryoablation.

Tissue damage caused by heat depends on the tissue temperature achieved and the duration of heating. After 4 to 6 minutes at 50° C to 55° C, irreversible cellular damage begins to occur. Irreversible damage to mitochondrial and cytosolic enzymes of the cells with tissue coagulation occurs at temperatures between 60° C and 100° C. Above 100° C to 110° C, tissue vaporizes and carbonizes. To achieve adequate tumor destruction, the entire target volume must be subject to cytotoxic temperatures. RFA, microwave, and laser ablation are three heat-based methods. In RFA, the patient is part of a closed-loop circuit, which includes an RF generator, an electrode needle (placed in the tumor), and a large dispersive electrode (ground pads placed on the patient). An alternating electric field is created within the tissue of the patient and frictional heat is produced around the needle electrode due to differences in electrical resistance. Microwave ablation uses electromagnetic energy at frequencies of 900 kHz or greater to rotate water molecules to create frictional heat. The microwave needle antenna radiates an energetic field into tissue, which creates an active zone of heating. Laser ablation uses light energy applied via laser fibers directly inserted into the tissue.

In cryoablation, hollow needle probes are inserted into the tumors and argon and helium gases are circulated in and out of the probe to respectively cool and thaw the probe tip. An ice ball is created around the probe tip, which causes tissue destruction by cellular dehydration, membrane rupture from intracellular ice crystal formation, and ischemic microvascular thrombosis at temperatures between −20° C and −40° C.

## 25. What are the advantages of RFA and other methods of percutaneous thermal ablation?

- Low mortality and complication rates. Multicenter surveys report mortality rates ranging from 0.1% to 0.5%, major complication rates ranging from 2.2% to 3.1%, and minor complication rates ranging from 5% to 8.9%.
- Repeatability
- Minimally invasive and shorter recovery times compared with surgery
- Can be used in combination with other treatment therapies
- Less destruction of nonneoplastic tissue than surgery

## 26. What are the contraindications of RFA or percutaneous thermal ablative techniques?

The only absolute contraindications are uncorrectable coagulopathy or a noncompliant patient. RFA and other percutaneous ablative techniques are local treatments and are usually not performed in patients with vascular invasion or extrahepatic metastases. Patients with colonization of the biliary tract from bilioenteric anastomoses, endoscopic sphincterotomy, or bilioenteric fistula are at increased risk of post ablation liver abscess. Some liver transplant centers may exclude patients from transplant consideration who have had percutaneous tumor ablation due to concerns of tumor recurrence from tract seeding so it is important to discuss treatment options with referral hepatologists and surgeons, who are expert in liver transplantation.

## 27. Describe the association of Childs-Pugh score and survival in patients with HCC treated with RFA.

Both univariate and multivariate analysis in multiple studies reveal that Childs-Pugh classification is a prognostic factor for survival. In a study of 266 patients with 392 HCCs by Yan and colleagues:

- Overall 1-, 3-, and 5-year survival rates were 82.9%, 57.9%, and 42.9%.
- 1-, 3-, and 5-year survival rates were 89.7%, 73.4%, and 62.8% in Childs-Pugh class A cirrhotics, versus
- 1-, 3-, and 5-year survival rates of 77.2%, 39.9%, and 27% in Childs-Pugh class B cirrhotics
- 1-, 3-, and 5-year survival rates of 58.3%, 25%, and 25% in Childs-Pugh class C cirrhotics

## 28. Describe the risks of RFA related to the anatomic location of the tumor?

Superficial tumors adjacent to the gastrointestinal tract are at risk for thermal injury to the bowel wall. The colon appears to be at greater risk for perforation than the stomach and small bowel due to the thinner wall thickness and its lesser mobility. The gallbladder and biliary tract are also at risk for thermal injury. Perforation of the gallbladder is rare but ablation of tumors adjacent to the gallbladder can be associated with iatrogenic cholecystitis, which is usually self-limited. Bilomas and biliary stenoses can also occur. Lesions in the dome of the liver can result in thermal injury to the diaphragm, pneumothorax, or hemothorax. Vessels in the vicinity or adjacent to lesions are usually protected because of the "heat sink" effect of flowing blood. However, if the vessel is very small or the flow is decreased for any reason, thrombosis can occur. The *heat sink* effect may also result in incomplete ablation of the neoplastic tissues adjacent to the vessel from heat loss.

## 29. In the treatment of HCC, how do survival outcomes of RFA compare to surgical resection?

Most studies evaluating surgical resection and RFA show similar long term outcomes. In a randomized control trial of 112 patients with a solitary HCC less than 5 cm by Chen et al., there were no significant differences in local recurrence, overall survival, or disease-free survival between the two groups.

## 30. Describe the advantages of combining RFA with transcatheter arterial chemoembolization (TACE) in the treatment of HCC?

The effectiveness of RFA is limited by the size of the tumor, decreases with lesions greater than 3 cm in diameter, and is likely due to incomplete ablation. Blood flow promotes heat loss and may be one of the factors responsible for this size limitation. During TACE, embolization material is often injected into the hepatic artery following the delivery of the chemotherapy agents/lipiodol cocktail to reduce arterial inflow and to prevent rapid chemotherapy washout. Even without the injection of additional embolization material, there is an embolization effect from the lipiodol deposition. The combination of tissue hypoxia/ischemia and chemotherapy results in tumor necrosis. By performing TACE prior to RFA, the heat loss from tissue perfusion should be reduced or eliminated. Therefore, the volume of tumor ablation should increase in size allowing for more effective treatment of larger HCCs compared with RFA alone.

## 31. What other liver cancers have been treated with percutaneous thermal ablative techniques?

Liver metastases from neuroendocrine, gastric, pancreatic, pulmonary, renal, uterine, or ovarian cancer and melanoma have all been successfully treated with RFA. Besides HCC, the majority of percutaneous thermal ablative procedures are performed for the treatment of colorectal liver metastases (Fig. 68-6).

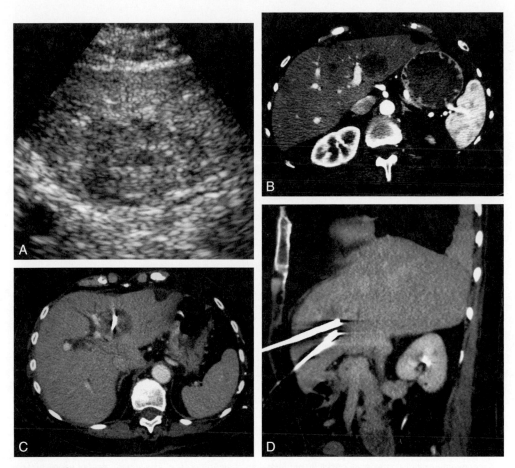

**Figure 68-6.** Ultrasound and computed tomography (CT) scan–guided microwave ablation of a colorectal liver metastasis. *A,* Ultrasound demonstrates a hypoechoic solid mass in the left lobe of the liver. *B,* Contrast-enhanced CT of the liver demonstrates a corresponding 3-cm hypodense solid mass in the lateral segment. *C,* At the time of the procedure, IV contrast was administered to enhance visualization of the mass for proper placement of the microwave antenna prior to ablation. Note the hyperdense metallic thermal probe at the center of the metastasis. The left portal vein abuts the mass but was protected from injury by the heat sink effect. *D,* Sagittal CT image depicts the two microwave antennas needed to create an adequate zone of ablation to treat the 3-cm mass to include a margin of tissue around the mass.

## SPLENIC INTERVENTIONS

### 32. What interventions are possible in the spleen?

Performance of percutaneous procedures in the spleen remains controversial. Some reports suggest that FNAs and catheter drainages of the spleen are possible. Although these procedures can be performed successfully, their overall risk is relatively high. Serious complications are estimated to occur in as many as 7% of cases (roughly 2 to 10 times more often than for other image-guided abdominal interventions). Uncontrolled hemorrhage necessitating emergency splenectomy is not uncommon. Therefore, the procedure should be clearly indicated, and its risks and benefits need to be thoroughly discussed with the patient and the referring physician. The possibility of emergency splenectomy must be emphasized. Surgical backup must be immediately available. If a percutaneous procedure is attempted, the size of the needle or catheter should be conservative. The lesion should be approached avoiding any intervening parenchyma (Fig. 68-7). Alternatives should be considered if the abnormality is not subcapsular and is surrounded by splenic tissue.

## PANCREATIC PROCEDURES

### 33. What procedures are appropriate for solid pancreatic masses?

Solid masses, usually suspected tumors, can be aspirated percutaneously (Fig. 68-8). Only FNAs should be performed; core biopsies should be avoided, because the use of cutting needles can result in severe pancreatitis. If a skinny needle is used and the lesion is solid, any organ, including the stomach, small bowel, and colon, can be traversed. Antibiotic

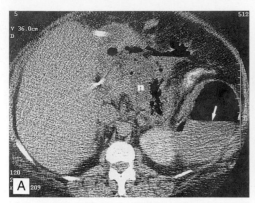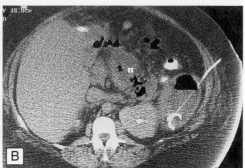

**Figure 68-7.** Percutaneous catheter drainage of a splenic abscess that developed after gastric bypass surgery. *A,* Diagnostic computed tomography scan shows a large-air-fluid level in the spleen (*arrow*). Although contained by the splenic capsule, the entire spleen is virtually suppurated. Note associated infected, acute pancreatic necrosis (n). *B,* An 8-Fr catheter placed into the splenic abscess drained a large volume of purulent material. No hemorrhagic complication occurred, probably because only the splenic capsule was traversed. The infected pancreatic necrosis (n) was drained separately.

coverage is recommended for procedures through the bowel. Major blood vessels should be avoided. The diagnosis of pancreatic adenocarcinoma often can be established by cytopathology alone; a negative result must be interpreted with caution and assumed to be a sampling error until proved otherwise. As noted previously, percutaneous biopsy of suspected cystadenomas or cystadenocarcinomas should be avoided.

**34. What procedures are used for pancreatic fluid collections?**

Various acute and chronic pancreatic fluid collections can be aspirated and drained. Fluid collections should be defined according to the classification system adopted by the International Symposium on Acute Pancreatitis. Pancreatic-related collections can be aspirated to determine whether they are sterile or infected (Fig. 68-9). In this setting, bowel should not be crossed with the aspiration needle to avoid contaminating and superinfecting otherwise sterile fluid.

**35. What precautions apply to percutaneous drainage of pancreatic fluid collections?**

If endoscopic internal drainage is not possible, percutaneous drainage of most sterile and infected pancreatic collections can be undertaken, if clinically indicated. The drainage of infected collections requires coverage with antibiotics. Routine techniques with 8-Fr catheters are usually adequate to treat focal pancreatic abscesses, which can be successfully drained in 7 to 10 days. Sterile acute or chronic pancreatic fluid collections and pseudocysts are more difficult to manage, and may require straight catheter drainage for 30 to 120 days. In these cases, concomitant endoscopic stenting of obstructing pancreatic duct pathology can facilitate catheter drainage and obviate pancreaticocutaneous fistula as a complication. Attempts at draining infected pancreatic necrosis may require aggressive treatment with multiple, large-bore, sump catheters. To prevent superinfection, percutaneous drains should be avoided in cases of sterile pancreatic necrosis.

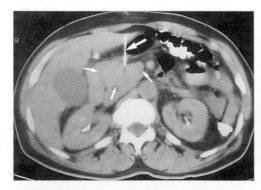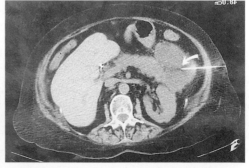

**Figure 68-8.** Fine-needle aspiration of pancreatic head carcinoma. Computed tomography scan shows mild fullness of the pancreative uncinate process (*small arrows*). A skinny needle (*large arrow*), passed through the liver and bowel wall without complication, was used to obtain cellular material diagnostic of pancreatic adenocarcinoma.

**Figure 68-9.** Aspiration of an acute pancreatic fluid collection associated with pancreatitis that occurred after lung transplantation. Computed tomography scan shows placement of a 20-gauge needle (*curved arrow*) into the collection. Withdrawn fluid was sterile; all cultures were negative for the growth of microorganisms.

# ADRENAL BIOPSY

## 36. What is the role of adrenal gland biopsy?

Because incidental adrenal gland adenomas can be characterized often with thin-section, dynamic CT and in-phase versus out-of-phase MR pulse sequences, fewer adrenal lesions need to be biopsied. Because of the risk of hypertensive crisis, possible pheochromocytomas should not be needled. FNA of other adrenal masses is usually sufficient for cytopathologic diagnosis. Approaching either adrenal gland can be difficult. Transhepatic access, decubitus positioning with the lesion-side down to elevate the adjacent hemidiaphragm, and angled routes may be necessary.

## BIBLIOGRAPHY

1. Beland MD, Gervais DA, Levis DA, et al. Complex abdominal and pelvic abscesses. Efficacy of adjunctive tissue type plasminogen activator for drainage. Radiology 2008;247:567–73.
2. Bergenfeldt M, Genell S, Lindholm K, et al. Needle-tract seeding after percutaneous fine-needle biopsy of pancreatic carcinoma. Case report. Acta Chir Scand 1988;154:77–9.
3. Bissonnette RT, Gibney RG, Berry BR, et al. Fatal carcinoid crisis after percutaneous fine-needle biopsy of hepatic metastasis: Case report and literature review. Radiology 1990;174:751–2.
4. Bradley III EL. A clinically based classification system for acute pancreatitis: Summary of the International Symposium on Acute Pancreatitis, Atlanta, September 11–13, 1992. Arch Surg 1993;128:586–90.
5. Casola G, Nicolet V, van Sonnenberg E, et al. Unsuspected pheochromocytoma: Risk of blood-pressure alterations during percutaneous adrenal biopsy. Radiology 1986;159:733–5.
6. Chen MS, Li JQ, Zheng Y, et al. A prospective randomized trial comparing local ablative therapy and partial hepatectomy for small hepatocellular carcinoma. Ann Surg 2006;243:321–8.
7. Cheng BQ, Jia CQ, Liu CT, et al. Chemoembolization combined with radiofrequency ablation for patients with hepatocellular carcinoma larger than 3 cm: A randomized controlled trial. JAMA 2008;299:1669–977.
8. del Pilar Fernandez M, Murphy FB. Hepatic biopsies and fluid drainages. Radiol Clin North Am 1991;29:1311–28.
9. Dodd III GD, Soulen MC, Kane RA, et al. Minimally invasive treatment of malignant hepatic tumors: At the threshold of a major breakthrough. Radiographics 2000;20:9–27.
10. Freeny PC, Hauptmann F, Althaus SJ, et al. Percutaneous CT-guided catheter drainage of infected acute necrotizing pancreatitis: Techniques and results. Am J Roentgenol AJR 1998;170:969–77.
11. Hanna RM, Dahniya MH, Badr SS, et al. Percutaneous catheter drainage in drug-resistant amoebic abscess. Trop Med Int Health 2000;5:578–81.
12. Hariri M, Slivka A, Carr-Locke DL, et al. Pseudocyst drainage predisposes to infection when pancreatic necrosis is unrecognized. Am J Gastroenterol 1994;89:1781–4.
13. Price RB, Bernardino ME, Berkman WA, et al. Biopsy of the right adrenal gland by the transhepatic approach. Radiology 1983;148:566.
14. Quinn SF, van Sonnenberg E, Casola G, et al. Interventional radiology in the spleen. Radiology 1986;161:289–91.
15. Silverman SG, Mueller PR, Pfister RC. Hemostatic evaluation before abdominal interventions: An overview and proposal. Am J Roentgenol AJR 1990;154:233–8.
16. Stigliano R, Marelli L, Yu D, et al. Seeding following percutaneous diagnostic and therapeutic approaches for hepatocellular carcinoma. What is the risk and outcome? Seeding risk for percutaneous approach of HCC. Cancer Treat Rev 2007;33:437–47.
17. van Sonnenberg E, D'Agostino HB, Casola G, et al. Percutaneous abscess drainage: Current concepts. Radiology 1991;181:617–26.
18. van Sonnenberg E, Wittich GR, Casola G, et al. Percutaneous drainage of infected and noninfected pancreatic pseudocysts: Experience in 101 cases. Radiology 1981;170:757–76.
19. van Sonnenberg E, Wroblicka JT, D'Agostino HB, et al. Symptomatic hepatic cysts: Percutaneous drainage and sclerosis. Radiology 1994;190:387–92.
20. Yan K, Chen MH, Yang W, et al. Radiofrequency ablation of hepatocellular carcinoma: Long-term outcome and prognostic factors. Eur J Radiol 2008;67:336–67.

# INTERVENTIONAL RADIOLOGY: FLUOROSCOPIC AND ANGIOGRAPHIC PROCEDURES

**69** CHAPTER

*Kimi L. Kondo, DO, Paul D. Russ, MD,*
*Stephen W. Subber, MD*

## HEPATIC TRANSARTERIAL CHEMOEMBOLIZATION

### 1. Define *hepatic transarterial chemoembolization.*

Hepatic transarterial chemoembolization (TACE) is a treatment for unresectable primary and secondary hepatic malignancies (Fig. 69-1). This procedure combines the intra-arterial infusion of chemotherapeutic agents with subsequent embolization of the blood vessel supplying the tumor, a combination that leads to high local drug concentrations and tumor ischemia while decreasing systemic toxicity.

### 2. How safe is hepatic TACE?

TACE is a relatively safe therapy because liver tumors derive most of their blood supply from the hepatic artery. The unique dual blood supply to the background liver (hepatic artery and portal vein) allows safe embolization of the neoplasm's arterial blood supply with little risk of hepatic ischemia.

### 3. Why would TACE be used to treat patients with hepatic malignancy?

Surgical resection or transplantation each is an optimal treatment for patients with hepatic malignancy. Unfortunately, many patients are not surgical candidates because of tumor extent, invasion of blood vessels, associated liver dysfunction, or distant metastases. Response to conventional treatments, such as systemic chemotherapy or radiation therapy, has been poor, although new drugs like sorafenib (Nexavar) show promise.

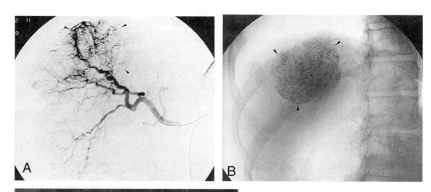

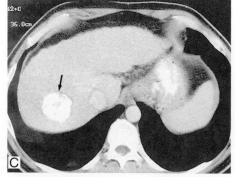

**Figure 69-1.** Chemoembolization of a hepatocellular carcinoma. *A,* Hepatic arteriogram demonstrates a hypervascular mass (*black arrowheads*) in the posterior segment of the right lobe. *B,* Angiographic image of the stained tumor (*black arrowheads*) after embolization with Ethiodol/chemotherapeutic drug emulsion and particles. *C,* Postembolization CT scan shows persistent, dense uptake and retention of Ethiodol in the lesion (*black arrow*). Complete tumor staining results in tumor necrosis and, possibly, longer patient survival.

### 4. How effective is TACE?

Response rates are encouraging for hepatocellular carcinoma (HCC) as well as for metastatic carcinoid and islet cell tumors but less promising for colorectal metastases. There is level I evidence that TACE prolongs survival in patients with well-compensated liver disease and intermediate HCC, but TACE is still considered palliative treatment.

## YTTRIUM-90 ($^{90}$Y)-RADIOEMBOLIZATION

### 5. Describe $^{90}$Y-radioembolization.

Yttrium-90 radioembolization is a form of interarterial brachytherapy. Microspheres containing $^{90}$Y are injected into the hepatic arteries via a catheter. The primary mode of action is the emission of radiation and the second mode of action is the embolization of the vasculature. $^{90}$Y is a beta emitter and has a mean tissue penetration of 2.5 mm and a maximum penetration of 10 mm. Radiation essentially ceases after 10 days.

### 6. Name the two FDA-approved and commercially available radioactive microspheres and describe their differences.

SIR-Spheres are nonbiodegradable *resin* beads, 35 μm in diameter and FDA approved for the treatment of unresectable colorectal liver metastases with concomitant use of floxuridine (FUDR). Theraspheres are nonbiodegradable *glass* beads, 25 μm in diameter and FDA approved for the treatment of unresectable HCC (Fig. 69-2). The activity per particle is higher with Theraspheres, measuring 2500 Bq as opposed to 50 Bq for SIR-Spheres. The number of particles delivered per treatment and the embolization effect with Theraspheres is less compared with SIR-Spheres.

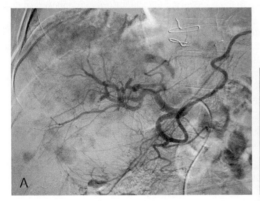
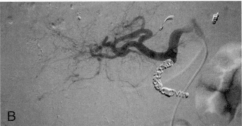
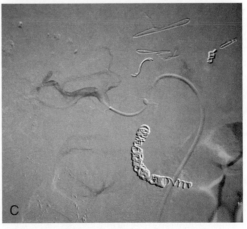

**Figure 69-2.** Therasphere $^{90}$Y-radioembolization of multifocal HCC. *A,* Common hepatic arteriogram demonstrates multiple hypervascular masses throughout the liver. *B,* Postembolization arteriogram confirms complete occlusion of the right gastric artery and gastroduodenal artery prior to radioembolization of the right hepatic lobe. Prophylactic embolization is performed to avoid complications of nontarget embolization via intestinal vessels. *C,* Injection of Therasphere $^{90}$Y glass beads through a microcatheter in the distal right hepatic artery.

### 7. Compare and contrast radioembolization and TACE.

Both radioembolization and TACE rely on hepatic arterial blood flow to deliver the therapeutic agents to the tumors. Nontarget embolization can occur with both procedures but with radioembolization, the physical sphere itself also serves as the radiotherapeutic and therefore the potency of locoregional delivery is greater. Complications associated with nontarget embolization are mainly due to embolization of the gastrointestinal system, which results in ulcerations. Prior to radioembolization, diagnostic arteriography and selective embolization of extrahepatic vessels arising from hepatic vessels, intestinal collaterals, and variant anatomy, must be performed. Technetium-99 macroaggregated albumin (MAA) is injected into the hepatic artery after embolization of extrahepatic pathways and nuclear medicine scanning is performed to determine pulmonary shunt fraction and nontarget embolization. If the percentage of pulmonary shunting is high, there is a risk of radiation pneumonitis.

Radioembolization has a significantly decreased incidence and severity of postembolization syndrome and thus can be performed as an outpatient procedure without the need for hospitalization. Preservation of arterial and portal inflow is desirable in radioembolization as opposed to chemoembolization since the locoregional radiotherapeutic effect is dependent on an oxygenated environment to promote free radical generation.

### 8. What are the contraindications of radioembolization?
- Uncorrectable coagulopathy
- Severe anaphylactoid contrast reaction
- Severe liver or renal dysfunction
- Predicted risk of greater than 30 Gray (Gy) from a single treatment or accumulated dose of 50 Gy to be delivered to the lungs
- Granulocyte count less than $1.5 \times 10^9$/L
- Greater than 70% tumor replacement of liver or greater than 50% tumor replacement of liver with an albumin level less than 3.0 g/dL
- Bilirubin greater than 2.0 mg/dL

## BILIARY PROCEDURES

### 9. Is percutaneous transhepatic biliary drainage the primary method to treat biliary obstruction?
The role of percutaneous transhepatic biliary drainage (PTBD) in the management of benign and malignant biliary disease has diminished significantly with the advancement of interventional endoscopy. Currently, endoscopic drainage is the primary method for biliary decompression, because of its relative lack of complications and better patient tolerance compared with the transhepatic approach. However, not all endoscopic drainages are successful, and PTBD continues to play an important role in the management of biliary disease. Biliary disease is best managed by a team that includes an endoscopist, interventional radiologist, and surgeon.

### 10. What are the indications for PTBD?
- Unsuccessful endoscopic drainage
- Biliary obstruction at or above the level of the porta hepatis
- Biliary obstruction following biliary-enteric anastomosis
- Bile duct injuries after laparoscopic cholecystectomy

The most common of these indications is failed endoscopic drainage for any reason.

### 11. What particular problems are involved in the treatment of hilar obstruction?
Hilar obstruction is difficult to treat for both endoscopists and interventionalists. Usually it is secondary to cholangiocarcinoma or metastatic disease that involves the left and right bile ducts, with frequent occlusion of intrahepatic segmental ducts. The multisegmental nature of these obstructions makes them difficult to drain by the endoscopist; in general, drainage is better accomplished by PTBD. Bilateral drains may be required.

### 12. Why is endoscopic drainage difficult in patients with biliary obstruction after biliary-enteric anastomosis?
The success rate for endoscopic drainage in patients with biliary obstruction after biliary-enteric anastomosis is less than 50%, because of the technical difficulty of negotiating the endoscope through the afferent loop. PTBD may be necessary to evaluate for recurrent disease or anastomotic stricture.

### 13. Describe the approach to bile duct injuries due to laparoscopic cholecystectomy.
Bile duct injuries due to laparoscopic cholecystectomy result from inadvertent laceration or ligation of the biliary system. PTBD is directed at relieving the obstruction or, in patients with a bile leak, diverting the bile and stenting the injury. This procedure allows healing and may be curative. Otherwise, elective surgery is performed once the patient's condition stabilizes. Endoscopic drainage can be difficult because the bile duct may be severed.

### 14. Explain the advantages and disadvantages of using metallic stents for the treatment of biliary obstruction.
Metallic stents have supplanted plastic endoprostheses in the percutaneous treatment of malignant biliary obstructions for palliation (Fig. 69-3). Their primary advantage is the smaller-sized catheter used to deliver the stent compared with the much larger plastic endoprosthesis, thus decreasing patient discomfort and liver complications. In addition, metallic stents expand to larger internal diameters (up to 12 mm or larger), affording better drainage and longer patency rates. A major disadvantage is the high cost; moreover, if they occlude because of tumor overgrowth, epithelial hyperplasia, or inspissated bile, reintervention is necessary.

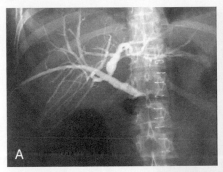
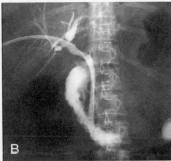
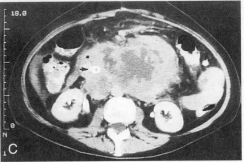

**Figure 69-3.** A 58-year-old woman presented with jaundice and an abdominal mass. **A,** A cholangiogram performed after percutaneous transhepatic biliary drainage shows complete obstruction of the common bile duct. **B,** After placement of a metallic stent, the common bile duct is widely patent. **C,** CT scan of the abdomen shows the large, poorly differentiated lymphoma encasing the biliary stent (*arrow head*).

## 15. What are the indications for percutaneous cholecystostomy?

Percutaneous placement of a drainage catheter into the gallbladder is a well-established technique. Its two primary indications are:

- Persistent and unexplained sepsis in critically ill patients with acalculous cholecystitis
- Acute cholecystitis in patients too ill to undergo surgery. In unstable patients, it can be performed at the bedside, if necessary.

Less frequent indications include temporary treatment for gallbladder perforation, drainage for distant malignant biliary obstruction, and transcholecystic biliary intervention.

## GASTROINTESTINAL BLEEDING

## 16. When do diagnostic angiography and percutaneous transcatheter therapy play a role in the management of gastrointestinal (GI) bleeding?

Acute GI bleeding that is refractory to conservative management or invasive endoscopic techniques requires angiographic evaluation. For the interventional radiologist to identify the bleeding site, the following conditions must be met:

- The patient must be actively bleeding at the time of the study.
- The bleeding must be brisk enough to be detectable during the angiogram, usually 1.5 to 2.0 mL/min.

GI bleeding at lower rates is difficult to detect angiographically. Once the bleeding site is identified, transcatheter embolization is a treatment option.

## 17. How important is localization of the bleeding site before angiography?

Preangiographic localization of the GI bleeding site is extremely helpful. A visceral angiogram involves evaluation of the celiac, superior mesenteric, and inferior mesenteric arteries; selective catheterization of these vessels and the multiple angiographic projections needed when looking for a bleeding site can make this a tedious and time-consuming procedure, requiring large contrast volumes. If the preangiographic endoscopy has localized and failed to treat the bleeding, the vessel supplying this region should be studied first to shorten the procedure. If the exact site of bleeding is not known, distinguishing an upper from a lower GI source is helpful and can guide the interventionalist in choosing which vessel should be studied first. A technetium 99m–labeled red blood cell study may provide localizing information; the procedure may be repeated after 12 hours if no bleeding is demonstrated initially.

## 18. What two types of transcatheter therapy are used for GI bleeding?

Selective embolization and vasopressin (Pitressin) infusion. Vasopressin infusion is rarely used today because of the cardiovascular complications (myocardial ischemia, arrhythmias, visceral ischemia), high rate of rebleeding after discontinuation of the infusion, difficulty in maintaining catheter position, and the long treatment times of 12 to 24 hours. Modern coaxial systems and microcatheters permit superselective catheterization with accurate deposition of embolic material at the bleeding site (Fig. 69-4). These advances have decreased the risk of bowel infarction, making transcatheter embolization a relatively safe procedure even in the small bowel and colon.

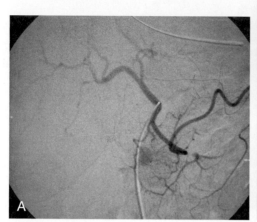 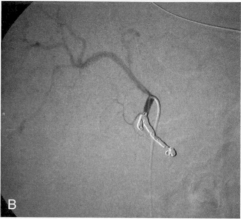

**Figure 69-4.** A 52-year-old man with upper GI bleeding from a duodenal ulcer after failed endoscopic treatment. **A,** Selective gastroduodenal artery (GDA) arteriogram demonstrates active bleeding and contrast extravasation from a branch of the superior pancreaticoduodenal arcade. **B,** Cessation of bleeding after particle and coil embolization of the GDA and superior pancreaticoduodenal arcade.

## 19. What agents are used for transcatheter embolization?

Embolic agents include Gelfoam, polyvinyl alcohol (PVA) particles, metallic coils, and *n*-butyl cyanoacrylate (NBCA). PVA particles and metallic coils are the most common agents used for GI bleeding.

# TRANSJUGULAR LIVER BIOPSY

## 20. What are the specific indications for transjugular liver biopsy?

- Coagulopathy
- Need for hepatic venous pressure gradient (HVPG)
- Massive obesity
- Massive ascites? Ascites is often listed as an indication for transjugular liver biopsy and a contraindication for percutaneous liver biopsy. However, several studies have demonstrated no significant difference in minor or major complication rates with percutaneous liver biopsies in patients with or without ascites and normal coagulation.

## 21. How is it performed?

Access is obtained in the right internal jugular vein. Using fluoroscopy and an angled catheter, the right hepatic vein is selected. Contrast is injected to confirm selection of the appropriate hepatic vein. A guidewire is advanced through the catheter and into the hepatic vein. The catheter is then removed and exchanged over the wire for the 7-Fr curved sheath with an inner stiffening metal cannula. The sheath is directed anteriorly and the biopsy needle is advanced into the sheath until the tip is a few millimeters beyond the sheath and into the liver parenchyma. The semiautomated spring-fire mechanism is depressed and the biopsy obtained. A minimum of two or three specimens are obtained. Both 18-gauge and 19-gauge devices are available.

## 22. Why is it important to biopsy via the right hepatic vein and not the middle hepatic vein?

The right hepatic vein is posterior to the middle hepatic vein, and thus when an anterior biopsy is performed, there is a maximum volume of liver parenchyma to avoid inadvertent capsular perforation. In the anteroposterior projection, it is often difficult to differentiate the right hepatic vein from the middle hepatic vein. In the lateral projection, the catheter will be directed posteriorly if it is in the right hepatic vein.

# TRANSJUGULAR INTRAHEPATIC PORTOSYSTEMIC SHUNT

### 23. What is TIPS? How is it performed?

Transjugular intrahepatic portosystemic shunt (TIPS) is a percutaneous technique that creates a shunt within the liver between the portal and hepatic veins to treat variceal bleeding or ascites, complications of portal hypertension (Fig. 69-5). The procedure is performed by accessing the hepatic venous system, usually the right hepatic vein, via the right internal jugular vein. A 16-gauge Colapinto transjugular needle is used to puncture through the liver from the hepatic vein into the portal vein. The transhepatic tract is dilated with a balloon catheter, followed by placement of a partially polytetrafluoroethylene (ePTFE)-covered nitinol stent (Viatorr).

### 24. What are the benefits of successful TIPS?

Successful TIPS result in a reduction of the portosystemic pressure gradient (PSG) to 8 to 12 mm Hg (bleeding from varices is rare in patients with a PSG less than 12 mm Hg), and the stent is dilated until this goal is reached. If the PSG cannot be reduced sufficiently, parallel shunts may be necessary. Esophageal and gastric varices usually decompress once the TIPS has been placed. If the varices continue to fill at portal venography, the interventionalist may elect to embolize them.

### 25. What are the indications for TIPS?

The most important and frequent indication for TIPS is refractory variceal hemorrhage (Fig. 69-6), either acute (bleeding not controlled with sclerotherapy or pharmacotherapy) or chronic (recurrent major hemorrhage despite a course of sclerotherapy). TIPS is particularly helpful with bleeding from inaccessible intestinal or gastric varices and bleeding due to portal hypertensive gastropathy. Additional indications for TIPS include refractory ascites, refractory hepatic hydrothorax, and Budd-Chiari syndrome or other veno-occlusive diseases. TIPS is not indicated for the initial therapy of acute variceal bleeding, as a bridge to transplantation to reduce intraoperative morbidity, or for treatment of hepatopulmonary syndrome.

### 26. What are the contraindications to performing the TIPS procedure?

There are few absolute contraindications to TIPS. Because it is a portosystemic shunt, TIPS increases right-sided heart pressures and should not be performed in patients with right heart failure. It should not be performed in patients with polycystic liver disease, in whom the risk of hemorrhage is significantly increased because the shunt tract may traverse the cysts rather than be contained by hepatic parenchyma. TIPS is also precluded, if diversion of hepatic blood flow is likely to exacerbate hepatic dysfunction and cause severe hepatic failure. Exceptions include cases of variceal bleeding or fulminant Budd-Chiari syndrome. Relative contraindications include systemic infection, portal vein thrombosis, biliary obstruction, and severe hepatic encephalopathy.

### 27. What is the technical success rate for TIPS? What are the most common causes of a failed procedure?

TIPS is one of the more technically challenging procedures performed by the interventional radiologist. Nonetheless, the technical success rate is greater than 90%. Most failures are due to portal vein occlusion, when the occluded segment of portal vein cannot be catheterized from the transjugular approach.

### 28. How effective is the TIPS procedure for controlling variceal hemorrhage?

TIPS is extremely effective in controlling acute variceal hemorrhage. It appears to be as effective as a surgical portacaval shunt without the added risk of hepatic injury from general anesthesia. Mid-term studies have found the rate of recurrent variceal bleeding after TIPS to be less than 10%. Nearly all patients with recurrent bleeding were found to have shunt abnormalities, either stenosis or occlusion. Angiographic reevaluation with shunt revision (balloon dilatation or additional stent placement) or placement of a second TIPS nearly always controls bleeding.

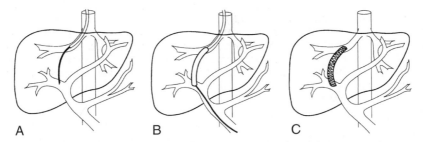

A          B          C

**Figure 69-5.** Transjugular intrahepatic portosystemic shunt procedure. *A,* After placement of a sheath in the right hepatic vein, a Colapinto needle is used to puncture through the liver to the portal vein. *B,* The liver parenchyma is dilated with a balloon catheter. *C,* A metallic stent is placed across the transhepatic tract.

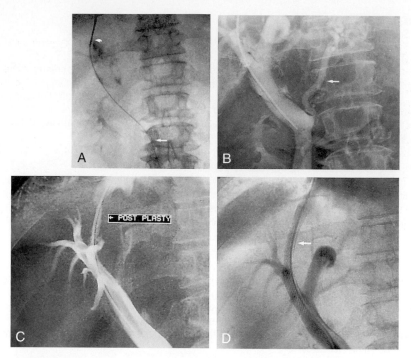

**Figure 69-6.** Transjugular intrahepatic portosystemic shunt in a 52-year-old woman with cryptogenic cirrhosis and refractory variceal bleeding. **A,** The portal vein has been punctured with a Colapinto needle (*arrowhead*) and a guidewire placed into the superior mesenteric vein (*arrow*). The portosystemic gradient (PSG) was 28 mm Hg. **B,** Portal venogram shows a large cardiac vein and esophageal varices (*arrow*). **C,** After balloon dilation of the transhepatic tract, a suboptimal portosystemic shunt is shown. **D,** A metallic stent (*arrow*) has been deployed across the transhepatic tract, allowing greater luminal diameter. Postprocedural PSG was 10 mm Hg.

## 29. What are the morbidity and mortality rates for TIPS?

TIPS is generally accepted to have lower morbidity and mortality rates than surgically created portacaval shunts. Published series show a 30-day mortality rate of 3% to 15%. Most deaths are in Child-Pugh class C patients. The direct procedure-related mortality rate is 2% to 5%. Procedure-related deaths are due predominantly to intraprocedural cardiac events or intraperitoneal hemorrhage after puncture through the liver capsule. Serious procedural complications, which occur in less than 10% of patients, include self-limited intraperitoneal hemorrhage, myocardial infarction, transient renal failure, hepatic arterial injury, hepatic infarction, and pulmonary edema.

## 30. Describe the major long-term complication of TIPS. How is it treated?

The most significant long-term complication of TIPS is hepatic encephalopathy. New or worsened encephalopathy is seen in about 25% of patients after TIPS. Usually it can be treated with diet, oral neomycin, and lactulose administration. Clinical variables associated with increased risk for developing post-TIPS encephalopathy include an etiology of liver disease other than alcohol, female gender, increasing age, and prior history of encephalopathy. Severe encephalopathy may require complete or partial occlusion of the shunt.

## 31. How is shunt patency followed?

Shunt patency can be followed noninvasively by color Doppler ultrasound or venography. Protocols differ among institutions. Prior to the availability of the ePTFE-covered Viatorr stent graft, a baseline study was obtained 24 hours after the procedure. In asymptomatic patients, routine follow-up was performed at 3 and 6 months after TIPS, then at 6-month intervals because bare stent malfunction ranged from 23% to 87% at 1 year. Reported 1-year patency rates with the use of the Viatorr stent graft are 81% to 84% and thus the need for frequent routine ultrasound surveillance is in question. If an early ultrasound evaluation is performed, it should be done at least 5 days after TIPS creation because air bubbles in the ePTFE fabric create gas artifacts, which do not allow complete visualization and evaluation in the first 2 to 4 days. If the patient becomes symptomatic (e.g., variceal bleeding or ascites) or if significant interval change is demonstrated by ultrasound, venography with therapeutic intervention should be performed to restore normal shunt function.

## BIBLIOGRAPHY

1. Camma C, Schepis F, Orlando A, et al. Transarterial chemoembolization for unresectable hepatocellular carcinoma: Meta-analysis of randomized controlled trials. Radiology 2002;224:47–54.
2. Chan AO, Yuen MF, Hui CK, et al. A prospective study regarding the complications of transcatheter intraarterial lipiodol chemoembolization in patients with hepatocellular carcinoma. Cancer 2002;94:1747–52.
3. Gordon RL, Ring EJ. Combined radiologic and retrograde endoscopic and biliary interventions. Radiol Clin North Am 1990;28:1289–95.
4. Kerlan RK, LaBerge JM, Gordon RL, et al. Transjugular intrahepatic portosystemic shunts: Current status. Am J Roentgenol AJR 1995;164:1059–66.
5. Laberge J, Ring E, Gordon R, et al. Creation of transjugular intrahepatic portosystemic shunts with the Wallstent endoprosthesis: Results in 100 patients. Radiology 1993;187:413–20.
6. Lee BH, Choe DH, Lee JH, et al. Metallic stents in malignant biliary obstruction: Prospective long-term clinical results. Am J Roentgenol AJR 1997;168:741–5.
7. Lee KH, Sung KB, Lee DY, et al. Transcatheter arterial chemoembolization for hepatocellular carcinoma: Anatomic and hemodynamic considerations in the hepatic artery and portal vein. Radiographics 2002;22:1077–91.
8. Llovet JM, Ricci S, Mazzaferro V, et al. Sorafenib in advanced hepatocellular carcinoma. N Engl J Med 2008;359:378.
9. Mauro MA, Murphy KP, Thomson KR, et al. Image-Guided Interventions. Philadelphia: Saunders; 2008.
10. Mammen T, Shyamkumar NK, Eapen CE, et al. Transjugular liver biopsy: A retrospective analysis of 601 cases. J Vasc Interv Radiol 2008;19:351–8.
11. Ong JP, Sands M, Younossi ZM. Transjugular intrahepatic portosystemic shunts (TIPS): A decade later. J Clin Gastroenterol 2000;30:14–28.
12. Peck DJ, McLoughlin RF, Hughson MN, et al. Percutaneous embolization of lower gastrointestinal hemorrhage. J Vasc Interv Radiol 1998;9:747–51.
13. Rosen RJ, Sanchez G. Angiographic diagnosis and management of gastrointestinal hemorrhage: Current concepts. Radiol Clin North Am 1994;32:951–67.
14. Salem R, Thurston KG. Radioembolization with $^{90}$yttrium microspheres: A state-of-the-art brachytherapy treatment for primary and secondary liver malignancies. Part 1: Technical and methodologic considerations. J Vasc Interv Radiol 2006;17:1251–78.
15. Salem R, Thurston KG. Radioembolization with $^{90}$yttrium microspheres: A state-of-the-art brachytherapy treatment for primary and secondary liver malignancies Part 2: Special topics. J Vasc Interv Radiol 2006;17:1425–39.
16. Soulen MC. Chemoembolization of hepatic malignancies. Semin Interv Radiol 1997;14:305–11.

# NONIVASIVE GASTROINTESTINAL IMAGING: ULTRASOUND, COMPUTED TOMOGRAPHY, MAGNETIC RESONANCE IMAGING

*Michael G. Fox, MD, Ryan Kaliney, MD, David W. Bean, Jr, MD, and Kevin M. Rak, MD*

## LIVER IMAGING

**1. How is segmental liver anatomy defined?**

Early descriptions of liver anatomy divided the organ into four lobes based on the surface configuration and the vasculature, primarily the hepatic veins. The different hepatic segments are divided by intersegmental fissures, which are traversed or are in the same plane as the hepatic veins.

The main lobar fissure divides the right and left lobes of the liver and is represented by a line extending from the gallbladder recess through the inferior vena cava (IVC). In the liver, it is represented by the middle hepatic vein. The right intersegmental fissure divides the anterior and posterior segments of the right lobe of the liver and is approximated by the right hepatic vein. The left intersegmental fissure divides the medial and lateral segments of the left lobe of the liver. It is marked on the external liver margin by the falciform ligament, and internally the ligamentum teres runs within it. In the liver, it is represented by the left hepatic vein. The caudate lobe is the portion of liver located between the IVC and the fissure of the ligamentum venosum.

More recently, Couinaud's anatomy has become widely used as a method to further subdivide the liver into eight segments, each of which has its own blood supply (see Chapter 27, Fig. 27-1).

**2. How has the advent of multidetector computed tomography (MDCT) changed the evaluation of the liver, pancreas and biliary system?**

MDCT using either a 16-detector or a 64-detector computed tomography (CT) device allows for scanning the abdomen with very thin collimation (0.6 mm) and even thinner (0.5 mm) reconstruction intervals, which allow for true isotropic volumetric data sets. This allows the creation of exquisite multiplanar reformatations (MPRs), without *stair-step* artifacts, and demonstration of the anatomy in the coronal, sagittal or any other imaging plane. In addition, the exams are performed much quicker than with single-slice CT.

The liver parenchyma has a dual blood supply with 75% of its blood flow from the portal vein and 25% from the hepatic artery. As a result, the images can be obtained in either a noncontrast phase (NCCT), or late hepatic arterial phase (HAP), portal vein inflow or late HA phase, portal venous phase (PVP), or any combination of these phases depending on the clinical indication. The early HAP is usually 15 to 20 seconds after injection, the portal vein inflow phase or late HAP is 30 to 40 seconds after injection, and the PVP is 60 to 70 seconds after injection. The dominant contrast effect in the liver is in the PVP.

Since MDCT improves the imaging of the hepatic vasculature, it is very helpful in preoperative or pre–intra-arterial chemotherapy planning as well as in the detection of hepatic infarctions, aneurysms/pseudoaneurysms, portal vein thrombosis, or strictures. Liver volumes prior to hepatic resection can also be estimated using volume-rendered images.

**3. What is CT arterial portography?**

To increase liver enhancement, some medical centers place a catheter in the superior mesenteric artery for contrast injection during CT scanning. This technique, called CT arterial portography (CTAP), can increase the sensitivity of lesion detection to 91%, which is higher than that of single-slice contrast-enhanced CT even with triple-phase imaging. However, a recent paper suggests that MDCT combined with superparamagnetic iron oxide (SPIO)–enhanced magnetic resonance imaging (MRI) is similar in accuracy to CTAP for hepatocellular carcinoma (HCC) lesions greater than 10 mm in diameter in cirrhotic livers.

**4. What causes fatty filtration of the liver?**

Fatty infiltration of the liver is due to deposition of triglycerides within the hepatocytes and is most commonly associated with obesity but is also present in other disorders such as ethanol abuse, diabetes, excessive steroids, hyperlipidemia, hyperalimentation, radiation therapy or chemotherapy, and glycogen storage disease. It may be reversible, and it can cause slightly abnormal liver function tests (LFTs) and hepatomegaly. Fatty infiltration may be diffuse or focal. Fatty infiltration or sparing typically occurs around the gallbladder fossa and along the liver margin, in the medial segment of the left lobe near the fissure for the ligamentum teres, anterior to the porta hepatis and around the IVC.

## 5. Describe the imaging findings of fatty infiltration of the liver.

- *Ultrasound (US):* Fatty infiltration is seen as a focal or diffuse area of increased echogenicity. Depending on the degree of involvement, there can be decreased visualization or nonvisualization of intrahepatic vessels, the deeper posterior portions of the liver, and the diaphragm posterior to the liver. US does not show any mass effect on adjacent biliary structures or blood vessels. The finding of diffusely increased echogenicity of the liver is nonspecific and can be seen in hepatitis or cirrhosis.

- *CT:* Fatty infiltration is seen as an area of decreased attenuation, which is easier to appreciate in the focal form with adjacent normal liver. On NCCT scan, the normal liver is usually 8 HU greater in density than the spleen, but in fatty infiltration it is less dense than the spleen by 10 HU or more. However, other lesions may appear as an area of decreased density on NCCT, such as HCC and metastatic disease. In fatty infiltration, the hepatic vessels stand out and may appear as if they contain contrast on an unenhanced scan. In focal fatty infiltration, the normal hepatic vessels traverse the area of decreased attenuation, a finding not seen in a malignant mass. Focal fatty infiltration tends to have linear margins and to be in a lobar distribution (Fig. 70-1).

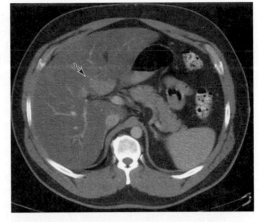

**Figure 70-1.** Computed tomography image of fatty infiltration. Focal fatty sparing (*arrow*) adjacent to the gallbladder fossa with fatty replacement of the remainder of the liver parenchyma is noted on this axial CT image. There is no evidence of mass effect on the liver vasculature.

- *MRI:* Signal differences in focal fatty infiltration of the liver usually are not as dramatic as those seen in subcutaneous fat; in fact, the signal changes may be quite subtle. As with CT, it is important to see normal vessels in the area of signal abnormality and no mass effect on adjacent structures. Fat-suppression MRI scans are more sensitive than routine T1-weighted (T1W) and T2-weighted (T2W) scans and show fatty infiltration as areas of decreased signal intensity compared with normal liver. Fatty areas will demonstrate decreased signal on out-of-phase images, which are very reliable in diagnosing this condition.

## 6. Describe the imaging findings in cirrhosis.

- *US:* Cirrhosis is characterized by abnormal echotexture. The hepatic parenchyma is typically hyperechoic with *coarsened* echoes, making the liver somewhat heterogeneous, and the intrahepatic vasculature is poorly defined. Unfortunately, these findings are nonspecific. Increased parenchymal echogenicity also is seen in fatty infiltration, and heterogeneity may be due to infiltrating neoplasm. Furthermore, no direct correlation exists between degree of hepatic dysfunction and sonographic appearance. More specific sonographic features of cirrhosis include nodularity of the liver surface and selective enlargement of the caudate lobe. A caudate–right lobe volume ratio greater than 0.65 is highly specific but not sensitive in diagnosing cirrhosis. In cirrhosis, the Doppler waveform may demonstrate either decreased amplitude of phasic oscillations with loss of reversed flow or a flattened waveform.

- *MDCT:* Although early parenchymal changes may not be visible on CT, the initial manifestation of alcoholic liver disease, fatty infiltration, is well seen. The attenuation of the liver becomes heterogeneous and abnormally lower than that of the spleen. The presence of regenerating nodules, which are isodense with liver, can often only be inferred from the nodular contour of the liver edge. The caudate lobe and lateral-segment left lobe typically enlarge, and the right lobe and medial segment of the left lobe typically atrophy. In advanced cirrhosis, liver volume usually decreases and periportal fibrosis and regenerative nodules can compress the portal and hepatic venous structures which may result in altered hepatic perfusion and portal hypertension. The complications of portal hypertension, especially varices, are exquisitely demonstrated with MDCT; however, unlike sonography, CT cannot determine the direction of vascular flow. Increased attenuation of the mesenteric fat is also noted (Fig. 70-2).

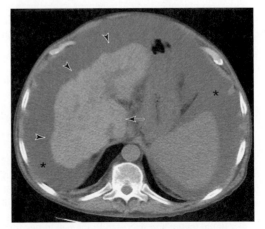

**Figure 70-2.** Computed tomography image of cirrhosis. The liver margin is nodular in contour (*arrowheads*). The caudate lobe (*arrow*) is hypertrophied as compared with the right and left lobes. Perihepatic and perisplenic ascites (*) is present.

- *MR:* Early MR changes of cirrhosis include enlargement of the hilar periportal space in up to 98% of patients due to atrophy of the medial segment of the left hepatic lobe. Later findings include a caudate–right hepatic lobe ratio of greater than 0.65, which has a specificity for cirrhosis of up to 90%. An even more specific sign of cirrhosis (98%) is the expanded gallbladder fossa sign. Imaging findings of portal hypertension are similar to those on MDCT and initially include dilatation of the portal and splenic veins with later occlusion and cavernous transformation of the portal vein, and the development of portosystemic collaterals and ascites.

7. **Define *primary* and *secondary hemochromatosis*.**
   - *Primary hemochromatosis* is an autosomal recessive disease in which patients absorb excessive amounts of dietary iron that accumulate in the parenchymal cells
     of the liver, heart, pituitary gland and pancreas. HCC appears hyperintense to the background of a
     low intensity liver.
   - *Secondary hemochromatosis*, caused by multiple blood transfusions, results in iron deposition in the reticuloendothelial cells of primarily the liver and spleen and not typically in the pancreas. Neither MR nor CT can distinguish which cells of a particular organ are overloaded with iron. Therefore, the organ distribution of imaging abnormalities can provide valuable information.

   Many patients with untreated hemochromatosis will develop cirrhosis and 25% will develop HCC.

8. **Which is the most sensitive exam in detecting hemochromatosis?**
   MR is more sensitive and specific than CT in detecting hemochromatosis. US of the liver is normal despite iron deposition unless underlying cirrhosis exists. The attenuation of the liver on noncontrast CT scans is typically greater than 85 HU in hemochromatosis, compared with a normal attenuation of about 60 HU. On MR, the iron deposition causes decreased signal intensity compared with the paraspinal muscles because of paramagnetic effects. The findings are most striking on T2W images but can be seen to a lesser extent on T1W images. MR quantification in the future may eliminate the need for some liver biopsies.

9. **How do liver metastases appear on different imaging modalities?**
   - *US:* Variable. Gastrointestinal (GI) and more vascular tumors (e.g., islet cell, carcinoid, choriocarcinoma, renal cell carcinomas) tend to produce hyperechoic metastases, which may mimic a hemangioma. Hypoechoic lesions are also common, particularly with lymphoma, breast, lung, and cystic or necrotic metastases. Hypoechoic halos surrounding liver masses produce the nonspecific but common *bull's-eye* appearance, which is often seen with malignant lesions and requires additional workup. The sensitivity of US for detecting metastases is about 61%; however, intraoperative US can increase the sensitivity to 96% and may be the most sensitive modality available.
   - *MDCT:* On NCCT images, most liver metastases are of low attenuation compared with the surrounding parenchyma. Branches of the hepatic artery supply liver metastases, and their detection is based on the timing of the contrast bolus and the vascularity of the lesions. Hypovascular metastases, such as colon adenocarcinoma, are most common and are best imaged in the PVP. Hypervascular metastases—renal cell, breast, thyroid, melanoma, and neuroendocrine tumors—are the exception. Imaging during the HAP should be added to PVP imaging to detect more of these lesions (Fig. 70-3).
   - *MRI:* Recent studies have demonstrated increased sensitivity of dynamic gadolinium-enhanced MRI compared with single-slice CT for the detection of liver metastasis. In addition, MRI has a much greater sensitivity for characterizing liver lesions than CT. In general, metastases are hypointense on T1W images and hyperintense on T2W images. Exceptions occur with hemorrhagic and malignant melanoma metastases, which are hyperintense to varying degrees on T1W images. Imaging with MRI contrast agents approaches the sensitivity of CTAP for detecting metastasis.

10. **What MRI contrast agents are available for use in hepatobiliary imaging?**
    The two main categories of MRI contrast agents used in hepatobiliary imaging are hepatocyte-selective and reticuloendothelial system–selective agents. Hepatocyte-selective agents include mangafodipir trisodium (Mn-DPDP), gadobenate diglumine (Gd-BOPTA), and gadolinium-ethoxybenzyle diethylenetriaminepentaacetic acid (Gd-EOB-DTPA). The reticuloendothelial system–selective agents are iron-containing compounds.

    Mn-DPDP is a hepatobiliary agent that is taken up by hepatocytes and excreted in the bile. It has a long (up to 10 hours) imaging window. On T1W images, Mn-DPDP causes increased signal in the normal liver. Therefore, lesions not of hepatocellular origin do not enhance. Examples include metastases, cholangiocarcinoma, lymphoma, hemangioma, and cysts. However, lesions that are of hepatocellular origin (HCC, focal nodular hyperplasia [FNH], adenomas, and regenerating nodules) do enhance. Gd-BOPTA is taken up by functioning hepatocytes and excreted in the bile in addition to being in the extracellular space. The maximal benefit in the detection of lesions with this agent occurs with imaging 1 to 2 hours after injection, which is the time of peak liver-to-lesion contrast. Imaging in the hepatobiliary phase can differentiate between FNH (with biliary ducts) and HA. Gd-EOB-DTPA is similar to Gd-BOPTA except that the time of peak liver-to-lesion contrast occurs 20 to 45 minutes after injection.

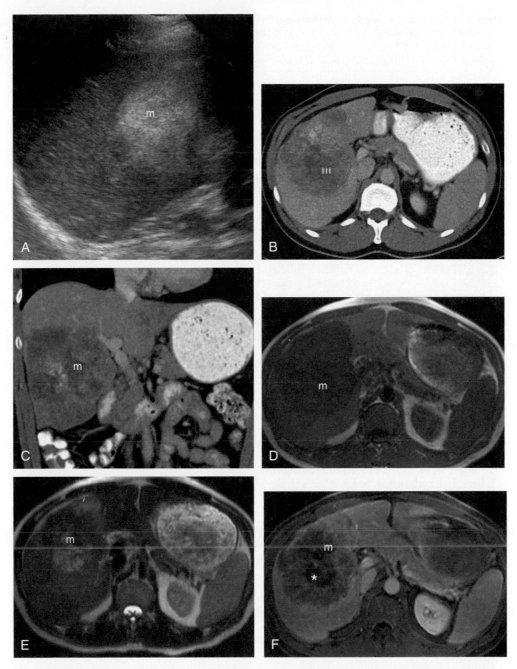

**Figure 70-3.** Ultrasound, computed tomography (CT), and magnetic resonance images of hepatic metastases (m) from colonic adenocarcinoma. *A,* Rounded, hyperechoic mass (m) on this longitudinal ultrasound image is a typical appearance for a metastatic lesion from a gastrointestinal tract malignancy or other hypervascular metastatic lesion (neuroendocrine tumors, choreocarcinoma, renal cell carcinoma, melanoma, etc.). *B,* Axial CT image of heterogeneous metastasis (m) with hypodense areas of necrosis centrally and coronal (*C*) CT image. *D,* Axial T1W image demonstrating low signal within the metastasis (m) with (*E*) axial T2W image demonstrating heterogeneously increased signal. *F,* Commonly seen with colonic adenocarcinoma metastases (m) are nonenhancing areas of central necrosis (*) as demonstrated on this postcontrast T1W image.

Reticuloendothelial system–selective agents contain iron oxide particles. Two SPIO-containing formulations, SPIO ferumoxides and carboxydextran-coated SPIO particles, are available. They are taken up primarily by Kupffer cells and result in decreased T2W signal. Lesions that do not have reticuloendothelial elements, such as metastases and cysts, do not take up the agent and remain hyperintense on T2W images. They can improve the detection of HCC but are limited in severe cases of cirrhosis. Limitations of SPIOs include lack of effectiveness at characterizing lesions smaller than 1 to 2 cm, long infusion time (30 minutes), and dose-related toxicity.

**11. What are the three growth patterns of HCC?**
1. Large solitary mass (50%)
2. Multifocal HCC (40%)
3. Diffuse infiltration (10%)

In North America, underlying liver disease is present in 60% to 80% of patients with HCC. HCC arising in noncirrhotic livers tends to occur at a younger age (fibrolamellar HCC) and typically presents as a solitary, well-circumscribed mass.

**12. How does HCC appear on different imaging modalities?**
- *US:* Variable, sometimes simulating metastatic disease. HCCs less than 5 cm are often hypoechoic, whereas larger lesions have mixed echogenicity. Fat within the tumor may cause internal hyperechoic foci. Vascular invasion is common, with invasion of the portal veins more frequent than the hepatic veins. Tumor thrombus can be demonstrated with Doppler ultrasound and typically has an arterial waveform.
- *MDCT:* Underlying cirrhotic or hemochromatotic changes are commonly seen, and 7% to 10% of HCCs demonstrate calcification. Tumors are typically hypodense on NCCT but may appear hyperdense in fatty livers. Small HCCs (less than 3 cm) typically demonstrate homogeneous enhancement in the HAP, which may detect up to 30% more tumor nodules than imaging in the PVP. Larger tumors have heterogeneous enhancement, and central necrotic areas of low attenuation are common. The tumor demonstrates low attenuation on the PVP. Using the late HAP and the PVP, more than 95% to 98% of lesions are reportedly detected. Even so, sometimes contour deformity, mass effect, or vascular, especially venous, invasion might be the only clues to detection. Hemoperitoneum, due to rare spontaneous rupture, and hemorrhage within the tumor may also occur. CTAP increases sensitivity, especially in detecting small lesions (Fig. 70-4).
- *MR:* MRI can help to distinguish between regenerative nodules, dysplastic nodules and HCC.
  A. Regenerative nodules are usually less than 1 cm in diameter and are variable in signal on the T1W images. They are usually iso to decreased in signal to normal liver on the T2W sequences, especially when they contain iron, which causes markedly decreased signal on gradient echo (GRE) and T2W images. These nodules usually do not enhance.
  B. Dysplastic nodules are considered premalignant and are usually larger than regenerative nodules. They often demonstrate increased T1W and decreased T2W signal; however, there is overlap with HCC.
  C. HCC is usually hypointense on T1W images but may be iso- or hyperintense, depending on the degree of fatty change and internal fibrosis. Findings which suggest HCC include increased T2W signal and a diameter greater than 2 to 3 cm. The addition of gadolinium enhanced images increases the detection of HCC. There is marked HAP enhancement with late washout and the presence of a peripherally enhancing pseudocapsule on PVP images. As the degree of malignancy increases, there is increased hepatic arterial flow to the nodules with decreased portal flow. A nodule within a nodule appearance is highly suggestive of a foci of HCC within a dysplastic nodule (Fig. 70-5).

Encapsulated HCC typically has a hypointense rim on T1W and T2W images. Fibrolamellar HCC appears somewhat similar to FNH as both have a central scar with multiple fibrous septa. However, fibrolamellar HCC has a high prevalence of calcification, and the central scar is typically hypointense on T2W images, whereas it is hyperintense in FNH.

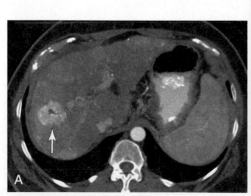
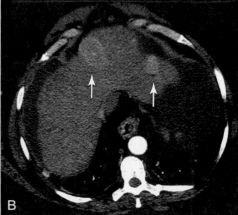

**Figure 70-4.** Computed tomography images of hepatocellular carcinoma. *A,* During the arterial phase of contrast enhancement, a hepatoma appears as a focus of early arterial enhancement (*arrow*) and can be delineated from the surrounding hepatic parenchyma. *B,* Detecting early arterial enhancing foci of hepatocellular carcinoma requires accurate timing of the intravenous contrast bolus. Lesions (*arrows*) are often subtle on the arterial phase images.

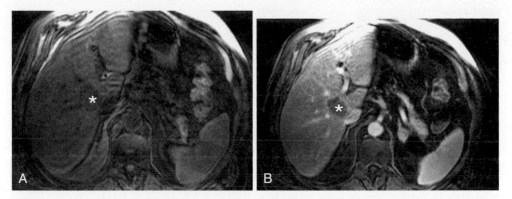

**Figure 70-5.** MR images of hepatocellular carcinoma. **A,** Rounded intrahepatic mass (*) near the inferior vena cava demonstrates low signal intensity on unenhanced T1W images. **B,** On delayed contrast enhanced imaging, there is persistent peripheral enhancement of the lesion (*) with central washout.

### 13. What is the most common benign neoplasm of the liver?
Cavernous hemangiomas. Most are less than 3 cm in size, solitary, and occurring in females. Blood flow within cavernous hemangiomas is usually very slow, which accounts for some of its imaging characteristics.

### 14. Describe the imaging characteristics of hepatic hemangiomas.
- *US:* Cavernous hemangiomas appear as well-defined hyperechoic masses in a normal liver. Doppler and color flow imaging usually demonstrate no detectable flow within the mass, but a feeding vessel may sometimes be detected. Occasionally hemangiomas have a mixed or hypoechoic appearance, especially in the setting of a fatty liver.
- *MDCT:* On NCCT, hemangiomas are usually isodense to blood vessels and 20% have calcifications. HAP imaging reveals a characteristic peripheral nodular enhancement pattern, that is isodense to the aorta initially followed by slow filling of the center of the lesion, which is isodense to the blood pool in the PVP. The enhancement does not typically washout, and large lesions may not completely enhance. Hemangiomas less frequently may demonstrate initial central or uniform enhancement; however, this pattern is also seen in malignant lesions.
- *MRI:* A typical hemangioma is well defined and has decreased signal intensity relative to normal liver on T1-weighted images. On T2-weighted images, hemangiomas have increased signal compared with the liver. The signal is equal to or greater than the signal of bile within the gallbladder and should continue to increase with greater T2 weighting. Using fast-scanning techniques and Gd-DTPA, a similar enhancement pattern can be seen on MRI and CT, which is nearly pathognomonic (Fig. 70-6).

### 15. Outline the workup for a suspected cavernous hemangioma.
If a lesion has the typical US findings of a cavernous hemangioma, and if the patient has normal liver function tests (LFTs and αFP) and no history of a malignancy that may metastasize to the liver or a risk factor for HCC such as cirrhosis, follow-up US in 3 to 6 months is appropriate. If the lesion is atypical on US or if the patient has a known primary neoplasm or abnormal LFTs, further workup is warranted. Microbubble-enhanced sonography has demonstrated promise in diagnosing nearly 100% of hemangiomas. The decision to obtain a $^{99m}$Tc-tagged red blood cell (RBC) scan, MRI, or multiphase CT varies with the facility and the preference of the radiologists. $^{99m}$Tc-tagged RBC scan is highly sensitive and specific for lesions greater than 2 cm. If the lesion is less than 2 cm, the RBC scan can be attempted, but sensitivity and specificity decrease as the size of the lesion decreases. MRI, preferably with heavily T2-weighted and gadolinium enhanced T1 imaging, and MDCT are also very effective, even with smaller lesions.

If the initial lesion is found by CT and follows the strict criteria of a hemangioma (a well-defined, low-density lesion on unenhanced images, with peripheral enhancement followed by complete filling of the lesion), further workup is probably not necessary. If the diagnosis needs confirmation, a tagged RBC study or US is a good choice. If the initial CT scan does not meet the strict criteria or the patient has abnormal LFTs, a confirmatory nuclear medicine or MRI scan is appropriate. If the CT criteria are not met, it is typically due to incomplete filling of the lesion.

If these different studies do not confirm that the lesion is a cavernous hemangioma, biopsy may be necessary for the final diagnosis.

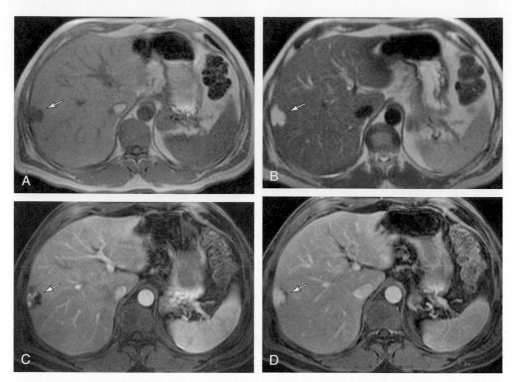

**Figure 70-6.** Magnetic resonance images of a hepatic cavernous hemangioma. *A,* Cavernous hemangioma (*arrow*) has decreased signal compared with liver parenchyma on unenhanced T1W image. *B,* Increased T2W signal, classic for cavernous hemangioma, is evident within the lobulated mass. (*arrow*). *C, D,* Serial images of the mass (*arrow*) following administration of intravenous gadolinium contrast material demonstrates the progressive centripetal enhancement of the hemangioma, from the classic appearance of peripheral, nodular discontinuous enhancement (*C*) to near complete enhancement on the more delayed image (*D*).

## 16. How can FNH and hepatocellular adenoma (HCA) be differentiated?

Hepatic adenomas and FNH are more common in women, and both, particularly HCA, are associated with oral contraceptive use. FNH is benign, whereas HCA can cause morbidity and mortality because of its propensity for hemorrhage and rare malignant degeneration to HCC. FNH is typically less than 5 cm when diagnosed and HCAs are often 8 to 15 cm in diameter. FNH contains all of the normal liver elements in an abnormal arrangement; however, HCAs contain few if any bile ducts or Kupffer cells. Hepatic adenomas are more likely to demonstrate calcification or fat than FNH. If a lesion is hyperintense on T1W sequences, has a pseudocapsule, and lacks a central scar, an HCA is favored over FNH. However, in smaller lesions without hemorrhage, biopsy may be required for differentiation.

## 17. Describe the appearance of FNH on imaging modalities.

The characteristic feature is the central scar, containing radiating fibrous tissue with vascular and biliary elements. However, the central scar is nonspecific and may be seen with fibrolamellar HCC, hemangioma, and other lesions.

- On *US*, FNH is often a subtle lesion. Therefore, minimal contour abnormalities and vascular displacement should raise the possibility of FNH. A well-demarcated hypo- to isoechoic mass, possibly demonstrating a central scar, may be identified. Doppler images, especially demonstrating a stellate arterial pattern, are helpful in confirming a lesion and are suggestive of FNH. The use of microbubble contrast agents demonstrates hypervascularity in the lesion in the arterial phase with stellate vessels and/or a tortuous feeding artery with persistent enhancement in the portal venous phase.
- On *NCCT* images, FNH is hypo- to isodense without calcification. FNH is hyperdense on HAP images, because it is supplied by the hepatic artery. On PVP images, it commonly isodense to normal liver with a hyperdense pseudocapsule. When the central low-density scar is present—35% cases if lesion is less than 3 cm and 65% cases if lesion is greater than 3 cm, it has a lower attenuation than the normal liver on HAP and PVP images. On 5- to 10-minute delayed images, the scar usually appears hyperdense. Enlarged feeding arteries and draining veins may be seen, especially with the use of MPRs. Thus, if no central scar is seen, FNH may be missed on CT or seen only as a deformity of the liver contour.
- On *MR*, FNH is hypo- to isointense on T1W and iso- to hyperintense on T2W images with the central scar hypointense on T1W and hyperintense on T2W images. The lesion demonstrates diffuse early enhancement with the exception of the central scar, which usually demonstrates delayed enhancement due to the fibrous tissue. Unlike HCC and adenomas, no capsular enhancement is identified in FNH.

Because of the presence of Kupffer cells, sulfur-colloid scintigraphy demonstrates normal uptake in 50%, decreased uptake in 40%, and increased uptake or hot-spots in 10%. However, HCA also may show normal sulfur colloid uptake in 20%.

### 18. How does HCA appear on imaging modalities?

- *US* typically shows a heterogeneous mass due to areas of internal hemorrhage; however, the mass may be hyperechoic because of the high lipid content.
- On *NCCT*, a hypodense mass is typically seen due to intratumoral fat; however, internal areas of higher attenuation may be present due to recent hemorrhage. Hemorrhage is a key distinguishing feature from FNH. Contrast-enhanced CT may show centripetal enhancement similar to that in hemangiomas, although this enhancement does not persist in adenomas.
- On *MR*, HCA is iso- to slightly hyperintense on T2W images and has variable signal on T1W images. It may be hyperintense on T1W images due to internal fat/glycogen, although similar findings may be seen in HCC. HCA can demonstrate decreased signal on out-of-phase imaging due to the high lipid content. Enhancement is most pronounced in the HAP with rapid washout in the PVP. HCA is commonly heterogeneous as a result of necrosis and internal hemorrhage, and the presence of hemorrhage helps differentiate HCA from HCC.

Because of the absence of Kupffer cells, *sulfur-colloid scintigraphy* usually demonstrates decreased uptake; however, HCA may show normal sulfur colloid uptake in 20% and occasionally even increased uptake.

### 19. Describe the appearance of a hepatic abscess on imaging.

- *US:* On US, a hepatic abscess appears as a complex fluid collection, typically with septations, an irregular wall, and debris or air within the fluid. Air is seen as a focal area of echogenicity with posterior shadowing. An abscess can also appear as a simple fluid collection, similar to a cyst.
- *CT:* CT is the most sensitive imaging modality; however, the CT findings vary with the size and age of the abscess. Generally, an abscess appears as a well-defined low-attenuating mass that may be uni- or multilocular and contain internal septations. It typically has a well-defined enhancing wall. The most specific sign for an abscess is air bubbles within the abscess cavity, although this sign is not present in the majority of cases.
- *MRI:* An abscess appears as a well-defined lesion of low signal intensity on T1W images and high signal intensity on T2W images. The cavity may contain septations and have homogeneous or heterogeneous signal. The capsule has a low-signal rim and may enhance with gadolinium.

Other causes of complex cysts, such as a focal hematoma, and necrotic or hemorrhagic neoplasm, may have similar appearances.

## DOPPLER IMAGING OF THE LIVER

### 20. What is a normal Doppler waveform?

A *normal* Doppler waveform is different for each artery or vein of the body. Veins have continuous low-velocity flow that frequently varies with respiration. In the portal vein, flow is normally hepatopedal, toward the liver, and generally ranges from 15 to 18 cm/sec. Flow in the hepatic veins is triphasic and pulsatile and directed away from the liver into the IVC. Arterial flow varies dramatically with the cardiac cycle, showing high-velocity flow during systole and relatively high flow (i.e., low resistance) during diastole.

The change in frequency of reflected sound waves from flowing blood, also known as the Doppler frequency shift, and the angle at which the US beam interfaces with the flowing blood, the Doppler angle, are utilized by US to calculate the velocity and direction of blood flow. It is important to remember that the Doppler angle should be less than 60 degrees to avoid erroneous velocity calculations. In grey scale, these data are presented on a graph with the baseline representing no flow and the operator determining whether to display flow toward the transducer as either above or below the baseline.

Color Doppler can also be used to verify the presence and direction of flow. The operator determines whether blood flowing toward the transducer is blue or red, and blood flowing away from the transducer takes on the other color. Therefore, flow in arteries and veins normally is assigned a different color.

### 21. Describe the sonographic findings of portal hypertension on Doppler waveforms.

Portal hypertension can be suggested on US by a portal vein (PV) diameter of greater than 13 mm, an increase of less than 20% in the PV diameter with deep inspiration, a monophasic waveform, and decreased flow velocity. However, the portal vein size is so variable that specific measurements are unreliable and, in fact, the size of the portal vein may decrease with the development of portosystemic collaterals, which develop later with portal hypertension. The easiest collateral to detect by US is the recanalized paraumbilical vein, which drains the left portal vein as it travels through the ligamentum teres to the abdominal wall. The coronary (left gastric) vein, another collateral vessel, connects with the portosplenic confluence and ascends to the gastroesophageal junction, producing esophageal varices. Other portosystemic collaterals include splenorenal shunts, retroperitoneal veins, and hemorrhoidal veins. Retrograde (hepatofugal) flow in the portal vein indicates advanced disease and is a useful but late finding (Fig. 70-7).

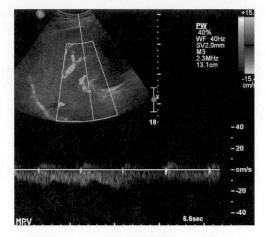

**Figure 70-7.** Hepatofugal flow. Doppler ultrasound image of the main portal vein in the setting of cirrhosis and portal hypertension demonstrates the waveform being below the baseline indicating flow away from the transducer and away from the periphery of the liver.

### 22. How are Doppler waveforms altered in portal vein thrombosis?

In more acute portal vein thrombosis, flow in the portal vein is markedly diminished or absent. In most instances, echogenic material is seen in the portal vein, although in a few cases the portal vein may appear normal. Doppler analysis yields no waveform, and with color imaging, no color is seen in the vessel. In cavernous transformation of the portal vein, which may take 12 months to develop, the portal vein is not identified; however, there are multiple tubular channels in the porta hepatis with demonstrable flow by color imaging or Doppler evaluation. An arterial waveform within the thrombus has a high specificity for malignancy.

### 23. How does Budd-Chiari syndrome affect Doppler waveforms?

Budd-Chiari syndrome refers to obstruction of hepatic venous outflow. It can occur at a number of levels, from the small hepatic venules to the IVC. Typically, the liver parenchyma is diffusely heterogeneous, but to make the diagnosis, one must observe echogenic thrombus or absent flow in one or more of the hepatic veins or the suprahepatic IVC. Intrahepatic collaterals extending from the hepatic veins to the liver surface are common. Twenty percent of patients have associated portal vein thrombosis, and many have ascites. The caudate lobe is frequently spared as it has separate drainage to the IVC.

### 24. Discuss the role of US in the evaluation of transjugular intrahepatic portosystemic shunts (TIPS).

A baseline sonographic examination, documenting flow within the shunt and determining velocity measurements in the middle and both ends of the shunt, is obtained 24 to 48 hours after the procedure. The flow is usually of high velocity and turbulent; however, there is a wide range of normal velocities in patent, well-functioning shunts. A minimum velocity less than 90 cm/sec and certainly less than 50 to 60 cm/sec, a peak velocity of greater than 190 cm/sec, or a gradient (difference between maximum and minimum velocity) of greater than 100 cm/sec should prompt a portogram for further evaluation. Additional signs of a failing shunt include reaccumulation of ascites, reappearance or increased size of varices, and blood flow away from the shunt. Routine follow-up imaging is recommended in 3 months, 6 months, 12 months, and then annually.

## BILIARY TRACT IMAGING

### 25. Describe the sonographic findings in acute cholecystitis

A wall thickness greater than 3 mm in a distended gallbladder is abnormal and must be explained. Acute cholecystitis commonly demonstrates gallbladder wall thickening, pericholecystic fluid, a sonographic Murphy sign, and gallstones. Hyperemia within and around the wall and a prominent cystic artery are more specific findings in acute cholecystitis. Overall, sonography has a sensitivity and specificity of 88% and 80%, respectively, for diagnosing acute cholecystitis.

### 26. What other conditions can result in gallbladder wall thickening?

Many other conditions can cause gallbladder wall thickening. Congestive heart failure, constrictive pericarditis, hypoalbuminemia, renal failure, portal venous congestion from portal hypertension, and hepatic veno-occlusive disease can produce gallbladder wall thickening. Inflammation of the gallbladder from nearby hepatitis, pancreatitis, and colitis may also produce wall thickening. Chronic cholecystitis, acquired immunodeficiency syndrome (AIDS)-related cholangitis, adenomyomatosis, primary sclerosing cholangitis, and leukemic infiltration are additional causes of wall thickening. Gallbladder carcinoma also causes wall thickening but is usually easily differentiated by its masslike appearance and association with adenopathy and liver metastases.

## 27. Describe the radiologic workup of suspected biliary tree obstruction.

US is the screening examination of choice when biliary ductal disease is suspected. The size of the common bile duct (CBD) is more sensitive than dilated intrahepatic ducts in assessing early or partial biliary obstruction. A CBD diameter greater than 6 mm indicates ductal dilatation; however, the extrahepatic ductal diameter may increase with age and following cholecystectomy or resolved obstruction. In complicated cases, Doppler examination can readily differentiate the biliary ducts from vasculature in the portal triad. Normal nondilated intrahepatic ducts are less than 2 mm in diameter and less than 40% of the diameter of the adjacent portal vein. With intrahepatic ductal dilatation, tubular low-echogenicity structures are seen to parallel the portal veins, producing the *too many tubes* sign (Fig. 70-8A).

Once biliary disease is detected, MDCT is more efficacious in depicting the degree, site, and cause of obstruction because bowel gas commonly obscures sonographic visualization of the distal CBD (Fig. 70-8B). In addition, MDCT provides more complete delineation of the full length of the CBD, especially with the use of coronal MPRs.

Endoscopic retrograde cholangiopancreatography (ERCP) or percutaneous transhepatic cholangiography provides a more detailed evaluation than US or CT but both modalities are invasive. Newer techniques allow the diagnosis of biliary ductal dilatation by MRI and MR cholangiopancreatography (MRCP).

## 28. What is MRCP? What advantages does it have compared with ERCP?

MRCP is a noninvasive way to evaluate the hepatobiliary tract using heavily T2W images. MRCP can reliably demonstrate the common bile duct, the pancreatic duct, the cystic duct and aberrant hepatic ducts. It can differentiate dilated from normal ducts, and it exceeds the accuracy of CT and US in detecting choledocholithiasis. It is comparable to ERCP in detecting choledocholithiasis and in detecting extrahepatic strictures (Fig. 70-9).

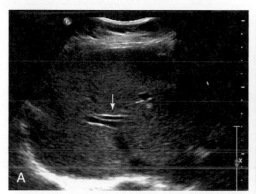
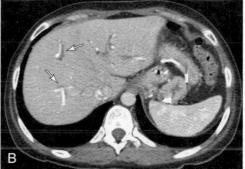

**Figure 70-8.** Intrahepatic ductal dilatation. *A,* Sonographic image demonstrates the double duct sign (*arrow*) consistent with intrahepatic ductal dilatation. *B,* Contrast-enhanced axial computed tomography image demonstrates nonenhancing dilated ducts (*open arrows*).

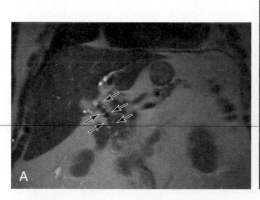
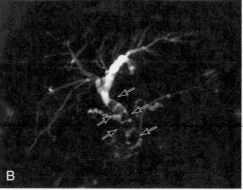

**Figure 70-9.** Choledocholithiasis. *A,* Coronal T2-weighted magnetic resonance image demonstrates numerous gallstones (*open arrows*) within the common bile duct. *B,* MRCP depicts choledocholithiasis (*open arrows*) in same patient.

The advantages of MRCP over ERCP are that it is noninvasive, less expensive, does not require radiation or sedation, can detect extraductal pathology, better visualizes ducts proximal to an obstruction and visualizes the ducts in their *native* state. In addition, MRCP can be performed in patients in which ERCP has been unsuccessful. The main drawback of MRCP is that it may delay therapeutic intervention in patients with a high clinical suspicion of bile duct obstruction. Other drawbacks of MRCP relate to decreased spatial resolution which limits the evaluation of nondilated, peripheral intrahepatic or side ducts.

MRCP is comparable to ERCP in diagnosing extrahepatic biliary and pancreatic duct abnormalities, and it is the modality of choice for imaging patients with biliary-enteric anastomoses. It is more sensitive than ERCP in detecting pseudocysts and is potentially more accurate in evaluating biliary cystadenomas and cystadenocarcinomas.

## 29. Describe the differential imaging features seen in the common causes of biliary obstruction.

- Biliary obstruction may be related to biliary (choledocholithiasis, cholangitis, cholangiocarcinoma) or extrabiliary disease (pancreatitis, periampullary carcinoma). Intrahepatic ductal dilatation with a normal CBD suggests an intrahepatic mass or abnormality. Dilatation of the pancreatic duct typically localizes the obstruction to the pancreatic or ampullary level.
- An abrupt transition from a dilated CBD to a narrowed or obliterated duct is more characteristic of a neoplasm or stone, whereas a gradual tapering of the CBD at the pancreatic head is typical of fibrosis associated with chronic pancreatitis. However, chronic pancreatitis also can present as a focal mass, and, biopsy may be required for differentiation.
- US is 60% to 70% accurate in detecting common duct stones; unlike gallbladder calculi, CBD stones do not necessarily cause acoustic shadowing. CT detection requires thin-section (3-mm) acquisition. Depending on their composition, stones may be seen as soft tissue or calcific intraluminal densities (Fig. 70-10).

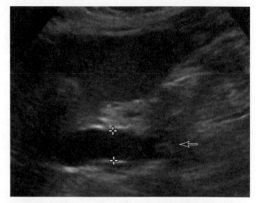

**Figure 70-10.** Sonographic image demonstrates markedly dilated common bile duct (calipers) with obstructing echogenic stone (*arrow*).

- Cholangiocarcinoma should be suspected in patients with abrupt biliary obstruction but no visualized mass or stone. The primary mass is difficult to identify by US. Because cholangiocarcinoma often arises near or at the liver hilum (Klatskin tumor), it commonly presents with dilated intrahepatic ducts and normal-sized extrahepatic ducts. On MDCT, the tumor is typically a low-attenuating mass with mild peripheral enhancement on images obtained 10 to 20 minutes after injection. Unlike HCC, the tumor typically encases and does not invade the adjacent vessels. MRCP and MRI with a hepatobiliary agent or gadolinium is beneficial in the diagnosis. Cholangiocarcinoma typically presents with low T1W and high T2W signal and demonstrates progressive delayed enhancement on MRI due to fibrous tissue within the tumor. This can be helpful in determining the area to biopsy.

## PANCREATIC IMAGING

## 30. How can acute pancreatitis be distinguished from chronic pancreatitis on imaging?

### *ACUTE*

US is limited in the initial evaluation of acute pancreatitis for several reasons:

1. Overlying bowel gas frequently limits complete visualization of the gland.
2. Evaluating the extent of peripancreatic fluid collections is inferior to that of CT.
3. Unlike CT, US cannot diagnose pancreatic necrosis. However, US is effective in the follow-up of pseudocysts, which may be echo-free or have internal echogenicity due to hemorrhage or debris.

CT is the preferred study in patients with clinically severe pancreatitis. An initial unenhanced scan is typically performed to detect calculi, pancreatic calcifications, and hemorrhage. Imaging in the pancreatic phase (35 to 40 seconds after intravenous contrast injection) and in the PVP is performed. MPRs are helpful to better depict the anatomy. CT is not performed to make the diagnosis of pancreas, as the exam may be normal in mild cases of pancreatitis, but rather to evaluate for necrosis or other complications. When CT abnormalities are present, the pancreas appears enlarged and slightly heterogeneous, with inflammation causing peripancreatic fat to have a higher attenuation (*dirty fat*). With more *severe* disease, intraglandular intravasation of pancreatic fluid causes intrapancreatic fluid collections, and

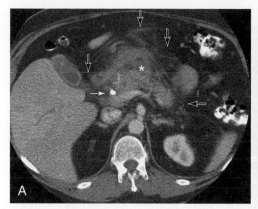
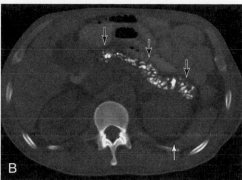

**Figure 70-11.** Pancreatitis. *A,* Contrast-enhanced computed tomography (CT) image in patient with acute pancreatitis due to obstruction from pancreatic carcinoma. Extensive stranding in the peripancreatic fat (*open arrows*), a nonenhancing pseudocyst anterior to the pancreatic body (*) and a common bile duct stent (*arrow*) are noted. *B,* Noncontrast CT image demonstrates numerous calcifications within the pancreas consistent with chronic pancreatitis (*black or upper arrows*). Left perinephric fat stranding (*arrow*) due to pyelonephritis.

extravasation causes peripancreatic fluid collections, peripancreatic inflammation, and thickened fascial planes. Fluid collections are most common in the anterior pararenal space and lesser sac but may have wide extension (Fig. 70-11*A*).

### CHRONIC

US may demonstrate calcifications, ductal dilatation, heterogeneous echotexture, focal mass lesions, and pseudocysts in chronic pancreatitis. The gland may be diffusely enlarged early in the disease but become atrophic with focally enlarged areas later.

Similar findings are noted with CT. The gland size is variable, and focal enlargement due to a chronic inflammatory mass may necessitate biopsy to exclude carcinoma. The pancreatic duct can be dilated (greater than 3 mm) to the level of the papilla and may appear beaded, irregular, or smooth. Intraductal calcifications are the most reliable CT indicator of chronic pancreatitis (Fig. 70-11*B*). Pseudocysts may be seen within or adjacent to the gland.

**31. Describe the role of CT and US in assessing the complications of pancreatitis.**
- *Pseudocysts* evolve from fluid collections in about 10% to 20% of patients with acute pancreatitis. The development of a pseudocyst requires 4 to 6 weeks. More than half of those measuring less than 5 cm regress spontaneously. Pseudocysts failing to resolve after 6 weeks, those remaining larger than 5 cm in diameter and those causing symptoms (pain, infection, hemorrhage, GI obstruction, or fistula) require drainage. US typically demonstrates an anechoic fluid collection with or without internal debris surrounded by a thin wall; however, a complex or even solid appearance can occur early in formation. On enhanced CT, a pseudocyst appears as a well-defined fluid collection with a uniformly thin, enhancing wall. Gas bubbles inside a pseudocyst relate to infection or fistula formation within the bowel.
- *Acute peritonitis* may occur after a pseudocyst ruptures into the peritoneal cavity. Pancreatic ascites, which also presents as free intraperitoneal fluid from leakage of fluid anteriorly, does not present with peritonitis. Posterior leakage of fluid can present with a pleural effusion, classically on the left.
- CT can detect *necrosis* with an accuracy of about 85%. Necrosis is defined as a lack of contrast enhancement in the expected location of pancreatic tissue, and it can develop early or late in the course of the illness. It is best demonstrated by CT, 2 to 3 days after the onset of symptoms. The degree of necrosis is an important prognostic factor. Patients with no CT evidence of necrosis have a 0% mortality rate and a morbidity rate of only 6%. Patients with mild necrosis (less than 30% of the total gland) exhibit a 0% mortality rate but have a rate of complications of 40%, and patients with more severe necrosis (greater than 50%) have a mortality rate of 11% to 25% and a morbidity rate of 75% to 100%. Necrotic tissue can become secondarily infected, which is recognized on CT as gas bubbles within areas of pancreatic gland necrosis (i.e., emphysematous pancreatitis). More commonly, infected areas do not contain gas, and a culture of a percutaneous aspirate is needed to verify the diagnosis and identify the organism.
- *Pancreatic abscesses* result from liquefactive necrosis with subsequent infection. US shows a hypo to anechoic mass with a surrounding thickened wall. CT shows a focal low-attenuation fluid collection with thick enhancing walls. If gas bubbles are present, an abscess needs to be excluded. Rates of abscess formation vary with the amount of pancreatic necrosis. Abscesses usually occur 4 weeks after the onset of acute pancreatitis. The distinction between abscess and infected necrosis can be difficult, but it is an important one because a pancreatic abscess usually requires more aggressive treatment.

- *Pseudoaneurysms,* resulting from enzymatic breakdown of the arterial wall, most commonly involve the splenic artery, followed by the gastroduodenal and pancreaticoduodenal arteries. Rupture of the pseudoaneurysm can occur in up to 10% of cases resulting in massive hemorrhage usually into a pseudocyst but can occur into the retroperitoneum, peritoneal cavity, pancreatic duct, or bowel, resulting in a GI bleed. MDCT is probably best for identifying pseudoaneurysms, which present as densely enhancing structures, usually in close proximity to a pseudocyst. US with color Doppler can be just as sensitive in detecting pseudoaneurysms and their complications, provided that there is no overlying bowel gas. Angiography can be performed for embolization, which is successful in at least 75% of cases.
- *Splenic vein thrombosis* is detected by lack of normal enhancement in the expected region of the splenic vein on MDCT and is present in up to 45% of cases of chronic pancreatitis. Color Doppler can be used to make the same diagnosis. Thrombosis of the portal and superior mesenteric veins, although less common, is also well imaged by both modalities. The presence of splenic vein thrombosis increases the risk of bleeding gastric varices.

## 32. What are the imaging findings of pancreatic ductal adenocarcinoma?

- *Pancreatic enlargement.* Although enlargement may be focal or diffuse, focal enlargement is more common. Diffuse enlargement is often secondary to pancreatitis caused by the neoplasm. Focal enlargement is better appreciated in the body and tail of the pancreas.
- *Distortion of the pancreatic contour or shape.* Enlargement and contour distortion are the most frequent findings of pancreatic cancer.
- *Difference in density or echogenicity.* On US pancreatic cancer tends to be hypoechoic compared with normal pancreas; however, it also may appear isoechoic compared with normal pancreas. On CT, it is usually hypodense in comparison with normal pancreas; a finding better demonstrated with the use of intravenous contrast.
- *Pancreatic duct dilatation* can be an important clue of a small neoplasm that may not be appreciated otherwise. It is more common when the neoplasm is located in the pancreatic head.
- *Biliary tract dilatation.* Bile duct dilatation is more commonly seen with a neoplasm in the head of the pancreas. Isolated intrahepatic biliary ductal dilatation may be seen with pancreatic cancer that has spread to the porta hepatis.
- *Local invasion* into the peripancreatic fat is most commonly seen, but invasion into the porta hepatis, stomach, spleen, and adjacent bowel loops also may occur.
- *Regional lymph node enlargement.* Pancreatic cancer may spread to the nodes in the porta hepatis, para-aortic region, and area around the celiac and superior mesenteric artery axis.
- *Liver metastasis.* The liver is a common site of metastasis for pancreatic cancer. Metastases appear as low-density lesions.

## 33. Which imaging modality is best for detecting and staging pancreatic cancer?

MDCT with MPRs is the best imaging modality. MDCT is better at evaluating adjacent spread or nodal involvement than US, and it does not have the problem of incomplete evaluation of the pancreas due to overlying bowel gas. However, if the pancreas is completely evaluated with sonography, carcinoma can reliably be excluded. Dynamic MRI with gadolinium can be performed in patients with iodine contrast allergy.

## 34. What are the CT criteria for unresectability of pancreatic carcinoma?

If there is peripancreatic vascular invasion or involvement of greater than 50% of the vascular circumference with tumor, lymph node metastases remote to the peripancreatic chain, malignant ascites, or metastatic disease, the tumor is considered unresectable. MDCT has a negative predictive value (NPV) of 87% for resectability and 100% for vascular invasion.

## 35. What are the characteristic features of the major cystic pancreatic neoplasms?

Serous (microcystic) and mucinous (macrocystic) cystic, intraductal papillary mucinous, and solid papillary epithelial neoplasms are the most common.

Serous tumors are more common in women aged 60 years or older. They are almost always benign and predominate in the pancreatic head. Serous tumors calcify more commonly than any other pancreatic tumors and are typified by a central stellate scar, which may calcify. They comprise numerous less than 2-cm cysts and on US are often hyperechoic because the multiple small cysts may not be individually resolved. The hyperechoic central stellate scar and calcifications suggest the diagnosis and may be seen on US or CT. The CT appearance is also varied; innumerable minute cysts may appear as a solid tumor, whereas multiple small but visible cysts have a honeycomb or *Swiss-cheese* appearance.

Mucinous cystic neoplasms also have a strong female predominance but tend to occur in somewhat younger patients. They have a strong predilection for the pancreatic tail (85%), peripherally calcify in 10% to 25% of cases, and must be considered malignant. They are larger lesions, averaging 5 cm, and are composed of unilocular or multilocular cysts greater than 2 cm. US demonstrates internal septations that have variable number and thickness but are typically thicker than those in microcystic tumors. The tumor wall and organ of origin are better demonstrated with CT, whereas internal septations and solid excrescences are better seen by US.

Intraductal papillary mucinous tumors are rare but are most prevalent in men over 60 years of age. They are characterized by the production of large amounts of mucin and ductal dilatation may result from mucin plugs. From 40% to 80% of the tumors are malignant. The presence of intraductal papillary nodules and a prominent duodenal papilla help separate this tumor from chronic pancreatis. ERCP is best for diagnosis. Findings associated with malignancy include: ductal dilatation greater than 10 mm, large mural nodules, intraductal calcifications, bulging duodenal papilla, and diffuse or multifocal involvement.

Solid papillary epithelial neoplasm is most often seen in younger black or Asian females and is characteristically present in the tail of the pancreas. They are often large at presentation (9 cm) and have a low malignant potential.

## ABDOMINAL AND PELVIC IMAGING

### 36. How is simple ascites distinguished from complicated ascites?

* *Simple ascites* is a watery transudate that is usually secondary to major organ system failure (i.e., hepatic, renal, or cardiac failure). Because it is a transudate, simple ascites has a CT density similar to water (0 to 20 HU). In general, as the protein content of the fluid increases, so do the HU. By US, simple ascites is anechoic, without internal echoes or septations, and demonstrates increased through transmission. Simple ascites is *free-flowing* and located in the dependent portions of the abdomen and pelvis. It is often found in Morison pouch, paracolic gutters, and the pelvis. With large amounts of ascites, the bowel seems to float within the fluid, usually in the center of the abdomen. Simple ascites also has a sharp, smooth interface with other intra-abdominal contents (Fig. 70-12).
* *Loculated ascites* is not a *simple* fluid collection, because it indicates the presence of adhesions. The adhesions may be due to benign causes (e.g., prior surgery) or an infectious or malignant process. Loculated ascites is typically located in nondependent portions of the abdomen, does not move when the patient is scanned in a different position, and often displaces adjacent bowel loops.
* *Complex ascites* is usually secondary to an infectious, hemorrhagic, or neoplastic process. Usually, the density measurements must be greater than 20 HU to be considered complex, reflecting the increased protein content. Other findings of complex ascites include internal debris or septations or a thick or nodular border or capsule. The presence of air bubbles within the collection suggests an abscess. Some complex fluid collections do not have these findings and aspiration may be required to confirm whether a collection is simple.

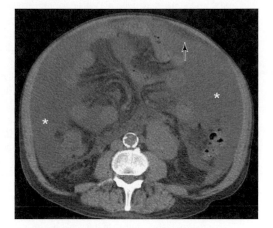

**Figure 70-12.** Ascites. Noncontrast CT image demonstrates marked ascites (*) with elevation of the omental fat (*white open arrow*).

### 37. How do you differentiate abdominal fluid from pleural fluid?

Both US and CT are good modalities to ascertain whether a collection is intra-abdominal or pleural. If the collection can be seen by US, it usually outlines the diaphragm, making the determination less confusing. Certain signs have been described to make this differentiation on CT:

1. Ascites is located anterior or medial to the diaphragmatic crus, whereas pleural fluid is located posterior or lateral to the crus.
2. Pleural effusion can appear to touch the spine or aorta.
3. Abdominal fluid is often contiguous with other abdominal fluid collections.
4. Ascites has a sharp interface with intra-abdominal organs such as the liver and spleen. Pleural fluid has a less sharp interface because the diaphragm lies between the fluid and abdominal organs.
5. Ascitic fluid spares the bare area of the liver, which lies between the left and right coronary ligaments along the posterior border of the right lobe of the liver. The bare area is formed by peritoneal reflections that suspend the liver from the diaphragm. Peritoneal fluid cannot pass through these ligaments to accumulate in the bare area; however, because the bare area is in contact with the diaphragm, pleural fluid can accumulate behind the bare area.

### 38. How has MDCT changed evaluation of the small bowel?

The standard for small bowel imaging has been fluoroscopic small bowel follow-through (SBFT) and enteroclysis. However, the advent of MDCT allows imaging of the entire abdomen in a single breath-hold acquisition, and the creation of MPRs in coronal and sagittal imaging planes facilitates the evaluation of the small bowel. Ideal imaging of the small bowel requires intraluminal contrast, bowel distention, and intravenous contrast to best evaluate the mucosa and bowel wall as well as imaging of the surrounding structures, such as adjacent fat. The use of neutral contrast agents such as Volumen is becoming more common as it allows better depiction of the bowel wall and mucosa compared with positive contrast agents such as meglumine diatrizoate (Gastrografin). This technique is called CT enterography as the intraluminal contrast is administered orally. Alternatively, CT enteroclysis, in which the intraluminal contrast is administered via a nasojejunal tube, can be performed. The latter procedure is invasive; however, some studies indicate that this technique is the best method for diagnosing low-grade small bowel obstruction, often indicating the cause of obstruction, and is a good technique to evaluate for Crohn's disease. One study reported an accuracy of 97% in detecting small bowel pathology with CT enteroclysis.

With adequate distention, the thickness of the bowel wall is usually 4 mm or less on MDCT. Smooth and concentric thickening of the bowel wall is a typical appearance for nonmalignant disease (e.g., Crohn, ulcerative colitis, and ischemic, infectious, or radiation enteritis). Extraintestinal findings are an important part of the exam. In Crohn's disease, MDCT is the best initial exam in the acute setting, and one should look for associated abscesses, fibrofatty proliferation, fistulas, and inflammation of the mesentery. However, SBFT remains more sensitive for subtle mucosal changes compared with MDCT (Fig. 70-13).

**Figure 70-13.** Crohn's disease. Computed tomography image depicts small bowel wall thickening (*open arrows*) in this patient with Crohn's disease. Adjacent fluid within the mesentery is noted. (*).

*Eccentric and irregular bowel wall thickening* greater than 2 cm is suspicious for carcinoma, especially if confined to a short segment with adenocarcinoma being the most common primary small bowel malignancy. Adenocarcinoma should be considered in the presence of associated liver lesions. Small bowel carcinoids are the next most common primary small bowel malignancy and are typically located in the ileum, usually contain calcification, and have a surrounding desmoplastic reaction. Lymphoma should be considered if there is associated massive mesenteric or retroperitoneal adenopathy; most benign small bowel tumors, such as neurofibromas and leiomyomas, are difficult to distinguish from malignant tumors; however, lipomas are the exception. They are easily recognized by their low attenuation (−90 to −120 HU). The most common metastatic tumor to the small bowel is colon carcinoma.

MDCT is a useful tool in the evaluation of *small bowel obstruction*, especially when the diagnosis is in doubt; however, supine and erect abdominal radiographs should remain the initial diagnostic exam. In addition to determining if the bowel is obstructed, MDCT, particularly when MPRs are used, can determine the cause and level of obstruction, especially when the obstruction is high grade. The site of obstruction or *transition zone* is the location in which the proximal bowel is dilated and the distal bowel is decompressed. MDCT can also determine if there is a closed-loop obstruction or bowel ischemia. Bowel ischemia should be considered when wall thickening, mesenteric stranding, and mesenteric fluid are present. Pneumatosis, portal venous gas, and intramural hemorrhage are present in more severe cases. *Enteroenteric intussusception* is easily defined by the invaginated low-density mesenteric fat situated between the higher density of the inner intussusceptum and the outer intussuscipiens. (Fig. 70-14).

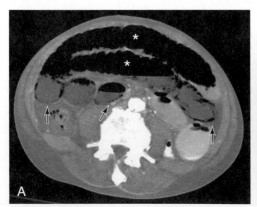
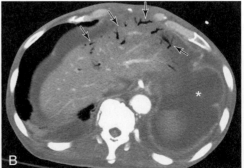

**Figure 70-14.** Ischemia. *A,* Computed tomography (CT) image demonstrates dilated air and fluid filled small bowel loops (*). Air is present in the nondependent walls of multiple small bowel loops (*open arrows*). *B,* CT image demonstrates intrahepatic air within multiple branches of the portal vein (*open arrows*). Ascites is also noted (*).

## 39. How is CT used to evaluate the large bowel?

Optimal evaluation of the colon requires bowel preparation and luminal distention with rectal contrast or air to evaluate the true wall thickness. Normal wall thickness of a distended colon is less than 3 mm, 3 to 6 mm is indeterminate, and greater than 6 mm is abnormal. The addition of intravenous contrast facilitates the evaluation of the bowel wall and improves the evaluation of solid organs and vascular structures.

Wall thickening is present in numerous conditions including Crohn's disease, ischemic colitis, pseudomembranous colitis, radiation colitis, neutropenic colitis, and inflammatory colitis due to cytomegalovirus (CMV) or *Campylobacter* infection. On contrast-enhanced CT, wall thickening can present either as homogeneous enhancing soft tissue density or as concentric rings of high attenuation from hyperemic enhancement of the mucosa and serosa surrounding the low attenuation of the nonenhancing submucosa termed the *halo* or *target* sign (Fig. 70-15).

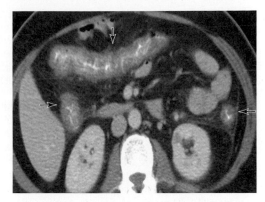

**Figure 70-15.** Colitis. Computed tomography image demonstrates marked circumferential wall thickening of the colon (*open arrows*) in patient with pseudomembranous colitis.

The cause of wall thickening sometimes can be determined by location or associated findings. For example, bowel wall thickening in the region of the splenic flexure suggests ischemic disease from hypoperfusion in the watershed area between the superior mesenteric artery (SMA) and inferior mesenteric artery (IMA) distribution. Inflammation from a ruptured appendix can produce wall thickening mimicking a primary cecal process, and a severe episode of pancreatitis can cause thickening of the transverse colon if inflammatory changes spread through the transverse mesocolon.

Irregular, eccentric, or lobulated wall thickening is suggestive of *adenocarcinoma*. In some cases, an intraluminal polypoid mass can be seen. Findings of regional adenopathy, retroperitoneal adenopathy or liver metastases help to confirm the diagnosis of carcinoma. Signs of extracolonic extension include strands of soft tissue extending into the pericolonic fat, loss of fat planes between the colon and surrounding structures and a masslike appearance. CT is useful in evaluating anastomotic recurrence from colorectal carcinoma, which can occur in the serosa beyond the reach of the endoscope. PET (positron emission tomography) imaging is used to stage colorectal carcinoma.

## 40. Describe the optimal radiographic workup of diverticulitis.

MDCT is greater than 95% accurate in the diagnosis of diverticulitis. It is superior to other modalities because it directly depicts the severity of the pericolic inflammation and the full degree of intraperitoneal or retroperitoneal extension. It is more sensitive than a barium study in detecting abscesses and fistulas.

The hallmark of acute diverticulitis on CT is increased attenuation in the pericolic fat or *dirty fat*. With greater degrees of inflammation, a soft tissue phlegmon or a fluid- and occasionally air-containing abscess may be seen. With free perforation, air bubbles may be seen in the peritoneal cavity or retroperitoneum. Diverticula and a thickened bowel wall are usually present, but these findings are nonspecific. The bowel wall thickening occasionally may be difficult to distinguish from colon cancer. Findings that suggest tumor include: a short segment (less than 10 cm), an abrupt transition zone, wall thickness greater than 2 cm, lymphadenopathy and metastases (Fig. 70-16).

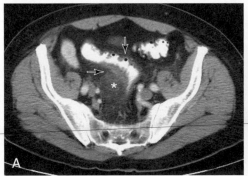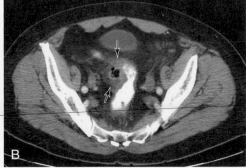

**Figure 70-16.** Diverticulitis. *A,* Computed tomography (CT) image demonstrates thickened wall of the sigmoid colon (*open arrows*) with stranding in the adjacent fat (*) indicative of diverticulitis. *B,* CT image slightly more caudal demonstrates an air-filled abscess cavity (*open arrows*) with adjacent thickened sigmoid colon wall.

The assessment of the colon by CT is greatly improved with adequate colonic opacification or distention with oral contrast or, if the patient has no peritoneal signs, with rectal air insufflation or water-soluble contrast administration.

## 41. What are the CT and US findings of acute appendicitis?

- *US:* Findings of acute appendicitis include a distended (greater than 6 mm) and noncompressible appendix with or without an adjacent fluid collection, an appendicolith, peritoneal fluid, abnormal flow in the wall of the appendix and a focal mass representing a phlegmon or abscess.
- *CT:* The hallmark finding is a distended (greater than 6 mm), thick-walled appendix with abnormal enhancement. An appendicolith may be seen in one-fourth of cases. Local signs of inflammation include increased density or stranding in the adjacent fat tissue, focal thickening of adjacent fascia, focal fluid collections, and adjacent phlegmon or abscess (Fig. 70-17).

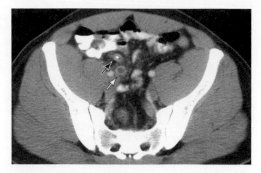

**Figure 70-17.** Appendicitis. Computed tomography image demonstrates dilated fluid filled appendix (*bottom arrow*) with minimal surrounding fat-stranding and an appendicolith (*top arrow*).

## 42. Which examination is better for diagnosing acute appendicitis?

The sensitivity and specificity of CT are slightly superior to those of US, and CT is better at demonstrating both a normal appendix and the extent of adjacent inflammatory changes. The disadvantages of CT are its higher cost, use of ionizing radiation, and use of contrast material. US is highly operator dependent but is usually a good first choice in children, pregnant women, and thin people. CT should be used for all other types of patients and is more effective in obese patients.

## 43. Discuss the role of imaging in the assessment of intra-abdominal abscess

- *US:* US is best suited for evaluation of abscesses in the pelvis and right and left upper quadrants, where the bladder, liver, and spleen, respectively, provide acoustic windows for sound transmission. Abscesses have a varied appearance but commonly are irregularly marginated and primarily hypoechoic, with internal areas of increased echogenicity. US can also be performed at the patient's bedside, unlike other modalities.
- *MDCT:* CT is the first choice for detecting abscess in acutely ill patients. The CT appearance of an abscess depends on its maturity. Initially, an abscess may appear as a soft-tissue density mass. As it matures and undergoes liquefactive necrosis, the central region develops a near-water attenuation, possibly with internal air bubbles or an air-fluid level. Granulation tissue forming the wall of the abscess typically enhances with intravenous contrast, providing a higher attenuation rim. Mass effect with displacement of surrounding structures may be seen, and increased density in the adjacent fat is common.

## 44. What is CT or *virtual colonoscopy* and how effective is it in screening for polyps?

CT colonoscopy (CTC) requires a thin-section MDCT and dedicated CT colonography software. Bowel preparation requires catharsis usually with magnesium citrate or sodium phosphate. The addition of dilute 2% CT barium to tag residual stool and/or diatrizoate (Gastrografin) to opacify luminal fluid helps differentiate stool from polyps. Distension is performed with either room air or automated $CO_2$ delivery via a small-caliber flexible catheter. Advantages over optical colonoscopy are that sedation is NOT required and other areas of the abdomen can be evaluated; however, CTC exposes the patient to radiation. Most studies suggest that the accuracy of CTC is greater than barium enemas and approaches optical colonoscopy, especially for polyps greater than 10 mm if the colon is properly prepped and distended. However, there is a steep learning curve for the interpretation of the exams, which requires the review of both two- and three-dimensional images and only very well-trained and experienced radiologists should interpret the exams.

# AIDS-RELATED DISORDERS

## 45. What characteristic features of AIDS are seen in the biliary system?

There are three main categories of biliary disease in AIDS patients: non–HIV-associated pathology, acalculous cholecystitis, and AIDS cholangiopathy.

Gallstones and benign bile duct strictures can also be seen in AIDS patients and should be excluded.

Acalculous cholecystitis, which manifests with gallbladder wall thickening, pericholecystic fluid, and a sonographic Murphy sign, is usually seen in patients with concurrent CMV or *Cryptosporidium* infection as well as sclerosing cholangitis or papillary stenosis. Cholecystectomy is usually an effective treatment.

HIV or AIDS-related cholangiopathy is usually secondary to infection with *Cryptosporidium* or less commonly CMV and typically occurs in patients with CD4 counts less than 100. US is often initially performed, and a negative exam virtually excludes the diagnosis. ERCP or MRCP displays the morphologic appearance of the entire ductal system better than US or CT. Irregular extrahepatic and intrahepatic (left greater than right) dilated ducts, beading of the mucosa, wall thickening, papillary narrowing, diffuse intrahepatic or extrahepatic strictures, intraductal debris, or any combination of these findings can be seen in AIDS-related cholangitis. These findings may mimic those of sclerosing cholangitis, papillary stenosis, or both. With the advent of newer antiretroviral therapy, the incidence has decreased substantially.

Biliary ductal dilatation can also be caused by obstruction from enlarged lymph nodes in the porta hepatis from *Kaposi sarcoma (KS)* or *lymphoma*. Non–AIDS-related conditions, such as biliary calculi, cholangiocarcinoma, or pancreatic carcinoma, also may be a consideration. A search for these entities should be made in the appropriate clinical setting.

### 46. Describe the imaging features of AIDS in the liver.

*Hepatomegaly* is seen in nearly 67% of patients with AIDS with most hepatic disorders present when there is advanced immunosuppression. *Mycobacterium avium-intracellulare* complex (MAC) is the most common opportunistic pathogen found on liver biopsy in patients with HIV. On US, multiple small echogenic foci can be seen with MAC; however, focal lesions in the liver are seen more commonly with *Mycobacterium tuberculosis* (MTB) as MTB infection usually occurs when the patient has a higher CD4 count and can more effectively mount an immune response. MAC may present with multiple low-attenuating lesions on CT due to granuloma formation. Diffusely increased liver echogenicity on US is often caused by fatty infiltration; however, *hepatic granulomata* caused by *MAC, MTB, Cryptococcus,* histoplasmosis, CMV, toxoplasmosis, or drug toxicity can also produce an echogenic liver. Infection in the liver also can take the form of single or multiple liver abscesses, especially in intravenous drug users with AIDS, with *Staphylococcus aureus* as the most common organism. Liver calcifications are noted classically in *Pneumocystis carinii* infection but may also be seen with MAC and CMV infection.

KS is the most common neoplasm in AIDS. It is an aggressive tumor in this population, involving any portion of the GI tract. The findings are variable because the tumor is multifocal. US shows hepatomegaly and hyperechoic lesions in the parenchyma. KS can also present with bulky hyperattenuating, markedly enhancing lymphadenopathy on CT in the retroperitoneum and mesentery.

*Non-Hodgkin lymphoma (NHL)* is the second most common AIDS-related neoplasm. NHL in AIDS patients tends to be more aggressive, malignant, and more commonly extranodal and involves the GI tract with greater frequency than in the general population. Usually NHL is associated with bulky adenopathy of the retroperitoneum, mesentery, or mediastinum sometimes in isolation but often with splenic or hepatic masses. On US, lesions are usually hypoechoic, whereas on CT they are generally low in attenuation.

### 47. What extrahepatic manifestations of AIDS in the GI tract can be noted by imaging?

Submucosal nodules with or without ulceration may be seen with barium studies anywhere in the GI tract in patients with KS, but most commonly in the duodenum. CT often demonstrates nodular mural thickening and large focal masses. Lymphadenopathy is usually absent or mild in KS, unlike lymphoma.

NHL in AIDS is usually of B-cell type and aggressive, with a propensity for extranodal distribution. Lymphadenopathy is usually bulky, but an isolated node may be involved. Bowel wall thickening may be a manifestation of GI tract involvement, most commonly involving the stomach, distal ileum, and rectum.

Many opportunistic infections are manifested in patients with AIDS. *Candida albicans,* herpes simplex (HSV), or CMV may cause esophagitis. CT may demonstrate thick-walled bowel with enhancing serosa and mucosa. MTB may involve the ileocecal region, with wall thickening and low-density lymph nodes in the right lower quadrant typical on CT. MAC usually involves the small bowel. *Cryptosporidium* infection on CT has a nonspecific appearance, but mildly dilated, fluid-filled small bowel contents are characteristic.

Imaging of HIV-positive patients often reveals multiple diffuse lymph nodes, located in the retroperitoneum, mesentery, and pelvis. Proctitis may be seen as a thickened rectal wall with increased attenuation of perirectal fat. Patients with clinical AIDS often demonstrate an opportunistic infection or tumor on CT or US. Enlargement of lymph nodes suggests AIDS rather than HIV disease, and focal defects in solid organs suggest either abscess or tumor infiltration.

## BIBLIOGRAPHY

1. Balci NC, Semelka RC. Contrast agents for MR imaging. Radiol Clin N Am 2005;43:887–98.
2. Barish MA, Rocha TC. Multislice CT colonography: Current status and limitations. Radiol Clin N Am 2005;43:1049–62.
3. Federle MP, Jeffrey RB, Desser TS, et al. editors. Diagnostic imaging abdomen. Salt Lake City, UT: Amirsys; 2004.
4. Kamel IR, Liapi E, Fishman EK. Liver and biliary system: Evaluation by multidetector CT. Radiol Clin N Am 2005;43:977–97.

5. Lee JKT, Sagel SS, Stanley RJ, et al. editors. Computed body tomography with MRI. 3rd ed. Philadelphia: Lippincott-Raven; 1998.
6. Martin DR, Danrad R, Hussain SH. MR imaging of the liver. Radiol Clin N Am 2005;43:861–86.
7. Middleton WD, Teefey SA, Darcy MD. Doppler evaluation of transjugular intrahepatic portosystemic shunts. Ultrasound Q 2003;19:56–70.
8. Motohara T, Semelka RC, Bader TR. MR Cholangiopancreatography. Radiol Clin N Am 2003;41:89–96.
9. Oto A, Tamm EP, Szklaruk J. Multidetector row CT of the liver. Radiol Clin N Am 2005;43:827–48.
10. Paspulati RM. Multidetector CT of the pancreas. Radiol Clin N Am 2005;43:999–1020.
11. Patak MA, Mortele KJ, Ros PR. Multidetector row CT of the small bowel. Radiol Clin N Am 2005;43:1063–77.
12. Reeders JWAJ, Yee J, Gore RM, et al. Gastrointestinal infection in the immunocompromised (AIDS) patient. Eur Radiol 2004;14:E84–102.
13. Rumack CM, Wilson SR, Charboneau JW, editors. Diagnostic ultrasound. 3rd ed. St. Louis: Mosby; 2005.
14. Wu CM, Davis F, Fishman EK. Radiologic evaluation of the acute abdomen in the patient with acquired immune immunodeficiency syndrome (AIDS): The role of CT scanning. Semin Ultrasound CT MR 1998;19:190–9.
15. Yukisawa S, Okugawa H, Masuya Y, et al. Multidetector helical CT plus superparamagnetic iron oxide-enhanced MR imaging for focal hepatic lesions in cirrhotic liver: A comparison with multi-phase CT during hepatic arteriography. Eur J Radiol 2007;61:279–89.

# NUCLEAR IMAGING

CHAPTER 71

*Cyrus W. Partington, MD, FACNM, FACR, and
Won Song, MD*

---

1. **Outline the general advantages of nuclear medicine procedures compared with other imaging modalities.**
   - Provide functional information that either is not available by other modalities or is obtained at greater expense or patient risk.
   - High contrast (target-to-background ratio) can be achieved in many instances by nuclear medicine techniques, allowing diagnostic studies despite poor spatial resolution.
   - Relatively noninvasive studies are the rule in nuclear medicine. They require only injection of a radioactive dose or swallowing of a substance, followed by imaging.

2. **What are the disadvantages of nuclear medicine procedures compared with other radiographic studies?**
   - Spatial resolution, usually on the order of 1 to 2 cm, is inferior to that of other imaging modalities.
   - Imaging times can be long, sometimes up to 1 hour or more.
   - Radiation risk is obviously greater than with magnetic resonance imaging (MRI) or ultrasound (US). However, the radiation risk from most nuclear medicine studies is usually significantly less than that of an average computed tomography (CT) study. Gallium-67 and indium-111 white blood cell studies are the exceptions; they involve an average of 2 to 4 times more radiation exposure than other nuclear medicine studies. Positron emission tomography with CT (PET/CT) has the radiation dose of a CT in addition to the radiation from the PET scan. In some studies, such as gastric emptying and esophageal transit studies, radiation risk is insignificant compared with traditional imaging methods, such as fluoroscopy.
   - Availability may be limited. Specialized procedures require radiopharmaceuticals or interpretive expertise not available in all centers.

3. **What nuclear medicine tests are most helpful in gastrointestinal (GI) medicine?**
   Nuclear medicine procedures have been used in the evaluation of nearly every GI problem (Table 71-1). Current improvements in and widespread use of endoscopy, manometry, pH monitoring, and diagnostic radiologic imaging techniques (CT, MRI, US) have limited the use of nuclear medicine to specific clinical problems.

4. **How is cholescintigraphy (hepatobiliary imaging) performed? What is a normal study?**
   The technique for a basic cholescintigraphic study is the same for nearly all of its clinical indications (see Question 3). The patient is injected with a technetium-99m–labeled iminodiacetic acid (IDA) derivative. Although commonly referred to as a HIDA scan, *hepatic IDA* is no longer used in imaging. Disofenin and mebrofenin are used currently because of improved pharmacokinetics. High bilirubin levels (greater than 5 for disofenin and greater than 10 for mebrofenin) can cause a competitive inhibition of radiopharmaceutical uptake; however, administering a higher dose can overcome this impediment.

   After injection, sequential images, usually 1 minute in duration, are routinely obtained for 60 minutes. Normally, the liver rapidly clears the radiopharmaceutical. On images displayed at normal intensity, blood pool activity in the heart is faint or indiscernible by 5 minutes after injection. Persistent blood pool activity and poor liver uptake are indications of hepatocellular dysfunction. Right and left hepatic ducts, the common bile duct, and small bowel are typically visualized within 30 minutes. The gallbladder usually is seen within 30 minutes but can still be considered normal if visualized within 1 hour, provided the patient has not eaten within 4 hours. By 1 hour, nearly all the activity is in the bile ducts, gallbladder, and bowel; the liver is seen faintly or not at all. In all of the studies listed in Question 3, failure to see an expected structure at 1 hour (e.g., gallbladder in acute cholecystitis, small bowel in biliary atresia) requires delayed imaging (4 hours for evaluation for acute cholecystitis, 24 hours for biliary atresia). In some cases, various manipulations, such as sincalide infusion or morphine injection, are performed after the initial 60-minute images.

5. **How should patients with acute cholecystitis be prepared? What manipulations are used to shorten the study or increase its reliability?**
   Traditionally, acute cholecystitis is diagnosed on functional cholescintigraphy by noting a lack of filling of the gallbladder on both the initial 60-minute study and subsequent 4-hour delayed images. Patient preparation is vital in ensuring that lack of gallbladder visualization is a true-positive finding. Use of morphine can also shorten the time needed to complete this study.

527

**Table 71-1.** Uses of Nuclear Medicine Procedures in GI Diseases

| TEST/STUDY | USEFUL IN DIAGNOSIS/EVALUATION |
| --- | --- |
| Cholescintigraphy (hepatobiliary imaging) | Acute cholecystitis<br>Gallbladder dyskinesis<br>Common duct obstruction<br>Biliary atresia<br>Sphincter of Oddi dysfunction<br>Hepatic mass<br>Biliary leak<br>Choleangiointestinal anastomosis patency |
| Gastric emptying | Quantification of gastric motility |
| Esophageal motility/transit | Quantification of esophageal transit<br>Evaluation/detection of reflux<br>Detection of pulmonary aspiration |
| $^{14}$C-urea breath test | Identification of *Helicobacter pylori* infection |
| Liver/spleen scan | Hepatic mass lesions<br>Accessory spleen/splenosis |
| Heat-damaged RBC scan | Accessory spleen/splenosis |
| $^{67}$Gallium scan | Staging of abdominal malignancies<br>Abdominal abscess |
| $^{111}$In-pentetreotide (OctreoScan) | Neuroendocrine tumor staging/recurrence |
| $^{111}$In WBC scan | Evaluation of abdominal infection/abscess<br>Evaluation of active inflammatory bowel disease |
| $^{99m}$Tc-HMPAO WBC scan | Evaluation of active inflammatory bowel disease |
| $^{99m}$Tc-RBC scan | GI bleeding localization<br>Hepatic hemangiomas |
| Pertechnetate (NaTcO4) scanning | Meckel diverticulum |
| $^{99m}$Tc-sulfur colloid dynamic imaging | GI bleeding localization |
| Hepatic arterial perfusion with $^{99m}$Tc MAA | Hepatic intra-arterial catheter perfusion |
| $^{90}$Y microspheres | Treatment of unresectable hepatocellular carcinoma<br>Treatment of hepatic metastatic lesions |
| $^{18}$F-FDG PET and PET/CT | Evaluation of various malignancies<br>Assessment of inflammatory bowel disease |

$^{14}$C, carbon-14; RBC, red blood cell; $^{111}$In, indium-111; $^{99m}$Tc, technetium-99m; HMPAO, hexamethyl-propyleneamine-oxime; WBC, white blood cell; $^{90}$Y, yttrium-90; $^{18}$F-FDG, 18F-fluorodeoxyglucose; PET, positron emission tomography.

Because food is a potent and long-lasting stimulus for endogenous cholecystokinin (CCK) release, the patient should not eat for 4 hours prior to the study because endogenous CCK will prevent normal gallbladder relaxation and consequently impair normal filling. These patients should wait 4 hours to ensure an optimal study. On the other hand, patients who have had a prolonged fast (longer than 24 hours), are receiving intravenous hyperalimentation, or are severely ill can develop viscous bile formation, which cannot be adequately emptied out of a normal gallbladder. This can impair radiopharmaceutical filling of the gallbladder, which in turn can also cause a false-positive study. In these patients at risk for viscous bile formation, the short-acting CCK analog sincalide can be administered (0.02 µg/kg intravenously over 5 minutes), 30 minutes prior to cholescintigraphy. This ensures proper emptying of the gallbladder before the radiopharmaceutical is administered and will prevent a false-positive event from occurring.

Despite these manipulations, the gallbladder may not be visualized during the initial 60 minutes of the study. Rather than re-image at 4 hours, the study can be expedited using morphine (0.04 mg/kg intravenously), provided small bowel activity is seen within the initial 60 minutes. After morphine administration, imaging is continued for another 30 minutes. Because morphine causes sphincter of Oddi contraction, the resultant increased biliary tree pressure will overcome a functional obstruction of the cystic duct. If the gallbladder is still not seen, delayed imaging is not necessary and acute cholecystitis is diagnosed (Fig. 71-1). Overall, the sensitivity for acute calculous cholecystitis is 97% with a specificity of 85%. The sensitivity and specificity are slightly lower in acute acalculous cholecystitis with a sensitivity and specificity of 79% and 87%, respectively. If there is pericholecysitic hepatic activity with a subsequent *rim sign*, the potential for a complicated cholecystitis (i.e., gangrenous or perforated gallbladder) is significantly higher (Fig. 71-2).

### 6. How is cholescintigraphy used to diagnose and manage biliary leak?
Cholescintigraphy is highly sensitive and specific for detecting biliary leak. Nonbile fluid collections are common after surgery and can significantly limit the specificity of anatomic studies. In cases of a post cholecystectomy bile leak, cholescintigraphy can demonstrate accumulation of activity in the gallbladder fossa with progressive activity in dependent regions, commonly the right paracolic gutter (Fig. 71-3). Additional delayed images up to 24 hours after

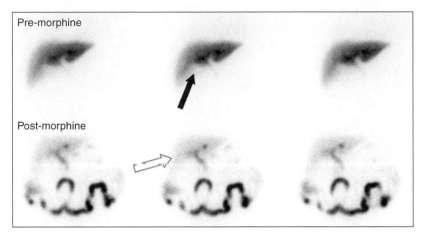

**Figure 71-1.** Acute cholecystitis. Premorphine images: After injection with $^{99m}$Tc mebrofenin, selected 1 minute static images during the initial 60 minute images demonstrate absence of radiotracer in the expected location of the gallbladder (*black arrow*). Despite 60 minutes of imaging, the gallbladder was not visualized. Postmorphine images: To expedite the examination, morphine was administered; however, continued imaging for 30 minutes did not demonstrate gallbladder filling (*white arrow*).

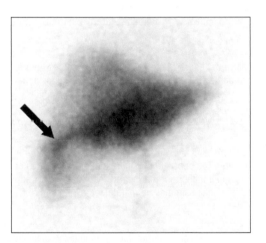

**Figure 71-2.** Acute gangrenous cholecystitis. During the initial 60 minutes of hepatobiliary imaging, pericholecystic hepatic activity (rim sign) is noted without visualization of the gallbladder. The rim sign is thought to be secondary to regional hyperemia, which increases delivery of the radiopharmaceutical to this area, in addition to localized hepatic dysfunction, which prevents efficient excretion of the radiopharmaceutical. Approximately 40% of patients with this type of activity have a perforated or gangrenous gallbladder.

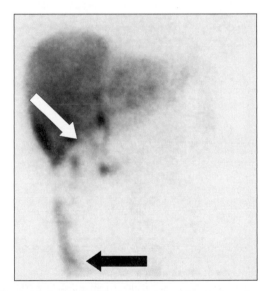

**Figure 71-3.** Bile leak. After laparoscopic cholecystectomy, the patient developed severe right upper quadrant pain. Injection of $^{99m}$Tc mebrofenin was followed with acquisition of 1 minute sequential images. There is accumulation of the radiopharmaceutical in the gallbladder fossa (*white arrow*) as well as activity in the right paracolic gutter "tail sign" (*black arrow*) consistent with bile leak.

injection can demonstrate small leaks. Because cholescintigraphy has poor spatial resolution, the exact origin of the leak may not be determined and endoscopic retrograde cholangiopancreatography (ERCP) or percutaneous transhepatic cholangiography (PTC) may be necessary for anatomic definition. Cholescintigraphy can also be used noninvasively to document resolution of a bile leak. Bilomas can also be detected if there is a focus of increased activity that correlates with a fluid collection noted on previous cross-sectional imaging.

**7. What is the role of cholescintigraphy in diagnosing biliary atresia?**
If the patient is properly prepared for the examination, cholescintigraphy can be helpful in excluding the diagnosis of biliary atresia. The primary differential diagnostic possibility in neonates is severe neonatal hepatitis. The role of scintigraphy is not to diagnose biliary atresia but rather to rule out biliary atresia as a possible diagnosis. To improve the sensitivity of the study, premedication of the neonate with oral phenobarbital (5 mg/kg/day in divided doses for 5 days)

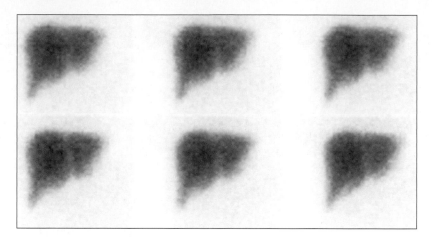

**Figure 71-4.** High-grade biliary obstruction. After injection of $^{99m}$Tc mebrofenin, there is no visible activity in the intrahepatic ducts or small bowel in the initial 60 minutes of images. Additional 4- and 24-hour images (not shown) did not demonstrate activity in the small bowel activity.

is vital, because it stimulates hepatic activity and increases the ability of the liver to extract the radiopharmaceutical. The importance of therapeutic serum levels of phenobarbital cannot be overemphasized because a scan due to poor preparation is indistinguishable from a scan consistent with biliary atresia or neonatal hepatitis. If radioactivity is not seen in the small bowel, delayed images must be obtained and if small bowel is visualized, biliary atresia is ruled out. In adults, absence of activity in the intrahepatic ducts or small bowel can represent a high grade obstruction (Fig. 71-4). In the early stages, conventional imaging will be normal. Fortunately, scintigraphy will demonstrate abnormal excretion before anatomic abnormalities are detectable.

Unfortunately, similar to biliary atresia, severe hepatic dysfunction/hepatitis may have a similar appearance. Additional delayed images should be obtained to assess for activity in the small bowel, which would exclude the diagnosis of a high grade obstruction.

## 8. What is gallbladder dyskinesia? How does cholescintigraphy evaluate the emptying of the gallbladder?

A significant number of patients with normal conventional imaging and clinical evaluation have pain referable to the gallbladder, as evidenced by relief of symptoms after cholecystectomy. The poorly understood and heterogeneous entity of gallbladder dyskinesia has been proposed as the cause of this pain. It is thought that poorly coordinated contractions between the gallbladder and cystic duct can cause pain. Gallbladder dyskinesia may be manifested by an abnormally low ejection of bile under the stimulus of cholecystokinin (sincalide).

After the gallbladder has filled during cholescintigraphy, gallbladder contraction is stimulated by an infusion of sincalide, 0.02 μg/kg over 30 minutes. The amount of gallbladder emptying over 30 minutes reflects the gallbladder ejection fraction (GBEF), normal being greater than 35%. This protocol has demonstrated correlation of both normal and abnormal GBEF with surgical and medical follow-up.

## 9. What nuclear medicine esophageal studies are available? How are they used?

- *Esophageal motility study.* The evaluation of esophageal dysmotility should begin with assessment for anatomic abnormalities using endoscopy, barium swallowing study or computed tomography. This is typically followed by manometry if an anatomic cause is not identified. A nuclear medicine study is performed if a diagnosis is still uncertain. Rapid sequential imaging in either the supine or upright position after ingestion of $^{99m}$Tc-colloid in water is performed with additional subsequent dry swallows during imaging. Esophageal motility studies are also useful in evaluation of response to therapy for dysmotility and achalasia.
- *Esophageal reflux study.* This study is performed by serial imaging of the esophagus after the patient drinks acidified orange juice containing $^{99m}$Tc-sulfur colloid with subsequent serial inflation of an abdominal binder. Although less sensitive than 24-hour pH monitoring, the test is more sensitive than barium studies and can be used as a screening study or evaluation of response to therapy.
- *Pulmonary aspiration studies.* These studies are performed by imaging the chest after oral administration of $^{99m}$Tc-colloid in water or formula in infants. Activity in the lungs is diagnostic of aspiration. Although sensitivity is low, it is likely higher than that of radiographic contrast studies. The test has the advantage of easy serial imaging to detect intermittent aspiration.

## 10. What is a nuclear medicine gastric emptying study?

Either liquid or solid-phase gastric emptying studies can be performed. Liquid studies are typically conducted on infants. After the infant receives a mixture of $^{99m}$Tc-sulfur colloid with milk or formula at the normal feeding time, imaging is performed and an emptying half-time is calculated. In adults, a solid-phase emptying study usually is performed after an overnight fast and subsequent ingestion of $^{99m}$Tc-sulfur colloid–labeled scrambled eggs as part of a standard meal. Anterior and posterior imaging is obtained with either dynamic imaging over 90 minutes or static images at 0, 1, 2, and 4 hours. The percentage of emptying is calculated based on the geometric mean of the anterior and posterior counts. A consensus statement by the Society of Nuclear Medicine has recommended the use of a low-fat, egg-white meal, although this is not necessarily used at every clinic and normal values are institution dependent and will obviously vary with different meal compositions. Using a 285-calorie meal of scrambled eggs, bread, and jam, normal $t_{\frac{1}{2}}$ (time at which 50% of the gastric contents is emptied) gastric emptying time is less than 135 minutes (Fig. 71-5).

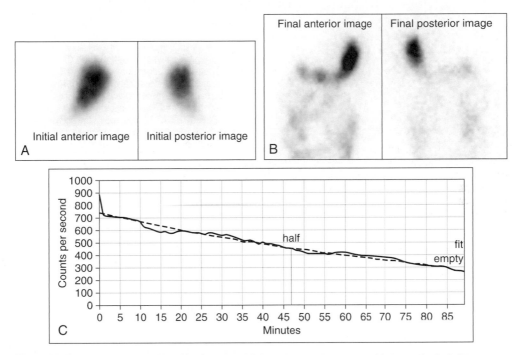

**Figure 71-5.** Normal gastric emptying. After ingestion of $^{99m}$Tc sulfur colloid in two scrambled eggs, 1-minute images were obtained for 90 minutes in the anterior (**A**) and posterior (**B**) projections. Gastric emptying is calculated using the decay correct geometric mean of the counts on the anterior and posterior images. **C,** The emptying curve demonstrates normal gastric emptying with $t_{\frac{1}{2}}$ = 47 minutes and 60% emptying at 90 minutes.

## 11. What is the role for nuclear medicine studies in evaluating hepatic mass lesions?

The traditional liver/spleen scan using an intravenous injection of $^{99m}$Tc-sulfur colloid has largely been replaced by US and dynamic multiphase CT and MRI. In addition to superior resolution with CT and MRI, adjacent structures can also be evaluated. If results are inconclusive, nuclear medicine testing can provide additional information, which can lead to the proper diagnosis.

Sulfur colloid is comprised of small particles (0.3 to 1.0 micrometers) that are phagocytosed by the reticuloendothelial systems, including Kupffer cells in the liver. Lesions that lack Kupffer cells in the liver will not accumulate sulfur colloid. Virtually all neoplasms, including metastasis, focal inflammatory and infectious diseases of the liver, and vascular malformations, manifest as decreased radionuclide activity (*cold*) on both liver-spleen and hepatobiliary imaging. However, focal nodular hyperplasia (FNH) can demonstrate a nonspecific appearance on CT, MRI, and US. If a lesion appears isointense (*warm*) or hyperintense (*hot*) compared with the rest of the liver, it can be presumed to be FNH because no other hepatic lesion contains a sufficient number of Kupffer cells to concentrate sulfur colloid. Occasionally, FNH can appear cold if there are not enough Kupffer cells to accumulate a sufficient amount of sulfur colloid, which unfortunately does not differentiate it from other hepatic masses. Additional imaging with cholescintigraphy will demonstrate early and prolonged uptake of the radiopharmaceutical due to the presence of hepatocytes in FNH with impaired clearance of the radiopharmaceutical from these lesions.

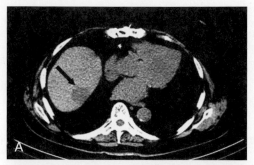

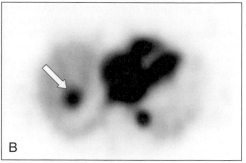

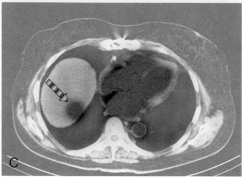

**Figure 71-6.** Evaluation of mass lesion. SPECT/CT scan of the liver using in vitro tagged [99m]Tc RBC. **A,** Initial CT evaluation of the hepatic mass (*black arrow*) demonstrated findings that were suggestive of an atypical hemangioma. Additional evaluation was suggested. **B,** SPECT imaging (using CT attenuation correction from SPECT/CT) demonstrates normal blood pool activity of [99m]Tc RBC with an additional intense focus (*white arrow*) that corresponds to the hepatic mass. **C,** Fused images of simultaneously acquired SPECT and CT images reveals the intense focus to be in the exact region of the hepatic mass consistent with hemangioma.

The evaluation of hepatic lesions is limited on planar imaging to approximately 1 to 2 cm. To evaluate smaller lesions, single-photon emission computed tomography (SPECT) imaging, which is produced using rotating gamma camera heads and reconstructing the data into three dimensions, can be used in the evaluation of lesions in the subcentimeter range.

Utilizing multiphasic imaging with CT or MRI, evaluation for hepatic hemangiomas is excellent. However, if atypical features are noted, imaging using SPECT with [99m]Tc-labeled red blood cells can provide additional information for hemangiomas larger than 2 cm and close to the hepatic surface (Fig. 71-6), frequently at lower cost and without intravenous contrast injection. Additional SPECT imaging also improves the ability to evaluate smaller hemangiomas.

### 12. How can nuclear medicine procedures assist in detecting ectopic gastric tissue?

As a source of pediatric GI bleeding, a Meckel diverticulum invariably contains ectopic gastric mucosal tissue. Because [99m]Tc-pertechnetate is concentrated and extracted by gastric tissue, it is an ideal agent to localize sources of GI bleeding due to a Meckel diverticulum, which can be difficult to detect with traditional radiographic studies.

The study is performed by injecting pertechnetate intravenously and imaging the abdomen for 60 minutes. Typically, ectopic gastric mucosa appears at the same time as gastric mucosa and does not move during imaging. Sensitivity is 85% for detection of bleeding from a Meckel diverticulum. Manipulations to increase the sensitivity of the study may include additional pharmaceuticals such as cimetidine (to block pertechnetate release from ectopic mucosa), pentagastrin (to enhance mucosal uptake), and glucagon (to inhibit bowel motility and prevent movement of the radiopharmaceutical).

### 13. Can accessory splenic tissue or splenosis be detected via nuclear medicine procedures?

After splenectomy as treatment of idiopathic thrombocytopenia, approximately 30% of adult patients can result in treatment failure, which may be secondary to an accessory spleen or splenosis. Unrecognized splenosis may also be a cause of unexplained abdominal pain or present as an abdominal or pelvic mass on CT. The most sensitive imaging procedure for localization of small foci of splenic tissue is the heat-damaged [99m]Tc–red blood cell (RBC) scan, because damaged RBCs localize in splenic tissue intensely and specifically. This is the procedure of choice, especially if SPECT is used. However, the RBC-damaging process requires additional laboratory manipulation and may not be readily available in many clinics. It is therefore reasonable to perform a liver-spleen scan as an initial study and, if it is positive for splenic tissue, to institute appropriate therapy (Fig. 71-7). If it is negative or inconclusive, a heat-damaged RBC study should be performed.

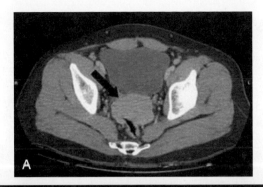

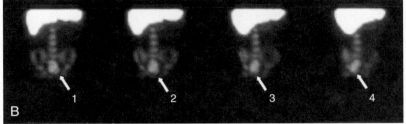

**Figure 71-7.** Splenosis. **A,** CT image of the pelvis demonstrates a large soft tissue mass (*black arrow*) in the pelvis of a patient with a remote history of trauma that eventually led to splenectomy. **B,** SPECT imaging with $^{99m}$Tc sulfur colloid demonstrates increased activity in the pelvis (*white arrows*) that correlates with the pelvic mass, consistent with splenosis.

## 14. Which nuclear medicine procedures are useful in localizing lower GI bleeding?

The difficulty of localizing acute lower GI bleeding is well recognized. Even acute and rapid bleeding can be intermittent and frequently not detected on angiography or the culprit lesion is obscured by luminal blood during endoscopy. Small bowel bleeding distal to areas accessible by upper endoscopy is notoriously difficult to localize.

Two nuclear procedures have been used to localize GI bleeding sources: short-term imaging with $^{99m}$Tc-sulfur colloid injection and extended imaging using $^{99m}$Tc-tagged RBC injection. Despite the theoretical advantage of $^{99m}$Tc-sulfur colloid in being able to detect smaller bleeds, this technique shares the limitation of angiography: a short intravascular residence time, which mandates the bleed to be active at the exact point of imaging. In addition, the normal biodistribution of sulfur colloid to the liver and spleen limits the evaluation of possible bleeds around the hepatic and splenic flexures. $^{99m}$Tc-RBC imaging has assumed dominance because the long intravascular residence time allows detection of intraluminal radioactive blood accumulation if extended imaging is necessary.

The first step is performing an in vitro tagging of RBCs with $^{99m}$Tc-pertechnetate, which provides the highest RBC tagging efficiency. In vitro tagging of radiolabeled RBCs involves obtaining a small blood sample (1 to 3 mL) from the patient and using $^{99m}$Tc-pertechnetate to label the RBCs in reaction vials. The labeled RBCs are injected back into the patient and dynamic 1- or 2-second flow images are obtained over 60 seconds. In the case of a brisk bleed, the flow images will allow for better localization because delayed images will demonstrate significant radiotracer spread through the bowel (Fig. 71-8). Immediately after dynamic flow images are obtained, sequential 1-minute images are acquired for 90 minutes. The use of dynamic imaging is important because sensitivity for localization is higher when the study is displayed in a cine-loop. If the patient has an intermittent bleed and the initial study is negative, images can be acquired up to 24 hours later if the patient actively bleeds again without reinjecting additional tagged RBCs. Unfortunately, delayed images will have a significant disadvantage in localizing the area of active bleeding because of normal peristaltic activity and the additional time from the beginning of the bleed to the time of imaging.

## 15. Are nuclear medicine procedures clinically useful in localizing GI bleeding, or are simpler techniques adequate?

$^{99m}$Tc-RBC studies are more sensitive than both colonoscopy and angiography in detecting intermittent bleeding. Upper endoscopy would be a better choice if an upper GI bleed is suspected because tagged RBC studies are limited in the assessment of the stomach due to physiologic splenic activity. In addition to better visualization, upper endoscopy can also provide therapeutic options. One advantage of the tagged RBC study is that it allows for a survey of both the small and large bowel over a much longer time frame. Once the bleed is localized, therapeutic options with interventional radiology can be facilitated, because less time is required to find which vessel to treat.

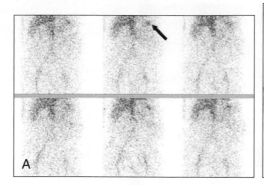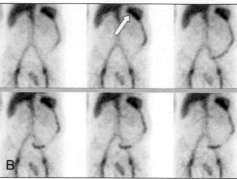

**Figure 71-8.** Gastrointestinal bleed. *A,* After injection of in vitro labeled $^{99m}$Tc RBCs, 1-second per frame flow images were obtained, which demonstrate a focus of increasing activity (*black arrow*) at the splenic flexure. Due to the brisk nature of this bleed, the flow images were useful in localizing the origin of the bleed. *B,* Additional 1-minute-per-frame images demonstrate significant radiotracer uptake at the splenic flexure (*white arrow*) and extending activity moving anterograde down the descending colon and into the sigmoid colon. The patient subsequently had a colectomy performed.

## 16. Is nuclear medicine helpful in placement of arterial perfusion catheters?

The use of hepatic arterial infusion chemotherapy can serve as an adjuvant treatment following surgery or may be used for patients with unresectable disease. Occasional unrecognized systemic shunting, catheter dislodgment, and unintended perfusion of an area not suitable for highly toxic chemotherapeutic drugs hamper placement of hepatic arterial perfusion catheters. Arterial catheter injection of $^{99m}$Tc-macroaggregated albumin (MAA) results in temporary microembolization and provides an imaging map of the true area of perfusion of the catheter. After a baseline scan, if there has been a significant change in perfusion, further therapy with chemotherapy would entail significant risk for gastrointestinal toxicity.

## 17. Are there additional minimally invasive treatments for unresectable malignant liver masses?

Use of yttrium-90 microspheres is a newer treatment option that delivers concentrated radiation to unresectable hepatocellular carcinoma and metastatic disease. $^{90}$Y, with a half-life of 64.5 hours, releases beta particles that radiate adjacent soft tissue with an average penetration of 2.5 mm. $^{90}$Y microspheres have a diameter of approximate 30 μm, which become trapped in the capillary beds of the intended masses and delivery a substantial dose of radiation specifically to these regions without the dangers of systemic radiation.

To safely deliver the dose of radiation to the targeted disease, hepatic angiography via the femoral artery is performed first. To safely map the perfusion and subsequent delivery area of $^{90}$Y microspheres, $^{99m}$Tc-MAA is administered directly to the hepatic artery in the identical manner that the $^{90}$Y microspheres will be delivered. Because $^{99m}$Tc-MAA particles are similarly sized compared to $^{90}$Y microspheres, the biodistribution of these radiopharmaceuticals should be nearly identical. Using the images from $^{99m}$Tc-MAA, the biodistribution is assessed and a shunt fraction is calculated to assess potential unwanted systemic distribution, particularly to the lungs. If these images and calculations demonstrate a safe delivery of $^{99m}$Tc-MAA, then treatment with $^{90}$Y microspheres is possible.

## 18. Can abdominal malignancies be evaluated with nuclear medicine studies?

$^{111}$In pentetreotide (OctreoScan, Mallinckrodt Medical) is a somatostatin analog that targets a variety of neuroendocrine tumors including carcinoid tumors, pancreatic islet cell neoplasm, gastrinoma, pheochromocytoma, neuroblastoma, and paraganglioma. Whole body planar and SPECT imaging are performed at 4 and 24 hours. The additional anatomic information provided by CT images, by fusion software, or with simultaneous acquisition with SPECT/CT provides localization of disease. In addition, if performed with SPECT/CT, the use of attenuation correction can improve detection of lesions deep within the body (Fig. 71-9).

## 19. What is PET and how does it work?

Positron emission tomography (PET) uses specialized positron-emitting radiopharmaceuticals and equipment to detect areas of increased metabolic activity, a characteristic commonly seen in malignancies. The most commonly used radiopharmaceutical in PET imaging is $^{18}$F-fluorodeoxyglucose ($^{18}$F-FDG), which is a marker for glucose metabolism. Unlike other commonly used radiopharmaceuticals in nuclear medicine, $^{18}$F-FDG has a short half-life (110 minutes) and requires a cyclotron for production. Due to the complexity and cost of operating a cyclotron, the vast majority of nuclear medicine clinics do not have an on-site cyclotron and require the use of a separate PET radiopharmacy to provide the PET radiopharmaceutical. In addition, the short half-life of $^{18}$F-FDG and the need to transport the $^{18}$F-FDG from an outside facility to the imaging site can limit the overall accessibility of PET imaging

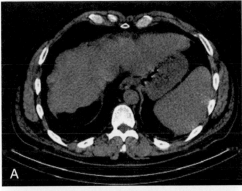
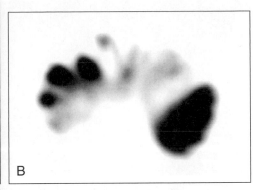
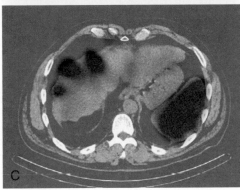

**Figure 71-9.** Metastatic carcinoid. SPECT/CT images were obtained after injection of 6 mCi ¹¹¹In-pentetreotide (OctreoScan). **A,** Noncontrast CT image demonstrates a nodular appearance of the hepatic dome. **B,** Multiple areas of increased uptake are noted in the reconstructed axial image from the CT attenuation corrected SPECT images of ¹¹¹In-pentetreotide. **C,** Fusion of the SPECT and CT images demonstrates anatomic and metabolic correlation of the metastatic carcinoid tumors.

Tumors demonstrate increased ¹⁸F-FDG avidity due to increased expression of glucose transporters (GLUT-1) and hexokinase, which is responsible for phosphorylating glucose and also ¹⁸F-FDG. After ¹⁸F-FDG is phosphorylated, it is not metabolized any further and becomes effectively trapped intracellularly.

Patient preparation for a study using ¹⁸F-FDG entails fasting for 4 to 6 hours prior the examination to optimize the uptake of ¹⁸F-FDG into malignant cells. At the time of the administration of ¹⁸F-FDG, blood glucose levels less than 150 mg/dL are optimal, although images obtained in patients with blood glucose levels up to 200 mg/dL can still yield diagnostic results. Use of insulin can interfere with the biodistribution of ¹⁸F-FDG, which can complicate the preparation of insulin-dependent diabetics.

### 20. What malignancies can PET and PET/CT be used for?

PET has been a proved modality in the evaluation of various malignancies including esophageal, gastric, pancreatic, and colon cancers as well as gastrointestinal stromal tumors (GISTs), carcinoid tumors, and lymphoma. In addition, PET/CT has demonstrated utility in the assessment of inflammatory bowel disease.

Combined with CT, PET/CT exemplifies the value of combined metabolic and anatomic imaging. The most common scenarios in which PET and PET/CT have been useful are staging/surveillance of malignancies and evaluation of postoperative sites.

Although routine staging of colon cancer is not recommended, ¹⁸F-FDG PET/CT has demonstrated significant benefit in assessing recurrence and restaging (Fig. 71-10). Studies with ¹⁸F-FDG have been useful in patients with increasing carcinoembryonic antigen (CEA) levels without anatomic abnormalities and in the evaluation of liver metastases, which are often underestimated with other radiologic modalities.

Detection of primary and metastatic pancreatic cancer using ¹⁸F-FDG PET/CT has been proven as well. Unfortunately, there are some lesions that are not ¹⁸F-FDG avid and the sensitivity of this test has been limited in detecting cystic pancreatic malignancies, mucinous tumors, and low cellular density lesions. In addition, pancreatitis and inflammatory pseudotumors will also demonstrate FDG avidity.

GISTs typically have a rounded, exophytic appearance with well-defined borders on CT imaging. ¹⁸F-FDG PET imaging demonstrates intense activity in malignant GIST, with lower metabolic activity in non-malignant GIST. ¹⁸F-FDG PET can also serve in predicting response to therapy.

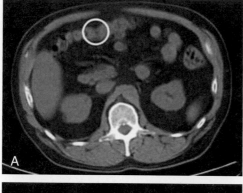
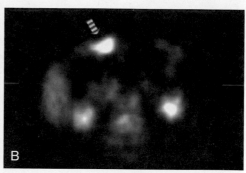
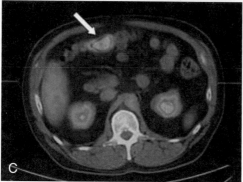

**Figure 71-10.** Colon cancer imaged with [18]F-FDG PET/CT. **A,** CT image demonstrate a soft tissue lesion in the transverse colon (*white circle*). **B,** Simultaneously acquired PET images reveals focal increased FDG activity (*striped arrow*). **C,** Fusion of these two images demonstrates that the increased FDG activity overlies the transverse colon soft tissue lesion (*white arrow*), consistent with malignancy.

One malignancy that has a low sensitivity on [18]F-FDG PET is hepatocellular carcinoma. Typically, poorly differentiated HCC will be [18]F-FDG avid. Well-differentiated HCC can have higher levels of glucose-6-phosphatase, which will dephosphorylate the phosphorylated [18]F-FDG and permit it to leach out of the cell. Alternative PET radiotracers such as [11]C-choline and [11]C-acetate have been shown to have better avidity for well-differentiated HCC but are not as widely available as [18]F-FDG.

## BIBLIOGRAPHY

1. Annovazzi A, Bagni B, Burroni L, et al. Nuclear medicine imaging of inflammatory/infective disorders of the abdomen. Nucl Med Commun 2005;26:657–64.
2. Biancone L, Schillaci O, Capoccetti F, et al. Technetium-99m-HMPAO labeled leukocyte single photon emission computerized tomography (SPECT) for assessing Crohn's disease extent and intestinal infiltration. Am J Gastroenterol 2005;100:344–54.
3. Choi B, Nguyen M. The diagnosis and management of benign hepatic tumors. J Clin Gastroenterol 2005;39:401–12.
4. Ell PJ, Gambhir SS. In: Nuclear medicine in clinical diagnosis and treatment. 3rd ed. Edinburgh: Churchill Livingstone; 2004. pp. 789–818, 837–846.
5. Howarth D. The role of nuclear medicine in the detection of acute gastrointestinal bleeding. Semin Nucl Med 2006;36:133–46.
6. Huynh L, Kim S, Murphy T. The typical appearance of focal nodular hyperplasia in triple-phase CT scan, hepatobiliary scan, and Tc-99m sulfur colloid scan with SPECT. Clin Nucl Med 2005;30:736–9.
7. Ikeda O, Kusunoki S, Nakaura T, et al. Comparison of fusion imaging using a combined SPECT/CT system and intra-arterial CT: assessment of drug distribution by an implantable port system in patients undergoing hepatic arterial infusion chemotherapy. Cardiovasc Intervent Radiol 2006;29:371–9.
8. Kehagias D, Moulopoulos L, Antoniou A, et al. Focal nodular hyperplasia: Imaging findings. Eur Radiol 2001;11:202–12.
9. Malfertheiner P, Megraud F, O'Morain C, et al. Current concepts in the management of *Helicobacter pylori* infection: The Maastricht III consensus report. Gut 2006;56:772–81.
10. Mariani G, Pauwels E, AlSharif A, et al. Radionuclide evaluation of the lower gastrointestinal tract. J Nucl Med 2008;49:776–87.
11. Maurer A. Consensus report on gastric emptying: What's needed to prevent tarnishing a gold standard? J Nucl Med 2008;49:339.
12. Maurer A, Parkman H. Update on gastrointestinal scintigraphy. Semin Nucl Med 2006;36:110–8.
13. Mettler FA, Guiberteau MJ. Essentials of nuclear medicine. 5th ed. Philadelphia: WB Saunders, 2006. pp. 203–10, 215–220.
14. Pelosi E, Masaneo I, Clara R, et al. Technetium-99m labeled macroaggregated albumin arterial catheter perfusion scintigraphy: Prediction of gastrointestinal toxicity in hepatic arterial chemotherapy. Eur J Nucl Med 2000;27:668–75.
15. Stasi R, Evangelista M, Stipa E, et al. Idiopathic thrombocytopenic purpura: Current concepts in pathophysiology and management. Thromb Haemost 2008;99:4–13.
16. Vilaichone R, Varocha M, Graham D. *Helicobacter pylori* diagnosis and management. Gastroenterol Clin N Am 2006;35:229–47.
17. Ziessman H. Acute cholecystitis, biliary obstruction, and biliary leakage. Semin Nucl Med 2003;33:279–96.

# ENDOSCOPIC ULTRASOUND

*Peter R. McNally, DO*

CHAPTER 72

**1. When was intraluminal gastrointestinal (GI) ultrasound (US) first performed?**

Wild and Reid performed the first US (rectal) in 1956. For the past decade, interest in the use of GI US has been revitalized. Intraluminal US permits precise definition of the gut wall layers and examination of adjacent structures of the chest and abdomen. The proximity of the US transducer and the high scanning frequencies provide incomparable morphologic detail of the gut wall and extraintestinal anatomy. The instrumentation used in endoscopic ultrasound (EUS) includes linear- and radial-array echoendoscopes, with some capable of Doppler flow analysis. Introduction of miniature US probes allow the endoscopist to evaluate near obstructing lesions and ductal structures of the pancreatobiliary tree.

**2. How do US waves visualize the GI tract?**

Ultrasound pulses represent longitudinal waves that are propagated through soft tissues or fluid by motion of molecules within the conducting media. The US wavelength is the distance between two waves of compression and rarefaction. Ultrasound is defined as frequency greater than 20,000 cycles/sec (20 Hz); most diagnostic US uses frequencies ranging from 2 to 20 million cycles/sec (2 to 20 MHz). The velocity of sound transmission through soft tissues is a constant 1540 m/sec and is independent of frequency. Transmission of US within a medium depends on the compressibility and density of the medium, two properties that tend to be inversely proportional. Because US power is diminished as it traverses tissue, the intensity of the returning echo, when related to the original echo is expressed in negative terms.

**3. How does the frequency of the US beam influence the depth of beam penetration and image resolution?**

For maximal resolution of US, the transmitted waves should be parallel. If the target of interest is too close or too far from the transducer, divergence of the wavelength causes distortion of the image. Hence, proper positioning of the US transducer and use of the appropriate frequency are essential to provide maximal resolution (Table 72-1).

**Table 72-1.** Proper Positioning of the Ultrasound Transducer and Use of the Appropriate Frequency

| ULTRASOUND FREQUENCY (MHZ) | PENETRATION (CM) | AXIAL RESOLUTION (MM) |
|---|---|---|
| 5 | 8 | 0.8 |
| 10 | 4 | 0.4 |
| 20 | 2 | 0.2 |

**4. What are the ultrasonographic properties of the common structures of the body?**

| | |
|---|---|
| Water/blood | Echo poor (black) |
| Collagen | Echo rich (white) |
| Air | Reflection (reverberation echoes) |
| Bone | Reflection (reverberation echoes) |
| Muscle | Echo poor (black) |

## NORMAL ANATOMY

**5. What determines the thickness of the echosonographic layer visualized? What is the normal endosonographic anatomy of the intestinal wall?**

The thickness of the intraluminal US image of the intestinal wall does not equal the total thickness of a histologic section. Kimmey and colleagues hypothesized that the overall appearance of the US image is determined by a combination of echoes from two sources: those created at interfaces between tissue layers with different acoustic impedances and those created within the internal structures of the tissue layer. Using 5- to 12-MHz scanning frequencies, the intestinal wall has five sonographic layers (Fig. 72-1).

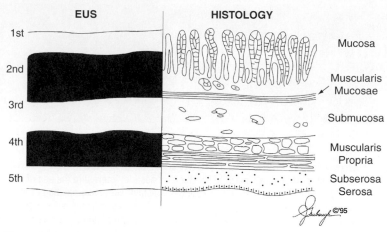

**Figure 72-1.** Correlation of endoscopic ultrasound image to the histologic composition of the bowel wall.

### 6. What are the imaging characteristics of normal and malignant lymph nodes on EUS?

The high resolution of EUS imaging allows even normal lymph nodes to be visualized. Normal lymph nodes are characterized by the presence of internal echoes, a beanlike shape, and size less than 1 cm. Malignant lymph nodes tend to be hypoechoic, rounded, and larger than 1 cm; they exhibit distinct margins.

### 7. How are blood vessels distinguished from lymph nodes on EUS?

Blood vessels generally appear as anechoic, curvilinear structures that often branch. Branching and posterior wall enhancement (hyperechoic) are helpful in distinguishing paraluminal vessels from hypoechoic lymph nodes.

### 8. Describe the normal EUS anatomy of the retroperitoneum. What are its major landmarks?

The pancreas and retroperitoneum are the most challenging and difficult areas to examine with intraluminal US. Familiarity with the gross and US anatomy is essential. The examination begins with the echoendoscope at the level of the duodenal ampulla. Antimotility agents, such as glucagon, are frequently necessary. The US examination usually is conducted with a 7.5-MHz scanning frequency. The normal paraduodenal anatomy is shown in Figure 72-2. The normal pancreas has a homogeneous echo pattern, usually slightly more hyperechoic than the liver. There is considerable interobserver variation in measurement of the head of the pancreas, probably due to variations in the angle of view. The remainder of the pancreas is examined from a paragastric position. In the stomach, the water-filled lumen method is used.

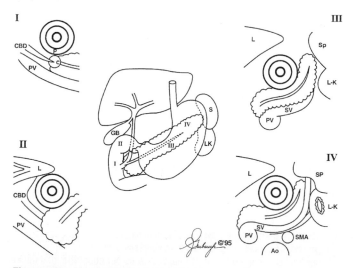

**Figure 72-2.** Four commonly used positions to examine the pancreas by EUS. I, transverse section at the level of the ampulla. II, Sagittal section near the duodenal bulb. III, Transverse section of the pancreatic body through the posterior wall of the stomach. IV, Transverse section of the body and tail of the pancreas from the proximal stomach. A, ampulla; CBD, common bile duct; L-K, left kidney; PV, portal vein; SV, splenic vein; L, liver; Sp, spleen; SA, superior mesenteric artery, Ao, aorta.

## 9. What are the indications for EUS examination?

### STAGING OF GASTROINTESTINAL TUMORS

| | |
|---|---|
| Esophageal carcinoma | Ampullary tumors |
| Gastric carcinoma | Biliary tract carcinoma |
| Gastric lymphoma (non-Hodgkin lymphoma) | Colorectal carcinoma |
| Pancreatic lymphoma | Colorectal adenoma |
| Pancreatic endocrine tumors | Submucosal tumors |

### EVALUATION OF NONNEOPLASTIC DISEASE

| | |
|---|---|
| Reflux esophagitis | Portal hypertension |
| Achalasia | Chronic pancreatitis |
| Gastric ulcer | Common bile duct stones |
| Giant gastric folds | Inflammatory bowel disease |

## 10. How is EUS used in the clinical evaluation of esophageal cancer?

Currently, EUS has no role in the diagnosis of esophageal cancer. Findings from EUS provide morphologic staging but do not supplant the need for histologic diagnosis of malignancy. EUS has not been shown to be helpful in differentiating malignant from inflammatory strictures. It is not sufficiently sensitive to use as a screening test for cancer (i.e., in Barrett's esophagus with dysplasia). Combined EUS with or without fine-needle aspiration (FNA) and computed tomography (CT) scanning provides the most accurate method of tumor node metastasis (TNM) staging for esophageal cancer. CT should be performed first to exclude distant metastasis (M stage), followed by EUS-FNA for precise T and N staging. During the conduct of the EUS examination, it is especially important to identify the aorta and then trace it to the celiac axis. Identification of a malignant celiac lymph node carries an ominous prognosis, since it represents M1 or distant metastasis (Table 72-2).

## 11. How can EUS findings affect clinical management of esophageal carcinoma?

- Direct stage-dependent treatment decisions
- More accurate pretreatment prognosis
- Preoperative assessment of tumor resectability

EUS exclusion of occult cancer, submucosal invasion, and malignant adenopathy for high-grade dysplasia/Barrett's esophagus has promise in guiding selection of patients for new endoscopic ablation techniques.

## 12. What are the problematic areas for EUS in the staging of esophageal cancer?

- At presentation, 25% to 50% of esophageal cancers are so advanced that passage of the echoendoscope beyond the cancer is prohibited. Wallace and others recently showed that obstructing malignant esophageal strictures can be safely dilated to permit EUS with FNA in about 90% of such patients.
- Accurate T1 staging is difficult, and overstaging is common.
- EUS features cannot accurately distinguish between malignant and inflammatory lymph nodes. Only about 25% of patients with nodal metastasis exhibit the four characteristic EUS features: round shape, size greater than 1 cm, hypoechoic, and distinct margins. EUS-FNA of suspicious lymph nodes should be done to improve staging accuracy.
- EUS does not accurately stage esophageal cancer after chemoradiation.

### Table 72-2. TNM Staging for Esophageal Carcinoma

| PRIMARY TUMOR (T) | | REGIONAL LYMPH NODES (N) | |
|---|---|---|---|
| Tx | Primary tumor cannot be assessed | Nx | Regional lymph nodes cannot be assessed |
| T0 | No evidence of primary tumor | N0 | No regional lymph node metastasis |
| Tis | Carcinoma in situ | N1 | Regional lymph node metastasis |
| T1 | Tumor invades lamina propria or submucosa | Distant metastasis (M) | |
| T2 | Tumor invades muscularis propria | Mx | Presence of distant metastasis |
| T3 | Tumor invades the adventitia | M0 | No distant metastasis |
| T4 | Tumor invades adjacent structures | M1 | Distant metastasis |

## 13. Does EUS have a role in the evaluation of gastric cancer?

EUS has no role in the initial diagnosis of gastric cancer and should not be used as a screening tool in patients at risk for this disease. However, in patients where the suspicion of linitis plastica is not confirmed by biopsy, identification of the typical EUS pattern of this cancer contributes significantly to the correct diagnosis (Fig. 72-3). Radial sector scanning in the region of the pylorus and proximal fundus can be technically difficult. If stage-dependent treatment protocols are employed, then EUS is indicated when CT shows no metastasis (M0). EUS appears to be reliable in predicting stages T1-3, which are surgically resectable (R0).

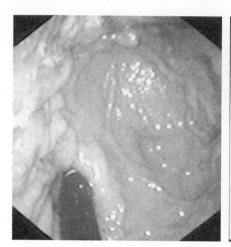 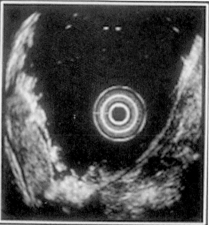

**Figure 72-3.** Endoscopic view of a gastric adenocarcinoma (*left*) compared with EUS findings (*right*) of a thickened tumor involving the first three echo layers, from the 7 o'clock to the 9 o'clock position. The echoendoscope is located in the center of the water-filled stomach.

## 14. What are the problematic areas for EUS staging of gastric malignancy?

1. Overstaging of 20% to 30%, mainly in T2 lesions, is partly due to the peculiar histopathologic definition of stage T2 (infiltration into the submucosa) versus T3 (invasion of the serosa), a differentiation that cannot be made by EUS. Also, portions of the stomach are not covered by serosa.

2. Differentiation of gastric cancer confined to the mucosa (and therefore amenable to endoscopic treatment) from cancer involving the submucosa (with an attendant increase in the incidence of lymph node metastasis) is relatively inaccurate (60% to 70%). Small lesions that are flat, slightly depressed, or elevated at endoscopy and cancerous on biopsy can be assumed to be confined to the mucosa if EUS shows no abnormality of the gastric wall in relation to the tumor. Overstaging occurs predominantly with ulcerating, early carcinomas, because EUS cannot differentiate malignancy from ulcer-related fibrosis and inflammation.

3. Distinguishing inflammatory from malignant lymph nodes requires EUS-FNA sampling.

## 15. Summarize the TNM staging classification for gastric malignancy.

### PRIMARY TUMOR (T)

Tx Primary tumor cannot be assessed

T0 No evidence of primary tumor

T1 Tumor confined to mucosa or submucosa

T2 Tumor invades muscularis propria or subserosa

T3 Tumor invades serosa without invasion into adjacent structures

T4 Tumor invades adjacent structures

### REGIONAL LYMPH NODES (N)

Nx Regional lymph nodes cannot be assessed

N0 No regional lymph node metastasis

N1 Positive perigastric lymph nodes, 3 cm from the tumor edge

N2 Positive perigastric lymph nodes, 3 cm from the tumor edge or positive lymph nodes along the gastric, common hepatic, splenic, or celiac arteries

### DISTANT METASTASIS (M)

Mx Presence of distant metastasis
M0 No distant metastasis
M1 Distant metastasis

**16. How does staging affect treatment?**
Resectable tumors (R0) = stages T1-T3. Chemotherapy is used for stage T4.

**17. Is EUS helpful in the evaluation of gastric lymphoma?**
Yes. Unlike gastric adenocarcinoma, gastric lymphoma has a highly characteristic pattern of horizontal extension. EUS is quite accurate in determining the T and N stage for gastric lymphoma and helps to select the most appropriate medical or surgical treatment (Fig. 72-4). Low-grade mucosa-associated lymphoid tissue (MALT) lymphoma often is associated with *Helicobacter pylori* and may regress with antibiotic eradication of the infection. When antibiotic treatment fails to reverse the malignant process or if *H. pylori* is absent, EUS is helpful in staging and guiding treatment.

**18. How is EUS helpful in evaluating pancreatic neoplasms?**
The introduction of EUS-FNA has greatly advanced the role of EUS in the management of suspected pancreatic neoplasms. Organ-preserving pancreatic resections can be performed when tumors of low malignant potential, such as cystadenomas and neuroendocrine tumors, are diagnosed. Erickson and Carza showed that EUS-FNA is superior to CT-FNA for the diagnosis of pancreatic cancer. In their hands, the incidence of peritoneal carcinomatosis is lower than CT-FNA and decreased the need for operative staging by 75%.

**19. Neuroendocrine tumors (NETs) of the pancreas and peripancreas are often difficult to localize by conventional CT, US, and angiography. Does EUS examination offer any value in localizing these tumors?**
Yes. EUS is the most accurate imaging method available for the localization of pancreatic NETs. When CT and sonographic findings are negative, EUS remains more than 90% accurate. However, EUS fails to detect up to 50% of extrapancreatic NETs; either transabdominal US or CT remains the preferred first test. One needs considerable experience with EUS of the pancreas to achieve this accuracy rate.

**20. Describe the use of EUS in the evaluation of colon malignancy.**
Advances in laparoscopic and endoscopic surgical techniques provide alternatives to conventional exploratory laparotomy and segmental colonic resection for patients diagnosed with early-stage colon cancer. Studies are under way to evaluate the utility of colonoscopic EUS for accurate staging and selection of patients suitable for minimal access surgery and endoscopic mucosal resection.

**21. Describe the use of EUS in the evaluation of rectal malignancy.**
EUS is highly accurate in determining the T and N stage and superior to CT scanning. The combination of EUS and CT provides the most practical and accurate approach to staging rectal cancers, and the results of both tests should be

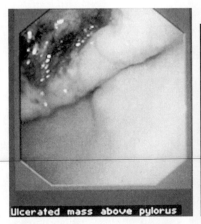
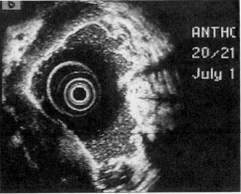

**Figure 72-4.** Endoscopic view of a gastric lymphoma (*left*) compared with EUS findings of a thickened hypoechoic tumor with foot-like extensions (pseudopodia) into the fourth echogenic layer at the 9 o'clock position. The echoendoscope is located in the center of the water-filled stomach (*right*).

considered in treatment planning. The endoscopic and surgical options are largely determined by the tumor stage: for T1 stage large polyp or small rectal cancer endoscopic mucosal resection or transanal resection is appropriate; whereas a T2 lesion should undergo radical resection, and a T3-4 or N1 lesion requires preoperative chemoradiation followed by radical resection.

## 22. Summarize the EUS characteristics of submucosal tumors (SMTs).

| | |
|---|---|
| Aberrant pancreas | Submucosal; similar in echogenicity to the pancreas; hypoechoic ductular structure may be present |
| Bronchogenic carcinoma | Hypoechoic; disrupts submucosa and muscularis propria; usually irregular outer margin |
| Breast cancer | Metastatic; same as bronchogenic cancer |
| Carcinoid | Mucosal; hypoechoic (Fig. 72-5) |
| Fibrovascular polyp | Submucosal; mixed echogenicity (Fig. 72-6) |
| Gastric cyst | Anechoic; smooth border; submucosal |
| Granular cell tumors | Hypoechoic; submucosal; smooth margin |
| Lipoma | Hyperechoic; submucosal (Fig. 72-7) |
| Leiomyoma | Hypoechoic; contiguous with muscularis propria; smooth outer margin (Fig. 72-8) |
| Leiomyosarcoma | Hypoechoic; contiguous with muscularis propria; large lesions may have irregular outer margin; adenopathy; small lesions identical to leiomyoma |
| Lymphoma | Hypoechoic; may disrupt submucosa; muscularis propria and adenopathy |
| Pancreatic pseudocyst | Anechoic; smooth margin; compresses normal wall |
| Varices | Anechoic; submucosal serpentine |
| Vessels | Anechoic; curvilinear branching; often with through-penetration enhancement of the posterior wall |

Smooth muscle tumors comprise the majority (53%) of SMTs encountered in the GI tract. The National Institutes of Health (NIH) Consensus Conference in 2001 redefined the group of smooth muscle tumors (leiomyomas, leiomyoblastomas, and leiomyosarcomas) into gastrointestinal stromal tumors (GISTs) that express tyrosine kinase (KIT). Endosonographic features of SMT suggestive of malignancy include size (larger than 30 mm), irregular margins, and possibly the presence of internal cystic spaces. Immunohistochemical staining of EUS-FNA sample is helpful in distinguishing GIST (CD117 and CD34) from true smooth muscle tumors and schwannomas (smooth muscle actin, desmin, and S-100). Often, surgical sections or EUS-core biopsies with Ki67 labeling index or mutational analysis is necessary to make the diagnosis of malignancy.

## 23. Is EUS useful in the evaluation of nonneoplastic disease?

Preliminary studies of EUS in the evaluation of reflux esophagitis, achalasia, and gastric ulcer have not shown EUS to be clinically important. EUS evaluation of enlarged gastric folds can determine the safety of large-particle biopsy devices and exclude the presence of intramural vascular structures. EUS findings contribute to the characterization of the cause of the process. Thickening of the first two layers is characteristic of inflammation, Ménétrier disease, and lymphoma; large-particle biopsies should be safe and diagnostic. Thickening of all layers suggests lymphoma or linitis plastica. If biopsy findings are still equivocal, laparoscopy/ laparotomy may be indicated.

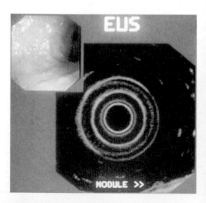

**Figure 72-5.** EUS finding of a mucosal hypoechoic carcinoid tumor and endoscopic findings.

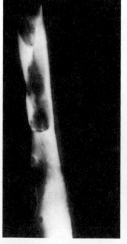

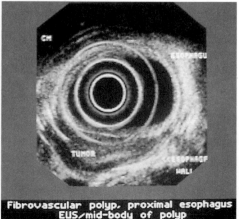

**Figure 72-6.** Esophageal fibrovascular polyp seen on barium swallow radiograph (*left*) and EUS findings (*right*).

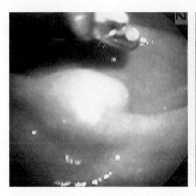
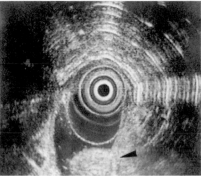

**Figure 72-7.** Endoscopic finding of a soft submucosal tumor (*left*) and EUS findings of a hyperechoic lipoma (*right*).

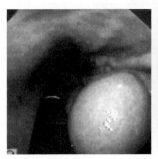
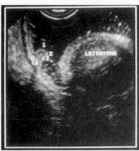

**Figure 72-8.** Endoscopic view of a submucosal tumor (*left*), confirmed to be a leiomyoma, arising from the fourth hyperechoic layer (*right*).

## 24. How is EUS used in the evaluation of patients with portal hypertension?

EUS can demonstrate fundal varices when endoscopic results are equivocal and define the vascular patency of the splenic vein. Some authorities suggest that intramural vessel enlargement can be detected in patients with portal hypertensive gastropathy. Faigel and colleagues determined that EUS identification of large paraesophageal varices greater than 5 mm was predictive of variceal hemorrhage. Others have shown that EUS can guide treatment of esophageal varices and facilitate treatment of bleeding gastric varices with injection of cyanoacrylate glue.

## 25. Does EUS have a role in the evaluation of recurrent idiopathic pancreatitis?

Yes. When endoscopic retrograde cholangiopancreatography (ERCP) fails to detect the anatomic cause of recurrent idiopathic pancreatitis (e.g., choledocolithiasis, microlithiasis, sphincter of Oddi dysfunction, pancreatic divism), EUS should be performed. EUS detects stones in the gallbladder and/or common bile duct in 77% of patients with recurrent idiopathic pancreatitis and negative results with previous CT, US, or ERCP.

## 26. What is the stack sign? Does it have clinical significance?

The stack sign refers to a characteristic view of the bile and pancreatic ducts. The view is obtained by positioning the echoendoscope in the long scope position with the transducer in the duodenal bulb. The balloon is inflated and advanced snugly into the apex of the bulb. From this position, the bile duct (closest to the transducer) and pancreatic duct can be seen to run parallel through the pancreatic head. The absence of the stack sign may suggest pancreatic divism.

## 27. Describe the role of EUS in the evaluation of chronic pancreatitis.

EUS is more sensitive than CT in detection of early chronic pancreatitis. Its role in monitoring for neoplastic change in patients with hereditary or chronic alcoholic pancreatitis is under evaluation. EUS-guided celiac block appears to be superior to CT-guided block in terms of pain control and cost. EUS features of chronic pancreatitis include:

### PARENCHYMAL ABNORMALITIES

- Hyperechoic foci (distinct 1- to 2-mm hyperechoic points)
- Hyperechoic strands (hyperechoic irregular lines)
- Lobularity (2- to 5-mm lobules)
- Cysts (thin-walled, round, anechoic structures larger than 2 mm in diameter within the pancreatic parenchyma)
- Shadowing calcifications

### DUCTAL ABNORMALITIES

- Dilation (head larger than 3 mm, body larger than 2 mm, and tail larger than 1 mm)
- Irregular duct

- Hyperechoic duct margins (duct wall visible as a distinct, hyperechoic structure)
- Visible side branches (anechoic structures budding from the main pancreatic duct)

## 28. Summarize the EUS criteria for chronic pancreatitis.

Mild chronic pancreatitis: 1 or 2 abnormal features

Moderate chronic pancreatitis: 3 to 5 abnormal features

Severe chronic pancreatitis: more than 5 abnormal features

## 29. What is the role of EUS in the evaluation of autoimmune pancreatitis (AIP)?

AIP is a fibroinflammatory disorder that is difficult to distinguish from pancreatic cancer. CT findings include diffuse enlargement of pancreas with low-density, capsule-like rim. EUS-FNA reveals a lymphocytic or plasma cell infiltrate in up to 73% of patients.

## 30. Discuss the role of EUS in evaluating patients with common bile duct stones.

A recent study of patients with choledocholithiasis found EUS to be superior to magnetic resonance cholangiopancreatography (MRCP), but both are highly accurate (96.9% and 82.2%, respectively). However, in most hospitals extracorporeal US will continue to be the most cost-effective first test to evaluate for choledocholithiasis. When the patient is too obese to permit diagnostic extracorporeal US, MRCP is the most accurate noninvasive test. The about 5% risk of pancreatitis with ERCP increases the appeal of EUS for evaluation of choledocholithiasis in high-risk patients.

# WEBSITES

http://www.simbionix.com/EUS.html

http://www.vhjoe.com

# BIBLIOGRAPHY

1. Ahmad NA, Kochman ML, Lewis JD, et al. Can EUS alone differentiate between malignant and benign cystic lesions of the pancreas? Am J Gastroenterol 2001;96:3295–300.
2. Anderson MA, Carpenter S, Thompson NW, et al. Endoscopic ultrasound is highly accurate and directs management in patients with neuroendocrine tumors of the pancreas. Am J Gastroenterol 2000;95:2271–7.
3. Barbour AP, Rizk NP, Gerdes H, et al. EUS predicts outcomes for patients with adenocarcinoma of the gastroesophageal junction. J Am Coll Surg. 2007;205:593–601.
4. Beseth BD, Bedford R, Isacoff WH, et al. Endoscopic ultrasound does not accurately assess pathologic stage of esophageal cancer after neoadjuvant chemoradiation. Am Surg 2000;66:827–31.
5. Bhutani MS. EUS in the diagnosis, staging and management of colorectal tumors. Gastroenterol Clin N Am 2008;37:215–27.
6. Caletti GC, Fusaroli P, Togliani T, et al. Endosonography in gastric lymphoma and large gastric folds. Eur J Ultrasound 2000;11:31–40.
7. Chari ST, Smyrk TC, Levey MJ, et al. Diagnosis of autoimmune pancreatitis: The Mayo Clinic experience. Clin Gastroenterol Hepatol 2006;4:1010–6.
8. Erickson RA, Garza AA. Impact of endoscopic ultrasound on the management and outcome of pancreatic carcinoma. Am J Gastroenterol 2000;95:2248–54.
9. Fletcher CD, Bermann JJ, Corless C, et al. Diagnosis of gastrointestinal stromal tumors: A consensus approach. Hum Pathol 2002;33:459–65.
10. Gan SI, Rajan E, Adler DG, et al. ASGE Guideline: Role of EUS. Gastrointest Endosc 2007;66:425–34.
11. Hussain N, Hawes RH. Principles of endosonography and imaging. Gastrointest Endosc Clin N Am 2005;15:1–12.
12. Jacobson BC, Hirota W, Baron TH, et al. The role of endoscopy in the assessment and treatment of esophageal cancer. Gastrointest Endosc 2003;57:817–22.
13. Lahoti S, Catalano MF, Alcocer E, et al. Obliteration of esophageal varices using EUS-guided sclerotherapy with color Doppler. Gastrointest Endosc 2000;51:331–43.
14. Levey MJ, Wiersema MJ. Pancreatic neoplasms. Gastrointest Endosc Clin N Am 2005;15:117–42.
15. Lui J, Carpenter S, Chuttani R, et al. ASGE: Technology Status Evaluation Report: Endoscopic ultrasound probes. Gastrointest Endosc 2006;63:751–4.
16. Micames C, Jowell PS, White R, et al. Lower frequency of peritoneal carcinomatosis in patients with pancreatic cancer diagnosed by EUS-guided FNA vs. percutaneous FNA. Gastrointest Endosc 2003;58:690–5.
17. Polkowski M, Butrk E. Submucosal lesions. Gastrointest Endosc Clin N Am 2005;15:33–54.
18. Savoy AD, Wallace MB. EUS in the management of the patient with dysplasia in Barrett's esophagus. J Clin Gastroenterol 2005;39:263–7.
19. Schechter NR, Yahalom J. Low-grade MALT lymphoma of the stomach: A review of treatment options. Int J Radiat Oncol Biol Phys 2000;46:1093–103.
20. Shah JN, Muthusamy VR. Minimizing complications of EUS and EUS-FNA. Gastrointest Endosc Clin N Am 2007;17:129–43.
21. Sheth S, Bedford A, Chopra S. Primary gallbladder cancer: Recognition of risk factors and role of prophylactic cholecystectomy. Am J Gastroenterol 2000;95:1402–10.
22. Tse F, Liu L, Barkun AN, et al. EUS: A meta-analysis of test performance in suspected choledocholithiasis. Gastrointest Endosc 2008;67:235–44.
23. Wallace MB, Hawes EH, Sahai AV, et al. Dilation of malignant esophageal stenosis to allow EUS guided fine-needle aspiration: Safety and effect on patient management. Gastrointest Endosc 2000;51:309–13.

# ADVANCED THERAPEUTIC ENDOSCOPY

*Wilson P. Pais, MD, MBA, FRCP, and*
*Mainor Antillon, MD, MBA, MPH*

# CHAPTER 73

### 1. What is advanced therapeutic endoscopy?

It is a group of techniques that are minimally invasive and organ sparing and yet can be used to diagnose, remove, and treat benign lesions and early malignancies of the gastrointestinal (GI) tract without need of traditional surgery using endoscopy.

### 2. What are the major advanced therapeutic endoscopy techniques?

- *Endoscopic mucosal resection* (EMR): This technique can remove mucosal lesions of the GI tract en bloc that are less than 2 cm (or piecemeal if larger lesions). It may use a cap at the tip of the scope and suction to retract the lesion into the cap and subsequent removal by electrocautery snare. Submucosal injections with various solutions (Table 73-1) are used to raise the lesions to provide cushion for dissection.

**Table 73-1.** Various Submucosal Injection Solutions Used in Endoscopic Mucosal Resection/Endoscopic Submucosal Dissection (EMR/ESD)

| SOLUTION | CUSHION DURABILITY | COMMENTS |
| --- | --- | --- |
| Normal saline | Short | Easy to inject, cheap, dissipates quickly |
| Hypertonic saline 3% | Moderate | Easy to inject, cheap, tissue damage |
| Hydroxypropyl methylcellulose 0.83% to 1.25% | Extended | Long lasting, relatively cheap, safe and effective, may cause tissue damage |
| Hyaluronic acid 1% | Extended | Long lasting, expensive, safe and effective, special storage |
| Dextrose 50% | Moderate | Easy to inject, cheap, tissue damage |
| Albumin 25% | Moderate | Easy to inject, expensive, safe |

- *Endoscopic submucosal dissection* (ESD): This technique can remove mucosal lesions on bloc that are larger than 2 cm and/or flat and/or in the deeper layers (submucosa) of the GI tract that cannot be removed by other endoscopic methods. It uses an electrocautery needle knife with high cutting power to make circumferential cut around the lesion and dissect the base of the lesion through the deeper submucosal layer. Submucosal injections are used provide cushion for dissection. Adding dye (indigo carmine or methylene blue) to injection solutions help in identifying the submucosal layer to determine margins of dissection.
- *Advanced endoscopic ultrasound* (EUS): This technique is used to diagnoses and treat lesion in the GI tract and in close proximity to the GI tract by making use of ultrasound for guidance. Some examples include sampling of suspected malignant lesions or lymph nodes with EUS-guided fine-needle aspiration (EUS-FNA), drainage of pancreatic or peripancreatic fluid collections, such as pancreatic pseudocysts, and celiac plexus neurolysis/block for pain control of pancreatic cancer or chronic pancreatitis (Figs. 73-1 through 73-5).

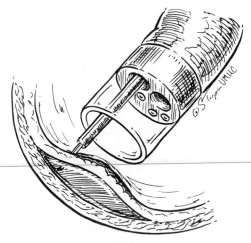

**Figure 73-1.** EMR cap with submucosal injection

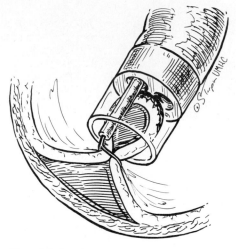

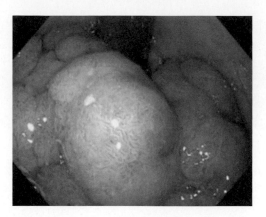

**Figure 73-2.** EMR technique to remove lesion with snare

**Figure 73-3.** Giant 14 cm rectal mass planned for ESD. (From Antillon MR, Bartalos CR, Miller ML, et al: En bloc endoscopic submucosal dissection of a 14 cm laterally spreading adenoma of the rectum with involvement to the anal canal: Expanding the frontiers of endoscopic surgery [with video]. Gastrointest Endosc 67:332–7, 2008.)

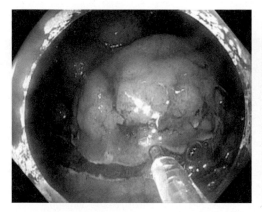

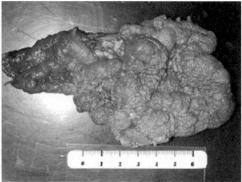

**Figure 73-4.** Dissection of mass with needle knife during endoscopic submucosal dissection. (From Antillon MR, Bartalos CR, Miller ML, et al: En bloc endoscopic submucosal dissection of a 14 cm laterally spreading adenoma of the rectum with involvement to the anal canal: Expanding the frontiers of endoscopic surgery [with video]. Gastrointest Endosc 67:332–7, 2008.)

**Figure 73-5.** Mass removed en bloc by endoscopic submucosal dissection. (From Antillon MR, Bartalos CR, Miller ML, et al: En bloc endoscopic submucosal dissection of a 14 cm laterally spreading adenoma of the rectum with involvement to the anal canal: Expanding the frontiers of endoscopic surgery [with video]. Gastrointest Endosc 67:332–7, 2008.)

### 3. What are the applications of EMR and ESD?

These techniques provide definite therapy for benign lesions, premalignant lesions, and early malignancies (Tis and T1 M0 N0). EUS and Kudo pit pattern analysis may be used to assess the tumor-node-metastasis (TMN) staging and invasiveness/removability of the lesion. Lesions in the mucosa and minimal submucosal invasion up to 1000 microns with tumor-free margins; well-differentiated and moderately differentiated lesions without lymphovascular involvement can be considered cured. The rationale for EMR and ESD in early malignancy is based on the fact that there is very low probability for lymph node involvement in Tis and T1 stage. See Table 73-2. Further, when accessible, EUS can determine status of Tis and T1 with 91% to 94% accuracy. A few examples include adenocarcinoma of the esophagus and colon, flat polyps, gastric nodules, and duodenal adenomas.

**Table 73-2.** Stage of Cancer and Lymph Node Status

| STAGE | NO. | % N1 |
|---|---|---|
| Tis | 29 | 0% |
| T1 mucosal | 38 | 2.6% |
| T1 submucosal | 27 | 22.2% |
| T2 | 37 | 42.3% |
| T3 | 219 | 77.2% |

### 4. How is EMR performed?

There are various commercially available EMR kits that can be used. The EMR cap is made of clear plastic that can be soft or hard and straight or oblique in various sizes up to 18 mm. Larger caps are soft to allow easier passage in to the GI tract. The oblique caps are helpful in esophagus and straight caps are helpful in stomach. The target lesion is raised with submucosal injection to form a cushion. The EMR cap of desired size is affixed to the tip of the endoscope. The electrocautery snare is opened and positioned on the distal internal circumferential ridge of the cap. The scope is advanced and placed over the lesion. Suction is applied to retract the lesion in to the cap. Once the lesion is well positioned in the cap the snare is closed and the lesion is captured with the snare. The suction is released. The lesion is then resected like a polyp. The lesion can be retrieved in the cap using suction. In addition to the above-discussed EMR-cap technique, there are several variations to the EMR techniques such as *inject-lift-and-cut* and a newer banding device for mucosectomy that can be used. See the website link about how to perform EMR.

### 5. How is ESD performed?

Even though various modified needle knives are available, only the conventional (straight fine tip with regulated length) needle knife is commercially available in the United States. The lesion is located and raised with submucosal injections. The borders of the lesion are defined using NBI (narrow band imaging) or adding a dye to the surface of the lesion (chromoendoscopy). The needle knife is passed through the instrument channel of the scope, and a circumferential submucosal cut is first made using fine movements and maneuvers. Subsequently, the base of the lesion is dissected with multiple cuts. Multiple submucosal injections are needed as the submucosal cushion tends to dissipate with time. Once the lesion is freed from the base, it can be retrieved with a Roth net or spider net. The specimen is immediately mounted onto Styrofoam with pins and oriented for pathologic examination. In addition to the above-discussed technique, there are other variations to the ESD such as magnetic-anchor–guided ESD. See the website link about how to perform ESD.

### 6. What are the differences/limitations of the EMR and ESD?

The ability of the EMR is limited by the largest suction cap size of 18 mm to accommodate the narrow passages in the GI tract. This is can be overcome by ESD. EMR and ESD cannot be performed in areas such as distal small bowel that are not accessible by traditional endoscopes. These procedures are technically difficult, time consuming, and labor intensive, and specialized training is needed.

### 7. What are the complications of EMR/ESD?

The major complications include bleeding (average 10% in various series) and perforation (4% to 10% for ESD and 0.3% to 0.5% for EMR). (See Table 73-3 for gastric ESD complications.) Most bleeding can be handled endoscopically using coagulation graspers and endoscopic clips without surgery. Most perforations can be handled endoscopically using endoscopic clips and loops without surgery. (See Table 73-4 for nonsurgical treatment of ESD perforations.) In certain instances, especially when the perforation is large, surgical repair is needed. In our own series for colorectal ESD (N = 54), the bleeding rate was 3.7% and the perforation rate was 7.4%. Other complications include stricture (esophageal or pyloric) and infections (Box 73-1).

**Table 73-3.** Gastric Endoscopic Submucosal Dissection Complications

| STUDY AUTHOR | NO. | LESION SIZE (mm) | EN BLOC RATE (%) | BLEED RATE (%) | PERFORATION (%) |
|---|---|---|---|---|---|
| Kakushima | 334 | 3 to 85 | 95 | 3.4 | 3.9 |
| Imagawa | 185 | 5 to 70 | 84 | 0 | 6.1 |
| Onozato | 160 | 24 | 94 | 7.6 | 0 |
| Imaeda | 25 | 10 to 25 | 100 | 0 | 0 |
| Yonezawa | 20 | 18 | 95 | 2.5 | 2.5 |
| Neuhaus | 10 | 20 to 45 | 100 | 0 | 20 |

**Table 73-4.** Sensitivity and Specificity of Endoscopic Ultrasound to Fine Needle Aspiration

| TISSUE | SENSITIVITY | SPECIFICITY |
|---|---|---|
| Pancreatic cancer | 90% to 95% | 90% to 100% |
| Mediastinal lymphadenopathy | 88% | 90% to 100% |
| Peri-intestinal lymphadenopathy | 70% to 90% | 93% to 100% |
| Mucosal/submucosal lesions | 50% to 90% | 80% to 100% |

**Box 73-1.** Nonsurgical Treatment of Endoscopic Submucosal Dissection Perforations

- A total of 27 perforations in 528 resections (5.1%)
- Various regions: esophagus, 4; gastric, 14; colon, 9
- Nonsurgical methods: clips in most, nasogastric tube, intravenous antibiotics, and pneumoperitoneum relieved by 18-gauge needle
- Mean antibiotic duration, 6.7 days
- Mean NPO period of 5.3 days
- Mean admission time, 12.1 days after ESD
- Median follow-up duration for no sequels/tumor spread for 36 months

From Fijushiro M. Endosc 2006.[E1]

### 8. What are some investigational applications of EMR/ESD?

These techniques along with EUS will aid in accessing the lesions outside of the GI tract such as mediastinal lymph nodes and intra-abdominal organs such as the gallbladder once the technique to create a perforation and close them effectively is mastered. Thereby, EMR/ESD will facilitate the development of other techniques such as natural orifice transluminal endoscopic surgery (NOTES) and mediastinoscopy.

### 9. What are some investigational applications of advanced endoscopic ultrasound?

- EUS-guided pancreatic necrosectomy and drains with large-bore plastic or metal stents
- EUS-guided antitumor therapy
- EUS-guided nonpapillary pancreatic and bile duct drainage

### 10. What is the role of EUS-guided fine-needle aspiration (FNA) biopsy in tissue sampling? Sampling of nodes?

EUS-FNA has been shown to aid in the diagnosis of primary lesions within or close to the gastrointestinal tract such as rectal, esophageal, pancreatic, and lung cancers. The EUS-FNA of lymph nodes has overall sensitivity of 84%, specificity of 92%, positive predictive value of 88%, and negative predictive value of 89%. The sensitivity and specificity vary with the type/location of lesion being evaluated. The sensitivity and specificity of EUS-FNA are higher for lesions such as pancreatic neuroendocrine tumors and pancreatic cancer and lower for submucosal lesions such as gastrointestinal stromal tumors (GISTs). The main utility of EUS-FNA is in nodal staging of these lesions, not only allowing imaging of lymph nodes but also providing samples of these nodes (Fig. 73-6).

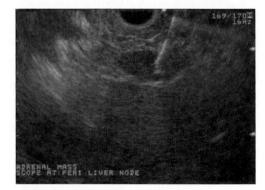

**Figure 73-6.** EUS-FNA of a lymph node.

### 11. How is EUS-FNA performed?

EUS is performed with a linear array scope, which provides an image along the long axis of the scope. This allows the endoscopist to visualize the exact position and action of the needle in sonographic real time. The flow and Doppler capability of this instrument allow for visualization of vascular structures that need to be avoided to perform safe tissue sampling. The 19- to 24-gauge aspiration needle, with a stylet, is introduced through the scope channel and under direct ultrasound visualization is advanced into the area to be sampled. Once the lesion has been entered, the stylet is advanced to the original position to clear any nonlesional tissue possibly adherent from the passage of the needle through the gastrointestinal tract. Suction is then applied with a syringe to the proximal end of the needle. Sometimes several *passes* are performed to ensure that enough material is obtained.

### 12. What are the advantages of EUS-FNA over other sampling modalities?

EUS-FNA allows definitive cytologic diagnosis of both primary and metastatic lesions and thus permits staging of the primary tumor, regional lymph nodes, and metastatic lesions (the TNM system). First, the patients undergoing evaluation of a suspected GI wall malignancy often require a EUS exam to obtain:

- (T) staging information (depth of penetration of lesion through the GI wall) of the lesion
- (N) Nodal staging with tissue acquisition can be performed in the same setting.
- (M) EUS-FNA can also be useful in determining the presence of distal metastasis, such as to the liver.

In addition, EUS-FNA allows the sampling of extremely small lesions including pleural and ascitic fluid collections that cannot be obtained by other means (such as CT-guided biopsy). In general, EUS staging accuracy appears to be better than all modalities except surgical exploration (Fig. 73-7).

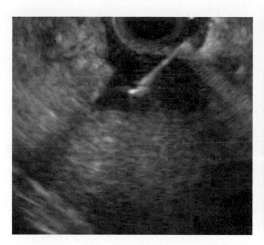

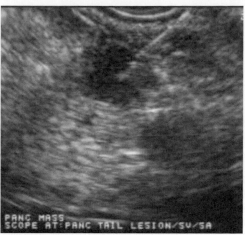

**Figure 73-7.** EUS-FNA of malignant ascites (not seen on CT scan).

**Figure 73-8.** EUS-FNA of neuroendocrine tumor in the tail of the pancreas.

### 13. What are the sensitivity and specificity of EUS-FNA for the diagnosis of malignancy?

The sensitivity and specificity of EUS-FNA for diagnosis of malignancy depend on the type of tissue being sampled (Table 73-4, Fig. 73-8).

### 14. What is the role of EUS-FNA in the evaluation of mediastinal lymphadenopathy?

EUS with FNA is the diagnostic test of choice for evaluating mediastinal lymphadenopathy. It has been found to be particularly useful in patients who have non–small cell lung cancer (NSCLC). In patients with NSCLC, the most significant predictor of long-term survival is the presence of metastasis within regional bronchopulmonary or mediastinal lymph nodes. In a large meta-analysis, EUS-FNA sensitivity in mediastinal nodes was 88.0% (95% CI, 85.8 to 90.0), and specificity was 96.4% (95% CI, 95.3 to 97.4). EUS-FNA is safer and more cost-effective than other more invasive methods of sampling, such as mediastinoscopy or thoracotomy (Fig. 73-9).

### 15. What are the risks of EUS-FNA?

The risks of EUS-FNA are thought to be extremely low, given the small diameter of the aspiration needle. In addition to the usual risks of any endoscopic procedure (bleeding, perforation, sedation risk), a 0.5% overall complication rate was reported in a multicenter trial predominantly from infectious or hemorrhagic events. EUS-FNA of the pancreas has a very small risk of acute pancreatitis, probably less than 1%.

### 16. What is the role of EUS in sampling pancreatic cystic neoplasms?

EUS with FNA can be used to obtain diagnosis in the case of suspected cystic neoplasms. Additional analysis of aspirated fluid can also be of value, such as a mucin stain (positive in intraductal papillary mucinous tumor, mucinous cystadenoma, and mucinous cystadenocarcinoma), determination of amylase level (suggestive of a pseudocyst), and CEA level. (A high CEA level would suggest the presence of mucinous cystadenoma with malignant potential, but a normal CEA level would suggest the presence of a serous cystadenoma or pseudocyst with no malignant potential [Fig. 73-10]).

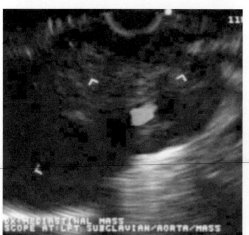

**Figure 73-9.** Mediastinal mass invading the left subclavian artery.

### 17. Is there a risk of biopsy tract seeding when EUS-FNA of a suspected malignancy is sampled?

Yes, although the amount of risk has been found to be very low. Comparative studies have found that there is less risk of seeding with EUS-FNA compared with percutaneous CT-guided FNA biopsy.

### 18. How is EUS-guided transmural pseudocyst drainage performed?

Transmural EUS-guided pseudocyst drainage can be performed by a multistep or single-step procedure. The multistep procedure involves EUS localization of the pseudocyst, followed by transmural drainage using a side-viewing endoscope (duodenoscope). Presence of gastric

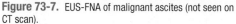

or duodenal varices and lack of bulging of the stomach/duodenum produced by the pseudocyst are contraindications to using a duodenoscope for transmural drainage.

The single-step procedure allows the endoscopist to achieve drainage of the pseudocyst with a single linear array EUS scope. This technique allows continued EUS imaging during the whole procedure. Presence of varices or the lack of a bulge does not preclude the performance of transmural drainage with this technique.

The placement of large-bore endoprostheses (10-Fr double-pigtail stents) requires the use of a therapeutic EUS scope. After the needle pathway is found to be safe (flow or Doppler interrogation), a 19-gauge FNA needle is advanced into the pseudocyst and cyst fluid is aspirated. A 0.035-inch guide wire is subsequently introduced through the needle into the pseudocyst cavity. Fluoroscopy can be used for guidance. After the guide-wire is coiled into the cyst, the FNA needle is removed, leaving the guide-wire in place. Opening of the gut-cyst wall is performed by cutting with needle knife, which is subsequently removed, leaving the guide-wire in place. Dilatation of the gut-cyst opening is performed, using a 10-mm biliary balloon dilator over the guide-wire. Dilation is followed by the placement of the first 10-Fr 2 to 3 cm double pigtail stent into the cyst. The original guide-wire is removed from the cyst. Placement of the second 10-Fr 2- to 3-cm double pigtail stent is performed over the wire after recannulation of the opening next to the first stent with the sphincterotome (Figs. 73-11 through 73-16).

19. **What are the indications for EUS-guided celiac plexus block (CPB) and celiac plexus neurolysis (CPN)? What is the difference? Why do they work?**
The celiac plexus transmits pain sensations from the pancreas and most of the abdominal organs. As a result, blockage of this transmission has been found to be effective in the therapy of pain.

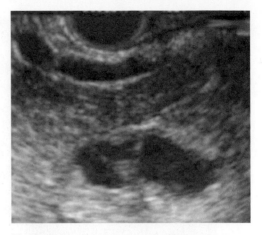

**Figure 73-10.** Septated cystic mass in the pancreas: biopsy positive for cystadenocarcinoma.

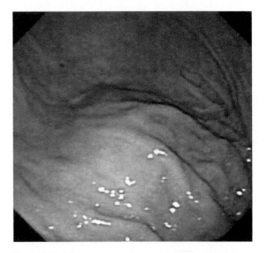

**Figure 73-11.** Bulge in gastric wall from pseudocyst seen endoscopically (bulge visualization is not necessary for single-step EUS-guided pseudocyst drainage).

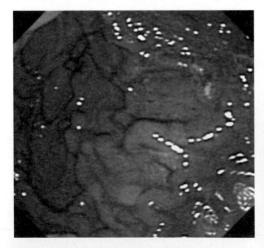

**Figure 73-12.** No bulge, but endoscopic presence of gastric varices in a patient with pseudocyst. EUS-guided pseudocyst drainage can still safely be performed.

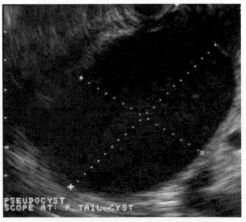

**Figure 73-13.** Visualization of pseudocyst with EUS.

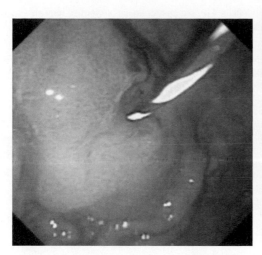

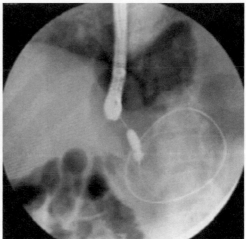

**Figure 73-14.** Transgastric placement of wire into cyst cavity.

**Figure 73-15.** Fluoroscopic view of wire in cyst cavity and dilation of tract.

- *CPB* refers to the use of steroid and /or local anesthetics to temporarily inhibit celiac plexus function in patients with uncontrolled pain secondary to chronic pancreatitis.
- *CPN* refers to the use of alcohol or phenol to produce neurolysis in patients with uncontrolled pain secondary to pancreatic cancer.

### 20. How are EUS-guided celiac plexus block and neurolysis performed?

The celiac trunk is easily identified with EUS, since it is located in close proximity to the posterior gastric wall. Due to its close proximity, EUS–fine-needle injection (FNI) is easily performed. A 22-gauge needle is advanced into the area and bupivacaine (an anesthetic) is injected to reduce discomfort. Next, alcohol (for pancreatic cancer) or steroids (for chronic pancreatitis) are injected to the plexus (Fig. 73-17).

### 21. What is the success rate of CPN? CPB?

The success rates of CPN and CPB differ. CPN performed for pain from pancreatic cancer has a reported sustained response of 78% at 2 weeks with a sustained response for up to 24 weeks independent of narcotic use or adjuvant therapy. CPB performed for pain secondary to chronic pancreatitis has a lower success rate.

### 22. What are the potential complications of CPN?

There is a 1% to 2% risk of major complications. Neurologic complications include lower extremity weakness, paresthesia, or paralysis. The artery of Adamkiewicz runs along the spine between T8 and L4 and perfuses the lower two thirds of the spinal cord. Spasm or thrombosis of this artery can lead to spinal cord ischemia. In addition, direct damage

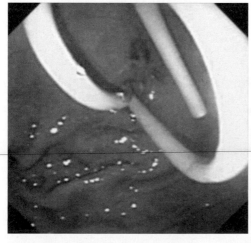

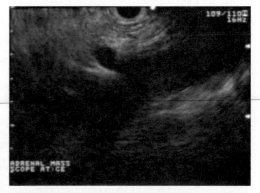

**Figure 73-16.** Final view of drainage stents.

**Figure 73-17.** Celiac axis identified by EUS

to the spinal cord or somatic nerves can cause neurologic deficits. Chronic gastroparesis or diarrhea may also occur. Bleeding, infection, and inadvertent organ puncture are also recognized complications.

**23. Is EUS-guided cholangiography or pancreatography possible? When are they indicated?**

Yes. EUS-guided pancreatography and cholangiography can be easily achieved due to the ability of EUS to image the common bile duct and pancreatic duct. Injection of contrast into the ducts can be performed. These techniques are used when endoscopic retrograde cholangiopancreatic tomography (ERCP) fails to gain access. This might be an issue in the case of tumor obstruction or surgically altered anatomy (Billroth II or gastrectomy with oux-en-Y). EUS-guided transduodenal and transgastric placement of the stents into the PD or biliary system is possible. This can be a viable alternative to percutaneous biliary drainage. EUS-guided pancreatic duct drainage has been performed via a transgastric route (pancreaticogastrostomy) to alleviate pain associated with chronic pancreatitis and ductal disruption/obstruction.

**24. What is high-frequency US-probe sonography-assisted EMR?**

A high-frequency ultrasound probe uses a frequency of 20 or 30 mHz, rather than 7.5- or 12-mHz frequencies used in a conventional EUS transducer. The probe is introduced through the working channel of a standard therapeutic endoscope. The advantage of this probe is that it can be placed directly on a lesion with direct endoscopic guidance. This allows one to evaluate the depth of invasion of a mucosal lesion, whether in the esophagus, stomach, or colon, and determine whether it can be appropriately and safely removed by EMR after submucosal injection (Fig. 73-18).

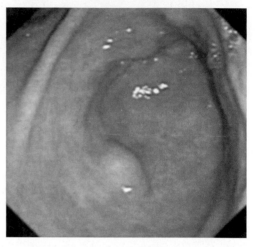

**Figure 73-18.** Submucosal mass seen on endoscopy.

## WEBSITES

http://daveproject.org/ViewFilms.cfm?Film_id=327

http://daveproject.org/viewfilms.cfm?film_id=597

## BIBLIOGRAPHY

1. Antillon MR, Bartalos CR, Miller ML, et al. En bloc endoscopic submucosal dissection of a 14-cm laterally spreading adenoma of the rectum with involvement to the anal canal: Expanding the frontiers of endoscopic surgery [with video]. Gastrointest Endosc 2008;67:332–7.
2. Antillon MR, Shah RJ, Stiegmann G, et al. Single-step EUS-guided transmural drainage of simple and complicated pancreatic pseudocysts. Gastrointest Endosc 2006;63:797–803.
3. Burmester E, Niehaus J, Leineweber T, et al. EUS-cholangio-drainage of the bile duct: Report of 4 cases. Gastrointest Endosc 2003;57(2).
4. Francois E, Kahaleh M, Giovannini M, et al. EUS-guided pancreaticogastrostomy. Gastrointest Endosc 2002;51:128–33.
5. Gotoda T, Oda I, Tamakawa K, et al. Prospective clinical trial of magnetic-anchor-guided endoscopic submucosal dissection for large early gastric cancer [with videos]. Gastrointest Endosc 2009;69:10–5.
6. Gunaratnam NT, Sarma AV, Norton ID, et al. A prospective study of EUS-guided celiac plexus neurolysis for pancreatic cancer pain. Gastrointest Endosc 2001;54:316–24.
7. Hawes RH, Fockens P. Endosonography. Philadelphia: WB Saunders; 2006. pp. 265–71.
8. Ho JM, Darcy SJ, Eysselein VE, et al. Evolution of fine needle aspiration cytology in the accurate diagnosis of pancreatic neoplasms. Am Surg 2007;73:941–4.
9. Kantsevoy SV, Alder DG, Conway JD, et al. Endoscopic mucosal resection and endoscopic submucosal dissection. Gastrointest Endosc 2008;68:11–8.
10. Levy MJ, Wiersema MJ. EUS-guided celiac plexus neurolysis and celiac plexus block. Gastrointest Endosc 2003;57:923–30.
11. Levy MJ, Topazian MD, Wiersema MJ, et al. Initial evaluation of the efficacy and safety of endoscopic ultrasound-guided direct ganglia neurolysis and block. Am J Gastroenterol 2008;103:98–103.
12. Naini BV, Apple SK, Presley M, et al. A correlation study on diagnostic endoscopic ultrasound-guided fine-needle aspiration of lymph nodes with histological and clinical diagnoses: The UCLA Medical Center experience. Diagn Cytopathol 2008;36:460–6.
13. Peng HQ, Greenwald BD, Tavora FR, et al. Evaluation of performance of EUS-FNA in preoperative lymph node staging of cancers of esophagus, lung, and pancreas. Diagn Cytopathol 2008;36:290–6.
14. Prasad P, Wittmann J, Pereira SP. Endoscopic ultrasound of the upper gastrointestinal tract and mediastinum: Diagnosis and therapy. Cardiovasc Intervent Radiol 2006;29:947–57.
15. Puli SR, Batapati Krishna Reddy J, Bechtold ML, et al. Endoscopic ultrasound: Its accuracy in evaluating mediastinal lymphadenopathy? A meta-analysis and systematic review. World J Gastroenterol 2008;21:3028–37.

# SURGERY: GASTROESOPHAGEAL REFLUX AND ESOPHAGEAL HERNIAS

Theodore N. Pappas, MD, and
James Padussis, MD

**CHAPTER 74**

## GASTROESOPHAGEAL REFLUX DISEASE

1. **Define *gastroesophageal reflux disease* (GERD).**
   GERD is defined as symptoms and/or mucosal injury due to the abnormal reflux of gastric contents into the esophagus. One third of the U.S. population suffers from symptoms of GERD at least once monthly, and 4% to 7% experience daily symptoms. Although there is a high prevalence of heartburn, not everyone with heartburn has GERD.

2. **Describe the typical and atypical symptoms of GERD.**
   The typical symptoms of GERD include heartburn, regurgitation, or water brash (in which the oral cavity suddenly fills with fluid, usually clear and perhaps acidic) or dysphagia (the blockage to the passage of food in the lower substernal area). Classic heartburn is defined as the substernal burning that lasts for a few moments to several minutes, that is relieved by antacids or food, and that occurs a half hour or an hour after meals. Atypical or extraesophageal symptoms include cough, asthma, hoarseness, and noncardiac chest pain. Atypical symptoms are the primary complaint in 20% to 25% of patients with GERD and are secondarily associated with heartburn and regurgitation in many more. Nearly 50% of patients with chest pain and negative coronary angiograms, 75% with chronic hoarseness, and up to 80% with asthma have a positive 24-hour esophageal pH test, indicating abnormal acid reflux into the esophagus. While many patients with atypical symptoms benefit from antireflux surgery, it is not as effective as for those patients with typical symptoms.

3. **What factors play a role in altering the gastroesophageal (GE) barrier?**
   The two most important are hypotension of the lower esophageal sphincter (LES) and loss of the angle of His due to hiatal hernia. Either may contribute to loss of competency of the sphincter and thus abnormal reflux. Physiologic reflux or reflux in early disease result from the transient loss of the high-pressure zone normally created by the tonic contraction of the smooth fibers of the LES. In severe GERD, the high-pressure zone is permanently reduced or nonexistent.

   A large hiatal hernia alters the geometry of the GE junction, and the angle of His is lost. There is a close relationship between the degree of gastric distention necessary to overcome the high-pressure zone and the morphology of the gastric cardia. In patients with an intact angle of His, more gastric dilatation and higher intragastric pressure are necessary to overcome the sphincter than in patients with a hiatal hernia. Furthermore, a hiatal hernia may also result in hypotension of the LES. However, every patient with a hiatal hernia does not have GERD, and the presence of a small, sliding hiatal hernia without GERD is not an indication for medical or surgical intervention.

4. **Describe the workup of patients with suspected GERD.**
   Because reoperations for GERD are associated with poorer results than an initial repair, every effort should be made to obtain a complete and thorough evaluation before surgical repair. The four recommended tests are barium swallow and upper gastrointestinal series, esophagogastroduodenoscopy (EGD), esophageal manometry, and 24-hour pH test.

   - *Barium esophagram* is most useful in assessing the size and reducibility of a hiatal hernia and presence of esophageal shortening. A large, fixed hiatal hernia or paraesophageal hernia and a short esophagus are evidence of advanced disease and may predict a long, difficult operation.
   - *EGD* helps to identify the presence of esophagitis and Barrett's esophagus. It can be also used to evaluate response to treatment and to detect complications of GERD, including peptic stricture and shortened esophagus. Furthermore, endoscopy provides valuable information about the absence of other lesions in the upper gastrointestinal tract that can produce symptoms identical to those of GERD.
   - *Esophageal manometry* evaluates the peristaltic function of the esophagus and the pressure and relaxation of the LES. It is not a diagnostic test but provides information about the severity of the underlying physiologic defects of the LES and esophageal body. It also determines the location of the LES for proper placement of 24-hour pH probes, 5 cm above the LES. Furthermore, manometry helps rule out achalasia or other esophageal motility problems.

- *Esophageal pH monitoring* is the most direct method for assessing the presence and severity of GERD and, because it has the highest sensitivity and specificity of all available tests, has become the gold standard for the diagnosis of GERD. It is especially useful in the evaluation of patients with atypical symptoms and patients with typical symptoms but with no evidence of esophagitis on endoscopy. The test also measures the correlation between symptoms and episodes of reflux. It should be performed in every patient before surgical repair and with patients off acid suppression. A new device, the BRAVO probe, is a miniaturized pH probe that is attached to the lower esophagus via EGD and transmits pH data to a recording device that the patient wears. It stays in the esophagus for 5 days and is then excreted in the stool. The advantage of the probe is that it is much better tolerated than the standard nasoesophageal probes.

### 5. What is the significance of a defective LES?

The finding of a permanently defective LES (pressure less than 6 mm Hg) has several implications. First, it is almost always associated with esophageal mucosal injury and predicts that symptoms will be difficult to control with medical therapy alone. It is a signal that surgical therapy is probably needed for consistent, long-term control as the condition is irreversible, even when the associated esophagitis has healed. The worse the esophageal injury, the more likely it is that the LES is defective. Approximately 40% of patients with pH-positive GERD and no mucosal injury have a mechanically defective LES, whereas nearly 100% of patients with long-segment Barrett's esophagus have a defective LES.

### 6. What is the significance of abnormal esophageal motility in patients with GERD?

Long-standing, severe GERD can lead to deterioration of esophageal body function. Abnormalities of esophageal body function include a lack of peristalsis, severely disordered peristalsis (more than 50% simultaneous contractions), or ineffective peristalsis (the amplitude of the contractions in one or more of the lower esophageal segments is less than 30 mm Hg) also called ineffective esophageal motility (IEM). Dysphagia is generally a prominent symptom in patients with defective peristalsis.

### 7. What is Barrett's esophagus and what are the risk factors?

Barrett's esophagus is defined as the metaplasia of the normally squamous epithelium of the esophagus into columnar epithelium with intestinal metaplasia. Barrett's esophagus is a premalignant condition and the incidence of esophageal adenocarcinoma increases nearly 40-fold in patients with Barrett metaplasia. Please see Chapter 7.

### 8. What are the indications for an antireflux operation?

The introduction of minimally invasive procedures to surgically treat GERD has increased the frequency of these operations. The ability to permanently stop gastroesophageal reflux and rid patients of dependence on expensive medications has prompted gastroenterologists to refer patients for surgical therapy more readily. Indications for surgery include complications of the disease including erosive esophagitis, peptic stricture, Cameron ulcer (chronic iron-deficiency anemia caused by slow bleeding from the point where the herniated stomach rubs against the diaphragm), and Barrett's esophagus. However, the most common indication for surgery is persistent symptoms despite maximal medical therapy and reluctance to take medication for life, or for whom medications are a financial burden. Surgery may be the treatment of choice in patients who are at high risk of progression despite medical therapy, the risk factors for which include:

- Nocturnal reflux on 24-hour esophageal pH study
- Structurally deficient LES (pressure less than 6 mm Hg)
- Mixed reflux of gastric and duodenal juice
- Mucosal injury at presentation

### 9. What are the surgical options to relieve GERD?

All of the successful surgical procedures for GERD have certain characteristics in common. All obtain an intra-abdominal segment of esophagus, prevent recurrence of the hiatal hernia if present, and create an antireflux valve.

- Dor fundoplication—partial 270-degree anterior fundoplication.
- Belsey Mark IV—partial 270-degree anterior fundoplication via thoracic approach.
- Toupet fundoplication—partial 270-degree posterior fundoplication.
- Nissen fundoplication—total 360-degree fundoplication.

The approach to the repair can be abdominal (open or laparoscopic), thoracic (open or video-assisted thoracic surgery), and even thoracoabdominal. None of the operations or approaches is perfect for all patients. If the esophagus is shortened, consider approaching from the chest and performing a Collis gastroplasty in which a portion of the lesser curvature is stapled and divided to create extra esophageal length (Fig. 74-1). If esophageal motility is an issue, consider a partial wrap so as not to produce severe dysphagia.

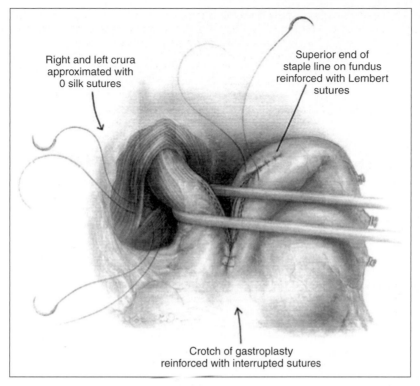

Right and left crura
approximated with
0 silk sutures

Superior end of
staple line on fundus
reinforced with Lembert
sutures

Crotch of gastroplasty
reinforced with interrupted sutures

**Figure 74-1.** Thoracoscopic view of Collis gastroplasty, which is necessary in patients with a short esophagus. (From Cameron JL: Current Surgical Therapy. Philadelphia, Mosby, 2004.)

**10. What are the important technical steps of a Nissen fundoplication?**

Despite the caveats in the previous paragraph, laparoscopic Nissen fundoplication is now the procedure of choice for most patients with all other operations compared to the best Nissen results. Five trocars are inserted in the upper abdomen to provide access for the laparoscope and instruments. The short gastric vessels are divided in the proximal part of the stomach, and the fundus of the stomach is mobilized so that it can be placed around the distal esophagus without tension. Dissection is performed to identify the right and left crura of the diaphragm. The distal esophagus is mobilized so that at least 3 cm of the distal esophagus lies without tension in the abdomen. The crura are approximated with nonabsorbable sutures, and the fundoplication is constructed around the distal esophagus (Fig. 74-2). A bougie (range, 48- to 60-Fr depending on the size of the patient) is placed in the esophagus to prevent an excessively tight fundoplication. Some surgeons anchor the wrap to the crura of the diaphragm and to the esophagus to help prevent it from slipping into the chest.

**11. What are the predictors of successful antireflux surgery?**

Predictors of successful antireflux surgery include typical symptoms of GERD (heartburn and regurgitation), an abnormal score on 24-hour esophageal pH monitor, and symptomatic improvement in response to acid suppression therapy before surgery. Each of these factors helps to establish that GERD is the cause of the symptoms and they have little to do with the severity of the disease.

**12. What are the predictors of poor outcome after antireflux surgery?**

Most patients with documented GERD, normal esophageal body function, and length without stricture or scarring have excellent outcomes. The presence of gastrointestinal (GI) symptoms other than typical GERD symptoms predicts less than optimal results. A large hiatal hernia, stricture with persistent dysphagia, and Barrett are characteristics of advanced GERD and may predict less than ideal results.

**13. Explain the benefits of surgical treatment of GERD.**

Antireflux procedures performed by experienced esophageal surgeons provide several benefits that cannot be accomplished with antacid medications. A successful operation augments the LES and repairs the hiatal hernia if present. It prevents the reflux of both gastric and duodenal juice, thus preventing aspiration. Antireflux operations also improve esophageal body motility and speed gastric emptying, which is often subclinically delayed in patients with GERD. More than 90% of patients are relieved of symptoms, eat unrestricted diets, and are satisfied with the surgical outcome.

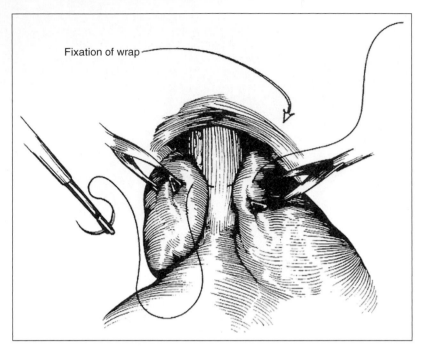

**Figure 74-2.** Laparoscopic view of the placement of the first fundoplication stitch. (From Cameron JL: Current Surgical Therapy. Philadelphia, Mosby, 2004.)

## 14. What are the complications of laparoscopic fundoplication?

A laparoscopic antireflux operation is associated with significantly reduced postoperative pain, shorter hospitalization, quicker recovery, and improved cosmesis when compared with the open approach. The overall incidence of complications after laparoscopic Nissen fundoplication is between 2% and 13%. Most complications are minor and include urinary retention, postoperative gastric distention, and superficial wound infections. Mild early dysphagia may be found in 15% to 20% of patients, but the incidence of residual dysphagia after 3 months is less than 5%. Less than 1% of these patients need intervention to treat dysphagia. The incidence of serious complications and mortality are both less than 1%.

## PARAESOPHAGEAL HERNIAS

## 15. Define the four types of hernias occurring at the hiatus.

* *Type I* is a sliding hiatal hernia in which the GE junction migrates through the hiatus into the posterior mediastinum. This is the most common type of hiatal hernia.
* *Type II* is a true paraesophageal hernia, characterized by an upward dislocation of the fundus of the stomach alongside a normally positioned GE junction. This is the least common type of hiatal hernia.
* *Type III* is a combination of types I and II, characterized by cephalad displacement of both the GE junction and typically a large portion of the fundus and body of the stomach into the chest. Type III hernias probably start as a sliding hernia, and as the hiatus enlarges over time a progressively greater portion of the fundus and body of the stomach herniate through the defect.
* *Type IV* are type III hernias in which other viscera such as the colon or spleen are included in the hernia sac. These are quite uncommon and represent only (2% to 5%) of all paraesophageal hernias (Table 74-1).

**Table 74-1.** Types of Hernias Occurring at the Hiatus

| HERNIA TYPE | LOCATION OF GASTROESOPHAGEAL JUNCTION | HERNIA CONTENTS | SPONTANEOUS REDUCIBILITY |
|---|---|---|---|
| Type I (Sliding) | Intrathoracic | Fundus | Usually reducible |
| Type II (True paraesophageal) | Intra-abdominal | Fundus ± body | Often fixed |
| Type III (Mixed) | Intrathoracic | Fundus + body | Fixed |
| Type IV (Type III with other viscera included) | Intrathoracic | Fundus + body + other organ | Fixed |

## 16. What causes a hiatal hernia?

The precise cause of a hiatal hernia is unknown. Its pathogenesis is thought to involve at least two important factors including increased intra-abdominal pressure and a progressive enlargement of the diaphragmatic hiatus. The increased incidence with age suggests that these hernias are acquired.

## 17. What are the signs and symptoms of a paraesophageal hernia?

Many hiatal hernias are asymptomatic and are first recognized on chest radiography. Type I is often associated with reflux but does not cause direct symptoms. Paraesophageal hernias classically cause symptoms of chest pain and shortness of breath after eating. Shortness of breath is secondary to loss of vital capacity due to impingement of hernia contents on the lung. Other symptoms, which may or may not be present, include early satiety, abdominal bloating, and gastroesophageal reflux. Cameron ulcers are often the cause of unexplained microcytic anemia in the elderly with otherwise normal upper and lower endoscopy. Rarely, acute herniation occurs, causing sudden pain and symptoms of gastric outlet obstruction. Strangulation can cause gastric necrosis, resulting in rapid decompensation, shock, and death.

## 18. How are hiatal and paraesophageal hernias diagnosed and evaluated?

Paraesophageal hernias are often first suspected because of a chest radiograph abnormality. Classically a retrocardiac air bubble with or without an air-fluid level will be present. Confirmation can be obtained with a barium swallow, which shows the typical appearance of a large intrathoracic stomach. Upper endoscopy is useful to evaluate the distal esophagus and stomach for ulcers, erosions, Barrett's esophagus, or neoplasms in this generally elderly population. An esophageal motility study is recommended in patients being considered for elective surgical correction of a paraesophageal hernia both to determine the status of the lower esophageal sphincter and to assess the function of the esophageal body. This is particularly true in any patient with symptoms of dysphagia. A 24-hour pH test is usually not necessary because a fundoplication is recommended as part of the procedure to correct this defect.

## 19. What are the indications for surgical repair of paraesophageal hernias?

In most patients with a paraesophageal hernia, it is the hernia itself that is responsible for symptoms and imparts the risk of life-threatening complications. The only therapy for the hernia is surgical, and currently there is controversy about which patients should have an operation and which procedure and approach are most appropriate. It was once widely recommended that any medically fit patient found to have a paraesophageal hernia undergo surgical correction regardless of symptoms or the age of the patient. This was based on information suggesting that there is a 30% risk of developing a life-threatening complication with these hernias, and that mortality for elective repair is significantly reduced compared with emergent surgery for complications of a paraesophageal hernia. Recent studies have suggested that the frequency of life-threatening complications is lower than previously reported and elective repair in truly asymptomatic patients is no longer recommended. However, all patients with symptoms or signs should undergo repair in the absence of prohibitive surgical risk.

## 20. What is the operative strategy of a paraesophageal hernia repair?

The key steps of paraesophageal hernia repair are:

- Return stomach and esophagus to their normal intra-abdominal positions.
- Remove the hernia sac.
- Close the hiatus.
- Anchor the stomach below the diaphragm.

In most circumstances, a fundoplication is added both to augment the lower esophageal sphincter and to aid in stabilizing the repair below the diaphragm. There are three approaches for the surgical repair of paraesophageal hernias: transabdominal, transthoracic, and laparoscopic. Traditionally, a transthoracic repair has been advocated because of the relative ease of mobilizing the esophagus and dissecting out the hernia sac and its contents. However, as the stomach is reduced blindly into the abdomen, an organoaxial rotation of the stomach could persist or redevelop and lead to an intra-abdominal gastric volvulus. The abdominal approach is now preferred with the main advantage being the ability to place the stomach into the appropriate anatomic orientation. Laparoscopic repair offers the advantages of decreased length of postoperative discomfort, earlier return to regular activities, and shorter hospital stay.

## WEBSITE

http://www.vhjoe.com

## BIBLIOGRAPHY

## Gastroesophageal Reflux Disease

1. Allen CJ, Anvari M. Gastro-oesophageal reflux related cough and its response to laparoscopic fundoplication. Thorax 1998;53:963–8.
2. Bredenoord AJ, Smout AJ. High resolution manometry. Dig Liver Dis 2008;40:174–81.
3. Campos GM, Peters JH, DeMeester TR, et al. Multivariate analysis of factors predicting outcome after laparoscopic Nissen fundoplication. J Gastrointest Surg 1999;3:292–300.
4. Campos GM, Peters JH, DeMeester TR, et al. The pattern of esophageal acid exposure in gastroesophageal reflux disease influences the severity of the disease. Arch Surg 1999;134:882–7; discussion, 887–888.
5. Castel DO. Management of gastroesophageal reflux disease. Maintenance medical therapy of gastroesophageal reflux? Which drugs, how long? Dis Esophagus 1994;7:230–3.
6. Collet D, Cadiere GB. Conversions and complications of laparoscopic treatment of gastroesophageal reflux disease. Formation for the Development of Laparoscopic Surgery for Gastroesophageal Reflux Disease Group. Am J Surg 1995;169:622–6.
7. Constantini M, Zaninotto G, Anselmino M, et al. The role of a defective lower esophageal sphincter in the clinical outcome of treatment for gastroesophageal reflux disease. Arch Surg 1996;131:655–9.
8. Fein M, Ritter MP, DeMeester TR, et al. Role of the lower esophageal sphincter and hiatal hernia in the pathogenesis of gastroesophageal reflux disease. J Gastrointest Surg 1999;3:405–10.
9. Fry LC, Monkemuller K, Malfertheiner P. Endoluminal therapy for gastro-oesophageal reflux disease: Evidence from clinical trials. Eur J Gastroen Hepat 2007;19:1125–39.
10. Hinder RA, Filipi CJ, Wetscher G, et al. Laparoscopic Nissen fundoplication is an effective treatment for gastroesophageal reflux disease. Ann Surg 1994;220:472–81; discussion, 481–483.
11. Hunter JG, Trus TL, Branum GD, et al. A physiologic approach to laparoscopic fundoplication for gastroesophageal reflux disease. Ann Surg 1996;223:673–85; discussion, 685–687.
12. Lundell L. Therapy of gastroesophageal reflux: evidence-based approach to antireflux surgery. Dig Dis 2007;25:188–96.
13. Nehra D, Howell P, Williams CP, et al. Toxic bile acids in gastro-oesophageal disease: Influence of gastric acidity. Gut 1999;44:598–602.
14. Oelschlager BK, Eubanks T, Oleynikov D, et al. Symptomatic and physiologic outcomes after operative treatment for extraesophageal reflux. Surg Endosc 2002;16:1032–6.
15. Pace F, Costamagna G, Penagini R, et al. Endoscopic antireflux procedures—An unfulfilled promise? Aliment Pharm Therap 2008;27:375–84.
16. Peters JH. The surgical management of Barrett's esophagus. Gastroenterol Clin North Am 1997;26:647–68.
17. Richter JE. Gastrooesophageal reflux disease. Best Pract Res Clin Ga 2007;21:609–31.
18. Schwartz MP, Smout AJ. The endoscopic treatment of gastro-oesophageal reflux disease. Aliment Pharm Ther 2007;26:1–6.
19. Sifrim D, Fornari F. Esophageal impedance-pH monitoring. Dig Liv Dis 2008;40:161–6.
20. So JB, Zeitels SM, Rattner DW. Outcomes of atypical symptoms attributed to gastroesophageal reflux treated by laparoscopic fundoplication. Surgery 1998;124:28–32.
21. Triadafilopoulos G. Endotherapy and surgery for GERD. J Clin Gastroenterol 2007;41:S87–96.
22. Vakil N. The role of surgery in gastro-oesophageal reflux disease. Aliment Pharm Ther 2007;25:1365–72.

## Paraesophageal Hernias

23. Draaisma WA, Gooszen HG, Tournoij E, Broeders IA. Controversies in paraesophageal hernia repair: A review of literature. Surg Endosc 2005;19:1300–8.
24. Kelty CJ, Falk GL. Mesh Repairs in hiatal surgery. The case against mesh repairs in hiatal surgery. Ann R Coll Surg Engl 2007;89:479–81.
25. Lal DR, Pellegrini CA, Oelschlager BK. Laparoscopic repair of paraesophageal hernia. Surg Clin North Am 2005;85:105–18.
26. Landreneau RJ, Del Pino M, Santos R. Management of paraesophageal hernias. Surg Clin North Am 2005;85:411–32.
27. Mehta S, Boddy A, Rhodes M. Review of outcome after laparoscopic paraesophageal hiatal hernia repair. Surg Laparosc Endosc Percutan 2006;16:301–6.
28. Oelschlager BK, Pelligrini CA. Paraesophageal hernias: Open, laparoscopic, or thoracic repair? Chest Surg Clin N Am 2001;11:589–603.
29. Smith G. Mesh repairs in hiatal surgery. The case for mesh repairs in hiatal surgery. Ann R Coll Surg Engl 2007;89:481–3.
30. Sytopoulos N, Gazelle GS, Rattner DW. Paraesophageal hernia: Operation or observation? Ann Surg 2002;236:492–501.
31. Wolf PS, Oeschlager BK. Laparoscopic paraesophageal hernia repair. Adv Surg 2007;41:199–210.

# SURGERY: ACHALASIA AND ESOPHAGEAL CANCER

*Theodore N. Pappas, MD, and*
*James Padussis, MD*

# CHAPTER 75

## ACHALASIA

**1. Define *achalasia*. What are the classic findings of esophageal achalasia?**
Achalasia is a primary motility disorder of the esophagus characterized by a loss of peristaltic waveform in the body and failure of the lower sphincter to relax in response to swallowing. The condition is relatively rare, occurring at an incidence of 0.5 to 1 per 100,000 of the population per year. Achalasia can occur at any age and typically has an insidious onset.

**2. What are the most common symptoms of achalasia?**
The nonrelaxing lower esophageal sphincter (LES) causes a functional outflow obstruction to the lower esophagus, resulting in progressive dysphagia, regurgitation, weight loss, and chest pain. Please see Chapter 4 for more discussion about the diagnosis of achalasia.

**3. What is pseudoachalasia? How is it diagnosed?**
Characteristic manometric and radiologic findings of achalasia may, occasionally, be seen in patients with distal esophageal obstruction from an infiltrating tumor. Such patients have a local tumor that may directly intrinsically or extrinsically compress the esophagus. Endoscopy helps rule out the possibility of pseudoachalasia but cannot diagnosis a mural or extramural tumor. When this is suspected based on a history of substantial weight loss (more than 20 lb in 6 months), endoscopic ultrasonography (EUS) and/or computed tomography (CT) is recommended.

**4. What is vigorous achalasia?**
Is a variant of achalasia where the esophageal body responds to a swallow with normal or less often high-amplitude contractions that may be multiphasic, but as with classic achalasia, there are no progressive peristaltic waves. Patients with vigorous achalasia are usually younger and have chest pain as a prominent symptom. Most investigators believe that vigorous achalasia is an early form of the disease that presents in some patients.

**5. What are the nonsurgical options for treatment of achalasia?**
- Smooth muscle relaxants
- Botulinum
- Pneumatic dilatation of the LES

Please see Chapter 4 for more discussion of medical management of achalasia.

**6. What are the basic components of laparoscopic Heller myotomy for achalasia?**
Surgical treatment of achalasia consists of a longitudinal myotomy of the distal esophagus and gastroesophageal (GE) junction. Most myotomies were performed through the chest before the advent of minimally invasive surgery. The transabdominal laparoscopic approach is currently the procedure of choice with good long-term results in 84% to 94% of patients.

Five trocars are placed in the upper abdomen in an arrangement similar to that of a laparoscopic antireflux operation. A myotomy roughly 6 to 8 cm in length is performed, with 3 cm below the GE junction. The myotomy is carried down to the level of the mucosa. A partial fundoplication is performed after the completion of the myotomy around a 52-Fr bougie. There is a general consensus that a complete 360-dgree wrap may cause significant obstruction at the distal end of the esophagus and lead to worsening of esophageal function in patients with already impaired peristalsis. The Toupet fundoplication (partial posterior wrap) and Dor fundoplication (partial anterior wrap) are equally popular among surgeons. With the addition of an antireflux wrap, the incidence of gastroesophageal reflux disease (GERD) decreases from 25% to 48% to 5% to 20%. Most of these patients have mild-to-moderate reflux and can be easily managed medically.

### 7. How do long-term results of Heller myotomy compare with mechanical esophageal dilatation?

In the only randomized controlled trial with long-term follow-up that compared pneumatic dilatation and surgical myotomy, dysphagia was relieved in 91% of patients after surgical myotomy and 65% after pneumatic dilatation. In addition, several large retrospective series have compared the two treatments and favor operative myotomy over pneumatic dilatation. With the introduction of the laparoscope, the historical concerns about the morbidity associated with open surgical techniques have essentially disappeared and the morbidity and mortality of both surgical and nonsurgical options are now nearly identical. The long-term success and safety of laparoscopic myotomy have completed the shift in favor of surgery as the primary therapeutic option for patients with achalasia.

### 8. Describe the complications of Heller myotomy.

The most common complication of a surgical myotomy is esophageal perforation, which is reported in less than 5% of patients. While the rate of perforation is not increased, it has been reported that previous pneumatic dilatation and botulinum toxin injection increase the technical difficulty in performing a myotomy. Mucosal injuries detected during surgery may be repaired primarily. An unrecognized esophageal perforation may present as persistent fever, tachycardia and/or left-sided pleural effusion. These patients require close observation and may necessitate reoperation if conservative measures fail.

Early postoperative dysphagia results usually from an incomplete myotomy while causes of late dysphagia also include healing of the myotomy or, more rarely, a reflux-induced peptic stricture. Incomplete myotomy responds usually to extension of the myotomy. However, in patients where the first myotomy was complete, a second myotomy is less likely to be successful and such patients may require esophageal resection.

### 9. Summarize the treatment algorithm for patients with achalasia.

Laparoscopic surgical myotomy has replaced pneumatic dilatation as the treatment of choice for achalasia. Heller myotomy should be offered as early as possible to young patients with achalasia. They have a higher incidence of failure with dilatation and botulinum toxin injections, and early surgery is recommended to avoid long-term complications. Pneumatic dilatation may be offered once or twice to patients with mild-to-moderate disease. However, superior long-term results after surgical myotomy argue strongly for surgery in any patient who is fit enough to undergo general anesthesia. Botulinum toxin injection should be reserved for patients who are unable to tolerate surgery because of significant comorbidities or whose clinical presentation is complicated and the diagnosis of achalasia is in doubt.

### 10. What is the association between achalasia and esophageal cancer?

Patients with achalasia are thought to be at increased risk for the development of squamous cell carcinoma. Tumors develop at an age 10 years younger than in the general population and carry a worse prognosis because of late diagnosis. The effect of surgical treatment on the incidence of cancer is not known and surveillance endoscopy is recommended every 2 years.

## ESOPHAGEAL CANCER

### 11. What is the incidence of esophageal cancer?

Cancer of the esophagus accounts for 1% of all newly diagnosed cancers in the United States, and the incidence has continued to rise in the last 30 years. An estimated 13,200 new cases of carcinomas of the esophagus were diagnosed in 2001, with 12,500 deaths due to the disease. It is seven times more common in men than women and is the seventh leading cause of death from cancer among men. Whereas squamous cell carcinoma accounted for most cancers of the esophagus 40 years ago, adenocarcinoma now represents more than 70% of such tumors in the United States. This is primarily caused by the striking increase in incidence of adenocarcinoma among white men older than 60 years. The cause for the rising incidence and changing demographics is unknown.

### 12. What are the risk factors of esophageal cancer?

Risk factors for squamous cell carcinoma have been well described. Tobacco and excessive alcohol consumption appear to have a synergistic effect in its pathogenesis. Risk factors for the development of distal esophageal adenocarcinoma are less clear. The presence of Barrett's esophagus is associated with an increased risk of developing adenocarcinoma, and recently a population-based case-control study from Sweden has demonstrated that symptomatic chronic gastroesophageal reflux is also a risk factor. For a discussion of the diagnosis and staging of esophageal cancer, please see Chapters 5 and 7.

### 13. Describe the relationship of Barrett's esophagus to esophageal cancer.

Barrett columnar-lined esophagus is an acquired condition of the distal esophagus associated with chronic gastroesophageal reflux. The incidence of adenocarcinoma increases nearly 40-fold in patients with Barrett's esophagus.

It is estimated that 5% of patients with Barrett's esophagus will eventually develop invasive cancer, and patients with histologically proven Barrett's esophagus require lifelong surveillance because of this risk. It is generally believed that disease progresses from Barrett metaplasia to low-grade dysplasia to high-grade dysplasia to adenocarcinoma.

## 14. Can Barrett's esophagus regress after antireflux therapy?
Recent publications have strongly suggested that curtailing reflux decreases the tendency of GERD patients without Barrett to develop Barrett's esophagus. In addition, reflux control diminishes, if not eliminates completely, the tendency toward dysplastic and/or malignant degeneration of existing Barrett epithelium. This effect is manifested by:

- Inducing actual regression of dysplastic to nondysplastic Barrett epithelium
- Stabilizing the Barrett epithelium in a nondysplastic state
- Allowing a return to normal squamous epithelium. The majority of regression occurs within 5 years after surgery.

## 15. Discuss the surgical management of patients with high-grade dysplasia.
*High-grade dysplasia* is defined as the detection in the Barrett epithelium of epithelial abnormalities that could equally be described as carcinoma in situ. Multiple large surgical series document that following esophageal resection, between 20% and 40% of patients with Barrett's esophagus who have severe dysplasia will be found to actually have invasive carcinoma in the specimen. Although this means that the majority of the patients will not have invasive carcinoma, the inability to reliably distinguish the two groups preoperatively means that every patient should be thought of as having a probably carcinoma. In addition, the likelihood of developing cancer in the first 3 to 5 years once severe dysplasia has been identified is 25% to 50%. This increases to 80% risk of adenocarcinoma development in 8 years. Therefore, the finding of severe dysplasia is an extremely strong indication for surgical resection.

## 16. What are the surgical approaches to the patient with esophageal cancer?
Surgery is the primary treatment modality for esophageal cancer. In the United States, esophageal resection is most commonly performed, using one of the following approaches:

- *Transhiatal esophagectomy* involves both a midline laparotomy and left cervical incision. The short gastric and left gastric arteries are ligated, whereas the right gastric artery and right gastroepiploic arcade are carefully preserved. A cervical gastroesophageal anastomosis is performed through the cervical incision. The main advantage of this approach is avoidance of a thoracic anastomosis because a cervical leak carries much less morbidity than for a thoracic leak.
- *Ivor-Lewis esophagectomy* requires a midline laparotomy and a right posterolateral thoracotomy. En bloc resection is performed from the hiatus to the apex of the chest. A gastroesophageal anastomosis is performed in the right chest.
- *Multi-incision esophagectomy* is performed less often and requires a midline laparotomy, thoracotomy and a cervical incision.
- *Left thoracoabdominal esophagectomy* involves one incision extended across the abdomen and posterolateral chest.

Regardless of the incision approach, the same operative procedure is performed, that is, esophagogastrectomy with regional lymph node resection. Though each approach has its proponents, transhiatal esophagectomy is the most common procedure performed, with a decreased incidence of pulmonary complications, the reduced morbidity and mortality of an anastomotic leak, and no evidence that a radical lymphadenectomy benefits overall survival cited as the most compelling arguments.

## 17. When is neoadjuvant therapy appropriate in the treatment of patients with esophageal carcinoma?
The data on neoadjuvant therapy are mixed with some studies showing no statistical difference in outcomes and others demonstrating some benefit to chemoradiation followed by surgery. Potential advantages of neoadjuvant therapy include cancer down staging, increased resectability, and reduction in micrometastasis. In addition, the chemotherapeutic agents used (cisplastin, mitomycin, and 5-fluorouracil) all possess radiosensitizing properties. It is an accepted practice at many institutions to undergo resection alone in patients with clinical stage I and II disease, whereas patients with stage III disease are more commonly treated by neoadjuvant therapy. However, more studies are needed to verify the effectiveness of this treatment strategy.

## 18. Describe nonsurgical options for treatment of esophageal cancer.
Nonsurgical options for treatment of esophageal cancer can be divided into interventions for palliation and those for cure. Precancerous lesions or superficial cancers confined to the mucosa without evidence of metastatic spread can be cured with local therapy. Appropriate candidates include patients with limited high-grade dysplasia and superficial adenocarcinoma associated with Barrett's esophagus. In these cases, alternative therapies, such as endoscopic mucosal resection, endoscopically applied laser, photodynamic therapy, or argon plasma coagulation, are ablative therapies that have been curative in certain cases. When curative treatment is not possible, in addition to systemic chemotherapy,

palliative care measures have included external beam radiation, endoluminal brachytherapy, endoluminal stenting, laser ablation, and photodynamic therapy.

## 19. What is the survival of patients with esophageal cancer?

The overall 5-year survival in patients undergoing surgery varies, depending on stage. Those patients with stage I disease have an excellent 5-year survival, around 80%. The 5-year survival for stage II and stage III disease is 35% and 10%, respectively. Those with stage IV disease live rarely beyond 18 months. Unfortunately, most esophageal cancers present at later stages, when cure is not possible and palliation is the only treatment option.

## BIBLIOGRAPHY

### Achalasia

1. Annese V, Bassotti G. Non-surgical treatment of esophageal achalasia. World J Gastroenterol 2006;12:5763–6.
2. Bonavina L. Minimally invasive surgery for esophageal achalasia. World J Gastroenterol 2006;12:5921–5.
3. Bortolotti MM, Lopilato C, Porrazzo C, et al. Effects of sildenafil on esophageal motility of patients with idiopathic achalasia. Gastroenterology 2000;118:253–7.
4. Farrohki F, Vaezi MF. Idiopathic (primary) achalasia. Orphanet J Rare Dis 2007;2:38.
5. Finley RJ, Rattenberry J, Clifton JC, et al. Practical approaches to the surgical management of achalasia. Am Surg 2008;74:97–102.
6. Leyden JE, Moss AC, MacMathuna P. Endoscopic pneumatic dilation versus botulinum toxin injection in the management of primary achalasia. Cochrane Database Syst Rev 2006;4: CD005046.
7. Litle VR. Laparoscopic Heller myotomy for achalasia: A review of the controversies. Ann Thorac Surg 2008;85:S743–6.
8. Luckey AE, DeMeester SR. Complications of achalasia surgery. Thorac Surg Clin 2006;16:95–8.
9. Pehlivanov N, Pasricha PJ. Achalasia: Botox, dilatation or laparoscopic surgery in 2006. Neurogastroenterol Motil 2006;18:799–804.
10. Pohl D, Tatuian R. Achalasia: An overview of diagnosis and treatment. J Gastrointest Liver Dis 2007;16:297–303.

### Esophageal Cancer

11. Avidan B, Sonnenberg A, Schnell TG, et al. Hiatal hernia size, Barrett's length, and severity of acid reflux are all risk factors for esophageal adenocarcinoma. Am J Gastroenterol 2002;97:1930–6.
12. Barr H. High-grade dysplasia in Barrett's oesophagus. The case against oesophageal resection. Ann R Coll Surg Engl 2007;89:586–8.
13. Dyer SM, Levison DB, Chen RY, et al. Systematic review of the impact of endoscopic ultrasound on the management of patients with esophageal cancer. Int J Technol Assess Health Care 2008;24:25–35.
14. Gurski RR, Peters JH, Hagen JA, et al. Barrett's Esophagus can and does regress after antireflux surgery: A study of prevalence and predictive features. J Am Coll Surg 2003;195:706–12.
15. Ku GY, Ilson DH. Preoperative therapy in esophageal cancer. Clin Adv Hematol Oncol 2008;6:371–9.
16. Lagergren J, Bergstrom R, Lindgren A, et al. Symptomatic gastroesophageal reflux as a risk factor for esophageal adenocarcinoma. N Engl J Med 1999;340:825–31.
17. Mabrut J, Baulieux J, Adham M, et al. Impact of anti-reflux operation on columnar-lined esophagus. J Am Coll Surg 2003;196:60–7.
18. Oelschlager BK, Barreca M, Chang L, et al. Clinical and pathologic response of Barrett's esophagus to laparoscopic antireflux surgery. Ann Surg 2003;238:458–64.
19. Pennathur A, Luketich JD. Resection for esophageal cancer: Strategies for optimal management. Ann Thorac Surg 2008;85:S751–6.
20. Pondugula K, Wani S, Sharma P. Barrett's esophagus and esophageal adenocarcinoma in adults: Long-term GERD or something else? Curr Gastroenterol Rep 2007;9:468–74.
21. Rastogi A, Puli S, El-Serag HB, et al. Incidence of esophageal adenocarcinoma in patients with Barrett's esophagus and high-grade dysplasia: A meta-analysis. Gastrointest Endosc 2008;67:394–8.
22. Veuillez V, Rougier P, Seitz JF. The multidisciplinary management of gastrointestinal cancer. Multimodal treatment of oesophageal cancer. Best Pract Res Clin Gastroenterol 2007;21:947–63.

# SURGERY FOR PEPTIC ULCER DISEASE

# CHAPTER 76

*Theodore N. Pappas, MD, and*
*James Padussis, MD*

**1. Describe the five types of gastric ulcer in terms of location, gastric acid secretory status, incidence, and complications.**

A peptic ulcer may arise at various locations, including the stomach (gastric ulcer), duodenum (duodenal ulcer), and esophagus (esophageal ulcer). Gastric ulcers are further divided into five types based on location, secretory status, and cause (Table 76-1, Fig. 76-1).

**2. Describe the classic indications and goals for peptic ulcer surgery.**

Since the introduction of $H_2$-receptor antagonists and proton pump inhibitors (PPIs) and the identification of *Helicobacter pylori* as an ulcerogenic cofactor, the frequency of elective operations for peptic ulcer disease (PUD) has decreased by more than 90%. Currently, surgery for duodenal and gastric ulcers is generally reserved for the management of complications of PUD. The classic indications for peptic ulcer surgery are:

- Intractability of symptoms
- Perforation
- Bleeding
- Gastric outlet obstruction

The main goals of surgery are to:

- Treat any complications of PUD
- Eliminate the factors that contribute to ulcer occurrence

These goals should be accomplished with minimization of surgical side effects and complications.

**3. What are the three classic operations used for PUD?**
- Truncal vagotomy and drainage
- Truncal vagotomy and antrectomy
- Highly selective vagotomy (parietal cell vagotomy or proximal gastric vagotomy)

**4. Describe the truncal vagotomy, selective vagotomy, and highly selective vagotomy.**
- *Truncal vagotomy*—involves the division of both anterior and posterior vagal trunks at the esophageal hiatus above the origins of the hepatic and celiac branches. Periesophageal dissection must include the distal 6 to 8 cm of the esophagus to ensure division of gastric vagal branches that arise from the trunks above the level of the hiatus. Thus, truncal vagotomy results in denervation of all vagal nerve–supplied viscera. A drainage procedure, usually a pyloroplasty, must be performed with truncal vagotomy, because denervation of the pylorus results in impaired gastric emptying.

**Table 76-1.** The Five Types of Gastric Ulcer Defined by Location, Gastric Acid Secretory Status, Complications and Incidence

| TYPE | LOCATION | ACID HYPERSECRETION | COMPLICATIONS | INCIDENCE |
|------|----------|---------------------|---------------|-----------|
| I | Gastric body, lesser curvature | No | Bleeding uncommon | 55% |
| II | Body of stomach + duodenal ulcer | Yes | Bleeding, perforation, obstruction | 20% |
| III | Prepyloric | Yes | Bleeding, perforation | 20% |
| IV | High on lesser curvature | No | Bleeding | <5% |
| V | Anywhere (medication induced) | No | Bleeding, perforation | <5% |

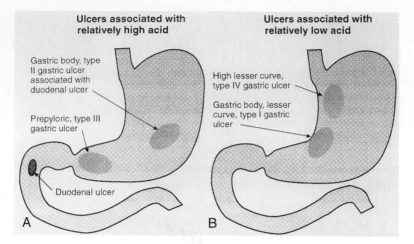

**Figure 76-1.** The four types of gastric ulcers and their association with either (**A**) high acid or (**B**) low acid. (From Sabiston DC Jr: Textbook of Surgery: The Biologic Basis of Modern Surgical Practice. Philadelphia, WB Saunders, 1997.)

- *Selective vagotomy*—involves division of the vagal trunks distal to the hepatic and celiac branches, thereby preserving vagal innervation to the gallbladder and celiac plexus. This reduces the incidence of gallbladder dysmotility, gallstones, and diarrhea. However, selective vagotomy also results in complete gastric vagotomy, necessitating a drainage procedure. Selective vagotomy is not the operation of choice, as it is needlessly complex and not superior to truncal vagotomy; it is rarely used and only of historic importance.
- *Highly selective vagotomy* (parietal cell vagotomy or proximal gastric vagotomy)—involves selective division of the vagal fibers to the acid-producing parietal cell mass of the gastric fundus, while maintaining vagal fibers to the antrum and distal gut. The anterior and posterior neurovascular attachments are divided along the lesser curvature of the stomach, beginning approximately 7 cm from the pylorus and progressing to the gastroesophageal junction, with additional skeletalization of the distal 6 to 8 cm of the esophagus to ensure division of the *criminal nerve of Grassi*. Innervation of the antrum and pylorus is maintained because the two terminal branches of the anterior and posterior nerves of Latarjet are left intact.

### 5. Why is an outlet or *drainage* procedure added to truncal vagotomy? What are the surgical options?

Truncal vagotomy involves division of both anterior and posterior vagal trunks at the esophageal hiatus. This procedure results in denervation of the acid-producing mucosa of the gastric fundus as well as the pylorus and antrum, causing an alteration of normal pyloric coordination and impaired gastric emptying. Thus, a procedure to eliminate function of the pyloric sphincter must be performed to allow gastric drainage. There are four primary options for an outlet procedure (Fig. 76-2):

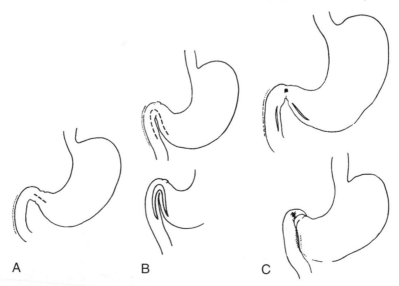

**Figure 76-2.** *A,* Heineke-Mikulicz pyloroplasty. *B,* Finney pyloroplasty. *C,* Jaboulay gastroduodenostomy are the primary options for an outlet or *drainage* procedure after truncal vagotomy. (From Zollinger RM: Atlas of Surgical Operations. New York, McGraw-Hill, 1993.)

- *Heineke-Mikulicz pyloroplasty*—a longitudinal incision of the pyloric sphincter, extending into the duodenum and antrum, is closed transversely
- Finney pyloroplasty—a U-shaped incision crossing the pylorus is made and a gastroduodenostomy is created; used in cases of extensive duodenal scarring to create a wider gastroduodenal opening
- Jaboulay gastroduodenostomy—a side-to-side gastroduodenostomy is created in which the incision does not cross the pyloric sphincter; used when severe pyloric scarring precludes division of the pyloric channel
- Gastrojejunostomy—Billroth II or Roux-en-Y anastomosis

## 6. What are the relative indications and contraindications to highly selective vagotomy?

Highly selective vagotomy is indicated for the treatment of intractable duodenal ulcers because, unlike truncal vagotomy, it does not require a drainage procedure. It has also been used in the emergent treatment of bleeding or perforated duodenal ulcers in stable patients. Highly selective vagotomy is contraindicated in patients with prepyloric ulcers or with gastric outlet obstruction because they demonstrate high rates of recurrent ulceration. The ulcer recurrence rate is closely tied to the surgeon's experience with this operation and in the PPI era should only be performed by an experienced gastrointestinal (GI) surgeon well versed in the technique.

## 7. What are the surgical options for reconstruction after antrectomy?

- Billroth I reconstruction consists of a gastroduodenostomy in which the anastomosis is created between the gastric remnant and the duodenum (Fig. 76-3).
- Billroth II reconstruction consists of a gastrojejunostomy in which a side-to-side anastomosis is created between the gastric remnant and a loop of jejunum, with closure of the duodenal stump (Fig. 76-4).
- Roux-en-Y reconstruction involves the creation of a jejunojejunostomy (forming a Y-shaped figure of small bowel) downstream from the anastomosis of the free jejunal end to the gastric remnant (gastrojejunostomy).

## 8. How is the type of reconstruction determined for a given patient?

The decision of which type of reconstruction to perform is determined, in large part, by the extent of duodenal scarring due to PUD. Severely scarred duodenum cannot be used for a Billroth I anastomosis. The Billroth I reconstruction, however, offers the most physiologic anastomosis because it restores normal continuity of the GI tract. The Billroth II reconstruction may be complicated by afferent loop syndrome in which obstruction of the afferent limb results in accumulation of bile and pancreatic secretions, causing right upper quadrant abdominal pain that is alleviated by bilious vomiting. Roux-en-Y reconstruction allows diversion of bile and pancreatic secretions away from the gastric outlet, thereby reducing the risk of bile reflux gastritis. However, it can result in a delay in gastric emptying.

## 9. Define *intractability* in terms of the medical treatment of PUD?

*Intractability* is defined as mucosal healing refractory to maximal medical therapy. The following three criteria define a refractory ulcer and are generally indications for operative intervention:

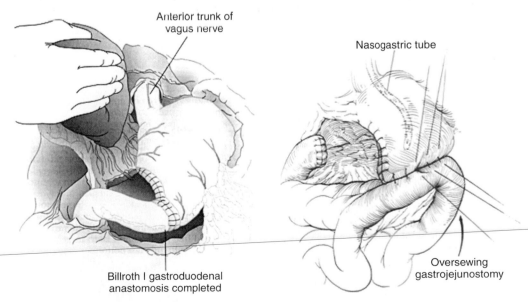

**Figure 76-3.** Hemigastrectomy with Billroth I anastomosis. (From Townsend CM: Sabiston Textbook of Surgery, ed 18. Philadelphia, WB Saunders, 2008.)

**Figure 76-4.** Hemigastrectomy with Billroth II anastomosis. (From Sabiston DC: Atlas of General Surgery. Philadelphia, WB Saunders, 1994.)

- Ulcer persistence after 3 months of medical therapy
- Ulcer recurrence within 1 year, despite maintenance medical therapy
- Ulcer disease in which cycles of prolonged activity are interrupted by brief or absent remissions

## 10. Describe the most appropriate elective operative procedure for duodenal ulcers and each type of gastric ulcer.

The choice of operation for gastric ulcers depends on several factors: ulcer location, acid secretory status, and presence of a coexistent duodenal ulcer. In general, gastric ulcers should be included with the resection while duodenal ulcers heal after acid suppression.

- *Type I:* antrectomy with inclusion of the ulcer and Billroth I or II reconstruction. Although type I gastric ulcers are associated with low to normal acid secretion, most surgeons include a truncal vagotomy, unless achlorhydria is demonstrated.
- *Type II and III:* truncal vagotomy, antrectomy with inclusion of the gastric ulcer and Billroth I reconstruction. Type II and III gastric ulcers are associated with high rates of acid secretion and therefore the goal of the surgery is removal of the gastric mucosa at risk for ulceration and reduction of acid secretion.
- *Type IV:* distal gastrectomy with resection proximally to include the ulcer high on the lesser curvature and Billroth I anastomosis. Because type IV ulcers are located high on the lesser curvature they are surgically challenging.
- *Type V:* surgery is reserved for treatment of complications. Type V gastric ulcers generally heal rapidly with cessation of aspirin or a nonsteroidal anti-inflammatory drug (NSAID) and institution of an $H_2$-receptor antagonist or PPI. An intractable type V gastric ulcer should raise suspicion for underlying malignancy.
- *Duodenal ulcer:* historically, the highly selective vagotomy has been the mainstay of treatment. However, the intractable duodenal ulcer is a rare entity in the PPI era and may represent a more resistant variant with a higher rate of recurrence. Therefore, truncal vagotomy with pyloroplasty is predominantly used today.

## 11. Describe the presentation of a patient with a perforated peptic ulcer.

Patients usually describe a prodrome of gnawing pain in the epigastric region prior to perforation. With acute perforation, the epigastric pain becomes diffuse and is often associated with fever, tachycardia, tachypnea, and hypotension. Patients with a perforated posterior duodenal ulcer will often present with upper GI bleeding secondary to erosion into the gastroduodenal artery. On examination, the patient with peptic ulcer perforation lies immobile. Bowel sounds are typically absent, and the abdomen is diffusely tender and rigid. The white blood cell count is elevated, and, in 70% of cases, free intraperitoneal air is found on upright abdominal radiographs. Although computed tomography (CT) scan is the most sensitive radiologic test for free intraperitoneal air, it is rarely indicated because patients with perforated peptic ulcer usually present with classic signs and symptoms, and CT scanning only serves to delay an operation.

## 12. Why do almost all perforated gastric ulcers require an operation?

- Perforated gastric ulcers usually fail to heal spontaneously.
- They are associated with a risk of adenocarcinoma.
- Gastric ulcer disease produces a hypoacidic environment with resultant bacterial overgrowth and abscess formation with perforation.
- On rare occasions, patients with a perforated duodenal ulcer may be managed medically, particularly if the ulcer has been perforated for longer than 24 hours, and a contrast study indicated that the perforation is contained.

## 13. What are the contraindications to medical management of perforated PUD?

- Concurrent use of corticosteroids, which makes healing unlikely
- Continued leak, as demonstrated by a contrast radiograph
- Perforation in a patient taking an $H_2$-receptor antagonist or a PPI. A definitive ulcer operation is necessary to allow ulcer healing and to reduce the risk of recurrence

## 14. What are the three major goals of operation for perforated PUD?

- Repair of the perforation—usually performed by suturing the perforation closed and buttressing the repair with omental fat as a Graham patch (Fig. 76-5).

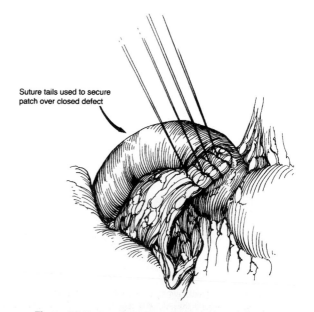

Suture tails used to secure patch over closed defect

**Figure 76-5.** Omental patching of a perforated peptic ulcer.

- Copious irrigation of the abdominal cavity
- Definitive ulcer operation—a patient who has had a perforation for less than 24 hours and is hemodynamically stable without significant comorbidities should undergo a definitive ulcer operation if he or she has known PUD, has been receiving medical therapy for PUD, or is taking medication that increases the risk of PUD.

## 15. What is the preferred operation for treatment of perforated gastric ulcer?

The major distinction between surgical management of perforated duodenal and perforated gastric ulcers is that in all cases of perforated gastric ulcers, carcinoma must be excluded. Thus, all perforated gastric ulcers must undergo biopsy or resection. One option is to perform a wedge resection as diagnostic biopsy. Controversy exists as to whether a definitive ulcer operation should be added to this procedure, with most surgeons in favor of a definitive acid-reducing procedure in type II or III variant. An alternative for perforated antral ulcers is antrectomy (with inclusion of the ulcer in the resection), to which truncal vagotomy may be added if the patient is an acid hypersecretor.

## 16. What is the preferred operation for treatment of a perforated duodenal ulcer?

In patients who have undergone medical therapy to eradicate *H. pylori*, the classic operation for a perforated duodenal ulcer is truncal vagotomy and pyloroplasty, with incorporation of the perforation into the pyloroplasty closure. This relatively simple procedure requires a short operative time. In the ideal surgical candidate, highly selective vagotomy with patch closure of the perforation is recommended, although this procedure requires a high degree of surgical expertise. Patients who have not been treated for *H. pylori* prior to perforation should undergo repair and Graham patch of a perforated duodenal ulcer with postoperative *H. pylori* eradication therapy, in lieu of a definitive ulcer operation.

## 17. What are the major risk factors for mortality in the surgical treatment of perforated PUD?

- Severe comorbidities
- Perforation present for longer than 24 hours
- Hemodynamic instability on presentation

Patients with one of these risk factors have a mortality rate of approximately 10%; with two risk factors, the mortality rate increases to 46%. Patients with all three risk factors have a mortality rate of nearly 100%. Thus, nonsurgical management of perforated PUD should be considered in elderly patients with any of these risk factors.

## 18. Discuss the role for laparoscopy in the management of perforated PUD and the indications for conversion to an open operation.

The surgical goals in the laparoscopic management of a perforated peptic ulcer are similar to those of open surgical management:

- Repair of the perforation
- Copious irrigation of the abdominal cavity
- Addition of a definitive ulcer operation, which depends on the skill of the surgeon and may involve either laparoscopic truncal vagotomy and pyloroplasty or a laparoscopic highly selective vagotomy

The relative indications for conversion to an open procedure include posterior location of the ulcer and inadequate localization. The presence of a perforated gastric ulcer with its suspicion for malignancy often necessitates conversion for definitive diagnosis.

## 19. In patients with GI bleeding caused by PUD, what are the predictors for rebleeding in the hospital? What is the Forrest classification?

- Hemodynamic instability
- Hematocrit less than 30
- Multiple comorbidities
- Coagulopathy
- Hematemesis
- Inability to clear the stomach with aggressive lavage

The Forrest classification describes endoscopic risk factors for rebleeding; see Chapter 51.

## 20. What are the classic indications for operation for rebleeding after endoscopic therapy?

After endoscopic therapy for a bleeding peptic ulcer, patients who require further resuscitation with 6 units of blood should be strongly considered for surgical intervention. In general, the indications for surgical treatment of a bleeding peptic ulcer are:

- Hemodynamic instability as a result of massive hemorrhage, although cardiovascular stabilization must precede surgery
- Need for multiple transfusions due to continued bleeding
- Failure of nonsurgical therapy to prevent bleeding

## 21. What are the operative options for control of a bleeding gastric ulcer?

Bleeding gastric ulcers require excision and biopsy to rule out malignancy. Small gastric ulcers (less than 2 cm) can usually be excised easily and safely, with the addition of an ulcer operation for patients who are acid hypersecretors. Large gastric ulcers, lesser curvature ulcers, bleeding ulcers associated with gastritis, and gastric ulcers that penetrate into the pancreas often require a more radical and technically demanding operation (subtotal, 75% resection, or near total, 95% resection, gastrectomy) to control hemorrhage.

## 22. What is the most appropriate surgical procedure for a bleeding duodenal ulcer?

Control of the ulcer bed is attained by performing a duodenotomy with direct ligation of the bleeding vessel or complete plication of the ulcer bed. If a posterior duodenal ulcer has eroded into the gastroduodenal artery, bleeding may be profuse. If a patient has ulcer disease refractory to medical management or is on chronic NSAID therapy, a definitive ulcer operation is then performed. This may consist of either truncal vagotomy and pyloroplasty or a truncal vagotomy and antrectomy. An alternative approach is to attain control of the bleeding duodenal ulcer through a pyloroplasty incision, in which case a truncal vagotomy completes the definitive ulcer operation. Patients who have not been treated for *H. pylori* prior to bleeding should undergo ligation of the bleeder only, with postoperative *H. pylori* eradication therapy, in lieu of a definitive ulcer operation.

## 23. How is gastric outlet obstruction due to PUD surgically managed?

Gastric outlet obstruction (GOO) can result from an acute exacerbation of PUD in the setting of chronic pyloric and duodenal scarring. Classically, patients with GOO present with nausea, emesis, early satiety, and weight loss. Although radiologic contrast studies are useful in evaluation, upper endoscopy is critical to rule out a malignant cause of the obstruction. While in *H. pylori*–positive patients a trial of medical management may be successful, operative intervention is necessary in over 75% of patients presenting with GOO. The two main goals of surgery are to relieve the obstruction and to perform a definitive ulcer operation. Truncal vagotomy and antrectomy with Billroth II reconstruction is performed if the duodenal stump can be safely closed. If the stump cannot be closed, a tube duodenostomy is left in place for control of secretions until the stump closes by secondary intention. An alternative is to perform a truncal vagotomy and pyloroplasty, which often requires the Finney pyloroplasty or Jaboulay gastroduodenostomy because of severe scarring. Truncal vagotomy and gastrojejunostomy may be performed, if the severe scarring precludes an adequate drainage procedure via the duodenum.

## 24. Discuss the role for endoscopic and laparoscopic management of GOO secondary to PUD.

In *H. pylori*–positive patients, endoscopic balloon dilatation combined with laparoscopic highly selective vagotomy and medical therapy has been associated with success rates as high as 75%. Patients treated with balloon dilatation, without treatment of *H. pylori* infection, however, have a higher rate of failure and recurrent obstruction. Patients who are negative for *H. pylori* do not respond favorably to balloon dilatation and should be considered for surgical treatment early in the process.

Laparoscopic truncal vagotomy and drainage procedure, either pyloroplasty or jejunostomy, has been described successfully in small case series with low morbidity. The choice of open or laparoscopic management depends on the skill and experience of the surgeon.

## 25. What are the long-term outcomes and risks for complications after truncal vagotomy and drainage, truncal vagotomy and antrectomy, and highly selective vagotomy?

Truncal vagotomy and antrectomy, while having the lowest recurrence rate, also has the highest morbidity and mortality (Table 76-2). Highly selective vagotomy, while having the lowest morbidity and mortality, has the highest recurrence rate. The surgeon must balance these issues, patient preference, and the pathophysiology of the ulcer type in question when choosing an operative plan.

**Table 76-2.** Comparison of Surgical Options for Peptic Ulcer Disease

| | TRUNCAL VAGOTOMY AND ANTRECTOMY | TRUNCAL VAGOTOMY AND DRAINAGE | HIGHLY SELECTIVE VAGOTOMY |
|---|---|---|---|
| Mortality rate | 1% to 2% | 0.5% to 0.8% | 0.05% |
| Recurrence rate | Low | Moderate | High |
| Dumping | 10% to 15% | 10% | 1% to 5% |
| Diarrhea | 20% | 25% | 1% to 5% |

## 26. What are the Visick criteria?

The Visick criteria are used to grade outcome after surgery for PUD:

- Grade I—No symptoms
- Grade II—Mild symptoms that do not affect daily life
- Grade III—Moderate symptoms that affect daily life and require treatment but are not disabling
- Grade IV—Recurrent ulceration or disabling symptoms

Grades I and II are considered adequate results. Most poor outcomes fall into grade III.

## 27. How should postoperative gastroparesis be managed?

Postoperative gastroparesis typically occurs in patients who undergo surgery for gastric outlet obstruction. Evaluation should begin with esophagogastroduodenoscopy (EGD), upper GI series with small bowel follow-through, and gastric emptying scan. Once mechanical obstruction has been ruled out, medical treatment is successful in most cases. Prokinetic agents such as erythromycin and metocloperamide may be helpful. The indications for reoperation are:

- Early marginal ulcers refractory to medical management
- Anatomic abnormalities of the gastric outlet
- Recurrent bezoar associated with weight loss

Intractable gastroparesis following vagotomy and drainage may be treated with subtotal gastrectomy. A Billroth II reconstruction may be preferable to Roux-en-Y reconstruction because the latter option may be associated with persistent gastric emptying problems.

## 28. Describe the management of duodenal stump disruption (*blow-out*) after truncal vagotomy, antrectomy, and Billroth II reconstruction.

Patients presenting with localized right upper quadrant tenderness are managed by aggressive percutaneous drainage of the abscess under radiologic guidance. An acute abdomen with free perforation and leakage of duodenal contents into the peritoneal cavity may require surgical management as a last resort. This includes re-closure of the duodenal stump over a tube duodenostomy as well as an external drain around the tube. Mortality from stump blowout approaches 10%.

## 29. What is dumping syndrome? Describe the pathophyoiology and treatment.

The dumping syndrome consists of tachycardia, diaphoresis, hypotension, and abdominal pain after meals in patients who have undergone ulcer operations, such as truncal vagotomy. Its pathophysiology is loss of receptive relaxation of the fundus in response to a gastric load. Thus, gastric pressure increases during a meal, and rapid decompression through the gastric outlet causes the classic signs and symptoms. Symptoms improve typically with time and can be alleviated in some patients by separation of solids and liquids during meals. Conversion of a Billroth II to a Billroth I or a Billroth operation to a Roux-en-Y reconstruction can improve symptoms. Octreotide, a somatostatin analog, has been used to alleviate symptoms.

## 30. Describe the pathophysiology of bile reflux gastritis. How is it managed?

Bile reflux gastritis occurs when ablation of the pylorus in a gastric ulcer operation results in stasis of bile in the stomach. The diagnosis is made with the following triad of findings:

1. Postprandial epigastric pain accompanied by nausea and bilious emesis
2. Evidence of bile reflux into the stomach or gastric remnant
3. Biopsy-proved gastritis

Bile reflux gastritis can occur after truncal vagotomy and pyloroplasty or truncal vagotomy and antrectomy with Billroth reconstruction. Although up to 20% of patients who undergo these operations may have transient bile reflux gastritis postoperatively, symptoms resolve in all but 1% to 2%.

Treatment of bile reflux gastritis requires revision of the pyloroplasty or the Billroth reconstruction to a Roux-en-Y gastrojejunostomy with a 50- to 60-cm limb (Fig. 76-6). Bilious emesis resolves in nearly 100% of patients who undergo revision. The symptoms of bile reflux gastritis may be indistinguishable from those of gastroparesis. Because the Roux-en-Y gastrojejunostomy worsens the symptoms of gastroparesis, care must be taken to exclude the diagnosis of gastroparesis preoperatively.

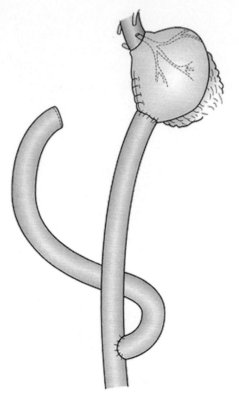

**Figure 76-6.** Conversion of Billroth I or Billroth II reconstruction to a Roux-en-Y anastomosis. (From Cameron JL: Current Surgical Therapy. Philadelphia, Mosby, 2004.)

## 31. What is the presentation of Zöllinger-Ellison syndrome?

Most patients with Zöllinger-Ellison syndrome present with PUD and/or diarrhea. Ulcers are typically duodenal. The diarrhea resembles steatorrhea and results from a combination of high volumes of acid and neutralization of pancreatic enzymes. In patients with Zöllinger-Ellison syndrome associated with multiple endocrine neoplasia (MEN) syndrome I, signs and symptoms may be related to parathyroid or pituitary disease.

## 32. How is Zöllinger-Ellison syndrome diagnosed?

A high level of suspicion is required for the diagnosis of gastrinoma. Serum gastrin should be measured in all patients undergoing peptic ulcer surgery. If the gastrin level is in the range of 1000 to 2000 pg/mL, gastric pH analysis demonstrating acid production confirms the diagnosis. If the gastrin level is minimally elevated, the patient should undergo gastric pH analysis and a secretin test. The secretin test is performed by comparison of basal serum gastrin level with gastrin level after the administration of secretin. Gastrinoma is suspected in patients with an increase in the serum gastrin level of 200 pg/mL after secretin administration. Normal patients have no change or a reduction in serum gastrin after secretin administration. Because achlorhydria is more common than gastrinoma, an elevation in serum gastrin is due more commonly to lack of acid as opposed to ectopic gastrin production. Therefore, measurement of acid production is also essential in making the appropriate diagnosis.

## 33. For which patients with Zöllinger-Ellison syndrome is operative intervention indicated?

Surgery is the treatment of choice for patients with nonmetastatic sporadic gastrinoma. In addition, patients with metastatic gastrinoma who are unable to tolerate or are refractory to medical management should be considered for operative intervention. The gastrinoma seen as part of MEN syndrome differs from sporadic gastrinomas. Sporadic gastrinomas are often solitary and located in the pancreas or duodenum, but not both, and are amenable to surgical resection and cure. Although gastrinomas seen with MEN syndrome are usually multiple, virtually always in the duodenum and often multicentric, they are also found in the pancreas and are more difficult to cure surgically. Gastrinoma associated with hypercalcemia should suggest MEN syndrome complicated by hyperparathyroidism, and parathyroidectomy is essential for management of gastric acid hypersecretion. Elevated serum gastrin levels postoperatively after gastrinoma surgery indicate residual gastrinoma(s) that should be treated medically. Medical management is also generally indicated for patients with metastatic gastrinoma. Medical management consists of high-dose PPIs with the goal of reducing gastric acid output to less than 10 mEq/hr for the hour that immediately precedes the next scheduled dose of antisecretory medication.

## 34. Describe the preoperative evaluation for gastrinoma.

CT scan with intravenous and oral contrast is routine in the preoperative evaluation for gastrinoma resection to rule out metastatic disease, and its accuracy is dependent on the size of the gastrinoma. In some cases, magnetic resonance imaging (MRI) is used because it is more sensitive than CT scan for liver metastases. Rarely, partial venous sampling for gastrin has been successful in localizing gastrinoma; however, this is an expensive and cumbersome technique with a risk of complications. The advent of somatostatin receptor scintigraphy (octreotide) scan has greatly improved the preoperative localization of gastrinomas. This study relies on the high density of somatostatin receptors on gastrinomas and uses the radiolabeled synthetic somatostatin analog, iodine-125—[125I]octreotide—to identify primary as well as metastatic gastrinomas.

Recent studies have demonstrated that somatostatin receptor scintigraphy has high sensitivity and specificity for detection of primary and metastatic gastrinomas and is the initial imaging modality of choice for localization. Endoscopic ultrasound has recently been used to localize gastrinomas; however, it is highly operator dependent and does not reliably identify small tumors in the duodenum. Intraoperative upper endoscopy with transillumination may also help to localize small duodenal gastrinomas. More recently, a modification of octreotide scanning has become available as an adjunct to intraoperative localization. A handheld gamma-detecting probe is used intraoperatively to localize gastrinomas after the injection of [125I]octreotide.

## 35. Where is the gastrinoma triangle? What percentage of tumors occur in this area?

The apex of the gastrinoma triangle is at the cystic duct–common bile duct junction, and the triangle is bounded by the border of the second and third portions of the duodenum and the junction of the neck and body of the pancreas (Fig. 76-7). Approximately 60% to 75% of gastrinomas are found within this triangle.

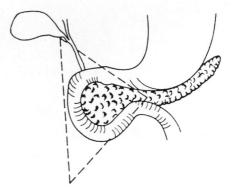

**Figure 76-7.** The gastrinoma triangle.

## 36. Describe the operative scheme for exploration, localization, and removal of gastrinoma.

If no tumor is obvious on preoperative CT scan, and other preoperative localization studies have failed, exploration begins with exposure of the anterior surface of the pancreas by mobilization of the transverse colon. A Kocher maneuver is then performed to mobilize the duodenum, allowing complete bimanual palpation of the pancreas. Intraoperative ultrasound is concentrated in the gastrinoma triangle. Biopsy of lymph nodes should be performed because, occasionally, the gastrinoma is localized to a solitary node. If ultrasound of the pancreas does not reveal the tumor, duodenal gastrinoma should be suspected. A pyloroplasty incision is made, and the duodenal wall is visually inspected and manually palpated. An alternative method of localizing duodenal gastrinomas is to transilluminate the wall with intraoperative endoscopy. Gastrinomas in the duodenal wall or pancreas may be enucleated, but solitary lesions in the pancreatic tail are often treated by distal pancreatectomy.

If no lesion is found or if the disease is found to be multicentric or metastatic, an ulcer operation may be performed as palliation. This procedure often consists of a truncal vagotomy and pyloroplasty. Alternatively, the patient may be maintained on a PPI. In rare cases, a total gastrectomy may be performed for control of acid production in patients who are refractory to medical therapy or unable to tolerate the side effects of the medication.

## 37. Describe the risk of gastric stump cancer after partial gastrectomy for duodenal and gastric ulcer.

*Gastric stump carcinoma* is defined as adenocarcinoma of the stomach that occurs at least 5 years after partial gastric resection for benign disease. In patients who have had a partial distal gastrectomy for gastric ulcer, the relative risk is no different than in the general population in the first 20 years but rises to 3.0 after 20 years. Annual screening gastroscopy and biopsy should be performed in patients who underwent gastric resection at least 15 years earlier and have moderate-to-severe dysplasia on biopsy.

### BIBLIOGRAPHY

1. Anlauf M, Gabrecht N, Henopp T, et al. Sporadic versus hereditary gastrinomas of the duodenum and pancreas: Distinct clinico-pathological and epidemiological features. World J Gastroenterol 2006;12:5440–6.
2. Azimuddin K, Chamberlain RS. The surgical management of pancreatic neuroendocrine tumors. Surg Clin North Am 2001;81:511–25.
3. Behrman SW. Management of complicated peptic ulcer disease. Arch Surg 2005;140:201–8.
4. Dubois F. New surgical strategy for gastroduodenal ulcer: Laparoscopic approach. World J Surg 2000;24:270–6.
5. Hansson L-E. Risk of stomach cancer in patients with peptic ulcer disease. World J Surg 2000;24:315–20.
6. Harbison SP, Dempsey DT. Peptic ulcer disease. Curr Probl Surg 2005;42:346–454.
7. Jamieson GG. Current status of indications for surgery for peptic ulcer disease. World J Surg 2000;24:256–8.
8. Johnson AG. Proximal gastric vagotomy: Does it have a place in the future management of peptic ulcer? World J Surg 2000;24:259–63.
9. Kleef J, Friess H, Buchler MW. How *Helicobacter pylori* changed the life of surgeons. Dig Surg 2003;20:93–102.
10. Klondo K. Duodenogastric reflux and gastric stump carcinoma. Gastric Cancer 2002;5:1–22.
11. Lipof T, Shapiro D, Kozol RA. Sporadic versus hereditary gastrinomas of the duodenum and pancreas: Distinct clinico-pathological and epidemiological features. World J Gastroenterol 2006;12:3248–52.
12. Millat B, Fingerhut A, Borie F. Surgical treatment of complicated duodenal ulcers: Controlled trials. World J Surg 2000;24:299–306.
13. Mercer DW, Robinson EK. The stomach. In: Sabiston Jr DC, editors. Textbook of surgery: The biological basis of modern surgical practice. 18th ed. Philadelphia: Saunders/Elsevier; 2008. pp. 1236–56.
14. Mulholland MW. Duodenal ulcer. In: Greenfield LJ, editor. Surgery: Scientific principles and practice. 3rd ed. Philadelphia: Lippincott Williams & Wilkins; 2001. pp. 750–66.
15. Noguiera C, Silva AS, Santos JN, et al. Perforated peptic ulcer: Main factors of morbidity and mortality. World J Surg 2003;27:782–7.
16. Norton JA, Fang TD, Jensen RT. Surgery for gastrinoma and insulinoma in multiple endocrine neoplasia type 1. J Natl Cancer Inst 2006;4:148–53.
17. Ohmann C, Imhof M, Roher HD. Trends in peptic ulcer bleeding and surgical treatment. World J Surg 2000;24:284–93.
18. Sabiston Jr DC. Atlas of general surgery. Philadelphia: WB Saunders; 1994.
19. Sanabria AE, Morales CH, Villegas MI. Laparoscopic repair for perforated peptic ulcer disease. Cochrane Database Syst Rev 2005;4: CD004778.
20. Simeone DM, Hassan A, Scheiman JM. Giant peptic ulcer: A surgical or medical disease? Surgery 1999;126:474–8.
21. Soreide K, Sarr MG, Soreide JA. Pyloroplasty for benign gastric outlet obstruction—Indications and techniques. Scand J Gastroenterol 2006;95:11–6.
22. Svanes C. Trends in perforated peptic ulcer: Incidence, etiology, treatment, and prognosis. World J Surg 2000;24:277–83.
23. Testini M, Portincasa P, Piccini G, et al. Significant factors associated with fatal outcome in emergency open surgery for perforated peptic ulcer. World J Gastroenterol 2003;9:2338–40.
24. Van Holstein CS. Long-term prognosis after partial gastrectomy for gastroduodenal ulcer. World J Surg 2000;24:307–14.
25. Zollinger FM. Atlas of surgical operations. New York: McGraw-Hill; 1993.

# CHAPTER 77

# SURGICAL APPROACH TO THE ACUTE ABDOMEN

*Kevin Rothchild, MD, and*
*Jonathan A. Schoen, MD*

**1. What is the significance of the term *acute abdomen*?**

Acute abdomen refers to any abdominal condition that requires prompt diagnosis. While many may ultimately require surgical intervention, it is not necessarily indicated by the term.

**2. What are the critical factors in the history of present illness?**

Age, location, character, and duration of pain; as well as associated problems.

**3. Which disorders are associated with specific age groups?**

- *Neonates:* intussusception, appendicitis, Meckel diverticulitis, mesenteric adenitis, midgut volvulus, malrotation, hypertrophic pyloric stenosis, small bowel atresia, annular pancreas
- *Adults:* cholecystitis, diverticulitis, gynecologic disorders, peptic ulcer disease, incarcerated hernia, ruptured spleen, renal or biliary stone, pancreatitis, small bowel obstruction
- *Elderly patients:* diverticulitis, colon cancer, appendicitis, aortic aneurysm, colonic (cecal/sigmoid) and small bowel volvulus, mesenteric ischemia

**4. Summarize the significance of pain location.**

- *Right upper quadrant:* biliary tract disease, hepatitis, peptic ulcer disease, pulmonary disease
- *Right flank:* hepatitis, pyelonephritis, appendicitis
- *Right lower quadrant:* appendicitis, ectopic pregnancy, incarcerated inguinal hernia, rectus sheath hematoma, ovarian torsion, pelvic inflammatory disease, ruptured ovarian cyst, Meckel diverticulitis, Crohn's disease
- *Epigastrium:* pancreatitis, peptic ulcer disease, cardiac disease, esophageal disease
- *Central abdomen:* bowel obstruction, bowel ischemia, midgut volvulus, appendicitis (early)
- *Left upper quadrant:* splenic rupture, peptic ulcer disease, pulmonary disease, leaking abdominal aortic aneurysm
- *Left lower quadrant:* diverticulitis, incarcerated inguinal hernia, ovarian torsion, pelvic inflammatory disease, colon cancer (perforated)

**5. What associated problems help to pinpoint the diagnosis?**

Past medical and surgical history are key. In premenopausal women, pelvic inflammatory disease and pregnancy-related issues must be screened as part of the initial assessment.

**6. What is the peritoneum and its pain innervation, and what are peritoneal signs?**

The peritoneum is derived from the mesoderm. It consists of two double-layered sheets of cells that form the visceral and parietal layers, each with their own neural innervation. The visceral layer covers the organs and has autonomic innervation. This innervation is both afferent as well as efferent, and pain from these nerves is perceived as midline pain. These are slow C fibers and produce dull, crampy pain of insidious nature. The parietal layer covers the inner surfaces of the abdominal parietes and has somatic innervation from the corresponding spinal nerves, each producing a sensation of pain in the local area from which it originates. These are fast transmitters and they rise to pain that is sharp and exquisite. Peritonitis refers to any inflammation of the peritoneal layers. This inflammation leads to guarding or spasm of the muscle when it is palpated. Voluntary guarding is described when the patient can consciously eliminate the muscular response, and involuntary guarding refers to a guarding response that cannot be repressed. The latter is more foreboding; a tense and boardlike abdomen often is associated with diffuse peritonitis.

**7. What is the significance of *rebound pain,* and should it be elicited?**

If one palpates deeply with the fingers and suddenly releases the manual pressure, often this may elicit severe pain on the rebound in patients with peritoneal irritation. Many surgeons believe that this sign does not convey any more information than can be obtained with gentle, deep palpation, and it often causes unexpected and *unnecessary* pain.

**8. What is the nature of intestinal pain?**

The intestines themselves are insensate to direct pain from traumatic injury or inflammation. However, intense pain can be elicited from stretching or distention, as well as contraction against resistance, as is seen in colicky pain from obstruction.

**9. How does the duration of pain help in making a diagnosis?**

Pain is often sudden with perforated ulcer, diverticulum, ruptured aneurysm, or renal stones. Intermittent pain is often seen with bowel obstruction or biliary colic. Gradually worsening pain can be seen with appendicitis or pyelonephritis.

**10. Is acute abdomen ruled out by absence of fever or leukocytosis?**

No. Fever and leukocytosis are often late occurrences. Elderly and immunocompromised patients may be unable to mount an immune response even late in the course of the disease process.

**11. What is the significance of bowel sounds?**

Bowel sounds are notoriously inaccurate in the surgical evaluation of the abdomen. Their absence may be indicative of ileus or peritonitis, whereas loud borborygmi, tinkling, or rushes may be suggestive of an obstructive process.

**12. What is the most important part of the abdominal examination?**

Palpation, which permits assessment of localized tenderness, guarding, or diffuse peritonitis. One should attempt to begin palpation away from the area of expected maximal tenderness. Rectal exam is also essential. A pelvic exam can also be invaluable in female patients of childbearing age with abdominal pain.

**13. What are the psoas and obturator signs?**

Inflammation of the psoas muscle causes pain on hip flexion-extension, whereas inflammation of the internal obturator muscle causes pain on internal rotation and flexion of the hip. Retrocecal appendicitis or, on occasion, diverticulitis may be responsible for these signs.

**14. What is Rovsing sign?**

Palpation of the *left* lower quadrant can elicit pain in the *right* lower quadrant, often seen in appendicitis.

**15. What is Kehr's sign?**

Pain in the left upper quadrant radiates to the *top* of the left shoulder secondary to diaphragmatic irritation. Kehr's sign often indicates hematoma from splenic injury or can be seen in perforated peptic ulcer.

**16. Define *mittelschmerz*.**

Pain in the middle of the menstrual cycle secondary to ovulation, often perceived in the lower midline.

**17. How does urinalysis help in the assessment?**

White blood cells in the urine may indicate urinary tract infection. Hematuria may suggest ureteral stones or tumor. Glucose or ketones may reveal diabetic ketoacidosis. An inflamed appendix abutting an adjacent ureter may lead to the finding of white and/or red blood cells in the analysis.

**18. What should be the first imaging study obtained?**

An acute abdominal series consists of an upright, supine, and lateral decubitus abdominal film. It is quick and inexpensive, yet can provide vital information. Upright chest radiograph may reveal free air under the diaphragm or suggest a pulmonary process. Free air may also be seen over the liver in a left lateral decubitus abdominal film. Air-fluid levels on the upright film may suggest bowel obstruction, while lack of air in the rectum may indicate a complete obstruction. Only 10% of gallstones are radiopaque, but 90% of ureteral calculi are visualized. Appendiceal fecalith may suggest appendicitis in the setting of right lower quadrant pain. Air in the biliary tree may be seen with biliary-enteric fistula or pelvic pyelophlebitis.

**19. How is ultrasound (US) used?**

US helps to evaluate the gallbladder and biliary tree and to assess for free peritoneal fluid and can visualize the female adnexa (in the setting of possible ectopic pregnancy or ovarian cyst/mass). Unfortunately, abdominal US exam is limited in the setting of obesity as well as bowel distention from obstruction.

**20. What additional imaging studies may help in the diagnosis?**

Computed tomography (CT) scan of the abdomen and pelvis with oral and intravenous contrast is useful in the setting of intra-abdominal abscess, pancreatitis, aortic aneurysm or dissection, arterial and venous occlusive disease, hepatic, splenic, retroperitoneal, and renal disorders. Upper and lower gastrointestinal (GI) series may pinpoint the level of bowel obstruction or establish the diagnosis if CT is inconclusive. Angiography or US (less sensitive) can be used to assess mesenteric arterial flow.

**21. If the diagnosis is in doubt, what other procedure should be done?**

Surgical exploration (via laparotomy or laparoscopy) of the abdomen is the next step if diagnostic studies are equivocal, and it is mandatory when the patient's condition worsens despite aggressive resuscitation.

**22. Is exploratory laparotomy justified, even if it produces no significant findings?**

Yes. Despite the risk of general anesthesia, postoperative pain, risk of wound infection, and a small lifetime risk of bowel obstruction from adhesions (less than 5%), it is still safer to undergo an exploration than to miss the diagnosis of appendicitis or bowel infarction.

**23. Is exploratory laparoscopy useful in the setting of acute abdomen?**

Laparoscopy is useful only when it provides a positive pathologic finding. If the exam is negative, the next step is conversion to laparotomy. In the setting of a distended abdomen with dilated intestine from bowel obstruction, its use is limited; however, its use is helpful and expanding in the setting of possible appendicitis, Meckel diverticulum, inflammatory bowel disease, or possible adnexal disease.

**24. In blunt trauma, CT scan of the abdomen and pelvis reveals free peritoneal fluid collections. When is observation appropriate instead of immediate surgical exploration?**

In the setting of trauma, any free fluid seen on CT should be concerning for possible bowel injury, for which CT is notoriously insensitive. Any patient must be hemodynamically stable for observation to be appropriate. Small lacerations to the liver or spleen are readily identifiable and should be treated with aggressive resuscitation. Escalating pain, fluid requirements, or need for blood transfusion should prompt an immediate exploration.

**25. Do all penetrating injuries to the abdomen require laparotomy?**

No. In the era of CT scanning, a hemodynamically stable patient with a negative CT can be observed. Many stab wounds and low-velocity firearm injuries are tangential and do not penetrate the abdominal fascia. However, observation in the setting of multiple trauma can be time-consuming and immediate exploration to rule out injury can be beneficial at times. High-velocity bullet wounds almost always require exploration due to the high likelihood of associated bowel and adjacent organ injury.

**26. What is the role of laparoscopy in trauma?**

Laparoscopy can be a useful adjunct to assess for diaphragmatic injuries or when penetration of the abdominal fascia cannot be ascertained. The classic example is a stab wound to the left upper quadrant.

**27. When is surgery indicated for peptic ulcer disease (PUD)?**

- *Perforation:* Closure with an omental or a Graham patch is acceptable for patients without previous history of PUD and for hemodynamically unstable patients. Definitive antiulcer surgery is indicated in hemodynamically stable patients with a prior history or chronic PUD. Resection of the ulcer crater with adequate margins should be performed for gastric ulcers. Definitive gastrectomy is undertaken after recovery if carcinoma is found in the specimen.
- *Obstruction:* If duodenal obstruction from an ulcer is not relieved by 7 days, surgery is generally indicated. Balloon dilation and/or stenting is an alternative in patients who are poor surgical candidates.
- *Bleeding:* Surgery is indicated in any hemodynamically unstable patient or in those requiring greater than 6 units of packed red blood cells within a 24-hour period. EGD as well as angiography can be very useful in this setting prior to operative intervention.
- *Intractability:* Despite benign biopsies, recurrent or nonhealing gastric ulcers should be resected due to risk of underlying carcinoma.

**28. When is cholecystectomy optimal for acute pancreatitis, presumably due to gallstone disease?**

Classically patients with gallstone pancreatitis would undergo cholecystectomy 4 to 6 weeks following their initial hospitalization; however, more recent studies show high recurrence rates with this delay. In addition, early surgery (i.e., during the same hospitalization, after pain has resolved) has shown similar complication and conversion rates compared with the delayed approach.

**29. When is surgery indicated for severe acute pancreatitis?**

Patients with progressively hemorrhagic or necrotizing, infected pancreatitis should undergo surgery when resuscitative measures fail. CT-guided catheter drainage of well-localized pancreatic abscesses may be an option in some cases.

Despite aggressive surgery, mortality rates are still in excess of 40% in some series. The impact of surgery on survival is still debatable.

**30. Describe treatment for a pancreatic pseudocyst.**

Many small (less than 6 cm) pseudocysts are asymptomatic, regress on their own, and should be followed. Larger cysts with symptoms or infected cysts should be drained, via either CT-guided drainage, endoscopy (generally transgastric), or surgery. Surgery can consist of either resection or drainage (via the stomach or small bowel). Patients with an isolated history of pancreatic cyst and no history of pancreatitis should have the entire cyst resected due to suspicion of cystadenocarcinoma.

**31. What is the best method to diagnose pain secondary to mesenteric ischemia?**

Despite multiple modalities (CT, US, angiography) to assess intestinal vascular flow, high index of suspicion, a careful history, and physical exam remain the best method to diagnose mesenteric ischemia. Pain out of proportion to physical exam is a classic finding. Atrial fibrillation, recent cardiac surgery, and any hypercoagulable state should arouse suspicion. Base deficit from arterial blood gas may reflect ischemia and/or necrosis, but a normal blood gas or lactate should not delay exploration. Laparoscopy can be helpful if there is not excessive bowel dilation.

**32. Describe the surgical strategy for the treatment of Crohn's disease.**

Due to the chronicity of the disease, any surgical strategy should be to maximize small bowel length. Strictureplasty has been shown to be an effective measure with multiple Crohn's strictures and maintains small bowel length. In the setting of long segments of disease, resection is generally limited to areas of grossly diseased bowel (not microscopically normal).

**33. When should surgery be offered for uncomplicated acute diverticulitis?**

Due to the risk of recurrence (as high as 40% to 50%), surgery is generally indicated after two episodes. Age less than 50 is a relative rather than absolute indication. Free perforation with peritonitis, bowel obstruction, and severe bleeding are indications for immediate surgery. Catheter drainage of a localized abscess can often postpone surgery and may often obviate the need for acute colostomy formation (Hartmann procedure).

**34. Should elderly patients with sigmoid or cecal volvulus undergo surgery?**

Yes. After immediate reduction with barium enema or endoscopy, the recurrence rate may be as high as 50% to 90%. Unless the patient cannot tolerate an operation or is in a moribund state, surgery should be offered during the same hospitalization.

**35. How should toxic megacolon in the setting of ulcerative colitis be managed?**

Aggressive fluid resuscitation, bowel rest, broad-spectrum antibiotics, and intravenous corticosteroids are the mainstays of medical therapy. Serial abdominal exams and plain films are mandatory to assess for colonic distention or impending perforation. Total abdominal colectomy with end-ileostomy is often required if there is no improvement in 48 hours.

**36. How should Ogilvie's syndrome be managed?**

The vast majority of patients improve with bowel rest and removal of narcotics; however, colonic decompression is indicated in the presence of pain or significant distention (more than 12 cm). Intravenous neostigmine as a prokinetic agent has a high success rate (greater than 80% to 90% in some small series), although the patient must be an acceptable candidate from a cardiac standpoint. Tube cecostomy can be considered in moribund patients.

**37. After endoscopic retrograde cholangiopancreatography (ERCP), a patient develops upper abdominal and back pain. What steps should be considered?**

CT scan and/or repeat esophagogastroduodenoscopy (EGD) usually reveal the source of the injury. The main focus should be on the location of the leak—is it the biliary-pancreatic system or the duodenum? Bile duct injury may be treated by endoscopic stent placement with percutaneous drainage of intra-abdominal collection or surgery if the injury is complex. Pancreatitis is not uncommon and should be treated expectantly. A *contained*, small leak in the posterior duodenum (retroperitoneal) may be treated with bowel rest and gastric decompression; however, laparotomy is indicated in the presence of ongoing pain or signs of diffuse peritonitis.

**38. How should esophageal perforation be managed after endoscopy? What if the patient has achalasia? Esophageal carcinoma?**

Small, contained leaks in the mediastinum (noted on upper GI or CT) may be treated by having the patient take nothing by mouth (NPO) and antibiotics, although chest tube decompression is often required. More extensive leaks require surgical repair. The type of repair (reconstruction versus diversion) is often based on the timing of the injury (early versus late). In the setting of achalasia, concomitant Heller myotomy with fundoplication can be performed. In the presence of carcinoma, the tumor as well as the area of injury should be resected, followed by an esophagogastrostomy at the same procedure.

**39. How should colonic perforation be managed after colonoscopy?**

The risk of perforation of the colon is 0.2% to 0.4% after diagnostic colonoscopy and 0.3% to 1.0% with polypectomy. In a well-prepped colon, bowel rest, antibiotics, and observation are often appropriate, provided there is no evidence of diffuse peritonitis. For small perforations, immediate laparoscopic repair is a viable alternative. Other complications such as bleeding or even splenic rupture have been seen after colonoscopy, but these are rarer.

## BIBLIOGRAPHY

1. Ahmed A, Eller PM, Schiffman FJ. Splenic rupture: An unusual complication of colonoscopy. Am J Gastroenterol 1997;92:1201–4.
2. Boyd WP, Nord HJ. Diagnostic laparoscopy. Endoscopy 2000;32:153–8.
3. Chae FH, Stiegmann GV. Current laparoscopic gastrointestinal surgery. Gastrointest Endosc 1998;47:500–11.
4. Cope Z. Cope's early diagnosis of the acute abdomen. New York: Oxford University Press; 1921.
5. Marco CA, Schoenfeld CN, Keyl PM, et al. Abdominal pain in geriatric emergency patients: Variables associated with adverse outcomes. Acad Emerg Med 1998;5:1163–8.
6. McKellar DP, Reilling RB, Eiseman B. Prognosis and outcomes in surgical disease. St. Louis: Quality Medical Publishing; 1999.
7. Mindelzun RE, Jeffrey RB. The acute abdomen: Current CT imaging techniques. Semin Ultrasound CT MR 1999;20:63–7.
8. Norton LW, Stiegmann GV, Eiseman B. Surgical decision making. Philadelphia: WB Saunders; 2000.
9. Ponec RJ, Saunders MD, Kimmey MB. Neostigmine for the treatment of acute colonic pseudo-obstruction. N Engl J Med 1999;341:137–41.
10. Pritchard JR, Schoetz DJ. Strictureplasty of the small bowel in patients with Crohn's disease. An effective surgical option. Arch Surg 1999;125.
11. Simic O, Strathausen S, Hess W, et al. Incidence and prognosis of abdominal complications after cardiopulmonary bypass. Cardiovasc Surg 1999;7:419–24.

# COLORECTAL SURGERY: POLYPOSIS SYNDROMES AND INFLAMMATORY BOWEL DISEASE

# CHAPTER 78

*Martin D. McCarter, MD, FACS*

### 1. Name four different types of intestinal polyps.
- Neoplastic (adenomatous, tubular, villous, tubulovillous)
- Hamartomatous
- Inflammatory/lymphoid
- Hyperplastic

### 2. What is a hamartoma?
A hamartoma is an exuberant growth of normal tissue in an abnormal amount or location. An isolated hamartomatous polyp has no malignant potential.

### 3. Which intestinal polyposis syndromes are associated with hamartomatous polyps?
- Peutz-Jeghers syndrome
- Juvenile polyposis (familial or generalized)
- Cronkhite-Canada syndrome (hamartomatous polyps with alopecia, cutaneous pigmentation, and toenail and fingernail atrophy)
- Intestinal ganglioneuromatosis (isolated or with von Recklinghausen disease or multiple endocrine neoplasia type 2)
- Ruvalcaba-Myhre-Smith syndrome (polyps of colon and tongue, macrocephaly, retardation, unique facies, pigmented penile macules)
- Cowden disease (gastrointestinal [GI] polyps with oral and cutaneous verrucous papules [tricholemmomas], associated with breast cancer, thyroid neoplasia, and ovarian cysts)

### 4. How is Peutz-Jeghers syndrome manifest?
This autosomal dominant trait is often heralded by the presence of melanin spots on the lips and buccal mucosa. Hamartomas are almost always present on the small intestine and occasionally on the stomach and colon. Previously considered a benign process, patients with Peutz-Jeghers syndrome are at increased risk for cancer.

### 5. Describe the manifestation of familial adenomatous polyposis (FAP).
FAP is a mendelian-dominant, non–sex-linked disease in which more than 100 adenomatous polyps affect the colon and rectum. FAP is caused by mutation in the adenomatous polyposis coli (*APC*) gene on the long arm of chromosome 5 at the *5q21-q22* locus. The APC protein is a tumor suppressor that, when mutated, fails to bind beta-catenin and allows for unregulated cellular growth. One-third of patients present as the propositus case (presumed mutation) with no prior family history. The disease invariably leads to invasive colon cancer if not treated. The average age at diagnosis of colon cancer is 39 years compared with 65 years for routine colon cancer.

### 6. What is Gardner syndrome?
FAP plus fibromas of the skin, osteomas (typically of the mandible, maxilla, and skull), epidermoid cysts, desmoid tumors, and extra dentition.

### 7. How does one screen for FAP?
When family history is positive, children should undergo annual sigmoidoscopic surveillance beginning at age 10 to 12 years. When polyps are identified, a full colonoscopy is recommended. Once multiple adenomas are documented, colectomy is recommended. State-of-the-art presymptomatic detection uses molecular genetic screening. Direct mutational analysis of the *APC* gene, restrictive fragment length polymorphism linkage analysis, or protein truncation assay can determine whether a person is affected with 95% to 99% certainty if genetic material is available from affected and unaffected members of the kindred. Ophthalmoscopic exam for congenital hypertrophy of the retinal pigment epithelium (CHRPE) can detect involved patients as early as 3 months of age with a 97% positive predictive value for developing FAP. CHRPE is present in 55% to 100% of FAP patients and is documented with wide-angle fundus photography.

## 8. What are the surgical indications for ulcerative colitis?
- Intractability or failure of medical management
- Fulminant colitis (toxic megacolon, bleeding, diarrhea)
- Prophylaxis of carcinoma (presence of high-grade dysplasia)
- Treatment of carcinoma

## 9. What are the elective surgical options for FAP and chronic ulcerative colitis?
- Total proctocolectomy with end (Brooke) ileostomy
- Total proctocolectomy with continent ileostomy reservoir (Kock pouch)
- Abdominal colectomy with ileorectal anastomosis
- Near-total proctocolectomy ± rectal mucosectomy and ileal pouch-anal anastomosis (IPAA)

## 10. Can one always tell the difference between Crohn's disease and ulcerative colitis?
No. Colitis that cannot be categorized as definitely Crohn or ulcerative colitis is called indeterminate colitis and may account for 5% to 10% of cases referred for surgical consideration.

## 11. What is pouchitis? How is it treated?
Pouchitis, one of the most frequent long-term complications of IPAA, is a nonspecific acute and/or chronic inflammation of the reservoir. Pouchitis is found in 7% to 44% of patients with IPAA; it presents with watery, bloody stools, urgency, frequency, abdominal pain, fever, malaise, and possible exacerbation of extraintestinal manifestations of inflammatory bowel disease. The cause is uncertain, but the risk is greater in chronic ulcerative colitis than in familial polyposis. Pouch stasis, bacterial overgrowth, colonification of ileal mucosa, ischemia, pelvic sepsis, oxygen-derived free radicals, altered immune status, and lack of mucosal trophic factors have been proposed as etiologies.

Successful treatment regimens include metronidazole and other antianaerobic antibiotics as well as steroid or 5-aminosalicylate enemas. Topical volatile fatty acids and glutamine have been used with variable success. Although half of patients with pouchitis at some time suffer a recurrence, very few develop intractable involvement requiring pouch excision.

## 12. Does a defunctionalized colon develop colitis?
Although controversial, some patients with a portion or the entire colon out of the fecal stream develop an inflammation difficult to distinguish from ulcerative colitis on biopsy. The diagnosis of diversion colitis is suggested when bloody mucopus is passed from the separate colorectal segment. The colon may be isolated by diverting ileostomy, end or loop colostomy, mucous fistula, or Hartmann procedure. It is believed that short-chain fatty acids normally produced by anaerobic bacteria serve as a trophic factor for the colonocytes. The diversion colitis quickly resolves on restoration of intestinal continuity; when restoration is not possible, the administration of short-chain fatty acid enemas is beneficial.

## 13. What type of ileal pouches are used?
Higher-volume pouches are advocated. W (quadruplicated) pouches have a greater capacity than S (triplicate) and J (two-limbed) pouches. The functional results may not be all that different. Shorter efferent limbs (for S pouches) are also used to avoid outlet obstruction. The author prefers a long (15 cm) J pouch (when feasible in one stage) preserving the anal transition zone. The procedure has classically been two-staged, with construction of a temporary ileostomy followed at an interval by ileostomy takedown. Recent experience has shown that the morbidity of a one-stage IPAA may be less if the patient is taking no or low-dose steroids and the operation is performed without complication. Because there is really only *one shot* at getting it right (pelvic sepsis significantly diminishes ultimate pouch function), intraoperative judgment is at a premium.

# ANORECTAL DISEASE

## 14. What are anal fissures?
A generally painful rip or tear in the sensitive anoderm of the anal canal. Most anal fissures are located in the posterior (90%) or anterior (10%) midline of the anal canal.

## 15. What disorders should be considered in patients with laterally situated anal fissures?
Crohn's disease, ulcerative colitis, syphilis, tuberculosis, leukemia, carcinoma, and acquired immunodeficiency syndrome (AIDS).

## 16. How are acute fissures managed?
Conservative treatment consists of stool softeners and bulk agents to avoid hard bowel movements, sitz baths to help decrease sphincter spasm, topical anesthetics, and topical steroids. Suppositories generally should be avoided because they may induce anal spasm. Topical nitroglycerin or nifedipine ointment reduces anal spasm. Injection of botulinum toxin also has been used to relax the anal sphincter.

**17. What are the signs of a chronic anal fissure? What do they imply?**

A chronic anal fissure can be identified by the presence of a sentinel pile (skin tag or hemorrhoid), anal ulcer (with fibropurulent material or visible internal sphincter muscle in the base), and a hypertrophied anal papilla arising from the dentate line. A chronic anal fissure usually does not respond to conservative treatment, and surgical intervention is in order.

**18. Which surgical procedures are available for treatment of a chronic anal fissure?**

Open or closed lateral internal sphincterotomy, excision (ulcerectomy), excision and Y-V or other anoplasty, or anal dilation.

**19. How are hemorrhoids classified?**

- *External hemorrhoids* originate distal to the dentate line of the anus and are covered by squamous epithelium. External hemorrhoids may thrombose or become filled with clotted blood. Typically these are painful involving the anoderm.
- *Internal hemorrhoids* arise above (proximal to) the dentate line and are covered with transitional and columnar epithelium. First-degree hemorrhoids swell and bleed. Second-degree hemorrhoids prolapse and spontaneously reduce. Third-degree hemorrhoids prolapse and can be manually reduced, whereas fourth-degree hemorrhoids are irreducible. Typically these are not painful above the anoderm.

**20. How are acute hemorrhoids treated?**

- *Topical medicines:* anesthetics, hydrocortisone preparations, astringents (witch hazel, glycerin, magnesium sulfate).
- *Emergency hemorrhoidectomy* requires 2 weeks of recovery time. Circular stapling devices have been used to treat larger hemorrhoids.

**21. List several minimally invasive outpatient treatments of internal hemorrhoids.**

Rubber band ligation, bipolar cautery, direct current electrical therapy, infrared coagulation, sclerotherapy, and cryotherapy.

**22. Who is the patron saint of hemorrhoid sufferers?**

Fiachra (Irish), Fiacre (French), or Fiacrius (Latin). An Irish holy man famed for cures of such less desirable maladies, he died in France on August 30, 670 AD.

**23. How is an acute thrombosed external hemorrhoid best treated?**

Excision of the clot and involved hemorrhoidal complex (as opposed to incision alone) best prevent future recurrence at the same site.

**24. Explain the cause of anorectal abscesses and fistulas.**

A cryptoglandular origin seems to provide the best explanation. Four to 10 anal glands enter the anal canal at the level of the crypts in the dentate line. The glands extend back into the internal sphincter two-thirds of the time and into the intersphincteric space half the time. Blockage of the gland leads to an overgrowth of bacteria with resultant pressure necrosis and abscess formation. An abscess or infection that causes an abnormal communication between two surfaces (such as the anal canal and perianal skin) creates a fistula.

**25. List the various types and locations of anorectal abscesses.**

Submucosal, intersphincteric, perianal (anal verge), ischiorectal (perirectal), and supralevator.

**26. What is the best treatment for an anorectal abscess?**

Prompt incision and drainage. There is little or no role for antibiotics (exceptions are immunocompromised patients and patients with prosthetic heart valves or severe cellulitis) and no reason to wait for the abscess to *point* or become fluctuant before surgical treatment.

**27. What is the Goodsall rule?**

See Figure 78-1.

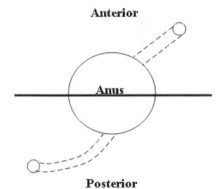

**Figure 78-1.** The Goodsall rule helps predict the location of the internal opening of an anal fistula based on the site of its external opening. Accurately determining the *criminal crypt* of fistula origin on the dentate line is important at the time of surgical treatment, generally fistulotomy. If the anus is divided into imaginary anterior and posterior halves in the coronal plane, posterior fistulas tend to curve into the posterior midline. Anterior fistulas shorter than 3 cm tend to proceed radially to the dentate line, whereas anterior fistulas longer than 3 cm may track back to the posterior midline.

## 28. What is a seton?

A drainage device used to control and treat an anal fistulous abscess. It is inserted through and through a fistula tract and secured to itself, thus making a circle about some portion of the anal sphincter muscle. It serves as a cutting device to exteriorize the fistula slowly. Typical setons are Penrose drains, Silastic *vessel loops*, or silk sutures.

## 29. What are the common indications for inserting a seton?

- High fistulous abscesses involving greater than one-half the length of the anal canal muscle
- Anterior fistulas in a woman
- Inflammatory bowel disease
- Elderly patients or patients with multiple previous anorectal surgeries

## 30. List new developments for treatment of anorectal fistulas.

- Fibrin sealant glues
- Collagen plug
- Monoclonal anti–tumor necrosis factor antibodies for Crohn's fistulas
- Park fistulotomy procedure, with excision/debridement of the fistula tract, muscle repair, advancement flap coverage of the internal opening, and drainage of the external portion of the fistula tract

## 31. When is anorectal suppurative disease especially dangerous?

In the presence of neutropenia, as associated with chemotherapy, the mortality at 1 month may approach 50%. Unfortunately, surgery and even anorectal digital examination may be contraindicated. Often bacterial infection is widespread without formation of purulence or a classic abscess.

## 32. What is Fournier gangrene?

Fournier gangrene is a necrotizing soft tissue infection of the perineum. Although rare, it can present as a suspected perirectal abscess so a high index of suspicion must be maintained. Treatment is prompt surgical debridement.

- *Local signs*—crepitence, bullea, cellulitis
- *Systemic signs*—altered mental status, hypotension, oliguria

## 33. Describe perianal Paget disease.

Perianal (extramammary) Paget disease is characterized by a scaly inflamed dermis resembling eczema. Biopsy reveals typical Paget cells with round, pale, vacuolated mucin-positive cytoplasm with an eccentric reticular nucleus. It is often a chronic condition, but underlying carcinoma must be ruled out as cancer is associated with Paget disease.

## 34. Which patient characteristics are associated with rectal prolapse?

| | |
|---|---|
| Chronic constipation | Deep pouch of Douglas |
| Neurologic disease | Patulous anus |
| Female sex | Diastasis of the levator ani muscles |
| Nulliparity | Lack of fixation of the rectum to the sacrum |
| Redundant rectosigmoid colon | Previous anorectal surgery |

## 35. What surgical options are available for rectal prolapse?

In general, procedures can narrow the anal orifice (Thiersch operation), obliterate the pouch of Douglas (Moschcowitz procedure), restore the condition of the pelvic floor (levator plication), excise (abdominally or perineally) the excess rectosigmoid colon, and/or fixate or suspend the rectum. Combinations of these options are often used.

## 36. How is rectal prolapse handled in pediatric patients?

Most prolapses in children are mucosal prolapses alone. It is usually handled with a bowel management program to reduce constipation and straining. Surgical or invasive methods, such as sclerosis, encirclement, or excision, are rarely necessary.

# COLORECTAL MALIGNANCIES

## RECTAL CANCER

## 37. What is the best way to stage rectal cancer?

It has been said that an educated finger is the best instrument; however, the overall accuracy of staging depends on the information desired and the modality chosen. While the table provides some general guidelines, operator experience plays an important role in the overall accuracy (Table 78-1).

**Table 78-1.** Estimated Accuracy of Rectal Cancer Staging Modalities

|  | ENDOSCOPIC ULTRASOUND | MAGNETIC RESONANCE IMAGING | COMPUTED TOMOGRAPHY |
|---|---|---|---|
| T stage | 85% | 80% | 65% |
| N stage | 75% | 60% | 55% |
| Overall | 80% | 70% | 60% |

### 38. When is endoscopic mucosal resection (EMR) indicated?
Large benign polyps and some T1 tumors. Those with adverse features such as lymphovascular invasion and positive margins need additional therapy such as full-thickness (surgical) excision or radiotherapy.

### 39. What are the indications for neoadjuvant (before surgery) and adjuvant (after surgery) therapy?
Any N1 or T4 disease. Generally indicated for uT3 lesions and some uT2 lesions. Neoadjuvant therapy decreases local recurrence rates and improves chances for sphincter preservation.

### 40. What is an abdominal perineal resection (APR), and when is it indicated?
Removal of the entire anus and rectum with an end colostomy. It is generally indicated for total anal incontinence or tumors that invade the anal sphincter. Low rectal cancers that do not directly invade the anal sphincter can in certain situations be managed with sphincter preservation and colon J-pouch reconstruction.

## COLON CANCER

### 41. What are the fundamental principals of colon resection for cancer?
- A 5-cm margin on either side of the tumor
- Vascular supply taken at the origin of the closest named vessel (ileocolic, right colic, middle colic, left colic, inferior mesenteric artery)
- Adequate lymph node staging (generally aim for a minimum of 12 nodes evaluated)

### 42. Does laparoscopic surgery compromise the chance for a cure?
No. Several prospective randomized studies have demonstrated equivalent cancer survival from both open and laparoscopic approach. The key to achieving this is to conduct the same extent of resection either way. Initial concerns for excessive port site metastasis are unfounded.

### 43. What are the pros and cons of laparoscopic versus open colectomy?

#### Pro
- Smaller incisions
- Less pain medication
- Quicker recovery and return to work
- Possible earlier return of bowel function

#### Con
- Steep learning curve for technical proficiency
- Increased difficulty in reoperative setting or with acute inflammation (diverticulitis)

## BENIGN COLON AND SMALL BOWEL DISEASE

### 44. What are the findings of sigmoid volvulus on plain abdominal film and contrast enema?
The plain film demonstrates a *bent inner tube* or *coffee-bean* sign of massively dilated, air-filled sigmoid colon arising out of the pelvis. The contrast enema shows a *bird's beak* appearance as the colon narrows at the twist at the rectosigmoid junction.

### 45. How is a nonstrangulated sigmoid volvulus treated?
Rigid or flexible sigmoidoscopic or colonoscopic decompression, followed by elective sigmoid resection.

**46. Why should elective surgery be performed after a successful endoscopic detorsion and decompression of a sigmoid volvulus?**

Recurrence is the rule with sigmoid volvulus. Elective sigmoid resection of prepped and decompressed bowel generally can be accomplished with a mortality rate of less than 5%. Emergency operation for a sigmoid volvulus involves a mortality rate of 35% to 80%.

**47. Do colon perforations from colonoscopy mandate surgical repair?**

Not all perforations require surgery. Sound clinical judgment is critical. Limited controlled perforations with minimal contamination generally seal on their own. Signs of systemic illness (tachycardia, fever, hypotension, increasing abdominal pain) generally require surgery.

**48. What is Ogilvie syndrome?**

Colonic pseudo-obstruction presents with signs, symptoms, and radiologic findings suggestive of obstruction without a mechanical source. Most often seen in hospitalized patients with other underlying medical conditions found to have marked colonic air on abdominal radiograph. Treatments include managing the underlying medical issues, colonoscopic decompression, and neostigmine.

**49. What does plain radiographic study of the abdomen reveal in large bowel obstruction?**

Differential air-fluid levels (stair steps) of the small intestine or a massively dilated colon. The colon is identified by the presence of haustral folds, compared to the valvulae conniventes of the small intestine. The rectum is usually gasless, although gas distal with a colonic obstruction may not have completely cleared the distal colon. A picture resembling small bowel obstruction (SBO) alone may appear in a very proximal colon obstruction. Colonic pseudo-obstruction also may give a roentgenographic picture similar to true obstruction.

**50. What radiologic findings are associated with gallstone ileus?**

Air in gallbladder or biliary tree, SBO at the level of the ileocecal valve, large bowel obstruction at the sigmoid colon, and occasionally a calcified mass at the above points.

**51. What does endometriosis have to do with the alimentary system?**

Endometriosis is the presence of functioning endometrial tissue outside the uterus. When this hormonally active tissue implants on intestinal surfaces, it can cause pain, cyclical bleeding, and obstructive symptoms.

**52. What is a primary bowel obstruction?**

Refers to an intestinal obstruction without a known etiology such as adhesions or a prior cancer diagnosis. Primary bowel obstructions virtually always require an operation at some point.

**53. How is postoperative ileus differentiated from postoperative SBO?**

This distinction can be extremely difficult. Postoperative ileus generally occurs up to 1 week after operation, whereas postoperative SBO may last 7 to 30 days or longer. SBO is associated with nausea, vomiting, distention, and abdominal pain, whereas an ileus may be associated with painless failure to pass bowel movements. The radiographic picture may or may not include differential air-fluid levels in each disorder.

**54. Is treatment of postoperative SBO different from treatment of SBO remote from surgery?**

Yes. Generally, one waits out a postoperative obstruction for an indefinite period, as long as there is no evidence of strangulation or impending perforation. Approximately 80% resolve without surgery. Nasogastric suction is the mainstay of treatment for postoperative SBO, whereas "the sun never sets" on a suspected mechanical SBO remote from surgery; one generally operates as soon as the diagnosis of complete obstruction is made.

**55. What is the most common cause of SBO?**

Adhesions.

**56. Can adhesions be prevented?**

Absorbable hyaluronate and carboxymethylcellulose membranes lead to a statistically significant reduction in the number and severity of intra-abdominal adhesions, although it is unclear if this translates into a reduced future need for operative intervention.

**57. What are the pathologic findings of late radiation enteritis?**

Obliterative arteritis. Severe fibrosis commonly is accompanied by telangiectasia formation. The pelvis may be "frozen" because of incredibly dense adhesions and fibrosis.

## 58. What are general principles of managing radiation enteritis?

Medical management options are generally exhausted before surgery is contemplated or attempted. Cholestyramine, elemental diets, and total parenteral nutrition are commonly used. Although surgery is not withheld for urgent indications (complete obstruction, perforation, abscess not amenable to percutaneous drainage, bleeding, or unresponsive fistulas), it carries significant morbidity and mortality rates. Enterolysis, or separating of adhesions, in radiated bowel is associated with a high rate of fistula formation. Anastomosis can be performed safely if at least one end of bowel to be connected has not been radiated. Intestinal bypass procedures without resection may be necessary.

## 59. What treatments are available for bleeding radiation proctitis?

Topical anti-inflammatory drugs (steroids, mesalamine enemas, or suppositories), laser ablation of telangiectasias, and application of 4% formaldehyde solutions (under controlled situations in the operating room).

## WEBSITES

http://www.fascrs.org

http://www.nccn.org

### BIBLIOGRAPHY

1. Church JM. The ASCRS textbook of colon and rectal surgery. New York: Springer Science and Business Media LLC; 2006.
2. Collins EE, Lund JN. A review of chronic anal fissure management. Tech Coloproctol 2007;11:209–23.
3. Fleshman J, Sargent DJ, Green E, et al. Laparoscopic colectomy for cancer is not inferior to open surgery based on 5-year data from the COST Study Group trial. Ann Surg 2007;246:655–62.
4. Knudsen AL, Bisgaard ML, Bulow S. Attenuated familial adenomatous polyposis (AFAP): A review of the literature. Fam Cancer 2003;2:43–55.
5. Lacy BE, Weiser K. Gastrointestinal motility disorders: An update. Dig Dis 2006;24:228–42.
6. McCarter MD, Quan SH, Busam K, et al. Long-term outcome of perianal Paget's disease. Dis Colon Rectum 2003;46:612–6.
7. McGuire BB, Brannigan AE, O'Connell PR. Ileal pouch-anal anastomosis. Br J Surg 2007;94:812–23.
8. Scaldeferri F, Fiocchi C. Inflammatory bowel disease: Progress and current concepts of etiopathogenesis. J Dig Dis 2007;8:171–8.
9. Vasen HF, Möslein G, Alonso A. Guidelines for the clinical management of familial adenomatous polyposis (FAP). Gut 2008;57:704–13.
10. Vrijland WW, Tseng LN, Eijkman HJ, et al. Fewer intraperitoneal adhesions with use of hyaluronic acid-carboxymethylcellulose membrane: A randomized clinical trial. Ann Surg 2002;235:193–9.
11. Yu ED, Shou Z, Shen B. Pouchitis. World J Gastroenterol 2007;13:5598–604.

# BARIATRIC SURGERY

*Jonathan A. Schoen, MD*

**1. What is the definition of *obesity*?**
Excess body fat.

**2. How is body fat relative to weight usually measured?**
By calculating the body mass index (BMI). This is simply $kg/m^2$.

**3. Describe the BMI classification system.**
- $<18$ $kg/m^2$ = underweight
- 18 to 24 $kg/m^2$ = healthy weight
- 25 to 29 $kg/m^2$ = overweight
- 30 to 39 $kg/m^2$ = obese
- $\geq40$ $kg/m^2$ = morbidly obese

**4. What are the limitations of BMI?**
- In those with a higher proportion of fat relative to muscle—the elderly
- Or in those with an unusually high proportion of muscle—bodybuilders

**5. What proportion of the U.S. adult population is considered overweight?**
64%, or 127 million adults.

**6. What proportion of the U.S. adult population is considered obese?**
31%, or 60 million adults. Obesity is now considered a national epidemic.

**7. Are there health implications associated with a BMI of 30 $kg/m^2$?**
Obesity is considered a major factor contributing to many health problems, including diabetes mellitus (DM), hypertension, sleep apnea and pickwickian syndromes, asthma, coronary artery disease, cardiomyopathy and cardiac failure, gastroesophageal reflux disease (GERD), degenerative joint disease, hypercholesterolemia, fatty liver, gout, urinary incontinence, gallbladder disease, psychological disorders, menstrual irregularities, and certain cancers (endometrial, colon, postmenopausal breast, esophageal, hepatocellular, prostate, and kidney).

**8. Can obesity lead to premature death?**
Yes. Individuals who have a BMI greater than 30 $kg/m^2$ have a 50% to 100% increased risk of premature death from all causes compared to individuals with a BMI of 20 to 25 $kg/m^2$.

This increased mortality is directly proportional to increasing BMI. Obesity causes 400,000 preventable deaths in the United States and is a close second to smoking as the leading cause of preventable death.

**9. How successful is nonsurgical treatment of obesity?**
Evidence suggests that nonsurgical treatment (diet/behavior modification, exercise programs, and psychological support) for morbid obesity has a more than 90% failure rate. Similarly, pharmacologic therapy for morbid obesity has been hampered by serious side effects and, overall, has met with disappointing results.

**10. How is obesity best treated?**
The National Institutes of Health (NIH) Consensus Statement in 1991 concluded that medical therapy was ineffective for severe clinical obesity and that surgery was indicated for this population of patients.

## 11. What was the NIH Consensus Statement?

Those with severe clinical obesity defined as a BMI of 40 kg/m² (morbid obesity) or a BMI of 35 to 39 kg/m² with severe, debilitating comorbidities are best treated with a surgical weight loss procedure.

## 12. List the contraindications to bariatric surgery.

- Endocrine disorders that cause morbid obesity
- Psychological instability
- Alcohol or drug abuse
- End-stage organ disease or terminal cancer

## 13. Categorize the surgical options for weight reduction.

- Restrictive
- Combination restrictive/malabsorptive
- Malabsorptive
- Other

## 14. List the options for restrictive surgery.

- *Vertical-banded gastroplasty.* A stapling device is used to divide the stomach vertically along the lesser curve starting at the angle of His to create a small (20 mL) pouch. A prosthetic device is then wrapped around the outlet of the pouch to prevent it from dilating over time. This operation has fallen out of favor due to poor long-term success and is only rarely performed.
- *Gastric banding.* This procedure is performed laparoscopically and involves placement of an adjustable band around the top of the stomach to create a small (15-mL) pouch. The band is connected to a reservoir placed in the subcutaneous tissue that enables band adjustment.
- *Sleeve gastrectomy.* This procedure is gaining in popularity and involves stapling and removing a majority of the gastric body and fundus leaving the lesser curvature and a small amount of antrum. The pylorus remains intact.

## 15. Describe the combined restrictive/malabsorptive option.

Known as the Roux-en-Y gastric bypass, it has been performed in the United States for nearly 50 years. It has been performed laparoscopically for the past 15 years and historically is the gold standard and most common operation for weight loss in this country. The procedure is the performed in the following way:

- A 15- to 30-mL gastric pouch is created by completely dividing the proximal stomach (the restrictive part).
- The proximal jejunum is divided 15 to 50 om from the ligament of Treitz (length depends on surgeon preference).
- The distal end of this divided proximal jejunum is measured out between 75 and 150 cm, and this Roux limb is anastomosed to the gastric pouch. The varying length of Roux limb is thought to affect absorption of calories; however, this likely has a small role in weight loss unless the Roux limb is made very long (a distal gastric bypass).
- The proximal end of divided jejunum (biliopancreatic limb) is anastomosed to Roux limb at the previously measured length, creating the Y configuration (Fig. 79-1).

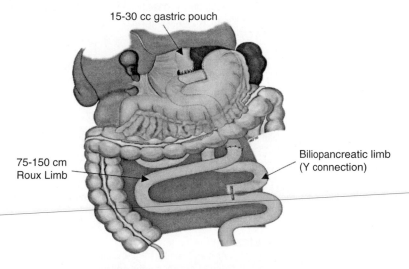

15-30 cc gastric pouch

75-150 cm
Roux Limb

Biliopancreatic limb
(Y connection)

**Figure 79-1.** The laparoscopic Roux-en-Y gastric bypass.

#### 16. What is the option for malabsorptive surgery?

Biliopancreatic diversion with and without a duodenal switch. A subtotal gastrectomy is performed, leaving a gastric remnant of 250 to 500 mL. The small bowel is divided 200 to 300 cm proximal to the ileocecal valve and the ileum is anastomosed to the stomach. The jejunum is connected to the side of the ileum approximately 50 to 100 cm from the ileocecal valve. This procedure results in malabsorption by creating a short common channel for digestion and absorption of food.

#### 17. The other category includes which procedures?

The intragastric balloon, the gastric pacer, the intraluminal sleeve. These are being studied for efficacy and may have a limited role in the future.

#### 18. What are the weight loss expectations after each procedure?

Success following bariatric surgery is determined by both weight lost and improvement in obesity-related comorbidities. Most surgical studies report outcome as percent excess weight loss (excess weight = [preoperative weight − ideal weight]). The lap band typically produces 40% to 60% evaporation weight loss (EWL) over 2 to 3 years but has a 20% failure rate. The gastric bypass has long-term data showing a 50% loss of excess body weight maintained after 14 years. Most current laparoscopic literature shows up to 5-year excess weight loss in the 60% to 80% range. There is typically some recidivism after 2 years and it has a 10% failure rate. The biliopancreatic diversion is the most effective weight loss procedure and results in the loss of 80% excess weight maintained over the long term. The sleeve gastrectomy is currently being studied for long-term success and so far comes close to the gastric bypass in terms of weight loss efficacy.

#### 19. Are these just cosmetic operations?

No. Depending on the procedure, with the lap band being the least effective but the safest and the biliopancreatic diversion carrying the greatest risks but the most efficacy, nearly all of the patient's obesity-induced comorbid conditions are improved or resolved within 1 year.

#### 20. Does surgical weight loss translate to improved long-term survival?

Yes. Recent studies have shown an up to a 40% reduction in long-term mortality in a surgical group compared with a nonsurgical group.

#### 21. Which comorbidity can have the most dramatic improvement?

Type 2 DM. In fact, there is much discussion about the surgical treatment for type 2 DM given the very impressive results after the gastric bypass and biliopancreatic diversion. About 90% of diabetics are resolved of their hyperglycemia after these two operations even prior to weight loss.

#### 22. How does the gastric bypass and biliopancreatic diversion *cure* diabetes prior to weight loss?

This is more complex than calorie restriction and involves changes in gut hormones. Bypassing the duodenum and proximal jejunum (the proximal gut theory) changes GIP hormone levels and likely other as-of-yet-unknown hormonal levels that play a role in the incretin effect. The hindgut theory is based on the hypothesis that food now reaches the terminal ileum and colon faster, resulting in a greater activation and release of other hormones, namely GLP-1 and PYY 3-36, which result in greater insulin secretion and sensitivity.

#### 23. Can these changes in the gut hormonal milieu have a detrimental effect?

Although these changes are only beginning to be understood, the rare hyperinsulinemic hypoglycemia and apparent beta cell hyperplasia seen years after a gastric bypass may be due to hormonal overstimulation of the pancreas.

#### 24. What are other complications after a gastric bypass?

Complications can be divided into early (within 30 days) and late.

- Early complications include mortality (0.2%), anastomotic leaks (2%), GI bleeding (2%), pulmonary embolus (0.4%), and wound infection (3.0%).
- Late complications include anastomotic stenosis (5%), small bowel obstruction from internal hernias (3%), marginal ulceration (10%), cholelithiasis (10%), and vitamin/mineral deficiencies.

#### 25. How are anastomotic leaks handled?

These are usually at the gastrojejunostomy anastomosis and can be treated conservatively with total parenteral nutrition (TPN), nothing by mouth (NPO), and percutaneous catheter drainage if the patient is stable. An unstable patient or a nonhealing fistula requires surgical repair.

### 26. How is an anastomotic stenosis treated?

Many surgeons purposely make the gastrojejunostomy anastomosis small (about 1 cm) to enhance the restrictive aspect of the operation. If this anastomosis becomes too small for the patient to tolerate, endoscopic balloon dilatation is usually successful.

### 27. What is a marginal ulcer, and how is it treated?

This is an ulcer usually found on the jejunal side of the gastrojejunostomy. It is often related to local ischemia, smoking, or nonsteroidal anti-inflammatory drug (NSAID) use and usually heals with a proton pump inhibitor (PPI) and Carafate therapy.

### 28. What are the vitamin/mineral deficiencies and potential long-term risks?

Vitamin $B_{12}$, folate, and iron deficiency anemia can occur in up to 40% of patients without lifelong supplementation. Hypocalcemia with or without vitamin D deficiency and resulting osteoporosis can also occur without lifelong supplementation. The deficiencies are a result of bypassing most of the stomach, all of the duodenum, and the proximal jejunum.

### 29. What is the most common surgical weight loss procedure in Europe and Australia?

The laparoscopic adjustable gastric band (lap band). There does appear to be a recent trend toward the gastric bypass given the higher failure rate after the lap band.

### 30. Why would someone choose a lap band over a Roux-en-Y gastric bypass?

It is safer. It is simple to place and reversible as there is no anatomical reconfiguration. It also avoids vitamin and mineral deficiencies. It requires close follow-up for best results.

### 31. What are the specific complications after a lap band procedure?

- Erosion (1%)
- Slip or prolapse (5%)
- Pouch or esophageal dilatation (less than 5%)
- Port or tubing break/infection (less than 5%)
- Need for reoperation (10%)

### 32. How does the biliopancreatic diversion work?

It creates a fixed amount of malabsorption whereby all fat and most starch can only be absorbed in 50 to 100 cm of terminal ileum.

### 33. Is there malnutrition, and how problematic is it?

Protein has only 200 to 300 cm of ileum to be absorbed. Up to 30% of patients end up with protein-calorie malnutrition requiring hospitalization and TPN or surgical revision. A high–protein/lower carbohydrate diet is required to avoid inducing a state of starvation mimicking kwashiorkor disease.

### 34. Are there other health risks associated with biliopancreatic diversion?

Yes. The risks are similar to those of gastric bypass except they are higher. Mortality is 1% to 2%. Leaks, obstructions, and ulcers can occur. Vitamin $B_{12}$, folate, and iron deficiency anemia are common without lifelong supplementation. Hypocalcemia and bone demineralization are common, leading to bone pain and osteoporosis if calcium and vitamin D are not administered in high doses lifelong. Patients also complain of frequent diarrhea, foul-smelling stool and flatulence, and halitosis.

### 35. Why would one choose biliopancreatic diversion?

Aside from being arguably the most effective weight loss procedure, patients can eat as much as they want. This may be the best procedure for the binge-eater or compulsive snacker who classically fails the other weight loss procedures. The biliopancreatic diversion has also been proved to be effective for the so-called super morbid obese (BMI = 50 kg/m$^2$) who may not lose as much with the other procedures.

### 36. What does preoperative surgical counseling entail with any procedure?

All patients undergo extensive preoperative education and counseling and must attend a required nutritional class and pass a psychological evaluation. Although this is practice dependent, all patients should be taught that these procedures are just tools—the most effective tools for weight loss to date—and for long-term success they must combine the operation with diet compliance, daily exercise, support groups, and close follow-up.

# BIBLIOGRAPHY

1. Adams TD, Gress RE, Smith SC, et al. Long-term mortality after gastric bypass surgery. N Engl J Med 2007;357:753.
2. Belachew M, Legrand M, Vincent V, et al. Laparoscopic adjustable gastric banding. World J Surg 1998;22:955–63.
3. Biertho L, Steffen R, Ricklin T, et al. Laparoscopic gastric bypass versus laparoscopic adjustable gastric banding: A comparative study of 1,200 cases. J Am Coll Surg 2003;197:536–47.
4. Buchwald H, Avidor Y, Braunwald E, et al. Bariatric surgery: A systematic review and meta-analysis. JAMA 2004;292:1724–37.
5. Buchwald H, Estok R, Fahrbach K, et al. Trends in mortality in bariatric surgery: A systematic review and meta-analysis. Surgery 2007;142:621.
6. Demaria EJ, Sugerman HJ, Meador JG, et al. High failure rate after laparoscopic adjustable silicone gastric banding for treatment of morbid obesity. Ann Surg 2001;233:809–18.
7. Hess DS, Hess DW. Biliopancreatic diversion with a duodenal switch. Obes Surg 1998;8:267–82.
8. Higa KD, Boone KB, Ho T, et al. Laparoscopic Roux-en-Y gastric bypass for morbid obesity. Arch Surg 2000;135:1029–34.
9. NIH Consensus Conference. Gastrointestinal surgery for severe obesity. Ann Intern Med 1991;115:956–61.
10. Podnos Y, Jimenez JC, Wilson SE, et al. Complications after laparoscopic gastric bypass. Arch Surg 2003;138:957–61.
11. Pories W, Swanson MS, MacDonald KG, et al. Who would have thought it? An operation proves to be the most effective therapy for adult-onset diabetes mellitus. Ann Surg 1995;222:339–51.
12. Schauer PR, Burguera B, Ikramuddin S, et al. Effect of laparoscopic Roux-en Y gastric bypass on type 2 diabetes mellitus. Ann Surg 2003;238:467.
13. Schauer PR, Ikramuddin S, Gourash W, et al. Outcomes after laparoscopic Roux-en-Y gastric bypass for morbid obesity. Ann Surg 2000;232:515–29.
14. Scopinaro N, Adami GF, Marinari GM, et al. Biliopancreatic diversion. World J Surg 1998;22:936–46.
15. Sjöström L, Narbro K, Sjöström CD, et al. Effects of bariatric surgery on mortality in Swedish obese subjects. N Engl J Med 2007;357:741.
16. Wittgrove AC, Clark GW. Laparoscopic gastric bypass, Roux-en-Y—500 Patients: Technique and results, with 3-60 month follow-up. Obes Surg 2000;10:233–9.

# LAPAROSCOPIC SURGERY

*John J. Tiedeken, MD, and*
*Anthony J. LaPorta, MD*

# CHAPTER 80

### 1. When did laparoscopic surgery become a credible surgical option?

Mouret initiated laparoscopic cholecystectomy in France in 1987. Reddick and Olsen are credited with the first laparoscopic cholecystectomy in the United States. At first denounced, this procedure quickly became the standard of care and by 1991 was considered the treatment of choice for symptomatic cholelithiasis. Since then, the field of laparoscopic surgery has explored virtually every surgical disease, and laparoscopic surgery has become the standard approach for a multitude of procedures.

### 2. What are the advantages of laparoscopic surgery compared with open procedures?

Laparoscopic procedures are less invasive. As a result, they cause less trauma to tissues and organs, less postoperative discomfort, and more rapid return to baseline functions. The laparoscopic approach has replaced the open approach for certain procedures. The most notable example is laparoscopic cholecystectomy for symptomatic cholelithiasis. This is also becoming the case with laparoscopic appendectomy, laparoscopic bariatric procedures, and laparoscopic antireflux surgery. Video-assisted thorascopic surgery has largely replaced open thoracotomy for smaller lesions. Minimally invasive techniques have also become common in pediatric surgery.

### 3. What are the contraindications to laparoscopic surgery?

- The patient's inability to tolerate general anesthesia or a pneumoperitoneum, usually due to advanced cardiopulmonary disease.
- An uncorrectable coagulopathy
- The inability to safely place ports and create a working space
- Portal hypertension due to the risk of rapid, fatal hemorrhage
- Surgeon experience is a consideration for all operative procedures, open and laparoscopic. The experience required varies depending on the complexity of the procedure. Credentialing standards have been established for the more common laparoscopic procedures.

### 4. Does laparoscopic surgery preserve immune function?

Yes. Both human and animal studies have shown that laparoscopy preserves immune function. In contrast, open surgery causes a reduction in lymphocyte and neutrophil chemotaxis, killer cell activity, and lymphocyte and macrophage interactions as well as delayed hypersensitivity responses. Bessler and Whelan demonstrated that immune depression is directly related to incision length. Although adequate exposure is important, smaller incisions might independently decrease morbidity and mortality.

### 5. What are the respiratory effects of pneumoperitoneum (planned intra-abdominal hypertension)?

Pneumoperitoneum alters respiratory mechanics. Intra-abdominal hypertension results in elevation of the diaphragm, decreases in functional residual capacity and total lung volume, ventilation-perfusion inequalities, and atelectasis. Some patients may require increased peak inspiratory pressure to compensate for decreased respiratory compliance. No significant change occurs in arterial oxygenation in healthy patients under pneumoperitoneum, but in patients with cardiopulmonary compromise, arterial oxygen desaturation has been reported, presumably secondary to mechanical pulmonary dysfunction.

### 6. What are the hemodynamic effects?

Mean arterial blood pressure (MAP) and systemic peripheral resistance are increased (up to 35% and 160%, respectively) at operative levels of pneumoperitoneum (12 to 15 mm Hg), presumably as a result of sympathetic vasoconstriction from hypercarbia. Cardiac index may increase 20%. As intra-abdominal pressure increases more than 20 mm Hg, cardiac output falls and abdominal venous compliance decreases, reaching a point at which effective Trendelenburg position and higher pneumoperitoneum can combine in patients with preexisting cardiopulmonary disease to produce potential hemodynamic compromise. Portal venous blood flow is reduced by 70% when intra-abdominal pressure reaches 25 mm Hg. Many workers believe that renal blood flow and therefore glomerular filtration rate also decrease with pneumoperitoneum greater than 12 to 15 mm Hg, although this phenomenon has not been well documented.

In summary, intra-abdominal hypertension greater than 15 mm Hg can result in significant changes in central hemodynamics and even more pronounced changes in splanchnic circulation.

**7. At 24 hours after open upper abdominal surgery using subcostal incisions, patients show a decrease in pulmonary function tests of nearly 50%. What decreases should be expected at 24 hours after laparoscopic cholecystectomy?**
See Table 80-1.

**Table 80-1.** Postoperative Pulmonary Function Tests: Open versus Laparoscopic Surgery

| | PERCENTAGE OF PREOPERATIVE VALUE | |
| --- | --- | --- |
| MEASUREMENT AT 24 HOURS AFTER SURGERY | OPEN SURGERY | LAPAROSCOPIC SURGERY |
| Forced vital capacity (FVC) | 54% | 73% |
| Forced expiratory volume at 1 sec (FEV$_1$) | 52% | 72% |
| Forced expiratory flow at 25% to 75% (FEF$_{25-75}$) | 53% | 81% |

In one study, the decrease in pulmonary function measured at 24 hours after laparoscopic cholecystectomy was approximately one-half of that seen with open surgery. In a related study, age-, gender-, and size-matched patients were randomized prospectively to open versus laparoscopic cholecystectomy, and pulmonary function tests were measured preoperatively and postoperatively. FVC and FEV$_1$ were similarly decreased, but less so with laparoscopic than with open surgery. Functional residual capacity was significantly higher at 72 hours after laparoscopic than after open surgery. Respiratory function is less impaired and recovery is improved after laparoscopic surgery compared with open surgery.

**8. Should we routinely use prophylactic antibiotics for laparoscopic cholecystectomy?**
Yes, for the following reasons:

- Bile spills during laparoscopic cholecystectomy occur in 30% to 50% of cases
- Normal bile is often colonized with bacteria (30% to 40% of patients).
- Acute cholecystitis is associated with a 60% rate of bacterbilia after the first 24 hours of inflammation.

For routine laparoscopic cholecystectomies, a first-generation cephalosporin should provide adequate prophylaxis for most common organisms, although many surgeons use a second-generation cephalosporin.

**9. What is the difference between the hepatocystic triangle and the triangle of Calot?**
To avoid major biliary tract injury, knowledge of the hepatocystic triangle and Calot triangle is essential. Lateral inferior retraction of the gallbladder at the infundibulum (Hartman pouch) with cephalad retraction at the dome facilitates the identification of both. Dissection for laparoscopic cholecystectomy should start at the gallbladder neck (Hartman's pouch) and proceed to the cystic duct, followed by dissection of the cystic artery. Excessive dissection toward the common bile duct is fraught with danger and may result in inadvertent injury to the common hepatic duct or an aberrant right hepatic artery (seen in 10% of cases). Identification of the hepatocystic triangle (cystic duct, common hepatic duct, and border of the liver) avoids injury to the common hepatic duct (Fig. 80-1).

**10. Which alternative gases can be used for laparoscopy?**
Room air, oxygen, nitrous oxide, helium, and CO$_2$ have been used to create the pneumoperitoneum needed for laparoscopy, but CO$_2$ is the most commonly used. Research is ongoing to identify alternative gases for pneumoperitoneum. Helium shows promise in an experimental animal model of chronic obstructive pulmonary disease, in which helium compared with CO$_2$ pneumoperitoneum showed far less arterial CO$_2$ retention.

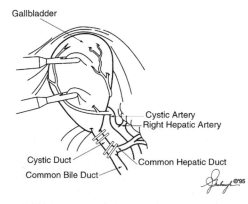

Figure 80-1. The Calot triangle, formed by the cystic duct, cystic artery, and common hepatic duct, is essential for dissection in laparoscopic cholecystectomy. The hepatocystic triangle is defined as the area between the cystic duct, common hepatic duct, and border of the liver.

**11. List the advantages and disadvantages of using carbon dioxide ($CO_2$) as an insufflation gas instead of other gases.**
See Table 80-2.

**Table 80-2.** Advantages and Disadvantages of Carbon Dioxide as an Insufflation Gas

| ADVANTAGES | DISADVANTAGES |
|---|---|
| $CO_2$ suppresses combustion and therefore is believed to be ideal for operative laparoscopy. | $CO_2$ is rapidly absorbed and thus can raise the arterial partial pressure of $CO_2$ and lower pH, with adverse potential metabolic and hemo-dynamic consequences in susceptible patients. |
| $CO_2$ has a high diffusion coefficient, reducing the risk of a serious gas embolism. Up to 100 mL/min of $CO_2$ can be injected directly into the bloodstream of animals without adverse outcome. | Insufflation of cold $CO_2$ (0.3° C), especially in high-flow systems or long procedures, can result in a drop in core temperature with resultant hypothermia. |
| $CO_2$ is safely absorbed and can be effectively eliminated by the lungs with moderate hyperventilation. | Tension $CO_2$ pneumothorax, either from occult defects in the diaphragm or in the absence of diaphragmatic injury (typically in subhiatal laparoscopic surgery), has been reported. |
| $CO_2$ is inexpensive and readily available. | $CO_2$ gas embolism can occur, even without direct insufflation into mesenteric veins. |

**12. A 9-year-old girl presents with a 2-month history of right upper quadrant abdominal pain that most commonly occurs after eating fatty foods and usually resolves in 30 minutes. She is afebrile, and the physical exam is unremarkable. Laboratory values, including complete blood count and biliary panel, are normal. An abdominal ultrasound of the right upper quadrant demonstrates no evidence of cholelithiasis, gallbladder wall thickening, or pericholecystic fluid. What should be the next step in your evaluation?**
The history is consistent with biliary colic. Typical symptoms of biliary colic include right upper quadrant or epigastric pain, which may radiate to the right scapula. The pain is often aggravated by eating, especially fatty foods. The cause of biliary dyskinesia is unknown. An initial diagnosis of cholelithiasis was not demonstrated by ultrasound. An upper gastrointestinal (UGI) series or esophagogastroduodenoscopy (EGD) would demonstrate possible gastric pathology but would not evaluate the biliary system. A computed tomography (CT) scan is less sensitive than ultrasound for detection of gallstones and would not be helpful. Because the history points toward a biliary etiology, a hepatoiminodiacetic acid (HIDA) scan should be the next step in the evaluation.

**13. The HIDA scan demonstrated rapid filling of the gallbladder and unobstructed flow into the duodenum. Cholecystokinin (CCK) is administered, and the gallbladder ejection fraction (EF) is calculated at 30%. What is the most likely diagnosis? How should the patient be treated?**
The most likely diagnosis is biliary dyskinesia, which is defined as the presence of symptoms of typical biliary colic without evidence of cholelithiasis and a gallbladder ejection fraction less than 35% to 50%. Cholecystectomy is successful in 85% of patients with typical symptoms of colic and gallbladder EF less than 35% to 50%. A study by Gollin demonstrated that children with biliary dyskinesia characterized by typical biliary colic and a gallbladder EF less than 40% respond equally well to cholecystectomy (about 79% success rate).

**14. Summarize the key strategies for safe laparoscopic cholecystectomy.**
- Dissection from the infundibulum down toward the cystic duct
- Dissection from lateral to medial
- Adequate inferolateral traction to open the triangle of Calot
- Dissection to develop continuity both laterally and medially from the neck of the gallbladder onto the cystic duct
- Divide no structure unless you are certain about its identity

**15. Compare the rate of conversion from laparoscopic cholecystectomy to open cholecystectomy in patients with acute versus chronic cholecystitis.**
The rate of conversion from laparoscopic cholecystectomy to open cholecystectomy is 2 to 4 times higher for acute cholecystitis than for chronic cholecystitis (typically reported at 3% to 5%) among experienced laparoscopic surgeons.

**16. What pathophysiologic features of acute cholecystitis increase the likelihood of technical difficulties?**
- Distended, inflamed, thick-walled gallbladder (GB)
- Intrahepatic gallbladder
- Inflammation of cystic duct and cystic artery

**17. How does laparoscopic gastric bypass compare to open gastric bypass?**
Laparoscopic patients have a shorter length of stay and also a lower 30-day morbidity.

The number of laparoscopic bariatric procedures performed in the United States has increased significantly since 1999. Laparoscopic procedures for morbid obesity are now more common than open procedures. The American Society for Metabolic and Bariatric Surgery reports an estimated 177,600 people in the United States had bariatric surgery in 2006. Most of these were performed laparoscopically (see Chapter 79).

**18. Is there any clearly defined benefit to laparoscopic appendectomy?**
No. Most studies have shown no benefit for laparoscopic appendectomy over open appendectomy in hospital length of stay, total hospital charges, operative time, recovery time or return to work, or postoperative pain. However, the false diagnosis rate for appendicitis is four times higher among females. For young women, the laparoscopic approach has a clear advantage because gynecologic disorders (ectopic pregnancy, pelvic inflammatory disease, ovarian cysts, and endometriosis) may mimic appendicitis.

**19. Is gangrenous or perforated appendicitis a contraindication to laparoscopic appendectomy?**
No. Although conversion rates vary between 6% and 50%, reportedly related to surgical experience, laparoscopic appendectomy is associated with a decreased wound infection rate, quicker return of bowel function, and no difference in intra-abdominal abscess rate.

**20. Is laparoscopic antireflux surgery (LARS) justified for chronic gastroesophageal reflux disease (GERD)?**
Yes. Medical treatment costs $6 billion a year. Several prospective randomized trials have shown surgery to be more effective in the properly selected patient. The overall success rate at 10 years is 90%.

**21. A 46-year-old woman with a BMI of 44 kg/m² is referred for a laparoscopic antireflux procedure. She has been taking proton pump inhibitors for 20 years. Her symptoms are well controlled with medication; however, she prefers a surgical procedure if it will allow her to stop taking medication. Her past medical history includes hypertension and non–insulin-dependent diabetes. She recently had an EGD, which was normal. Esophageal manometry is also normal. What is your recommendation?**
A laparoscopic Roux-en-Y gastric bypass. Morbid obesity is a relative contraindication for LARS in patients with morbid obesity since they would probably benefit more from a bariatric procedure.

**22. What are the benefits and drawbacks of laparoscopic versus open inguinal hernia repair?**
Laparoscopic hernia repair:

- Is more expensive
- Is technically more demanding
- Requires longer operative time
- Is associated with increased risk of visceral and vascular injuries (especially transabdominal peritoneal repair [TAP]).

However, recurrence rates are similar between the two approaches. Additionally, laparoscopic repair allows the surgeon to evaluate, and possibly repair, a contralateral hernia at the time of the operation. It is also noteworthy that laparoscopic repair is associated with less acute and chronic groin pain; thus allowing patients to return to their normal activities sooner.

**23. What is the role of laparoscopic surgery for curable colon cancer?**
Laparoscopic surgery for benign diseases of the colon and rectum has been accepted for well over a decade. There were real concerns about the adequacy of resection in laparoscopic surgery from an oncologic perspective. The COST Study Group trial has demonstrated that the laparoscopic colectomy for curable colon

cancer is not inferior to open surgery based on 5-year prospective outcome data. Several prospective studies have further shown that laparoscopic colon resection results in less use of narcotics and oral analgesics, quicker return of bowel function, and shorter length of stay. The role of laparoscopic surgery in rectal cancer is not yet defined.

24. **A thin, 68-year-old woman with chronic obstructive pulmonary disease from 52 years of smoking undergoes laparoscopic cholecystectomy for acute cholecystitis. Because she has had a previous lower midline abdominal incision, you choose the *open* Hasson technique for initial trocar placement and have no difficulties with access to the peritoneal cavity. You immediately insufflate with a flow rate of 10 L/min to a pneumoperitoneum of 15 mm Hg and then proceed with laparoscopic cholecystectomy. Fifteen minutes into the procedure, the anesthesiologist observes that the patient's end-tidal $CO_2$ is elevated and plans to draw an arterial blood gas. Before he can do so, the patient experiences several episodes of ventricular tachycardia and arrests. What is the pathophysiology behind these events?**

Insufflated $CO_2$ is directly absorbed through the peritoneum into the capillary bed and bloodstream. Typically, the partial pressure of $CO_2$ ($P_{CO_2}$) and end-tidal $CO_2$ increase only slightly, but in certain circumstances the $P_{CO_2}$ can rise dramatically, causing a significant drop in pH. The resulting acidemia aggravates any preexisting cardiac condition. Most patients adapt to the absorbed $CO_2$ by maximizing plasma and intracellular buffering systems and accelerating $CO_2$ transport and elimination with mild hyperventilation, but some patients have impaired $CO_2$ clearance mechanisms. Patients who cannot handle an acute change in $P_{CO_2}$ are those with high metabolic and cellular respiratory rates (e.g., septic patients), those with large ventilatory dead space (e.g., patients with chronic obstructive pulmonary disease [COPD]), and those with poor cardiac output (e.g., patients with cardiac failure).

During laparoscopy, special care and monitoring should be provided to prevent significant hypercarbia and acidemia. Rapid shifts in intra-abdominal pressure (with attendant $P_{CO_2}$ absorption gradients) should be avoided, such as those that follow initial insufflation at a high rate with a resultant sudden large gradient between intra-abdominal $CO_2$ pressure and $P_{CO_2}$. Equilibrium between $CO_2$ pressure in blood and tissues occurs at about 20 minutes. After initial insufflation, arterial $P_{CO_2}$ steadily rises for about 20 minutes, then plateaus.

This septic patient with preexisting COPD was subjected to rapid $CO_2$ insufflation, which resulted in hypercarbia, peaking 15 to 20 minutes after rapid insufflation, and consequent acidemia, triggering ventricular irritability and arrest.

25. **Can laparoscopic cholecystectomy be done safely in the pregnant patient?**

Yes. Laparoscopic cholecystectomy can be performed safely in the pregnant patient, in all trimesters. Indications are the same as an open operation including repeated attacks of biliary colic, acute cholecystitis, obstructive jaundice, gallstone pancreatitis, and peritonitis. Laparoscopic cholecystectomy is superior to nonoperative management for patients presenting in the first and second trimesters with bilious tract disease.

26. **Can laparoscopic appendectomy be performed safely during pregnancy?**

Yes. Notably, appendicitis is the most common nonobstetric surgery during pregnancy. When performed by an experienced laparoscopic surgeon, there is no difference in preterm delivery (12% to 16%), uterine injuries, or neonatal outcomes.

27. **What are some technical considerations when performing laparoscopy on the pregnant patient?**

Utilize the left lateral decubitus position, when possible, to minimize uterine compression of the inferior vena cava (IVC). Minimize reverse Trendelenburg and insufflation pressures to help reduce decreased venous return. Always use sequential compression device (SCD) or other deep venous thrombosis (DVT) prophylaxis.

28. **What percentage of patients have free intra-abdominal air on upright radiograph 24 hours after laparoscopic procedure?**

In the nonpostoperative state, the presence of subdiaphragmatic free air on upright chest radiograph is diagnostic of intra-abdominal perforation. After an open abdominal or laparoscopic procedure the significance of free intra-abdominal air is less clear. Nonpathologic subdiaphragmatic air may be seen in 24% to 39% of patients after laparoscopic surgery and in 60% of patients after open surgical procedures. The difference relates to the solubility of $CO_2$ used in laparoscopy versus the solubility of trapped room air within the abdominal cavity. $CO_2$ is more soluble in serum than room air and is absorbed 32 times more quickly.

### 29. What are the indications and contraindications for laparoscopic adrenalectomy? What are the advantages of laparoscopic adrenalectomy?

Adrenal masses can be divided into functioning, nonfunctioning, and malignant tumors. Functioning or hormonally active tumors (e.g., pheochromocytoma, aldosteronoma, androgen-producing adenoma, glucocorticoid-producing adenoma, bilateral adrenal hyperplasia) should be resected. Studies have shown that tumors as large as 10 cm can be resected laparoscopically. Nonfunctioning or hormonally inactive adrenal tumors greater than 4 cm or tumors greater than 3 cm that have grown over the course of serial studies should be resected. The risk of malignancy increases with size; most adrenal cancers measure greater than 6 cm. Laparoscopic resection of adrenocortical cancer is controversial. If the tumor is confined to the adrenal gland, laparoscopic resection may be possible. The need for clear surgical margins may necessitate conversion to an open procedure if direct extension of tumor involves surrounding structures. The contraindications to laparoscopic resection of adrenal tumors are based on the surgeon's clinical judgment and laparoscopic abilities. Radiographic imaging aids the surgeon in determining laparoscopic resectability. Studies have demonstrated that laparoscopic adrenalectomy is a safe and beneficial alternative to an open procedure. Patients who undergo laparoscopic adrenalectomy have less operative blood loss, lower transfusion requirements, fewer admissions to intensive care, decreased use of pain medication, quicker return of bowel function, and decreased hospital stay. In some studies, however, operative times were significantly longer for laparoscopic surgery.

### 30. How are bile spills managed?

Despite the best efforts by experienced surgeons, bile spill is seen in 30% to 50% of laparoscopic cholecystectomies. Sterile laparoscopic specimen bags are indicated to retrieve lost gallstones, to remove a friable, disrupted gallbladder, or to remove detached, necrotic tissue. Use of closed suction drains should follow the same guidelines used at open surgery.

## WEBSITES

http://www.laparoscopyhospital.com/lap_app.htm

http://www.vhjoe.org/Volume2Issue3/2-3-3.htm

## BIBLIOGRAPHY

1. Abuzeid AW, Banerjea A, et al. Gastric slippage as an emergency: Diagnosis and management. Obes Surg 2007;17:559–61.
2. Affleck D, Handrahan D, et al. The laparascopic management of appendicitis and cholelithiasis during pregnancy. American Journal of Surgery 1999;178:523–9.
3. Allendorf JD, Bessler M, Whelan RL, et al. Postoperative immune function varies inversely with the degree of surgical trauma in a murine model. Surg Endosc 1997;11:427–30.
4. Barone J, Bears S, et al. Outcome study of cholecystectomy during pregnancy. American Journal of Surgery 1999;177:232–6.
5. Boller AM, Nelson H. Colon and rectal cancer: Laparoscopic or open? Clin Canc Res 2007;13:6894s–6s.
6. Cameron J. Current surgical therapy. 9th ed. St. Louis: Mosby; 2008.
7. Curet M. Special problems in laparoscopic surgery. Surg Clin N Am 2000;80:1093–111.
8. EU Hernia Trialists Collaboration. Laparoscopic compared with open methods of groin hernia repair: Systematic review of randomized controlled trials. Br J Surg 2000;87:860–7.
9. Fleshman J, Sargent DJ, et al. Laparoscopic colectomy for cancer is not inferior to open surgery based on 5-year data from the COST Study Group trial. Ann Surg 2007;245:655–62.
10. Gollin G, Raschbaum GR, et al. Cholecystectomy for suspected biliary dyskinesia in children with chronic abdominal pain. J Pediatr Surg 1999;34:854–7.
11. Gravante G, Araco A, et al. Laparoscopic adjustable gastric bandings: A prospective randomized study of 400 operations performed with 2 different devices. Arch Surg 2007;142:958–61.
12. Greene FL. The impact of laparoscopy on cancer management. Surg Endosc 2000;14:217–8.
13. Ishibashi S, Takechi H, et al. Length of laparotomy incision and surgical stress assessed by serum IL-6 level. Injury 2006;37:247–51.
14. Kumar S, Wilson R, et al. Chronic pain after laparoscopic and open mesh repair of groin hernia. Br J Surg 2002;89:1476–9.
15. Lee SW, Southall JC, Gleason NR, et al. Lymphocyte proliferation in mice after full laparotomy is the same whether performed in a sealed carbon dioxide chamber or room air. Surg Endosc 2000;14:235–8.
16. Nadler EP, Young HA, et al. An update on 73 U.S. obese pediatric patients treated with laparoscopic adjustable gastric banding: Comorbidity resolution and compliance data. J Pediatr Surg 2008;43:141–6.
17. Tolonen P, Victorzon M, Makela J. 11-Year experience with laparoscopic adjustable gastric banding for morbid obesity: What happened to the first 123 patients? Obes Surg 2008;18:251–5.

# INDEX

Page numbers followed by *b*, indicate boxes; *f*, figures; *t*, tables.